D1060239

SYSTEMIC PATHOLOGY / THIRD EDITION

General Editor W. St C. Symmers

Volume 9

The Skin

EDITED BY

David Weedon
MD(Qld), FRCPA

Visiting Pathologist, Royal Brisbane Hospital and Princess Alexandra Hospital,
Brisbane, Queensland, Australia;
formerly Professor of Clinical Anatomical Pathology,
University of Queensland, Brisbane, Australia

CONTRIBUTORS

Geoffrey Strutton MB BS(Qld), FRCPA
Visiting Pathologist, Royal Brisbane Hospital, Brisbane, Queensland, Australia

Kurt S. Stenn MD,
Professor of Dermatology and Pathology, School of Medicine,
Yale University, New Haven, Connecticut, USA

Michael A. Goldenhersh MD and *Richard W. Trepeta* MD
School of Medicine, Yale University, New Haven, Connecticut, USA

CHURCHILL LIVINGSTONE
EDINBURGH LONDON MADRID MELBOURNE NEW YORK AND TOKYO 1992

CHURCHILL LIVINGSTONE
Medical Division of Longman Group UK Limited

Distributed in the United States of America by Churchill
Livingstone Inc., 650 Avenue of the Americas, New York, N.Y. 10011, and
by associated companies, branches and representatives
throughout the world.

©Longman Group UK Limited 1992

All rights reserved. No part of this publication may be
reproduced, stored in a retrieval system, or transmitted in any
form or by any means, electronic, mechanical, photocopying,
recording or otherwise, without either the prior permission of the
publishers (Churchill Livingstone, Robert Stevenson House,
1–3 Baxter's Place, Leith Walk, Edinburgh EH1 3AF), or a licence
permitting restricted copying in the United Kingdom issued by the
Copyright Licensing Agency Ltd, 90 Tottenham Court Road, London,
WIP 9HE.

First published 1992

ISBN 0-443-03201-7

British Library Cataloguing in Publication Data
CIP catalogue record for this book is available
from the British Library.

Library of Congress Cataloging in Publication Data
The Skin / edited by David Weedon; with contributions by Geoffrey
  Strutton ... [et al .]. -- 3rd ed.
            p. cm. -- (Systemic pathology ; v. 8)
   Include index.
   1. Skin--Histopathology. 2. Skin--Biopsy, Needle.   I. Weedon, David.
   II. Strutton, Geoffrey.   III. Series.
   [DNLM: 1. Skin--pathology. 2. Skin Diseases--pathology.   QZ 4
S995 1986 v. 8]
RB111.S97 1987 vol. 8
[RL95]
616. 07 s--dc20
[616. 5'07}
DNLM/DLC
for Library of Congress   91–23096
                                                 CIP

The
publisher's
policy is to use
**paper manufactured
from sustainable forests**

Printed and bound in Great Britain by
William Clowes Limited, Beccles and London

Preface

The histopathology of the skin occupies an important place in both general pathology and dermatology. Skin diseases, because of their ready accessibility to clinical inspection and biopsy, can be studied throughout their natural course. While this has contributed to our understanding of many skin diseases, it has also led to a proliferation of diagnoses in dermatology, some of which merely represent different stages or clinical expressions of the one basic disease process. The many clinical variants of cutaneous tuberculosis — lupus vulgaris, tuberculosis verrucosa, scrofuloderma to name just a few — are testimony to this. Little wonder that the skin has become a bewildering subject to many trainees in pathology and dermatology.

Attempts have been made over the past two decades to make dermatopathology a less formidable subject by the adoption of a morphological approach to the categorization of skin diseases rather than the aetiological one that has been used in the past. The morphological classification of skin diseases can be based on the pattern of inflammation present in a biopsy from a particular disease, or based on 'tissue reaction patterns', which group together those cutaneous diseases that share certain histopathological features. The latter approach has been adopted, where possible, in this book, although an inevitable consequence of this approach is some duplication. The infectious diseases and infestations are discussed under their traditional aetiological headings.

It cannot be stressed too strongly that clinical dermatology and dermatopathology are interrelated subjects and, accordingly, close clinicopathological correlation is essential in the study of diseases of the skin. For this reason, clinical aspects of each disease have been included.

This book would not have been possible without the help and encouragement of many colleagues. The General Editor, Professor W. St C. Symmers, has been of great personal assistance throughout the long gestation period of this book with his helpful comments and guidance. The contributions of Geoffrey Strutton and Kurt Stenn have also been most welcome. Special mention must be made of John Sullivan, who stimulated my initial interest in dermatopathology over 20 years ago, John Kerr, whose brilliant concept of 'apoptosis' encouraged me to look at its role in various skin diseases, and Bernard Ackerman, whose detailed morphological observations on so many skin diseases provided the intellectual stimulation which has maintained my interest in this challenging subject. Finally, my thanks are due to Dawn Dean who typed all of the manuscript, to Graham Dean for his assistance with the technical aspects of word processing and computer typesetting, and the staff of Churchill Livingstone who gave helpful advice throughout this project.

Southport, Queensland
Australia, October 1992   David Weedon

Contents

Kurt S. Stenn, Michael A. Goldenhersh and Richard W. Trepeta

Structure and functions of the skin

INTRODUCTION

The skin is the external covering of an animal, separating its body from the surroundings. As a buffer, the skin must provide the organism with protective, perceptive and communicative functions. It must protect against trauma, microbial penetration, toxic agents, electromagnetic radiation, temperature fluctuation, and body fluid loss; it must perceive changes of the temperature and of the texture of the environment, and it must communicate to other organisms by odour and visible embellishment. The skin serves these functions by its unique primary and associated structures. Its external surface is a highly impermeable, laminated, but shedding epithelial product, keratin, formed by a multilayered epithelium, the epidermis. The epidermis is moored to an elastic but tough, relatively acellular collagenous layer, the dermis, which contains within it a rich vascular supply and adnexa. The adnexa of the skin include hair and nails, which are protective keratinous redundancies, sebaceous and apocrine glands, which are secretory organs serving to moisten the skin surface, and eccrine glands, whose watery secretions help regulate body temperature. Underlying the dermis is a fibrofatty cushion/insulating layer, the subcutis. As skin function varies with body location, so does skin structure. Therefore, there is a range of cutaneous morphologies: for example, while palmar-plantar skin has a thick epidermis with a prominent keratin layer, eyelid skin has a thin epidermis with a delicate keratin layer; while scalp dermis is rich in large hair follicles, nasal dermis contains small hair follicles; while abdominal skin shows a thick subcutis made of adipose tissue, finger skin subcutis is thin and collagenous.

EMBRYOLOGY OF THE SKIN

By two weeks of gestation the embryo is covered by a primitive skin consisting of an outer ectodermally derived single cuboidal epithelial layer, the epidermis, which sits upon a loosely packed connective tissue dermis.[1] In general the epidermis matures earlier than the dermis. By four weeks the epidermis acquires a second layer, the outer one called *periderm*. The periderm is a transient, non-keratinizing epidermal covering which sloughs as soon as maturation of the underlying epidermis is complete. The surface microvilli and blebs of the periderm cells imply, by analogy, that these cells have a function of transport or secretion; indeed, evidence has been presented to support the idea that periderm modifies or secretes amniotic fluid.[2]

By about the eighth week an *intermediate layer* appears between the periderm and the basal layer which increases in thickness and cell number during the next 12–20 weeks. By 24 weeks the periderm sloughs, the granular and keratin layers form, and the intermediate layer assumes the morphology of the squamous layer.

By the 12th week both types of dendritic immigrant cells — the melanocytes and Langerhans cells — can be identified within the epidermis. The Merkel cell appears later, between 16 and 28 weeks.

As the epidermis becomes multilayered it extends focal proliferations into the dermis which mature to form the pilosebaceous, eccrine and nail structures.

The dermis arises from the somite mesoderm.[3] By 4–8 weeks the dermis is made of stellate mesenchymal cells embedded in a matrix of hyaluronic acid and glycogen. With maturation, the dermal content of water, glycosaminoglycans and cells decreases and the fibrous content increases. By 16–20 weeks the two dermal compartments — papillary and reticular — can be distinguished by the size and orientation of the collagen fibres in these regions. Much of the maturation of the dermis occurs postnatally, long after the mature epidermis appears. Indeed, dermal elastic fibres which appear initially during the first 12 weeks

of development do not mature fully before the first or second postnatal year.

THE EPIDERMIS

While the epidermis is composed predominantly of keratinocytes, at least three other resident cells are also present: the Merkel cell (epithelium derived), the Langerhans cell (bone marrow derived) and the melanocyte (neural crest derived).

KERATINOCYTES

The epidermis is a stratified squamous epithelial sheet covering the total external surface of the body. It is not only the most cellular but also the most dynamic layer of the skin: it continuously sheds (and thereby cleanses) and regenerates itself. The epidermis forms a broadly undulating interface with the dermis. It extends into the dermis as broad folds (the *rete ridges*) and the dermis projects into the epidermis in finger-like projections, the *dermal papillae*. The epidermis regenerates itself by means of a population of dividing stem cells restricted, in general, to regions of the *basal layer*. The basal cells are cuboidal and rest directly on the *basement membrane* zone. The dividing basal cells are not evenly distributed along the epidermis but are localized predominantly in the tips of the rete ridges and are relatively rare among the basal cells overlying the dermal papillae.[4,5] Normally, only about 17% of the basal cells make up the dividing cell population. On average, one daughter cell of each division leaves the basal layer and enters the next layer of the epidermis, the squamous or *prickle cell layer*. As the cells develop in this layer they acquire more cytoplasm, cytoplasmic filaments and characteristic intercellular attachments, the prickles, or *desmosomes*. As the cells mature, they flatten, and in the slower growing regions move outwards in well-organized, hexagonally packed columns. The prickle layer varies in thickness from 4–10 cells. Above it the maturing cells acquire irregular basophilic cytoplasmic granules, the *keratohyaline granules*, which give the identifying characteristic to the *stratum granulosum* or *granular layer*. The granular layer is 1–3 cells thick. The cells of this layer differentiate further by losing all cytoplasmic detail, flattening further, and packing into a dense keratinous sheet, the *stratum corneum* or *keratin layer*. The outer portion of the latter is composed of flake-like squames, which eventually desquamate. The total epidermal renewal time is roughly 2 months. The cells take 26–42 days to transit through the living epidermis (from basal to granular layer) and then 14 more days to pass through the keratin layer to desquamate.

The structure of the epidermis has been likened to that of a brick wall in which the protein-rich cells (the bricks) are embedded in a lipid-rich adhesive (mortar-like) environment (see Table 1.1).[6] The predominant cell of the epidermis, the *keratinocyte*, is so named for the filamentous

Table 1.1 Protein constituents of the epidermis

Tonofilaments (keratin filaments)

Basal layer keratin: types 5 and 14 (K5 and K14)
Suprabasal layer: K1 and K10
Proliferative epidermis (psoriasis): K6 and K16

Keratohyaline granule

Filaggrin
Loricrin

Cornified envelope

Loricrin
Involucrin
Keratolinin
Pancornulins

product it produces. *Keratin filaments* (or *tonofilaments*) literally fill the cytoplasm of the upper epidermal keratinocytes. Individual fibres appear to extend from one desmosome through the cytoplasm, around the nucleus and on to the other distant desmosomes. Each keratin filament is assembled from a protofilament made of two different keratin molecules. Keratin is an alpha-helical non-glycosylated protein molecule. Heretofore 29 different keratin molecules, ranging in molecular weight from 40–67 kd, have been identified. These keratins are catalogued into two groups according to acid-basic properties and molecular weight. Type I keratins are more acidic and of lower molecular weight, type II are more basic and of higher molecular weight. Although it has been found that the specific keratins in any one

region of the skin or any one level of the epidermis (or adnexa) vary, the reason for any given distribution or even for the large number of different keratins is not yet apparent. We recognize that the keratin pair K5/K14 is found in basal cells and K1/K10 in the differentiated upper epidermal cells. Current concepts of the mechanism of epidermal differentiation have been reviewed recently.[7]

The keratohyaline granules which are prominent in the granular layer contain elements which appear to assist the packing and cross-linking of keratin. Arising from a large molecular weight polyphosphorylated precursor within the granule is *filaggrin*, a cationic, histidine-rich protein of approximately 50 kd molecular weight.[8,9] When mixed in vitro with purified keratin filaments filaggrin causes filament aggregation. It is thought that the filaggrin in keratohyaline granules helps aggregate, orient and stabilize the keratin filaments of the upper epidermal cells. In the upper epidermis the keratin filaments are stabilized by disulphide bond cross-links which make this intracytoplasmic structural mesh highly insoluble. A second stable, resistant proteinaceous intracytoplasmic structure, the *cornified envelope*, forms in the outer epidermis. This structure polymerizes from at least two protein monomers, *loricrin* (45kd) and *involucrin* (92 kd).[10] These two proteins are cross-linked into an envelope underlying the plasma membrane by an *epidermal transglutaminase*.[11] This enzyme joins the lysyl residues of one polypeptide chain with glutamyl residues of a second, resulting in a cross-linked mesh insoluble even to reducing reagents. Thus, there are two important insoluble proteinaceous structures formed within the cytoplasm of the maturing keratinocyte:

1. cables of cross-linked keratin filaments coursing from desmosome to desmosome, and
2. a rigid enclosure, the cornified envelope, which forms just beneath the cell membrane.

In all layers the keratinocytes are attached to one another by both defined and ill-defined cell contacts (Table 1.2). Most of these cells have desmosomal attachments: these are prominent and easily seen in the spinous or mid-epidermal layer. The desmosome is a round, plaque-like point contact

Table 1.2 Epidermal cell attachment molecules

Desmosome — The primary epithelial cell attachment structure which provides anchorage for tonofilaments.

Desmoplakins (DPI–IV) : Nonglycosylated cytoplasmic proteins.

Plakoglobulin: Nonglycosylated protein found within the plaque of desmosomes and other intermediate junction.

Desmogleins (DGI–IV): Extracellular glycosylated proteins. DGI is the pemphigus foliaceous antigen.

Desmocollins (I & II): Glycoproteins found in the desmoglea.

Focal adherens plaque

Integrins — A family of membrane glycoproteins consisting of 2 subunits (α and β) which mediate cell adhesion and are associated with focal adhesion plaques.[23, 24]

$6\beta4$ Mediates basal cell anchorage, associated with the hemidesmosome.

$\left. \begin{array}{l} 2\beta1 \\ 3\beta1 \end{array} \right\}$ Mediate intercellular adhesion mostly on basal cells but also found on suprabasal cells.

Hemidesmosome

Bullous pemphigoid antigen — Manifests extracellular and cytoplasmic domains. Its collagen-like domain serves to stabilize extracellular matrix interaction.[22]

Adherens junction

Cadherins

Epidermal cell membrane

I-CAM 1 — Expression induced by interferon and TNF-β.[25]

---

between two cells.[12] It is a complex structure consisting of:

1. the intercellular mesh which contains desmogleins (glycoproteins, one of which is the pemphigus foliaceous antigen),
2. the bilaminar cell membrane and
3. the cytoplasmic attachment plaque containing desmoplakins, plakoglobulin and other constituents.[12]

Keratin filaments form hair-pin loops in the region of the attachment plaques and appear to bind close to them. Another organized intercellular attachment found between epidermal cells is the *gap junction* which provides a low resistance channel between adjacent cells and serves as a passageway for ions and other small molecules; it provides a means of intercellular communication. Besides these two structures, epidermal cells adhere

by focal adhesion plaques and intercellular regions which are less well defined morphologically and chemically.

Recent work suggests that in the upper epidermis cholesterol esters are important components of cell adhesion. Indeed, in one form of ichthyosis (X-linked), a disease of keratin accumulation and decreased desquamation, there is an accumulation of epidermal cholesterol sulphate associated with a deficiency in the aryl sulphatase.[13] This discovery implicates not only one mechanism for interkeratinocyte adhesion but also a mechanism for keratinocyte dyshesion and desquamation. That dyshesion is an active inherent process of normal epidermis is evidenced by the desquamation that occurs in skin under protective dressings. Undoubtedly dyshesion is under exquisite control, modulated by the environment and the body; an example of a protective response is seen in the retarded dyshesion occurring within the tightly-packed keratin layer which accumulates over sites of chronic rubbing (lichen simplex chronicus).

Besides adhesion/dyshesion, lipids also play a role in the permeability barrier of the skin. This barrier excludes the transport of aqueous solution from the dermis outwards or from the keratin layer inwards. By experimentally perfusing aqueous dyes from either direction, the barrier is seen to reside in the region of the granular layer.[14] Electron microscopic studies reveal that small membrane-bound lipid-rich lamellated granules (100–500 nm in diameter), referred to as *membrane-coating granules* or *Odland bodies*, are secreted into the intercellular space at this level of the epidermis. Because of their location and their lipid-rich nature, the membrane-coating granules are thought to form the permeability barrier.[15]

MERKEL CELLS

Within mammalian skin are focal specialized thickenings called hair discs or Pinkus corpuscles. These dome-shaped elevations contain within their basal layer Merkel cells. Identified by electron microscopy, these round cells with lobulated irregular nuclei bulge into both the epidermis and the dermis. While they have desmosomal attachments to the surrounding keratinocytes,

Merkel cells have only loosely-packed keratin filaments. Because of the latter observation, Merkel cells are believed to be epithelium-derived. Localized to one of their cytoplasmic poles are numerous dense-core osmiophilic (neurosecretory) granules, 70–90 nm in diameter, which resemble the monoamine storage granules of nerve endings. At the same pole each Merkel cell contacts one neurite which inserts into the epidermis at this point. Merkel cells are believed to function as slow-adapting mechanoreceptors; nevertheless, since so few Pinkus corpuscles are found in man, it is considered unlikely that the corpuscle or the Merkel cell contributes a great deal to human sensory capacity. Although Merkel cells have not been found in normal dermis, an aggressive dermal tumour made of cells exhibiting cytoplasmic features of Merkel cells has been described.[16] The relationship between this Merkel cell tumour (also referred to as a trabecular carcinoma) and mature Merkel cells is not yet known (see p. 934).

LANGERHANS CELLS

More than a century ago Paul Langerhans discovered a dendritic, non-keratinocytic, non-melanocytic, gold-staining cell within the epidermis. Interdigitating among keratinocytes, the Langerhans cell (LC) can be identified by light microscopy, using special procedures such as gold or ATPase staining, or by electron microscopy. It is typically about the size of the surrounding keratinocytes but it is devoid of keratin filaments, desmosomes and melanosomes. Its nucleus is lobulated and often convoluted. The cell is identified by its unique cytoplasmic inclusion, the *Birbeck granule*, seen by electron microscopy as a racket-shaped membrane-bound vesicle of unknown function.

Langerhans cells make up 2–4% of the resident epidermal cells and are found within the epidermis above the basal layer. Although the density of LCs is rather constant per unit area of skin (in man ranging from 460–1000 cells/mm^2), between species and between different anatomical regions there are differences, e.g. mouse tail skin has very few LCs in contrast to mouse abdominal and ear skin. Although the largest number of LCs is found in the epidermis, they are also found in the adnexa (hair follicles and sebaceous and apocrine glands) and in other stratified squamous epithelia such as the lining of the oral cavity, oesophagus, vagina and cervix. Where they are found in smaller numbers, as in the thymus, lymphoid tissue and dermis, they are believed to be in transit between antigen-processing tissues.

Recently, it has been demonstrated that this cell originates in the bone marrow and is the only resident epidermal cell which bears receptors for the Fc portion of the IgG molecule and complement (C3) and expresses the Ia antigen, an antigen restricted to immunocomponent cells. It has been shown that this cell is required for antigen processing and for the induction of contact hypersensitivity and that it plays a role in graft rejection. It is currently accepted that the LC is a cell of the monocyte-macrophage series which serves as the most peripheral cellular component of the afferent immune system and that it acts as a cellular link, a sentinel, between the host and the environment. It plays a central role in a very important immunological organ.[17,18]

MELANOCYTES AND CUTANEOUS PIGMENTATION

Pigmentation of skin and hair provides a front-line defence against ultraviolet and visible electromagnetic radiation.[19] The pigment is produced by a resident epidermal dendritic cell, the melanocyte. This cell, derived from the neural crest, migrates to the epidermis during the third month of fetal life and rests in mature skin slightly below the basal cells in a dell of the basal lamina. The melanocyte synthesizes melanin pigment, packages it in *melanosomes*, and distributes it to keratinocytes by means of its dendritic extensions.

Many different pigments classified as melanin are found within animals and plants. Mammalian melanins are dense, insoluble polymers of high molecular weight, composed of indole-5,6-quinone units, the formation of which is catalysed by the action of a tyrosinase on tyrosine and dihydroxy-phenylalanine. The two melanins important to human hair and skin colour are the brown-black *eumelanin* and the yellow-red *phaeomelanin*. While both molecules are derived from tyrosine, phaeomelanin also contains the sulphur-amino acid cysteine. Melanin absorbs electromagnetic radiation over a broad spectrum covering the ultraviolet and visible wave lengths. In the melanocyte the pivotal enzyme tyrosinase is prepackaged into a Golgi-derived vesicle which over a series of maturation steps acquires melanin and becomes a highly organized ellipsoidal organelle, the melanosome. The melanosome is transported peripherally into the dendritic processes of the melanocyte and is then actively taken up by keratinocytes. Each melanocyte distributes melanosomes to a family of keratinocytes which constitutes the *epidermal melanin unit*. Once within the keratinocyte, melanosomes aggregate and become membrane-enclosed, thus forming the melanosome complex. While melanosome distribution is less localized in the upper epidermal cells the lower epidermal keratinocytes show perinuclear localization. In the latter cells the pigment is positioned to protect the cellular genome from incoming radiation.

What is perceived as normal cutaneous pigmentation depends only in small part on the cornified layer and the dermal blood supply — most of the colour of the skin is due to its melanin content. Pigmentation is a direct function of the quantity and the packaging of melanosomes in keratinocytes. In Caucasoid skin melanosomes are aggregated within keratinocytes into large complexes; in contrast, Negroid skin melanosomes are larger and within keratinocytes remain singly dispersed. The number of melanocytes varies from region to region of the skin but within the same mammalian species the melanocyte density is the same regardless of the skin colour.

The formation of melanin is influenced by a variety of endogenously secreted polypeptide and steroid hormones. Melanocyte-stimulating hormone (MSH) acting through intracellular cyclic adenosine monophosphate (cyclic AMP) stimulates tyrosinase activity. Melanocytic growth is stimulated by oestrogens and thus hyperoestrogenic states, such as pregnancy, are accompanied by hyperpigmentation.

THE EPIDERMO–DERMAL JUNCTION

Like other epithelial tissues the epidermis rests upon a basement membrane sheet which appears on light microscopy after sectioning and periodic acid–Schiff staining as a thin undulating homogeneous band. By electron microscopy the basement membrane zone is more complex. As described above, the downward projecting epidermal rete ridges interlock with the upward projecting dermal papillae. The epidermis folds over the dermal papillae and forms ridges in the dermal depressions. The plasma membranes of the basal cells covering the dermal papillae have a serrated surface while those cells of the deep epidermal ridges have a smooth lower surface.[4] In both areas the cells rest on an electron-lucent sheet, the *lamina lucida*, which contains proteoglycans and the large cruciate-shaped protein, laminin. Below this is an electron-opaque sheet, the *lamina densa*, which is structured by the unique collagen type IV. Thin *anchoring filaments* extend from the basal cell membrane through the lamina lucida. The basal epithelial cells are buttoned to the basement membrane zone by hemidesmosomes which contain within their structure bullous pemphigoid antigen, a protein with collagenous domains.[20–22] *Anchoring fibrils* which are made of type VII collagen extend from the lamina densa into the collagenous dermis. *Hemidesmosomes* which help anchor the basal cells to the basement membrane are most numerous within the basal cells adjacent to the top of the dermal papilla. Extending from the tips of the cellular invaginations below the hemidesmosomes are aggregates of fine filaments, the *dermal microfibrillary bundle*.

The specific molecules constituting the basement membrane zone (Table 1.3) are currently being identified.[26] Recognizing these moieties is important to the understanding of the vesiculobullous diseases. They are discussed further, with the vesiculobullous diseases, in Chapter 6 , page 140.

The basement membrane zone serves to moor the epidermis to the dermis, to support epidermal growth, and to act as a filtration barrier to epidermal–dermal traffic. Depending on the aetiology, in pathological states the skin may split at any level; e.g. suction, shear stress, and trypsin exposure cause a split within the lamina lucida; col-

Table 1.3 Molecules of the basement membrane zone

Microscopic structure	Molecular constituent
Hemidesmosome	
Tonofilament	Keratins (K5, K14)
Attachment plaque	Bullous pemphigoid antigen
	Integrin 6β4
Lamina Lucida	Laminin
	Heparan sulphate
	Cicatricial pemphigoid antigen
	GB-3 polypeptide
Lamina densa	Type IV collagen
	Nidogen/entactin
	KF-1
	LH7:2
	Heparan sulphate proteoglycan
Anchoring fibrils	Type VII collagen

lagenase causes a split at the level of the lamina densa; and elastase causes a split in the dermis beneath the lamina densa.

THE DERMIS

The supportive structure of the skin is provided by the dermis, a relatively hypocellular layer of varying thickness. It is composed of a structural collagen matrix, elastin and ground substance. Embedded within the dermis are epidermal appendages, nerve endings, resident cells and vessels.

COLLAGEN, ELASTIC TISSUE AND GROUND SUBSTANCE

With respect to the packing of collagen the dermis is divided into two compartments:

1. the *papillary dermis* which underlies the epidermis and extends about the adnexa (in which location it is also known as the *adventitial dermis*) and
2. the deeper lying *reticular dermis*. The papillary dermis is composed of fine fibres consisting predominantly of type III and type I collagen. It moors the epidermis, interdigitates with the reticular dermis, and surrounds the epidermal appendages. The reticular dermis is made of densely-packed coarse-fibred collagen which is predominantly type I. The collagen bundles traverse the dermis in a pattern that has not yet been defined. Associated with these two interstitial collagens are the finely-filamentous collagens type V and type VI.[27,28]

The elastic network of the dermis is not homogeneous but composed of three different but related varieties of fibres — *oxytalan, elaunin* and *elastin* — arranged into three interconnected layers (see p. 361). The oxytalan fibres, located within the papillary dermis and apparently consisting of a 350 kd protein fibrillin,[29,30] run perpendicular to the dermo-epidermal junction in an arborizing fashion. They join superficially with the epidermal basement membrane and take origin from the elaunin fibre plexus which runs parallel to the dermo–epidermal junction within the papillary dermis. The elaunin fibre plexus in turn takes origin from the elastin fibres of the reticular dermis. The elastin fibres form an inter-anastomosing three-dimensional plexus which extends down to the subcutaneous fat.

The ground substance of the dermis fills the spaces between the collagen fibres and collagen bundles. It is composed primarily of mucopolysaccharides, with the addition of water, salts and glycoproteins. The mucopolysaccharides, which compose only 0.1–0.3% of the dry weight of the skin, are all highly anionic due to their content of uronic acid or "uronic" sulphate, or both. They appear to maintain the salt and water balance of the dermis. The four major mucopolysaccharides of the skin are *hyaluronic acid, dermatan sulphate, chondroitin 6-sulphate* and *heparan sulphate*. Hyaluronic acid appears to be the predominant component of normal dermal ground substance and it is the mucopolysaccharide that accumulates in various disease states (see Ch. 13, pp. 385–400).

DERMAL BLOOD VESSELS AND LYMPHATICS

The blood vessels of the dermis are primarily arranged into two horizontal plexuses interconnected by arborizing vertical channels.[31] The *lower horizontal plexus* is situated at the dermal–subcutis interface and consists of a band-like network of intertwining arterioles and venules.

The arterioles have a homogeneous basement membrane, discontinuous subendothelial elastic lamina, and 4–5 layers of smooth muscle cells. In contrast, the venules have a multilayer basement membrane along with 5–6 layers of pericytes. In larger venules the pericytes take on the characteristics of smooth muscle cells and are separated by layers of elastic fibres. Bicuspid valves are present within the deep venules at the sites of junction of small venules with larger collecting venules.

Ascending arterioles and venules connect the lower horizontal plexus with the *upper horizontal plexus*. In addition, the ascending vessels arborize to form capillary networks which surround the sweat glands and hair bulbs.

The upper horizontal plexus is situated at the junction of the papillary dermis with the reticular dermis. It is a band-like network of intertwining and anastomosing arterioles and post-capillary venules, similar in arrangement to the deep horizontal plexus. The arterioles have the same meshwork internal elastic lamina and homogeneous basement membrane as are observed in the arterioles of the deep plexus, with only one or two layers of smooth muscle cells. These arterioles and post-capillary venules are connected by a capillary network, part of which produces the capillary loops of the dermal papillae. The capillary walls lack elastic fibres and contain a basement membrane which changes from homogeneous to multilayered as the capillary changes from an arteriolar capillary to a venous capillary. The post-capillary venules have a multilayer basement membrane and are surrounded by structurally supportive veil cells rather than smooth muscle cells. The most functionally active area of the dermal vasculature appears to be the post-capillary venule. Histamine, for example, acts on the endothelial cells of this region to produce cell gaps; this leads to increased vascular permeability and oedema (urticaria). The post-capillary venule is also the site of neutrophil and lymphocyte emigration during inflammation, the segment most sensitive to bradykinin and serotonin, and the almost exclusive depository of the circulating immune complexes in allergic vasculitis.

The *dermal lymphatic network* has an organization similar to that of the blood vessels. [32] The lymphatic capillaries begin as blind tubes within the dermal papillae and join an upper horizontal lymphatic plexus which intertwines with the upper dermal blood plexus. The vessels of the upper horizontal lymphatic plexus contain valves to prevent backflow of lymph. Descending lymphatics penetrate the dermis to the deep dermal horizontal lymphatic plexus which intertwines with the deep dermal blood plexus. In contrast to capillary blood vessels the lymphatic capillaries have a discontinuous basement membrane and no pericytes or closely related elastic fibres. Anchoring filaments, believed to be elastin, extend from the outer surface of the lymphatic into the surrounding interstitial collagen.

CUTANEOUS INNERVATION

The nerves of the dermis are both myelinated and unmyelinated, autonomic and sensory. [33,34] The autonomic nerves conduct efferent impulses from the central nervous system to the smooth muscle cells of the cutaneous vasculature and appendages while the sensory nerves transmit afferent impulses from the free nerve endings and special sensory organs back to the central nervous system. They ascend, along with the dermal blood supply, from the underlying subcutaneous tissue and form analogous superficial and deep plexuses. The deep nervous plexus is located at the dermal subcutaneous junction and is composed of multiple nerve branches, each of numerous nerve trunks. Nerve branches pass from the deep plexus to the deep receptors, appendages, and vasculature. They also cross over and reorganize into small mixed nerve bundles which ascend to the superficial nerve plexus located beneath the epidermal ridges. From the superficial plexus single axons pass into the superficial receptors of the dermal papillae and the epidermis. The density of the dermal and epidermal nerve fibres varies with body site as do the number and type of dermal sensory receptors.

The sensory receptors of the dermis can be divided into free and encapsulated nerve endings. The free nerve endings form the majority of the sensory receptors in the skin and are derived from small unmyelinated axons. Though primarily intraepidermal, free nerve endings are also present around appendages and at the dermo–epidermal junction. The epidermal free nerve endings are believed to be sensitive to touch and pain while the peritrichial and Merkel cell-associated free nerve endings are believed to be mechanoreceptors.

The encapsulated receptors of the skin are located within the dermis and are of five main types: Pacinian corpuscles, Meissner's corpuscles, Ruffini corpuscles, Krause end-bulbs and genital corpuscles. Of these, only the first two will be considered here. *Pacinian corpuscles* are distributed throughout the reticular dermis and subcutis, with greatest concentration in the palms, soles, digits, nipples and external genitalia. They are large (up to 4 mm long and 1 mm in diameter) and round to ovoid; they have a multilaminar structure resembling an onion and containing a central unmyelinated nerve fibre. The Pacinian corpuscles serve as mechanoreceptors sensitive to vibration, pressure and tension. It is believed that their structure amplifies any applied compressing or distorting force. *Meissner's corpuscles* are located just below and perpendicular to the dermo–epidermal junction in the papillary dermis. They are most numerous on the palmar and plantar surfaces, lips, eyelids, external genitalia and nipples. They are smaller than Pacinian corpuscles and composed of modified Schwann cells stacked transversely. One or more myelinated nerves enter the bottom of the corpuscle, demyelinate and give off multiple arborizing nerve branches which pursue an upward spiral course around and between the stacked cells of the corpuscle. Meissner's corpuscles are mechanoreceptors sensitive to touch and permit two-point tactile discrimination.

Of all the sensations transmitted by the sensory receptors of the skin, itching or pruritus is perhaps the most unusual and certainly the most important in the evolution of skin disease. The sensation of itching can be divided into spontaneous itch, such as that elicited by a light touch, and diffuse pathological itch, such as that associated with skin disease. Spontaneous itch is carried by the A delta fibres and is usually well localized temporally and spatially. In contrast, pathological itch is carried by C fibres and is both poorly localized and more persistent. The itch sensation, although inherent to the sensory network of the entire skin and palpebral conjunctiva, exhibits both regional and personal variation. Its receptors are located within the papillary dermis and show greater apparent density in the perianal and perigenital regions, ear canals, eyelids and nostrils. The itch receptors appear related to the pain receptors in that individuals congenitally lacking pain receptors do not experience itching. However, the two sensations, itch and pain, can be dissociated and are not identical. The itch sensation can be elicited by a wide variety of both physical and chemical stimuli including trypsin, papain, plasmin, epidermal protease, kallikrein and bradykinin. It is speculated that pathological itch is mediated by kinins formed by proteases released by tissue injury.

RESIDENT CELL POPULATION

In addition to the above components of the dermis there exists a relatively stable resident cell population. This population includes *fibroblasts, histiocytes, dermal dendrocytes, mast cells* and *lymphocytes.*

The fibroblast is the predominant cell of the dermis and is responsible for dermal synthesis, maintenance and repair. It produces dermal collagen, elastin and ground substance. It is recognized that the fibroblasts of the papillary dermis differ functionally from those of the reticular dermis.[35,36]

The histiocytes of the dermis are of both the fixed and the free type. Their function in the dermis is threefold. First, they serve as scavengers, phagocytosing free haemosiderin, melanin, lipid and miscellaneous cellular and non-cellular debris. Second, they participate in the body's immune response, both by elimination of potentially immunogenic molecules which prevent antigen overload and by concentration and retention of small quantities of antigen for presentation to lymphocytes. Third, through multiplication they contribute to granulomatous reactions.

A subgroup of phagohistiocytic cells has been identified and called the dermal dendrocyte. These highly dendritic cells phagocytose melanin and contain lysozyme but also bear coagulation factor XIIIa, HLA-DR, and OKM-1 surface markers. Moreover, they are S100 negative. They are thought to be one of the bone marrow-derived, immunologically competent cells in the skin. [37, 38]

Mast cells are primarily in a perivascular location. They function in the dermal inflammatory process through the release of various chemical mediators which attract additional cellular elements (eosinophils and neutrophils) and increase vascular permeability. The heterogeneity of mast cells is currently recognized. [39]

A small number of lymphocytes is scattered throughout the dermis in a predominantly perivascular distribution (see p. 1025). Cell typing reveals that the dermal lymphocyte population is approximately 80% T lymphocytes, equally divided between helper cells and suppressor cells, and 20% B lymphocytes. They are assumed to function in normal immunologic surveillance.

THE SUBCUTIS

The subcutis is composed of lobules of fat separated by fibrous trabeculae.[40] It extends from the lower dermis to the fibrous surface of muscle, bone or cartilage. The thickness and distribution of the subcutis varies with age, sex, and body location.

The smallest unit of organization of the subcutis is the primary microlobule. It is approximately 1 mm in diameter and composed of a grape-like aggregation of fat cells which are round to polygonal and contain a single peripheral crescent-shaped nucleus and one large central cytoplasmic lipid vacuole. In contrast, immature fat cells (normally found in the fetus) contain multiple small lipid droplets. Each microlobule of the subcutis is surrounded by thin collagenous fibres and is supplied by one terminal arteriole-venule pair. The arteriole enters the centre of the primary lobule and breaks up into numerous capillaries which surround each fat cell. The capillaries empty into the venule at the periphery of the primary lobule.

Secondary lobules are composed of grape-like clusters of primary lobules. Each measures approximately 1 cm in diameter, is surrounded by a distinct fibrous capsule, and is supplied by a single central arteriole and venule. The secondary microlobules are organized into the large lobules which compose the subcutis.

The large fibrous septa of the subcutis, which provide the organizational structure of the primary and secondary microlobules, are continuous with and similar in composition to the overlying dermis. Within them run the arterioles, veins, lymphatics and nerves which supply the overlying dermis and epidermis.

The subcutis functions as an insulation to prevent heat loss, as protection from trauma and as an energy reservoir. In addition the three-dimensional mobility of the skin is due in large part to the malleability of the subcutis.

THE SKIN ADNEXA

Supplementing its protective function, the skin has three specialized redundancies referred to as *epidermal appendages* or *adnexa*. These epidermis-derived structures consist of the *pilosebaceous apparatus* (with its *hair*, *sebaceous* and *apocrine* elements), the *eccrine glands* and the *nails*.

HAIRS

The human body is covered in most areas by a variably dense population of pilosebaceous structures. These derive from the primitive epidermis and consist of a centrally positioned hair follicle with an associated *arrector pili muscle*. Into the hair follicle canal open ducts from a mid-lying sebaceous gland and, in some body regions, a superior-lying apocrine gland. Except for palmar-plantar skin, pilosebaceous structures are found within the skin of all areas. Their density, size and components vary with body site; for example, many pilosebaceous structures are present in facial and scalp skin whereas few are found in the skin of the trunk; the hair follicles of the face, upper part of the back and upper part of the chest have uniquely large sebaceous glands, while those in axillary or inguinal skin have in addition prominent apocrine glands.

In general the pilosebaceous structure is positioned in the skin at an angle so that the growing hair shaft projects inferiorly and posteriorly. The hair shaft, an epithelial product, arises from the deep portion of the hair follicle. The size of the hair shaft is directly proportional to the size of the hair follicle. Two types of hair shafts are recognized over the body: *terminal hair*, a coarsely pigmented, thick shaft arising from a terminal hair follicle which projects into the deep dermis and even into the subcutis, and *vellus hair*, a fine, very thin, unpigmented shaft arising from a vellus hair follicle which projects only to the upper dermis (e.g. forehead hair). Both vellus and terminal follicles show similar growth patterns. Adjacent human hair follicles grow asynchronously and their growth cycle has three stages: active shaft growth (*anagen*), which on the scalp lasts for 2–6 years, an involutionary (regressing) stage (*catagen*), which lasts 2–4 weeks, and a resting stage (*telogen*), which lasts 2–4 months (see p. 455). Although the hair follicle grows from stem cells resting in its mid-portion (the bulge),[41] the hair shaft grows from the hair bulb, the inferior portion of the follicle, as an epithelial product showing a pattern of keratinization similar to epidermal cells. Growth pressure from the bulb apparently pushes the shaft upwards. The terminal hair shaft contains a central core, the *medulla*, surrounded by a thick cylinder of densely packed keratin, the *cortex*. The cortex is covered by a single row of overlapping cells, the *shaft cuticle*. The shaft is held and shaped in the follicle by another cylindrical structure, the internal *root sheath*, the inner surface of which is also lined by a cuticle, the *sheath cuticle*. In contrast to the cuticle of the shaft, the cells of which point inwards, the cells of the sheath cuticle point outwards. The two cuticular layers intermesh and moor the shaft to the sheath. Outside the cuticle of the internal root sheath are two additional cellular cylinders of the internal root sheath, *Huxley's layer* and *Henle's layer*. As the shaft moves outwards its associated cells keratinize. The first cells to keratinize completely are those of Henle's layer. The cells of the internal root sheath keratinize completely by the middle of the follicle (the *isthmus*). In this same region a smooth muscle, the *arrector pili*, situated on the side of the shaft and forming an obtuse angle with the epidermis, is inserted into the follicle. At about this level the outermost epithelial shell of the follicle, the *external root sheath*, becomes apparent. In its lower portion this layer is made up of cells rich in glycogen (the *trichilemma*); above the isthmus the cells of this layer assume epidermal characteristics. The upper third of the follicle (*infundibulum*) begins at the point of entrance of the sebaceous duct. At this level the internal root sheath, now called the infundibulum, is penetrated by the duct of the apocrine gland.

The infundibulum and the isthmus are permanent segment zones of the pilosebaceous structure. The growth cycle of the follicle involves changes in the inferior portion which atrophies during catagen and virtually disappears in telogen. During catagen the basement membrane about the lower part of the follicle becomes thick and wavy and the cells of the sheath show apoptosis (see p. 455).[42]

SEBACEOUS GLANDS

The sebaceous gland develops from the mid portion of the primitive hair follicle.[43] The take-off of the sebaceous duct demarcates the infundibulum and isthmus of the follicle. The sebaceous duct is short and serves as a passageway for the lipid-rich secretions of the glandular portions. The sebaceous gland is multilobular. The holosecretory product arises from the growth and differentiation of the peripheral basal cells. These basal cells move by growth pressure into the central lobule where they differentiate, accumulate cytoplasmic lipid, and eventually disintegrate at the level of the duct, releasing the mature sebaceous product, *sebum*. Sebum consists in large part of triglycerides, wax esters and squalene.

Sebaceous glands are present in skin regions wherever pilosebaceous structures are found; however, the size of the gland varies with location, e.g. they are largest in the skin of seborrhoeic areas (the face and the upper part of the trunk). Under androgenic stimulus these glands increase in size (e.g. at puberty) but they are small in childhood and atrophic in old age.

Although the actual role sebum plays in the health of skin is unknown, it has been postulated to act as emollient, bacteriostat, insulator and pheromone.

APOCRINE GLANDS

The apocrine gland[44] develops from the primitive hair follicle above the insertion of the sebaceous duct. The gland is of the simple tubular type. It sits as a coil in the deep dermis. The secretory portion consists of simple epithelium which shows a 'budding-type' (apocrine secretion) as well as a merocrine type of cytoplasmic secretion into the gland lumen. Because the gland stores its secretions it is expansile and shows variable width in tissue sections. Its secretions, released after a sympathetic stimulus, travel along an epithelium- and cuticle-lined duct through the upper infundibulum on to the skin surface. Mature apocrine glands are found regularly in the axilla, anogenital region, female breast, eyelids (Moll's glands) and external auditory canal.

Apocrine secretions are protein rich. The role that they play in normal skin physiology is not known. The bacterial breakdown of apocrine secretion has been identified as the source of axillary body odour.

ECCRINE GLANDS

Arising as a separate appendage of the primitive epidermis is the eccrine gland.[45] It is a coiled tubular structure in the deep dermis with a straight duct that then twists through the epidermis. The eccrine duct is morphologically identical to the apocrine duct. The eccrine glandular portion is made up of two cell types: the glycogen-containing *clear cells* (secretory cells) which are wider at their base, and the neutral mucopolysaccharide-containing *dark cells* (mucoid cells) which are wider towards the lumen. The secretory portions of the gland are enclosed by a layer of myoepithelial cells outside which is the basement membrane; the myoepithelial cells contract in response to acetylcholine.

Eccrine secretions consist predominantly of water and serve to dissipate body heat by means of surface evaporation. The watery secretions are produced in the glandular portion. In the proximal duct the salt content of the secretions is reduced, leading to the release of a hypotonic sweat on to the skin surface. A defective chloride ion channel in this region of the duct is found in patients with cystic fibrosis. Since the eccrine gland does not store its secretions, its lumen remains narrow. The eccrine gland is innervated by non-myelinated sympathetic post-ganglionic nerve fibres: their

neurochemical mediator is acetylcholine. These glands will secrete as long as the thermal or neural stimulus persists.

NAILS

The nail, another epidermis-derived appendage, covers the dorsal aspect of the distal part of the digits and serves as a protective cover and as a structural support for the extremity of the digit. The *nail plate* is composed of hard keratin, the differentiation product of the *nail matrix*. Except for its planar orientation, the relationship of the nail plate to the nail matrix is analogous to the relationship of the hair shaft to the matrix of the hair follicle. The nail plate is surrounded on three sides by folds of skin, the *lateral and proximal nail folds*, and it rests upon the *nail bed*.

The nail matrix begins proximally beneath the proximal nail fold and its distal boundary is demarcated by the distal aspect of the white half-moon, or *lunula*. The matrix is composed of small basaloid cells which keratinize without forming keratohyaline granules. Most of the nail plate is translucent because the keratinocytes composing it terminally differentiate to form orthokeratin. Over the lunula, however, keratinization is incomplete since the keratinocytes retain their nuclei and thus form opaque keratin. The nail matrix is the only source of the cells that form the nail plate. The superficial aspect of the nail plate is derived mainly from cells of the proximal part of the matrix, while the deep portion of the nail plate derives mainly from cells of the distal part of the matrix. It is the growth pressure of proliferation of new cells within the matrix which pushes the nail outwards. Normal finger-nails grow approximately 0.1 mm per day and toe-nails about half as fast.

The nail plate is supported by the underlying nail bed. The nail bed begins at the distal aspect of the lunula and extends outwards to the *hyponychium*. The nail bed has parallel longitudinal grooves and ridges comprised of squamous epithelium with a well-vascularized underlying dermis. Since the capillaries in the nail bed run parallel to the grooves, their rupture leads to longitudinal (splinter) haemorrhages. The nail bed epithelium differentiates without the formation of keratohyaline granules but with the process of parakeratosis. The parakeratotic elements adhere tightly to the overlying nail plate and are carried outwards with it. Because the nail plate and the nail bed epidermis are tightly adherent, nail avulsion leads to the separation of the nail bed from the underlying dermis.

The proximal and lateral nail folds keratinize like epidermis in general, with the formation of keratohyaline granules. The proximal nail fold is wedge-shaped, possessing dorsal and ventral surfaces. The stratum corneum contributing to the cuticle derives from the distal aspect of both the dorsal and ventral surfaces.

The *distal groove* is seen as a shallow, narrow, transverse depression just distal to a closely trimmed nail plate. The hyponychium is the region proximal to the distal groove and distal to the nail bed. Thus, from proximal to distal, the regions beneath the nail plate are: matrix, nail bed, hyponychium and distal groove. The hyponychium keratinizes with formation of keratohyaline granules and thick orthokeratin. Since it keratinizes without a granular layer and forms parakeratin, the nail bed can be readily distinguished from the hyponychium.

REFERENCES

Embryology of the skin

1. Holbrook KA, Wolff K. The structure and development of skin. In: Fitzpatrick TB, Eisen AZ, Wolff K et al, eds. Dermatology in general medicine. New York: McGraw-Hill, 1987; 93–124.
2. Parmley TH, Seeds AE. Fetal skin permeability to isotopic water (THO) in early pregnancy. Am J Obstet Gynecol 1970; 108: 128–131.
3. Smith LT, Holbrook KA. Embryogenesis of the dermis in human skin. Clin Lab Invest 1986; 3: 271–280.

The epidermis

4. Lavker RM, Sun T-T. Heterogeneity in epidermal basal keratinocytes: morphological and functional correlations. Science 1982; 215: 1239–1241.
5. Morris RJ, Fischer SM, Klein-Szanto AJP, Slaga TJ. Subpopulations of primary adult murine epidermal basal cells sedimented on density gradients. Cell Tissue Kinet 1990; 23: 587–602.
6. Elias PM. Epidermal lipids, barrier function, and desquamation. J Invest Dermatol 1983; 80: 44s–49s.
7. Fuchs E. Epidermal differentiation: the bare essentials. J Cell Biol 1990; 111: 2807–2814.
8. Dale BA, Resing KA, Haydock PV. Filaggrins. In: Goldman RD, Steinert PM, eds. Cellular and molecular biology of intermediate filaments. New York: Plenum, 1990; 393–409.
9. Haydock PV, Dale BA. Filaggrin, an intermediate filament-associated protein: structural and functional implications from the sequence of a cDNA from rat. DNA and Cell Biol 1990; 9: 251–261.
10. Mehrel T, Hohl D, Rothnagel JA et al. Identification of a major keratinocyte cell envelope protein, loricrin. Cell 1990; 61: 1103–1112.
11. Thacher SM, Rice RH. Keratinocyte-specific transglutaminase of cultured human epidermal cells: relation to cross-linked envelope formation and terminal differentiation. Cell 1985; 40: 685–695.
12. Schwarz MA, Owaribe K, Kartenbeck J, Franke WW. Desmosomes and hemidesmosomes: constitutive molecular components. Ann Rev Cell Biol 1990; 6: 461–491.
13. Williams ML. The ichthyoses — pathogenesis and prenatal diagnosis: a review of recent advances. Pediatr Dermatol 1983; 1: 1–24.
14. Squier CA. The permeability of keratinized and nonkeratinized oral epithelium to horseradish peroxidase. J Ultrastr Res 1973; 43: 160–177.
15. Odland GF, Holbrook KA. The lamellar granules of epidermis. Curr Probl Dermatol 1981; 9: 29–49.
16. Gould VE, Moll R, Moll I et al. Neuroendocrine (Merkel) cells of the skin: hyperplasias, dysplasias, and neoplasms. Lab Invest 1985; 52: 334–353.
17. Choi KL, Sauder DN. The role of Langerhans cells and keratinocytes in epidermal immunity. J Leukocyte Biol 1986; 39: 343–358.
18. Walsh LJ, Lavker RM, Murphy GF. Determinants of immune cell trafficking in skin. Lab Invest 1990; 63: 592–600.
19. Jimbow K, Fitzpatrick TB, Quevedo WC Jr. Formation, chemical composition and function of melanin pigments. In: Bereiter-Hahn J, Matoltsy AG, Richards KS, eds. Biology of the integument. Vol II. Vertebrates. Berlin: Springer Verlag, 1986; 278–292.

The epidermo–dermal junction

20. Mutasim DF, Takahashi Y, Labib RS et al. A pool of bullous pemphigoid antigen(s) is intracellular and associated with the basal cell cytoskeleton-hemidesmosome complex. J Invest Dermatol 1985; 84: 47–53.
21. Westgate GE, Weaver AC, Couchman JR. Bullous pemphigoid antigen localization suggests an intracellular association with hemidesmosomes. J Invest Dermatol 1985; 84: 218–224.
22. Guidice GJ, Squiquera HL, Elias PM, Diaz LA.

Identification of two collagen domains within the bullous pemphigoid autoantigen, BP180. J Clin Invest 1991; 87: 734–738.

23. Ruoslahti E. Integrins. J Clin Invest 1991; 87: 1–5.

24. Larjava H. Expression of 1 integrins in normal human keratinocytes. Am J Med Sci 1991; 301: 63–68.

25. Krutmann J, Kock A, Schauer E et al. Tumor necrosis factor β and ultraviolet radiation are potent regulators of human keratinocyte ICAM-1 expression. J Invest Dermatol 1990; 95: 127–131.

26. Briggaman RA. Epidermal–dermal junction: structure, composition, function and disease relationships. Progress in Dermatol 1990; 24(2): 1–8.

The dermis

27. Keene DR, Engvall E, Glanville RW. Ultrastructure of type VI collagen in human skin and cartilage suggests an anchoring function for this filamentous network. J Cell Biol 1988; 107: 1995–2006.

28. Chanoki M, Ishii M, Fukai K et al. Immunohistochemical localization of type V collagen in human skin. Arch Dermatol Res 1988; 280: 145–151.

29. Sakai LY, Keene DR, Engvall E. Fibrillin, a new 350-kD glycoprotein, is a component of extracellular microfibrils. J Cell Biol 1986; 103: 2499–2509.

30. Dahlback K, Ljungquist A, Lofberg H et al. Fibrillin immunoreactive fibers constitute a unique network in the human dermis: immunohistochemical comparison of the distributions of fibrillin, vitronectin, amyloid P component and orcein stainable structures in normal skin and elastosis. J Invest Dermatol 1990; 94: 284–291.

31. Braverman IM. Ultrastructure and organization of the cutaneous microvasculature in normal and pathologic states. J Invest Dermatol 1989; 93: 2S–9S.

32. Ryan TJ. Structure and function of lymphatics. J Invest Dermatol 1989; 93: 18S–24S.

33. Sinclair D. Mechanism of cutaneous sensation. New York: Oxford University Press, 1981.

34. Munger BL, Ide C. The structure and function of cutaneous sensory receptors. Arch Histol Cytol 1988; 51: 1–34.

35. Buckingham RB, Prince RK, Rodnan GP, Taylor F. Increased collagen accumulation in dermal fibroblast cultures from patients with progressive systemic sclerosis (scleroderma). J Lab Clin Med 1978; 92: 5–21.

36. Azzarone B, Macieira-Coelho A. Heterogeneity of the kinetics of proliferation within human skin fibroblastic cell populations. J Cell Sci 1982; 57: 177–187.

37. Headington JT. The dermal dendrocyte. Adv Dermatol 1986; 1: 159–171.

38. Cerio R, Griffiths CEM, Cooper KD et al. Characterization of factor XIIIa positive dermal dendritic cells in normal and inflamed skin. Br J Dermatol 1989; 121: 421–431.

39. Galli SJ. New insights into "the riddle of the mast cells": microenvironmental regulation of mast cell development and phenotypic heterogeneity. Lab Invest 1990; 62: 5–33.

The subcutis

40. Spearman RIC. Structure and function of subcutaneous tissue. The Physiology and Pathophysiology of the Skin 1982; 7: 2252–2281.

The skin adnexa

41. Cotsarelis G, Sun T–T, Lavker RM. Label-retaining cells reside in the bulge area of pilosebaceous unit: implications for follicular stem cells, hair cycle and skin carcinogenesis. Cell 1990; 61: 1329–1337.

42. Weedon D, Strutton G. Apoptosis as the mechanism of the involution of hair follicles in catagen transformation. Acta Derm Venereol 1981; 61: 335–339.

43. Wheatley VR. The sebaceous glands. The Physiology and Pathophysiology of the Skin 1986; 9: 2705–2971.

44. Craigmyle MBL. The apocrine glands and the breast. Chichester: J Wiley & Sons, 1984.

45. Hashimoto K, Hori K, Aso M. Sweat glands. In: Bereiter–Hahn J, Matoltsy AG, Richards KS, eds. Biology of the integument. Vol II. Vertebrates. Berlin: Springer Verlag, 1986; 339–373.

An approach to the interpretation of skin biopsies

INTRODUCTION

Trainees in dermatopathology usually experience difficulty in the interpretation of skin biopsies from inflammatory diseases of the skin. To the trainee, there seems to be an endless number of potential diagnoses in dermatopathology, with many bewildering names. However, if a logical approach is adopted, the great majority of skin biopsies can be diagnosed specifically and the remainder can be partly categorized into a particular group of diseases. It should not be forgotten that the histopathological features of some dermatoses are not diagnostically specific and it may only be possible in these circumstances to state that the histopathological features are 'consistent with' the clinical diagnosis.

The interpretation of many skin biopsies requires the identification and integration of two different, morphological features — the *tissue reaction pattern* and the *pattern of inflammation*.

Tissue reaction patterns are distinctive morphological patterns which categorize a group of cutaneous diseases. Within each of these histopathological categories there are diseases which may have similar or diverse clinical appearances and aetiologies. Some diseases may show histopathological features of more than one reaction pattern at a particular time, or during the course of their evolution.

The *pattern of inflammation* refers to the distribution of the inflammatory cell infiltrate within the dermis and/or the subcutaneous tissue. There are several distinctive patterns of inflammation (see below): their recognition assists in making a specific diagnosis.

Some dermatopathologists base their diagnostic approach on recognizing the inflammatory pattern, while others look first to see if the biopsy can be categorized into one of the 'tissue reactions', and use the pattern of inflammation to further categorize the biopsy. In practice, the experienced dermatopathologist sees these two aspects (tissue reaction pattern and inflammatory pattern) simultaneously, integrating and interpreting the findings in a matter of seconds.

The categorization of inflammatory dermatoses by their tissue reactions will be considered first.

Tissue reaction patterns

There are many different reaction patterns in the skin, but the majority of inflammatory dermatoses can be categorized into six different patterns. For convenience, these will be called the *major tissue reaction patterns*. There are a number of other diagnostic reaction patterns which occur much less commonly than the major group of six, but which are nevertheless specific for other groups of dermatoses. These patterns will be referred to as *minor tissue reaction patterns*. They will be considered after the major reaction patterns.

Patterns of inflammation

There are four patterns of cutaneous inflammation characterized on the basis of distribution of inflammatory cells within the skin:

1. Superficial perivascular inflammation
2. Superficial and deep dermal inflammation
3. Folliculitis and perifolliculitis
4. Panniculitis.

There are numerous dermatoses showing a superficial perivascular inflammatory infiltrate in the dermis and a limited number in the other categories. Sometimes panniculitis and folliculitis are regarded as minor tissue reaction patterns, because of their easily recognizable pattern.

MAJOR TISSUE REACTION PATTERNS

A significant number of inflammatory dermatoses can be categorized into one of the following six major reaction patterns, of which the key morphological feature is included in parentheses:

1. *Lichenoid* (basal cell damage)
2. *Psoriasiform* (regular epidermal hyperplasia)
3. *Spongiotic* (intraepidermal intercellular oedema)
4. *Vesiculobullous* (blistering within or beneath the epidermis)
5. *Granulomatous* (chronic granulomatous inflammation)
6. *Vasculopathic* (pathological changes in cutaneous blood vessels).

Each of these reaction patterns will be discussed in turn, together with a list of the dermatoses found in each category.

THE LICHENOID REACTION PATTERN

The lichenoid reaction pattern (see Ch.3, pp. 31–71) is characterized by *epidermal basal cell damage*, which may be manifested by cell death and/or basal vacuolar change (known in the past as 'liquefaction degeneration'). The basal cell death usually presents in the form of shrunken eosinophilic cells, with pyknotic nuclear remnants, scattered along the basal layer of the epidermis (Fig. 2.1). These cells are known as Civatte bodies. They are undergoing death by apoptosis, a

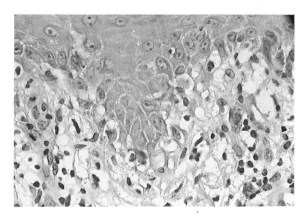

Fig. 2.1 The lichenoid reaction pattern. There are shrunken keratinocytes, with pyknotic nuclear remnants (Civatte bodies) in the basal layer. These cells are undergoing death by apoptosis. Haematoxylin — eosin

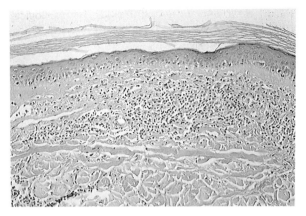

Fig. 2.2   The poikilodermatous variant of the lichenoid reaction pattern. It is characterized by mild vacuolar change of the basal layer of the epidermis, mild epidermal atrophy and dilatation of vessels in the papillary dermis. Haematoxylin — eosin

morphologically distinct type of cell death seen in both physiological and pathological circumstances (see p. 31). Sometimes the basal cell damage is quite subtle with only an occasional Civatte body and very focal vacuolar change. This is a feature of some drug reactions.

A distinctive subgroup of the lichenoid reaction pattern is the *poikilodermatous pattern*, characterized by mild basal damage, usually of vacuolar type, associated with epidermal atrophy, pigment incontinence and dilatation of vessels in the papillary dermis (Fig. 2.2). It is a feature of the various types of poikiloderma (see p. 54).

The specific diagnosis of a disease within the lichenoid tissue reaction requires an assessment of several other morphological features. These include:

1. the *type of basal damage* (vacuolar change is sometimes more prominent than cell death in lupus erythematosus, dermatomyositis, the poikilodermas and drug reactions);
2. the *distribution of the accompanying inflammatory cell infiltrate* (the infiltrate touches the undersurface of the basal layer in lichen planus and its variants, and in disseminated superficial actinic porokeratosis; it obscures the dermo–epidermal interface in erythema multiforme, fixed drug eruptions and acute pityriasis lichenoides (PLEVA); and it involves the deep as well as the superficial part of the dermis in lupus erythematosus, syphilis, photolichenoid eruptions and some drug reactions);

3. the presence of *prominent pigment incontinence* (as seen in drug reactions, the poikilodermas, lichenoid reactions in dark-skinned people and some of the solar exacerbated lichen planus variants, e.g. lichen planus actinicus); and
4. the presence of *satellite cell necrosis* (lymphocyte-associated apoptosis) — defined here as *two or more* lymphocytes in close proximity to a Civatte body (a feature of graft versus host reaction, regressing plane warts and erythema multiforme).

The diseases showing the lichenoid reaction pattern are listed in Table 2.1.

Table 2.1 Diseases showing the lichenoid reaction pattern

Lichen planus
Lichen planus variants
Lichen nitidus
Lichen striatus
Benign lichenoid keratosis
Lichenoid drug eruptions
Fixed drug eruptions
Erythema multiforme
Graft-versus-host disease
AIDS interface dermatitis
Lupus erythematosus
Dermatomyositis
Poikiloderma congenitale
Congenital telangiectatic erythema
Dyskeratosis congenita
Pityriasis lichenoides
Lichenoid purpura
Late secondary syphilis
Porokeratosis
Drug eruptions
Regressing warts and tumours
Lichen amyloidosus
Vitiligo
Lichenoid tattoo reaction

THE PSORIASIFORM REACTION PATTERN

This reaction pattern was originally defined as the cyclic formation of a suprapapillary exudate with focal parakeratosis related to it (see Ch. 4, pp.

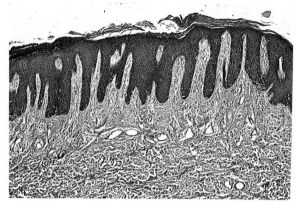

Fig. 2.3   The psoriasiform reaction pattern showing epidermal hyperplasia with regular elongation of the rete processes.
Haematoxylin — eosin

73–94). The concept of the 'squirting dermal papilla' was also put forward with the suggestion that serum and inflammatory cells escaped from the blood vessels in the papillary dermis and passed through the epidermis to form the suprapapillary exudate referred to above. The epidermal hyperplasia which also occurred was regarded as a phenomenon secondary to these other processes. From a morpho-

Table 2.2 Diseases showing the psoriasiform reaction pattern

Psoriasis
Pustular psoriasis
Reiter's syndrome
Pityriasis rubra pilaris
Parapsoriasis
Lichen simplex chronicus
Subacute and chronic spongiotic dermatitides
Erythroderma
Mycosis fungoides
Chronic candidosis and dermatophytoses
Inflammatory linear verrucous epidermal naevus (ILVEN)
Norwegian scabies
Bowen's disease (psoriasiform variant)
Clear cell acanthoma
Lamellar ichthyosis
Pityriasis rosea ('herald patch')
Pellagra
Acrodermatitis enteropathica
Glucagonoma syndrome
Secondary syphilis

logical viewpoint, the psoriasiform tissue reaction is defined as *epidermal hyperplasia in which there is elongation of the rete ridges, usually in a regular manner* (Fig. 2.3).

It is acknowledged that this latter approach has some shortcomings, as many of the diseases in this category, including psoriasis, show no significant epidermal hyperplasia in their early stages. Rather, dilated vessels in the papillary dermis and an overlying suprapapillary scale (indicative of the 'squirting papilla') may be the dominant features in early lesions of psoriasis.

Diseases showing the psoriasiform reaction pattern are listed in Table 2.2.

THE SPONGIOTIC REACTION PATTERN

The spongiotic reaction pattern (see Ch. 5, pp. 95–125) is characterized by *intraepidermal intercellular oedema (spongiosis)*. It is recognized by the presence of widened intercellular spaces between keratinocytes, with elongation of the intercellular bridges (Fig. 2.4). The spongiosis may vary from microscopic foci to grossly visible vesicles. This reaction pattern has been known in the past as the 'eczematous tissue reaction'. Inflammatory cells are present within the dermis, and their distribution and type may aid in making a specific diagnosis within this group. This is the most difficult reaction pattern in which to make a specific clinicopathological diag-

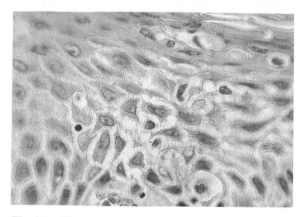

Fig. 2.4   The spongiotic reaction pattern. There is mild intercellular oedema with elongation of the intercellular bridges.
Haematoxylin — eosin

nosis; often a diagnosis of 'spongiotic reaction consistent with …' is all that can be made.

The major diseases with this tissue reaction pattern (atopic dermatitis, allergic and irritant contact dermatitis, nummular dermatitis and seborrhoeic dermatitis) all show progressive psoriasiform hyperplasia of the epidermis with chronicity (Fig. 2.5). This change is usually accompanied by diminishing spongiosis, but this will depend on the activity of the disease. Both patterns may be present in a single biopsy. The psoriasiform hyperplasia is, in part, a response to chronic rubbing and scratching. Four patterns of spongiosis can be recognized:

1. *eosinophilic spongiosis* (where there are numerous eosinophils within the foci of spongiosis);
2. *miliarial (acrosyringial) spongiosis* (where the oedema is related to the acrosyringium);
3. *follicular spongiosis* (where the spongiosis is centred on the follicular infundibulum); and

4. *haphazard spongiosis* (the other spongiotic disorders in which there is no particular pattern of spongiosis).

The diseases showing the spongiotic reaction pattern are listed in Table 2.3.

Table 2.3 Diseases showing the spongiotic reaction pattern

Eosinophilic spongiosis
    Pemphigus (precursor lesions)
    Pemphigus vegetans
    Bullous pemphigoid
    Idiopathic eosinophilic spongiosis
    Allergic contact dermatitis
    Arthropod bites
    Eosinophilic folliculitis
    Incontinentia pigmenti (first stage)
Miliarial spongiosis
    Miliaria
Follicular spongiosis
    Infundibulofolliculitis
    Atopic dermatitis (follicular lesions)
    Apocrine miliaria
    Eosinophilic folliculitis
Other spongiotic disorders
    Irritant contact dermatitis
    Allergic contact dermatitis
    Nummular dermatitis
    Sulzberger–Garbe syndrome
    Seborrhoeic dermatitis
    Atopic dermatitis
    Pompholyx
    Hyperkeratotic dermatitis of the hands
    Juvenile plantar dermatosis
    Stasis dermatitis
    Pityriasis rosea
    Papular acrodermatitis of childhood
    Spongiotic drug reactions
    Chronic superficial dermatitis
    Light reactions
    Dermatophytoses
    Arthropod bites
    Grover's disease (spongiotic variant)
    Toxic erythema of pregnancy
    Erythema annulare centrifugum
    Pigmented purpuric dermatoses
    Pityriasis alba
    Erythroderma
    Mycosis fungoides

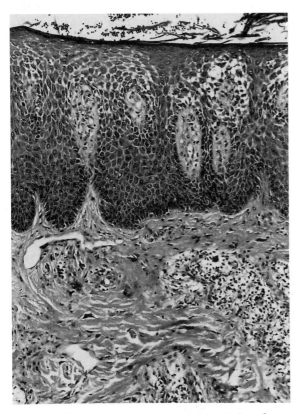

Fig. 2.5 The spongiotic reaction pattern in a lesion of some duration. Psoriasiform hyperplasia coexists with the spongiosis.
Haematoxylin — eosin

THE VESICULOBULLOUS REACTION PATTERN

In this reaction pattern, there are *vesicles or bullae at any level within the epidermis or at the dermo–epidermal junction* (see Ch. 6, pp. 127–180). A specific diagnosis can usually be made in a particular case by assessing three features — the anatomical level of the split, the underlying mechanism responsible for the split and, in the case of subepidermal lesions, the nature of the inflammatory infiltrate in the dermis.

The *anatomical level of the split* may be subcorneal, within the stratum malpighii, suprabasal or subepidermal. The *mechanism responsible* for vesiculation may be exaggerated spongiosis, intracellular oedema and ballooning (as occurs in viral infections such as herpes simplex), or acantholysis. Acantholysis is the loss of coherence between epidermal cells. It may be a primary phenomenon or secondary to inflammation, ballooning degeneration (as in viral infections of the skin) or epithelial dysplasia. In the case of subepidermal blisters, electron microscopy and

Table 2.4 Vesiculobullous diseases

Intracorneal and subcorneal blisters	Lichen sclerosus et atrophicus
Impetigo	Lichen planus pemphigoides
Staphylococcal 'scalded skin' syndrome	Polymorphous light eruption
Dermatophytosis	Fungal infections
Pemphigus foliaceus and erythematosus	Dermal allergic contact dermatitis
Subcorneal pustular dermatosis	Bullous leprosy
Infantile pustular dermatoses	Bullous mycosis fungoides
Miliaria crystallina	*Subepidermal blisters with eosinophils* [*]
Intraepidermal (stratum malpighii) blisters	Bullous pemphigoid
Spongiotic blistering diseases	Herpes gestationis
Palmoplantar pustulosis	Arthropod bites (in sensitized individuals)
Viral blistering diseases	Drug reactions
Epidermolysis bullosa (Weber–Cockayne type)	*Subepidermal blisters with neutrophils* [*]
Friction blister	Dermatitis herpetiformis
Suprabasilar blisters	Linear IgA bullous dermatosis
Pemphigus vulgaris and vegetans	Cicatricial pemphigoid
Familial benign chronic pemphigus	Localized cicatricial pemphigoid
Darier's disease	Bullous urticaria
Grover's disease	Bullous acute vasculitis
Acantholytic solar keratosis	Bullous lupus erythematosus
Subepidermal blisters with little inflammation	Erysipelas
Epidermolysis bullosa	Sweet's syndrome
Porphyria cutanea tarda	Epidermolysis bullosa acquisita
Bullous pemphigoid (cell-poor variant)	*Subepidermal blisters with mast cells*
Burns	Bullous urticaria pigmentosa
Toxic epidermal necrolysis	*Miscellaneous blistering diseases*
Suction blisters	Diabetes mellitus
Blisters overlying scars	Drug-overdose-related bullae
Bullous amyloidosis	Methyl-bromide-induced bullae
Drug reactions	Etretinate-induced bullae
Subepidermal blisters with lymphocytes	PUVA-induced bullae
Erythema multiforme	Cancer-related bullae
Bullous fixed drug eruption	Lymphatic bullae

[*]Varying admixtures of eosinophils and neutrophils may be seen in cicatricial pemphigoid and late lesions of dermatitis herpetiformis.

immunoelectron microscopy could be used to make a specific diagnosis in most cases. In practice, the subepidermal blisters are subdivided on the basis of the *inflammatory cell infiltrate within the dermis*. Knowledge of the immunofluorescence findings is often helpful in categorizing the subepidermal blistering diseases.

Table 2.4 lists the various vesiculobullous diseases, based on the anatomical level of the split and, in the case of subepidermal lesions, the predominant inflammatory cell within the dermis.

THE GRANULOMATOUS REACTION PATTERN

This group of diseases (see Ch.7, pp. 181–207) is characterized by the presence of *chronic granulomatous inflammation*; that is, localized collections of epithelioid cells usually admixed with giant cells, lymphocytes, plasma cells, fibroblasts and non-epithelioid macrophages (Fig. 2.6). Five histological types of granuloma can be identified on the basis of the con-

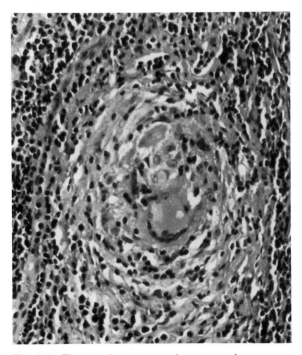

Fig. 2.6   The granulomatous reaction pattern. A tuberculoid granuloma is present in the dermis. Haematoxylin — eosin

stituent cells and other changes within the granulomas — sarcoidal, tuberculoid, necrobiotic, suppurative and foreign body.

Sarcoidal granulomas are composed of epithelioid cells and giant cells, some containing asteroid bodies or other inclusions. The granulomas are often referred to as 'naked granulomas', in that they have only a sparse 'clothing' of peripheral lymphocytes and plasma cells in contrast to tuberculoid granulomas that usually have more abundant lymphocytes. Some overlap occurs between sarcoidal and tuberculoid granulomas.

Tuberculoid granulomas resemble those seen in tuberculosis, although caseation necrosis is not always present. The giant cells that are present within the granuloma are usually of Langhans type.

Necrobiotic granulomas are composed of epithelioid cells, lymphocytes and occasional giant cells associated with areas of 'necrobiosis' of collagen. Sometimes the inflammatory cells are arranged in a palisade around the areas of necrobiosis. The term 'necrobiosis' has been criticized because it implies that the collagen (which is not a vital structure) is 'necrotic'. The process of necrobiosis is characterized by an accumulation of acid mucopolysaccharides between the collagen bundles and degeneration of some interstitial fibroblasts and histiocytes.

Suppurative granulomas have neutrophils within, and sometimes surrounding, the granuloma. The granulomatous component is not always well formed.

Foreign body granulomas have multinucleate, foreign body giant cells as a constituent of the granuloma. Foreign material can usually be visualized in sections stained with haematoxylin and eosin, although at other times it requires the use of polarized light for its detection.

The identification of organisms by the use of special stains (the periodic acid–Schiff and other stains for fungi, and stains for acid-fast bacilli), or by culture, may be necessary to make a specific diagnosis. Organisms are usually scanty in granulomas associated with infectious diseases. The distribution of the granulomas (they may be arranged along nerve fibres in tuberculoid leprosy) may assist in making a specific diagnosis.

It should also be noted that many of the infectious diseases listed in Table 2.5 as causing

Table 2.5 Diseases causing the granulomatous reaction pattern

Sarcoidal granulomas
   Sarcoidosis
   Reactions to foreign materials
Tuberculoid granulomas
   Tuberculosis
   Tuberculids
   Leprosy
   Late syphilis
   Leishmaniasis
   Protothecosis
   Papular rosacea
   Perioral dermatitis
   Lupus miliaris disseminatus faciei
   Crohn's disease
Necrobiotic granulomas
   Granuloma annulare
   Necrobiosis lipoidica
   Rheumatoid nodules
   Rheumatic fever nodules
   Reactions to foreign materials
Suppurative granulomas
   Chromomycosis and phaeohyphomycosis
   Sporotrichosis
   Mycobacterium marinum infection
   Blastomycosis
   Paracoccidioidomycosis
   Coccidioidomycosis
   Blastomycosis-like pyoderma
   Ruptured cysts and follicles
   Mycetoma, nocardiosis and actinomycosis
   Cat-scratch disease
   Lymphogranuloma venereum
   Pyoderma gangrenosum
Foreign body granulomas
   Exogenous material
   Endogenous material
Miscellaneous
   Orofacial granulomatosis
   Elastolytic granulomas
   Granulomatous T-cell lymphomas

the granulomatous tissue reaction can also produce inflammatory reactions that do not include granulomas, depending on the stage of the disease and the immune status of the individual.

THE VASCULOPATHIC REACTION PATTERN

The vasculopathic reaction pattern (see Ch.8, pp. 209–265) includes a clinically heterogeneous group of diseases which have in common *pathological changes in blood vessels*. The most important category within this tissue reaction pattern is *vasculitis*, which can be defined as an inflammatory process involving the walls of blood vessels of any size (Fig. 2.7). Some dermatopathologists insist on the presence of fibrin within the vessel wall before they will accept a diagnosis of vasculitis. This criterion is far too restrictive and it ignores the fact that exudative features, such as fibrin extravasation, are not prominent in chronic inflammation in any tissue of the body. On the other hand, a diagnosis of vasculitis should not be made simply because there is a perivascular infiltrate of inflammatory cells. Notwithstanding these comments, in resolving and late lesions of vasculitis there may only be a tight perivascular inflammatory cell infiltrate, making it difficult to make a diagnosis of vasculitis. The presence of endothelial swelling in small vessels and an increase in fibrohistiocytic cells (a 'busy dermis') and sometimes acid mucopolysaccharides in the dermis are further clues which assist in confirming that a resolving vasculitis is present. Although it is useful to categorize vasculitis into acute, chronic lymphocytic

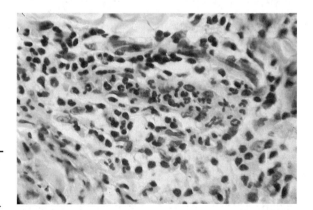

Fig. 2.7 Acute vasculitis. Neutrophils are present in the wall of a small vessel which also shows swelling of its endothelium.
Haematoxylin — eosin

Table 2.6 Diseases showing the vasculopathic reaction pattern

Non-inflammatory purpuras	*Neutrophilic dermatoses*
Senile purpura	Sweet's syndrome
Vascular occlusive diseases	Bowel-associated dermatosis-arthritis syndrome
Warfarin necrosis	Rheumatoid neutrophilic dermatosis
Atrophie blanche	Acute generalized pustulosis
Disseminated intravascular coagulation	Behçet's syndrome
Purpura fulminans	*Chronic lymphocytic vasculitis*
Thrombotic thrombocytopenic purpura	Toxic erythema
Cryoglobulinaemia	Toxic erythema of pregnancy
Cholesterol embolism	Prurigo of pregnancy
Miscellaneous conditions	Gyrate erythemas
Urticarias	Pityriasis lichenoides
Acute vasculitis	Pigmented purpuric dermatoses
Hypersensitivity vasculitis	Malignant atrophic papulosis (Degos)
Henoch–Schönlein purpura	Perniosis
Rheumatoid vasculitis	Rickettsial and viral infections
Urticarial vasculitis	Pyoderma gangrenosum
Mixed cryoglobulinaemia	Polymorphous light eruption (variant)
Hypergammaglobulinaemic purpura	Sclerosing lymphangitis of the penis
Septic vasculitis	*Vasculitis with granulomatosis*
Erythema elevatum diutinum	Wegener's granulomatosis
Granuloma faciale	Lymphomatoid granulomatosis
Polyarteritis nodosa	Allergic granulomatosis
Kawasaki disease	Lethal midline granuloma
Superficial thrombophlebitis	Giant cell (temporal) arteritis
Miscellaneous associations	Takayasu's arteritis

and granulomatous forms, it should be remembered that an acute vasculitis may progress with time to a chronic stage. Fibrin is rarely present in these late lesions.

Other categories of vascular disease include non-inflammatory purpuras, vascular occlusive diseases, and urticarias. The purpuras are characterized by extravasation of erythrocytes and the vascular occlusive diseases by fibrin and/or platelet thrombi or, rarely, other material in the lumen of small blood vessels. The urticarias are characterized by increased vascular permeability, with escape of oedema fluid and some cells into the dermis. The neutrophilic dermatoses are included also because they share some morphological features with the acute vasculitides.

The diseases showing the vasculopathic reaction pattern are listed in Table 2.6.

MINOR TISSUE REACTION PATTERNS

This is a term of convenience for a group of reaction patterns in the skin that are seen much less frequently than the six major patterns already discussed. Like the major reaction patterns, each of the patterns to be considered below is diagnostic of a certain group of diseases of the skin. Sometimes a knowledge of the clinical distribution of the lesions (e.g. whether they are localized, linear, zosteriform or generalized) is required before a specific clinicopathological diagnosis can be made. The minor tissue reaction patterns to be discussed, with their key morphological feature in parentheses, are:

1. *Epidermolytic hyperkeratosis* (hyperkeratosis with granular and vacuolar degeneration)

2. *Acantholytic dyskeratosis* (suprabasilar clefts with acantholytic and dyskeratotic cells)
3. *Cornoid lamellation* (a column of parakeratotic cells with absence of an underlying granular layer)
4. *Papillomatosis ('church-spiring')* (undulations and protrusions of the epidermis)
5. *Angiofibromas* (increased dermal vessels with surrounding fibrosis)
6. *Eosinophilic cellulitis with 'flame figures'* (dermal eosinophils and eosinophilic material adherent to collagen bundles)
7. *Transepithelial elimination* (elimination of material via the epidermis or hair follicles).

The first four patterns listed are all disorders of epidermal maturation and keratinization. They will be discussed briefly below and in further detail in Chapter 9 (pp. 267–301). Angiofibromas are included with tumours of fibrous tissue in Chapter 34 (pp. 873–903), while eosinophilic cellulitis is discussed with the cutaneous infiltrates in Chapter 40 (pp. 995–1074). Transepithelial elimination is a process which may occur as a secondary event in a wide range of skin diseases. It is discussed below.

EPIDERMOLYTIC HYPERKERATOSIS

The features of this reaction pattern are *compact hyperkeratosis accompanied by granular and vacuolar degeneration of the cells of the spinous and granular layers* (Fig. 2.8). This pattern may occur in diseases or lesions which are generalized (bullous ichthyosiform erythroderma), systematized (epidermal naevus variant), palmar-plantar (a variant of palmoplantar keratoderma), solitary (epidermolytic acanthoma), multiple and discrete (disseminated epidermolytic acanthoma) or follicular (naevoid follicular hyperkeratosis). Rarely, this pattern may be seen in solar keratoses. Not uncommonly, epidermolytic hyperkeratosis is an incidental finding in a biopsy taken because of the presence of some other lesion.

ACANTHOLYTIC DYSKERATOSIS

Acantholytic dyskeratosis is characterized by *suprabasilar clefting with acantholytic and dyskerato-*

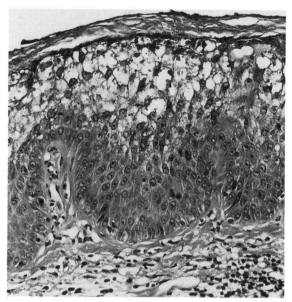

Fig. 2.8 Epidermolytic hyperkeratosis, characterized by granular and vacuolar degeneration of the upper layers of the epidermis and overlying hyperkeratosis. Haematoxylin — eosin

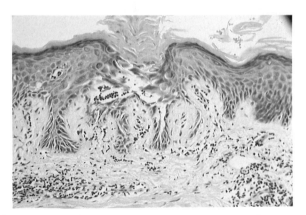

Fig. 2.9 Acantholytic dyskeratosis with suprabasal clefting and dyskeratotic cells in the overlying epidermis. Haematoxylin — eosin

tic cells at all levels of the epidermis (see p. 279) (Fig. 2.9). It may be a generalized process (Darier's disease), a systematized process (a variant of epidermal naevus), transient (Grover's disease), palmar-plantar (a very rare form of keratoderma), solitary (warty dyskeratoma), an incidental finding or a feature of a solar keratosis (acantholytic solar keratosis).

CORNOID LAMELLATION

Cornoid lamellation (Fig. 2.10) is localized faulty keratinization characterized by a *thin column of parakeratotic cells with an absent or decreased underlying granular zone and vacuolated or dyskeratotic cells in the spinous layer* (see p. 276). Although cornoid lamellation is a characteristic feature of porokeratosis and its clinical variants, it can be found as an incidental phenomenon in a range of inflammatory, hyperplastic and neoplastic conditions of the skin.

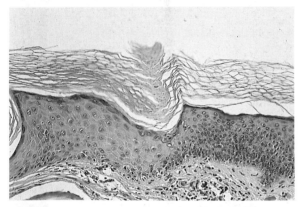

Fig. 2.10   A cornoid lamella in porokeratosis. A thin column of parakeratotic cells overlies a narrow zone in which the granular layer is absent.
Haematoxylin — eosin

PAPILLOMATOSIS ('CHURCH-SPIRING')

Papillomatosis refers to the presence of undulations or projections of the epidermal surface. This may vary from tall 'steeple-like' projections to quite small, somewhat broader elevations of the epidermal surface. The term 'church-spiring' is sometimes used to refer to these changes. The various lesions showing papillomatosis are listed in Table 2.7.

ACRAL ANGIOFIBROMAS

This reaction pattern is characterized by an *increase in the number of small vessels which is associated with perivascular and, sometimes, perifol-*

Table 2.7 Lesions showing papillomatosis

Seborrhoeic keratosis
Acrokeratosis verruciformis
Verruca vulgaris
Epidermodysplasia verruciformis
Verruca plana
Stucco keratosis
Tar keratosis
Arsenical keratosis
Solar keratosis
Acanthosis nigricans
Reticulated papillomatosis
Epidermal naevus
Verrucous carcinoma
Keratosis follicularis spinulosa
Disseminated spiked hyperkeratosis
Multiple digitate hyperkeratosis
Hyperkeratosis lenticularis

Table 2.8 Conditions showing an angiofibromatous pattern

Adenoma sebaceum
Subungual and periungual fibroma
Acquired acral fibrokeratoma
Fibrous papule of the nose
Pearly penile papules

licular fibrosis (see p. 873). The fibrous tissue usually contains stellate fibroblasts. The conditions showing this reaction pattern are listed in Table 2.8.

EOSINOPHILIC CELLULITIS WITH 'FLAME FIGURES'

In eosinophilic cellulitis with 'flame figures' there is *dermal oedema with an infiltration of eosinophils and some histiocytes, and scattered 'flame figures'* (Fig. 2.11). 'Flame figures' result from the adherence of amorphous or granular eosinophilic material to collagen bundles in the dermis. They are small, poorly circumscribed foci of apparent 'necrobiosis' of collagen, although they are eosinophilic rather than basophilic as seen in the usual 'necrobiotic' disorders.

Eosinophilic cellulitis with 'flame figures' can

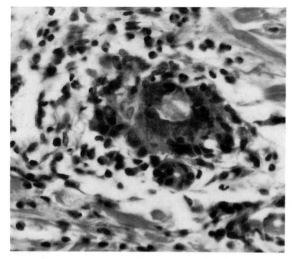

Fig. 2.11   Eosinophilic cellulitis with flame figures. Haematoxylin — eosin

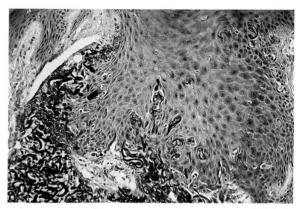

Fig. 2.12   Transepithelial elimination of solar-elastotic material is occurring through an enlarged follicular infundibulum.
Verhoeff — van Gieson

occur as part of a generalized cutaneous process known as Wells' syndrome (see p. 998). This reaction pattern, which may represent a severe urticarial hypersensitivity reaction to various stimuli, can also be seen, rarely, in biopsies from bullous pemphigoid, dermatitis herpetiformis, diffuse erythemas, and *Trichophyton rubrum* infections. The 'flame figures' of eosinophilic cellulitis resemble the Splendore–Hoeppli deposits which are sometimes found around parasites in tissues.

TRANSEPITHELIAL ELIMINATION

The term 'transepithelial elimination' was coined by Mehregan for a *biological phenomenon whereby materials foreign to the skin are eliminated through pores between cells of the epidermis or hair follicle, or are carried up between cells as a passive phenomenon, during maturation of the epidermal cells*.[1] The validity of this hypothesis has been confirmed using an animal model.[2] The process of transepithelial elimination can be recognized in tissue sections by the presence of pseudoepitheliomatous hyperplasia or expansion of hair follicles (Fig. 2.12). These downgrowths of the epidermis or follicle usually surround the material to be eliminated. Various tissues, substances or organisms can be eliminated from the dermis in this way, including elastic fibres, collagen, erythro-

cytes, amyloid, calcium salts, bone, foreign material, inflammatory cells and debris, fungi and mucin.[3-15] The various disorders (also known as 'perforating disorders') which may show transepithelial elimination are listed in Table 2.9.

The apparent transepithelial elimination of a

Table 2.9 Diseases in which transepithelial elimination may occur

Necrobiosis lipoidica
Necrobiotic xanthogranuloma
Perforating folliculitis
Pseudoxanthoma elasticum
Elastosis perforans serpiginosa
Reactive perforating collagenosis
Calcaneal petechiae ('black heel')
Amyloidosis
Chondrodermatitis nodularis helicis
Calcinosis cutis
Osteoma cutis
Deep mycoses
Cutaneous tuberculosis
Blastomycosis-like pyoderma
Sarcoidosis
Foreign body granulomas
Suture material
Lichen nitidus
Papular mucinosis
Acne keloidalis nuchae
Solar elastosis
Cutaneous tumours

sebaceous gland has been reported.[16] This process was probably an artefact of tissue sectioning.

PATTERNS OF INFLAMMATION

Four patterns of inflammation can be discerned in biopsies taken from the various inflammatory diseases of the skin — superficial perivascular inflammation, superficial and deep dermal inflammation, folliculitis and perifolliculitis, and panniculitis. Superficial band-like infiltrates are not included as a separate category as they are usually associated with the lichenoid reaction pattern, or the infiltrate is merely an extension of a superficial perivascular infiltrate.

SUPERFICIAL PERIVASCULAR INFLAMMATION

This pattern of inflammation is usually associated with the spongiotic, psoriasiform or lichenoid reaction patterns. On some occasions, diseases which are usually regarded as showing the spongiotic reaction pattern have only very mild spongiosis which may not always be evident on casual inspection of one level of a biopsy. This should be kept in mind when a superficial perivascular inflammatory reaction is present.

Causes of a superficial perivascular infiltrate, in the absence of spongiosis or another reaction pattern, include the following diseases:

Drug reactions
Dermatophytoses
Viral exanthems
Chronic urticaria
Erythrasma
Superficial annular erythemas
Pigmented purpuric dermatoses
Resolving dermatoses.

SUPERFICIAL AND DEEP DERMAL INFLAMMATION

This pattern of inflammation may accompany a major reaction pattern, as occurs in discoid lupus erythematosus in which there is a concomitant lichenoid reaction pattern, and in photocontact allergic dermatitis in which there is a spongiotic reaction pattern in addition to the dermal inflammation. This pattern of inflammation may also occur in the absence of any of the six major reaction patterns already discussed. The predominant cell type is usually the lymphocyte but there may be a variable admixture of other cell types. The usually-quoted mnemonic of diseases causing this pattern of inflammation is the eight 'L' diseases — light reactions, lymphoma (including pseudolymphomas), leprosy, lues (syphilis), lichen striatus, lupus erythematosus, lipoidica (includes necrobiosis lipoidica and incomplete forms of granuloma annulare) and lepidoptera (used incorrectly in the mnemonic to refer to arthropod bites and other parasitic infestations). To the eight 'L diseases' should be added 'DRUGS' — drug reactions, reticular erythematous mucinosis, urticaria (chronic urticaria and the urticarial stages of bullous pemphigoid and herpes gestationis), gyrate erythemas (deep type) and scleroderma (particularly the localized variants).

This list is obviously incomplete but it covers most of the important diseases having this pattern of inflammation. For example, the vasculitides and various granulomatous diseases have superficial and deep inflammation in the dermis but they have been excluded from the mnemonics because they constitute major reaction patterns. It is always worth keeping in mind the mnemonics (the eight 'L' diseases and 'DRUGS') when a superficial and deep infiltrate is present in tissue sections.

FOLLICULITIS AND PERIFOLLICULITIS

Inflammation of the hair follicle (folliculitis) usually extends into the adjacent dermis, producing a perifolliculitis. For this reason, these two patterns of inflammation are considered together. There are several ways of classifying the various folliculitides, the most common being based on the anatomical level of the follicle (superficial or deep) that is involved. This distinction is not always clear cut and in some cases of folliculitis due to an infectious agent the follicle may be inflamed throughout its entire length. The folliculitides are discussed in further detail in Chapter 15, pages 439–447.

Because infectious agents are an important cause of folliculitis and perifolliculitis the subclassification of diseases showing this pattern of inflammation into 'infective' and 'non-infective' groups is sometimes made. If this aetiological classification is used in conjunction with the anatomical level of the follicle most affected by the inflammation, four groups of folliculitides are produced. The important diseases in each of these groups are listed in parentheses:

1. *Superficial infective folliculitis* (impetigo, some fungal infections, herpes simplex folliculitis, folliculitis of secondary syphilis)
2. *Superficial non-infective folliculitis* (infundibulofolliculitis, actinic folliculitis, acne vulgaris (?), acne necrotica, eosinophilic pustular folliculitis)
3. *Deep infective folliculitis* (kerion, favus, pityrosporum folliculitis, Majocchi's granuloma, folliculitis decalvans, furuncle, herpes simplex folliculitis)
4. *Deep non-infective folliculitis* (hidradenitis suppurativa, dissecting cellulitis of the scalp, acne conglobata, perforating folliculitis).

In sections stained with haematoxylin and eosin, the division into superficial or deep folliculitis can usually be made, except in cases with overlap features. Further subdivision into infective and non-infective types may require the use of special stains for organisms.

PANNICULITIS

Inflammatory lesions of the subcutaneous fat can be divided into three distinct categories: *septal panniculitis*, in which the inflammation is confined to the interlobular septa of the subcutis; *lobular panniculitis*, in which the inflammation involves the entire fat lobule and often the septa as well; and *panniculitis secondary to vasculitis involving large vessels in the subcutis*, in which the inflammation is usually restricted to the immediate vicinity of the involved vessel. The various panniculitides are listed in Table 2.10. They are discussed further in Chapter 17, pages 499–516.

Table 2.10 Diseases causing a panniculitis

Septal panniculitis
  Erythema nodosum
  Necrobiosis lipoidica
  Scleroderma
Lobular panniculitis
  Nodular vasculitis
  Erythema induratum
  Subcutaneous fat necrosis of the newborn
  Sclerema neonatorum
  Cold panniculitis
  Weber–Christian disease
  α_1–antitrypsin deficiency
  Cytophagic histiocytic panniculitis
  Pancreatic panniculitis
  Lupus panniculitis
  Connective tissue panniculitis
  Post-steroid panniculitis
  Lipodystrophy syndromes
  Factitial panniculitis
  Traumatic fat necrosis
  Infective panniculitis
  Eosinophilic panniculitis
Panniculitis secondary to large vessel vasculitis
  Cutaneous polyarteritis nodosa
  Superficial migratory thrombophlebitis

REFERENCES

1. Mehregan AH. Elastosis perforans serpiginosa. A review of the literature and report of 11 cases. Arch Dermatol 1968; 97: 381–393.
2. Bayoumi A-HM, Gaskell S, Marks R. Development of a model for transepidermal elimination. Br J Dermatol 1978; 99: 611–620.
3. Woo TY, Rasmussen JE. Disorders of transepidermal elimination. Part 1. Int J Dermatol 1985; 24: 267–279.
4. Woo TY, Rasmussen JE. Disorders of transepidermal elimination. Part 2. Int J Dermatol 1985; 24: 337–348.
5. Patterson JW. The perforating disorders. J Am Acad Dermatol 1984; 10: 561–581.

6. Jones RE Jr. Questions to the Editorial Board and other authorities. Am J Dermatopathol 1984; 6: 89–94.
7. Goette DK. Transepithelial elimination of altered collagen after intralesional adrenal steroid injections. Arch Dermatol 1984; 120: 539–540.
8. Goette DK, Berger TG. Acne keloidalis nuchae. A transepidermal elimination disorder. Int J Dermatol 1987; 26: 442–444.
9. Goette DK. Transepidermal elimination of actinically damaged connective tissue. Int J Dermatol 1984; 23: 669–672.
10. Goette DK, Odom RB. Transepithelial elimination of granulomas in cutaneous tuberculosis and sarcoidosis. J Am Acad Dermatol 1986; 14: 126–128.
11. Goette DK. Transepithelial elimination of Monsel's solution-induced granuloma. J Cutan Pathol 1984; 11: 158–161.
12. Goette DK, Robertson D. Transepithelial elimination in chromomycosis. Arch Dermatol 1984; 120: 400–401.
13. Batres E, Klima M, Tschen J. Transepithelial elimination in cutaneous sarcoidosis. J Cutan Pathol 1982; 9: 50–54.
14. Goette DK. Transepithelial elimination of suture material. Arch Dermatol 1984; 120: 1137–1138.
15. Goette DK. Transepithelial elimination of benign and malignant tumors. J Dermatol Surg Oncol 1987; 13: 68–73.
16. Weigand DA. Transfollicular extrusion of sebaceous glands: natural phenomenon or artifact? A case report. J Cutan Pathol 1976; 3: 239–244.

The lichenoid reaction pattern

INTRODUCTION

The lichenoid reaction pattern (lichenoid tissue reaction) is characterized histologically by epidermal basal cell damage.[1,2] This takes the form of cell death and/or vacuolar change (liquefaction degeneration). The cell death usually involves only scattered cells in the basal layer which become shrunken with eosinophilic cytoplasm. These cells, which have been called Civatte bodies, often contain pyknotic nuclear remnants. Sometimes, fine focussing up and down will reveal smaller cell fragments, often without nuclear remnants, adjacent to the more obvious Civatte bodies.[3] These smaller fragments have separated from the larger bodies during the process of cell death. Ultrastructural studies have shown that the basal cells in the lichenoid reaction pattern usually die by apoptosis, a comparatively recently described form of cell death, which is quite distinct morphologically from necrosis.[4,4a]

In *apoptosis*, single cells become condensed and then fragment into small bodies by an active budding process (Fig. 3.1). In the skin, these condensed apoptotic bodies are known as Civatte bodies (see above). The smaller apoptotic bodies, some of which are beyond the resolution of the light microscope, are usually phagocytosed quickly by adjacent parenchymal cells, or by tissue macrophages.[4] Cell membranes and organelles remain intact for some time in apoptosis, in contradistinction to necrosis where breakdown of these structures is an integral and prominent part of the process. Because keratinocytes contain tonofilaments which act as a 'straight-jacket' within the cell, budding and fragmentation are

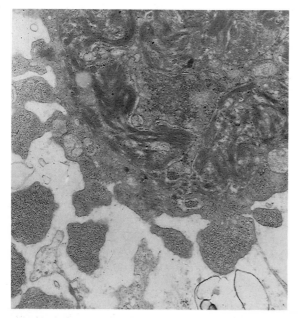

Fig. 3.1 Apoptosis of a basal keratinocyte in lichen planus. There is surface budding and some redistribution of organelles within the cytoplasm. Electron micrograph × 12 000

less complete in the skin than they are in most other cells in the body undergoing death by apoptosis. This is particularly so if the keratinocyte accumulates filaments in its cytoplasm, immediately preceding its death. The apoptotic bodies that are rich in tonofilaments are usually larger than the others; they tend to 'resist' phagocytosis by parenchymal cells, although some are phagocytosed by macrophages. Others are extruded into the papillary dermis, where they are known as *colloid bodies*.[5] These bodies appear to trap immunoglobulins non-specifically, particularly the IgM molecule, which is larger than the others.

Some of the diseases included within the lichenoid reaction pattern show necrosis of the epidermis rather than apoptosis; in others, the cells have accumulated so many cytoplasmic filaments prior to death, that the actual mechanism — apoptosis or necrosis — cannot be discerned by light or electron microscopy. The term 'filamentous degeneration', introduced by Hashimoto, seems appropriate in these circumstances.[6] It should be noted that apoptotic keratinocytes have been seen in normal skin,

suggesting that cell deletion also occurs as a normal physiological phenomenon.[7]

Vacuolar change (liquefaction degeneration) is often an integral part of the basal damage in the lichenoid reaction. Sometimes it is more prominent than the cell death. It results from intracellular vacuole formation and oedema, as well as from separation of the lamina densa from the plasma membrane of the basal cells. Vacuolar change is usually prominent in lupus erythematosus, particularly the acute systemic form, and in dermatomyositis and some drug reactions.

As a consequence of the basal cell damage, there is variable *melanin incontinence* resulting from interference with melanin transfer from melanocytes to keratinocytes, as well as from the death of cells in the basal layer.[1] Melanin incontinence is particularly prominent in some drug-induced and solar-related lichenoid lesions, as well as in patients with marked racial pigmentation.

Another feature of the lichenoid reaction pattern is a variable *inflammatory cell infiltrate*. This varies in composition, density and distribution according to the disease. An assessment of these characteristics is important in distinguishing the various lichenoid dermatoses. As apoptosis, unlike necrosis, does not itself evoke an inflammatory response, it can be surmised that the infiltrate in those diseases with prominent apoptosis is of pathogenetic significance, and not a secondary event.[4] Furthermore, apoptosis is the usual method of cell death resulting from cell-mediated mechanisms, whereas necrosis and possibly vacuolar change result from humoral factors, including the deposition of immune complexes.

In summary, the lichenoid reaction pattern includes a heterogeneous group of diseases which have in common basal cell damage.[7a] The histogenesis is also diverse and includes cell-mediated and humoral immune reactions, and possibly ischaemia in one condition. Scattered apoptotic keratinocytes can also be seen in the sunburn reaction in response to ultraviolet radiation; these cells are known as 'sunburn cells'.[7b] A specific histological diagnosis can usually be made by attention to such factors as:

1. the nature and extent of the basal damage,

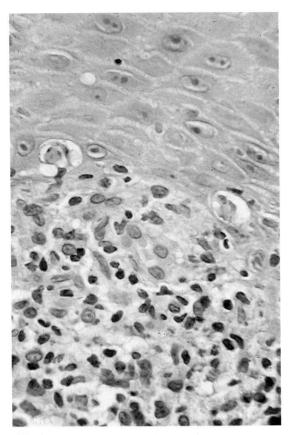

Fig. 3.2 Lichen planus. Two apoptotic keratinocytes (Civatte bodies) are present in the basal layer of the epidermis. An infiltrate of lymphocytes touches the undersurface of the epidermis.
Haematoxylin — eosin

2. the nature, composition and distribution of the inflammatory reaction,
3. the amount of melanin incontinence which results from the basal damage, and
4. other individual characteristics.[2]

These points are considered further in Tables 3.1 and 3.2 on pages 57 and 58.

A discussion of the various dermatoses within this group follows. The conditions listed as 'other lichenoid diseases' are discussed only briefly as they are considered in detail in other chapters.

LICHENOID DERMATOSES

LICHEN PLANUS

Lichen planus, a relatively common eruption of unknown aetiology, displays violaceous, flat-topped papules, which are usually pruritic. A network of fine white lines (Wickham's striae) may be seen on the surface of the papules. There is a predilection for the flexor surface of the wrists, the trunk, the thighs and the genitalia. Oral lesions are common; rarely the oesophagus is also involved.[8] Nail changes occur[9,10] and, as with oral lesions,[11] these may be the only manifestations of the disease.[12,13] Spontaneous resolution of lichen planus is usual within 12 months, although post-inflammatory pigmentation may persist for some time afterwards.

Familial cases are uncommon, and rarely these are associated with HLA-D7.[14–17] An association with HLA-DR1 has been found in non-familial cases.[18] Lichen planus has been reported in association with immunodeficiency states,[19] primary biliary cirrhosis,[20,21] pemphigus,[22] ulcerative colitis[23] and lichen sclerosus et atrophicus with coexisting morphoea.[24] Squamous cell carcinoma is a rare complication of the oral cases of lichen planus and of the hypertrophic and ulcerative variants (see below).[25–27]

Cell-mediated immune reactions appear to be important in the pathogenesis of lichen planus.[28] It has been suggested that these reactions are precipitated by an alteration in the antigenicity of epidermal keratinocytes, possibly caused by a virus or a drug or by an allogeneic cell.[29] Recent transplantation experiments do not support this view.[29a] Keratinocytes in lichen planus express HLA-DR on their surface and this may be one of the antigens which has an inductive or perpetuating role in the process.[30–33] The cellular response consists of many activated T lymphocytes.[34,35] There is an increase in helper T cells in the infiltrate[36,37] and an elevated helper/suppressor T-cell ratio in the peripheral blood.[38] Lymphokines produced by these T lymphocytes, including interferon-γ and tumour necrosis factor, may have an effector role in producing the destruction of keratinocytes;[38a,38b] suppressor/cytotoxic cells possibly play a role also.[3,39] Langerhans cells are increased, and it has been suggested that these cells process the foreign antigen initially.[31]

Most studies have found no autoantibodies and no alteration in serum immunoglobulins in lichen planus.[40] However, a lichen planus-specific antigen has been detected recently in the epidermis, and a circulating antibody to it has been found in the serum of individuals with lichen planus.[41] Its pathogenetic significance remains uncertain.

Replacement of the damaged basal cells is achieved by an increase in actively dividing keratinocytes in both the epidermis and the skin appendages.[42,43]

Histopathology[44]

The basal cell damage in lichen planus takes the form of multiple, scattered Civatte bodies (Fig. 3.2). Eosinophilic colloid bodies, which are PAS positive and diastase resistant, are found in the papillary dermis (Fig. 3.3). They measure approximately 20 μm in diameter. The basal damage is associated with a band-like infiltrate of lymphocytes and some macrophages which presses against the undersurface of the epidermis (Fig. 3.4). Occasional lymphocytes extend into the basal layer, where they may be found in close contact with basal cells and sometimes with Civatte bodies. The infiltrate does not obscure the interface or extend into the mid-epidermis as in erythema multiforme and fixed drug eruptions (see pp. 41 and 43). Plasma cells are occasionally present in the skin lesions;[45] they are invariably present in lesions adjacent to or on mucous membranes. There is variable melanin incontinence but this is most conspicuous in

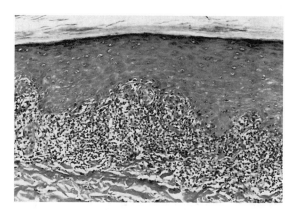

Fig. 3.4 Lichen planus. A band-like infiltrate of lymphocytes fills the papillary dermis and touches the undersurface of the epidermis.
Haematoxylin — eosin

lesions of long duration, and in dark-skinned people.

Other characteristic epidermal changes include hyperkeratosis, wedge-shaped areas of hypergranulosis related to the acrosyringia and acrotrichia, and variable acanthosis. At times the rete ridges become pointed, imparting a 'saw tooth' appearance to the lower epidermis. There is sometimes mild hypereosinophilia of keratinocytes in the malpighian layer. Small clefts (Caspary–Joseph[46] spaces) may form at the dermo–epidermal junction secondary to the basal damage. A variant in which the lichenoid changes are localized to the acrosyringium has been reported.[47] Transepidermal elimination with perforation is another rare finding.[48]

Ragaz and Ackerman have studied the evolution of lesions in lichen planus.[44] They found an increased number of Langerhans cells in the epidermis in the very earliest lesions, before there was any significant infiltrate of inflammatory cells in the dermis. In resolving lesions, the infiltrate is less dense, and there may be minimal extension of the inflammatory infiltrate into the reticular dermis.

Direct immunofluorescence of involved skin shows colloid bodies in the papillary dermis, staining for complement and immunoglobulins, particularly IgM.[49] An irregular band of fibrin is present along the basal layer in most cases.[50] Often there is irregular extension of the fibrin into the underlying papillary dermis (Fig. 3.5).

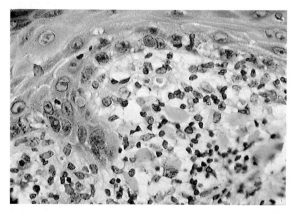

Fig. 3.3 Lichen planus. There are numerous colloid bodies in the papillary dermis.
Haematoxylin — eosin

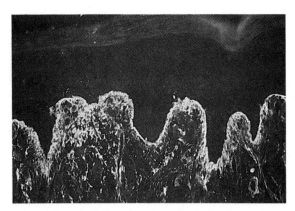

Fig. 3.5 Lichen planus. A band of fibrin involves the basement membrane zone and extends into the papillary dermis.
Direct immunofluorescence

Electron microscopy. Ultrastructural studies have confirmed that lymphocytes attach to basal keratinocytes, resulting in their death by apoptosis.[3,4,51] Many cell fragments, beyond the limit of resolution of the light microscope, are formed during the budding of the dying cells. The cell fragments are phagocytosed by adjacent keratinocytes and macrophages. The large tonofilament-rich bodies that result from redistribution of tonofilaments during cell fragmentation appear to resist phagocytosis and are extruded into the upper dermis, where they are recognized on light microscopy as colloid bodies.[52-55] Various studies have confirmed the epidermal origin of these colloid bodies.[56,57] There is a suggestion from some experimental work that sublethal injury to keratinocytes may lead to the accumulation of tonofilaments in their cytoplasm.[58] Some apoptotic bodies contain more filaments than would be accounted for by a simple redistribution of the usual tonofilament content of the cell.

LICHEN PLANUS VARIANTS

A number of clinical variants of lichen planus occur. In some, typical lesions of lichen planus are also present. These variants are discussed in further detail below.

Atrophic lichen planus

Atrophic lesions may resemble porokeratosis clinically. Typical papules of lichen planus are usually present at the margins. Experimentally, there is an impaired capacity of the atrophic epithelium to maintain a regenerative steady state.[59]

Histopathology

The epidermis is thin and there is loss of the normal rete ridge pattern. The infiltrate is usually less dense than in typical lichen planus.

Hypertrophic lichen planus

Hypertrophic lesions are usually confined to the shins, although sometimes they are more generalized. They appear as single or multiple, pruritic plaques, which may have a verrucous appearance;[60] they usually persist for many years. Rarely, squamous cell carcinoma develops in lesions of long standing.[61]

Histopathology

The epidermis shows prominent hyperplasia and overlying orthokeratosis (Fig. 3.6). At the margins there is usually psoriasiform hyperplasia representing concomitant changes of lichen sim-

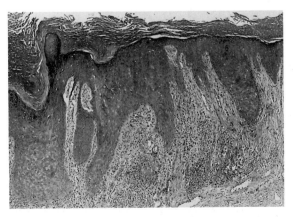

Fig. 3.6 Hypertrophic lichen planus. The epidermis shows irregular hyperplasia. The dermal infiltrate is concentrated near the tips of the rete ridges.
Haematoxylin — eosin

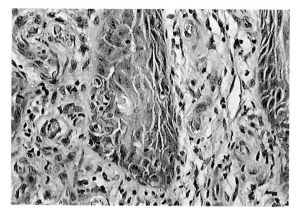

Fig. 3.7   Hypertrophic lichen planus. There are a number of Civatte bodies near the tips of the rete ridges. Haematoxylin — eosin

plex chronicus secondary to the rubbing and scratching (see p. 84). Vertically oriented collagen ('vertical-streaked collagen') is present in the papillary dermis in association with the changes of lichen simplex chronicus.

The basal cell damage is usually confined to the tips of the rete ridges, and may be missed on casual observation (Fig. 3.7). The infiltrate is not as dense or as band-like as in the usual lesions of lichen planus. A few eosinophils and plasma cells may be seen in some cases, in which the ingestion of beta blockers can sometimes be incriminated.

Xanthoma cells have been found in the dermis, localized to a plaque of hypertrophic lichen planus, in a patient with secondary hyperlipidaemia.[62]

Linear lichen planus

This rare variant must be distinguished from linear naevi and other dermatoses with linear variants. Linear lichen planus usually involves the limbs.

Ulcerative lichen planus

Ulcerative lichen planus (erosive lichen planus) is characterized by ulcerated and bullous lesions on the feet.[63] Mucosal lesions, alopecia, and more typical lesions of lichen planus are sometimes present. Squamous cell carcinoma may develop in lesions of long standing. Variants of ulcerative lichen planus involving the penis[64] or the vulva, vagina and mouth[64a] have been reported.

Castleman's tumour (giant lymph node hyperplasia) is a rare association of erosive lichen planus.[64b]

Antibodies directed against a nuclear antigen of epithelial cells have been reported in patients with erosive lichen planus of the oral mucosa.[64c]

Histopathology

There is epidermal ulceration with more typical changes of lichen planus at the margins of the ulcer. Plasma cells are invariably present in cases involving mucosal surfaces. Eosinophils were prominent in the oral lesions of a case associated with methyldopa therapy.

Lichen planus erythematosus

This has been challenged as an entity. Non-pruritic, red papules, with a predilection for the forearms, have been described.[60]

Histopathology

A proliferation of blood vessels may be seen in the upper dermis in addition to the usual features of lichen planus.

Erythema dyschromicum perstans

Erythema dyschromicum perstans (ashy dermatosis, lichen planus pigmentosus)[65] is a slowly progressive, asymptomatic, ash-coloured or brown macular hyperpigmentation[66-68] which has been reported from most parts of the world;[69-71] it is most prevalent in Latin America.[72] Lesions are often quite widespread, although there is a predilection for the trunk.[73] Unilateral[74] and linear lesions[75] have been described. Activity of the disease may cease after several years.

Lichen planus pigmentosus, originally reported from India, is thought by some to be the same condition,[67,76] although this has been disputed.[77] Erythema dyschromicum perstans has been regarded as a macular variant of lichen planus[76,78] on the basis of the simultaneous occurrence of both conditions in several patients[68,79,79a] and similar immunopathological findings.[79b] Paraphenylenediamine has been incriminated in its aetiology,[76] although this has not been confirmed.

Histopathology[66]

In the active phase, there is a lichenoid tissue reaction with basal vacuolar change and occasional Civatte bodies (Fig. 3.8). The infiltrate is usually quite mild in comparison to lichen planus. Furthermore, there may be deeper extension of the infiltrate. There is prominent melanin incontinence, and this is the only significant feature in older lesions. The pigment usually extends deeper in the dermis than in post-inflammatory pigmentation of other causes.[77]

Immunofluorescence has shown IgM, IgG and complement-containing colloid bodies in the dermis, as in lichen planus.[78] Apoptosis and residual filamentous bodies are present on electron microscopy.[66]

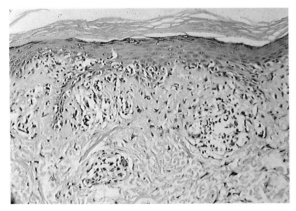

Fig. 3.8 Erythema dyschromicum perstans. There is patchy basal cell damage and some pigment incontinence. Haematoxylin — eosin

Lichen planus actinicus

This is a distinct clinical variant of lichen planus in which lesions are limited to sun-exposed areas of the body.[80–81] It has a predilection for dark-skinned races.[82] There is some variability in the clinical expression of the disease in different countries, and this has contributed to the proliferation of terms used — lichen planus tropicus,[83] lichen planus subtropicus,[84] lichenoid melanodermatitis[85] and summertime actinic lichenoid eruption (SALE).[81,86] The development of pigmentation in some cases[87] has also led to the suggestion that there is overlap with erythema dyschromicum perstans (see above).[79] Lesions have been induced by repeated exposure to ultraviolet radiation.[88]

Histopathology[84]

The appearances resemble lichen planus quite closely,[88a] although there is usually more marked melanin incontinence[81,88] and there may be focal parakeratosis.[80a] The inflammatory cell infiltrate in lichen planus actinicus is not always as heavy as it is in typical lesions of lichen planus.

Lichen planopilaris

Lichen planopilaris is a clinical variant of lichen planus in which keratotic follicular lesions are present, usually in association with other manifestations of lichen planus.[89–90] The Graham Little–Piccardi–Lassueur syndrome is a closely related entity in which there is cicatricial alopecia of the scalp, follicular keratotic lesions of glabrous skin and variable alopecia of the axillae and groins.[90] A linear variant of lichen planopilaris has also been reported.[90a]

Histopathology[89,89a]

In *follicular lesions* a lichenoid reaction pattern, which involves the basal layer of the follicular epithelium, is accompanied by a dense perifollicular infiltrate of lymphocytes and a few macrophages (Fig. 3.9). Unlike lupus erythematosus, the infiltrate does not extend around blood vessels of the mid and deep plexus. In *non-follicular lesions*, the infiltrate extends beneath the epidermis, as in lichen planus. If scarring alopecia develops there is variable perifollicular fibrosis and loss of hair follicles.

Direct immunofluorescence shows colloid bodies containing IgG and IgM in the dermis

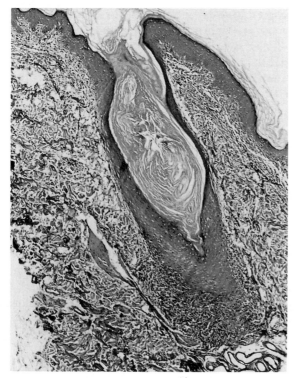

Fig. 3.9 Lichen planopilaris. The lichenoid infiltrate is confined to a perifollicular location and to the adjacent basal layer of the epidermis.
Haematoxylin — eosin

adjacent to the upper portion of the involved follicles.[90]

Lichen planus pemphigoides

This is a controversial entity which has, until recently, been regarded by many as the coexistence of lichen planus and bullous pemphigoid.[91] It is characterized by the development of tense blisters, often on the extremities, in someone with lichen planus. The bullae may develop on normal or erythematous skin, or in the papular lesions of lichen planus.[92,93] They do not necessarily recur with subsequent exacerbations of the lichen planus.[94,95] Similar lesions have been induced by the anti-motion-sickness drug cinnarizine.[96]

Recent immunohistochemical studies suggest that the bullous pemphigoid and lichen planus pemphigoides antigens are antigenetically diffe-

rent.[93,97–97b] This has resulted in the theory that damage to the basal layer in lichen planus may expose or release a basement membrane zone antigen, different to that of bullous pemphigoid, which leads to the formation of circulating antibodies and consequent blister formation.[97] Lichen planus pemphigoides is therefore different from *bullous lichen planus*[98] in which vesicles or bullae develop only in the lichenoid papules, probably as a result of unusually severe basal damage and accompanying dermal oedema.[99,99a]

Histopathology

A typical lesion of lichen planus pemphigoides consists of a subepidermal bulla which is cell poor, with only a mild, perivascular infiltrate of lymphocytes and eosinophils.[100,101] The presence of eosinophils has not been mentioned in all reports. Sometimes a lichenoid infiltrate is present at the margins of the blister[99] and there are occasional degenerate keratinocytes in the epidermis overlying the blister.[93] Lesions which arise in papules of lichen planus show predominantly the features of lichen planus; a few eosinophils are usually present, in contrast to bullous lichen planus in which they are absent.[93] In one report, a pemphigus-vulgaris-like pattern was present in the bullous areas.[102]

Direct immunofluorescence of the bullae usually shows IgG, C3, and C9 neoantigen in the basement membrane zone, and there is often a circulating antibody to the basement membrane zone.[103–104a] Recent studies have shown that the immunoreactants are deposited in the lamina lucida.[97–97b] Indirect split-skin immunofluorescence has shown binding to the roof of the split.[97a]

Electron microscopy. In lichen planus pemphigoides the split occurs in the lamina lucida, as it does in bullous pemphigoid.[97a,104b]

Keratosis lichenoides chronica

This dermatosis is characterized by violaceous, papular and nodular lesions in a linear and reticulate pattern on the extremities, and a seborrhoeic-dermatitis-like facial eruption.[105–106] Oral ulceration and nail involvement may occur.[107,108] The condition is possibly an unusual chronic variant of lichen planus.[109] The earlier literature on this and related entities was reviewed several years ago.[110]

Histopathology

There is a lichenoid reaction pattern with prominent basal cell death and focal basal vacuolar change.[109] The inflammatory infiltrate usually includes a few plasma cells, and sometimes there is deeper perivascular and periappendageal cuffing.[111] Telangiectasia of superficial dermal vessels is sometimes noted.[111a] Epidermal changes are variable, with alternating areas of atrophy and acanthosis sometimes present, as well as focal parakeratosis. Numerous IgM-containing colloid bodies are usually found on direct immunofluorescence.[107]

Lupus erythematosus/lichen planus overlap syndrome

This is a heterogeneous entity in which one or more of the clinical, histological and immunopathological features of both diseases are present.[112–115] Some cases may represent the coexistence of lichen planus and lupus erythematosus, while in others the ultimate diagnosis may depend on the course of the disease.[116,117] Before the diagnosis of an overlap syndrome is entertained, it should be remembered that some lesions of cutaneous lupus erythematosus may have numerous Civatte bodies and a rather superficial inflammatory cell infiltrate which at first glance may be mistaken for lichen planus. The use of an immunofluorescent technique using patient's serum and autologous lesional skin as a substrate may assist in the future in elucidating the correct diagnosis in some of these cases.[118]

LICHEN NITIDUS

Lichen nitidus is a rare, usually asymptomatic chronic eruption characterized by the presence of multiple, small flesh-coloured papules, 1–2 mm in diameter.[119] The lesions have a predilection for the upper extremities, chest, abdomen and genitalia of children and young adult males.[119] Nail changes[120] and involvement of the palms and soles[121,121a] have rarely been reported.

Although regarded originally as a variant of lichen planus,[122] lichen nitidus is now considered a distinct entity of unknown aetiology.

Histopathology

A papule of lichen nitidus shows a dense, well circumscribed, subepidermal infiltrate, sharply limited to one or two adjacent dermal papillae.[119] Claw-like, acanthotic rete ridges, which appear to grasp the infiltrate, are present at the periphery of the papule (Fig. 3.10). The inflammatory cells push against the undersurface of the epidermis, which may be thinned and show overlying parakeratosis. Occasional Civatte bodies are present in the basal layer.

In addition to lymphocytes, histiocytes and melanocytes there are also epithelioid cells and occasional multinucleate giant cells in the inflammatory infiltrate.[123] Rarely, plasma cells are conspicuous.[124] The appearances are sometimes frankly granulomatous, and these lesions must be distinguished from disseminated granuloma

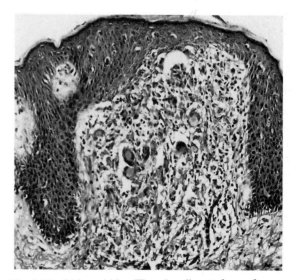

Fig. 3.10 Lichen nitidus. There is a discrete focus of inflammation involving the superficial dermis. Claw-like downgrowths of the rete ridges are present at its margin. Haematoxylin — eosin

annulare in which the infiltrate may be superficial and the necrobiosis sometimes quite subtle.

Rare changes that have been reported include subepidermal vesiculation,[125] transepidermal elimination of the inflammatory infiltrate,[123,126] and the presence of perifollicular granulomas.[126a]

Direct immunofluorescence is usually negative,[127] a distinguishing feature from lichen planus.

Electron microscopy. The ultrastructural changes in lichen nitidus are similar to those of lichen planus.[128]

LICHEN STRIATUS

Lichen striatus is a linear, papular eruption of unknown aetiology which may extend in continuous or interrupted fashion along one side of the body, usually the length of an extremity.[129] Annular,[130] and bilateral forms[131] have been reported. It has a predilection for female children and adolescents. Spontaneous resolution usually occurs after one or two years. A history of atopy is sometimes present in affected individuals.[132]

Histopathology[133–134]

There is a lichenoid reaction pattern with an infiltrate of lymphocytes, histiocytes and melanophages occupying three or four adjacent dermal papillae.[134] The overlying epidermis is acanthotic with mild spongiosis associated with exocytosis of inflammatory cells. The dermal papillae are mildly oedematous. The infiltrate is usually less dense than in lichen planus and it may extend around hair follicles or vessels in the mid-plexus. Eccrine extension of the infiltrate is sometimes present.[133,133a]

Electron microscopy. Dyskeratotic cells similar to the corps ronds of Darier's disease (see p. 281) have been described in the upper epidermis.[133a] The Civatte bodies in the basal layer show the usual changes of apoptosis on electron microscopy.

LICHEN PLANUS-LIKE KERATOSIS

Lichen planus-like keratosis is a commonly encountered entity in routine histopathology.[135–142] Synonyms used for this entity include solitary lichen planus,[135,136] benign lichenoid keratosis,[139] lichenoid benign keratosis[140,141] and involuting lichenoid plaque.[142] It should not be confused with lichenoid actinic (solar) keratosis[143,144] in which epithelial atypia is a prerequisite for diagnosis (see p. 739). Lichen planus-like keratoses are usually solitary, discrete, slightly raised lesions of short duration, measuring 3–10 mm in diameter. Lesions are violaceous or pink, often with a rusty tinge.[138] There may be a thin, overlying scale. There is a predilection for the arms and presternal area of middle-aged and elderly women. Lesions are sometimes mildly pruritic or 'burning'.[139] Clinically, lichen planus-like keratosis is usually misdiagnosed as a basal cell carcinoma or Bowen's disease.[136]

Lichen planus-like keratosis is probably a heterogeneous condition which represents the attempted cell-mediated immune rejection of any of several different types of epidermal lesion. In most instances this is a solar lentigo,[138,145,146] but in some lesions there is a suggestion of an underlying seborrhoeic keratosis or even a viral wart.

Histopathology[140,141,146]

There is a florid lichenoid reaction pattern with numerous Civatte bodies in the basal layer and accompanying mild vacuolar change (Fig. 3.11). The infiltrate is usually quite dense and often includes a few plasma cells and eosinophils, in addition to the lymphocytes and macrophages. The infiltrate may obscure the dermo–epidermal interface. Pigment incontinence may be prominent.

There is often mild hyperkeratosis and focal parakeratosis. Hypergranulosis is not as pronounced as in lichen planus. A contiguous solar lentigo is sometimes seen.[147]

Direct immunofluorescence shows colloid bodies containing IgM and some basement membrane fibrin.[140]

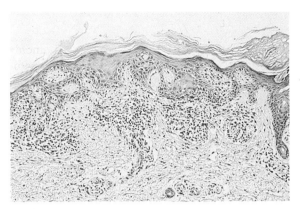

Fig. 3.11 Lichen planus-like keratosis. There is a lichenoid reaction pattern with deeper extension of the infiltrate than is usual in lichen planus.
Haematoxylin — eosin

Histopathology[148,156]

Lichenoid drug eruptions usually differ from lichen planus by the presence of focal parakeratosis and mild basal vacuolar change, as well as a few eosinophils and sometimes plasma cells in the infiltrate. There is often more melanin incontinence than in lichen planus. The infiltrate is often less dense and less band-like than in lichen planus itself. A few inflammatory cells may extend around vessels in the mid and lower dermis. This is particularly so in lesions which are photorelated. Sometimes the histological features closely simulate those of lichen planus. A few eosinophils in the infiltrate may be the only clue to the diagnosis. An unusual lichenoid reaction with epidermotropic multinucleate giant cells in the inflammatory infiltrate has been reported in a patient taking both methyldopa and chlorothiazide.[167]

LICHENOID DRUG ERUPTIONS

A lichenoid eruption has been reported following the ingestion of a wide range of chemical substances and drugs. The eruption may closely mimic lichen planus clinically, although at other times there is eczematization and more pronounced residual hyperpigmentation.[148] Some of the beta-adrenergic blocking agents produce a psoriasiform pattern clinically but lichenoid features histologically.[149,150] Discontinuation of the drug usually leads to clearing of the rash over a period of several weeks.[148]

Lichenoid eruptions have been produced by gold,[151–153] methyldopa,[154,155] beta-adrenergic blocking agents,[156,157] penicillamine,[158] quinine,[159] quinidine,[160] synthetic antimalarials,[161] and ethambutol.[162] Less common causes of a lichenoid reaction are captopril,[162a] naproxen,[163] dapsone, arsenicals, iodides, phenothiazine derivatives, chlorpropamide[163a] and streptomycin.[164] Thiazides and some tetracyclines may produce lesions in a photodistribution.[165] A lichenoid stomatitis, which may take time to clear after cessation of the drug, can be produced by methyldopa and rarely by lithium carbonate[166] or propanolol. Contact with colour film developer may produce a lichenoid photodermatitis.[148]

FIXED DRUG ERUPTIONS

A fixed drug eruption is a round or oval erythematous lesion which develops within hours of taking the offending drug, and which recurs at the same site with subsequent exposure to the drug.[168–170] Lesions may be solitary or multiple. A bullous variant with widespread lesions also occurs.[171,171a] Fixed eruptions subside on withdrawal of the drug, leaving a hyperpigmented macule.[172] Non-pigmenting lesions have been described,[173] and depigmented areas may be the result in patients whose skin is naturally heavily pigmented. Sometimes there is a burning sensation in the erythematous lesions, but systemic manifestations such as malaise and fever are uncommon.[169] Rare clinical variants include eczematous, urticarial, linear,[173a] and 'wandering'[174] types. Common sites of involvement include the face, lips,[175] buttocks and genitals.[176]

In one series of 446 cases of drug eruption, 92 (21%) were instances of fixed drug eruptions, and of these 16 were bullous and generalized.[177] Over 100 drugs have been incriminated, but the major offenders are sulphonamides,[178] tetracyclines,[179–181] tranquillizers, quinine, phenolphthalein (in laxatives), and some analgesics.[171,182,183] Specific drugs to be incriminated in some recent reports in the literature include minocycline,[184] nystatin,[185] penicillin,[186] erythromycin,[187,188] griseofulvin,[189] dimenhydrinate (Gravol),[189a] sulphamethoxazole,[190] trimethoprim,[191] temazepam,[191a] carbamazepine[192] and paracetamol (acetaminophen).[193–194] More complete lists are included in several reviews of the subject.[169,182,195] Two different drugs were involved in one patient.[196]

Numerous studies have attempted to elucidate the pathogenesis of fixed eruptions. It appears that the offending drug acts as a hapten and binds to a protein in basal keratinocytes, and sometimes melanocytes.[169] As a consequence, an immunological reaction is stimulated, which probably takes the form of an antibody-dependent, cellular cytotoxic response. Lymphocytes attack the drug-altered epidermal cells. Suppressor/cytotoxic lymphocytes play a major role in this process, and in preserving the cutaneous memory function which characterizes a fixed eruption.[197] Keratinocytes at the site of a fixed drug eruption express one of the cell adhesion molecules (intercellular adhesion molecule-1) that is involved in the adherence reaction between lymphocytes and epidermal keratinocytes.[197a] It has been suggested that localized expression of this adhesion antigen may be one factor that explains the site-specificity of fixed drug eruptions.[197a]

Histopathology[169,198]

Established lesions show a lichenoid reaction pattern with prominent vacuolar change and Civatte body formation (Fig. 3.12). The degenerate keratinocytes usually show less shrinkage than in lichen planus (Fig. 3.13). The inflammatory infiltrate tends to obscure the dermo-epidermal interface, as in erythema multiforme and some cases of pityriasis lichenoides et varioliformis acuta (PLEVA) (see pp. 42 and 56). The infiltrate may extend into the mid and upper epidermis producing death of keratinocytes above the basal layer (Fig. 3.14). Fixed drug eruptions can usually be distinguished from erythema multiforme by the deeper extension of the infiltrate, the presence of

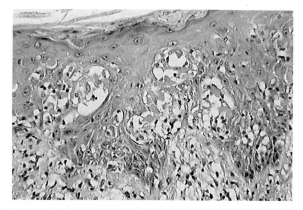

Fig. 3.12 Fixed drug eruption. Dead keratinocytes are present in the basal layer and at higher levels of the epidermis. Lymphocytes extend into the epidermis. Haematoxylin — eosin

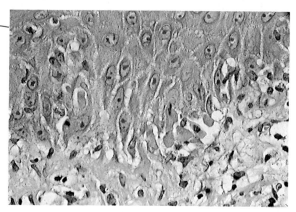

Fig. 3.13 Fixed drug eruption. There are many degenerate keratinocytes in the basal layer. They show less shrinkage than the Civatte bodies in lichen planus. In this field, the lymphocytic infiltrate is relatively sparse. Haematoxylin — eosin

a few neutrophils, and the more prominent melanin incontinence in fixed eruptions.

Based on one study,[198] it appears that very early lesions may show epidermal spongiosis, dermal oedema, and neutrophil microabscesses and numerous eosinophils in the dermis. These features have usually disappeared after several days, although some eosinophils persist.

The clinical variants of fixed drug eruption have not been documented very well, except for the bullous form which results when subepidermal clefting occurs. This may be misdiagnosed as

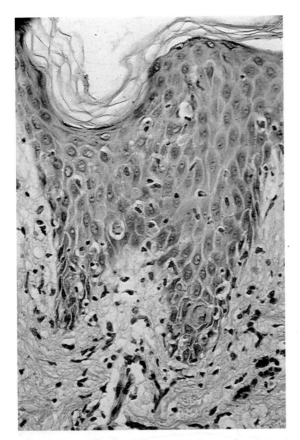

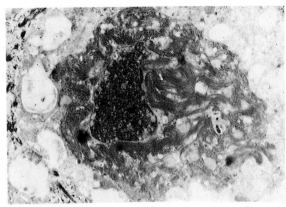

Fig. 3.15 Fixed drug eruption. There are thick clumps of cytoplasmic tonofilaments in a degenerate keratinocyte in the basal layer.
Electron micrograph × 7000

Fig. 3.14 Fixed drug eruption. The infiltrate of lymphocytes extends some distance into the epidermis resulting in cell death in the basal layer and above. Haematoxylin — eosin

erythema multiforme. Spongiotic vesiculation is present in the eczematous variant, and a picture resembling an urticarial reaction is seen in others. Presumably, the reaction in the non-pigmenting variant is in the dermis,[173] although no biopsy results have been reported.

Electron microscopy. There is prominent clumping of tonofilaments in the cytoplasm of basal keratinocytes (Fig. 3.15), which provides an explanation for the bright eosinophilic cytoplasm and the comparatively small amount of shrinkage that these cells undergo during cell death.[172] There is also condensation of nuclear chromatin. Intracytoplasmic desmosomes are sometimes seen.[199] Filamentous bodies composed of filaments which are less electron dense than in

the intact cells are quite numerous.[200] The bodies contain some melanosomes and sometimes nuclear remnants.[172] They are sometimes phagocytosed by adjacent keratinocytes or macrophages.[172] The accumulation of tonofilaments may represent a response by keratinocytes to sublethal injury or some other stimulus. It has the effect of masking the exact mode of death — apoptosis or necrosis. The term 'filamentous degeneration' (see p. 32) has some merit in these circumstances.

ERYTHEMA MULTIFORME

Erythema multiforme is a self-limited, sometimes episodic disease of the skin, which may also involve the mucous membranes. It is characterized by a pleomorphic eruption consisting of erythematous macules, papules, urticarial plaques, vesicles and bullae.[201,201a] Individual lesions may evolve through a papular, vesicular and target (iris) stage in which bullae surmount an erythematous maculopapule.[202] Lesions tend to be distributed symmetrically with a predilection for the extremities, particularly the hands.

The usual forms of erythema multiforme are sometimes called *erythema multiforme minor* to distinguish them from *erythema multiforme major* (Stevens–Johnson syndrome), a severe and sometimes fatal illness in which fever, systemic symptoms and severe oral lesions are usually present.[202–205] There may also be massive epidermal necrosis and peeling of large areas of the skin. In the past, these severe cases with disseminated epidermal necrosis[206] were regarded as a separate entity, *toxic epidermal necrolysis*. Many authors now regard toxic epidermal necrolysis as representing the severe end of the spectrum of erythema multiforme major.[207]

Unusual clinical presentations include the limitation of lesions to areas of lymphatic obstruction,[208] a photosensitive eruption,[208a] and the development of eruptive naevocellular naevi following severe erythema multiforme.[209] An increased association with HLA-B15 has been documented.[210]

Although the pathogenesis of erythema multiforme has been controversial, it is now generally regarded as resulting from a cell-mediated immune reaction to a variety of agents.[211] The lymphocyte is the predominant effector cell,[212] and the venule is one target,[213] although how this relates to the epidermal damage is still speculative. Immune complexes have been demonstrated in some cases, particularly those with recurrent or continuous lesions.[214] Over 100 different causal factors have been implicated, including viral and bacterial infections, drugs, and several associated neoplastic conditions.[215,216] Infection with herpes simplex virus type 1 is a common precipitating factor for minor forms, while *Mycoplasma pneumoniae* infection[217] and drugs[218] are often incriminated in the more severe cases.[204,219] Numerous drugs have been involved, most commonly the sulphonamides and non-steroidal anti-inflammatory drugs.[216,219a] Some other commonly prescribed drugs such as doxycycline,[219b,219c] cimetidine, theophylline,[219d] allopurinol, etretinate[219e] and griseofulvin[219f] have been incriminated but very rarely. Drugs are usually responsible for those cases designated as toxic epidermal necrolysis (see below).

Recently, herpes simplex virus DNA has been detected in cutaneous lesions of herpes-associated and idiopathic erythema multiforme, supporting the theory that erythema multiforme in these circumstances is an immunological process directed towards persistent virus.[219g]

Histopathology[204,220,221]

In established lesions, there is a lichenoid reaction pattern with a mild to moderate infiltrate of lymphocytes, some of which move into the basal layer, thereby obscuring the dermo-epidermal interface (Fig. 3.16). This is associated with prominent epidermal cell death, which is not always confined to the basal layer. There is also basal vacuolar change and some epidermal spongiosis.[220]

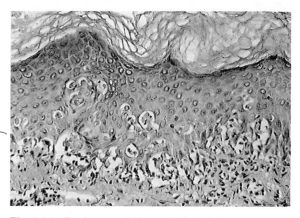

Fig. 3.16   Erythema multiforme. Cell death involves keratinocytes within and above the basal layer. The infiltrate of lymphocytes tends to obscure the dermo-epidermal interface.
Haematoxylin — eosin

Vesicular lesions are characterized by clefting at the dermo-epidermal junction and prominent epidermal cell death in the overlying roof (Fig. 3.17). This may involve single cells or groups of cells, or take the form of confluent necrosis.

The dermal infiltrate in erythema multiforme is composed of lymphocytes and a few macrophages involving the superficial and mid-dermal vessels and a more dispersed infiltrate along and within the basal layer. In severe cases of erythema multiforme showing overlap features with toxic epidermal necrolysis (see below) the infiltrate may be quite sparse with confluent necrosis of the detached overlying epidermis. Eosinophils are not usually prominent in erythema multiforme, although they have been specifically mentioned as an important feature in some reports.[220,221a] Likewise a vasculitis has been noted by some,[222]

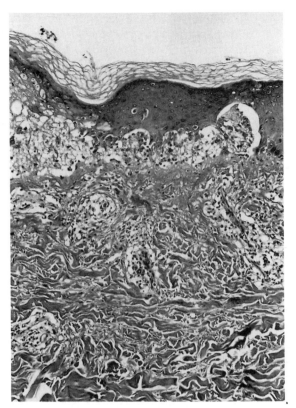

Fig. 3.17 Erythema multiforme with subepidermal vesiculation. A lichenoid reaction pattern is present at the margins of the blister.
Haematoxylin — eosin

but specifically excluded by most.[220,221,223] Nuclear dusting, not related to blood vessels, is sometimes present.[224]

Erythema multiforme has been divided into epidermal, dermal and mixed types based on the corresponding predominant histological features.[224] In the epidermal type there is prominent epidermal damage. In the dermal type there is pronounced dermal papillary oedema leading to subepidermal vesiculation; some basal epidermal damage is to be seen in some areas of the biopsy. It seems likely that diseases other than erythema multiforme — severe urticarias and urticarial vasculitis — have been included in this category of dermal erythema multiforme. There is little merit in the continued separation of these three histological subtypes.[225]

Direct immunofluorescence shows intraepidermal cytoid bodies, representing degenerate keratinocytes, which stain in a homogeneous pattern usually with IgM and sometimes C3.[226] Frequently, there is granular staining for C3 along the dermo–epidermal junction and, in early lesions, also in papillary dermal vessels.[227,228] The presence of properdin suggests activation of the alternate complement pathway.[228] Circulating pemphigus-like antibodies have been reported in one case.[228a]

Toxic epidermal necrolysis

Toxic epidermal necrolysis, now regarded as a variant of erythema multiforme major, presents with generalized tender erythema which rapidly progresses into a blistering phase with extensive shedding of skin.[228–232a] Erosive mucosal lesions are usually present. The mortality approaches 25%.[233]

Drugs are incriminated in the aetiology in the majority of cases, particularly sulphonamides,[233a] anticonvulsants[234,234a] and non-steroidal anti-inflammatory drugs, such as phenylbutazone and piroxicam.[235,235a] Allopurinol has been implicated in several cases.[236] The pathogenesis is uncertain. Cytotoxic lymphokines might explain the apparent discrepancy between the extent of the damage and the paucity of the dermal infiltrate. Macrophage-mediated cytotoxicity is another possible explanation, as the majority of non-keratinocytic cells in the epidermis are from the monocyte series.[237] The small number of T lymphocytes in the dermis is mainly of helper/inducer type.[238] Some genetic susceptibility is suggested by the increased incidence of HLA-B12 in affected individuals.[239]

There is increasing acceptance that toxic epidermal necrolysis is a severe variant of erythema multiforme, although an arbitrary figure of respectively more than 10% and 10% or less of body surface involvement has been used by others to separate toxic epidermal necrolysis from erythema multiforme.[233] Another group has suggested the term 'acute disseminated epidermal necrosis' for cases of toxic epidermal necrolysis and erythema multiforme with skin necrosis.[206]

Histopathology[230,240]

There is a subepidermal bulla with overlying confluent necrosis of the epidermis and a sparse perivascular infiltrate of lymphocytes. In early lesions there is some individual cell necrosis which may take the form of satellite cell necrosis with an adjacent lymphocyte or macrophage. This has been likened to the changes of graft-versus-host disease (see below).[229] A more prominent dermal infiltrate is seen in those cases which overlap with erythema multiforme.

GRAFT-VERSUS-HOST DISEASE

Graft-versus-host disease (GVHD) is a systemic syndrome with important cutaneous manifestations. It is usually seen in patients receiving allogeneic immunocompetent lymphocytes in the course of bone marrow transplants used in the treatment of aplastic anaemia,[241] leukaemia, or in immunodeficiency states.[242–243] It may also occur following maternofetal blood transfusions in utero,[244] intrauterine exchange transfusions, and following the administration of non-irradiated blood products to patients with disseminated malignancy and a depressed immune system. The acute stage can be precipitated in some individuals by autologous and syngeneic bone marrow transplantation.[245,246]

There is an early acute phase with vomiting, diarrhoea, hepatic manifestations and an erythematous macular rash.[243,247,247a] Uncommonly, there are follicular papules[247b] or blisters; rarely, toxic epidermal necrolysis ensues.[243] The chronic stage develops some months or more after the transplant. A preceding acute stage is present in 80% of these patients.[243,248] Chronic GVHD has an early lichenoid phase which resembles lichen planus, and includes oral lesions.[249,250] A poikilodermatous phase may precede the eventual sclerodermoid phase. The lesions of the latter may be localized[250a] or generalized.[243,251] Other late manifestations include alopecia, a lupus-erythematosus-like eruption, wasting, oesophagitis, liver disease, and the sicca syndrome.[252]

The pathogenesis appears to be complex,[253] but the essential factor is the interaction of donor cytotoxic T lymphocytes with recipient minor histocompatibility antigens.[254–256] Young rete ridge keratinocytes[257] and Langerhans cells[256,258] are preferred targets. The acute stage is associated with HLA-DR expression of keratinocytes.[259,260]

Histopathology[243,261]

In early acute lesions there is a sparse superficial perivascular lymphocytic infiltrate with exocytosis of some inflammatory cells into the epidermis. The number of these cells correlates positively with the probability of developing more severe, acute GVHD.[262] This is accompanied by basal vacuolation. Established lesions are characterized by more extensive vacuolation and lymphocytic infiltration of the dermis and scattered, shrunken, eosinophilic keratinocytes with pyknotic nuclei, at all levels of the epidermis.[243] These damaged cells are often accompanied by two or more lymphocytes, producing the picture known as 'satellite cell necrosis' (lymphocyte-associated apoptosis) (Fig. 3.18). A similar picture is sometimes seen in subacute radiation dermatitis (see p. 575).[262a] Fulminant lesions in the acute stage resemble those seen in toxic epidermal necrolysis with subepidermal clefting and full thickness epidermal necrosis.

In the early chronic phase, the lichenoid lesions closely resemble those of lichen planus, although the infiltrate is not usually as dense.[263] Pigment incontinence may be prominent. Biopsies taken from follicular papules resemble lichen planopilaris.[247b,249] Immunofluorescence shows a small amount of IgM and C3 in colloid bodies in the papillary dermis and some immunoglobulins on necrotic keratinocytes.[249,250]

In the late sclerodermoid phase, there are mild epidermal changes such as atrophy and basal vacuolation. There is thickening of dermal collagen bundles which assume a parallel arrangement. The dermal fibrosis, which may result in atrophy of skin appendages, usually extends into the subcutis, resulting in septal hyalinization.[261] Subepidermal bullae were present in one reported case.[264]

Electron microscopy. Ultrastructural examination shows 'satellite cell necrosis' in both stages

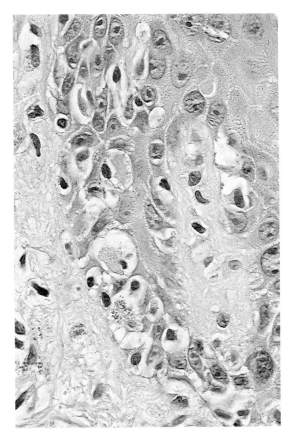

Fig. 3.18 Graft-versus-host disease. Lymphocytes are in close apposition to apoptotic keratinocytes. Haematoxylin — eosin

with lymphocytes in close contact with occasional keratinocytes,[265] some of which show the changes of apoptosis. The term 'lymphocyte-associated apoptosis' is therefore more appropriate than 'satellite cell necrosis'.[265a] Lymphocytes are also in contact with melanocytes[266] and Langerhans cells, the latter being reduced in number. Melanosomes may be increased in the melanocytes.[267] The late sclerotic phase is distinct from scleroderma with some apoptotic cells in the epidermis and numerous active fibroblasts in the upper dermis.[268]

AIDS INTERFACE DERMATITIS

A lichenoid reaction pattern with interface changes resembling those seen in erythema multiforme or fixed drug eruptions has been reported in some patients with the acquired immunodeficiency syndrome and in whom the clinical presentation suggested a drug reaction.[269] The patients had numerous opportunistic infections, and all had received at least one medication prior to the onset of the rash. It has been suggested that systemic and cutaneous immune abnormalities may be relevant in the pathogenesis.[269]

LUPUS ERYTHEMATOSUS

Lupus erythematosus is a chronic inflammatory disease of unknown aetiology which principally affects middle-aged women. It has traditionally been regarded as an immune disorder of connective tissue, along with scleroderma and dermatomyositis. However, a striking feature of cutaneous biopsies is the presence in all cases of the lichenoid reaction pattern.

Three major clinical variants are recognized — chronic discoid lupus erythematosus which involves only the skin, systemic lupus erythematosus which is a multisystem disease, and subacute lupus erythematosus in which distinct cutaneous lesions are sometimes associated with mild systemic illness.[270,271] Some overlap exists between the histological changes seen in these various clinical subsets.[272] There are several less common clinical variants which will be considered after a discussion of the major types.

Discoid lupus erythematosus

The typical lesions of discoid lupus erythematosus are sharply demarcated, erythematous, scaly patches with follicular plugging. They usually involve the skin of the face, often in a butterfly distribution on the cheeks and bridge of the nose. The neck, scalp, lips,[273] oral mucosa[274] and hands are sometimes involved. The lesions may undergo atrophy and scarring. Cicatricial alopecia may result from scalp involvement. Squamous cell carcinoma is a rare complication in any site.[275–277]

Because discoid lesions may be seen in up to

20% of individuals with systemic lupus erythematosus,[278] often as a presenting manifestation, it is difficult to estimate accurately the incidence of the progression of the discoid to the systemic form. It is in the order of 5%,[279,280] and is most likely in those who present abnormal laboratory findings, such as a high titre of antinuclear antibody (ANA) and antibodies to DNA, from the beginning of their illness.[281] Visceral manifestations are absent in uncomplicated discoid lupus erythematosus, although low titre ANA is present in some.[282] An increased incidence of HLA-DRw6 has been found.[283] Lesions resembling discoid lupus erythematosus can be found in the female carriers of X-linked chronic granulomatous disease,[284–286] and rarely in an autosomal form of that disease.[287]

A *hypertrophic variant* of discoid lupus erythematosus in which verrucous lesions develop, usually on the arms, has been reported.[288–291] Lupus erythematosus hypertrophicus et profundus is a very rare destructive variant of hypertrophic discoid lupus erythematosus with a verrucous surface and eventual subcutaneous necrosis.[292]

Annular lesions, resembling erythema multiforme, may rarely develop acutely in patients with discoid lupus erythematosus or systemic lupus erythematosus.[292a] This syndrome, known as Rowell's syndrome, is also characterized by a positive test for rheumatoid factor and speckled antinuclear antibodies.[292a]

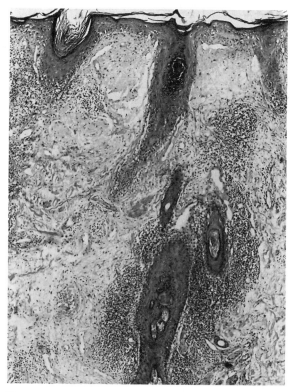

Fig. 3.19   Discoid lupus erythematosus. The dermal infiltrate is both superficial and deep. Haematoxylin — eosin

Histopathology[272,293]

Discoid lupus erythematosus is characterized by a lichenoid reaction pattern and a superficial and deep dermal infiltrate of inflammatory cells which have a tendency to accumulate around the pilosebaceous follicles (Fig. 3.19). The lichenoid reaction takes the form of vacuolar change ('liquefaction degeneration'), although there are always scattered Civatte bodies. In lesions away from the face the number of Civatte bodies is always much greater, and a few colloid bodies may be found in the papillary dermis (Fig. 3.20). In older lesions, there is progressive thickening of the basement membrane, which is best seen with a PAS stain. Other epidermal changes include

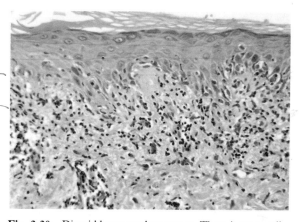

Fig. 3.20   Discoid lupus erythematosus. There is more cell death and less vacuolar change in the basal layer than usual. Distinction from the subacute form is difficult in these cases. Haematoxylin — eosin

hyperkeratosis, keratotic follicular plugging and some atrophy of the malpighian layer.

The dermal infiltrate is composed predominantly of lymphocytes with a few macrophages. Occasionally there are a few plasma cells, and rarely there are neutrophils and nuclear dust in the superficial dermis in active lesions. Plasma cells are prominent in oral lesions.[274] Fibrin extravasation and superficial oedema are also seen in the papillary dermis in some early lesions. Mucin is sometimes increased, but only rarely are there massive amounts.[294] Calcification has been reported on a few occasions.[295,296]

In hypertrophic lesions there is prominent hyperkeratosis and epidermal hyperplasia. There may be a vague resemblance to a superficial squamous cell carcinoma.[288] Elastic fibres are often present between epidermal cells at the tips of the epidermal downgrowths.

Direct immunofluorescence of involved skin in discoid lupus will show the deposition of immunoglobulins, particularly IgG and IgM, along the basement membrane zone in 50–90% of cases (Fig. 3.21).[297–298] Complement components are less frequently present. This so-called lupus band test is positive much less often in lesions from the trunk.[299] A positive lupus band test should always be interpreted in conjunction with the clinical and histological findings, as it may be obtained in chronic light-exposed skin[299a] and some other conditions.[300]

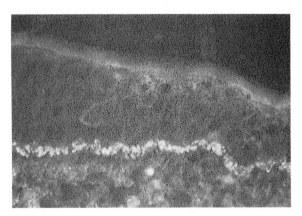

Fig. 3.21 Discoid lupus erythematosus. A broad band of C3 is present along the basement membrane zone. Direct immunofluorescence

Electron microscopy. There is some disorganization of the basal layer, scattered apoptotic keratinocytes and reduplication of the basement membrane.[290,301,302]

Subacute lupus erythematosus

This variant is characterized by recurring, photosensitive, non-scarring lesions which may be annular or papulosquamous in type.[303] They are widely distributed on the face, neck, upper trunk and extensor surfaces of the arms.[304] The patients frequently have a mild systemic illness with musculoskeletal complaints and serological abnormalities, but no renal or central nervous system disease.[305] Severe visceral involvement is most uncommon.[306] Rare clinical presentations have included erythroderma[306a] and an association with the ingestion of thiazide[306b] and of griseofulvin.[306c]

The test for ANA is often negative if mouse liver is used as the test substrate, but positive if human Hep-2 cells are used.[307] There is a high incidence of the anticytoplasmic antibody Ro/SSA;[308–312] it is also found in neonatal lupus erythematosus, in the lupus-like syndrome that may accompany homozygous C2 deficiency,[313,314] and in Sjögren's syndrome.[315,316] The Ro/SSA antigen is now known to be localized in the epidermis and it is thought that antibodies to this antigen are important in the initiation of tissue damage.[316a] However, the antibody titre does not correlate with the activity of the skin disease.[317]

Histopathology[318]

The histopathological features differ only in degree from those seen in discoid lupus.[305,318a] Usually there is more basal vacuolar change, epidermal atrophy and dermal oedema and superficial mucin than in discoid lupus, but less hyperkeratosis, pilosebaceous atrophy, follicular plugging, basement membrane thickening and cellular infiltrate.[318–318b] Apoptotic keratinocytes (Civatte bodies) are sometimes quite prominent in subacute lupus erythematosus (Fig. 3.22).[318c] Furthermore, the infiltrate is usually confined

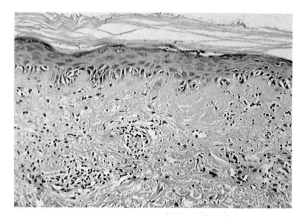

Fig. 3.22 Subacute lupus erythematosus with patchy basal vacuolar change and occasional Civatte bodies. Haematoxylin — eosin

more to the upper dermis than in discoid lupus.[318,318d]

The lupus band test (see above) shows immunoglobulins at the dermo–epidermal junction in approximately 60% of cases. The band is usually not as thick or as intensely staining as in discoid lupus erythematosus. Very fine, dust-like particles of IgG have been described within the epidermis in approximately one-third of cases;[318e] this observation remains to be confirmed.

Systemic lupus erythematosus

In systemic lupus erythematosus (SLE) the changes in the skin are part of a much more widespread disorder. Four clinical manifestations are particularly important as criteria for the diagnosis of SLE: skin lesions, renal involvement, joint involvement, and serositis.[270] The coexistence of the first two of these manifestations is sufficient to justify a strong presumption of the diagnosis.

Cutaneous lesions take the form of erythematous, slightly indurated patches with only a little scale. They are most common on the face, particularly the malar areas. The lesions are usually more extensive and less well defined than those of discoid lupus erythematosus, and devoid of atrophy. They may spread to the chest and other parts of the body. In some instances, they may be urticarial,[319] bullous,[320–323] purpuric or, rarely, ulcerated. It is important to remember that skin lesions do not develop at all in about 20% of patients with SLE; approximately the same proportion have discoid lesions of the type seen in chronic discoid lupus erythematosus, but usually without scarring. This latter group often has less severe disease.[278] The digits, calves and heels are involved in the rare chilblain (perniotic) lupus which results from microvascular injury in the course of SLE.[324]

SLE may coexist with other diseases such as rheumatoid arthritis, scleroderma, dermatomyositis, Sjögren's syndrome, autoimmune thyroiditis,[325] myasthenia gravis,[326] pemphigus,[326] gout,[327] sarcoidosis,[328] porphyria cutanea tarda,[329] Sweet's syndrome,[330] psoriasis,[331,332] dermatitis herpetiformis,[333] acanthosis nigricans,[270] and various complement deficiencies.[334,335] Many of these cases represent the chance coexistence of the two diseases, although the concurrence of SLE with diseases such as scleroderma, dermatomyositis and rheumatoid arthritis has been included in the concept of mixed connective disease, an ill-defined condition with various overlap features and the presence of ribonucleoprotein antibody (see p. 331).[336–339]

Joint symptoms, serositis and renal disease are frequent.[270,340] Rare manifestations include vegetations on the valve leaflets in the heart, vasculitis,[341] diffuse pulmonary interstitial fibrosis, peripheral neuropathy and ocular involvement.[270] Neurological manifestations are not uncommon, and occasionally these are thromboembolic in nature, related to the presence of circulating anticardiolipin antibodies (the 'lupus anticoagulant', see p. 215).[342,343] Cutaneous infarction[344] and ulceration[345] are other rare manifestations of this circulating antibody.

SLE usually runs a chronic course with a series of remissions and exacerbations. The commonest causes of death are renal failure and vascular lesions of the central nervous system. The 10 year survival rate currently exceeds 90%.[270]

Investigations. Various laboratory investigations are undertaken in the diagnostic study of patients with suspected lupus erythematosus.[346,347] The LE cell preparation is now of historical interest only, and it has been replaced as a screening test by the immunofluorescent detection of circulating antinuclear antibodies (ANA).[348] Various patterns of immunofluorescence, corresponding to different circulating antibodies, can be seen; the incidence of positivity depends on the substrate used.[349] A homogeneous staining pattern is usually obtained. This test is positive in more than 90% of untreated patients, many of the negative cases belonging to the subset with anti-Ro/SSA antibodies (see p. 49).

Much more specific for the diagnosis is the detection of antibodies to double-stranded DNA. They are found in over 50% of cases and the titre may be used to monitor the progress of treatment.[270] The presence of these antibodies is often associated with renal disease. They are usually assayed by an indirect immunofluorescence method using the trypanosomatid organism *Crithidia luciliae* as the substrate, although this may contain antigens other than double-stranded DNA.[350]

Other antibodies may also be detected, including rheumatoid factor and antibodies to extractable nuclear antigen (ENA). False positive serological tests for syphilis are sometimes present.[270]

Aetiology. Altered immunity, drugs, viruses, genetic predisposition, hormones, and ultraviolet light may all contribute to the aetiology and pathogenesis of lupus erythematosus.[270] Immunological abnormalities are a key feature. Various autoantibodies are often present, and high levels of antibodies against double-stranded DNA have been considered specific for SLE. Immune complexes are found in about 50% of affected individuals,[279] and those containing DNA appear to be responsible for renal injury. There have been conflicting reports on the role of the various T-cell subsets.[351,352] Other immunological findings include a reduction in epidermal Langerhans cells, loss of HLA-DR surface antigens on dermal capillaries and a small percentage of Leu 8-positive cells in the dermal infiltrate.[352,353]

In a small but important proportion of cases the onset of systemic lupus is quite clearly related to the ingestion of drugs.[270] Those incriminated include procainamide,[354] isoniazid, hydralazine,[354,355] quinidine,[356] penicillamine,[357] sulphonamides,[358] chlorpromazine,[359] phenylbutazone, practolol, phenobarbitone and phenytoin. Oral contraceptives may sometimes result in a flare-up of the disease. Withdrawal of the drug is usually followed by slow resolution of the process. Procainamide-induced SLE, which is the best studied of the drug-related cases, has a low incidence of renal involvement.[270] High titres of leucocyte-specific ANA are present in those with clinical disease.[360]

The role of viruses is still controversial. Structures resembling paramyxovirus have been demonstrated on electron microscopy, particularly in endothelial cells, in SLE and also in discoid lupus erythematosus.[301,361] There is doubt about the nature of these inclusions.

Familial cases have been recorded, usually in siblings, but also in successive generations. The disease has been observed in numerous pairs of identical twins. Several HLA types have been incriminated.[362]

The role of sunlight in inducing and exacerbating cutaneous lupus of all types is well documented.[363–364] Sunlight-induced damage of cellular DNA contributes ultimately to the formation of immune complexes which may be of pathogenetic significance.

Histopathology[272]

The cutaneous lesions of systemic lupus erythematosus show prominent vacuolar change involving the basal layer (Fig. 3.23). Civatte body formation is not usually a feature. Oedema, small haemorrhages and a mild infiltrate of inflammatory cells, principally lymphocytes, are present in the upper dermis. Fibrinoid material is deposited in the dermis around capillary blood vessels, on collagen and in the interstitium. It sometimes contributes to thickening of the basement membrane zone (Fig. 3.24). Hyaluronic acid can be demonstrated by special stains,[365,366] and its presence may be helpful in distinguishing the lesions of SLE from polymorphous light eruption.[367]

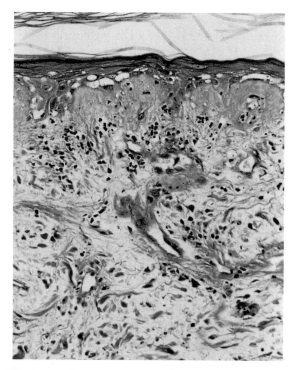

Fig. 3.23 Acute lupus erythematosus. Basal vacuolar change is present but Civatte bodies are sparse. Haematoxylin — eosin

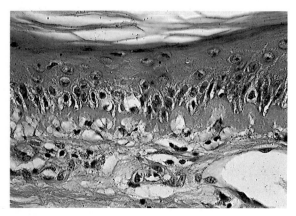

Fig. 3.24 Acute lupus erythematosus. There is thickening of the basement membrane zone and subtle basal vacuolar change. Haematoxylin — eosin

Haematoxyphile bodies — altered nuclei that are the tissue equivalent of the LE cells in the blood — are found rarely in the skin, in contrast to visceral lesions in which they are not infrequent.

The incidence of a positive lupus band test (see p. 49) will depend on the site biopsied.[368] Involved skin is positive in almost 100% of cases, while uninvolved skin from sun-exposed areas is positive in about 90% of cases.[369] Biopsies of uninvolved skin from sun-protected areas are positive in only one–third of cases. Immunoreactants are also deposited in the basement membrane zone of the conjunctiva and the lip.[369a] The lupus band test may be negative in remissions, very early lesions, and some cases of drug-induced lupus erythematosus.[370] Immuno-electron microscopy has shown that the immunoglobulin deposits are predominantly in the papillary dermis, just beneath the basal lamina.[371] DNA is a major component of the complexes.

Variants of lupus erythematosus

Neonatal lupus erythematosus. This is a rare syndrome[372–376] characterized by a transient lupus dermatitis developing in the neonatal period, accompanied by a variety of haematological and systemic abnormalities,[377,377a] including congenital heart block.[378] Approximately 20% of the mothers have SLE at the time of the birth, and a similar percentage will subsequently develop it.[378] The Ro/SSA antibody is present in infants and mothers in nearly all cases,[379,380] and it has been suggested that this is of maternal origin and crosses the placenta, where it is subsequently destroyed by the infant.[381] The anticardiolipin antibody has been reported in a baby with neonatal lupus erythematosus.[381a] Successive siblings may be affected with this condition.[382]

Bullous lupus erythematosus. This is a rare form of SLE, with a skin eruption which clinically and histologically closely resembles dermatitis herpetiformis.[383–385] The blisters are subepidermal with neutrophils in the papillary dermis and some lymphocytes around vessels in the superficial plexus.[385a] Bullae have been reported in a case of discoid lupus erythematosus[386] and also following steroid withdrawal in SLE.[323] Linear IgA has been found in addition to IgG in the basement membrane zone.[387] The immunoreactants are deposited beneath the lamina densa.[385a] Antibodies to the epidermolysis bullosa acquisita antigen were noted in one report.[320] Evidence supporting a role for immune complex-mediated inflammation in the pathogenesis of bullous lesions has been presented.[388]

Lupus panniculitis. Lupus panniculitis (lupus profundus) presents clinically as firm subcutaneous inflammatory nodules, from 1–4 cm or more in diameter, situated on the head, neck, arms, abdominal wall, thighs or buttocks.[389] It is a rare complication which may precede the development of overt systemic or discoid lupus erythematosus.[390] In some cases the lesions subside without any other sign of the disease. It is discussed in more detail with the panniculitides (Ch. 17).

DERMATOMYOSITIS

Dermatomyositis is characterized by the coexistence of a non-suppurative myositis (polymyositis) and inflammatory changes in the skin.[391,392] Cutaneous lesions may precede the development of muscle involvement.[393,393a] Dermatomyositis may occur in either sex, and at any age. Those cases commencing in childhood are sometimes considered as a separate clinical group, because of the greater incidence in them of multi-organ disease.[394,395] Rarely this includes a necrotizing vasculitis that may involve the gut and other organs with a fatal outcome.[394]

The skin lesions are violaceous or erythematous, slightly scaly lesions with a predisposition for the face, shoulders, the extensor surfaces of the forearms, and the thighs.[396] Poikilodermatous features (telangiectasia, hyperpigmentation and hypopigmentation) may be present.[397] Other characteristic findings are nail fold changes,[398] purplish discoloration and oedema of the periorbital tissues (heliotrope rash), and atrophic papules or plaques over the knuckles (Gottron's papules).[397] Plaques of calcification sometimes develop.[399,400]

Other clinical features include the presence of proximal muscle weakness and elevation of certain serum enzymes such as creatine phosphokinase.[396,401] Raynaud's phenomenon, dysphagia, Sjögren's syndrome, retinopathy, and overlap features with scleroderma[402,403] and with lupus erythematosus sometimes occur.[397,404] Fibrosing alveolitis is a rare, but debilitating complication which is usually associated with the presence of the anti-Jo-1 antibody.[405] Other autoantibodies are sometimes present.

An underlying malignancy is present in 10% or more of cases.[406–409] The cutaneous manifestations may precede the diagnosis of the malignancy by up to a year or more.

The aetiology and pathogenesis are unknown but immunological mechanisms are probably involved. In addition to the various autoantibodies that are often present, activated T cells and natural killer cells have been demonstrated in biopsied muscle.[396] A dermatomyositis-like syndrome has been associated with certain viral illnesses and with toxoplasmosis,[410] and has followed administration of hydroxyurea[410a] and of penicillamine.[396] Cytoplasmic inclusions resembling the paramyxovirus-like structures seen in lupus erythematosus (see p. 51) have also been found in blood vessels in cases of dermatomyositis.[411]

Histopathology[412]

The histological changes are quite variable. At times the changes are subtle (Fig. 3.25) with only a sparse superficial perivascular infiltrate of lymphocytes, associated with variable oedema and mucinous change in the upper dermis.[412] More often, there are the features of a lichenoid tissue reaction consisting of vacuolar change in the basal layer. Only occasional Civatte bodies are present, if any (Fig. 3.26). A few neutrophils are sometimes present in the infiltrate, particularly in those cases with fibrinoid material in the papillary dermis and around superficial vessels. The basement membrane is often thickened. These appearances are indistinguishable from those of acute lupus erythematosus.

At other times, there are additional features of epidermal atrophy, melanin incontinence and dilatation of superficial vessels (poikilodermatous

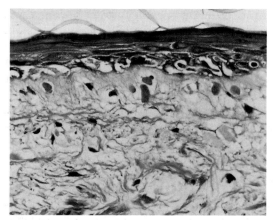

Fig. 3.25 Dermatomyositis. The changes are quite subtle with mild basal vacuolar change and several colloid bodies in the papillary dermis. The appearances may be indistinguishable from acute lupus erythematosus although in the latter disease basement membrane thickening may be more pronounced and colloid bodies less frequent than in dermatomyositis.
Haematoxylin — eosin

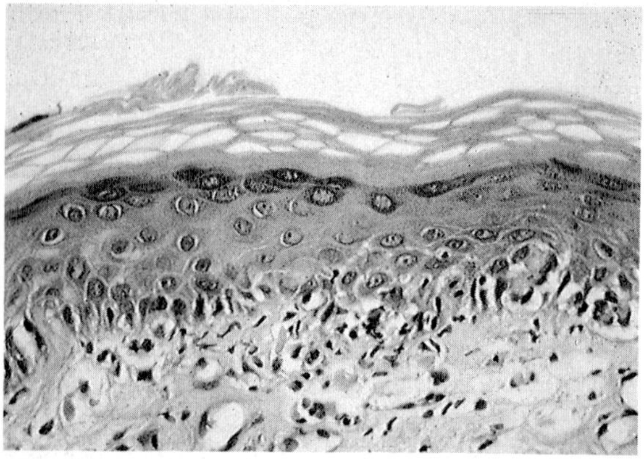

Fig. 3.26 Dermatomyositis. The lichenoid reaction pattern is more obvious in this case. The appearances are indistinguishable from cutaneous lupus erythematosus.
Haematoxylin — eosin

changes).[412] A biopsy from a Gottron's papule will show mild hyperkeratosis and some acanthosis, in addition to the basal vacuolar change.[413]

Unusual findings include subepidermal vesiculation, a non-specific panniculitis and dystrophic calcification. An osteogenic sarcoma developed in an area of heterotopic ossification in one case of dermatomyositis.[414]

Intercellular deposits of immunoglobulins have been reported in the epidermis of nail fold biopsies.[415] Colloid bodies containing IgM are sometimes quite prominent in the papillary dermis. The lupus band test is usually negative. Immunoglobulins, including IgA, have been reported in muscle biopsies in dermatomyositis.[416]

POIKILODERMAS

The poikilodermas are a heterogeneous group of dermatoses characterized clinically by erythema, mottled pigmentation and, later, epidermal atrophy. These changes result from basal vacuolar change with consequent melanin incontinence and variable telangiectasia of blood vessels in the superficial dermis (Fig. 3.27). For this reason, Pinkus included the poikilodermatous pattern as a subgroup of the lichenoid tissue reaction.[1]

Four distinct groups of poikilodermatous dermatoses are found:

1. the genodermatoses poikiloderma congenitale (Rothmund–Thomson syndrome), congenital telangiectatic erythema (Bloom's syndrome) and dyskeratosis congenita;
2. a stage in the evolution of early mycosis fungoides;
3. a variant of dermatomyositis and less frequently of SLE; and

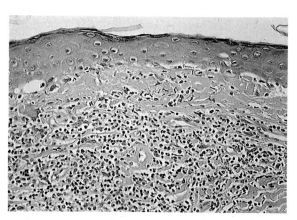

Fig. 3.27 The poikilodermatous reaction pattern in a case of early mycosis fungoides.
Haematoxylin — eosin

4. a miscellaneous group which may follow radiation, cold and heat injury, prolonged exposure to sunlight (poikiloderma of Civatte), and ingestion of drugs (arsenicals and busulphan) or which may occur in the evolution of chronic graft–versus–host reaction.[417]

The three genodermatoses mentioned above are distinct clinical entities, but the poikiloderma which may precede mycosis fungoides (poikiloderma atrophicans vasculare) is regarded by many as an early stage in the evolution of mycosis fungoides. It is therefore considered in Chapter 40. Likewise, poikilodermatomyositis represents a clinicopathological variant of dermatomyositis rather than a disease sui generis. Poikiloderma of Civatte is probably not a distinct entity.[418] It has been suggested that some poikilodermas are possibly related in some way to a graft-versus-host reaction.[417]

POIKILODERMA CONGENITALE

Over 100 cases of poikiloderma congenitale (Rothmund–Thomson syndrome) have been reported in the literature in English.[419,419a] It is an autosomal recessive, multisystem disorder which affects principally the skin, eyes and skeletal system.[420,420a] A reticular erythematous eruption commences in the first year of life, and this is followed by the development of areas of hyperpigmentation. Warty keratoses may appear on the hands, elbows, knees and feet. Other clinical features[421] include a short stature, cataracts, hypogonadism, mental retardation, photosensitivity to ultraviolet A radiation[419,421a] and, rarely, the development of skin cancers[422] and osteogenic sarcoma.[423]

Hereditary sclerosing poikiloderma is an autosomal dominant disorder with many similar clinical features.[424,425] However, there are linear hyperkeratotic and sclerotic bands in the flexural areas, sclerosis of the palms and soles, and clubbing of the nails.[424,425]

Kindler's syndrome, initially thought to represent the association of poikiloderma congenitale with dystrophic epidermolysis bullosa,[426,427] is now regarded as a distinct, but related entity.[427a]

Similar cases have been reported under the title *hereditary acrokeratotic poikiloderma*.[428,429] Both groups of cases are characterized by acral bullae and keratoses with poikilodermatous changes.[427a] Photosensitivity is often present in Kindler's syndrome.[429a]

Another variant with poikiloderma, traumatic bulla formation and pitted palmoplantar keratoderma has been reported.[430]

Histopathology

There are the usual poikilodermatous features of hyperkeratosis, epidermal atrophy, basal vacuolar change, numerous telangiectatic vessels, scattered dermal melanophages, and a variable upper dermal inflammatory cell infiltrate.[431,432]

The keratotic (warty) lesions show hyperkeratosis, a normal or thickened epidermis, and some loss of cell polarity, with dyskeratotic cells present as well.[420]

The bullae in Kindler's syndrome are subepidermal and cell-poor, although ultrastructural studies have shown the split can occur at several levels within the dermo–epidermal junction zone.[429a]

CONGENITAL TELANGIECTATIC ERYTHEMA

This rare autosomal recessive disorder is usually known by the eponymous designation Bloom's syndrome. In addition to the telangiectatic, sunsensitive facial rash, there is stunted growth, proneness to respiratory and gastrointestinal infections, chromosomal abnormalities, and a variety of congenital malformations.[433,434] Various chromosomal breakages are found in cultured lymphocytes, the most characteristic being a high rate of sister chromatid exchanges during metaphase.[435] As a consequence, there is a significant tendency to develop various malignancies,[436] particularly acute leukaemia and lymphoma.[433,437]

Histopathology

The facial rash consistently shows dilatation of dermal capillaries. There is usually only a mild perivascular infiltrate of lymphocytes. Basal vacuolar change may occur but does not usually result in pigment incontinence.

DYSKERATOSIS CONGENITA

Dyskeratosis congenita is a rare, sometimes fatal genodermatosis characterized primarily by the triad of reticulate hyperpigmentation, nail dystrophy and leucokeratosis of mucous membranes.[438,439] Other less constant features include a Fanconi-type pancytopenia,[440] eye and dental changes, mental deficiency, deafness,[441] intracranial calcification,[442] palmoplantar hyperkeratosis, scarring alopecia[443] and an increased incidence of malignancy, particularly related to the mucous membranes.[441,444]

Although found predominantly in Caucasian males, it has been reported in several races,[438,443] and occasionally in females.[445] Most cases are inherited as a sex-linked recessive trait,[441] but several kindreds with autosomal dominant inheritance have been reported.[446]

The skin changes, which may resemble poikiloderma, usually develop on the face, neck and upper trunk in childhood.[447] It has been suggested recently that there may be pathogenetic features in common with graft-versus-host disease (see p. 46).[439] Chromosomal breakages are another feature of dyskeratosis congenita.[448]

Histopathology

Usually there are mild hyperkeratosis, epidermal atrophy, prominent telangiectasia of superficial vessels, and numerous melanophages in the papillary dermis. Less constant features include mild basal vacuolar change, fibrosis of the upper dermis and a mild lymphocytic infiltrate beneath the epidermis.[439,445,447] Civatte bodies have not been recorded.

OTHER LICHENOID DISEASES

In addition to the dermatoses discussed above, a number of other important diseases may also show features of the lichenoid reaction pattern.

They are discussed more fully in other chapters, but they are also included here for completeness. Only the salient histological features are mentioned.

PITYRIASIS LICHENOIDES

In the acute form of pityriasis lichenoides, pityriasis lichenoides et varioliformis acuta (PLEVA), there is a heavy lymphocytic infiltrate which obscures the dermo–epidermal interface in much the same way that it does in erythema multiforme and fixed drug eruption (Fig. 3.28). This may be associated with focal epidermal cell death and overlying parakeratosis, or confluent epidermal necrosis. The dermal infiltrate varies from a mild lymphocytic vasculitis to a heavy infiltrate which also extends between the vessels and is accompanied by variable haemorrhage. The dermal infiltrate is often wedge-shaped in distribution with the apex towards the deep dermis. PLEVA is considered further with the lymphocytic vasculitides in Chapter 8 (p. 237).

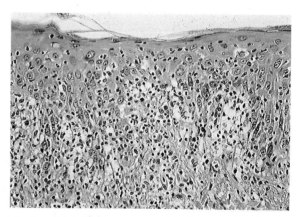

Fig. 3.28   Pityriasis lichenoides (acute form). The dermo-epidermal interface is obscured by the inflammatory cell infiltrate.
Haematoxylin — eosin

LICHENOID PURPURA

Some lesions of pigmented purpuric dermatosis may show lichenoid as well as purpuric and chronic vasculitic features. The presence of purpura and haemosiderin are important clues to the diagnosis.

LATE SECONDARY SYPHILIS

Some lesions of late secondary syphilis show a lichenoid reaction pattern (see p. 610). There is usually extension of the inflammatory infiltrate into the mid and deep dermis. Plasma cells are usually present in the infiltrate.

POROKERATOSIS

In lesions of porokeratosis, particularly the disseminated superficial actinic form, a lichenoid tissue reaction associated with a heavy superficial lymphocytic infiltrate can occur. A careful search will reveal the diagnostic cornoid lamella at the periphery of the infiltrate. The lichenoid infiltrate may be directed against the abnormal epidermal clones which emerge in this condition. Poroker-

atosis is considered in detail in Chapter 9 (p. 276).

DRUG ERUPTIONS

The lichenoid reaction pattern is a prominent feature in lichenoid and fixed drug eruptions. In many other drug-induced cutaneous reactions, a very occasional Civatte body (apoptotic keratinocyte) may be seen in the basal layer or at a higher level within the epidermis. There may be an associated exocytosis of a few lymphocytes. Apoptotic cells are a valuable clue to the drug aetiology of an otherwise non-specific spongiotic tissue reaction (see p. 114). These cells are usually easier to find in morbilliform drug eruptions (see p. 562).

REGRESSING WARTS AND TUMOURS

The regression of viral warts, particularly plane warts, is associated with a lichenoid reaction pat-

Table 3.1 Key histopathological features of various lichenoid diseases

Disease	Histopathological features
Lichen planus	Prominent Civatte bodies, band-like inflammatory infiltrate, wedge-shaped hypergranulosis. Hypertrophic form has changes limited to the tips of the acanthotic downgrowths and often superadded lichen simplex chronicus. The infiltrate extends around hair follicles in lichen planopilaris. Pigment incontinence is conspicuous in erythema dyschromicum perstans.
Lichen nitidus	Focal (papular) lichenoid lesions; some giant cells; dermal infiltrate often 'clasped' by acanthotic downgrowths.
Lichen striatus	Clinically linear; irregular and discontinuous lichenoid reaction; infiltrate sometimes around follicles and sweat glands.
Lichen planus-like keratosis	Solitary; prominent Civatte body formation; solar lentigo often at margins.
Lichenoid drug eruptions	Focal parakeratosis; eosinophils, plasma cells and melanin incontinence may be features. Deep extension of the infiltrate occurs in photolichenoid lesions.
Fixed drug eruptions	Interface-obscuring infiltrate, often extends deeper than erythema multiforme; cell death often above basal layer. Neutrophils often present.
Erythema multiforme	Interface-obscuring infiltrate; sometimes subepidermal vesiculation and variable epidermal cell death.
Lupus erythematosus	Mixed vacuolar change and Civatte bodies. SLE has prominent vacuolar change and minimal cell death. Discoid lupus away from the face has more cell death and superficial and deep infiltrate; follicular plugging; basement membrane thickening.
Dermatomyositis	May resemble acute lupus with vacuolar change, epidermal atrophy, some dermal mucin; infiltrate usually superficial and often sparse.
Poikilodermas	Vacuolar change; telangiectasia; pigment incontinence; late dermal sclerosis.
Pityriasis lichenoides	Acute form combines lymphocytic vasculitis with epidermal cell death; interface-obscuring infiltrate; focal haemorrhage; focal parakeratosis.

Table 3.2 Diagnoses associated with various pathological changes in the lichenoid reaction pattern

Pathological change	Possible diagnoses
Vacuolar change	Lupus erythematosus, dermatomyositis, drugs and poikiloderma
Interface-obscuring infiltrate	Erythema multiforme, fixed drug eruption, pityriasis lichenoides (acute)
Purpura	Lichenoid purpura
Cornoid lamella	Porokeratosis
Deep dermal infiltrate	Lupus erythematosus, syphilis, drugs, photolichenoid eruption
'Satellite cell necrosis'	Graft-versus-host disease, erythema multiforme, regressing plane warts
Prominent pigment incontinence	Poikiloderma, drugs, 'racial pigmentation' and an associated lichenoid reaction, erythema dyschromicum perstans and related entities

tern and exocytosis of cells into the epidermis. Keratinocytes in the stratum malpighii, presumably expressing viral antigen, are attacked by lymphocytes, resulting in death of the keratinocytes by apoptosis. Sometimes two or more lymphocytes 'surround' a keratinocyte, similar to the 'satellite cell necrosis' (lymphocyte-associated apoptosis) of graft-versus-host disease (see p. 46).

A lichenoid reaction pattern can be associated with a variety of epidermal tumours, where it appears to represent the attempted immunological regression of those lesions. It may be seen in seborrhoeic keratoses (the so-called 'irritated' seborrhoeic keratosis — see p. 735), solar keratoses (lichenoid solar keratoses — see p. 739)

and intraepidermal carcinomas (see p. 741). The lichen planus-like keratosis, which has already been discussed (see p. 40), represents a similar reaction in a solar lentigo and probably some other epithelial lesions.

A similar mechanism is involved in the partial regression of basal and squamous cell carcinomas and other cutaneous tumours. However, these circumstances do not conform to the definition of the lichenoid reaction pattern, namely basal epidermal cell damage. Accordingly they will not be considered further in this section.

LICHEN AMYLOIDOSIS

In lichen amyloidosis there is an accumulation of filamentous material in basal cells, with their eventual death. The filamentous material is extruded into the dermis in a manner similar to the formation of colloid bodies. The basal cells possibly die by apoptosis but the accumulation of the filamentous material obscures this basic process (see p. 410).

VITILIGO

In active lesions of vitiligo, careful search will often reveal an occasional lymphocyte in contact with a melanocyte. The destruction of melanocytes by lymphocyte-mediated apoptosis would explain the features of vitiligo (see p. 306).

LICHENOID TATTOO REACTION

A lichenoid reaction, localized to the red areas, is a rare complication in a tattoo.

REFERENCES

Introduction

1. Pinkus H. Lichenoid tissue reactions. Arch Dermatol 1973; 107: 840–846.
2. Weedon D. The lichenoid tissue reaction. Int J Dermatol 1982; 21: 203–206.
3. Weedon D. Apoptosis in lichen planus. Clin Exp Dermatol 1980; 5: 425–430.
4. Weedon D, Searle J, Kerr JFR. Apoptosis. Its nature and implications for dermatopathology. Am J Dermatopathol 1979; 1: 133–144.
4a. Weedon D. Apoptosis. Adv Dermatol 1990; 5: 243–256.
5. Sumegi I. Colloid bodies in dermatoses other than lichen planus. Acta Derm Venereol 1982; 62: 125–131.
6. Hashimoto K. Apoptosis in lichen planus and several

other dermatoses. Acta Derm Venereol 1976; 56: 187–210.

7. Grubauer G, Romani N, Kofler H et al. Apoptotic keratin bodies as autoantigen causing the production of IgM-anti-keratin intermediate filament autoantibodies. J Invest Dermatol 1986; 87: 466–471.

7a. Oliver GF, Winkelmann RK, Muller SA. Lichenoid dermatitis: A clinicopathologic and immunopathologic review of sixty-two cases. J Am Acad Dermatol 1989; 21: 284–292.

7b. Gilchrest BA, Soter NA, Stoff JS, Mihm MC Jr. The human sunburn reaction: Histologic and biochemical studies. J Am Acad Dermatol 1981; 5: 411–422.

Lichenoid dermatoses

8. Jobard-Drobacheff C, Blanc D, Quencez E et al. Lichen planus of the oesophagus. Clin Exp Dermatol 1988; 13: 38–41.

9. Scott MJ Jr, Scott MK Sr. Ungual lichen planus. Arch Dermatol 1979; 115: 1197–1199.

10. Zaias N. The nail in lichen planus. Arch Dermatol 1970; 101: 264–271.

11. Shklar G. Erosive and bullous oral lesions of lichen planus. Histologic studies. Arch Dermatol 1968; 97: 411–416.

12. Colver GB, Dawber RPR. Is childhood idiopathic atrophy of the nails due to lichen planus? Br J Dermatol 1987; 116: 709–712.

13. Wilkinson JD, Dawber RPR, Bowers RP, Fleming K. Twenty-nail dystrophy of childhood. Br J Dermatol 1979; 100: 217–221.

14. Sodaify M, Vollum DI. Familial lichen planus. A case report. Br J Dermatol 1978; 98: 579–581.

15. Copeman PWM, Tan RS-H, Timlin D, Samman PD. Familial lichen planus. Another disease or a distinct people? Br J Dermatol 1978; 98: 573–577.

16. Mahood JM. Familial lichen planus. A report of nine cases from four families with a brief review of the literature. Arch Dermatol 1983; 119: 292–294.

17. Kofoed ML, Wantzin GL. Familial lichen planus. J Am Acad Dermatol 1985; 13: 50–54.

18. Powell FC, Rogers RS, Dickson ER, Moore SB. An association between HLA DR1 and lichen planus. Br J Dermatol 1986; 114: 473–478.

19. Flamenbaum HS, Safai B, Siegal FP, Pahwa S. Lichen planus in two immunodeficient hosts. J Am Acad Dermatol 1982; 6: 918–920.

20. Graham-Brown RAC, Sarkany I, Sherlock S. Lichen planus and primary biliary cirrhosis. Br J Dermatol 1982; 106: 699–703.

21. Epstein O. Lichen planus and liver disease. Br J Dermatol 1984; 111: 473–475.

22. Neumann-Jensen B, Worsaae N, Dabelsteen E, Ullman S. Pemphigus vulgaris and pemphigus foliaceus coexisting with oral lichen planus. Br J Dermatol 1980; 102: 585–590.

23. Davies MG, Gorkiewicz A, Knight A, Marks R. Is there a relationship between lupus erythematosus and lichen planus? Br J Dermatol 1977; 96: 145–154.

24. Connelly MG, Winkelmann RK. Coexistence of lichen sclerosus, morphea, and lichen planus. Report of four cases and review of the literature. J Am Acad Dermatol 1985; 12: 844–851.

25. Yesudian P, Rao R. Malignant transformation of hypertrophic lichen planus. Int J Dermatol 1985; 24: 177–178.

26. Odukoya O, Gallagher G, Shklar G. A histologic study of epithelial dysplasia in oral lichen planus. Arch Dermatol 1985; 121: 1132–1136.

27. Fulling H-J. Cancer development in oral lichen planus. A follow-up study of 327 patients. Arch Dermatol 1973; 108: 667–669.

28. Black MM. What is going on in lichen planus? Clin Exp Dermatol 1977; 2: 303–310.

29. Morhenn VB. The etiology of lichen planus. A hypothesis. Am J Dermatopathol 1986; 8: 154–156.

29a. Gilhar A, Pillar T, Winterstein G, Etzioni A. The pathogenesis of lichen planus. Br J Dermatol 1989; 120: 541–544.

30. Shiohara T, Moriya N, Tanake Y et al. Immunopathologic study of lichenoid skin diseases: Correlation between HLA-DR-positive keratinocytes or Langerhans cells and epidermotropic T cells. J Am Acad Dermatol 1988; 18: 67–74.

31. Shiohara T, Moriya N, Tsuchiya K et al. Lichenoid tissue reaction induced by local transfer of Ia-reactive T-cell clones. J Invest Dermatol 1986; 87: 33–38.

32. Shiohara T, Moriya N, Mochizuki T, Nagashima M. Lichenoid tissue reaction (LTR) induced by local transfer of Ia-reactive T-cell clones. II. LTR by epidermal invasion of cytotoxic lymphokine-producing autoreactive T cells. J Invest Dermatol 1987; 89: 8–14.

33. Tjernlund UM. Ia-like antigens in lichen planus. Acta Derm Venereol 1980; 60: 309–314.

34. MacDonald DM, Schmitt D, Germain D, Thivolet J. Ultrastructural demonstration of T cells in cutaneous tissue sections using specific anti-human T cell antiserum. Br J Dermatol 1978; 99: 641–646.

35. Ebner H, Jurecka W. Cell proliferation in the lichen planus infiltrate. J Cutan Pathol 1977; 4: 185–190.

36. McMillan EM, Martin D, Wasik R, Everett MA. Demonstration in situ of "T" cells and "T" cell subsets in lichen planus using monoclonal antibodies. J Cutan Pathol 1981; 8: 228–234.

37. Bhan AK, Harrist TJ, Murphy GF, Mihm MC Jr. T cell subsets and Langerhans cells in lichen planus: in situ characterization using monoclonal antibodies. Br J Dermatol 1981; 105: 617–622.

38. Mauduit G, Fernandez-Bussy R, Thivolet J. Sequential enumeration of peripheral blood T cell subsets in lichen planus. Clin Exp Dermatol 1984; 9: 256–262.

38a. Shiohara T, Moriya N, Nagashima M. The lichenoid tissue reaction. A new concept of pathogenesis. Int J Dermatol 1988; 27: 365–374.

38b. Shiohara T. The lichenoid tissue reaction. An immunological perspective. Am J Dermatopathol 1988; 10: 252–256.

39. Gomes MA, Schmitt DS, Souteyrand P et al. Lichen planus and chronic graft-versus-host reaction. In situ identification of immunocompetent cell phenotypes. J Cutan Pathol 1982; 9: 249–257.

40. Shuttleworth D, Graham-Brown RAC, Campbell AC. The autoimmune background in lichen planus. Br J Dermatol 1986; 115: 199–203.

41. Olsen RG, du Plessis DP, Schultz EJ, Camisa C. Indirect immunofluorescence microscopy of lichen planus. Br J Dermatol 1984; 110: 9–15.

42. Ebner H, Gebhart W, Lassmann H, Jurecka W. The epidermal cell proliferation in lichen planus. Acta Derm Venereol 1977; 57: 133–136.

43. Eady RAJ, Cowen T. Epidermal repair in lichen planus: a light and electron microscopical study. Clin Exp Dermatol 1977; 2: 323–334.

44. Ragaz A, Ackerman AB. Evolution, maturation, and regression of lesions of lichen planus. New observations and correlations of clinical and histologic findings. Am J Dermatopathol 1981; 3: 5–25.

45. Lupton GP, Goette DK. Lichen planus with plasma cell infiltrate. Arch Dermatol 1981; 117: 124–125.

46. Ross TH. Caspary–Joseph spaces: a comment on priority. Int J Dermatol 1977; 16: 842–843.

47. Enhamre A, Lagerholm B. Acrosyringeal lichen planus. Acta Derm Venereol 1987; 67: 346–350.

48. Hanau D, Sengel D. Perforating lichen planus. J Cutan Pathol 1984; 11: 176–178.

49. Baart de la Faille-Kuyper EH, Baart de la Faille H. An immunofluorescence study of lichen planus. Br J Dermatol 1974; 90: 365–371.

50. Abell E, Presbury DGC, Marks R, Ramnarain D. The diagnostic significance of immunoglobulin and fibrin deposition in lichen planus. Br J Dermatol 1975; 93: 17–24.

51. Burkhart CG. Ultrastructural study of lichen planus: an evaluation of the colloid bodies. Int J Dermatol 1981; 20: 188–192.

52. Ebner H, Gebhart W. Light and electron microscopic differentiation of amyloid and colloid or hyaline bodies. Br J Dermatol 1975; 92: 637–645.

53. Ebner H, Gebhart W. Epidermal changes in lichen planus. J Cutan Pathol 1976; 3: 167–174.

54. Medenica M, Lorincz A. Lichen planus: an ultrastructural study. Acta Derm Venereol 1977; 57: 55–62.

55. El-Labban NG, Kramer IRH. Civatte bodies and the actively dividing epithelial cells in oral lichen planus. Br J Dermatol 1974; 90: 13–23.

56. Danno K, Horio T. Sulphydryl crosslinking in cutaneous apoptosis: A review. J Cutan Pathol 1982; 9: 123–132.

57. Gomes MA, Staquet MJ, Thivolet J. Staining of colloid bodies by keratin antisera in lichen planus. Am J Dermatopathol 1981; 3: 341–347.

58. Eady RAJ, Cowen T. Half-and-half cells in lichen planus. A possible clue to the origin and early formation of colloid bodies. Br J Dermatol 1978; 98: 417–423.

59. Maidhof R, Hornstein OP, Bauer G et al. Cell proliferation in lichen planus of the buccal mucosa. Acta Derm Venereol 1981; 61: 17–22.

60. Fox BJ, Odom RB. Papulosquamous diseases: A review. J Am Acad Dermatol 1985; 12: 597–624.

61. Kronenberg K, Fretzin D, Potter B. Malignant degeneration of lichen planus. Arch Dermatol 1971; 104: 304–307.

62. Weedon D, Robertson I. Lichen planus and xanthoma. Arch Dermatol 1977; 113: 519.

63. Crotty CP, Su WPD, Winkelmann RK. Ulcerative lichen planus. Follow-up of surgical excision and grafting. Arch Dermatol 1980; 116: 1252–1256.

64. Alinovi A, Barella PA, Benoldi D. Erosive lichen planus involving the glans penis alone. Int J Dermatol 1983; 22: 37–38.

64a. Pelisse M. The vulvo-vaginal-gingival syndrome. A new form of erosive lichen planus. Int J Dermatol 1989; 28: 381–384.

64b. Ashinoff R, Cohen R, Lipkin G. Castleman's tumor and erosive lichen planus: Coincidence or association? J Am Acad Dermatol 1989; 21: 1076–1080.

64c. Parodi A, Cardo PP. Patients with erosive lichen planus may have antibodies directed to a nuclear antigen of epithelial cells: a study of the antigen nature. J Invest Dermatol 1990; 94: 689–693.

65. Bhutani LK, Bedi TR, Pandhi RK, Nayak NC. Lichen planus pigmentosus. Dermatologica 1974; 149: 43–50.

66. Person JR, Rogers RS III. Ashy dermatosis. An apoptotic disease? Arch Dermatol 1981; 117: 701–704.

67. Tschen JA, Tschen EA, McGavran MH. Erythema dyschromicum perstans. J Am Acad Dermatol 1980; 2: 295–302.

68. Novick NL, Phelps R. Erythema dyschromicum perstans. Int J Dermatol 1985; 24: 630–633.

69. Stevenson JR, Miura M. Erythema dyschromicum perstans. Arch Dermatol 1966; 94: 196–199.

70. Knox JM, Dodge BG, Freeman RG. Erythema dyschromicum perstans. Arch Dermatol 1968; 97: 262–272.

71. Byrne DA, Berger RS. Erythema dyschromicum perstans. A report of two cases in fair-skinned patients. Acta Derm Venereol 1974; 54: 65–68.

72. Convit J, Kerdel-Vegas F, Rodriguez G. Erythema dyschromicum perstans. A hitherto undescribed skin disease. J Invest Dermatol 1961; 36: 457–462.

73. Holst R, Mobacken H. Erythema dyschromicum perstans (ashy dermatosis). A report of two cases from Scandinavia. Acta Derm Venereol 1974; 54: 69–72.

74. Urano-Suehisa S, Tagami H, Iwatsuki K. Unilateral ashy dermatosis occurring in a child. Arch Dermatol 1984; 120: 1491–1493.

75. Palatsi R. Erythema dyschromicum perstans. A follow-up study from Northern Finland. Dermatologica 1977; 155: 40–44.

76. Bhutani LK. Ashy dermatosis or lichen planus pigmentosus: What is in a name? Arch Dermatol 1986; 122: 133.

77. Sanchez NP, Pathak MA, Sato SS, et al. Circumscribed dermal melaninoses: classification, light, histochemical, and electron microscopic studies on three patients with the erythema dyschromicum perstans type. Int J Dermatol 1982; 21: 25–31.

78. Kark EC, Litt JZ. Ashy dermatosis — a variant of lichen planus? Cutis 1980; 25: 631–633.

79. Naidorf KF, Cohen SR. Erythema dyschromicum perstans and lichen planus. Arch Dermatol 1982; 118: 683–685.

79a. Berger RS, Hayes TJ, Dixon SL. Erythema dyschromicum perstans and lichen planus: Are they related? J Am Acad Dermatol 1989; 21: 438–442.

79b. Miyagawa S, Komatsu M, Okuchi T et al. Erythema dyschromicum perstans. Immunopathologic studies. J Am Acad Dermatol 1989; 20: 882–886.

80. Katzenellenbogen I. Lichen planus actinicus (lichen planus in subtropical countries). Dermatologica 1962; 124: 10–20.

80a. Salman SM, Kibbi A-G, Zaynoun S. Actinic lichen planus. A clinicopathologic study of 16 patients. J Am Acad Dermatol 1989; 20: 226–231.

81. Isaacson D, Turner ML, Elgart ML. Summertime actinic lichenoid eruption (lichen planus actinicus). J Am Acad Dermatol 1981; 4: 404–411.

82. Singh OP, Kanwar AJ. Lichen planus in India: an

appraisal of 441 cases. Int J Dermatol 1976; 15: 752–756.

83. El Zawahry M. Lichen planus tropicus. Dermatol Int 1965; 4: 92–95.

84. Dilaimy M. Lichen planus subtropicus. Arch Dermatol 1976; 112: 1251–1253.

85. Verhagen ARHB, Koten JW. Lichenoid melanodermatitis. A clinicopathological study of fifty-one Kenyan patients with so-called tropical lichen planus. Br J Dermatol 1979; 101: 651–658.

86. Bedi TR. Summertime actinic lichenoid eruption. Dermatologica 1978; 157: 115–125.

87. Salman SM, Khallouf R, Zaynoun S. Actinic lichen planus mimicking melasma. A clinical and histopathologic study of three cases. J Am Acad Dermatol 1988; 18: 275–278.

88. van der Schroeff JG, Schothorst AA, Kanaar P. Induction of actinic lichen planus with artificial UV sources. Arch Dermatol 1983; 119: 498–500.

88a. Macfarlane AW. A case of actinic lichen planus. Clin Exp Dermatol 1989; 14: 65–68.

89. Waldorf DS. Lichen planopilaris. Arch Dermatol 1966; 93: 684–691.

89a. Matta M, Kibbi A-G, Khattar J et al. Lichen planopilaris: A clinicopathologic study. J Am Acad Dermatol 1990; 22: 594–598.

90. Horn RT Jr, Goette DK, Odom RB et al. Immunofluorescent findings and clinical overlap in two cases of follicular lichen planus. J Am Acad Dermatol 1982; 7: 203–207.

90a. Kuster W, Kind P, Holzle E, Plewig G. Linear lichen planopilaris of the face. J Am Acad Dermatol 1989; 21: 131–132.

91. Hintner H, Tappeiner G, Honigsman H, Wolff K. Lichen planus and bullous pemphigoid. Acta Derm Venereol (Suppl) 1979; 89: 71–76.

92. Collins NJ, Dowling JP. Lichen planus and bullous pemphigoid. Australas J Dermatol 1982; 23: 9–13.

93. Lang PG Jr, Maize JC. Coexisting lichen planus and bullous pemphigoid or lichen planus pemphigoides? J Am Acad Dermatol 1983; 9: 133–140.

94. Saurat J-H. Does the bullous eruption of lichen planus pemphigoides recur when the LP relapses? J Am Acad Dermatol 1984; 10: 290.

95. Mora RG, Nesbitt LT Jr. Reply. J Am Acad Dermatol 1984; 10: 290.

96. Miyagawa S, Ohi H, Muramatsu T et al. Lichen planus pemphigoides-like lesions induced by cinnarizine. Br J Dermatol 1985; 112: 607–613.

97. Prost C, Tesserand F, Laroche L et al. Lichen planus pemphigoides: an immuno-electron microscopic study. Br J Dermatol 1985; 113: 31–36.

97a. Bhogal BS, McKee PH, Wonjnarowska F et al. Lichen planus pemphigoides: an immunopathological study. J Cutan Pathol 1989; 16: 297 (abstract).

97b. Okochi H, Nashiro K, Tsuchida T et al. Lichen planus pemphigoides: Case report and results of immunofluorescence and immunoelectron microscopic study. J Am Acad Dermatol 1990; 22: 626–631.

98. Camisa C, Neff JC, Rossana C, Barrett JL. Bullous lichen planus: Diagnosis by indirect immunofluorescence and treatment with dapsone. J Am Acad Dermatol 1986; 14: 464–469.

99. Oomen C, Temmerman L, Kint A. Lichen planus pemphigoides. Clin Exp Dermatol 1986; 11: 92–96.

99a. Gawkrodger DJ, Stavropoulos PG, McLaren KM, Buxton PK. Bullous lichen planus and lichen planus pemphigoides — clinico-pathological comparisons. Clin Exp Dermatol 1989; 14: 150–153.

100. Stingl G, Holubar K. Coexistence of lichen planus and bullous pemphigoid. An immunopathological study. Br J Dermatol 1975; 93: 313–320.

101. Mora RG, Nesbitt LT Jr, Brantley JB. Lichen planus pemphigoides: Clinical and immunofluorescent findings in four cases. J Am Acad Dermatol 1983; 8: 331–336.

102. Feuerman EJ, Sandbank M. Lichen planus pemphigoides with extensive melanosis. Arch Dermatol 1971; 104: 61–67.

103. Souteyrand P, Pierini AM, Bussy RF et al. Lichen planus pemphigoides: entity or association? Dermatologica 1981; 162: 414–416.

104. Sobel S, Miller R, Shatin H. Lichen planus pemphigoides. Immunofluorescence findings. Arch Dermatol 1976; 112: 1280–1283.

104a. Hintner H, Sepp N, Dahlback K et al. Deposition of C3, C9 neoantigen and vitronectin (S-protein of complement) in lichen planus pemphigoides. Br J Dermatol 1990; 123: 39–47.

104b. Murphy GM, Cronin E. Lichen planus pemphigoides. Clin Exp Dermatol 1989; 14: 322–324.

105. Nabai H, Mehregan AH. Keratosis lichenoides chronica. Report of a case. J Am Acad Dermatol 1980; 2: 217–220.

106. Ryatt KS, Greenwood R, Cotterill JA. Keratosis lichenoides chronica. Br J Dermatol 1982; 106: 223–225.

107. Kersey P, Ive FA. Keratosis lichenoides chronica is synonymous with lichen planus. Clin Exp Dermatol 1982; 7: 49–54.

108. Lang PG Jr. Keratosis lichenoides chronica. Successful treatment with psoralen-ultraviolet-A therapy. Arch Dermatol 1981; 117: 105–108.

109. Petrozzi JW. Keratosis lichenoides chronica. Possible variant of lichen planus. Arch Dermatol 1976; 112: 709–711.

110. Mehregan AH, Heath LE, Pinkus H. Lichen ruber moniliformis and lichen ruber verrucosus et reticularis of Kaposi. J Cutan Pathol 1984; 11: 2–11.

111. Margolis MH, Cooper GA, Johnson SAM. Keratosis lichenoides chronica. Arch Dermatol 1972; 105: 739–741.

111a. David M, Filhaber A, Rotem A et al. Keratosis lichenoides chronica with prominent telangiectasia: Response to etretinate. J Am Acad Dermatol 1989; 21: 1112–1114.

112. Copeman PWM, Schroeter AL, Kierland RR. An unusual variant of lupus erythematosus or lichen planus. Br J Dermatol 1970; 83: 269–272.

113. Romero RW, Nesbitt LT Jr, Reed RJ. An unusual variant of lupus erythematosus or lichen planus. Clinical, histopathologic, and immunofluorescent studies. Arch Dermatol 1977; 113: 741–748.

114. van der Horst JC, Cirkel PKS, Nieboer C. Mixed lichen planus-lupus erythematosus disease: a distinct entity? Clinical, histopathological and immunopathological studies in six patients. Clin Exp Dermatol 1983; 8: 631–640.

115. Piamphongsant T, Sawannapreecha S, Gritiyarangson

P et al. Mixed lichen planus-lupus erythematosus disease. J Cutan Pathol 1978; 5: 209–215.

116. Ahmed AR, Schreiber P, Abramovits W et al. Coexistence of lichen planus and systemic lupus erythematosus. J Am Acad Dermatol 1982; 7: 478–483.

117. Plotnick H, Burnham TK. Lichen planus and coexisting lupus erythematosus versus lichen planus-like lupus erythematosus. J Am Acad Dermatol 1986; 14: 931–938.

118. Camisa C, Neff JC, Olsen RG. Use of direct immunofluorescence in the lupus erythematosus/lichen planus overlap syndrome: An additional diagnostic clue. J Am Acad Dermatol 1984; 11: 1050–1059.

119. Lapins NA, Willoughby C, Helwig EB. Lichen nitidus. A study of forty-three cases. Cutis 1978; 21: 634–637.

120. Kellett JK, Beck MH. Lichen nitidus associated with distinctive nail changes. Clin Exp Dermatol 1984; 9: 201–204.

121. Weiss RM, Cohen AD. Lichen nitidus of the palms and soles. Arch Dermatol 1971; 104: 538–540.

121a. Coulson IH, Marsden RA, Cook MG. Purpuric palmar lichen nitidus — an unusual though distinctive eruption. Clin Exp Dermatol 1988; 13: 347–349.

122. Stankler L. The identity of lichen planus and lichen nitidus. Br J Dermatol 1967; 79: 125–126.

123. Bardach H. Perforating lichen nitidus. J Cutan Pathol 1981; 8: 111–116.

124. Eisen RF, Stenn J, Kahn SM, Bhawan J. Lichen nitidus with plasma cell infiltrate. Arch Dermatol 1985; 121: 1193–1194.

125. Jetton RL, Eby CS, Freeman RG. Vesicular and hemorrhagic lichen nitidus. Arch Dermatol 1972; 105: 430–431.

126. Banse-Kupin L, Morales A, Kleinsmith D. Perforating lichen nitidus. J Am Acad Dermatol 1983; 9: 452–456.

126a. Madhok R, Winkelmann RK. Spinous, follicular lichen nitidus associated with perifollicular granulomas. J Cutan Pathol 1988; 15: 245–248.

127. Waisman M, Dundon BC, Michel B. Immunofluorescent studies in lichen nitidus. Arch Dermatol 1973; 107: 200–203.

128. Clausen J, Jacobsen FK, Brandrup F. Lichen nitidus: electron microscopic and immunofluorescent studies. Acta Derm Venereol 1982; 62: 15–19.

129. Staricco RG. Lichen striatus. Arch Dermatol 1959; 79: 311–324.

130. Nutter AF, Champion RH. Lichen striatus occurring as an annular eruption: an acquired 'locus minoris resistentiae'. Br J Dermatol 1979; 101: 351–352.

131. Mopper C, Horwitz DC. Bilateral lichen striatus. Cutis 1971; 8: 140–141.

132. Toda K-I, Okamoto H, Horio T. Lichen striatus. Int J Dermatol 1986; 25: 584–585.

133. Reed RJ, Meek T, Ichinose H. Lichen striatus: a model for the histologic spectrum of lichenoid reactions. J Cutan Pathol 1975; 2: 1–18.

133a. Charles CR, Johnson BL, Robinson TA. Lichen striatus. A clinical, histologic and electron microscopic study of an unusual case. J Cutan Pathol 1974; 1: 265–274.

134. Stewart WM. Pathology of lichen striatus. Br J Dermatol (Suppl) 1976; 14: 18–19.

135. Lumpkin LR, Helwig EB. Solitary lichen planus. Arch Dermatol 1966; 93: 54–55.

136. Tegner E. Solitary lichen planus simulating malignant lesions. Acta Derm Venereol 1979; 59: 263–266.

137. Shapiro L, Ackerman AB. Solitary lichen planus-like keratosis. Dermatologica 1966; 132: 386–392.

138. Laur WE, Posey RE, Waller JD. Lichen planus-like keratosis. A clinicohistopathologic correlation. J Am Acad Dermatol 1981; 4: 329–336.

139. Goette DK. Benign lichenoid keratosis. Arch Dermatol 1980; 116: 780–782.

140. Berger TG, Graham JH, Goette DK. Lichenoid benign keratosis. J Am Acad Dermatol 1984; 11: 635–638.

141. Scott MA, Johnson WC. Lichenoid benign keratosis. J Cutan Pathol 1976; 3: 217–221.

142. Berman A, Herszenson S, Winkelmann RK. The involuting lichenoid plaque. Arch Dermatol 1982; 118: 93–96.

143. Hirsch P, Marmelzat WL. Lichenoid actinic keratosis. Dermatol Int 1967; 6: 101–103.

144. Tan CY, Marks R. Lichenoid solar keratosis — prevalence and immunologic findings. J Invest Dermatol 1982; 79: 365–367.

145. Goldenhersh MA, Barnhill RL, Rosenbaum HM, Stenn KS. Documented evolution of a solar lentigo into a solitary lichen planus-like keratosis. J Cutan Pathol 1986; 13: 308–311.

146. Barranco VP. Multiple benign lichenoid keratoses simulating photodermatoses: Evolution from senile lentigines and their spontaneous regression. J Am Acad Dermatol 1985; 13: 201–206.

147. Frigy AF, Cooper PH. Benign lichenoid keratosis. Am J Clin Pathol 1985; 83: 439–443.

148. Almeyda J, Levantine A. Lichenoid drug eruptions. Br J Dermatol 1971; 85: 604–607.

149. Gange RW, Levene GM. A distinctive eruption in patients receiving oxprenolol. Clin Exp Dermatol 1979; 4: 87–97.

150. Cochran REI, Thomson J, Fleming K, McQueen A. The psoriasiform eruption induced by practolol. J Cutan Pathol 1975; 2: 314–319.

151. Hjortshoj A. Lichen planus and acne provoked by gold. Acta Derm Venereol 1977; 57: 165–167.

152. Penneys NS, Ackerman AB, Gottlieb NL. Gold dermatitis. A clinical and histopathological study. Arch Dermatol 1974; 109: 372–376.

153. Penneys NS. Gold therapy: Dermatologic uses and toxicities. J Am Acad Dermatol 1979; 1: 315–320.

154. Burry JN. Ulcerative lichenoid eruption from methyldopa. Arch Dermatol 1976; 112: 880.

155. Burry JN, Kirk J. Lichenoid drug reaction from methyldopa. Br J Dermatol 1974; 91: 475–476.

156. Hawk JLM. Lichenoid drug eruption induced by propanolol. Clin Exp Dermatol 1980; 5: 93–96.

157. Cochran REI, Thomson J, McQueen A, Beevers DG. Skin reactions associated with propanolol. Arch Dermatol 1976; 112: 1173–1174.

158. Van Hecke E, Kint A, Temmerman L. A lichenoid eruption induced by penicillamine. Arch Dermatol 1981; 117: 676–677.

159. Meyrick Thomas RH, Munro DD. Lichen planus in a photosensitive distribution due to quinine. Clin Exp Dermatol 1986; 11: 97–101.

160. Maltz BL, Becker LE. Quinidine-induced lichen planus. Int J Dermatol 1980; 19: 96–97.
161. Bauer F. Quinacrine hydrochloride drug eruption (tropical lichenoid dermatitis). J Am Acad Dermatol 1981; 4: 239–248.
162. Frentz G, Wadskov S, Kassis V. Ethambutol-induced lichenoid eruption. Acta Derm Venereol 1981; 61: 89–91.
162a. Cox NH, Tapson JS, Farr PM. Lichen planus associated with captopril: a further disorder demonstrating the 'tin-tack' sign. Br J Dermatol 1989; 120: 319–321.
163. Heymann WR, Lerman JS, Luftschein S. Naproxen-induced lichen planus. J Am Acad Dermatol 1984; 10: 299–301.
163a. Franz CB, Massullo RE, Welton WA. Lichenoid drug eruption from chlorpropamide and tolazamide. J Am Acad Dermatol 1990; 22: 128–129.
164. Fellner MJ. Lichen planus. Int J Dermatol 1980; 19: 71–75.
165. Jones HE, Lewis CW, Reisner JE. Photosensitive lichenoid eruption associated with demeclocycline. Arch Dermatol 1971; 106: 58–63.
166. Hogan DJ, Murphy F, Burgess WR et al. Lichenoid stomatitis associated with lithium carbonate. J Am Acad Dermatol 1985; 13: 243–246.
167. Gonzalez JG, Marcus MD, Santa Cruz DJ. Giant cell lichenoid dermatitis. J Am Acad Dermatol 1986; 15: 87–92.
168. Sehgal VN, Gangwani OP. Fixed drug eruption. Current concepts. Int J Dermatol 1987; 26: 67–74.
169. Korkij W, Soltani K. Fixed drug eruption. A brief review. Arch Dermatol 1984; 120: 520–524.
170. Commens C. Fixed drug eruption. Australas J Dermatol 1983; 24: 1–8.
171. Kauppinen K. Cutaneous reactions to drugs with special reference to severe bullous mucocutaneous eruptions and sulphonamides. Acta Derm Venereol (Suppl) 1972; 68: 7–29.
171a. Baird BJ, De Villez RL. Widespread bullous fixed drug eruption mimicking toxic epidermal necrolysis. Int J Dermatol 1988; 27: 170–174.
172. Masu S, Seiji M. Pigmentary incontinence in fixed drug eruptions. Histologic and electron microscopic findings. J Am Acad Dermatol 1983; 8: 525–532.
173. Shelley WB, Shelley ED. Non pigmenting fixed drug eruption as a distinctive reaction pattern: Examples caused by sensitivity to pseudoephedrine hydrochloride and tetrahydrozoline. J Am Acad Dermatol 1987; 17: 403–407.
173a. Sigal-Nahum M, Konqui A, Gaulier A, Sigal S. Linear fixed drug eruption. Br J Dermatol 1988; 118: 849–851.
174. Guin JD, Haynie LS, Jackson D, Baker GF. Wandering fixed drug eruption: A mucocutaneous reaction to acetaminophen. J Am Acad Dermatol 1987; 17: 399–402.
175. Chan HL. Fixed drug eruptions. A study of 20 occurrences in Singapore. Int J Dermatol 1984; 23: 607–609.
176. Kuokkanen K. Erythema fixum of the genitals and the mucous membranes. Int J Dermatol 1974; 13: 4–8.
177. Kauppinen K, Stubb S. Drug eruptions: causative agents and clinical types. Acta Derm Venereol 1984; 64: 320–324.
178. Shukla SR. Drugs causing fixed drug eruptions. Dermatologica 1981; 163: 160–163.
179. Jolly HW Jr, Sherman IJ Jr, Carpenter CL Jr et al. Fixed drug eruptions to tetracyclines. Arch Dermatol 1978; 114: 1484–1485.
180. Minkin W, Cohen HJ, Frank SB. Fixed-drug eruption due to tetracycline. Report of a case. Arch Dermatol 1969; 100: 749.
181. Parish LC, Witkowski JA. Pulsating fixed drug eruption due to tetracycline. Acta Derm Venereol 1978; 58: 545–547.
182. Kauppinen K, Stubb S. Fixed eruptions: Causative drugs and challenge tests. Br J Dermatol 1985; 112: 575–578.
183. Sehgal VN, Rege VL, Kharangate VN. Fixed drug eruptions caused by medications: a report from India. Int J Dermatol 1978; 17: 78–81.
184. LePaw MI. Fixed drug eruption due to minocycline — report of one case. J Am Acad Dermatol 1983; 8: 263–264.
185. Pareek SS. Nystatin-induced fixed eruption. Br J Dermatol 1980; 103: 679–680.
186. Coskey RJ, Bryan HG. Fixed drug eruption due to penicillin. Arch Dermatol 1975; 111: 791–792.
187. Pigatto PD, Riboldi A, Riva F, Altomare GF. Fixed drug eruption to erythromycin. Acta Derm Venereol 1984; 64: 272–273.
188. Naik RPC, Singh G. Bullous fixed drug eruption presumably due to erythromycin. Dermatologica 1976; 152: 177–180.
189. Savage J. Fixed drug eruption to griseofulvin. Br J Dermatol 1977; 97: 107–108.
189a. Hogan DJ, Rooney ME. Fixed drug eruption due to dimenhydrinate. J Am Acad Dermatol 1989; 20: 503–504.
190. Verbov J. Fixed drug eruption owing to sulfamethoxazole. Arch Dermatol 1978; 114: 963–964.
191. Hughes BR, Holt PJA, Marks R. Trimethoprim associated fixed drug eruption. Br J Dermatol 1987; 116: 241–242.
191a. Archer CB, English JSC. Extensive fixed drug eruption induced by temazepam. Clin Exp Dermatol 1988; 13: 336–338.
192. Shuttleworth D, Graham-Brown RAC. Fixed drug eruption due to carbamazepine. Clin Exp Dermatol 1974; 9: 424–426.
193. Wilson HTH. A fixed drug eruption due to paracetamol. Br J Dermatol 1975; 92: 213–214.
193a. Duhra P, Porter DI. Paracetamol-induced fixed drug eruption with positive immunofluorescence findings. Clin Exp Dermatol 1990; 15: 296–297.
194. Meyrick Thomas RH, Munro DD. Fixed drug eruption due to paracetamol. Br J Dermatol 1986; 115: 357–359.
195. Pasricha JS. Drugs causing fixed drug eruptions. Br J Dermatol 1979; 100: 183–185.
196. Kanwar AJ, Majid A, Singh M, Malhotra YK. An unusual presentation of fixed drug eruption. Dermatologica 1982; 164: 115–116.
197. Hindsen M, Christensen OB, Gruic V, Lofberg H. Fixed drug eruption: an immunohistochemical investigation of the acute and healing phase. Br J Dermatol 1987; 116: 351–360.
197a. Shiohara T, Nickoloff BJ, Sagawa Y et al. Fixed drug

eruption. Expression of epidermal keratinocyte intercellular adhesion molecule-1 (ICAM-1). Arch Dermatol 1989; 125: 1371–1376.

198. Van Voorhees A, Stenn KS. Histological phases of bactrim-induced fixed drug eruption. The report of one case. Am J Dermatopathol 1987; 9: 528–532.

199. De Dobbeleer G, Achten G. Fixed drug eruption: ultrastructural study of dyskeratotic cells. Br J Dermatol 1977; 96: 239–244.

200. Komura J, Yamada M, Ofuji S. Ultrastructure of eosinophilic staining epidermal cells in toxic epidermal necrolysis and fixed drug eruption. Dermatologica 1969; 139: 41–48.

201. Tonnesen MG, Soter NA. Erythema multiforme. J Am Acad Dermatol 1979; 1: 357–364.

201a. Ledesma GN, McCormack PC. Erythema multiforme. Clin Dermatol 1986; 4: 70–80.

202. Huff JC, Weston WL, Tonnesen MG. Erythema multiforme: A critical review of characteristics, diagnostic criteria, and causes. J Am Acad Dermatol 1983; 8: 763–775.

203. Rasmussen JE. Erythema multiforme in children. Response to treatment with systemic corticosteroids. Br J Dermatol 1976; 95: 181–186.

204. Howland WW, Golitz LE, Weston WL, Huff JC. Erythema multiforme: Clinical, histopathologic, and immunologic study. J Am Acad Dermatol 1984; 10: 438–446.

205. Ting HC, Adam BA. Stevens-Johnson syndrome. A review of 34 cases. Int J Dermatol 1985; 24: 587–591.

206. Ruiz-Maldonado R. Acute disseminated epidermal necrosis types 1, 2, and 3: Study of sixty cases. J Am Acad Dermatol 1985; 13: 623–635.

207. Lever WF. My concept of erythema multiforme. Am J Dermatopathol 1985; 7: 141–142.

208. Heng MCY, Feinberg M. Localized erythema multiforme due to lymphatic obstruction. Br J Dermatol 1982; 106: 95–97.

208a. Shiohara T, Chiba M, Tanaka Y, Nagashima M. Drug-induced, photosensitive, erythema-multiforme-like eruption: Possible role for cell adhesion molecules in a flare induced by *Rhus* dermatitis. J Am Acad Dermatol 1990; 22: 647–650.

209. Soltani K, Bernstein JE, Lorincz AL. Eruptive nevocytic nevi following erythema multiforme. J Am Acad Dermatol 1979; 1: 503–505.

210. Duvic M, Reisner EG, Dawson DV, Ciftan E. HLA-B15 association with erythema multiforme. J Am Acad Dermatol 1983; 8: 493–496.

211. Zaim MT, Giorno RC, Golitz LE et al. An immunopathological study of herpes-associated erythema multiforme. J Cutan Pathol 1987; 14: 257–262.

212. Margolis RJ, Tonnesen MG, Harrist TJ et al. Lymphocyte subsets and Langerhans cells/indeterminate cells in erythema multiforme. J Invest Dermatol 1983; 81: 403–406.

213. Tonnesen MG, Harrist TJ, Wintroub BU et al. Erythema multiforme: microvascular damage and infiltration of lymphocytes and basophils. J Invest Dermatol 1983; 80: 282–286.

214. Leigh IM, Mowbray JF, Levene GM, Sutherland S. Recurrent and continuous erythema multiforme — a clinical and immunological study. Clin Exp Dermatol 1985; 10: 58–67.

215. Margolis RJ, Bhan A, Mihm MC Jr, Bernhardt M. Erythema multiforme in a patient with T cell chronic lymphocytic leukemia. J Am Acad Dermatol 1986; 14: 618–627.

216. Ledesma GN, McCormack PC. Erythema multiforme. Clin Dermatol 1986; 4: 70–80.

217. Sontheimer RD, Garibaldi RA, Krueger GG. Stevens-Johnson syndrome associated with *Mycoplasma pneumoniae* infections. Arch Dermatol 1978; 114: 241–244.

218. Curley RK, Verbov JL. Stevens-Johnson syndrome due to tetracyclines — a case report (doxycycline) and review of the literature. Clin Exp Dermatol 1987; 12: 124–125.

219. Dikland WJ, Orange AP, Stolz E, Van Joost T. Erythema multiforme in childhood and early infancy. Pediatr Dermatol 1986; 3: 135–139.

219a. Chan H-L, Stern RS, Arndt KA et al. The incidence of erythema multiforme, Stevens-Johnson syndrome, and toxic epidermal necrolysis. Arch Dermatol 1990; 126: 43–47.

219b. Curley RK, Verbov JL. Stevens-Johnson syndrome due to tetracyclines — a case report (doxycycline) and review of the literature. Clin Exp Dermatol 1987; 12: 124–125.

219c. Lewis-Jones MS, Evans S, Thompson CM. Erythema multiforme occurring in association with lupus erythematosus during therapy with doxycycline. Clin Exp Dermatol 1988; 13: 245–247.

219d. Brook U, Singer L, Fried D. Development of severe Stevens-Johnson syndrome after administration of slow-release theophylline. Pediatr Dermatol 1989; 6: 126–129.

219e. David M, Sandbank M, Lowe NJ. Erythema multiforme-like eruptions associated with etretinate therapy. Clin Exp Dermatol 1989; 14: 230–232.

219f. Rustin MHA, Bunker CB, Dowd PM, Robinson TWE. Erythema multiforme due to griseofulvin. Br J Dermatol 1989; 120: 455–458.

219g. Brice SL, Krzemien D, Weston WL, Huff JC. Detection of herpes simplex virus DNA in cutaneous lesions of erythema multiforme. J Invest Dermatol 1989; 93: 183–187.

220. Bedi TR, Pinkus H. Histopathological spectrum of erythema multiforme. Br J Dermatol 1976; 95: 243–250.

221. Ackerman AB, Penneys NS, Clark WH. Erythema multiforme exudativum: distinctive pathological process. Br J Dermatol 1971; 84: 554–566.

221a. Patterson JW, Parsons JM, Blaylock WK, Mills AS. Eosinophils in skin lesions of erythema multiforme. Arch Pathol Lab Med 1989; 113: 36–39.

222. Reed RJ. Erythema multiforme. A clinical syndrome and a histologic complex. Am J Dermatopathol 1985; 7: 143–152.

223. Ackerman AB. Erythema multiforme. Am J Dermatopathol 1985; 7: 133–139 (Editor's note).

224. Orfanos CE, Schaumburg-Lever G, Lever WF. Dermal and epidermal types of erythema multiforme. A histopathologic study of 24 cases. Arch Dermatol 1974; 109: 682–688.

225. Ackerman AB. Dermal and epidermal types of erythema multiforme. Arch Dermatol 1975; 111: 795.

226. Finan MC, Schroeter AL. Cutaneous immunofluorescence study of erythema multiforme:

Correlation with light microscopic patterns and etiologic agents. J Am Acad Dermatol 1984; 10: 497–506.

227. Imamura S, Yanase K, Taniguchi S et al. Erythema multiforme: demonstration of immune complexes in the sera and skin lesions. Br J Dermatol 1980; 102: 161–166.

228. Grimwood R, Huff JC, Weston WL. Complement deposition in the skin of patients with herpes-associated erythema multiforme. J Am Acad Dermatol 1983; 9: 199–203.

228a. Matsuoka LY, Wortsnan J, Stanley JR. Epidermal autoantibodies in erythema multiforme. J Am Acad Dermatol 1989; 21: 677–680.

229. Merot Y, Saurat JH. Clues to pathogenesis of toxic epidermal necrolysis. Int J Dermatol 1985; 24: 165–168.

230. Goldstein SM, Wintroub BW, Elias PM. Toxic epidermal necrolysis. Unmuddying the waters. Arch Dermatol 1987; 123: 1153–1156.

231. Rasmussen J. Toxic epidermal necrolysis. Med Clin North Am 1980; 64: 901–920.

232. Lyell A. Toxic epidermal necrolysis (the scalded skin syndrome): A reappraisal. Br J Dermatol 1979; 100: 69–86.

232a. Lyell A. Requiem for toxic epidermal necrolysis. Br J Dermatol 1990; 122: 837–838.

233. Revuz J, Penso D, Roujeau J-C et al. Toxic epidermal necrolysis. Clinical findings and prognosis factors in 87 patients. Arch Dermatol 1987; 123: 1160–1165.

233a. Roujeau J-C, Guillaume J-C, Fabre J-P et al. Toxic epidermal necrolysis (Lyell syndrome). Incidence and drug etiology in France, 1981–1985. Arch Dermatol 1990; 126: 37–42.

234. Stuttgen G. Toxic epidermal necrolysis provoked by barbiturates. Br J Dermatol 1973; 88: 291–293.

234a. Sherertz EF, Jegasothy BV, Lazarus GS. Phenytoin hypersensitivity reaction presenting with toxic epidermal necrolysis and severe hepatitis. Report of a patient treated with corticosteroid "pulse therapy". J Am Acad Dermatol 1985; 12: 178–181.

235. Guillaume J-C, Roujeau J-C, Revuz J et al. The culprit drugs in 87 cases of toxic epidermal necrolysis (Lyell's syndrome). Arch Dermatol 1987; 123: 1166–1170.

235a. Stotts JS, Fang ML, Dannaker CJ, Steinman HK. Fenoprofen-induced toxic epidermal necrolysis. J Am Acad Dermatol 1988; 18: 755–757.

236. Dan M, Jedwab M, Peled M, Shibolet S. Allopurinol-induced toxic epidermal necrolysis. Int J Dermatol 1984; 23: 142–144.

237. Roujeau JC, Dubertret L, Moritz S et al. Involvement of macrophages in the pathology of toxic epidermal necrolysis. Br J Dermatol 1985; 113: 425–430.

238. Merot Y, Gravallese E, Guillen FJ, Murphy GF. Lymphocyte subsets and Langerhans cells in toxic epidermal necrolysis. Report of a case. Arch Dermatol 1986; 122: 455–458.

239. Roujeau J-C, Huynh TN, Bracq C et al. Genetic susceptibility to toxic epidermal necrolysis. Arch Dermatol 1987; 123: 1171–1173.

240. Westly ED, Wechsler HL. Toxic epidermal necrolysis. Granulocytic leukopenia as a prognostic indicator. Arch Dermatol 1984; 120: 721–726.

241. Hood AF, Soter NA, Rappeport J, Gigli I. Graft-versus-host reaction. Cutaneous manifestations following bone marrow transplantation. Arch Dermatol 1977; 113: 1087–1091.

242. Breathnach SM, Katz SI. Immunopathology of cutaneous graft-versus-host disease. Am J Dermatopathol 1987; 9: 343–348.

242a. Tawfik N, Jimbow K. Acute graft-vs-host disease in an immunodeficient newborn possibly due to cytomegalovirus infection. Arch Dermatol 1989; 125: 1685–1688.

243. Harper JI. Graft versus host reaction: etiological and clinical aspects in connective tissue diseases. Semin Dermatol 1985; 4: 144–151.

244. Grogan TM, Broughton DD, Doyle WF. Graft-versus-host reaction (GVHR). A case report suggesting GVHR occurred as a result of maternofetal cell transfer. Arch Pathol 1975; 99: 330–334.

245. Hood AF, Vogelsang GB, Black LP et al. Acute graft-vs-host disease. Development following autologous and syngeneic bone marrow transplantation. Arch Dermatol 1987; 123: 745–750.

246. Ferrara JLM. Syngeneic graft-vs-host disease. Arch Dermatol 1987; 123: 741–742.

247. Mascaro JM, Rozman C, Palou J et al. Acute and chronic graft-vs-host reaction in skin: report of two cases. Br J Dermatol 1980; 102: 461–466.

247a. Mauduit G, Claudy A. Cutaneous expression of graft-v-host disease in man. Semin Dermatol 1988; 7: 149–155.

247b. Friedman KJ, LeBoit PE, Farmer ER. Acute follicular graft-vs-host reaction. Arch Dermatol 1988; 124: 688–691.

248. Matsuoka LY. Graft versus host disease. J Am Acad Dermatol 1981; 5: 595–599.

249. Saurat JH, Gluckman E. Lichen-planus-like eruption following bone marrow transplantation: a manifestation of the graft-versus-host disease. Clin Exp Dermatol 1977; 2: 335–344.

250. Saurat JH. Cutaneous manifestations of graft-versus-host disease. Int J Dermatol 1981; 20: 249–256.

250a. Van Vloten WA, Scheffer E, Dooren LJ. Localized scleroderma-like lesions after bone marrow transplantation in man. A chronic graft versus host reaction. Br J Dermatol 1977; 96: 337–341.

251. Spielvogel RL, Goltz RW, Kersey JH. Scleroderma-like changes in chronic graft vs host disease. Arch Dermatol 1977; 113: 1424–1428.

252. Sale GE, Shulman HM, Schubert MM et al. Oral and ophthalmic pathology of graft versus host disease in man: predictive value of the lip biopsy. Hum Pathol 1981; 12: 1022–1030.

253. Snover DC. Acute and chronic graft versus host disease: histopathological evidence for two distinct pathogenetic mechanisms. Hum Pathol 1984; 15: 202–205.

254. Breathnach SM. Current understanding of the aetiology and clinical implications of cutaneous graft-versus-host disease. Br J Dermatol 1986; 114: 139–143.

255. Gomes MA, Schmitt DS, Souteyrand P et al. Lichen planus and chronic graft-versus-host reaction. In situ identification of immunocompetent cell phenotypes. J Cutan Pathol 1982; 9: 249–257.

256. Breathnach SM, Katz SI. Cell-mediated immunity in cutaneous disease. Hum Pathol 1986; 17: 162–167.

257. Sale GE, Shulman HM, Gallucci BB, Thomas ED. Young rete ridge keratinocytes are preferred targets in cutaneous graft-versus-host disease. Am J Pathol 1985; 118: 278–287.

258. Sloane JP, Thomas JA, Imrie SF et al. Morphological and immunohistological changes in the skin in allogeneic bone marrow recipients. J Clin Pathol 1984; 37: 919–930.

259. Dreno B, Milpied N, Harousseau JL et al. Cutaneous immunological studies in diagnosis of acute graft-versus-host disease. Br J Dermatol 1986; 114: 7–15.

260. Lever R, Turbitt M, Mackie R et al. A perspective study of the histological changes in the skin in patients receiving bone marrow transplants. Br J Dermatol 1986; 114: 161–170.

261. Wick MR, Moore SB, Gastineau DA, Hoagland HC. Immunologic, clinical, and pathologic aspects of human graft-versus-host disease. Mayo Clin Proc 1983; 58: 603–612.

262. Hymes SR, Farmer ER, Lewis PG et al. Cutaneous graft-versus-host reaction: Prognostic features seen by light microscopy. J Am Acad Dermatol 1985; 12: 468–474.

262a. LeBoit PE. Subacute radiation dermatitis: A histologic imitator of acute cutaneous graft-versus-host disease. J Am Acad Dermatol 1989; 20: 236–241.

263. Saurat JH, Gluckman E, Bussel A et al. The lichen planus-like eruption after bone marrow transplantation. Br J Dermatol 1975; 92: 675–681.

264. Hymes SR, Farmer ER, Burns WH et al. Bullous sclerodermalike changes in chronic graft-vs-host disease. Arch Dermatol 1985; 121: 1189–1192.

265. Rozman C, Mascaro JM, Granena A et al. Ultrastructural findings in acute and chronic graft-vs-host reaction of the skin. J Cutan Pathol 1980; 7: 354–363.

265a. Slavin RE. Lymphocyte-associated apoptosis in AIDS, in bone-marrow transplantation, and other conditions. Am J Surg Pathol 1987; 11: 235–238.

266. Claudy AL, Schmitt D, Freycon F, Boucheron S. Melanocyte-lymphocyte interaction in human graft-versus-host disease. J Cutan Pathol 1983; 10: 305–311.

267. Gallucci BB, Shulman HM, Sale GE et al. The ultrastructure of the human epidermis in chronic graft-versus-host disease. Am J Pathol 1979; 95: 643–662.

268. Janin-Mercier A, Saurat JH, Bourges M et al. The lichen planus like and sclerotic phases of the graft versus host disease in man: an ultrastructural study of six cases. Acta Derm Venereol 1981; 61: 187–193.

269. Rico MJ, Kory WP, Gould EW, Penneys NS. Interface dermatitis in patients with the acquired immunodeficiency syndrome. J Am Acad Dermatol 1987; 16: 1209–1218.

270. Tuffanelli DL. Lupus erythematosus. J Am Acad Dermatol 1981; 4: 127–142.

271. Gilliam JN, Sontheimer RD. Distinctive cutaneous subsets in the spectrum of lupus erythematosus. J Am Acad Dermatol 1981; 4: 471–475.

272. Clark WH, Reed RJ, Mihm MC. Lupus erythematosus. Histopathology of cutaneous lesions. Hum Pathol 1973; 4: 157–163.

273. Coulson IH, Marsden RA. Lupus erythematosus

274. Shklar G, McCarthy PL. Histopathology of oral lesions of discoid lupus erythematosus. A review of 25 cases. Arch Dermatol 1978; 114: 1031–1035.

275. Sulica VI, Kao GF. Squamous-cell carcinoma of the scalp arising in lesions of discoid lupus erythematosus. Am J Dermatopathol 1988; 10: 137–141.

276. Keith D, Kelly AP, Sumrall AJ, Chhabra A. Squamous cell carcinoma arising in lesions of discoid lupus erythematosus. Arch Dermatol 1980; 116: 315–317.

277. Millard LG, Barker DJ. Development of squamous cell carcinoma in chronic discoid lupus erythematosus. Clin Exp Dermatol 1978; 3: 161–166.

278. Callen JP. Systemic lupus erythematosus in patients with chronic cutaneous (discoid) lupus erythematosus. Clinical and laboratory findings in seventeen patients. J Am Acad Dermatol 1985; 12: 278–288.

279. Rowell NR. The natural history of lupus erythematosus. Clin Exp Dermatol 1984; 9: 217–231.

280. Millard LG, Rowell NR. Abnormal laboratory test results and their relationship to prognosis in discoid lupus erythematosus. A long-term follow-up of 92 patients. Arch Dermatol 1979; 115: 1055–1058.

281. Callen JP, Fowler JF, Kulick KB. Serologic and clinical features of patients with discoid lupus erythematosus: Relationship of antibodies to single-stranded deoxyribonucleic acid and of other antinuclear antibody subsets to clinical manifestations. J Am Acad Dermatol 1985; 13: 748–755.

282. Prystowsky SD, Gilliam JN. Discoid lupus erythematosus as part of a larger disease spectrum. Arch Dermatol 1975; 111: 1448–1452.

283. Fowler JF, Callen JP, Stelzer GT, Cotter PK. Human histocompatibility antigen associations in patients with chronic cutaneous lupus erythematosus. J Am Acad Dermatol 1985; 12: 73–77.

284. Lindskov R, Munkvad JM, Valerius NH. Discoid lupus erythematosus and carrier status of x-linked chronic granulomatous disease. Dermatologica 1983; 167: 231–233.

285. Brandrup F, Koch C, Petri M et al. Discoid lupus erythematosus-like lesions and stomatitis in female carriers of X-linked chronic granulomatous disease. Br J Dermatol 1981; 104: 495–505.

285a. Garioch JJ, Sampson JR, Seywright M, Thomson J. Dermatoses in five related female carriers of X-linked chronic granulomatous disease. Br J Dermatol 1989; 121: 391–396.

286. Barton LL, Johnson CR. Discoid lupus erythematosus and X-linked chronic granulomatous disease. Pediatr Dermatol 1986; 3: 376–379.

287. Stalder JF, Dreno B, Bureau B, Hakim J. Discoid lupus erythematosus-like lesions in an autosomal form of chronic granulomatous disease. Br J Dermatol 1986; 114: 251–254.

288. Uitto J, Santa-Cruz DJ, Eisen AZ, Leone P. Verrucous lesions in patients with discoid lupus erythematosus. Clinical, histopathological and immunofluorescence studies. Br J Dermatol 1978; 98: 507–520.

289. Rubenstein DJ, Huntley AC. Keratotic lupus

erythematosus: Treatment with isotretinoin. J Am Acad Dermatol 1986; 14: 910–914.

290. Santa Cruz DJ, Uitto J, Eisen AZ, Prioleau PG. Verrucous lupus erythematosus: Ultrastructural studies on a distinct variant of chronic discoid lupus erythematosus. J Am Acad Dermatol 1983; 9: 82–90.

291. Vinciullo C. Hypertrophic lupus erythematosus: differentiation from squamous cell carcinoma. Australas J Dermatol 1986; 27: 76–82.

292. Otani A. Lupus erythematosus hypertrophicus et profundus. Br J Dermatol 1977; 96: 75–78.

292a. Parodi A, Drago EF, Varaldo G, Rebora A. Rowell's syndrome. Report of a case. J Am Acad Dermatol 1989; 21: 374–377.

293. Winkelmann RK. Spectrum of lupus erythematosus. J Cutan Pathol 1979; 6: 457–462.

294. Weigand DA, Burgdorf WHC, Gregg LJ. Dermal mucinosis in discoid lupus erythematosus. Report of two cases. Arch Dermatol 1981; 117: 735–738.

295. Ueki H, Takei Y, Nakagawa S. Cutaneous calcinosis in localized discoid lupus erythematosus. Arch Dermatol 1980; 116: 196–197.

296. Kabir DI, Malkinson FD. Lupus erythematosus and calcinosis cutis. Arch Dermatol 1969; 100: 17–22.

297. Weigand DA. The lupus band test: A re-evaluation. J Am Acad Dermatol 1984; 11: 230–234.

297a. Williams REA, Mackie RM, O'Keefe R, Thomson W. The contribution of direct immunofluorescence to the diagnosis of lupus erythematosus. J Cutan Pathol 1989; 16: 122–125.

298. Provost TT. Lupus band test. Int J Dermatol 1981; 20: 475–481.

299. Weigand DA. Lupus band test: Anatomical regional variations in discoid lupus erythematosus. J Am Acad Dermatol 1986; 14: 426–428.

299a. Gruschwitz M, Keller J, Hornstein OP. Deposits of immunoglobulins at the dermo-epidermal junction in chronic light-exposed skin: what is the value of the lupus band test? Clin Exp Dermatol 1988; 13: 303–308.

300. Wojnarowska F, Bhogal B, Black MM. The significance of an IgM band at the dermo-epidermal junction. J Cutan Pathol 1986; 13: 359–362.

301. Hashimoto K, Thompson DF. Discoid lupus erythematosus. Electron microscopic studies of paramyxovirus-like structures. Arch Dermatol 1970; 101: 565–577.

302. Schiodt M, Andersen L. Ultrastructural features of oral discoid lupus erythematosus. Acta Derm Venereol 1980; 60: 99–107.

303. Callen JP, Kulick KB, Stelzer G, Fowler JF. Subacute cutaneous lupus erythematosus. Clinical, serologic, and immunogenetic studies of forty-nine patients seen in a nonreferral setting. J Am Acad Dermatol 1986; 15: 1227–1237.

304. Harper JI. Subacute cutaneous lupus erythematosus (SCLE): a distinct subset of LE. Clin Exp Dermatol 1982; 7: 209–212.

305. Sontheimer RD, Thomas JR, Gilliam JN. Subacute cutaneous lupus erythematosus. A cutaneous marker for a distinct lupus erythematosus subset. Arch Dermatol 1979; 115: 1409–1415.

306. Weinstein CL, Littlejohn GO, Thomson NM, Hall S. Severe visceral disease in subacute cutaneous lupus erythematosus. Arch Dermatol 1987; 123: 638–648.

306a. DeSpain J, Clark DP. Subacute cutaneous lupus erythematosus presenting as erythroderma. J Am Acad Dermatol 1988; 19: 388–392.

306b. Fine RM. Subacute cutaneous lupus erythematosus associated with hydrochlorothiazide therapy. Int J Dermatol 1989; 28: 375–376.

306c. Miyagawa S, Okuchi T, Shiomi Y, Sakamoto K. Subacute cutaneous lupus erythematosus lesions precipitated by griseofulvin. J Am Acad Dermatol 1989; 21: 343–346.

307. Deng J-S, Sontheimer RD, Gilliam JN. Relationship between antinuclear and anti-Ro/SS-A antibodies in subacute cutaneous lupus erythematosus. J Am Acad Dermatol 1984; 11: 494–499.

308. Wechsler HL, Stavrides A. Systemic lupus erythematosus with anti-Ro antibodies: Clinical, histologic, and immunologic findings. Report of three cases. J Am Acad Dermatol 1982; 6: 73–83.

309. Wermuth DJ, Geoghegan WD, Jordon RE. Anti-Ro/SS antibodies. Association with a particulate (large speckledlike thread) immunofluorescent nuclear staining pattern. Arch Dermatol 1985; 121: 335–338.

310. Dore N, Synkowski D, Provost TT. Antinuclear antibody determinations in Ro(SSA)-positive, antinuclear antibody-negative lupus and Sjogren's syndrome patients. J Am Acad Dermatol 1983; 8: 611–615.

311. Sontheimer RD. Questions pertaining to the true frequencies with which anti-Ro/SS-A autoantibody and the HLA-DR3 phenotype occur in subacute cutaneous lupus erythematosus patients. J Am Acad Dermatol 1987; 16: 130–134.

312. Hymes SR, Russell TJ, Jordon RE. The anti-Ro antibody system. Int J Dermatol 1986; 25: 1–7.

313. Sontheimer RD. Immunological significance of the Ro/SSA antigen-antibody system. Arch Dermatol 1985; 121: 327–330.

314. Callen JP, Hodge SJ, Kulick KB et al. Subacute cutaneous lupus erythematosus in multiple members of a family with C2 deficiency. Arch Dermatol 1987; 123: 66–70.

315. Provost TT, Talal N, Harley JB et al. The relationship between anti-Ro (SS-A) antibody-positive Sjogren's syndrome and anti-Ro (SS-A) antibody-positive lupus erythematosus. Arch Dermatol 1988; 124: 63–71.

316. Lee LA. Anti-Ro (SSA) and anti-La (SSB) antibodies in lupus erythematosus and in Sjögren's syndrome. Arch Dermatol 1988; 124: 61–62.

316a. Jones SK, Coulter S, Harmon C et al. Ro/SSA antigen in human epidermis. Br J Dermatol 1988; 118: 363–367.

317. Purcell SM, Lieu TS, Davis BM, Sontheimer RD. Relationship between circulating anti-Ro/SS-A antibody levels and skin disease activity in subacute cutaneous lupus erythematosus. Br J Dermatol 1987; 117: 277–287.

318. Bangert JL, Freeman RG, Sontheimer RD, Gilliam JN. Subacute cutaneous lupus erythematosus and discoid lupus erythematosus. Comparative histopathologic findings. Arch Dermatol 1984; 120: 332–337.

318a. Jerdan JS, Hood AF, Moore GW, Callen JP. Histopathologic comparison of the subsets of lupus erythematosus. Arch Dermatol 1990; 126: 52–55.

318b. Tuthill RJ, Guitart J, Helm T, Camisa C.

Histopathology of subacute cutaneous lupus erythematosus. J Cutan Pathol 1989; 16: 328 (abstract).

318c. Herrero C, Bielsa I, Font J et al. Subacute cutaneous lupus erythematosus: Clinicopathologic findings in thirteen cases. J Am Acad Dermatol 1988; 19: 1057–1062.

318d. DeSpain JD, David KM, Bennion SD et al. Histologic findings in subsets of cutaneous lupus erythematosus. J Cutan Pathol 1989; 16: 300 (abstract).

318e. Nieboer C, Tak-Diamand Z, van Leeuwen-Wallau HE. Dust-like particles: a specific direct immunofluorescence pattern in sub-acute cutaneous lupus erythematosus. Br J Dermatol 1988; 118: 725–729.

319. Matthews CNA, Saihan EM, Warin RP. Urticaria-like lesions associated with systemic lupus erythematosus: response to dapsone. Br J Dermatol 1978; 99: 455–457.

320. Barton DD, Fine J-D, Gammon WR, Sams WM Jr. Bullous systemic lupus erythematosus: An unusual clinical course and detectable circulating autoantibodies to the epidermolysis bullosa acquisita antigen. J Am Acad Dermatol 1986; 15: 369–373.

321. Camisa C, Sharma HM. Vesiculobullous systemic lupus erythematosus. Report of two cases and a review of the literature. J Am Acad Dermatol 1983; 9: 924–933.

322. Penneys NS, Wiley HE III. Herpetiform blisters in systemic lupus erythematosus. Arch Dermatol 1979; 115: 1427–1428.

323. Callen JP. Cutaneous bullae following acute steroid withdrawal in systemic lupus erythematosus. Br J Dermatol 1981; 105: 603–606.

324. Millard LG, Rowell NR. Chilblain lupus erythematosus (Hutchinson). A clinical and laboratory study of 17 patients. Br J Dermatol 1978; 98: 497–506.

325. Van der Meer-Roosen CH, Maes EPJ, Faber WR. Cutaneous lupus erythematosus and autoimmune thyroiditis. Br J Dermatol 1979; 101: 91–92.

326. Cruz PD Jr, Coldiron BM, Sontheimer RD. Concurrent features of cutaneous lupus erythematosus and pemphigus erythematosus following myasthenia gravis and thymoma. J Am Acad Dermatol 1987; 16: 472–480.

327. DeCastro P, Jorizzo JL, Solomon AR et al. Coexistent systemic lupus erythematosus and tophaceous gout. J Am Acad Dermatol 1985; 13: 650–654.

328. Aronson PJ, Fretzin DF, Morgan NE. A unique case of sarcoidosis with coexistent collagen vascular disease. J Am Acad Dermatol 1985; 13: 886–891.

329. Cram DL, Epstein JH, Tuffanelli DL. Lupus erythematosus and porphyria. Coexistence in seven patients. Arch Dermatol 1973; 108: 779–784.

330. Goette DK. Sweet's syndrome in subacute cutaneous lupus erythematosus. Arch Dermatol 1985; 121: 789–791.

331. Kulick KB, Mogavero H Jr, Provost TT, Reichlin M. Serologic studies in patients with lupus erythematosus and psoriasis. J Am Acad Dermatol 1983; 8: 631–634.

332. Hays SB, Camisa C, Luzar MJ. The coexistence of systemic lupus erythematosus and psoriasis. J Am Acad Dermatol 1984; 10: 619–622.

333. Thomas JR III, Su WPD. Concurrence of lupus erythematosus and dermatitis herpetiformis. A report of nine cases. Arch Dermatol 1983; 119: 740–745.

334. Taieb A, Hehunstre J-P, Goetz J et al. Lupus erythematosus panniculitis with partial genetic deficiency of C2 and C4 in a child. Arch Dermatol 1986; 122: 576–582.

335. Massa MC, Connolly SM. An association between C1 esterase inhibitor deficiency and lupus erythematosus: Report of two cases and review of the literature. J Am Acad Dermatol 1982; 7: 255–264.

336. Rasmussen EK, Ullman S, Hoier-Madsen M et al. Clinical implications of ribonucleoprotein antibody. Arch Dermatol 1987; 123: 601–605.

337. Sharp GC, Anderson PC. Current concepts in the classification of connective tissue diseases. Overlap syndromes and mixed connective tissue disease (MCTD). J Am Acad Dermatol 1980; 2: 269–279.

338. Gilliam JN, Prystowsky SD. Mixed connective tissue disease syndrome. Arch Dermatol 1977; 113: 583–587.

339. Bentley-Phillips CB, Geake TMS. Mixed connective tissue disease characterized by speckled epidermal nuclear IgG deposition in normal skin. Br J Dermatol 1980; 102: 529–533.

340. Wechsler HL. Lupus erythematosus. A clinician's coign of vantage. Arch Dermatol 1983; 119: 877–882.

341. Callen JP, Kingman J. Cutaneous vasculitis in systemic lupus erythematosus. A poor prognostic indicator. Cutis 1983; 32: 433–436.

342. Yasue T. Livedoid vasculitis and central nervous system involvement in systemic lupus erythematosus. Arch Dermatol 1986; 122: 66–70.

343. Weinstein C, Miller MH, Axtens R et al. Livedo reticularis associated with increased titers of anticardiolipin antibodies in systemic lupus erythematosus. Arch Dermatol 1987; 123: 596–600.

344. Dodd HJ, Sarkany I, O'Shaughnessy D. Widespread cutaneous necrosis associated with the lupus anticoagulant. Clin Exp Dermatol 1985; 10: 581–586.

345. Grob J-J, Bonerandi J-J. Cutaneous manifestations associated with the presence of the lupus anticoagulant. J Am Acad Dermatol 1986; 15: 211–219.

346. Deegan MJ. Systemic lupus erythematosus. Some contemporary laboratory aspects. Arch Pathol Lab Med 1980; 104: 399–404.

347. Hochberg MC, Boyd RE, Ahearn JM et al. Systemic lupus erythematosus: a review of clinico-laboratory features and immunogenetic markers in 150 patients with emphasis on demographic subsets. Medicine (Baltimore) 1985; 64: 285–295.

348. Lerner EA, Lerner MR. Whither the ANA? Arch Dermatol 1987; 123: 358–362.

349. Sontheimer RD, Deng J-S, Gilliam JN. Antinuclear and anticytoplasmic antibodies. Concepts and misconceptions. J Am Acad Dermatol 1983; 9: 335–343.

350. Steinmetz SE, Deng J-S, Rubin RL et al. Reevaluation of specificity of Crithidia luciliae kinetoplast as a substrate for detecting antibodies to double-stranded deoxyribonucleic acid. J Am Acad Dermatol 1984; 11: 490–493.

351. Kohchiyama A, Oka D, Ueki H. T-cell subsets in

lesions of systemic and discoid lupus erythematosus. J Cutan Pathol 1985; 12: 493–499.

352. Andrews BS, Schenk A, Barr R et al. Immunopathology of cutaneous human lupus erythematosus defined by murine monoclonal antibodies. J Am Acad Dermatol 1986; 15: 474–481.

353. Ashworth J, Turbitt M, MacKie R. A comparison of the dermal lymphoid infiltrates in discoid lupus erythematosus and Jessner's lymphocytic infiltrate of the skin using the monoclonal antibody Leu 8. J Cutan Pathol 1987; 14: 198–201.

354. Ullman S, Wiik A, Kobayasi T, Halberg P. Drug-induced lupus erythematosus syndrome. Acta Derm Venereol 1974; 54: 387–390.

355. Peterson LL. Hydralazine-induced systemic lupus erythematosus presenting as pyoderma gangrenosum-like ulcers. J Am Acad Dermatol 1984; 10: 379–384.

356. Lavie CJ, Biundo J, Quinet RJ et al. Systemic lupus erythematosus (SLE) induced by quinidine. Arch Intern Med 1985; 145: 446–448.

357. Burns DA, Sarkany I. Penicillamine induced discoid lupus erythematosus. Clin Exp Dermatol 1979; 4: 389–392.

358. Adams JD. Drug induced lupus erythematosus — a case report. Australas J Dermatol 1978; 19: 31–32.

359. Pavlidakey GP, Hashimoto K, Heller GL, Daneshvar S. Chlorpromazine-induced lupuslike disease. Case report and review of the literature. J Am Acad

360. Gorsulowsky DC, Bank PW, Goldberg AD et al. Antinuclear antibodies as indicators for the procainamide-induced systemic lupus erythematosus-like syndrome and its clinical presentations. J Am Acad Dermatol 1985; 12: 245–253.

361. Haustein U-F. Tubular structures in affected and normal skin in chronic discoid and systemic lupus erythematosus: electron microscopic studies. Br J Dermatol 1973; 89: 1–13.

362. Arnett FC. HLA and genetic predisposition to lupus erythematosus and other dermatologic disorders. J Am Acad Dermatol 1985; 13: 472–481.

363. Farmer ER, Provost TT. Immunologic studies of skin biopsy specimens in connective tissue diseases. Hum Pathol 1983; 14: 316–325.

363a. Lehmann P, Holzle E, Kind P et al. Experimental reproduction of skin lesions in lupus erythematosus by UVA and UVB radiation. J Am Acad Dermatol 1990; 22: 181–187.

364. Zamansky GB. Sunlight-induced pathogenesis in systemic lupus erythematosus. J Invest Dermatol 1985; 85: 179–180.

365. Rongioletti F, Rebora A. Papular and nodular mucinosis associated with systemic lupus erythematosus. Br J Dermatol 1986; 115: 631–636.

366. Gammon WR, Caro I, Long JC, Wheeler CE Jr. Secondary cutaneous mucinosis with systemic lupus erythematosus. Arch Dermatol 1978; 114: 432–435.

367. Panet-Raymond G, Johnson WC. Lupus erythematosus and polymorphous light eruption. Differentiation by histochemical procedures. Arch Dermatol 1973; 108: 785–787.

368. Jacobs MI, Schned ES, Bystryn J-C. Variability of the lupus band test. Results in 18 patients with systemic lupus erythematosus. Arch Dermatol 1983; 119: 883–889.

369. Monroe EW. Lupus band test. Arch Dermatol 1977; 113: 830–834.

369a. Burge SM, Frith PA, Millard PR, Wojnarowska F. The lupus band test in oral mucosa, conjunctiva and skin. Br J Dermatol 1989; 121: 743–752.

370. Dahl MV. Usefulness of direct immunofluorescence in patients with lupus erythematosus. Arch Dermatol 1983; 119: 1010–1017.

371. Pehamberger H, Konrad K, Holubar K. Immunoelectron microscopy of skin in lupus erythematosus. J Cutan Pathol 1978; 5: 319–328.

372. Soltani K, Pacernick LJ, Lorincz AL. Lupus erythematosus-like lesions in newborn infants. Arch Dermatol 1974; 110: 435–437.

373. Rendall JRS, Wilkinson JD. Neonatal lupus erythematosus. Clin Exp Dermatol 1978; 3: 69–75.

374. Vonderheid EC, Koblenzer PJ, Ming PML, Burgoon CF Jr. Neonatal lupus erythematosus. Arch Dermatol 1976; 112: 698–705.

375. Lee LA, Weston WL. Neonatal lupus erythematosus. Semin Dermatol 1988; 7: 66–72.

376. Esterly NB. Neonatal lupus erythematosus. Pediatr Dermatol 1986; 3: 417–424.

377. Watson RM, Lane AT, Barnett NK et al. Neonatal lupus erythematosus. A clinical, serological and immunofluorescence study with review of the literature. Medicine (Baltimore) 1984; 63: 362–378.

377a. Watson R, Kang JE, May M et al. Thrombocytopenia in the neonatal lupus syndrome. Arch Dermatol 1988; 124: 560–563.

378. Draznin TH, Esterly NB, Furey NL, De Bofsky H. Neonatal lupus erythematosus. J Am Acad Dermatol 1979; 1: 437–442.

379. Lumpkin LR III, Hall J, Hogan JD et al. Neonatal lupus erythematosus. A report of three cases associated with anti-Ro/SSA antibodies. Arch Dermatol 1985; 121: 377–381.

380. Lin RY, Cohen-Addad N, Krey PR et al. Neonatal lupus erythematosus, multiple thromboses, and monoarthritis in a family with Ro antibody. J Am Acad Dermatol 1985; 12: 1022–1025.

381. Provost TT. Commentary: Neonatal lupus erythematosus. Arch Dermatol 1983; 119: 619–622.

381a. Katayama I, Kondo S, Kawana S et al. Neonatal lupus erythematosus with a high anticardiolipin antibody titer. J Am Acad Dermatol 1989; 21: 490–492.

382. Gawkrodger DJ, Beveridge GW. Neonatal lupus erythematosus in four successive siblings born to a mother with discoid lupus erythematosus. Br J Dermatol 1984; 111: 683–687.

383. Hall RP III, Lawley TJ, Katz SI. Bullous eruption of systemic lupus erythematosus. J Am Acad Dermatol 1982; 7: 797–799.

384. Olansky AJ, Briggaman RA, Gammon WR et al. Bullous systemic lupus erythematosus. J Am Acad Dermatol 1982; 7: 511–520.

385. Camisa C. Vesiculobullous systemic lupus erythematosus. J Am Acad Dermatol 1988; 18: 93–100.

385a. Rappersberger K, Tschachler E, Tani M, Wolff K. Bullous disease in systemic lupus erythematosus. J Am Acad Dermatol 1989; 21: 745–752.

386. Quirk CJ, Heenan PJ. Bullous discoid lupus

erythematosus: a case report. Australas J Dermatol 1979; 20: 85–87.

387. Tani M, Shimizu R, Ban M et al. Systemic lupus erythematosus with vesiculobullous lesions. Immunoelectron microscopic studies. Arch Dermatol 1984; 120: 1497–1501.

388. Gammon WR, Briggaman RA, Inman AO III et al. Evidence supporting a role for immune complex-mediated inflammation in the pathogenesis of bullous lesions of systemic lupus erythematosus. J Invest Dermatol 1983; 81: 320–325.

389. Feuerman EJ, Halevy S. Lupus erythematosus profundus (Kaposi-Irgang) with monoclonal gammopathy. Br J Dermatol 1977; 96: 79–82.

390. Marks R, Levene GM. Discoid lupus erythematosus and lupus erythematosus profundus in a child. Clin Exp Dermatol 1976; 1: 187–190.

391. Callen JP. Dermatomyositis. Int J Dermatol 1979; 18: 423–433.

392. Callen JP. Dermatomyositis and polymyositis update on current controversies. Australas J Dermatol 1987; 28: 62–67.

393. Kram LS. Dermatomyositis in six patients without initial muscle involvement. Arch Dermatol 1975; 111: 241–245.

393a. Rockerbie NR, Woo TY, Callen JP, Giustina T. Cutaneous changes of dermatomyositis precede muscle weakness. J Am Acad Dermatol 1989; 20: 629–632.

394. Winkelmann RK. Dermatomyositis in childhood. Clin Rheumat Dis 1982; 8: 353–381.

395. Woo TR, Rasmussen J, Callen JP. Recurrent photosensitive dermatitis preceding juvenile dermatomyositis. Pediatr Dermatol 1985; 2: 207–212.

396. Callen JP. Dermatomyositis. Dis Mon 1987; 33: 237–305.

397. Callen JP. Dermatomyositis — an update 1985. Semin Dermatol 1985; 4: 114–125.

398. Samitz MH. Clinical changes in dermatomyositis. A clinical sign. Arch Dermatol 1974; 110: 866–867.

399. Nielsen AO, Johnson E, Hentzer B, Kobayasi T. Dermatomyositis with universal calcinosis. A histopathological and electron optic study. J Cutan Pathol 1979; 6: 486–491.

400. Kawakami T, Nakamura C, Hasegawa H et al. Ultrastructural study of calcinosis universalis with dermatomyositis. J Cutan Pathol 1986; 13: 135–143.

401. Bohan A, Peter JB, Bowman RL, Pearson CM. A computer-assisted analysis of 153 patients with polymyositis and dermatomyositis. Medicine (Baltimore) 1977; 56: 255–286.

402. Mimori T. Scleroderma-polymyositis overlap syndrome. Clinical and serologic aspects. Int J Dermatol 1987; 26: 419–425.

403. Orihara T, Yanase S, Furuya T. A case of sclerodermatomyositis with cutaneous amyloidosis. Br J Dermatol 1985; 112: 213–219.

404. Rowell NR. Overlap in connective tissue diseases. Semin Dermatol 1985; 4: 136–143.

405. Phillips TJ, Leigh IM, Wright J. Dermatomyositis and pulmonary fibrosis associated with anti-Jo-1 antibody. J Am Acad Dermatol 1987; 17: 381–382.

406. Callen JP, Hyla JF, Bole GG Jr, Kay DR. The relationship of dermatomyositis and polymyositis to internal malignancy. Arch Dermatol 1980; 116: 295–298.

407. Vesterager L, Worm A-M, Thomsen K. Dermatomyositis and malignancy. Clin Exp Dermatol 1980; 5: 31–35.

407a. Basset-Seguin N, Roujeau J-C, Gherardi R et al. Prognostic factors and predictive signs of malignancy in adult dermatomyositis. A study of 32 cases. Arch Dermatol 1990; 126: 633–637.

408. Lakhanpal S, Bunch TW, Ilstrup DM, Melton LJ III. Polymyositis-dermatomyositis and malignant lesions: does an association exist? Mayo Clin Proc 1986; 61: 645–653.

408a. Cox NH, Lawrence CM, Langtry JAA, Ive FA. Dermatomyositis. Disease associations and an evaluation of screening investigations for malignancy. Arch Dermatol 1990; 126: 61–65.

409. Manchul LA, Jin A, Pritchard KI et al. The frequency of malignant neoplasms in patients with polymyositis-dermatomyositis. A controlled study. Arch Intern Med 1985; 145: 1835–1839.

410. Topi GC, D'Alessandro L, Catricala C, Zardi O. Dermatomyositis-like syndrome due to toxoplasma. Br J Dermatol 1979; 101: 589–591.

410a. Richard M, Truchetet F, Friedel J et al. Skin lesions simulating chronic dermatomyositis during long-term hydroxyurea therapy. J Am Acad Dermatol 1989; 21: 797–799.

411. Hashimoto K, Robinson L, Velayos E, Niizuma K. Dermatomyositis. Electron microscopic, immunologic, and tissue culture studies of paramyxovirus-like inclusions. Arch Dermatol 1971; 103: 120–135.

412. Janis JF, Winkelmann RK. Histopathology of the skin in dermatomyositis. Arch Dermatol 1968; 97: 640–650.

413. Hanno R, Callen JP. Histopathology of Gottron's papules. J Cutan Pathol 1985; 12: 389–394.

414. Eckardt JJ, Ivins JC, Perry HO, Unni KK. Osteosarcoma arising in heterotopic ossification of dermatomyositis: case report and review of the literature. Cancer 1981; 48: 1256–1261.

415. Chen Z, Maize JC, Silver RM et al. Direct and indirect immunofluorescent findings in dermatomyositis. J Cutan Pathol 1985; 12: 18–27.

416. Alexander CB, Croker BP, Bossen EH. Dermatomyositis associated with IgA deposition. Arch Pathol Lab Med 1982; 106: 449–451.

Poikilodermas

417. Person JR, Bishop GF. Is poikiloderma a graft-versus-host-like reaction? Am J Dermatopathol 1984; 6: 71–72.

418. Canizares O. Poikiloderma of Civatte. Arch Dermatol 1968; 98: 429–431.

419. Berg E, Chuang T-Y, Cripps D. Rothmund-Thomson syndrome. A case report, phototesting, and literature review. J Am Acad Dermatol 1987; 17: 332–338.

419a. Moss C. Rothmund-Thomson syndrome: a report of two patients and a review of the literature. Br J Dermatol 1990; 122: 821–829.

420. Shuttleworth D, Marks R. Epidermal dysplasia and skeletal deformity in congenital poikiloderma

(Rothmund-Thomson syndrome). Br J Dermatol 1987; 117: 377–384.

420a. Roth DE, Campisano LC, Callen JP et al. Rothmund-Thomson syndrome: a case report. Pediatr Dermatol 1989; 6: 321–324.

421. Rook A, Davis R, Stevanovic D. Poikiloderma congenitale. Rothmund-Thomson syndrome. Acta Derm Venereol 1959; 39: 392–420.

421a. Nanda A, Kanwar AJ, Kapoor MM et al. Rothmund-Thomson syndrome in two siblings. Pediatr Dermatol 1989; 6: 325–328.

422. Simmons IJ. Rothmund-Thomson syndrome: a case report. Australas J Dermatol 1980; 21: 96–99.

423. Dick DC, Morley WN, Watson JT. Rothmund-Thomson syndrome and osteogenic sarcoma. Clin Exp Dermatol 1982; 7: 119–123.

424. Weary PE, Hsu YT, Richardson DR et al. Hereditary sclerosing poikiloderma. Report of two families with an unusual and distinctive genodermatosis. Arch Dermatol 1969; 100: 413–422.

425. Greer KE, Weary PE, Nagy R, Robinow M. Hereditary sclerosing poikiloderma. Int J Dermatol 1978; 17: 316–322.

426. Bordas X, Palou J, Capdevila JM, Mascaro JM. Kindler's syndrome. Report of a case. J Am Acad Dermatol 1982; 6: 263–265.

427. Alper JC, Baden HP, Goldsmith LA. Kindler's syndrome. Arch Dermatol 1978; 114: 457.

427a. Forman AB, Prendiville JS, Esterly NB et al. Kindler syndrome: Report of two cases and review of the literature. Pediatr Dermatol 1989; 6: 91–101.

428. Weary PE, Manley WF Jr, Graham GF. Hereditary acrokeratotic poikiloderma. Arch Dermatol 1971; 103: 409–422.

429. Draznin MB, Esterly NB, Fretzin DF. Congenital poikiloderma with features of hereditary acrokeratotic poikiloderma. Arch Dermatol 1978; 114: 1207–1210.

429a. Hovnanian A, Blanchet–Bardon C, de Prost Y. Poikiloderma of Theresa Kindler: report of a case with ultrastructural study, and review of the literature. Pediatr Dermatol 1989; 6: 82–90.

430. Person JR, Perry HO. Congenital poikiloderma with traumatic bulla formation, anhidrosis, and keratoderma. Acta Derm Venereol 1979; 59: 347–351.

431. Blinstrub RS, Lehman R, Sternberg TH. Poilikoderma congenitale. Report of two cases. Arch Dermatol 1964; 89: 659–664.

432. Kristensen JK. Poikiloderma congenitale — an early case of Rothmund-Thomson's syndrome. Acta Derm Venereol 1975; 55: 316–318.

433. Gretzula JC, Hevia O, Weber PJ. Bloom's syndrome. J Am Acad Dermatol 1987; 17: 479–488.

434. Landau JW, Sasaki MS, Newcomer VD, Norman A. Bloom's syndrome. The syndrome of telangiectatic erythema and growth retardation. Arch Dermatol 1966; 94: 687–694.

435. Dicken CH, Dewald G, Gordon H. Sister chromatid exchanges in Bloom's syndrome. Arch Dermatol 1978; 114: 755–760.

436. Brothman AR, Cram LS, Bartholdi MF, Kraemer PM. Preneoplastic phenotype and chromosome changes of cultured human Bloom syndrome fibroblasts (strain GM 1492). Cancer Res 1986; 46: 791–797.

437. German J, Bloom D, Passarge E. Blooms syndrome XI. Progress report for 1983. Clin Genet 1984; 25: 166–174.

438. Wang SR, Wong CK. Dyskeratosis congenita. Dermatologica 1975; 150: 305–310.

439. Ling NS, Fenske NA, Julius RL et al. Dyskeratosis congenita in a girl simulating chronic graft-vs-host disease. Arch Dermatol 1985; 121: 1424–1428.

440. Gutman A, Frumkin A, Adam A et al. X-linked dyskeratosis congenita with pancytopenia. Arch Dermatol 1978; 114: 1667–1671.

441. Connor JM, Teague RH. Dyskeratosis congenita. Report of a large kindred. Br J Dermatol 1981; 105: 321–325.

442. Mills SE, Cooper PH, Beacham BE, Greer KE. Intracranial calcifications and dyskeratosis congenita. Arch Dermatol 1979; 115: 1437–1439.

443. Milgrom H, Stoll HL, Crissey JT. Dyskeratosis congenita. A case with new features. Arch Dermatol 1964; 89: 345–349.

444. Garb J. Dyskeratosis congenita with pigmentation, dystrophia unguium, and leukoplakia oris. Arch Dermatol 1958; 77: 704–712.

445. Sorrow JM, Hitch JM. Dyskeratosis congenita. First report of its occurrence in a female and a review of the literature. Arch Dermatol 1963; 88: 340–347.

446. Tchou P-K, Kohn T. Dyskeratosis congenita: An autosomal dominant disorder. J Am Acad Dermatol 1982; 6: 1034–1039.

447. Costello MJ, Buncke CM. Dyskeratosis congenita. Arch Dermatol 1956; 73: 123–132.

448. Aguilar-Martinez A, Lautre-Ecenarro MJ, Urbina-Gonzalez F et al. Cytogenetic abnormalities in dyskeratosis congenita — report of five cases. Clin Exp Dermatol 1988; 13: 100–104.

David Weedon

The psoriasiform reaction pattern

INTRODUCTION

The psoriasiform reaction pattern is defined morphologically as the presence of epidermal hyperplasia with elongation of the rete ridges in a regular manner. This definition encompasses a heterogeneous group of dermatological conditions. This morphological concept is much broader than the pathogenetic one outlined by Pinkus and Mehregan.[1] They considered the principal features of the psoriasiform tissue reaction to be the formation of a suprapapillary exudate with parakeratosis, secondary to the intermittent release of serum and leucocytes from dilated blood vessels in the papillary dermis (the so-called 'squirting papilla').

The increased mitotic activity of the epidermis which results in the elongated rete ridges and the psoriasiform epidermal hyperplasia is presumed to be secondary to the release of various mediators from the dilated vessels in the papillary dermis in psoriasis. These aspects are discussed in further detail below. The epidermal hyperplasia in lichen simplex chronicus may be related to chronic rubbing and irritation, while in Bowen's disease there is increased mitotic activity of the component cells. In many of the conditions listed the exact pathogenesis of the psoriasiform hyperplasia remains to be elucidated.

Psoriasis is the prototype of the psoriasiform reaction pattern, but it should be noted that early lesions of psoriasis and pustular psoriasis show no epidermal hyperplasia, although there is evidence of a 'squirting papilla' in the form of dilated vessels and exocytosis of inflammatory cells with neutrophils collecting in the overlying para-keratotic scale.

The major psoriasiform dermatoses — pso-riasis, pustular psoriasis, Reiter's syndrome, pity-riasis rubra pilaris, parapsoriasis and its variants and lichen simplex chronicus — will be con-sidered first.[2] The other dermatoses listed as causes of the psoriasiform reaction pattern have been discussed in detail in other chapters. They are included again here for completeness, with a brief outline of the features which distinguish them from the other psoriasiform dermatoses.

MAJOR PSORIASIFORM DERMATOSES

This group of dermatoses is characterized, as a rule, by regular epidermal hyperplasia, although in the early stages such features are usually absent. Psoriasis, which is the prototype for this tissue reaction, will be considered first.

PSORIASIS

Psoriasis (psoriasis vulgaris) is a chronic, relap-sing, papulosquamous dermatitis characterized by abnormal hyperproliferation of the epi-dermis.[2] It affects approximately 2% of the population and involves all racial groups, although it is rare in South American Indians.[3] There is a genetic proclivity to psoriasis, but no precise mode of inheritance is clear.[4] Con-cordance in monozygotic twins exceeds 70%.[4] Psoriasis is associated with HLA-CW6,[5] B13 and B17.[4]

Psoriasis typically consists of well circum-scribed erythematous patches with a silvery white scale (plaque form). Characteristic bleeding points develop when the scale is removed (Auspitz's sign).[6] Pruritus is sometimes present.[7] There is a predilection for the extensor surfaces of the extremities including the elbows and knees, and also the sacral region, scalp and nails.[8,9] The lips are not commonly involved,[10] and oral lesions in the form of whitish areas on the mucosa are quite rare.[11] Lesions may develop at sites of trauma.

In 5% or more of psoriatics, a seronegative polyarthritis develops.[3] Psoriasis has also been reported in association with vitiligo,[12] gout,[13] ankylosing spondylitis and inflammatory bowel disease.[14] Its association with bullous pemphi-goid and other bullous diseases,[15] perforating fol-liculitis,[16] lupus erythematosus,[17] epidermal naevi and surgical scars[18] and with AIDS[19] is probably a chance occurrence.

The mean age of onset of psoriasis is approxi-mately 25 years, although it also develops spo-radically in older persons, in whom it tends to have a milder course.[4,20] In Scandinavia, the disease commences in childhood in a high proportion of cases.[21] Congenital onset is a rare occurrence.[22] A family history of psoriasis and an association with HLA-CW6 are often present in those with early onset.[23,24] Psoriasis usually runs a chronic course, although spontaneous or treatment-induced remissions may occur.

Clinical variants. Several clinical variants of psoriasis have been recognized. *Guttate psoriasis* consists of 1–5 mm erythematous papules, which eventually develop a fine scale. It may be pre-ceded by a streptococcal pharyngitis.[25] There is a predilection for the trunk, and it is more com-mon in children.[26] Clearing may occur sponta-neously in weeks or months. Psoriasis begins as the guttate form in 15% or more of cases.[24] *Erythrodermic psoriasis* develops in approximately 2% of psoriatics and it accounts for 20% or more of erythrodermas.[27] It is a severe form with a high morbidity and an unpredictable course. Erythrodermic psoriasis may be precipitated by administration of systemic steroids, by the excess use of topical steroids or by a preceding illness; it may develop as a complication of photo-therapy.[27] *Sebopsoriasis* consists of yellowish-red, less well marginated lesions often distributed in seborrhoeic regions of the body.[28] Rare clinical variants include a naevoid form,[29] follicular psoriasis,[30] psoriasis spinulosa,[26,31] and linear psoriasis, although the occurrence of a linear form of psoriasis is not accepted by some authorities (see p. 731). Psoriasiform napkin dermatitis may also be a variant of psoriasis.[32] Pustular psoriasis is regarded as a discrete entity (see p. 78).

Trigger factors. Specific factors may trigger the onset or exacerbation of psoriasis. Trauma, infections[33] and drugs are accepted triggers, while the roles of climate, hormonal factors and stress are sometimes disputed.[4,34] The development of lesions in response to trauma (Koebner reaction) is present in approximately one-third of cases.[35] The role of infections has already been mentioned as a trigger factor in guttate psoriasis.[25] Various drugs may precipitate or exacerbate psoriasis, particularly lithium;[36,37] other drugs include quinidine,[38] clonidine, iodine, indomethacin,[38] various beta-blocker drugs,[39,40] terfenadine,[41] isotretinoin, interleukin[42] antimalarials and, rarely, the non-steroidal anti-inflammatory drugs. A psoriasiform eruption has been reported as a complication of several beta-blocker drugs and of the oral hypoglycaemic agent glibenclamide.[42a] The reactions caused by some of the beta-blocker drugs have a lichenoid histology despite their clinical appearance.

Pathogenesis of psoriasis

Psoriasis is a complex disease in which numerous abnormal findings have been reported.[43,44] Many of these changes, such as the increased epidermal proliferation, the dilatation of blood vessels in the papillary dermis,[45,46] and the increased neutrophil chemotaxis,[47] are probably secondary and tertiary events in the pathogenetic cascade.[48] The primary alteration in psoriasis is not known, although it is currently thought to involve either the immune system[49] or the signal-transducing system of epidermal keratinocytes.[48]

Many hormones and growth factors induce transmembrane signalling by activation of phospholipase C,[50] a substance which is increased in the epidermis in psoriasis. Furthermore, epidermal growth factor receptors, which are usually confined to the basal layer of the epidermis, are present in the suprabasal layers in psoriasis.[48] Abnormalities in cell surface glycoconjugates have also been found and these may have increased affinity for various immune mediators.[51]

Many immunological disturbances have been described in psoriasis, although it is acknowledged that some of these are of doubtful pathogenetic relevance.[49,52] The most important immunological findings are thought to be the presence of HLA-DR-positive keratinocytes in the epidermis, and the presence of activated T cells in the dermis.[53] These latter cells, which are predominantly of the CD4 phenotype, could possibly lead to the release of mediators of inflammation, some of which might also act as stimulators of epidermal growth.[53] Lymphocytes appear to aggregate in the dermis as a consequence of their selective adherence to the specialized endothelial cells that line the post-capillary venules in the papillary dermis of psoriatic lesions.[53a] The finding of immunoreactants in the stratum corneum[54–58] and dermis,[59,60] and the presence of circulating immune complexes in serum[43] are not thought to be of major pathogenetic significance.[53]

Polyamines[61] and by-products of arachidonic acid metabolism, especially prostaglandins and leucotrienes, are important mediators of inflammation, as well as regulators of epidermal growth.[48,62] Both leucotriene B_4 and interleukin 1 can cause a proliferation of keratinocytes.[53] Furthermore, interleukin 1 is a major chemotactic agent with possibly more activity than the various complement factors.[53] Exacerbations of psoriasis are preceded by a rapid increase in neutrophil chemotaxis.[63–65]

Epidermal hyperproliferation is one of the most important consequences of the pathogenetic events already discussed. There is an increase in the number of germinative cells and mitotic figures.[66] It has been estimated that there is a 12-fold increase in the number of basal and suprabasal keratinocytes in cell cycling.[48] There is also an alteration in the turnover time for the epidermis: three to four days in psoriasis compared with the usual 13 days in normal skin.[34] These changes in epidermal kinetics are accompanied by changes in the differentiation of the cells,[67] with alterations in the composition of keratin polypeptides, increased proteolytic activity and alterations in cell-surface glycoconjugates, as mentioned earlier.[68,69]

In summary, the key pathogenetic features in psoriasis appear to be the presence of an activated cellular immune system, an increase in polyamines and eiconasoids (arachidonic acid metabolites), abnormalities in the transmembranous signal-transducing system (including the presence of increased phospholipase C and the retention of growth factor receptors in suprabasal keratinocytes), and alterations in surface glycoproteins.[53,69] Alterations in epidermal kinetics are secondary to these other events.

Histopathology[2,70–73]

Psoriasis is a dynamic process, and consequently the histopathological picture varies during the evolution and subsequent resolution of individual lesions. The earliest changes, seen in lesions of less than 24 hours' duration, consist of dilatation and congestion of vessels in the papillary dermis and a mild, perivascular, lymphocytic infiltrate, with some adjacent oedema. There is also some exocytosis of lymphocytes into the epidermis overlying the vessels, and this is usually associated with mild spongiosis. The epidermis is otherwise normal. This is soon followed by the formation of mounds of parakeratosis, with exocytosis of

neutrophils through the epidermis to reach the summits of these parakeratotic foci (Fig. 4.1).[55,74,75] There is often overlying orthokeratosis of normal basket-weave type and loss of the underlying granular layer.[75] At this papular stage, increased mitotic activity can be seen in the basal layer of the epidermis associated with a modest amount of psoriasiform acanthosis (Fig. 4.2). Keratinocytes in the upper epidermis show some cytoplasmic pallor. Vessels in the papillary dermis are still dilated and somewhat tortuous and their lumen may contain neutrophils. Very few neutrophils are ever present in the perivascular infiltrate: this consists mainly of lymphocytes,

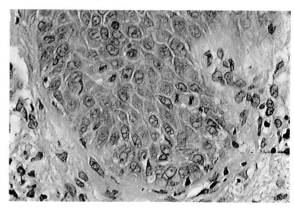

Fig. 4.2   Psoriasis. Mitoses are evident in keratinocytes within the epidermis.
Haematoxylin — eosin

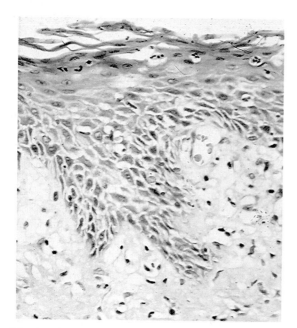

Fig. 4.1   Psoriasis. An early lesion with a few neutrophils collecting in the stratum corneum, some psoriasiform acanthosis and a dilated vessel in a dermal papilla.
Haematoxylin — eosin

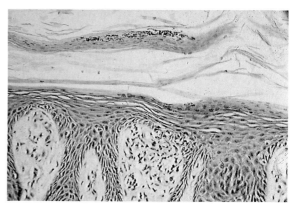

Fig. 4.3   Psoriasis. There is psoriasiform hyperplasia of the epidermis and neutrophils in the upper layers of the overlying parakeratotic scale.
Haematoxylin — eosin

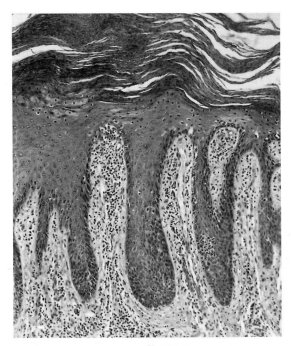

Fig. 4.4 Psoriasis. Confluent parakeratosis overlies an epidermis showing psoriasiform hyperplasia.
Haematoxylin — eosin

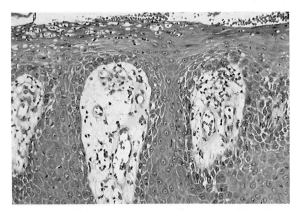

Fig. 4.5 Psoriasis. The dilated vessels in the papillary dermis are well shown. The suprapapillary epidermis ('plate') is relatively thin.
Haematoxylin — eosin

Langerhans cells and indeterminate cells.[76] A few extravasated erythrocytes may also be present. These changes can also be seen in guttate psoriasis although the epidermal hyperplasia is usually mild in this variant of psoriasis.[2]

In early plaques of psoriasis, and in 'hot spots' of more established plaques,[77] there are mounds of parakeratosis containing neutrophils, the neutrophils usually migrating to the upper layers (summits) of these mounds (Fig. 4.3). With time, confluent parakeratosis develops (Fig. 4.4). Several layers of parakeratosis containing neutrophils, with intervening layers of orthokeratosis, are sometimes present. While intracorneal collections of neutrophils (Munro microabscesses) are common, similar collections in the spinous layer (spongiform pustules of Kogoj) are less so. They are also much smaller than in pustular psoriasis. These pustules contain lymphocytes in addition to neutrophils. The epidermis now shows psoriasiform (regular) hyperplasia, with relatively thin suprapapillary plates overlying the dilated vessels of the papillary dermis (Fig. 4.5). A few mononuclear cells are usually present

in the lower layers of the suprapapillary epidermis. The dermal inflammatory cell infiltrate is usually a little heavier than in earlier lesions. It includes activated T lymphocytes,[78] fewer Langerhans cells than in earlier lesions and very occasional neutrophils.[76] Plasma cells and eosinophils are usually absent,[72] but eosinophil cationic protein has been identified, particularly in the upper third of the epidermis in psoriasis.[78a]

With time, there may be club-shaped thickening of the lower rete pegs with coalescence of these in some areas (Fig. 4.6).[71,72] Later lesions show orthokeratosis, an intact granular layer and some thickening of the suprapapillary plates. Exocytosis of inflammatory cells is usually mild. Differentiation of such lesions from lichen simplex chronicus may be difficult, although in the latter condition the suprapapillary plates and granular layer are usually more prominent and there may be vertically oriented collagen bundles in the papillary dermis (see p.84).[2] If psoriatic plaques are rubbed or scratched, the histopathological features of the underlying psoriasis may be obscured by these superimposed changes.

In resolving or treated plaques of psoriasis there is a progressive diminution in the inflammatory infiltrate, a reduction in the amount of epidermal hyperplasia and restoration of the granular layer.[70] Vessels in the papillary dermis are still dilated, although by now there is an

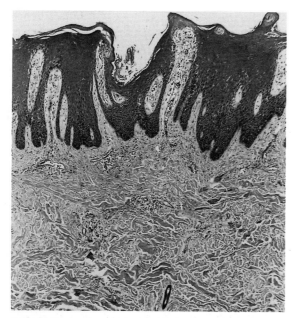

Fig. 4.6   Psoriasis. There is some coalescence of the tips of the rete pegs.
Haematoxylin — eosin

increase in fibroblasts in this region with mild fibrosis.[70] Only after 10–14 weeks of treatment do the histological appearances return to normal.[79]

Minor changes which have been reported in psoriasis of the scalp include mild sebaceous gland atrophy, a decrease in hair follicle size and thinner hair shafts.[80] Munro microabscesses are said to be uncommon in this region.[72] Another regional variation is the lessened epidermal hyperplasia in psoriasis of the penis and vulva.[72]

In *erythrodermic psoriasis*, the appearances may resemble those described in early lesions of psoriasis, a reflection of the early medical intervention that usually occurs in this condition. Dilatation of superficial vessels is usually quite prominent. Sometimes the histological changes do not resemble those of psoriasis at all.

In *follicular psoriasis*, there is follicular plugging with marked parakeratosis in the mid-zone of the ostium.[30] The dermal inflammatory infiltrate is both perivascular and perifollicular.

Skin tumours have rarely developed at sites treated with PUVA therapy,[81,82] although the use of coal tar does not produce any appreciable increase in skin cancers.[83] Variants of seborrhoeic keratosis have also been reported in

psoriatic patients receiving treatment with ultraviolet radiation.[83a] Of relevance is the controversy whether patients with psoriasis have an inherently low risk of developing skin cancer,[84] although recent studies suggest that this is not so.[85,86] Another rare complication of treatment is cutaneous ulceration, which has been reported following methotrexate therapy.[87]

Differential diagnosis. The histopathological differentiation of psoriasis from *chronic eczematous dermatitis*, particularly seborrhoeic dermatitis, is sometimes difficult. The presence of prominent spongiosis involving the rete ridges rules out psoriasis, while the presence of a leucocytic exudate, other than in a folliculocentric distribution, is quite uncommon in seborrhoeic dermatitis.[1] In seborrhoeic dermatitis there is often less epidermal hyperplasia than in psoriasis.

The features that distinguish psoriasis from *lichen simplex chronicus* have been discussed above. Spongiosis is sometimes present in the rete ridges in the latter condition if it is superimposed on an eczematous process.

In *pityriasis rubra pilaris*, there is mild to moderate psoriasiform hyperplasia, parakeratotic lipping of follicles and, in some lesions, alternating zones of orthokeratosis and parakeratosis in both horizontal and vertical directions.

Pustular psoriasis has more prominent spongiform pustulation than psoriasis vulgaris, particularly at the shoulders of the lesions.

Electron microscopy.[79] There are numerous cytoplasmic organelles in the keratinocytes, reflecting their hyperactivity. These are decreased with treatment.[88] Tonofilaments and desmosomes are reduced in number and size and there is also a reduction in the number of keratohyaline granules.[79] Vessels in the papillary dermis are dilated with abundant fenestrations.[79] Neutrophils are said to be polar in shape with ruffled cell membranes.[89,90]

PUSTULAR PSORIASIS

Pustular psoriasis is a rare, acute form of psoriasis characterized by the widespread eruption of numerous sterile pustules on an erythematous base, and associated with constitutional symptoms.[91] Skin tenderness, a neutrophil leucocytosis and an absolute lymphopenia[92] may precede the onset of the pustules. These may continue to develop in waves for several weeks or longer before remitting. Arthritis,[93] generalized erythroderma,[93] hypocalcaemia[94] and lesions of the mucous membranes, including fissured tongue and benign migratory glossitis (geographical tongue) may develop in the course of the disease.[95–98] Amyloidosis is an extremely rare complication.[99]

Several clinical variants of pustular psoriasis are recognized.[91,93] The *von Zumbusch type* is the most common variant. It has an explosive onset and a mortality as high as 30% in some of the earlier series. *Impetigo herpetiformis* is a controversial entity defined by some on the basis of flexural involvement with centripetal spread of the pustules,[100] and by others as a variant of pustular psoriasis occurring in pregnancy.[101,102] Onset in pregnancy is usually in the third trimester, although it develops earlier in subsequent pregnancies.[103–105] It usually remits post partum, but may flare with the use of oral contraceptives.[106] Fetal mortality is high as a consequence of placental insufficiency.[106] A subset related to hypoparathyroidism with hypocalcaemia is sometimes included in impetigo herpetiformis.[107] The *acral variant* arises in a setting of acrodermatitis continua which is a localized pustular eruption of one or more digits with displacement and dystrophy of the nails.[91,108] The development of generalized pustular psoriasis in acrodermatitis continua has a bad prognosis.[91,108] Other variants include an *exanthematic form*,[91,108] an *annular variant*[109–111] with some resemblance to subcorneal pustular dermatosis, and a *localized form* which consists of pustular psoriasis developing in pre-existing plaques of psoriasis.[91,93]

Generalized pustular psoriasis may develop in three main clinical settings.[91] In the first group there is a long history of psoriasis of early onset. In these cases the pustular psoriasis is often precipitated by some external provocative agent (see below). In the second group, there is preceding psoriasis of atypical form, in which the onset was relatively late in life. Precipitating factors are not usually present. In the third group, pustular pso-

riasis arises without pre-existing psoriasis. Pustular psoriasis may rarely develop as a consequence of persistent pustulosis of the palms and soles. Familial cases of pustular psoriasis[112,113] and onset in childhood have also been reported.[112–114]

Numerous factors have been implicated in precipitating pustular psoriasis.[115] These include infections, sunlight, alcohol, malignancy, metabolic and endocrine factors, emotional stress and drugs. The drugs include lithium,[116] iodides, non-steroidal anti-inflammatory agents, including phenylbutazone,[117] beta blockers,[118] penicillin and related drugs,[115] procaine, sulphonamides, morphine, hydroxychloroquine, progesterone[119] and nystatin. The withdrawal of steroids is a common precipitating factor which may be included in this category.[120]

One of the most striking features of pustular psoriasis is the enhanced chemotaxis of neutrophils, which is even more marked than in psoriasis.[121,122] The chemotactic factors in the affected areas of skin include leucotrienes, complement products and cathepsin 1.[123]

Histopathology[124,125]

The diagnostic feature is the presence of intraepidermal pustules at various stages of development (Fig. 4.7). The epidermis is usually only slightly acanthotic, while psoriasiform hyperplasia is seen only in older and persistent lesions (Fig. 4.8). Mitoses are usually present within the epidermis. Neutrophils migrate from dilated vessels in the papillary dermis into the epidermis. They aggregate beneath the stratum corneum and in the upper malpighian layer between degenerate and thinned keratinocytes to form the so-called spongiform pustules of Kogoj (Fig. 4.9).[126] The subcorneal pustules have a thin roof of stratum corneum. In later lesions these are replaced by scale crusts with collections of neutrophils trapped between parakeratotic layers. A few eosinophils may be present in the infiltrate.

The blood vessels in the papillary dermis are usually dilated and there is a perivascular infiltrate of lymphocytes and a few neutrophils. Large mononuclear cells were noted in the pustules and in the dermis in one report of impetigo herpetiformis.[127] They were thought to be specific for

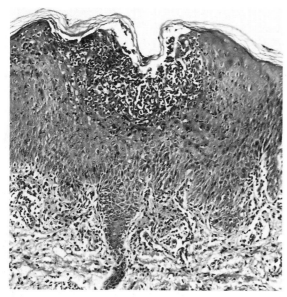

Fig. 4.7   Early pustular psoriasis. There is a heavy infiltrate of neutrophils in the upper layers of the epidermis near an acrosyringium.
Haematoxylin — eosin

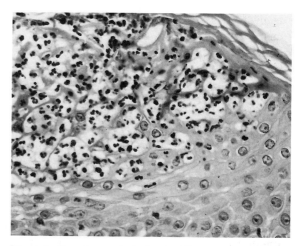

Fig. 4.9   Pustular psoriasis. A spongiform pustule of Kogoj is shown.
Haematoxylin — eosin

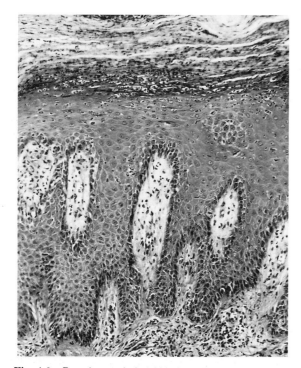

Fig. 4.8   Pustular psoriasis (old lesion). There is pronounced psoriasiform hyperplasia of the epidermis and mild spongiform pustulation in the upper layers.
Haematoxylin — eosin

this variant of pustular psoriasis, although they were specifically excluded in a subsequent report of this condition.[127]

Electron microscopy.[123] Multipolypoid herniations of basal keratinocytes have been described protruding into the dermis through large gaps in the basal lamina. Neutrophil proteases are probably responsible for this change. In another study there were gaps between the endothelial cells of dermal blood vessels.[128]

REITER'S SYNDROME

Reiter's syndrome is usually defined as the triad of non-gonococcal urethritis, ocular inflammation and arthritis.[129] The presence of mucocutaneous lesions is sometimes included as a fourth feature.[130] Reiter's syndrome occurs in approximately 30% of patients with reactive arthritis, which in turn develops in 1–3% of patients with sexually acquired, non-gonococcal infections of the genital tract.[129,131] Reiter's syndrome has also been associated with certain bacterial gut infections including those due to *Shigella flexneri*, *Yersinia enterocolitica*[132] and, rarely, *Campylobacter jejuni*.[133] The genital infectious agent which is usually incriminated is *Chlamydia trachomatosis*, but *Ureaplasma urealyticum* and species of *Mycoplasma* have also been isolated.[129,133] Recently, chlamydial elementary bodies have been detected by immunofluorescence and monoclonal antibodies in the synovium of patients with reactive arthritis, which to date has always been sterile by conventional cultures.[134]

There is genetic susceptibility to the development of reactive arthritis and Reiter's syndrome, and this is manifest by the presence of the histocompatibility antigen HLA-B27.[132,135] Other clinical features of Reiter's syndrome include a marked preponderance in males, a mean age of onset in the third decade of life, and a variable, often relapsing, course.[135–137] The arthritis most often involves the knees and ankles.

The mucocutaneous lesions, already alluded to, include a circinate balanitis with perimeatal erosions and mucosal ulcers.[138,139] In 10–30% of cases there are crusted erythematous papules and plaques with a predilection for the soles of the feet, genitalia, perineum, buttocks, scalp and extensor surfaces of the extremities.[137,140–142] Some lesions may be frankly pustular, resembling pustular psoriasis. These cutaneous lesions are known by the name keratoderma blennorrhagica. They usually heal after several weeks, without scarring.[141]

Histopathology

In most biopsies, the cutaneous lesions of Reiter's syndrome are indistinguishable from pustular psoriasis.[140] Accordingly, there is psoriasiform epidermal hyperplasia with a thick horny layer (Fig. 4.10). This is most prominent in lesions on the palms and soles and least prominent in penile and buccal lesions. Spongiform pustulation with exocytosis of neutrophils is another conspicuous feature.[143] A variable inflammatory cell infiltrate, usually including a few neutrophils, is present in the upper dermis.[144]

Various histological features have been claimed to be more suggestive of Reiter's syndrome than pustular psoriasis.[145] These include a thicker horny layer, larger spongiform pustules, eczematous changes, a thicker suprapapillary plate of epidermis, the presence of neutrophils in the dermis and the absence of clubbing of the

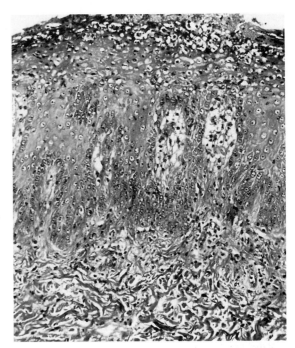

Fig. 4.10   Reiter's disease. The appearances may be indistinguishable from pustular psoriasis. Haematoxylin — eosin

rete ridges. The horny layer is sometimes more loosely attached than in pustular psoriasis, leading to its partial detachment during processing of the specimen. These various features are usually not sufficiently different from the findings in pustular psoriasis to allow a confident distinction to be made between the two conditions on biopsy material.

PITYRIASIS RUBRA PILARIS

Pityriasis rubra pilaris is a rare, erythematosquamous dermatosis of unknown aetiology characterized by small follicular papules with a central keratin plug, perifollicular erythema with a tendency to become confluent but with islands of sparing, palmoplantar hyperkeratosis, often with oedema, and pityriasis capitis.[146–149] The condition often begins with a seborrhoeic dermatitis-like rash on the face or scalp which rapidly spreads downwards.[150] In other patients, particularly juveniles, the disease starts on the lower half of the body.[151] Some patients may become erythrodermic.[152] Cases with localized lesions, restricted often to the elbows and knees, occur. Nail changes,[146,153] alopecia[147,148] and, rarely, multiple seborrhoeic keratoses may occur in patients with pityriasis rubra pilaris.[154] The age of onset and clinical course are variable.[155,156] Complete remission occurs within 6 months to 2 years in about 50% of cases.[155]

Although there is some resemblance to vitamin A deficiency (phrynoderma), serum vitamin A levels are normal.[152] Reduced levels of retinol-binding protein (the specific carrier of vitamin A) have been reported,[157] but the results of this work have not been confirmed.[158,159] Epidermal cell kinetics show an increased rate of cell proliferation.[160,161]

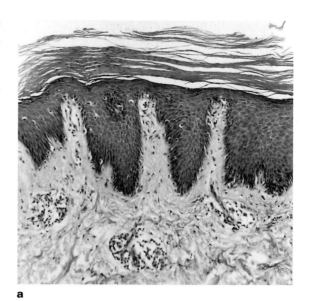

a

Histopathology[2,152,162]

The changes are most marked when erythema is greatest, and least impressive in biopsies of follicular papules.[149] There is diffuse orthokeratosis with spotted parakeratosis which also forms a collarette around the follicular ostia (Figs 4.11a,b). Parakeratosis is not prominent in early lesions. These changes may be described in another way — alternating orthokeratosis and parakeratosis in both vertical and horizontal directions (Fig. 4.12).[162] However, many cases will be missed if this criterion is too rigidly applied. There is also acanthosis: this is never as regular as that seen in psoriasis. There are broad rete ridges and thick suprapapillary plates. Hypergranulosis is often prominent and this may be focal or confluent.[162] An unusual perinuclear vacuolization is sometimes seen in cells in the malpighian layer and there may be some vacuolar change involving the pilary outer root sheath. There is a mild superficial perivascular and perifollicular lymphocytic infiltrate in the dermis. A rare histological finding is the presence of focal acantholytic dyskeratosis in the lesions of pityriasis rubra pilaris.[163]

In contrast to pityriasis rubra pilaris, vitamin A deficiency shows no focal parakeratosis, irregular acanthosis or dermal inflammatory infiltrate.[147]

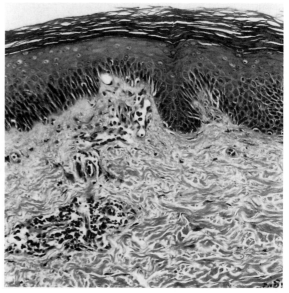

b

Fig. 4.11   Pityriasis rubra pilaris; **(a)**, as it should be, with psoriasiform hyperplasia and overlying 'geometric' parakeratosis; **(b)**, as it sometimes is, with atypical features. I have missed more cases of this disease (on the initial biopsy) than any other.
Haematoxylin — eosin

Electron microscopy. There are a decrease in tonofilaments and desmosomes, a large number of keratinosomes, and lipid-like vacuoles in the

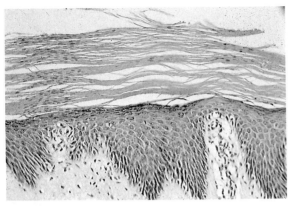

Fig. 4.12 Pityriasis rubra pilaris. There is alternating orthokeratosis and parakeratosis in both a horizontal and a vertical direction.
Haematoxylin — eosin

parakeratotic areas.[164] The basal lamina is focally split, containing gaps.[164]

PARAPSORIASIS

The term 'parapsoriasis', as originally introduced, referred to a heterogeneous group of asymptomatic, scaly dermatoses with some clinical resemblance to psoriasis.[165–167] These conditions were further characterized by chronicity and resistance to therapy. Three distinct entities are now recognized as having been included in the original concept of 'parapsoriasis' — pityriasis lichenoides, chronic superficial dermatitis (small plaque parapsoriasis, digitate dermatosis) and large plaque parapsoriasis (atrophic parapsoriasis, retiform parapsoriasis, patch stage mycosis fungoides).[166]

Confusion has arisen because of the retention of the term 'parapsoriasis' for two distinct conditions. In the United States, the term parapsoriasis en plaque is usually used to refer to the entity that in the United Kingdom is called chronic superficial dermatitis.[168] The term 'parapsoriasis' is also used for a condition with large plaques, which in 10–30% of cases progresses to a frank T-cell lymphoma of the skin.[169] Because of this potential progression, there has been a tendency in recent years to disparage the diagnosis of large plaque

parapsoriasis and to substitute terms such as 'premycosis fungoides' and 'patch stage mycosis fungoides'.[167,169] Our inability to identify from sections stained with haematoxylin and eosin those cases that will progress to cutaneous lymphoma does not seem sufficient justification for abandoning the concept of large plaque parapsoriasis, particularly when the use of nuclear DNA studies to select such cases is still at a comparatively early stage.

Brief mention will be made of the three entities included in the original concept of parapsoriasis.

Pityriasis lichenoides shows features of both chronic lymphocytic vasculitis and the lichenoid tissue reaction (see p. 236). It should no longer be considered as a variant of parapsoriasis.

Chronic superficial dermatitis (small plaque parapsoriasis) resembles a 'mild eczema', and is therefore discussed in detail on page 115, as part of the spongiotic tissue reaction. The spongiosis is often quite mild, and in chronic lesions may be absent. In these circumstances, the epidermal acanthosis may assume psoriasiform proportions, hence its mention here also. It differs from psoriasis by the absence of dilated vessels in the papillary dermis and the absence of neutrophil exocytosis. Furthermore, chronic superficial dermatitis lacks a thin suprapapillary plate and there is a paucity of mitoses in the keratinocytes (Fig. 4.13). Lymphocytes with a normal mature morphology are often found in the papillary dermis in chronic superficial dermatitis. This feature, combined with the regular acanthosis and focal parakeratosis, allows a diagnosis to be made in many cases with the scanning power of the light microscope.

Large plaque parapsoriasis, the third entity included originally as 'parapsoriasis', may also show features of psoriasiform epidermal hyperplasia, although in atrophic and poikilodermatous lesions the epidermis is thin, with loss of the rete ridge pattern. Basal vacuolar change and epidermotropism of lymphocytes are usually present. In lesions which progress to cutaneous T-cell lymphoma, atypical lymphoid cells eventually appear. Large plaque parapsoriasis is considered with other cutaneous lymphoid infiltrates on page 1032.

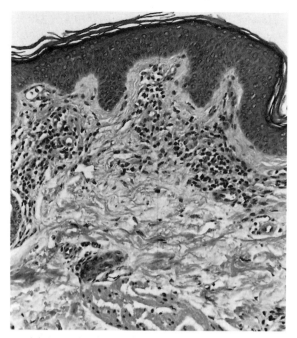

Fig. 4.13 Chronic superficial dermatitis with mild psoriasiform hyperplasia, thick suprapapillary 'plates' of epidermis and a mild, superficial lymphocytic infiltrate with some upward spread.
Haematoxylin — eosin

Finally, brief mention will be made of the term 'guttate parapsoriasis'. This term has been used in the past synonymously with both pityriasis lichenoides and chronic superficial dermatitis. It is best avoided.[167]

LICHEN SIMPLEX CHRONICUS

Lichen simplex chronicus ('circumscribed neurodermatitis') is an idiopathic disorder in which scaly, thickened plaques develop in response to persistent rubbing of pruritic sites.[170,171] There is a predilection for the nape of the neck, the ulnar border of the forearms, the wrists, the pretibial region, the dorsa of the feet and the perianal and genital region.[171,172] Atopic individuals are more prone than others to develop lichen simplex chronicus.[173]

Kinetic studies have shown epidermal cell proliferation similar to that seen in psoriasis although the transit time of the cells is not as fast.[172]

There is also an increase in mitochondrial enzymes in keratinocytes and an increase in the number of melanocytes in the basal layer.[174] Although these kinetic aspects are known, there is still no explanation for the pathogenesis of these plaques and the underlying pruritus, although it is apparent that self-induced trauma plays an important localizing role.[172]

Histopathology[171,175]

A thick layer of compact orthokeratosis (resembling that seen on normal palms and soles) is present, overlying hypergranulosis. Focal zones of parakeratosis are sometimes interspersed with the orthokeratosis, but there is not the confluent parakeratosis of psoriasis.[172] The epidermis shows psoriasiform hyperplasia with thicker rete ridges of less even length than in psoriasis (Fig. 4.14). Epidermal thickness and volume are

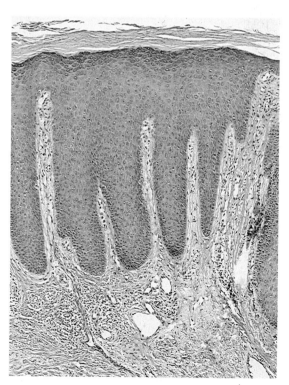

Fig. 4.14 Lichen simplex chronicus. Note the triad of psoriasiform epidermal hyperplasia, thick suprapapillary 'plates' and vertical orientation ('streaking') of collagen in the papillary dermis.
Haematoxylin — eosin

greater than in psoriasis.[172] Minimal papillomatosis is sometimes present in a few areas. Focal excoriation is another change that may be seen in lichen simplex chronicus.

There is marked thickening of the papillary dermis with bundles of collagen arranged in vertical streaks (Fig. 4.15).[175] Scattered inflammatory cells and some fibroblasts are usually present in this region of the dermis.

Regional variations occur in lichen simplex chronicus. Epidermal hyperplasia is usually quite mild in lesions on the lip, while vertical-streaked collagen is unusual in lesions on the scalp or in mucocutaneous regions such as the vulva and perianal area.[175]

Changes like those of lichen simplex chronicus may be superimposed on other dermatoses such as lichen planus (hypertrophic lichen planus), mycosis fungoides, actinic reticuloid and eczematous dermatitides including atopic dermatitis.[171,173] These changes are particularly prominent in some solar keratoses of the hands or forearms.

The term prurigo nodularis (see p. 732) is used for lesions with a nodular clinical appearance and prominent epidermal hyperplasia of pseudoepitheliomatous rather than psoriasiform type. At times, lesions with overlapping clinical and histopathological features of both lichen simplex chronicus and prurigo nodularis are found.

OTHER PSORIASIFORM DERMATOSES

This group of psoriasiform dermatoses has been arbitrarily separated from the so-called 'major psoriasiform dermatoses' because of their inclusion in various other chapters, on the basis of their aetiology or of other histopathological features.

SUBACUTE AND CHRONIC SPONGIOTIC DERMATITIDES

The various 'eczematous' dermatitides (allergic contact dermatitis, seborrhoeic dermatitis, nummular dermatitis and atopic dermatitis) may show prominent psoriasiform epidermal hyperplasia in their subacute and chronic stages.

Histopathology

In subacute lesions, spongiosis is usually sufficiently obvious to allow a correct diagnosis. In some chronic lesions, particularly if activity has been dampened by treatment prior to the taking of a biopsy, the spongiosis may be quite mild or even absent. The features which distinguish chronic seborrhoeic dermatitis from psoriasis have been discussed on page 78. In some cases of chronic atopic and nummular dermatitis the epidermal hyperplasia is not as regular and as even as that seen in psoriasis, although this is by no means invariable. The presence of eosinophils and plasma cells in the superficial dermis would

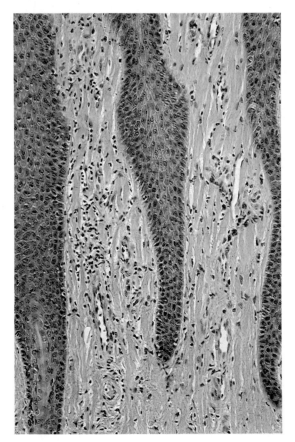

Fig. 4.15 Lichen simplex chronicus. The rete pegs are thinner than usual but the vertical 'streaking' of collagen in the papillary dermis is well developed.
Haematoxylin — eosin

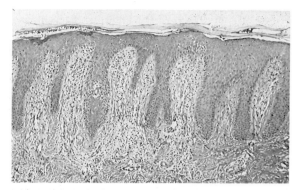

Fig. 4.16 Chronic allergic contact dermatitis with psoriasiform hyperplasia of the epidermis and small foci of spongiosis.
Haematoxylin — eosin

tend to exclude psoriasis. They may be found in any of the chronic spongiotic dermatitides that may simulate psoriasis histopathologically. The changes of lichen simplex chronicus may be superimposed on these chronic spongiotic dermatitides (Fig. 4.16).

ERYTHRODERMA

Erythroderma (exfoliative dermatitis) is a cutaneous reaction pattern characterized by erythema, oedema and scaling of all or most of the skin surface, often accompanied by pruritus (see p. 554). It may complicate a pre-existing dermatosis, follow the ingestion of a drug or be associated with an internal cancer or with cutaneous T-cell lymphoma.

Histopathology

The findings are variable and often non-specific. Psoriasiform hyperplasia, sometimes accompanied by mild spongiosis, may be present in cases of erythroderma not thought to be of psoriatic origin, while presumptive cases of erythrodermic psoriasis may show only non-specific changes in the epidermis. The difficulties encountered in an attempted histopathological diagnosis of erythroderma are mentioned on page 555.

MYCOSIS FUNGOIDES

Mycosis fungoides is a cutaneous T-cell lymphoma with three clinical stages — patch, plaque and tumour. Its varied clinical features are discussed on page 1033.

Histopathology

Psoriasiform hyperplasia of the epidermis is not uncommon in mycosis fungoides. It is usually of mild to moderate proportions. The presence of epidermotropism and variable cytological atypia of the lymphocytic infiltrate are features which distinguish this condition from other psoriasiform dermatoses (Fig. 4.17).

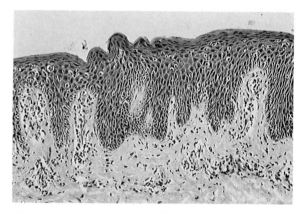

Fig. 4.17 Mycosis fungoides. There is psoriasiform hyperplasia of the epidermis and conspicuous epidermotropism of lymphocytes.
Haematoxylin — eosin

CHRONIC CANDIDOSIS AND DERMATOPHYTOSES

Psoriasiform epidermal hyperplasia may be present in lesions of chronic candidosis (see p. 646), and rarely in chronic dermatophyte infections, most notably in tinea imbricata.

Histopathology

The rete ridges are not unusually long in the psoriasiform hyperplasia of chronic candidosis. There are usually a few neutrophils and some serum in the overlying parakeratotic scale. Fungal elements, in the form of yeasts and pseudo-hyphae, may be sparse and difficult to find with the PAS stain. They are often more readily seen in methenamine silver preparations.

Hyphae and spores are usually abundant in the thick stratum corneum in tinea imbricata.

INFLAMMATORY LINEAR VERRUCOUS EPIDERMAL NAEVUS

The acronym ILVEN is often used in place of the more cumbersome inflammatory linear verrucous epidermal naevus. This condition is a variant of epidermal naevus which usually presents as a pruritic, linear eruption on the lower extremities (see p. 730). It must be distinguished from linear psoriasis.

Histopathology

The characteristic feature is the presence of alternating zones of orthokeratosis and parakeratosis in a horizontal direction, overlying a psoriasiform epidermis (Fig. 4.18). The zones of parakeratosis overlie areas of agranulosis. Focal mild spongiosis is often present as well.

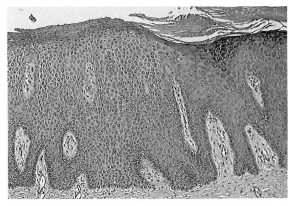

Fig. 4.18 Inflammatory linear verrucous epidermal naevus (ILVEN).   There are broad zones of parakeratosis alternating with orthokeratosis. The granular layer is absent beneath the parakeratotic zones.
Haematoxylin — eosin

NORWEGIAN SCABIES

Norwegian (crusted) scabies is a rare form of scabies which is usually found in the mentally and physically debilitated; it also occurs in immunosuppressed individuals (see p. 720). There are widespread crusted and secondarily infected hyperkeratotic lesions.

Histopathology

Overlying the psoriasiform epidermis there is a very thick layer of orthokeratosis and parakeratosis containing numerous scabies mites at all stages of development. The appearances are characteristic.

BOWEN'S DISEASE

There is a variant of Bowen's disease in which the epidermis shows psoriasiform hyperplasia (see p. 742). It has no distinguishing clinical features.

Histopathology

There is psoriasiform hyperplasia with a thick suprapapillary plate. Atypical keratinocytes usually involve the full thickness of the epidermis; sometimes there is sparing of the basal layer and the acrosyringium. Mitoses and dyskeratotic cells are usually present. Uncommonly, the psoriasiform variant of Bowen's disease is composed of pale pagetoid cells.

CLEAR CELL ACANTHOMA

The clear (pale) cell acanthoma presents as a papulonodular lesion, usually on the lower parts of the legs (see p. 737).

Histopathology

The characteristic feature is the presence of a well demarcated area of psoriasiform epidermal hyperplasia in which the cells have palely staining cytoplasm. Exocytosis of inflammatory cells may also be present. The pale keratinocytes contain abundant glycogen.

LAMELLAR ICHTHYOSIS

This is a rare, severe, autosomal recessive form of ichthyosis (see p. 268). It is usually manifest at birth.

Histopathology

There is prominent orthokeratosis and focal parakeratosis overlying a normal or thickened granular layer. Psoriasiform epidermal hyperplasia is sometimes present, although usually the epidermis shows only moderate acanthosis.

PITYRIASIS ROSEA

The 'herald patch' of pityriasis rosea may show the psoriasiform tissue reaction (see p. 111).

Histopathology

There is usually acanthosis and only mild psoriasiform hyperplasia. Small 'Pautrier-simulants', composed of inflammatory cells in a spongiotic focus, are often seen. There is usually focal parakeratosis overlying the epidermis.

PELLAGRA

Pellagra is caused by an inadequate amount of niacin (nicotinic acid) in the tissues. Skin lesions include a scaly erythematous rash in sun-exposed areas, sometimes with blistering, followed by hyperpigmentation and epithelial desquamation (see p. 519).

Histopathology

The findings are not usually diagnostic. Sometimes there is psoriasiform acanthosis with pallor of the upper epidermis and overlying orthokeratosis and focal parakeratosis. The psoriasiform acanthosis is more common in mixed nutritional deficiency states.

ACRODERMATITIS ENTEROPATHICA

Acrodermatitis enteropathica, a rare disorder resulting from zinc deficiency, presents with peri-orificial and acral lesions which may be eczematous, vesiculobullous, pustular or an admixture of these patterns (see p. 526).

Histopathology

In established lesions there is confluent parakeratosis overlying psoriasiform epidermal hyperplasia. The upper layers of the epidermis show a characteristic pallor, and sometimes there is focal necrosis or subcorneal clefting. The epidermal pallor disappears in late lesions.

GLUCAGONOMA SYNDROME

Necrolytic migratory erythema is the term used for the cutaneous lesions of the glucagonoma syndrome. This syndrome in most cases is a manifestation of a glucagon-secreting islet cell tumour of the pancreas (see p. 526).

Histopathology

The changes may resemble those seen in acrodermatitis enteropathica with psoriasiform hyperplasia, upper epidermal pallor, and overlying confluent parakeratosis. At other times there is focal or confluent necrosis of the upper epidermis with a preceding phase of pale, vacuolated keratinocytes. Subcorneal or intra-epidermal clefting and pustulation may develop. Psoriasiform epidermal hyperplasia of any significant degree is present in only a minority of cases.

SECONDARY SYPHILIS

The great imitator, syphilis, in the secondary

Table 4.1 Histopathological features of the various psoriasiform diseases

Disease	Histopathological features
Psoriasis	Progressive psoriasiform epidermal hyperplasia, initially mild; mitoses in basal keratinocytes; dilated vessels in dermal papillae; parakeratosis, initially focal and containing neutrophils, later confluent with few neutrophils; thinning of the suprapapillary epidermis.
Pustular psoriasis	Spongiform pustulation overshadows epidermal hyperplasia, except in lesions of some duration when both are present.
Reiter's syndrome	Closely resembles pustular psoriasis; the overlying, thick scale crust often detaches during processing.
Pityriasis rubra pilaris	Alternating orthokeratosis and parakeratosis, vertically and horizontally; follicular plugging with parafollicular (lipping) parakeratosis; mild to moderate epidermal hyperplasia; no neutrophil exocytosis.
Parapsoriasis	Variable epidermal hyperplasia; the superficial perivascular or band-like infiltrate involves the papillary dermis ('spills upwards'); some exocytosis/epidermotropism.
Lichen simplex chronicus	Conspicuous psoriasiform hyperplasia, sometimes irregular; prominent granular layer with patchy parakeratosis; thick suprapapillary epidermal plates; thick collagen in vertical streaks in papillary dermis; variable inflammatory infiltrate and plump fibroblasts.
Chronic spongiotic dermatitides	Progressive psoriasiform hyperplasia, usually with diminishing spongiosis eventually merging with picture of lichen simplex chronicus; chronic nummular lesions 'untidy' with mild exocytosis; eosinophils may be present in nummular and allergic contact lesions; chronic seborrhoeic dermatitis may mimic psoriasis but no neutrophils, less hyperplasia and sometimes perifollicular parakeratosis.
Erythroderma	Variable psoriasiform hyperplasia; usually focal spongiosis; no distinguishing features.
Mycosis fungoides	Epidermotropism; papillary dermal infiltrate of lymphocytes with variable cytological atypia.
Chronic candidosis and dermatophytoses	Psoriasiform hyperplasia not as regular or as marked as in psoriasis; spongiform pustules or neutrophils in parakeratotic scale; fungal elements may be sparse in candidosis.
ILVEN	Papillated psoriasiform hyperplasia with foci of parakeratosis overlying hypogranulosis; often focal mild spongiosis.
Norwegian scabies	Marked orthokeratosis and scale crust; numerous mites, larvae and ova in the keratinous layer.
Bowen's disease (psoriasiform type)	Full-thickness atypia of keratinocytes but basal layer sometimes spared; cells sometimes pale staining.
Clear cell acanthoma	Pallor of keratinocytes but no atypia; abundant glycogen; some exocytosis of inflammatory cells.
Lamellar ichthyosis	Mild psoriasiform hyperplasia with a thick compact or laminated orthokeratin layer overlying a prominent granular layer.
Pityriasis rosea (herald patch)	Mild psoriasiform hyperplasia; spongiosis and exocytosis of lymphocytes leading to 'mini-Pautrier simulants'; focal parakeratosis.
Pellagra, acrodermatitis enteropathica and glucagonoma syndrome	Mild to moderate psoriasiform hyperplasia; the upper epidermis shows pallor and ballooning progressing sometimes to necrosis, vesiculation or pustulation (not in pellagra); confluent parakeratosis overlying these changes; many cases of pellagra show mild, even non-specific changes.
Secondary syphilis	Superficial and deep dermal infiltrate which often includes plasma cells; may have lichenoid changes or granuloma formation in late stages.

phase, can sometimes present lesions with a psoriasiform pattern (see p. 633).

Histopathology

It should be stressed that there is considerable variation in the histopathological appearances of secondary syphilis. Psoriasiform hyperplasia is more often seen in late lesions of secondary syphilis. A lichenoid tissue reaction may also be present and this combination of tissue reactions is very suggestive of syphilis, particularly if the infiltrate in the dermis forms in both the superficial and deep parts. Plasma cells are commonly present, but they are not invariable.

REFERENCES

Introduction

1. Pinkus H, Mehregan AH. The primary histologic lesion of seborrhoeic dermatitis and psoriasis. J Invest Dermatol 1966; 46: 109–116.
2. Barr RJ, Young EM Jr. Psoriasiform and related papulosquamous disorders. J Cutan Pathol 1985; 12: 412–425.

Major psoriasiform dermatoses

3. Watson W. Psoriasis: Epidemiology and genetics. Dermatol Clin 1984; 2: 363–371.
4. Krueger GG, Eyre RW. Trigger factors in psoriasis. Dermatol Clin 1984; 2: 373–381.
5. Tiilikainen A, Lassus A, Karvonen J et al. Psoriasis and HLA–CW6. Br J Dermatol 1980; 102: 179–184.
6. Fry L. Psoriasis. Br J Dermatol 1988; 119: 445–461.
7. Gupta MA, Gupta AK, Kirkby S et al. Pruritus in psoriasis. Arch Dermatol 1988; 124: 1052–1057.
8. Farber EM, Nall ML. The natural history of psoriasis in 5,600 patients. Dermatologica 1974; 148: 1–18.
9. van der Kerkhof PCM. Clinical features. In: Mier PD, van der Kerkhof PCM, eds. Textbook of psoriasis. Edinburgh: Churchill Livingstone, 1986; 13–39.
10. Baumal A, Kantor I, Sachs P. Psoriasis of the lips. Report of a case. Arch Dermatol 1961; 84: 185–187.
11. Rudolph RI, Rudolph LP. Intraoral psoriasis vulgaris. Int J Dermatol 1975; 14: 101–104.
12. Koransky JS, Roenigk HH Jr. Vitiligo and psoriasis. J Am Acad Dermatol 1982; 7: 183–189.
13. Fordham JN, Storey GO. Psoriasis and gout. Postgrad Med J 1982; 58: 477–480.
14. Yates VM, Watkinson G, Kelman A. Further evidence for an association between psoriasis, Crohn's disease and ulcerative colitis. Br J Dermatol 1982; 106: 323–330.
15. Grunwald MH, David M, Feuerman EJ. Coexistence of psoriasis vulgaris and bullous diseases. J Am Acad Dermatol 1985; 13: 224–228.
16. Patterson JW, Graff GE, Eubanks SW. Perforating folliculitis and psoriasis. J Am Acad Dermatol 1982; 7: 369–376.
17. Millns JL, Muller SA. The coexistence of psoriasis and lupus erythematosus. An analysis of 27 cases. Arch Dermatol 1980; 116: 658–663.
18. Paslin DA. Psoriasis on scars. Arch Dermatol 1973; 108: 665–666.
19. Kaplan MH, Sadick NS, Wieder J, et al. Antipsoriatic effects of zidovudine in human immunodeficiency virus–associated psoriasis. J Am Acad Dermatol 1989; 20: 76–82.
20. Christophers E, Henseler T. Characterization of disease patterns in nonpustular psoriasis. Semin Dermatol 1985; 4: 271–275.
21. Nyfors A, Lemholt K. Psoriasis in children. A short review and a survey of 245 cases. Br J Dermatol 1975; 92: 437–442.
22. Lerner MR, Lerner AB. Congenital psoriasis. Report of three cases. Arch Dermatol 1972; 105: 598–601.
23. Farber EM, Mullen RH, Jacobs AH, Nall L. Infantile psoriasis: a follow-up study. Pediatr Dermatol 1986; 3: 237–243.

24. Lowe NJ. Psoriasis. Semin Dermatol 1988; 7: 43–47.
25. Whyte HJ, Baughman RD. Acute guttate psoriasis and streptococcal infection. Arch Dermatol 1964; 89: 350–356.
26. Beylot C, Puissant A, Bioulac P et al. Particular clinical features of psoriasis in infants and children. Acta Derm Venereol (Suppl) 1979; 87: 95–97.
27. Boyd AS, Menter A. Erythrodermic psoriasis. Precipitating factors, course and prognosis in 50 patients. J Am Acad Dermatol 1989; 21: 985–991.
28. Kerl H, Pachinger W. Psoriasis: odd varieties in the adult. Acta Derm Venereol (Suppl) 1979; 87: 90–94.
29. Atherton DJ, Kahana M, Russell-Jones R. Naevoid psoriasis. Br J Dermatol 1989; 120: 837–841.
30. Stankler L, Ewen SWB. Follicular psoriasis. Br J Dermatol 1981; 104: 153–156.
31. Lucky PA, Carter DM. Psoriasis presenting as cutaneous horns. J Am Acad Dermatol 1981; 5: 681–683.
32. Neville EA, Finn OA. Psoriasiform napkin dermatitis — a follow-up study. Br J Dermatol 1975; 92: 279–285.
33. Henderson CA, Highet AS. Acute psoriasis associated with Lancefield Group C and Group G cutaneous streptococcal infections. Br J Dermatol 1988; 118: 559–562.
34. Champion RH. Psoriasis. Br Med J 1986; 292: 1693–1696.
35. Melski JW, Bernhard JD, Stern RS. The Koebner (isomorphic) response in psoriasis. Arch Dermatol 1983; 119: 655–659.
36. Skott A, Mobacken H, Starmark JE. Exacerbation of psoriasis during lithium treatment. Br J Dermatol 1977; 96: 445–448.
37. Sarantidis D, Waters B. A review and controlled study of cutaneous conditions associated with lithium carbonate. Br J Psychiatry 1983; 143: 42–50.
38. Harwell WB. Quinidine-induced psoriasis. J Am Acad Dermatol 1983; 9: 278.
39. Gold MH, Holy AK, Roenigk HH Jr. Beta-blocking drugs and psoriasis. J Am Acad Dermatol 1988; 19: 837–841.
40. Gawkrodger DJ, Beveridge GW. Psoriasiform reaction to atenolol. Clin Exp Dermatol 1984; 9: 92–94.
41. Harrison PV, Stones RN. Severe exacerbation of psoriasis due to terfenadine. Clin Exp Dermatol 1988; 13: 275.
42. Lee RE, Gaspari AA, Lotze MT et al. Interleukin 2 and psoriasis. Arch Dermatol 1988; 124: 1811–1815.
42a. Goh CL. Psoriasiform drug eruption due to glibenclamide. Australas J Dermatol 1987; 28: 30–32.
43. Cram DL. Psoriasis: Current advances in etiology and treatment. J Am Acad Dermatol 1981; 4: 1–14.
44. Voorhees JJ. Leucotrienes and other lipoxygenase products in the pathogenesis and therapy of psoriasis and other dermatoses. Arch Dermatol 1983; 119: 541–547.
45. Mordovtsev VN, Albanova VI. Morphology of skin microvasculature in psoriasis. Am J Dermatopathol 1989; 11: 33–42.
46. Majewski S, Tigalonowa M, Jablonska S et al. Serum samples from patients with active psoriasis enhance

lymphocyte-induced angiogenesis and modulate endothelial cell proliferation. Arch Dermatol 1987; 123: 221–225.

47. Greaves MW. Neutrophil polymorphonuclears, mediators and the pathogenesis of psoriasis. Br J Dermatol 1983; 109: 115–118.

48. Bos JD. The pathomechanisms of psoriasis; the skin immune system and cyclosporin. Br J Dermatol 1988; 118: 141–155.

49. Kapp A, Gillitzer R, Kirchner H, Schopf E. Decreased production of interferon in whole blood cultures derived from patients with psoriasis. J Invest Dermatol 1988; 90: 511–514.

50. Pike MC, Lee CS, Elder JT et al. Increased phosphatidylinositol kinase activity in psoriatic epidermis. J Invest Dermatol 1989; 92: 791–797.

51. Schaumburg-Lever G, Alroy J, Ucci A et al. Cell surface carbohydrates in psoriasis. J Am Acad Dermatol 1984; 11: 1087–1094.

52. Wahba A. Immunological alterations in psoriasis. Int J Dermatol 1980; 19: 124–129.

53. Gottlieb AB. Immunologic mechanisms in psoriasis. J Am Acad Dermatol 1988; 18: 1376–1380.

53a. Chin Y-H, Falanga V, Taylor JR et al. Adherence of human helper/memory T-cell subsets to psoriatic dermal endothelium. J Invest Dermatol 1990; 94: 413–417.

54. Johannesson A, Hammar H, Sundqvist K-G. Deposition of immunoglobulins and complement in stratum corneum in microscopic lesions in patients with active psoriasis: the relationship to hyperproliferation. Acta Derm Venereol 1982; 62: 21–25.

55. Jablonska S, Chowaniec O, Beutner EH et al. Stripping of the stratum corneum in patients with psoriasis. Production of prepinpoint papules and psoriatic lesions. Arch Dermatol 1982; 118: 652–657.

56. Weiss VC, van den Broek H, Barrett S, West DP. Immunopathology of psoriasis: a comparison with other parakeratotic lesions. J Invest Dermatol 1982; 78: 256–260.

57. Takematsu H, Ohkohchi K, Tagami H. Demonstration of anaphylatoxins C3a and C4a and C5a in the scales of psoriasis and inflammatory pustular dermatoses. Br J Dermatol 1986; 114: 1–6.

58. Fattah AA, El Okby M, Ammar S et al. An immunologic study of psoriasis. Am J Dermatopathol 1986; 8: 309–313.

59. Ullman S, Halberg P, Hentzer B. Deposits of immunoglobulin and complement in psoriatic lesions. J Cutan Pathol 1980; 7: 271–275.

60. Doyle JA, Muller SA, Rogers RS III, Schroeter AL. Immunofluorescence in psoriasis: A clinical study in sixty patients. J Am Acad Dermatol 1981; 5: 655–660.

61. Lowe NJ, Breeding J, Russell D. Cutaneous polyamines in psoriasis. Br J Dermatol 1982; 107: 21–26.

62. McDonald CJ. Polyamines in psoriasis. J Invest Dermatol 1983; 81: 385–387.

63. Ternowitz T. Monocyte and neutrophil chemotaxis in psoriasis. J Am Acad Dermatol 1986; 15: 1191–1199.

64. Ternowitz T. The enhanced monocyte and neutrophil chemotaxis in psoriasis is normalized after treatment with psoralens plus ultraviolet A and anthralin. J Am Acad Dermatol 1987; 16: 1169–1175.

65. Preissner WC, Schroder J-M, Christophers E. Altered polymorphonuclear leukocyte responses in psoriasis: chemotaxis and degranulation. Br J Dermatol 1983; 109: 1–8.

66. Van Scott EJ, Ekel TM. Kinetics of hyperplasia in psoriasis. Arch Dermatol 1963; 88: 373–380.

67. Heenen M, Galand P. On cell kinetics in psoriasis. Br J Dermatol 1984; 110: 241–245.

68. Bernard BA, Asselineau D, Schaffar-Deshayes L, Darmon MY. Abnormal sequence of expression of differentiation markers in psoriatic epidermis: Inversion of two steps in the differentiation program? J Invest Dermatol 1988; 90: 801–805.

69. DiCicco LM, Fraki JE, Mansbridge JN. The plasma membrane in psoriasis. Int J Dermatol 1987; 26: 631–638.

70. Ragaz A, Ackerman AB. Evolution, maturation, and regression of lesions of psoriasis. Am J Dermatopathol 1979; 1: 199–214.

71. Gordon M, Johnson WC. Histopathology and histochemistry of psoriasis. I. The active lesion and clinically normal skin. Arch Dermatol 1967; 95: 402–407.

72. Stadler R, Schaumberg-Lever G, Orfanos CE. Histology. In: Mier PD, van de Kerkhof PCM, eds. Textbook of psoriasis. Edinburgh: Churchill Livingstone, 1986; 40–54.

73. Cox AJ, Watson W. Histological variations in lesions of psoriasis. Arch Dermatol 1972; 106: 503–506.

74. Chowaniec O, Jablonska S. Pre-pin-point lesions of psoriasis. Acta Derm Venereol (Suppl) 1979; 85: 39–45.

75. Chowaniec O, Jablonska S, Beutner EH et al. Earliest clinical and histological changes in psoriasis. Dermatologica 1981; 163: 42–51.

76. Bieber T, Braun-Falco O. Distribution of CD1a-positive cells in psoriatic skin during the evolution of the lesions. Acta Derm Venereol 1989; 69: 175–178.

77. Griffin TD, Lattanand A, Van Scott EJ. Clinical and histologic heterogeneity of psoriatic plaques. Therapeutic relevance. Arch Dermatol 1988; 124: 216–220.

78. De Panfilis G, Manara GC, Ferrari C et al. Further characterization of the "incipient lesion of chronic stationary type psoriasis vulgaris in exacerbation". Acta Derm Venereol (Suppl) 1989; 146: 26–30.

78a. Lundin A, Fredens K, Michaelsson G, Venge P. The eosinophil granulocyte in psoriasis. Br J Dermatol 1990; 122: 181–193.

79. Kanerva L, Lauharanta J, Niemi K-M, Lassus A. Light and electron microscopy of psoriatic skin before and during retinoid (Ro 10-9359) and retinoid-PUVA treatment. J Cutan Pathol 1982; 9: 175–188.

80. Headington JT, Gupta AK, Goldfarb MT et al. A morphometric and histologic study of the scalp in psoriasis. Arch Dermatol 1989; 125: 639–642.

81. Maddin WS, Wood WS. Multiple keratoacanthomas and squamous cell carcinomas occurring at psoriatic treatment sites. J Cutan Pathol 1979; 6: 96–100.

82. Kahn JR, Chalet MD, Lowe NJ. Eruptive squamous cell carcinomata following psoralen-UVA phototoxicity. Clin Exp Dermatol 1986; 11: 398–402.

83. Pittelkow MR, Perry HO, Muller SA et al. Skin cancer in patients with psoriasis treated with coal tar. Arch Dermatol 1981; 117: 465–468.

83a. Gupta AK, Siegel MT, Noble SC et al. Keratoses in patients with psoriasis: A prospective study in fifty-two inpatients. J Am Acad Dermatol 1990; 23: 52–55.

84. Kocsard E. The rarity of solar keratoses in psoriatic patients: preliminary report. Australas J Dermatol 1976; 17: 65–66.

85. Stern RS, Scotto J, Fears TR. Psoriasis and susceptibility to nonmelanoma skin cancer. J Am Acad Dermatol 1985; 12: 67–73.

86. Halprin KM, Comerford M, Taylor JR. Cancer in patients with psoriasis. J Am Acad Dermatol 1982; 7: 633–638.

87. Lawrence CM, Dahl MGC. Two patterns of skin ulceration induced by methotrexate in patients with psoriasis. J Am Acad Dermatol 1984; 11: 1059–1065.

88. Kanerva L. Electron microscopy of the effects of dithranol on healthy and on psoriatic skin. Am J Dermatopathol 1990; 12: 51–62.

89. Sedgwick JB, Hurd ER, Bergstresser PR. Abnormal granulocyte morphology in patients with psoriasis. Br J Dermatol 1982; 107: 165–172.

90. Cox NH. Morphological assessment of neutrophil leucocytes in psoriasis. Clin Exp Dermatol 1986; 11: 340–344.

91. Lyons JH III. Generalized pustular psoriasis. Int J Dermatol 1987; 26: 409–418.

92. Sauder DN, Steck WD, Bailin PB, Krakauer RS. Lymphocyte kinetics in pustular psoriasis. J Am Acad Dermatol 1981; 4: 458–460.

93. Baker H, Ryan TJ. Generalized pustular psoriasis. A clinical and epidemiological study of 104 cases. Br J Dermatol 1968; 80: 771–793.

94. Stewart AF, Battaglini–Sabetta J, Millstone L. Hypocalcemia-induced pustular psoriasis of von Zumbusch. Ann Intern Med 1984; 100: 677–680.

95. O'Keefe E, Braverman IM, Cohen I. Annulus migrans. Identical lesions in pustular psoriasis, Reiter's syndrome, and geographic tongue. Arch Dermatol 1973; 107: 240–244.

96. Wagner G, Luckasen JR, Goltz RW. Mucous membrane involvement in generalized pustular psoriasis. Report of three cases and review of the literature. Arch Dermatol 1976; 112: 1010–1014.

97. Dawson TAJ. Tongue lesions in generalized pustular psoriasis. Br J Dermatol 1974; 91: 419–424.

98. Hubler WR Jr. Lingual lesions of generalized pustular psoriasis. Report of five cases and a review of the literature. J Am Acad Dermatol 1984; 11: 1069–1076.

99. Mackie RM, Burton J. Pustular psoriasis in association with renal amyloidosis. Br J Dermatol 1974; 90: 567–571.

100. Katzenellenbogen I, Feuerman EJ. Psoriasis pustulosa and impetigo herpetiformis: single or dual entity? Acta Derm Venereol 1966; 46: 86–94.

101. Oosterling RJ, Nobrega RE, Du Boeuff JA, Van der Meer JB. Impetigo herpetiformis or generalized pustular psoriasis? Arch Dermatol 1978; 114: 1527–1529.

102. Lotem M, Katzenelson V, Rotem A et al. Impetigo herpetiformis: A variant of pustular psoriasis or a separate entity? J Am Acad Dermatol 1989; 20: 338–341.

103. Ott F, Krakowski A, Tur E et al. Impetigo herpetiformis with lowered serum level of vitamin D and its diminished intestinal absorption. Dermatologica 1982; 164: 360–365.

104. Beveridge GW, Harkness RA, Livingstone JRB. Impetigo herpetiformis in two successive pregnancies. Br J Dermatol 1966; 78: 106–112.

105. Bajaj AK, Swarup V, Gupta OP, Gupta SC. Impetigo herpetiformis. Dermatologica 1977; 155: 292–295.

106. Oumeish OY, Farraj SE, Bataineh AS. Some aspects of impetigo herpetiformis. Arch Dermatol 1982; 118: 103–105.

107. Moynihan GD, Ruppe JP Jr. Impetigo herpetiformis and hypoparathyroidism. Arch Dermatol 1985; 121: 1330–1331.

108. Ryan TJ, Baker H. The prognosis of generalized pustular psoriasis. Br J Dermatol 1971; 85: 407–411.

109. Resneck JS, Cram DL. Erythema annulare-like pustular psoriasis. Arch Dermatol 1973; 108: 687–688.

110. Rajka G, Thune PO. On erythema annulare centrifugum-type of psoriasis. Acta Derm Venereol (Suppl) 1979; 85: 143–145.

111. Adler DJ, Rower JM, Hashimoto K. Annular pustular psoriasis. Arch Dermatol 1981; 117: 313.

112. Hubler WR Jr. Familial juvenile generalized pustular psoriasis. Arch Dermatol 1984; 120: 1174–1178.

113. Khan SA, Peterkin GAG, Mitchell PC. Juvenile generalized pustular psoriasis. A report of five cases and a review of the literature. Arch Dermatol 1972; 105: 67–72.

114. McGibbon DH. Infantile pustular psoriasis. Clin Exp Dermatol 1979; 4: 115–118.

115. Katz M, Seidenbaum M, Weinrauch L. Penicillin-induced generalized pustular psoriasis. J Am Acad Dermatol 1987; 17: 918–920.

116. Lowe NJ, Ridgway HB. Generalized pustular psoriasis precipitated by lithium carbonate. Arch Dermatol 1978; 114: 1788–1789.

117. Reshad H, Hargreaves GK, Vickers CFH. Generalized pustular psoriasis precipitated by phenylbutazone and oxyphenbutazone. Br J Dermatol 1983; 108: 111–113.

118. Hu C-H, Miller AC, Peppercorn R, Farber EM. Generalized pustular psoriasis provoked by propanolol. Arch Dermatol 1985; 121: 1326–1327.

119. Murphy FR, Stolman LP. Generalized pustular psoriasis. Arch Dermatol 1979; 115: 1215–1216.

120. Lindgren S, Groth O. Generalized pustular psoriasis. Acta Derm Venereol 1976; 56: 139–147.

121. Kaminski M, Szmurlo A, Pawinska M, Jablonska S. Decreased natural killer cell activity in generalized pustular psoriasis (von Zumbusch type). Br J Dermatol 1984; 110: 565–568.

122. Ternowitz T, Thestrup-Pedersen K. Neutrophil and monocyte chemotaxis in pustulosis palmo-plantaris and pustular psoriasis. Br J Dermatol 1985; 113: 507–513.

123. Heng MCY, Heng JA, Allen SG. Electron microscopic features in generalized pustular psoriasis. J Invest Dermatol 1987; 89: 187–191.

124. Shelley WB, Kirschbaum JO. Generalized pustular psoriasis. Arch Dermatol 1961; 84: 123–128.

125. Kingery FAJ, Chinn HD, Saunders TS. Generalized pustular psoriasis. Arch Dermatol 1961; 84: 912–919.

126. Neumann E, Hard S. The significance of the epidermal sweat duct unit in the genesis of pustular psoriasis (Zumbusch) and the microabscess of Munro-Sabouraud. Acta Derm Venereol 1974; 54: 141–146.

127. Pierard GE, Pierard-Franchimont C, de la Brassinne M. Impetigo herpetiformis and pustular psoriasis during pregnancy. Am J Dermatopathol 1983; 5: 215–220.

128. Braverman IM, Cohen I, O'Keefe E. Metabolic and ultrastructural studies in a patient with pustular psoriasis (von Zumbusch). Arch Dermatol 1972; 105: 189–196.

129. Keat A. Reiter's syndrome and reactive arthritis in perspective. N Engl J Med 1983; 309: 1606–1615.

130. Calin A. Reiter's syndrome. Med Clin North Am 1977; 61: 365–376.

131. Editorial. Treating Reiter's syndrome. Lancet 1987; 2: 1125–1126.

132. Leirisalo M, Skylv G, Kousa M et al. Followup study on patients with Reiter's disease and reactive arthritis, with special reference to HLA-B27. Arthritis Rheum 1982; 25: 249–259.

133. Bengtsson A, Ahlstrand C, Lindstrom FD, Kihrstrom E. Bacteriological findings in 25 patients with Reiter's syndrome (reactive arthritis). Scand J Rheumatol 1983; 12: 157–160.

134. Keat A, Dixey J, Sonnex C et al. Chlamydia trachomatosis and reactive arthritis: the missing link. Lancet 1987; 1: 72–74.

135. Hart HH, McGuigan LE, Gow PJ, Grigor RR. Reiter's syndrome: chronicity of symptoms and employment. Aust NZ J Med 1986; 16: 452–456.

136. Butler MJ, Russell AS, Percy JS, Lentle BC. A follow-up study of 48 patients with Reiter's syndrome. Am J Med 1979; 67: 808–810.

137. Marks JS, Holt PJL. The natural history of Reiter's disease — 21 years of observations. Q J Med 1986; 60: 685–697.

138. Callen JP. The spectrum of Reiter's disease. J Am Acad Dermatol 1979; 1: 75–77.

139. Morton RS. Reiter's disease. Practitioner 1972; 209: 631–638.

140. Weinberger HW, Ropes MW, Kulka JP, Bauer W. Reiter's syndrome, clinical and pathologic observations. Medicine (Baltimore) 1962; 41: 35–91.

141. Hall WH, Finegold S. A study of 23 cases of Reiter's syndrome. Ann Intern Med 1953; 38: 533–550.

142. Montgomery MM, Poske RM, Barton EM et al. The mucocutaneous lesions of Reiter's syndrome. Ann Intern Med 1959; 51: 99–109.

143. Jaramillo D, Leon W, Cardenas V, Cortes A. Reiter's syndrome, immunodepression and strongyloidiasis. J Cutan Pathol 1978; 5: 200–208.

144. Shatin H, Canizares O, Ladany E. Reiter's syndrome and keratosis blennorrhagica. Arch Dermatol 1960; 81: 551–555.

145. Perry HO, Mayne JG. Psoriasis and Reiter's syndrome. Arch Dermatol 1965; 92: 129–136.

146. Gelmetti C, Schiuma AA, Cerri D, Gianotti F. Pityriasis rubra pilaris in childhood: a long term study of 29 cases. Pediatr Dermatol 1986; 3: 446–451.

147. Lamar LM, Gaethe G. Pityriasis rubra pilaris. Arch Dermatol 1964; 89: 515–522.

148. Griffiths WAD. Pityriasis rubra pilaris — an historical approach. 2. Clinical features. Clin Exp Dermatol 1976; 1: 37–50.

149. Griffiths WAD. Pityriasis rubra pilaris. Clin Exp Dermatol 1980; 5: 105–112.

150. Shvili D, David M, Mimouni M. Childhood-onset pityriasis rubra pilaris with immunologic abnormalities. Pediatr Dermatol 1987; 4: 21–23.

151. Griffiths A. Pityriasis rubra pilaris. Etiologic considerations. J Am Acad Dermatol 1984; 10: 1086-1088.

152. Niemi K-M, Kousa M, Storgards K, Karvonen J. Pityriasis rubra pilaris. A clinico-pathological study with a special reference to autoradiography and histocompatibility antigens. Dermatologica 1976; 152: 109–118.

153. Sonnex TS, Dawber RPR, Zachary CB et al. The nails in adult type 1 pityriasis rubra pilaris. J Am Acad Dermatol 1986; 15: 956–960.

154. Cohen PR, Prystowsky JH. Pityriasis rubra pilaris: A review of diagnosis and treatment. J Am Acad Dermatol 1989; 20: 801–807.

155. Davidson CL Jr, Winkelmann RK, Kierland RR. Pityriasis rubra pilaris. A follow-up study of 57 patients. Arch Dermatol 1969; 100: 175–178.

156. Gross DA, Landau JW, Newcomer VD. Pityriasis rubra pilaris. Report of a case and analysis of the literature. Arch Dermatol 1969; 99: 710–716.

157. Finzi AF, Altomare G, Bergamaschini L, Tucci A. Pityriasis rubra pilaris and retinol-binding protein. Br J Dermatol 1981; 104: 253–256.

158. van Voorst Vader PC, van Oostveen F, Houthoff HJ, Marrink J. Pityriasis rubra pilaris, vitamin A and retinol-binding protein: a case study. Acta Derm Venereol 1984; 64: 430–432.

159. Stoll DM, King LE, Chytil F. Serum levels of retinol binding protein in patients with pityriasis rubra pilaris. Br J Dermatol 1983; 108: 375.

160. Ralfs IG, Dawber RPR, Ryan TJ, Wright NA. Pityriasis rubra pilaris: epidermal cell kinetics. Br J Dermatol 1981; 104: 249–252.

161. Marks R, Griffiths A. The epidermis in pityriasis rubra pilaris: a comparison with psoriasis. Br J Dermatol (Suppl)1973; 9: 19-20.

162. Soeprono FF. Histologic criteria for the diagnosis of pityriasis rubra pilaris. Am J Dermatopathol 1986; 8: 277-283.

163. Kao GF, Sulica VI. Focal acantholytic dyskeratosis occurring in pityriasis rubra pilaris. Am J Dermatopathol 1989; 11: 172-176.

164. Kanerva L, Lauharanta J, Niemi K-M, Lassus A. Ultrastructure of pityriasis rubra pilaris with observations during retinoid (etretinate) treatment. Br J Dermatol 1983; 108: 653-663.

165. Everett MA, Headington JT. Parapsoriasis. JCE Dermatology 1978; 17 (12): 12-24.

166. Bennaman O, Sanchez JL. Comparative clinicopathological study on pityriasis lichenoides chronica and small plaque parapsoriasis. Am J Dermatopathol 1988; 10: 189-196.

167. Lambert WC, Everett MA. The nosology of parapsoriasis. J Am Acad Dermatol 1981; 5: 373-395.

168. Altman J. Parapsoriasis: a histopathologic review and classification. Semin Dermatol 1984; 3: 14-21.

169. Lazar AP, Caro WA, Roenigk HH Jr, Pinski KS. Parapsoriasis and mycosis fungoides: The Northwestern University experience, 1970 to 1985. J Am Acad Dermatol 1989; 21: 919-923.

170. Shaffer B, Beerman H. Lichen simplex chronicus and its variants. Arch Dermatol 1951; 64: 340-351.

171. Kouskoukis CE, Scher RK, Ackerman AB. The

problem of features of lichen simplex chronicus complicating the histology of diseases of the nail. Am J Dermatopathol 1984; 6: 45-49.

172. Marks R, Wells GC. Lichen simplex: morphodynamic correlates. Br J Dermatol 1973; 88: 249-256.

173. Singh G. Atopy in lichen simplex (neurodermatitis circumscripta). Br J Dermatol 1973; 89: 625-627.

174. Marks R, Wells GC. A histochemical profile of lichen simplex. Br J Dermatol 1973; 88: 557-562.

175. Ackerman AB. Marked compact hyperkeratosis as a sign of persistent rubbing. Am J Dermatopathol 1980; 2: 149-152.

The spongiotic reaction pattern

INTRODUCTION

The spongiotic tissue reaction is characterized by the presence of intraepidermal and intercellular oedema (spongiosis) (Fig. 5.1). It is recognized by the widened intercellular spaces between keratinocytes, with elongation of the intercellular bridges (Fig. 5.2).[1] The foci of spongiosis may vary from microscopic in size to grossly identifiable vesicles and even bullae. Mild spongiosis is well seen in semi-thin sections.[2] Inflammatory cells, usually lymphocytes, but sometimes eosinophils or even neutrophils, are also present.[1]

The spongiotic tissue reaction is a histopathological concept and not a clinical one, although several of the many diseases with this tissue reaction have been included, in the past,

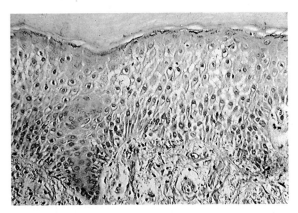

Fig. 5.1 The spongiotic reaction pattern. There is mild intracellular oedema leading to pallor of the keratinocytes, in addition to the intercellular oedema.
Haematoxylin — eosin

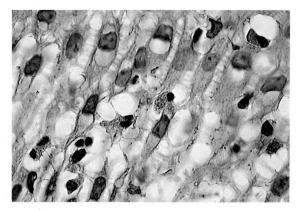

Fig. 5.2 The spongiotic reaction pattern. Note the elongation of the intercellular bridges resulting from the intercellular oedema. Occasional eosinophils are present within the epidermis.
Haematoxylin — eosin

in the category of 'eczemas'. This term (derived from Greek elements which mean 'boiling over') has fallen into some disrepute in recent years because it lacks preciseness.[3,4] The 'eczemas' all show epidermal spongiosis at some stage of their evolution, even though this has been disputed for atopic eczema. Clinically, the various spongiotic disorders may present with weeping, crusted patches and plaques as in the so-called eczemas, or as erythematous papules, papulovesicles and even vesiculobullous lesions. Resolving lesions, and those of some duration, may show a characteristic collarette of scale.

The mechanism involved in the collection of the intercellular fluid is controversial. It is generally accepted that the fluid comes from the dermis and, in turn, from blood vessels in the upper dermis. Various immunological reactions are involved in some of the diseases discussed in this chapter, but in others the aetiology of this fluid extravasation from vessels remains to be elucidated. The controversy also involves the mechanism by which the dermal oedema fluid enters the epidermis.[5,6] One concept is that an osmotic gradient develops towards the epidermis, drawing fluid into it.[5] The opposing view suggests that hydrostatic pressure leads to the epidermal elimination of dermal oedema.[7] The latter explanation does not satisfactorily explain the absence of spongiosis in pronounced urticarial reactions. Perhaps both mechanisms

are involved to a varying degree. The spongiotic tissue reaction is a dynamic process.[8] Vesicles come and go, and they can be situated at different levels in the epidermis.[8] Parakeratosis forms above areas of spongiosis, probably as a result of an acceleration in the movement of keratinocytes towards the surface, although disordered maturation may contribute.[9] Small droplets of plasma may accumulate in the mounds of parakeratosis contributing to the appearance of the collarettes of scale, mentioned above.[9]

Simulants of the spongiotic tissue reaction

There are several categories of disease in which casual histological examination may show a simulation of the spongiotic reaction pattern: they are excluded from consideration here.[1] Diseases that present a lichenoid reaction pattern with obscurement of the dermo–epidermal interface (such as pityriasis lichenoides, erythema multiforme and fixed drug eruption) or prominent vacuolar change (variants of lupus erythematosus) may show some spongiosis above the basal layer. They are not included among the diseases considered in this chapter.

Certain viral exanthems and morbilliform drug eruptions show mild epidermal spongiosis, but it is usually limited to the basal layer of the epidermis. Other viral diseases, such as herpes simplex and herpes zoster, show ballooning degeneration of keratinocytes with secondary acantholysis. Some spongiosis is invariably present but it is overshadowed by the other changes. Primary acantholytic disorders leading to vesiculation are also excluded. Mild spongiosis is seen overlying the dermal papillae in early lesions of psoriasis, but again this disease is not usually regarded as a spongiotic disorder.

The accumulation of acid mucopolysaccharides in the follicular infundibulum in follicular mucinosis may simulate spongiosis. Stains for mucin, such as the colloidal iron stain, will confirm the diagnosis, if any doubt exists.

Patterns of spongiosis

There are three special patterns of spongiosis which can be distinguished morphologically from the more usual type. These special patterns are *eosinophilic spongiosis*, characterized by the presence of numerous eosinophils within the spongiotic foci, *miliarial spongiosis* (acrosyringial spongiosis), in which the oedema is centred on the acrosyringium, and *follicular spongiosis*, in which there is involvement of the follicular infundibulum. Sometimes serial sections are required before it is appreciated that the spongiosis is related to the acrosyringium or acrotrichium. Diseases in these special categories will be discussed first, followed by a description of the more usual type of spongiotic disorders.

EOSINOPHILIC SPONGIOSIS

Eosinophilic spongiosis is a histological reaction pattern characterized by the presence of epidermal spongiosis associated with the exocytosis of eosinophils into the spongiotic foci.[10] Micro-abscesses, containing predominantly eosinophils, are formed.

Eosinophilic spongiosis is found in a heterogeneous group of dermatoses, most of which are considered elsewhere. It can be seen in the following conditions:

Pemphigus (precursor lesions)
Pemphigus vegetans
Bullous pemphigoid
Idiopathic eosinophilic spongiosis
Allergic contact dermatitis
Arthropod bites
Eosinophilic folliculitis (Ofuji's disease)
Incontinentia pigmenti (first stage).

PEMPHIGUS (PRECURSOR LESIONS)

Eosinophilic spongiosis may occur in the pre-acantholytic stage of both pemphigus foliaceus and pemphigus vulgaris (see p. 137).[10-13] In these early stages, direct immunofluorescence demonstrates the presence of IgG in the intercellular areas of the epidermis.[11] In those patients whose disease evolves into pemphigus foliaceus, the initial clinical presentation may resemble dermatitis herpetiformis.[12,14] Some of these cases have been reported in the literature as herpetiform pemphigus.[15,16]

Histopathology

The pattern is that described for eosinophilic spongiosis (Fig. 5.3). Acantholysis and transitional forms between eosinophilic spongiosis and the usual histological findings in pemphigus may be present.

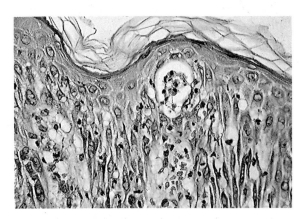

Fig. 5.3   Eosinophilic spongiosis as a precursor of pemphigus foliaceus.
Haematoxylin — eosin

PEMPHIGUS VEGETANS

Eosinophils are often prominent within the vesicles of pemphigus vegetans (see p. 138). Acantholysis, epidermal hyperplasia and the absence of spongiosis adjacent to the suprabasal vesicles usually allow the diagnosis of pemphigus vegetans to be made.

BULLOUS PEMPHIGOID

Eosinophilic spongiosis is an uncommon finding in the urticarial stage of bullous pemphigoid (see p. 151) and in erythematous patches adjacent to characteristic bullae in later stages of the disease.[17] There is usually a prominent dermal infiltrate of eosinophils and IgG is demonstrable along the basement membrane zone.

IDIOPATHIC EOSINOPHILIC SPONGIOSIS

Several cases have been recorded in which a localized, recurrent bullous eruption has been associated with the histological appearance of eosinophilic spongiosis.[18] Polycythaemia rubra vera was present in one case.[19]

ALLERGIC CONTACT DERMATITIS

Eosinophilic spongiosis may be seen in allergic contact dermatitis (see p. 104).

ARTHROPOD BITES

Eosinophilic spongiosis is occasionally seen in the reaction to the bite of certain arthropods, particularly the scabies mite (see p. 721).

EOSINOPHILIC FOLLICULITIS

In eosinophilic folliculitis (Ofuji's disease — see p. 440) the eosinophilic spongiosis involves the follicular infundibulum; sometimes the immediately adjacent epidermis is also involved.

INCONTINENTIA PIGMENTI

In the first stage of incontinentia pigmenti (see p. 317) there is prominent exocytosis of eosinophils into the epidermis and foci of eosinophilic spongiosis (Fig. 5.4). Occasional dyskeratotic keratinocytes may also be present.

MILIARIAL SPONGIOSIS

Miliarial spongiosis (acrosyringial spongiosis) is characterized by intraepidermal oedema centred on the acrosyringium. It is characteristic of the various clinical forms of miliaria.

MILIARIA

The miliarias are a clinically heterogeneous group of diseases which occur when the free flow

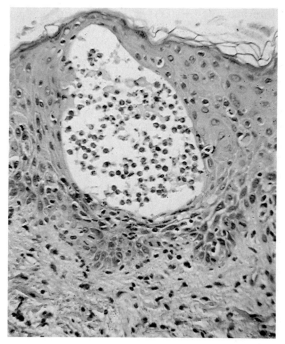

Fig. 5.4   Eosinophilic spongiosis in the first stage of incontinentia pigmenti. Haematoxylin — eosin

of eccrine sweat to the skin surface is impeded. Three variants of miliaria have been defined according to the depth at which this sweat duct obstruction occurs.

Miliaria crystallina (miliaria alba), which results from superficial obstruction in the stratum corneum, is characterized by asymptomatic, clear, 1–2 mm vesicles which rupture easily with gentle pressure.[20]

Miliaria rubra (prickly heat) consists of small, discrete, erythematous papulovesicles with a predilection for the clothed areas of the body.[21] The lesions are often pruritic. In severe cases, with recurrent crops of lesions, anhidrosis may result.[22] Occasionally, pustular lesions (miliaria pustulosa) may coexist.

Miliaria profunda refers to the development of flesh-coloured papules resembling goose-flesh, associated with obstruction of the sweat duct near the dermo–epidermal junction.[23] It usually follows severe miliaria rubra and is associated with anhidrosis.

Although it has been presumed since the last

century that obstruction of the eccrine duct is involved in the pathogenesis of the miliarias, the nature of this obstruction and its aetiology have been the subject of much debate.[23] The first demonstrable histological change is the accumulation of PAS-positive, diastase-resistant material in the distal pore,[23] although this has not always been found.[24] It is likely that there is an earlier stage of obstruction which cannot be demonstrated in tissue sections. After several days, a keratin plug forms as part of the repair process, leading to further obstruction of the duct, often at a deeper level. Various factors may contribute to the initial duct obstruction.[25,26] These include changes in the horny layer related to excess sweating, the presence of sodium chloride in more than isotonic concentration,[24] and lipoid depletion. In many cases there is an increase in the number of resident aerobic bacteria, particularly cocci.[23,27–29] These may alter in some way the terminal eccrine duct, although they may simply be a consequence of excess sweating and hydration of the horny layer. Miliaria has also developed at the site of previous radiotherapy, where it was associated with keratotic plugging of the eccrine orifices.[30]

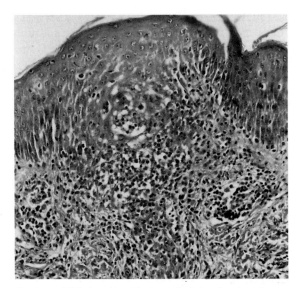

Fig. 5.5 Miliaria rubra. The spongiosis is related to the acrosyringium.
Haematoxylin — eosin

Histopathology

In *miliaria crystallina* there is a vesicle within, or directly beneath, the stratum corneum. There is often a thin, orthokeratotic layer forming the roof of the vesicle and a basket-weave layer of keratin in the base. A PAS-positive plug may be seen in the distal sweat pore.

Miliaria rubra is characterized by variable spongiosis and spongiotic vesiculation related to the epidermal sweat duct unit and the adjacent epidermis (Fig. 5.5). There is a small number of lymphocytes in the areas of spongiosis. An orthokeratotic or parakeratotic plug may overlie the spongiosis.[21] Sometimes there is oedema in the papillary dermis adjacent to the point of entry of the eccrine duct into the epidermis (Fig. 5.6). A mild lymphocytic infiltrate is usually present in this region. If the oedema is pronounced, leading to subepidermal vesiculation, then *miliaria profunda* is said to be present.

Less commonly, there is only slight spongiosis

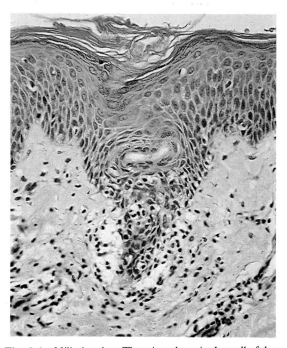

Fig. 5.6 Miliaria rubra. There is oedema in the wall of the eccrine duct as it enters the epidermis and also in the adjacent papillary dermis.
Haematoxylin — eosin

in the region of the acrosyringium in miliaria rubra associated with dilatation of the terminal eccrine duct.[21] It should be remembered that not all eccrine ducts are involved.

The secretory acini show few changes in the miliarias.[21] They may be mildly dilated. Often there is slight oedema of the connective tissue between the secretory units. Lymphocytes are not usually present, unless there is a prominent inflammatory cell infiltrate elsewhere in the dermis.

FOLLICULAR SPONGIOSIS

Follicular spongiosis refers to the presence of intercellular oedema in the follicular infundibulum (Fig. 5.7). It occurs in a limited number of circumstances:

Infundibulofolliculitis
Atopic dermatitis (follicular lesions)

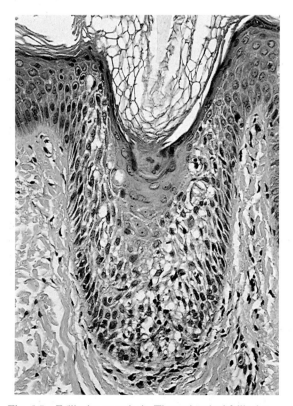

Fig. 5.7   Follicular spongiosis. The patient had follicular lesions on the trunk as a manifestation of atopic dermatitis. Haematoxylin — eosin

Apocrine miliaria
Eosinophilic folliculitis.

INFUNDIBULOFOLLICULITIS

This condition, also known as disseminate and recurrent infundibulofolliculitis, presents as a follicular, often pruritic, papular eruption with a predilection for the trunk and proximal parts of the extremities of young adult males.[31–34] It occurs almost exclusively in black patients. Although the lesions resemble those seen in some cases of atopic dermatitis, the individuals studied so far have not been atopic.[35]

Histopathology[31,33,35]

There is spongiosis of the follicular infundibulum with exocytosis of lymphocytes. A few neutrophils are sometimes present. There is widening of the follicular ostium and focal parakeratosis of the adjacent epidermis. Occasional follicles contain a keratin plug.[35] The follicular infundibulum is often hyperplastic. There is usually a slight infiltrate of lymphocytes around the follicles and around the blood vessels in the superficial part of the dermis. Mast cells may be increased.

ATOPIC DERMATITIS

Some patients with atopic dermatitis develop small follicular papules, often on the trunk.

Histopathology

There is spongiosis of the follicular infundibulum with exocytosis into this region of the epidermis. There are usually no neutrophils present. The adjacent epidermis may show mild acanthosis and sometimes focal parakeratosis. The histopathology resembles that seen in infundibulofolliculitis.

APOCRINE MILIARIA

Apocrine miliaria (Fox–Fordyce disease) presents as a chronic papular eruption, usually limited to the axilla (see p. 469). It results from rupture of the intraepidermal portion of the apocrine duct.

Histopathology

Serial sections may be required to demonstrate the spongiosis of the follicular infundibulum adjacent to the point of entry of the apocrine duct. There may be a few neutrophils in the associated inflammatory response.

EOSINOPHILIC FOLLICULITIS

Eosinophilic folliculitis (Ofuji's disease) is characterized by eosinophilic spongiosis centred on the follicular infundibulum. It is discussed in detail on page 440.

OTHER SPONGIOTIC DISEASES

Most of the other diseases in which the spongiotic reaction pattern occurs show spongiosis distributed randomly through the epidermis with no specific localization to the acrosyringium or follicular infundibulum, which indeed are often spared.

It is sometimes quite difficult to make a specific histopathological diagnosis of some of the diseases in this category. Often a diagnosis of 'spongiotic dermatitis consistent with ...' is as specific as one can be.

IRRITANT CONTACT DERMATITIS

Irritant contact dermatitis is an inflammatory condition of the skin produced in response to the direct toxic effect of an irritant substance.[36] The most commonly encountered of these irritants include detergents, solvents, acids and alkalis.[36-38] Other agents include wool fibres,[39] fibreglass,[39] and the milky sap of plants in the family Euphorbiaceae.[40,41] Even airborne substances in droplet, particulate or volatile form can cause this type of dermatitis.[42]

Our knowledge of irritant contact dermatitis is limited in spite of the fact that it is more common than allergic contact dermatitis, from which it may be difficult to distinguish.[43] Irritant reactions vary from simple erythema to purpura, eczematous reactions, vesiculobullous lesions and even epidermal necrosis with ulceration. Lesions are often more glazed than allergic reactions and subject to cracking, fissuring and frictional changes.[37] Irritant reactions occur at the site of contact with the irritant; in the case of airborne spread, the eyelids are a common site of involvement.[42] Pustular reactions have been reported with heavy metals, halogens and other substances.[44,45] These responses are assumed to be irritant in type. Acute ulceration is a severe reaction that may follow contact with alkalis, including cement.[46,47]

Susceptibility to irritant dermatitis is variable, although approximately 15% of the population have heightened sensitivity of their skin which appears to result from a thin, permeable stratum corneum.[43] Differences in skin sensitivity exist in different regions of the body.[48] Atopic individuals are also more susceptible[49] and both irritants and an atopic diathesis have been incriminated in the aetiology of occupational dermatitis of the hands.[43,50,51] Cumulative irritancy may also occur with agents in cosmetics, for example.[37] Susceptibility to irritants is also more common in winter months, apparently as a result of changes in the barrier functions of the stratum corneum.[52]

Irritants may act in several different ways. They may remove surface lipids and water-holding substances, damage cell membranes or denature epidermal keratins.[53] They may have a direct cytotoxic effect on cells. Some irritants are also chemotactic for neutrophils in vitro, while others may lead to the liberation of inflammatory mediators. The pathogenesis of irritant contact dermatitis continues to be poorly understood.[53]

Histopathology

The changes observed in irritant contact dermatitis vary with the nature of the irritant, including its mode of action and its concentration.[53,54] A knowledge of these factors helps to explain the conflicting descriptions in the literature.[55] Furthermore, many of the histopathological studies have been performed on animals, which are particularly liable to develop epidermal necrosis and dermo-epidermal separation with neutrophil infiltration when exposed to high concentrations of irritants.[54,56] In humans, high concentrations of an irritant will produce marked ballooning of keratinocytes in the upper epidermis with variable necrosis ranging from a few cells to confluent areas of the epidermis (Fig. 5.8).[57-59] Neutrophils are found in the areas of ballooning and necrosis, and mild spongiosis is also present in the adjacent epidermis (Fig. 5.9).[59]

If low and medium concentrations of an

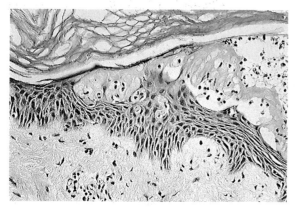

Fig. 5.8   Irritant contact dermatitis with superficial epidermal necrosis, oedema and some neutrophils. Haematoxylin — eosin

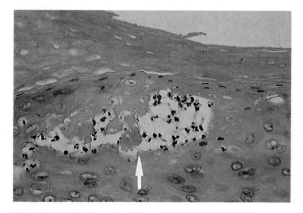

Fig. 5.9   Irritant contact dermatitis. There is focal ballooning and necrosis of keratinocytes in the upper epidermis together with spongiosis and a mild infiltrate of neutrophils. Haematoxylin — eosin
Photograph supplied by Dr J J Sullivan.

irritant are applied, the histopathological spectrum of the reactions produced often mimics that seen in allergic contact dermatitis, with epidermal spongiosis, mild superficial dermal oedema and a superficial, predominantly perivascular infiltrate of lymphocytes.[54,55,60] The lymphocytes are of helper/inducer type.[36] Langerhans cells are found diffusely through the upper dermis from day one to day four following contact with the irritant; this is in contrast to allergic contact dermatitis in which these cells are more perivascular in location and persist in the dermis for a longer period.[36] Occasional apoptotic keratinocytes may be seen in the epidermis in irritant reactions.[61,61a] In the recovery phase of irritant dermatitis mild epidermal hyperplasia is often present. Psoriasiform hyperplasia may develop in chronic irritant reactions.

Pustular reactions show subcorneal vesicles with neutrophils, cellular debris and a fibrinous exudate. There are also some neutrophils in the upper dermal infiltrate.

A recent detailed study using various irritants and human volunteers has confirmed the marked variability in histopathological responses, depending on the chemical used.[53] For example, propylene glycol produced hydration of corneal cells and a prominent basket-weave pattern.[53] Nonanoic acid resulted in tongues of eosinophilic keratinocytes with shrunken nuclei in the upper epidermis; croton oil caused a spongiotic tissue reaction resembling allergic contact dermatitis.[53] Sodium lauryl sulphate produced a thick zone of parakeratosis; dithranol caused some basal spongiosis and pallor of superficial keratinocytes; benzalkonium resulted in mild spongiosis, sometimes accompanied by foci of necrosis in the upper spinous layers.[53] The ultrastructural changes also varied widely with the different irritants.[53] Obviously, further studies are needed using other potential human irritants to increase our understanding of the diversity of irritant reactions.

ALLERGIC CONTACT DERMATITIS

Allergic contact dermatitis is an inflammatory

disorder which is initiated by contact with an allergen to which the person has previously been sensitized.[36] The prevalence of contact dermatitis (both irritant and allergic) in the general population in the United States has been variably estimated to be between 1.5 and 5.4%.[43] Allergic contact dermatitis is less frequent than irritant dermatitis, but both are a significant occupational problem.[62]

Clinically, there may be erythematous papules, small vesicles or weeping plaques, which are usually pruritic. The lesions develop 12–48 hours after exposure to the allergen. In the case of cosmetic reactions, the face, eyelids and neck are commonly involved, but the lesions may extend beyond the zone of contact, in contrast to irritant reactions.[63] Stasis dermatitis of the lower parts of the legs (see p. 110) is particularly susceptible to allergic contact reactions. Rarely reported allergic reactions include pustular lesions,[64] systemic contact reactions (see p. 113) and urticarial[65] or erythema multiforme-like lesions.[66] Resolution of allergic contact dermatitis occurs 2–3 weeks after the withdrawal of the relevant allergen or cross-sensitizing agent.

Numerous agents have been incriminated in the aetiology of allergic contact dermatitis.[67] They include cosmetics, foodstuffs, plants, topical medicaments and industrial chemicals. Reactions to cosmetics may result from the fragrances, preservatives or lanolin base.[63,68–70] Foodstuffs that have been implicated include flavourings, animal and fish proteins, flour additives, citrus fruits,[71] mangos, onions, garlic and chives.[72,73] The plants include poison ivy,[74,75] various members of the Compositae family,[74] tulips[75a] and *Alstroemeria* (Peruvian lily).[76,77] In the past, topical medicaments such as penicillin, sulphonamides, mercurials and antihistamines were the most common sensitizers.[78] Currently neomycin, benzocaine, ethylenediamine (a stabilizer), parabens preservatives and propylene glycol are common causes of such reactions.[78,78a] Other sensitizers include potassium dichromate, nickel salts,[79] formaldehyde, chemicals in rubber, acrylic resins, colouring agents, textile dyes,[80] cinnamic aldehyde, quarternium-15 and phenylenediamine.[81] Less common causes include vitamin E preparations,[78] topical corticosteroids,[82,83] bacitracin,[84] topical amide anaesthetics,[85] idoxuridine[86] and fluorouracil.[87] Allergic contact dermatitis can be provoked or intensified by chemically related substances. These cross-sensitization reactions are an important clinical problem.[78]

The specific allergen responsible for allergic contact dermatitis can be identified using a patch test.[88] However, these reactions are not always reproducible at sequential or concomitant testing.

Allergic contact dermatitis is a special type of delayed hypersensitivity reaction.[89,89a] The compound responsible for the allergic reaction is usually of low molecular weight (a hapten) and lipid soluble.[90] After penetrating the skin, the hapten becomes bound to a structural or cell surface protein, usually by a covalent bond, thus forming a complete antigen.[43,91] This antigen is processed by Langerhans cells, and possibly macrophages,[92] and then presented to T lymphocytes.[93] The actual way in which the Langerhans cells interact with the antigen and lymphocytes is not known, although the dendritic nature of Langerhans cells obviously assists in their antigen-presenting role.[43,94,95] This induction phase is followed by migration of T lymphocytes to the regional lymph nodes where there is clonal expansion of specifically sensitized lymphocytes.[79] On second and subsequent exposures to the allergen, the elicitant response occurs with proliferation of T lymphocytes both in the skin and regional lymph nodes.[84,90] Lymphocytes liberate various lymphokines in the affected area of skin,[89] leading to a further influx of inflammatory cells, particularly non-sensitized lymphocytes and some eosinophils. Basophils may play a role in a very limited group of circumstances.[91,96] The actual pathogenesis of the spongiosis still requires elucidation. Hypersensitivity to an allergen may persist for prolonged periods, although in a proportion of cases it subsides or disappears with time.[97]

Histopathology[58,59]

Allergic contact dermatitis is characterized in the very early stages by spongiosis which is most marked in the lower epidermis. This is followed

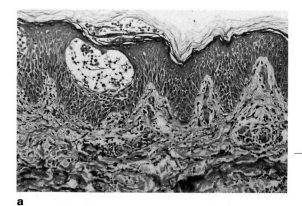

a

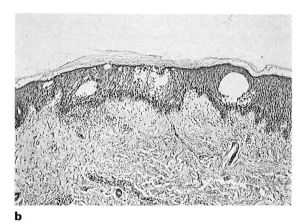

b

Figs. 5.10a,b Allergic contact dermatitis. The spongiosis and spongiotic vesiculation are at different levels of the epidermis.
Haematoxylin — eosin

cytes are predominantly helper T cells with Leu 3 (CD4) positivity.[98] The cells are often positive for Leu 8 and 9, markers which are uncommon in the lymphocytes in mycosis fungoides.[98]

Special variants of allergic contact reaction include the rare pustular form with exocytosis of neutrophils and subcorneal collections of these cells,[64] the purpuric form, which shows a lymphocytic vasculitis,[98a] and the secondary polymorphic reactions in which occasional degenerate basal keratinocytes have been reported.[65] Dermal contact sensitivity, another special variant of allergic contact reaction, has been poorly documented. It may result from exposure to neomycin and zinc and nickel salts. In this reaction pattern, the pronounced oedema of the papillary dermis overshadows the epidermal spongiosis (Fig. 5.11). In the papular lesions that result from penetration of the allergen into the dermis in 'bindii' (*Soliva pterosperma*) dermatitis, there is a mixed dermal infiltrate with some foreign body giant cells.[99] Marked oedema of the papillary dermis is usually present and draining sinuses may form.[99] Finally, lymphomatoid contact dermatitis is a poorly understood variant of allergic contact dermatitis in which the histological appearances may simulate mycosis fungoides.[99a–c] There is a heavy infiltrate of lymphocytes in the upper dermis in a so-called 'T-cell pattern' of distribution.

by the formation of spongiotic vesicles at different horizontal and vertical levels of the epidermis. This often has a very ordered pattern (Fig. 5.10). When present, it allows a distinction to be made from nummular dermatitis which may, at times, closely mimic allergic contact dermatitis histopathologically (see below).

The upper dermis contains a mild to moderately heavy infiltrate of lymphocytes, macrophages and Langerhans cells, with accentuation around the superficial plexus. Eosinophils are usually present, but in some cases only in small numbers. There is exocytosis of lymphocytes and sometimes eosinophils. Eosinophilic spongiosis is a rare pattern.

Marker studies have shown that the lympho-

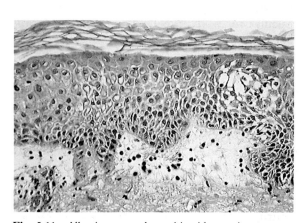

Fig. 5.11 Allergic contact dermatitis with prominent oedema of the papillary dermis. Certain specific contactants are usually associated with this pattern (see text).
Haematoxylin — eosin

NUMMULAR DERMATITIS

Nummular dermatitis (nummular eczema) commences with tiny papules and papulovesicles that become confluent and group themselves into coin-shaped patches which may be single or multiple.[100,101] The surface is usually weeping or crusted and the margins are flat. Central clearing may occur. Sites of predilection include the dorsum of the hands, the extensor surface of the forearms, the lower part of the legs, the outer aspect of the thighs and the posterior aspect of the trunk.[101] The course is usually chronic with remissions and exacerbations.[100,102]

The aetiology is unknown but numerous factors have been implicated over the years, often with very little basis. External irritants, cold, dry weather and a source of infection are factors which may aggravate nummular dermatitis.[102] In one series, all the cases were said to be related to varicose veins and/or oedema of the legs, suggesting stasis with autoeczematization as an aetiological factor.[103] Several drugs, such as methyldopa, gold, and antimycobacterial drugs in combination, appear to provoke nummular eczema.[104] There is no evidence for an atopic basis, as once thought.[100,101,105]

Histopathology[101,103,106]

The appearances vary with the chronicity and activity of the lesion. In early lesions there is epidermal spongiosis and sometimes spongiotic vesiculation associated with some acanthosis and exocytosis of inflammatory cells, including lymphocytes and occasional neutrophils. The spongiotic vesicles sometimes contain inflammatory cells.[103] There is progressive psoriasiform epidermal hyperplasia but this is not always as uniform as in allergic contact dermatitis (see above), which otherwise closely mimics nummular dermatitis. Scale crust often forms above this thickened epidermis. There is a superficial perivascular infiltrate in the dermis composed of lymphocytes, some eosinophils, and occasional neutrophils and plasma cells. Nummular dermatitis often has an 'untidy appearance' microscopically (Fig. 5.12).

Progressive rubbing and scratching of

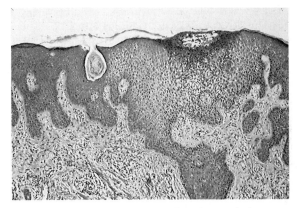

Fig. 5.12 Nummular dermatitis. There is spongiosis, irregular acanthosis and exocytosis of inflammatory cells. Haematoxylin — eosin

individual lesions lead to ulceration or the superimposed changes of lichen simplex chronicus.

SULZBERGER–GARBE SYNDROME

This rare entity, which is of doubtful status, is also known as 'the distinctive exudative discoid and lichenoid chronic dermatosis of Sulzberger and Garbe'.[107,108] It is regarded by some as a variant of nummular dermatitis,[106] although there are clinical differences. These include larger lesions, intense pruritus, a high prevalence of penile and facial lesions and a predilection for Jewish males.[109] Lesions vary in their clinical appearance throughout the course of the disease, and they often mimic many other dermatoses.[107]

Histopathology[106,109]

The histological changes are usually indistinguishable from those of nummular dermatitis. Dilatation of superficial vessels with endothelial swelling and perivascular oedema have been regarded as characteristic features,[107] although not accepted universally.[106]

SEBORRHOEIC DERMATITIS

Seborrhoeic dermatitis is a chronic dermatosis of disputed histogenesis, with a prevalence of 1–3%

in the general population.[110] It consists of erythematous, scaling papules and plaques, sometimes with a greasy yellow appearance with a characteristic distribution on the scalp, ears, eyebrows, eyelid margins and nasolabial area — the so-called 'seborrhoeic areas'.[110,111] Less commonly, it may involve other hair-bearing areas of the body, particularly the flexures and pectoral region. Males are more commonly affected.[110] Seborrhoeic dermatitis is not usually seen until after puberty; the exact nosological position of cases reported in infancy (infantile seborrhoeic eczema) is uncertain,[112] and their occurrence may represent another variant of the atopic tendency.[113–116]

Seborrhoeic dermatitis is one of the most common cutaneous manifestations of the acquired immunodeficiency syndrome (AIDS).[117,118] In these circumstances, it is often quite severe and atypical in distribution. Seborrhoeic dermatitis is also seen with increased frequency in association with a number of medical disorders which include Parkinson's disease,[119] epilepsy, congestive heart failure, obesity, chronic alcoholism, Leiner's disease (exfoliative dermatitis of infancy) and zinc deficiency.[111,117] It may occur as a reaction to arsenic, gold, chlorpromazine, methyldopa[111] and cimetidine.[120]

Pityriasis amiantacea. This condition consists of asbestos-like sticky scales, which bind down tufts of hair, involving localized areas of the scalp.[121,122] Seborrhoeic dermatitis is often present, although whether the two conditions are related is uncertain.[122]

Dandruff. This extremely common affliction of the scalp has been regarded as a mild expression of seborrhoeic dermatitis by some, and as a completely separate disorder by others.[110,123,124]

Traditionally, seborrhoeic dermatitis has been regarded as a dysfunction of sebaceous gland activity, often associated with an oily complexion. This view was supported by its localization to the 'seborrhoeic areas' of the body. However, a more recent study has shown that the sebum excretion rate is not increased in patients with seborrhoeic dermatitis.[125] The role of *Pityrosporum (Malassezia) ovale* in the aetiology is also controversial. This organism is quantitatively increased in both seborrhoeic dermatitis and dandruff but whether this is causal or a secondary event related to the increased keratin scale is disputed.[126–128] There is now increasing evidence favouring a primary role for *P. ovale*, and possibly other organisms as well.[111,126,129–130a]

Histopathology[131,132]

The changes are those of an acute, subacute or chronic spongiotic dermatitis depending on the age of the lesion biopsied (Figs 5.13 and 5.14). In *acute lesions* there is focal, usually mild, spongiosis with overlying scale-crust containing a few neutrophils; the crust is often centred on a follicle. The papillary dermis is mildly oedematous; the blood vessels in the superficial vascular plexus are dilated and there is a mild superficial perivascular infiltrate of lymphocytes, histiocytes and occasional neutrophils.[133] There is some exocytosis of inflammatory cells but this is not as prominent as it is in nummular dermatitis.

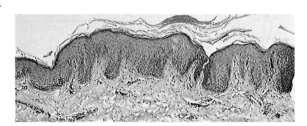

Fig. 5.13 Seborrhoeic dermatitis. Spongiosis is not a feature in this biopsy. There is psoriasiform hyperplasia of the epidermis and focal parakeratosis. Haematoxylin — eosin

In *subacute lesions* there is also psoriasiform hyperplasia, initially slight, with mild spongiosis and the other changes already mentioned. Numerous yeast-like organisms can usually be found in the surface keratin.

Chronic lesions show more pronounced psoriasiform hyperplasia and only minimal spongiosis. Sometimes the differentiation from psoriasis can be difficult but the presence of scale crusts in a folliculocentric distribution favours seborrhoeic dermatitis.

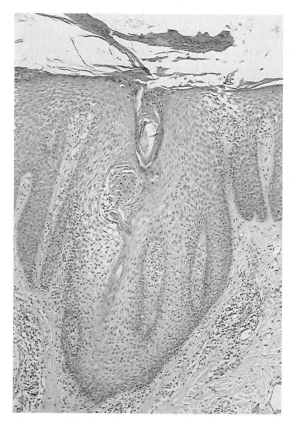

Fig. 5.14 Subacute seborrhoeic dermatitis with spongiosis and parakeratosis in a folliculocentric distribution. Haematoxylin — eosin

The seborrhoeic dermatitis related to AIDS shows spotty cell death of keratinocytes, increased exocytosis of leucocytes and some plasma cells and neutrophils in the superficial dermal infiltrate.[118]

Pityriasis amiantacea. There is spongiosis of both the follicular and surface epithelium with parakeratotic scale at the follicular ostia.[121] Parakeratotic scale is layered around the outer hair shafts in an 'onion skin' arrangement.[121] Sebaceous glands are sometimes shrunken.

Dandruff. There are no spongiotic or inflammatory changes in dandruff, but only minute foci of parakeratosis scattered within the thickened orthokeratotic scale.[133]

ATOPIC DERMATITIS

Atopic dermatitis (atopic eczema) is a chronic, pruritic, inflammatory disease of the skin which usually occurs in individuals with a personal and/or family history of atopy (asthma, allergic rhinitis and atopic dermatitis).[134-139] It is a common disorder with an incidence of approximately 1–2%.[135] Onset is usually in infancy or childhood.[137]

The diagnosis of atopic dermatitis is made on the basis of a constellation of major and minor clinical features.[134,136] Its distinction from infantile seborrhoeic dermatitis is sometimes difficult.[113,139] Major criteria for the diagnosis of atopic dermatitis include the presence of pruritus, chronicity, and a history of atopy, as well as lesions of typical morphology and distribution.[136] In infants and young children there is an erythematous, papulovesicular rash with erosions involving the face and extensor surfaces of the arms and legs.[140] This progresses with time to a scaly, lichenified dermatitis with a predilection for the flexures of the arms and legs.[141] Involvement of the hands and feet may occur at a later stage. Itchy follicular papules on the trunk are quite common in oriental and black patients.[142]

Minor clinical features[134,136] include xerosis, which may be focal or generalized, elevated IgE and IgG₄ in the serum,[141,143,144] increased colonization of the skin with *Staphylococcus aureus*,[145,146] a greater risk of viral and fungal infections of the skin,[147] pityriasis alba,[140] keratosis pilaris, cheilitis, nipple eczema, food intolerance, orbital darkening, white dermatographism and an increased incidence of dermatitis of the hands including pompholyx and irritant dermatitis.[148,149] Contact urticaria, particularly from contact with eggs, is not uncommon in those with atopic dermatitis.[150]

Atopic dermatitis-like skin lesions can be seen in a number of genodermatoses, the most important of which is ichthyosis vulgaris.[140] They also occur in the Wiskott–Aldrich syndrome, in ataxia telangiectasia, and in some patients with phenylketonuria.[140]

The course of atopic dermatitis is one of remissions and exacerbations; the symptom-free periods tend to increase with age.[136] There is also a tendency towards spontaneous remission in adult life.

Although the aetiology and pathogenesis of atopic dermatitis are still unclear, evidence suggests that IgE-mediated late phase responses as well as cell-mediated reactions contribute in some way.[151–155] Langerhans cells appear to be involved in antigen presentation.[156] The IgE-mediated reactions may be to ingested food[141,150] or to inhaled allergens such as human dander[157] and house dust mites.[158–160] The eiconasoids, prostaglandin E_2 and leucotriene B_4, both potent mediators of inflammation, are present in lesional skin in biologically active concentrations.[161] The pathways involved in their release have not been fully elucidated. Genetic factors also appear to be involved in the pathogenesis of atopic dermatitis in some way.[162] This is confirmed by the frequent presence of a family history of atopy and the high concordance in twins.[162]

Histopathology[135,163–166]

Atopic dermatitis presents the typical spectrum of acute, subacute and chronic phases as seen in some other spongiotic (eczematous) processes.[165] As such, the biopsy appearances may be indistinguishable from those seen in nummular dermatitis and allergic contact dermatitis. Subtle features, to be listed below, may sometimes allow the diagnosis to be made on biopsy, although most often the dermatopathologist is restricted to describing the findings as ' consistent with atopic dermatitis'.

Acute lesions show spongiosis and some spongiotic vesiculation,[166] even though some authorities deny the presence of spongiosis in atopic dermatitis. There is usually some intracellular oedema as well, leading to pallor of the cells in the lower epidermis.[164] Exocytosis of lymphocytes is usually present, although it is never a prominent feature. There is a perivascular infiltrate of lymphocytes and macrophages around vessels of the superficial plexus, but there is no significant increase in mast cells or basophils in acute lesions.[164] Occasional eosinophils may be present.

Subacute lesions show irregular acanthosis of the epidermis with eventual psoriasiform hyperplasia. With increasing chronicity of the lesion, the changes of rubbing and scratching become more obvious and the spongiosis less so.

Chronic lesions show hyperkeratosis, moderate to marked psoriasiform hyperplasia and variable, but usually only mild, spongiosis. Mast cells are now significantly increased in the superficial perivascular infiltrate.[163,164] Small vessels appear prominent due to an increase in their number and a thickening of their walls which involves both endothelial cells and the basement membrane.[164] Demyelination, focal vacuolation and fibrosis of cutaneous nerves are also observed.[163,164] Langerhans cells are increased in both the epidermis and the dermis.[167–169] With further lichenification of the lesions, there is prominent hyperkeratosis and some vertical streaking of collagen in the papillary dermis, the changes recognized as lichen simplex chronicus (see p. 84). Lichenified lesions have an increased number of mast cells in the dermis.[170]

If dry skin is biopsied in patients with atopic dermatitis there is usually focal parakeratosis, mild spongiosis and a mild perivascular infiltrate involving the superficial plexus.[171] There is focal hypergranulosis in those with dry skin alone,[172] but a reduced granular layer in those who have concurrent ichthyosis vulgaris.[171]

As already mentioned, there are several morphological features which, if present, favour the diagnosis of atopic dermatitis over the other spongiotic dermatitides which it closely resembles. The assessment of these features is somewhat subjective and, in some, it involves the use of techniques that are not routine. Features which favour the diagnosis of atopic dermatitis include prominence of small blood vessels in the papillary dermis, atrophy of sebaceous glands (this change is usually present only in those who have concomitant ichthyosis vulgaris),[171] and an increase in epidermal volume without psoriasiform folding of the dermo–epidermal interface (Fig. 5.15).[173] This latter change is a useful clue to the diagnosis of atopic dermatitis. Eosinophils and basophils are usually more prominent in the infiltrate of allergic contact dermatitis than in atopic dermatitis. Despite this relative paucity of eosinophils in atopic dermatitis, eosinophil

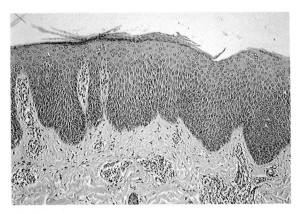

Fig. 5.15 Atopic dermatitis. There is an increase in epidermal volume which is associated with only partial psoriasiform folding. Focal parakeratosis is also present. Haematoxylin — eosin

major basic protein has been reported in the upper dermis in a fibrillar pattern.[174] The diagnostic value of this feature requires further study as do the findings of perivascular IgE[175] and intercellular epidermal staining for IgE, HLA-DR and CDIa in atopic dermatitis.[176] This also applies to the finding of a predominantly T helper-cell infiltrate in atopic dermatitis[168,169] and a T suppressor-cell infiltrate in allergic contact dermatitis;[175] the latter finding does not accord with the results of other studies.[98]

POMPHOLYX

Pompholyx (acral vesicular dermatitis, dyshidrotic eczema) is a common, recurrent, vesicular eruption of the palms and soles which is one of several clinical expressions of so-called 'chronic hand dermatitis'.[177,178] It consists of deep-seated vesicles, often with a burning or itching sensation, most commonly involving the palms, volar aspects of the fingers, and sometimes the sides of the fingers.[178] Lesions usually resolve after several weeks leading to localized areas of desquamation.

The term dyshidrotic eczema was introduced because of a mistaken belief that the pathogenesis of this condition involved hypersecretion of sweat and its retention in the acrosyringia.[179] The term should be avoided. Pompholyx is a

spongiotic dermatitis, the expression of which is modified by the thickened stratum corneum of palmar and plantar skin which reduces the possibility of rupture of the vesicles. Episodes may be precipitated by infections, including dermatophyte infections at other sites ('id reaction' — p. 111),[180] contact sensitivity to allergens such as medicaments and nickel,[180] and emotional stress.[181] An atopic diathesis is sometimes present.[182]

Histopathology[179]

Pompholyx is characterized by spongiosis of the lower malpighian layer with subsequent confluence of the spongiotic foci to form an intraepidermal vesicle (Fig. 5.16). The expanding vesicles displace acrosyringia at the outer margin of the vessels. There is a thick, overlying stratum corneum, characteristic of palms and soles. Other changes include a sparse, superficial perivascular infiltrate of lymphocytes with some exocytosis of these cells. Some persons develop pompholyx-like vesicles which soon evolve into pustules with histopathological features of pustulosis palmaris (see p. 134). A PAS stain should always be performed on vesicular lesions of the palms and soles, particularly if there are any neutrophils within the vesicles or stratum corneum, as dermatophyte infections may mimic the lesions of pompholyx (Fig. 5.17).

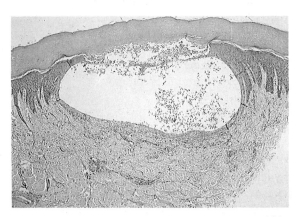

Fig. 5.16 Pompholyx. A unilocular vesicle is present within the epidermis. There is no spongiosis in the epidermis adjacent to the vesicle. Haematoxylin — eosin

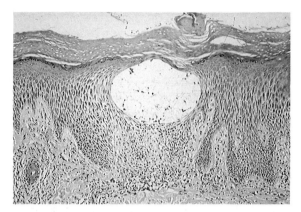

Fig. 5.17 Dermatophyte infection of the hands. There are only scattered neutrophils in the spongiotic vesicle, testimony to the necessity to keep a fungal infection in mind when the spongiotic reaction pattern is present on the hands or feet. Haematoxylin — eosin

Allergic contact dermatitis of the palms and soles may also be difficult to distinguish from pompholyx. In the former condition, mild spongiosis may be present adjacent to the vesicles and there are sometimes eosinophils in the inflammatory infiltrate.

HYPERKERATOTIC DERMATITIS OF THE PALMS

This somewhat neglected entity is a clinical variant of chronic hand dermatitis.[177,183] It presents as a sharply marginated, fissure-prone, hyperkeratotic dermatitis which is limited usually to the palms and occurs chiefly in adults. Involvement of the volar surfaces of the fingers is quite common. Plantar lesions are rare. The cause of the condition is unknown.

Histopathology

The appearances are those of a chronic spongiotic dermatitis with spongiosis and psoriasiform hyperplasia of the epidermis, although the elongation of the rete ridges is usually not as regular as in psoriasis. There is overlying compact orthokeratosis with small foci of parakeratosis. There is a moderately heavy chronic inflammatory cell infiltrate in the papillary

dermis, predominantly in a perivascular location. Lymphocyte exocytosis is quite prominent in the epidermis, but there are usually no neutrophils. The amount of spongiosis allows a distinction to be made from psoriasis.

JUVENILE PLANTAR DERMATOSIS

Juvenile plantar dermatosis is a condition which affects children between the ages of 3 and 14.[184] It presents as a shiny, scaly, erythematous disorder of weight-bearing areas of the feet.[185] Fissuring subsequently develops. Sometimes the hands, particularly the fingertips, are also affected. Most cases improve over the years.

The aetiology is uncertain, with conflicting evidence on the role of atopy and of footwear.[186–189] *Dermatitis palmaris sicca* is a related lesion of the palms.[190]

Histopathology[185,191,192]

Juvenile plantar dermatosis shows variable parakeratosis and hypogranulosis overlying psoriasiform acanthosis. A distinctive feature is the presence of spongiosis, mild spongiotic vesiculation, vacuolization of keratinocytes and exocytosis of lymphocytes, localized to the epidermis surrounding the acrosyringium.[185] Lymphocytes are present in the upper dermis around the sweat ducts at their point of entry into the acrosyringium.[185] Ducts and acrosyringia are not dilated.[191]

STASIS DERMATITIS

Stasis dermatitis (hypostatic dermatitis) is a common disorder of middle-aged and older individuals which is a consequence of impaired venous drainage of the legs.[193] In the early stages, there is oedema of the lower one-third of the legs which have a shiny and erythematous appearance. Subsequently, areas which are dry and scaly or crusted and weeping may develop.[193] Sometimes the changes are most prominent above the medial malleoli. Affected areas become discoloured, due in part to the deposition of haemosiderin in the dermis. Ulceration is a frequent complication of stasis dermatitis of long standing.[193]

Affected skin is unusually sensitive to contactants and, not infrequently, topical medications applied to these areas result in an eczematous reaction which can be quite widespread. This process of 'autoeczematization' is poorly understood.[194] It also encompasses the concept of 'id reactions' in which an eczematous reaction or pompholyx of the hands develops in response to a dermatophyte infection of the feet or allergic contact reaction at a site distant to the subsequent eczematous reaction.

Histopathology[193,195]

Stasis dermatitis is unlikely to be biopsied unless complications such as ulceration, allergic contact dermatitis or basal cell carcinoma arise. In stasis dermatitis, the spongiosis is usually mild, although spongiotic vesiculation may develop if there is a superimposed contact dermatitis. Focal parakeratosis and scale crusts may also be present.

The dermal changes are usually prominent and include a proliferation of small blood vessels in the papillary dermis. This neovascularization may lead occasionally to the formation of a discrete papule. There is variable fibrosis of the dermis which can be quite prominent in cases of long standing. Abundant haemosiderin is present throughout the dermis. It is not localized to the upper third of the dermis as occurs in the pigmented purpuric dermatoses (see p. 239). The veins in the deep dermis and subcutis are often thick-walled.

'Id reactions' on the palms resemble pompholyx (see above), although in several presumptive cases that I have studied there was moderate oedema of the papillary dermis, a change not associated with pompholyx of the more usual type.[195]

PITYRIASIS ROSEA

Pityriasis rosea is a common, acute, self-limited dermatosis in which oval, salmon-pink, papulo-squamous lesions develop on the trunk, neck and proximal extremities.[196] Lesions often follow the lines of skin cleavage. A scaly plaque 2–10 cm in diameter, the 'herald patch', may develop on the trunk 1–2 weeks before the other lesions. Pityriasis rosea has been reported at all ages,[197] but the majority of patients are between 10 and 35 years.[198] Clinical variants include those with acral or facial involvement,[197] oral lesions,[199] a unilateral distribution,[200] or the presence of purpuric or vesicular lesions.[196,201]

The aetiology is unknown, but an infectious aetiology, particularly a virus, has long been suspected. This is supported by a history of a preceding upper respiratory tract infection in some patients,[202] occasional involvement of close-contact pairs,[198] case clustering,[203] modification of the disease by the use of convalescent serum, and the development of a pityriasis rosea-like eruption in some cases of infection by ECHO 6 virus and by *Mycoplasma*.[196] Particles resembling togavirus or arenavirus have been found on electron microscopy of a herald patch,[204] suggesting that this might be the inoculation site. No viruses have ever been cultured.[205] Immunological reactions,[206] particularly cell-mediated, have also been regarded as important.[207]

A pityriasis-rosea-like eruption has been reported in association with the administration of many drugs,[196] including gold, bismuth, arsenicals, clonidine, barbiturates, methoxypromazine, pyribenzamine, penicillamine, isotretinoin, metronidazole[208] and captopril.[209]

Histopathology[207,210,211]

Although the lesions are clinically papulosquamous, microscopy shows a spongiotic tissue reaction. The histopathological features are not pathognomonic, although in most cases they are sufficiently characteristic to allow the diagnosis to be made, even without a clinical history (Fig. 5.18). The epidermis often has a vaguely undulating appearance. There is usually focal parakeratosis, sometimes with the formation of parakeratotic mounds. There is a diminution of the granular layer and focal spongiosis with lymphocyte exocytosis. Small spongiotic vesicles,

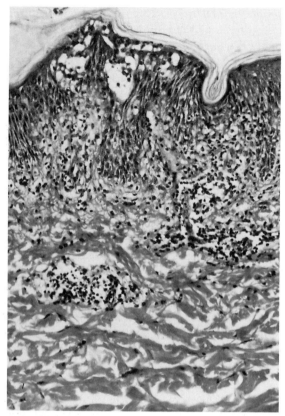

Fig. 5.18 Pityriasis rosea. Note the undulating epidermis and the small Pautrier-like foci.
Haematoxylin — eosin

sometimes simulating Pautrier microabscesses because of the aggregation of lymphocytes within them, are a characteristic feature; they are present in most cases if several levels are examined. Dyskeratotic cells may be seen at all levels of the epidermis; they are more common in the herald patch. Apoptotic keratinocytes are present in the lower epidermis in lesions undergoing involution. Multinucleate epidermal cells are uncommon. Focal acantholytic dyskeratosis has been reported once.[212]

The papillary dermis shows some oedema and sometimes homogenization of collagen. There may be some melanin incontinence. Red cell extravasation is common in the upper dermis, and this may extend into the lower layers of the epidermis. There is a mild to moderate lymphohistiocytic infiltrate in the upper dermis, with some eosinophils in the infiltrate in older lesions.

Electron microscopy. Ultrastructural examination has confirmed the presence of dyskeratotic cells in some patients.[213] These cells show aggregation of tonofilaments, some cytoplasmic vacuoles and intracytoplasmic desmosomes.[214] Cytolytic degeneration of keratinocytes adjacent to Langerhans cells has been reported in a herald patch.[215] Virus-like particles were seen in one recent study.[213]

PAPULAR ACRODERMATITIS OF CHILDHOOD

Papular acrodermatitis of childhood (Gianotti–Crosti syndrome) is an uncommon, self-limited disease of low infectivity characterized by the triad of an erythematous papular eruption of several weeks' duration, localized to the face and limbs, mild lymphadenopathy and acute hepatitis which is usually anicteric.[216,217] The skin lesions are flat-topped papules 1–2 mm in diameter, which sometimes coalesce. They may be mildly pruritic. Hepatitis B surface antigen is often present in the serum.[218–220]

It is now apparent that other viral infections, in particular infection with the Epstein–Barr virus,[221,222] coxsackie virus A16,[223] parainfluenza virus, hepatitis A virus,[224] hepatitis C virus[225] and cytomegalovirus,[226] are rarely associated with a similar acral dermatitis;[227,228] hepatitis and lymphadenopathy are not commonly present in these circumstances.[227,228] Gianotti used the term 'papulovesicular acro-related syndrome' for these cases.[229] Although infections associated with these other viruses often pursue a longer course, and may have tiny vesicular lesions, individual cases occur which closely resemble those associated with the hepatitis B virus. Accordingly it seems best to group all these virus-related disorders under the term Gianotti–Crosti syndrome.

Histopathology[230]

Although the changes are not diagnostically specific, they are often sufficiently characteristic at least to suggest the diagnosis. The appearances at low magnification often suggest that three tissue reactions — lichenoid, spongiotic and vasculitic are present simultaneously.[227] On closer inspection there is prominent exocytosis of mononuclear cells into the lower epidermis. This is usually associated with some basal vacuolar change, but cell death is not a conspicuous feature.[231] The spongiosis is usually mild, but small spongiotic vesicles containing a few inflammatory cells and resembling those of pityriasis rosea may be present (see above). Although most observers specifically deny the presence of a vasculitis, because of the absence of fibrin,[216] there is always a tight perivascular infiltrate of lymphocytes associated with variable endothelial swelling. In many instances the changes merit a diagnosis of lymphocytic vasculitis.[227] The inflammatory infiltrate not only fills the papillary dermis and extends into the epidermis, but it usually involves the mid and even the lower dermis to a lesser extent. There is often some oedema of the papillary dermis. Epidermal spongiosis is less prominent in cases related to the hepatitis B virus.

SPONGIOTIC DRUG REACTIONS

Spongiotic reactions to drugs occur in several different clinical and pathogenetic settings, although in some instances the precise mechanism that results in the spongiosis is unknown. A delayed hypersensitivity response is usually suspected.[232] The three major categories of spongiotic drug reactions are provocation of an endogenous dermatitis, systemic contact reactions and a miscellaneous group. Excluded from this discussion are the spongiotic reactions resembling pityriasis rosea produced by gold, captopril,[209] and other drugs (see p. 111), the phototoxic and photoallergic reactions produced by a variety of drugs[233] (see p. 579), and allergic contact dermatitis resulting from the topical application of various substances (see p. 103). Although there is mild spongiosis in the exanthematous (morbilliform) eruptions, these are histopathologically distinct from the other spongiotic reactions. They are discussed on page 562.

Reactions resembling seborrhoeic dermatitis or nummular dermatitis have been reported following the ingestion of various drugs including cimetidine, methyldopa,[104] and antituberculous therapy (see p. 105).[104] This is assumed to be a *provocation reaction* in an individual with a predisposition to the development of an endogenous dermatitis.[104]

Systemic contact dermatitis results from the administration of an allergen to an individual who has been sensitized to that agent by previous contact with it or with a related substance.[232] Systemic contact dermatitis may present as an exacerbation of vesicular hand dermatitis, as an eczematous flare at sites of previously positive patch tests, or as a systemic eczematous eruption with a predisposition for the buttocks, genital areas, elbow flexures, axillae, eyelids and side of the neck.[234] The term 'baboon syndrome' was coined for this eruption.[234] This is an important category of spongiotic drug reaction with numerous drugs incriminated. They include antibiotics used topically as well as systemically, such as neomycin and gentamicin, as well as procaine, quinine, chloral hydrate, clonidine, minoxidil, codeine, disulfiram, thiamine, isoniazid, cinnamon oil, aminophylline (cross-reacting with ethylenediamine, a stabilizer in creams)[235] and certain oral hypoglycaemic agents, diuretics and sweetening agents which cross-react with sulphonamides.[234,236,237]

The *miscellaneous category* of drugs producing the spongiotic tissue reaction undoubtedly includes agents which should be more appropriately included in other categories. For example, thiazide diuretics are usually included among the agents that produce photosensitive eruptions, but it appears that, on occasions, an eruption is produced which is not confined to exposed areas.[238,239] Other drugs in this miscellaneous category include sulphasalazine,[239] indomethacin,[239] allopurinol,[239] piroxicam[240] calcitonin and phenytoin sodium (sensitivity reaction).[241] The subcutaneous injection of heparin may produce an eczematous plaque.[242,243] Gold, in addition to causing a pityriasis-rosea-like reaction, also produces an eczematous eruption which may last for up to 12 months after the cessation of gold therapy.[244,245]

The incidence of spongiotic drug reactions is difficult to assess. Some reports make no mention of this type of reaction. One study reported that approximately 10% of cutaneous drug reactions were of 'eczematous' type.[246] In addition to generalized papules and eczematous plaques, a fixed eczematous eruption can also occur, the agents responsible usually being antibiotics.

Histopathology

By definition, there is epidermal spongiosis: this may occur at all levels of the epidermis. Spongiotic vesiculation is sometimes present. A characteristic feature is the presence of exocytosis of lymphocytes and occasionally of eosinophils. Often there is more exocytosis than would be expected for the amount of spongiosis in the

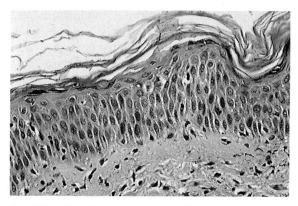

Fig. 5.20 Spongiotic drug reaction. The spongiosis is minimal in this area of the biopsy. Note the exocytosis of lymphocytes and an apoptotic keratinocyte. Haematoxylin — eosin

region (Fig. 5.19). Rare Civatte bodies (apoptotic cells) are almost invariably present, but a careful search is usually necessary to find these (Fig. 5.20). Small spongiotic vesicles containing lymphocytes are a characteristic feature of pityriasis-rosea-like eruptions (Fig. 5.21). In exanthematous eruptions the spongiosis and exocytosis are confined to the basal layers of the epidermis in a rather characteristic pattern.[247] Other epidermal changes in spongiotic drug reactions include variable parakeratosis and, in chronic lesions, some acanthosis.

The papillary dermis shows mild to moderate oedema and there is a predominantly perivascular infiltrate of lymphocytes. Occasional

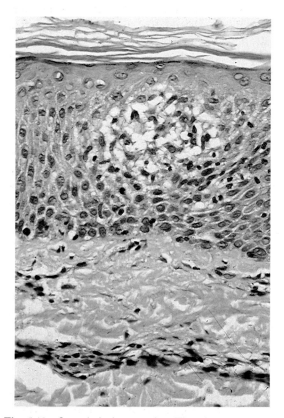

Fig. 5.19 Spongiotic drug reaction. There is more exocytosis of inflammatory cells in spongiotic drug reactions than in most other spongiotic diseases. Haematoxylin — eosin

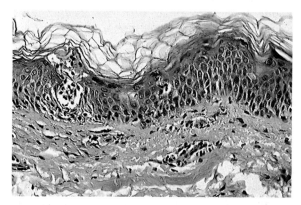

Fig. 5.21 Spongiotic drug reaction with pityriasis-rosea-like features. Captopril was implicated. Haematoxylin — eosin

eosinophils are often present, but this is not invariable. Some of the lymphoid cells appear to be larger than the usual mature lymphocyte. In a study of gold-induced reactions the lymphocytes were characterized as T helper cells.[245] Another feature of the infiltrate is its tendency to extend into the mid dermis, somewhat deeper than is usual with other spongiotic disorders. Red cell extravasation is sometimes present in the upper dermis.[245] Pigment incontinence is uncommon.

CHRONIC SUPERFICIAL DERMATITIS

Chronic superficial dermatitis (persistent superficial dermatitis, small plaque parapsoriasis,[248] digitate dermatosis[249]) is characterized by well-defined, round to oval patches with a fine 'cigarette-paper' scale, usually situated on the trunk and proximal parts of the extremities.[248,250] Individual lesions measure 2–5 cm in diameter, although larger patches, sometimes with a digitate pattern, may be found on the lower limbs, particularly the thighs.[251] The lesions usually have a reddish-brown colour, although the hue is yellowish in a small number of cases.[252] The term xanthoerythrodermia perstans was applied in the past to these latter cases.[249,253]

Onset of the disease is usually in middle life and there is a male predominance. The lesions are mostly asymptomatic and persistent, although a minority clears spontaneously.[254] Chronic superficial dermatitis, unlike large plaque parapsoriasis, with which it has been confused in the past, does not progress to lymphoma.[255] Its aetiology is unknown.

Histopathology[248,251,256]

Although classified with the spongiotic tissue reaction, it must be emphasized that the spongiosis in chronic superficial dermatitis is usually only focal and mild. There is usually focal parakeratosis or focal scale crust formation implying preceding spongiosis. The epidermis is usually acanthotic and, in older lesions, there may be psoriasiform hyperplasia.

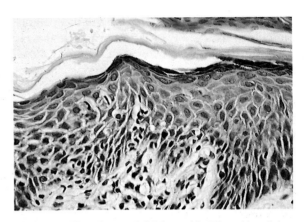

Fig. 5.22   Chronic superficial dermatitis. The epidermis is only mildly spongiotic and there is focal exocytosis of mature lymphocytes into the epidermis.
Haematoxylin — eosin

A mild infiltrate of lymphocytes and occasional histiocytes is present around blood vessels in the superficial plexus. Cells often extend high in the papillary dermis, a characteristic feature. Exocytosis of these cells is common, but mild (Fig. 5.22). There are no interface changes as in pityriasis lichenoides chronica[248] and no atypical lymphoid cells.

LIGHT REACTIONS

Epidermal spongiosis may be seen in photoallergic dermatitis (see p. 580), phototoxic dermatitis (see p. 579), the so-called eczematous form of polymorphous light eruption and in certain persistent light reactions such as actinic reticuloid (see p. 584).

Histopathology

Photoallergic and phototoxic reactions are akin to allergic contact and irritant contact reactions respectively. They may be morphologically indistinguishable, although in some photoallergic reactions the inflammatory cell infiltrate extends deeper in the dermis. There is usually a superficial and deep perivascular infiltrate of lymphocytes in the papulovesicular form (so-called 'eczematous' type) of polymorphous light eruption. The epidermis shows variable spongiosis leading to spongiotic vesiculation.

Actinic reticuloid may have a mildly spongiotic epidermis. However, the diagnosis is usually made on the basis of the dense, polymorphous infiltrate in the upper dermis which includes some large lymphoid cells with hyperchromatic nuclei and stellate fibroblasts.

DERMATOPHYTOSES

Dermatophyte infections can present with a spongiotic dermatitis and clinically they can mimic a range of 'eczematous' dermatitides (see p. 642).

Histopathology

In addition to the spongiosis, the stratum corneum is usually abnormal, with compact orthokeratosis, or parakeratosis sandwiched between orthokeratotic layers, or the presence of neutrophils in the stratum corneum (see p. 643). Sometimes spongiotic pustules are present. The presence of neutrophils within the epidermis or stratum corneum warrants a careful search for hyphae, including the use of the PAS stain.

ARTHROPOD BITES

Epidermal spongiosis is a common finding in certain arthropod bite reactions, particularly scabies. Vesicles and, rarely, bullous lesions may develop in response to some arthropods. Contact with moths of the genus *Hylesia* is said to cause vesicular lesions (see p. 726).

Histopathology

There is variable spongiosis, sometimes leading to spongiotic vesiculation. Exocytosis of eosinophils through the epidermis may be present, but eosinophilic spongiosis is quite uncommon. The dermis contains a superficial and deep perivascular infiltrate of lymphocytes and eosinophils; characteristically, there are interstitial eosinophils.

GROVER'S DISEASE

There is a rare variant of Grover's disease, clinically indistinguishable from the other histopathological variants, in which spongiosis is present (see p. 282).

Histopathology

Suprabasal clefting with some overlying dyskeratotic cells and grains will be found in addition to the spongiosis.

TOXIC ERYTHEMA OF PREGNANCY

Toxic erythema of pregnancy (see p. 234) presents as an intensely pruritic eruption of papules and urticarial plaques towards the end of pregnancy.

Histopathology

The tissue reaction is a subtle lymphocytic vasculitis with variable oedema of the papillary dermis. Epidermal spongiosis is present in one-third of cases. There may be focal parakeratosis as well.

ERYTHEMA ANNULARE CENTRIFUGUM

There are one or more annular, erythematous lesions which may spread outwards or remain stationary. A fine scale is sometimes present inside the advancing edge (see p. 235).

Histopathology

A biopsy through the advancing edge will show focal spongiosis and parakeratosis with an underlying superficial perivascular infiltrate of lymphocytes, often with a 'coat-sleeve' appearance. There are some similarities to pityriasis rosea, although a biopsy taken at right angles to the edge of erythema annulare centrifugum will show a much more localized process. A variant without spongiosis and with a deep as well as superficial inflammatory infiltrate also occurs.

Table 5.1 Histopathological features of the spongiotic diseases (excluding eosinophilic, miliarial and follicular variants)

Disease	Histopathological features
Irritant contact dermatitis	Superficial ballooning, necrosis and neutrophils; mild irritants produce spongiotic dermatitis mimicking allergic contact dermatitis, although superficial apoptotic keratinocytes may also be present.
Allergic contact dermatitis	Variable spongiosis and vesiculation at different horizontal and vertical levels, with an 'ordered' pattern; mild exocytosis; progressive psoriasiform hyperplasia with chronicity; usually eosinophils in superficial dermal infiltrate; superficial dermal oedema.
Nummular dermatitis	May mimic allergic contact dermatitis but usually more 'untidy'. Neutrophils may be in dermal infiltrate and even the epidermis; the psoriasiform hyperplasia in chronic cases may show variable thickening of adjacent rete pegs.
Seborrhoeic dermatitis	Variable spongiosis and psoriasiform hyperplasia depending on activity and chronicity. Scale crust and spongiosis may localize to follicular ostia.
Atopic dermatitis	Mimics other spongiotic diseases with variable spongiosis (usually quite mild) and psoriasiform hyperplasia; subtle features include prominence of vessels in the papillary dermis, increased epidermal volume without necessarily producing psoriasiform folding; eosinophil major basic protein present, sometimes disproportionate to eosinophils.
Pompholyx	Vesiculation with peripheral displacement of acrosyringia; process usually more sharply defined than allergic contact dermatitis of palms and soles; some evolve into picture of pustulosis palmaris with neutrophils (important to exclude fungi in these cases with PAS stain).
Stasis dermatitis	Mild spongiosis only; proliferation of superficial dermal vessels; extravasation of erythrocytes; abundant haemosiderin.
Pityriasis rosea	Undulating epidermis with focal parakeratosis and spongiotic vesicles, sometimes resembling small Pautrier microabscesses; lymphocyte exocytosis; sometimes erythrocyte extravasation in papillary dermis; 'herald patch' is more psoriasiform.
Papular acrodermatitis of childhood	Three tissue reaction patterns (lichenoid, spongiotic and lymphocytic vasculitis) often present; small spongiotic vesicles resembling pityriasis rosea may be present.
Spongiotic drug reactions	Spongiosis with conspicuous exocytosis of lymphocytes relative to the amount of spongiosis; rare apoptotic keratinocytes; eosinophils, plasma cells and activated lymphocytes may be in superficial dermal infiltrate; may show mid-dermal spillover; sometimes superficial dermal oedema.
Chronic superficial dermatitis	Only mild spongiosis and focal parakeratosis with variable psoriasiform hyperplasia; superficial perivascular infiltrate with characteristic upward extension and mild exocytosis.
Light reactions	Variable, usually mild spongiosis; superficial and deep perivascular dermal inflammation; a deep infiltrate is not invariable in lesions of short duration; subepidermal oedema in some cases of polymorphous light eruption; stellate fibroblasts, vertical collagen streaking, variable psoriasiform hyperplasia and some atypical lymphocytes with exocytosis in actinic reticuloid; scattered 'sunburn cells' in phototoxic lesions (sometimes with only mild other changes); deeply extending, straight, basophilic (elastotic) fibres in lesions of long duration.
Dermatophytoses	Neutrophils in stratum corneum, or compact orthokeratosis or 'sandwich sign' should alert observer to perform a PAS stain. Spongiotic vesicles may form on palms and soles.
Arthropod bites	Spongiotic vesicles containing variable numbers of eosinophils; superficial and deep dermal inflammation with interstitial eosinophils.
Grover's disease	Spongiosis with focal acantholysis in the spongiotic variant; untidy superficial dermal inflammation.
Toxic erythema of pregnancy	Spongiosis mild and inconstant; variable papillary dermal oedema; tight superficial perivascular infiltrate sometimes extending to mid dermis.
Erythema annulare centrifugum	Mild spongiosis and focal parakeratosis at periphery of lesion; mild perivascular cuffing with lymphocytes.
Pigmented purpuric dermatoses	Spongiosis mild and inconstant; lymphocytic vasculitis with variably dense infiltrate in the papillary dermis; haemosiderin in the upper dermis.
Pityriasis alba	Clinical diagnosis; mild focal spongiosis with minimal parakeratosis.
Erythroderma	Mild spongiosis; variable psoriasiform hyperplasia; appearances depend on underlying disease; a difficult diagnosis without clinical history.
Mycosis fungoides	Mild spongiosis, variable epidermal hyperplasia and epidermal mucinosis; epidermotropism, often with Pautrier microabscesses; variable cytological atypia of lymphocytes which extend upwards into the papillary dermis.

PIGMENTED PURPURIC DERMATOSES

Epidermal spongiosis, usually mild, may be present in several clinical variants of the pigmented purpuric dermatoses (see p. 238). The presence of a superficial, band-like infiltrate of inflammatory cells, often associated with a lymphocytic vasculitis, and the deposition of haemosiderin in the upper dermis usually overshadow the spongiosis.

PITYRIASIS ALBA

Pityriasis alba consists of variably hypopigmented, slightly scaly patches, usually on the head and neck of atopic individuals (see p. 310).

Histopathology

Pityriasis alba should be thought of if there is mild epidermal spongiosis with minimal exocytosis and focal parakeratosis in the clinical setting of hypopigmented lesions. There is a reduction in melanin in the basal layer of the epidermis.

ERYTHRODERMA

Erythroderma (exfoliative dermatitis) may complicate various spongiotic dermatitides, including atopic dermatitis, seborrhoeic dermatitis, photosensitive eczematous processes (for example, actinic reticuloid), nummular dermatitis, stasis dermatitis and contact dermatitis (see p. 554).

Histopathology

The underlying, pre-existing dermatosis is not always diagnosable when erythroderma supervenes. Often the amount of spongiosis is mild, even in cases with a pre-existing spongiotic dermatitis; there may even be psoriasiform hyperplasia of the epidermis without spongiosis in these circumstances.

MYCOSIS FUNGOIDES

Mycosis fungoides is a cutaneous T-cell lymphoma which evolves through several clinical stages (see p. 1033). An unequivocal diagnosis is sometimes difficult to make in the early stages of the disease.

Histopathology

There has been controversy in the past regarding the presence or absence of spongiosis in lesions of mycosis fungoides.[257,258] In one recent study slight spongiosis was found in 38% of lesions in the patch/plaque stage and moderate spongiosis in a further 17%.[258] There was no microvesiculation.[258] The epidermis appears to contain increased amounts of acid mucopolysaccharides. Other features which allow mycosis fungoides to be distinguished from other spongiotic disorders include the presence of a band-like infiltrate of lymphocytes (some atypical) and often eosinophils and plasma cells in the upper dermis associated with papillary dermal fibrosis. There is usually prominent epidermotropism of the lymphoid cells.

Spongiosis may also be found in the Sézary syndrome (see p. 1038).

REFERENCES

Introduction

1. Ackerman AB. More about spongiosis. Am J Dermatopathol 1984; 6: 419–420.
2. Russell Jones R. The histogenesis of eczema. Clin Exp Dermatol 1983; 8: 213–225.
3. Ackerman AB, Ragaz A. A plea to expunge the word "eczema" from the lexicon of dermatology and dermatopathology. Am J Dermatopathol 1982; 4: 315–326.
4. Sulzberger MB. Eczema viewed from the perspective of 60 years' experience. Am J Dermatopathol 1982; 4: 337–338.

5. Stenn KS, Balin AK, Higgins T, Stenn JO. Spongiosis. J Am Acad Dermatol 1981; 5: 213–214.
6. Russell Jones R. Spongiosis — a passive phenomenon? J Am Acad Dermatol 1982; 6: 547–549.
7. Russell Jones R. PEEPO: papular eruption with elimination of papillary oedema. Br J Dermatol 1982; 106: 393–400.
8. Russell Jones R, McDonald DM. Eczema. Immunopathogenesis and histogenesis. Am J Dermatopathol 1982; 4: 335–336.
9. Ackerman AB. Subtle clues to histopathologic findings from gross pathology (clinical lesions). Collarettes of scales as signs of spongiosis. Am J Dermatopathol 1979; 1: 267–272.

Eosinophilic spongiosis

10. Emmerson RW, Wilson-Jones E. Eosinophilic spongiosis in pemphigus. Arch Dermatol 1968; 97: 252–257.
11. Knight AG, Black MM, Delaney TJ. Eosinophilic spongiosis. A clinical histological and immunofluorescent correlation. Clin Exp Dermatol 1976; 1: 141–153.
12. Brodersen I, Frentz G, Thomsen K. Eosinophilic spongiosis in early pemphigus foliaceus. Acta Derm Venereol 1978; 58: 368–369.
13. Cooper A, Le Guay J, Wells JV. Childhood pemphigus initially seen as eosinophilic spongiosis. Arch Dermatol 1981; 117: 662–663.
14. Osteen FB, Wheeler CE Jr, Briggaman RA, Puritz EM. Pemphigus foliaceus. Early clinical appearance as dermatitis herpetiformis with eosinophilic spongiosis. Arch Dermatol 1976; 112: 1148–1152.
15. Jablonska S, Chorzelski TP, Beutner EH, Chorzelska J. Herpetiform pemphigus, a variable pattern of pemphigus. Int J Dermatol 1975; 14: 353–359.
16. Marsden RA, Dawber RPR, Millard PR, Mowat AG. Herpetiform pemphigus induced by penicillamine. Br J Dermatol 1977; 97: 451–452.
17. Nishioka K, Hashimoto K, Katayama I et al. Eosinophilic spongiosis in bullous pemphigoid. Arch Dermatol 1984; 120: 1166–1168.
18. Kennedy C, Hodge L, Sanderson KV. Eosinophilic spongiosis: a localized bullous dermatosis unassociated with pemphigus. Clin Exp Dermatol 1978; 3: 117–122.
19. Black MM. Eosinophilic spongiosis with polycythaemia rubra vera. Proc R Soc Med 1977; 70: 139–140.

Miliarial spongiosis

20. Gupta AK, Ellis CN, Madison KC, Voorhees JJ. Miliaria crystallina occurring in a patient treated with isotretinoin. Cutis 1986; 38: 275–276.
21. O'Brien JP. A study of miliaria rubra, tropical anhidrosis and anhidrotic asthenia. Br J Dermatol 1947; 59: 124–158.
22. O'Brien JP. Tropical anhidrotic asthenia. Its definition and relationship to other heat disorders. Arch Intern Med 1948; 81: 799–831.
23. Holzle E, Kligman AM. The pathogenesis of miliaria rubra. Role of the resident microflora. Br J Dermatol 1978; 99: 117–137.
24. Loewenthal LJA. The pathogenesis of miliaria. The role of sodium chloride. Arch Dermatol 1961; 84: 2–17.
25. O'Brien JP. The aetiology of poral closure. II. The role of staphylococcal infection in miliaria rubra and bullous impetigo. J Invest Dermatol 1950; 15: 102–133.
26. Sulzberger MB, Griffin TB. Induced miliaria, postmiliarial hypohidrosis, and some potential sequelae. Arch Dermatol 1969; 99: 145–149.
27. Henning DR, Griffin TB, Maibach HI. Studies on changes in skin surface bacteria in induced miliaria and associated hypohidrosis. Acta Derm Venereol 1972; 52: 371–375.
28. Lyons RE, Levine R, Auld D. Miliaria rubra. A manifestation of staphylococcal disease. Arch Dermatol 1962; 86: 282–286.
29. Singh E. The role of bacteria in anhidrosis. Dermatologica 1973; 146: 256–261.
30. Kossard S, Commens CA. Keratotic miliaria precipitated by radiotherapy. Arch Dermatol 1988; 124: 855–856.

Follicular spongiosis

31. Hitch JM, Lund HZ. Disseminate and recurrent infundibulo-folliculitis. Report of a case. Arch Dermatol 1968; 97: 432–435.
32. Hitch JM, Lund HZ. Disseminate and recurrent infundibulo-folliculitis. Arch Dermatol 1972; 105: 580–583.
33. Thew MA, Wood MG. Disseminate and recurrent infundibulo-folliculitis. Report of a second case. Arch Dermatol 1969; 100: 728–733.
34. Soyinka F. Recurrent disseminated infundibulofolliculitis. Int J Dermatol 1973; 12: 314–317.
35. Owen WR, Wood C. Disseminate and recurrent infundibulofolliculitis. Arch Dermatol 1979; 115: 174–175.

Other spongiotic disorders

36. Marks JG Jr, Zaino RJ, Bressler MF, Williams JV. Changes in lymphocyte and Langerhans cell populations in allergic and irritant contact dermatitis. Int J Dermatol 1987; 26: 354–357.
37. Rietschel RL. Irritant contact dermatitis. Dermatol Clin 1984; 2: 545–551.
38. Willis CM, Stephens CJM, Wilkinson JD. Experimentally-induced irritant contact dermatitis. Determination of optimum irritant concentrations. Contact Dermatitis 1988; 18: 20–24.
39. Hatch KL, Maibach HI. Textile fiber dermatitis. Contact Dermatitis 1985; 12: 1–11.
40. Webster GL. Irritant plants in the spurge family (Euphorbiaceae). Clin Dermatol 1986; 4: 36–45.
41. Worobec SM, Hickey TA, Kinghorn AD et al. Irritant contact dermatitis from an ornamental Euphorbia. Contact Dermatitis 1981; 7: 19–22.
42. Dooms-Goossens AE, Debusschere KM, Gevers DM et al. Contact dermatitis caused by airborne agents. A review and case reports. J Am Acad Dermatol 1986; 15: 1–10.
43. Andersen KE, Benezra C, Burrows D et al. Contact dermatitis. A review. Contact Dermatitis 1987; 16: 55–78.
44. Wahlberg JE, Maibach HI. Sterile cutaneous pustules: a manifestation of primary irritancy? Identification of

contact pustulogens. J Invest Dermatol 1981; 76: 381–383.

45. Dooms-Goossens A, Loncke J, Michiels JL et al. Pustular reactions to hexafluorosilicate in foam rubber. Contact Dermatitis 1985; 12: 42–47.

46. Rycroft RJG. Acute ulcerative contact dermatitis from Portland cement. Br J Dermatol 1980; 102: 487–489.

47. Fischer G, Commens C. Cement burns: rare or rarely reported? Australas J Dermatol 1986; 27: 8–10.

48. van der Valk PGM, Maibach HI. Potential for irritation increases from the wrist to the cubital fossa. Br J Dermatol 1989; 121: 709–712.

49. Shmunes E. Contact dermatitis in atopic individuals. Dermatol Clin 1984; 2: 561–566.

50. Rystedt I. Atopy, hand eczema, and contact dermatitis: summary of recent large scale studies. Semin Dermatol 1986; 5: 290–300.

51. Goh CL. An epidemiological comparison between hand eczema and non-hand eczema. Br J Dermatol 1988; 118: 797–801.

52. Agner T, Serup J. Seasonal variation of skin resistance to irritants. Br J Dermatol 1989; 121: 323–328.

53. Willis CM, Stephens CJM, Wilkinson JD. Epidermal damage induced by irritants in man: a light and electron microscopic study. J Invest Dermatol 1989; 93: 695–699.

54. Willis CM, Young E, Brandon DR, Wilkinson JD. Immunopathological and ultrastructural findings in human allergic and irritant contact dermatitis. Br J Dermatol 1986; 115: 305–316.

55. Nater JP, Hoedemaeker PJ. Histological differences between irritant and allergic patch test reactions in man. Contact Dermatitis 1976; 2: 247–253.

56. Mahmoud G, Lachapelle JM, van Neste D. Histological assessment of skin damage by irritants: its possible use in the evaluation of a 'barrier cream'. Contact Dermatitis 1984; 11: 179–185.

57. Nater JP, Baar AJM, Hoedemaeker PJ. Histological aspects of skin reactions to propylene glycol. Contact Dermatitis 1977; 3: 181–185.

58. Taylor RM. Histopathology of contact dermatitis. Clin Dermatol 1986; 4: 18–22.

59. Ackerman AB, Niven J, Grant-Kels JM. Differential diagnosis in dermatopathology. Philadelphia: Lea & Febiger, 1982; 14–17.

60. Reitamo S, Tolvanen E, Konttinen YT et al. Allergic and toxic contact dermatitis: inflammatory cell subtypes in epicutaneous test reactions. Br J Dermatol 1981; 105: 521–527.

61. Lindberg M. Studies on the cellular and subcellular reactions in epidermis at irritant and allergic dermatitis. Acta Derm Venereol (Suppl) 1982; 105: 1–45.

61a. Kanerva L. Electron microscopic observations of dyskeratosis, apoptosis, colloid bodies and fibrillar degeneration after skin irritation with dithranol. J Cutan Pathol 1990; 17: 37–44.

62. de Groot AC, Beverdam EGA, Ayong CT et al. The role of contact allergy in the spectrum of adverse effects caused by cosmetics and toiletries. Contact Dermatitis 1988; 19: 195–201.

63. Eiermann HJ, Larsen W, Maibach HI, Taylor JS. Prospective study of cosmetic reactions: 1977–1980. J Am Acad Dermatol 1982; 6: 909–917.

64. Burkhart CG. Pustular allergic contact dermatitis: a distinct clinical and pathological entity. Cutis 1981; 27: 630–638.

65. Goh CL. Urticarial papular and plaque eruptions. A noneczematous manifestation of allergic contact dermatitis. Int J Dermatol 1989; 28: 172–176.

66. Meneghini CL, Angelini G. Secondary polymorphic eruptions in allergic contact dermatitis. Dermatologica 1981; 163: 63–70.

67. Kuiters GRR, Sillevis Smitt JH, Cohen EB, Bos JD. Allergic contact dermatitis in children and young adults. Arch Dermatol 1989; 125: 1531–1533.

68. Larsen WG, Maibach HI. Fragrance contact allergy. Semin Dermatol 1982; 1: 85–90.

69. Larsen WG. Perfume dermatitis. J Am Acad Dermatol 1985; 12: 1–9.

70. Cronin E. "New" allergens of clinical importance. Semin Dermatol 1982; 1: 33–41.

71. Cardullo AC, Ruszkowski AM, DeLeo VA. Allergic contact dermatitis resulting from sensitivity to citrus peel, geraniol, and citral. J Am Acad Dermatol 1989; 21: 395–397.

72. Hausen BM, Hjorth N. Skin reactions to topical food exposure. Dermatol Clin 1984; 2: 567–578.

73. Nethercott JR, Holness DL. Occupational dermatitis in food handlers and bakers. J Am Acad Dermatol 1989; 21: 485–490.

74. Mitchell JC, Rook AJ. Diagnosis of contact dermatitis from plants. Semin Dermatol 1982; 1: 25–32.

75. Hurwitz RM, Rivera HP, Guin JD. Black-spot poison ivy dermatitis. An acute irritant contact dermatitis superimposed upon an allergic contact dermatitis. Am J Dermatopathol 1984; 6: 319–322.

75a. Gette MT, Marks JE Jr. Tulip fingers. Arch Dermatol 1990; 126: 203–205.

76. Marks JG Jr. Allergic contact dermatitis to *Alstroemeria*. Arch Dermatol 1988; 124: 914–916.

77. Thiboutot DM, Hamory BH, Marks JG Jr. Dermatoses among floral shop workers. J Am Acad Dermatol 1990; 22: 54–58.

78. Fisher AA. Contact dermatitis from topical medicaments. Semin Dermatol 1982; 1: 49–57.

78a. Hogan DJ. Allergic contact dermatitis to ethylenediamine. A continuing problem. Dermatol Clin 1990; 8: 133–136.

79. Benezra C, Foussereau J. Allergic contact dermatitis — a chemical-clinical approach. Semin Dermatol 1982; 1: 73–83.

80. Hatch KL, Maibach HI. Textile dye dermatitis. J Am Acad Dermatol 1985; 12: 1079–1092.

81. Storrs FJ, Rosenthal LE, Adams RM et al. Prevalence and relevance of allergic reactions in patients patch tested in North America — 1984 to 1985. J Am Acad Dermatol 1989; 20: 1038–1045.

82. Guin JD. Contact sensitivity to topical corticosteroids. J Am Acad Dermatol 1984; 10: 773–782.

83. Dooms-Goossens AE, Degreef HJ, Marien KJC, Coopman SA. Contact allergy to corticosteroids: A frequently missed diagnosis? J Am Acad Dermatol 1989; 21: 538–543.

84. Held JL, Kalb RE, Ruszkowski AM, DeLeo V. Allergic contact dermatitis from bacitracin. J Am Acad Dermatol 1987; 17: 592–594.

85. Curley RK, Macfarlane AW, King CM. Contact sensitivity to the amide anesthetics lidocaine, prilocaine, and mepivacaine. Case report and review of

the literature. Arch Dermatol 1986; 122: 924–926.

86. Amon RB, Lis AW, Hanifin JM. Allergic contact dermatitis caused by idoxuridine. Arch Dermatol 1975; 111: 1581–1584.
87. Goette DK, Odom RB. Allergic contact dermatitis to topical fluorouracil. Arch Dermatol 1977; 113: 1058–1061.
88. Fisher AA. New advances in contact dermatitis. Int J Dermatol 1977; 16: 552–568.
89. Nishioka K. Allergic contact dermatitis. Int J Dermatol 1985; 24: 1–8.
89a. Bergstresser PR. Immune mechanisms in contact allergic dermatitis. Dermatol Clin 1990; 8: 3–11.
90. Bergstresser PR. Immunologic mechanisms of contact hypersensitivity. Dermatol Clin 1984; 2: 523–532.
91. Bergstresser PR. Contact allergic dermatitis. Old problems and new techniques. Arch Dermatol 1989; 125: 276–279.
92. De Panfilis G, Giannotti B, Manara GC et al. Macrophage-T lymphocyte relationships in man's contact allergic reactions. Br J Dermatol 1983; 109: 183–189.
93. Breathnach SM. Immunologic aspects of contact dermatitis. Clin Dermatol 1986; 4: 5–17.
94. Giannotti B, De Panfilis G, Manara GC et al. Langerhans cells are not damaged in contact allergic reactions in humans. Am J Dermatopathol 1986; 8: 220–226.
95. Katz SI. The role of Langerhans cells in allergic contact dermatitis. Am J Dermatopathol 1986; 8: 232–233.
96. Mahapatro D, Mahapatro RC. Cutaneous basophil hypersensitivity. Am J Dermatopathol 1984; 6: 483–489.
97. Keczkes K, Basheer AM, Wyatt EH. The persistence of allergic contact sensitivity: a 10-year follow-up in 100 patients. Br J Dermatol 1982; 107: 461–465.
98. Wood GS, Volterra AS, Abel EA et al. Allergic contact dermatitis: novel immunohistologic features. J Invest Dermatol 1986; 87: 688–693.
98a. van Joost T, van Ulsen J, Vuzevski VD et al. Purpuric contact dermatitis to benzoyl peroxide. J Am Acad Dermatol 1990; 22: 359–361.
99. Commens C, McGeogh A, Bartlett B, Kossard S. Bindii (Jo Jo) dermatitis (Soliva pterosperma [Compositae]). J Am Acad Dermatol 1984; 10: 768–773.
99a. Orbaneja JG, Diez LI, Lozano JLS, Salazar LC. Lymphomatoid contact dermatitis. Contact Dermatitis 1976; 2: 139–143.
99b. Ecker RI, Winkelmann RK. Lymphomatoid contact dermatitis. Contact Dermatitis 1981; 7: 84–93.
99c. Wall LM. Lymphomatoid contact dermatitis due to ethylenediamine dihydrochloride. Contact Dermatitis 1982; 8: 51–54.
100. Hellgren L, Mobacken H. Nummular eczema — clinical and statistical data. Acta Derm Venereol 1969; 49: 189–196.
101. Sirot G. Nummular eczema. Semin Dermatol 1983; 2: 68–74.
102. Rietschel RL, Ray MC. Nonatopic eczemas. J Am Acad Dermatol 1988; 18: 569–573.
103. Bendl BJ. Nummular eczema of stasis origin. Int J Dermatol 1979; 18: 129–135.
104. Church R. Eczema provoked by methyl dopa. Br J Dermatol 1974; 91: 373–378.
105. Krueger GG, Kahn G, Weston WL, Mandel MJ. IgE levels in nummular eczema and ichthyosis. Arch Dermatol 1973; 107: 56–58.
106. Stevens DM, Ackerman AB. On the concept of distinctive exudative discoid and lichenoid chronic dermatosis (Sulzberger–Garbe). Is it nummular dermatitis? Am J Dermatopathol 1984; 6: 387–395.
107. Sulzberger MB. Distinctive exudative discoid and lichenoid chronic dermatosis (Sulzberger and Garbe) re-examined — 1978. Br J Dermatol 1979; 100: 13–20.
108. Rongioletti F, Corbella L, Rebora A. Exudative discoid and lichenoid chronic dermatosis (Sulzberger–Garbe). A fictional disease? Int J Dermatol 1989; 28: 40–43.
109. Freeman K, Hewitt M, Warin AP. Two cases of distinctive exudative discoid and lichenoid chronic dermatosis of Sulzberger and Garbe responding to azathioprine. Br J Dermatol 1984; 111: 215–220.
110. Kligman AM, Leyden JJ. Seborrheic dermatitis. Semin Dermatol 1983; 2: 57–59.
111. Fox BJ, Odom RB. Papulosquamous diseases: A review. J Am Acad Dermatol 1985; 12: 597–624.
112. Thomsen K. Seborrhoeic dermatitis and napkin dermatitis. Acta Derm Venereol (Suppl) 1981; 95: 40–42.
113. Podmore P, Burrows D, Eedy DJ, Stanford CF. Seborrhoeic eczema — a disease entity or a clinical variant of atopic eczema? Br J Dermatol 1986; 115: 341–350.
114. Podmore P, Burrows D, Eedy D. T-cell subset assay. A useful differentiating marker of atopic and seborrheic eczema in infancy? Arch Dermatol 1988; 124: 1235–1238.
115. Yates VM, Kerr REI, Mackie R. Early diagnosis of infantile seborrhoeic dermatitis and atopic dermatitis — clinical features. Br J Dermatol 1983; 108: 633–638.
116. Yates VM, Kerr REI, Frier K et al. Early diagnosis of infantile seborrhoeic dermatitis and atopic dermatitis — total and specific IgE levels. Br J Dermatol 1983; 108: 639–645.
117. Mathes BM, Douglass MC. Seborrheic dermatitis in patients with acquired immunodeficiency syndrome. J Am Acad Dermatol 1985; 13: 947–951
118. Soeprono FF, Schinella RA, Cockerell CJ, Comite SL. Seborrheic-like dermatitis of acquired immunodeficiency syndrome. A clinicopathologic study. J Am Acad Dermatol 1986; 14: 242–248.
119. Binder RL, Jonelis FJ. Seborrheic dermatitis in neuroleptic-induced Parkinsonism. Arch Dermatol 1983; 119: 473–475.
120. Kanwar AJ, Majid A, Garg MP, Singh G. Seborrheic dermatitis-like eruption caused by cimetidine. Arch Dermatol 1981; 117: 65–66.
121. Knight AG. Pityriasis amiantacea: a clinical and histopathological investigation. Clin Exp Dermatol 1977; 2: 137–143.
122. Hersle K, Lindholm A, Mobacken H, Sandberg L. Relationship of pityriasis amiantacea to psoriasis. A follow-up study. Dermatologica 1979; 159: 245–250.
123. Leyden JJ, McGinley KJ, Kligman AM. Role of microorganisms in dandruff. Arch Dermatol 1976; 112: 333–338.

124. Shuster S. The aetiology of dandruff and the mode of action of therapeutic agents. Br J Dermatol 1984; 111: 235–242.

125. Burton JL, Pye RJ. Seborrhoea is not a feature of seborrhoeic dermatitis. Br Med J 1983; 286: 1169–1170.

126. Ford GP, Farr PM, Ive FA, Shuster S. The response of seborrhoeic dermatitis to ketoconazole. Br J Dermatol 1984; 111: 603–607.

127. Faergemann J, Fredriksson T. Tinea versicolor with regard to seborrheic dermatitis. An epidemiological investigation. Arch Dermatol 1979; 115: 966–968.

128. Skinner RB Jr, Noah PW, Taylor RM et al. Double-blind treatment of seborrheic dermatitis with 2% ketoconazole cream. J Am Acad Dermatol 1985; 12: 852–856.

129. Bergbrant I-M, Faergemann J. Seborrhoeic dermatitis and Pityrosporum ovale: a cultural and immunological study. Acta Derm Venereol 1989; 69: 332–335.

130. Broberg A, Faergemann J. Infantile seborrhoeic dermatitis and Pityrosporum ovale. Br J Dermatol 1989; 120: 359–362.

130a. Heng MCY, Henderson CL, Barker DC, Haberfelde G. Correlation of Pityrosporum ovale density with clinical severity of seborrheic dermatitis as assessed by a simplified technique. J Am Acad Dermatol 1990; 23: 82–86.

131. Pinkus H, Mehregan AH. The primary histologic lesion of seborrheic dermatitis and psoriasis. J Invest Dermatol 1966; 46: 109–116.

132. Barr RJ, Young EM Jr. Psoriasiform and related papulosquamous disorders. J Cutan Pathol 1985; 12: 412–425.

133. Ackerman AB. Histologic diagnosis of inflammatory skin diseases. Philadelphia: Lea & Febiger, 1978; 239–240.

134. Hanifin JM, Rajka G. Diagnostic features of atopic dermatitis. Acta Derm Venereol (Suppl) 1980; 92: 44–47.

135. Hanifin JM. Atopic dermatitis. J Am Acad Dermatol 1982; 6: 1–13.

136. Hanifin JM. Clinical and basic aspects of atopic dermatitis. Semin Dermatol 1983; 2: 5–19.

137. Kang K, Tian R. Atopic dermatitis. An evaluation of clinical and laboratory findings. Int J Dermatol 1987; 26: 27–32.

138. Roth HL. Atopic dermatitis revisited. Int J Dermatol 1987; 26: 139–149.

139. Graham-Brown RAC. Atopic dermatitis. Semin Dermatol 1988; 7: 37–42.

140. Heskel N, Lobitz WC Jr. Atopic dermatitis in children: clinical features and management. Semin Dermatol 1983; 2: 39–44.

141. Sampson HA. The role of food allergy and mediator release in atopic dermatitis. J Allergy Clin Immunol 1988; 81: 635–645.

142. Ofuji S, Uehara M. Follicular eruptions of atopic dermatitis. Arch Dermatol 1973; 107: 54–55.

143. Gondo A, Saeki N, Tokuda Y. IgG_4 antibodies in patients with atopic dermatitis. Br J Dermatol 1987; 117: 301–310.

144. Shehade SA, Layton GT, Stanworth DR. IgG_4 and IgE antibodies in atopic dermatitis and urticaria. Clin Exp Dermatol 1988; 13: 393–396.

145. Lever R, Hadley K, Downey D, Mackie R. Staphylococcal colonization in atopic dermatitis and the effect of topical mupirocin therapy. Br J Dermatol 1988; 119: 189–198.

146. Higaki Y, Hauser C, Rilliet A, Saurat J-H. Increased in vitro cell-mediated immune response to staphylococcal antigens in atopic dermatitis. J Am Acad Dermatol 1986; 15: 1204–1209.

147. Bork K, Brauninger W. Increasing incidence of eczema herpeticum: Analysis of seventy-five cases. J Am Acad Dermatol 1988; 19: 1024–1029.

148. Norris PG, Levene GM. Pompholyx occurring during hospital admission for treatment of atopic dermatitis. Clin Exp Dermatol 1987; 12: 189–190.

149. Svensson A. Hand eczema: an evaluation of the frequency of atopic background and the difference in clinical pattern between patients with and without atopic dermatitis. Acta Derm Venereol 1988; 68: 509–513.

150. Esterly NB. Significance of food hypersensitivity in children with atopic dermatitis. Pediatr Dermatol 1986; 3: 161–174.

151. Zachary CB, MacDonald DM. Quantitative analysis of T-lymphocyte subsets in atopic eczema, using monoclonal antibodies and flow cytofluorimetry. Br J Dermatol 1983; 108: 411–422.

152. Hall TJ, Rycroft R, Brostoff J. Decreased natural killer cell activity in atopic eczema. Immunology 1985; 56: 337–344.

153. Uehara M, Sawai T. A longitudinal study of contact sensitivity in patients with atopic dermatitis. Arch Dermatol 1989; 125: 366–368.

154. Nicolas JF, Thivolet J. Immunologic features of atopic dermatitis. Semin Dermatol 1988; 7: 156–162.

155. Clark RAF. Cell-mediated and IgE-mediated immune responses in atopic dermatitis. Arch Dermatol 1989; 125: 413–416.

156. Najem N, Hull D. Langerhans cells in delayed skin reactions to inhalant allergens in atopic dermatitis — an electron microscopic study. Clin Exp Dermatol 1989; 14: 218–222.

157. Yu B, Sawai T, Uehara M et al. Immediate hypersensitivity skin reactions to human dander in atopic dermatitis. Arch Dermatol 1988; 124: 1530–1533.

158. Elliston WL, Heise EA, Huntley CC. Cell-mediated hypersensitivity to mite antigens in atopic dermatitis. Arch Dermatol 1982; 118: 26–29.

159. Beck H-I, Korsgaard J. Atopic dermatitis and house dust mites. Br J Dermatol 1989; 120: 245–251.

160. Norris PG, Schofield O, Camp RDR. A study of the role of house dust mite in atopic dermatitis. Br J Dermatol 1988; 118: 435–440.

161. Fogh K, Herlin T, Kragballe K. Eiconasoids in skin of patients with atopic dermatitis: Prostaglandin E_2 and leukotriene B_4 are present in biologically active concentrations. J Allergy Clin Immunol 1989; 83: 450–455.

162. Larsen FS, Holm NV, Henningsen K. Atopic dermatitis. A genetic-epidemiologic study in a population-based twin sample. J Am Acad Dermatol 1986; 15: 487–494.

163. Mihm MC Jr, Soter NA, Dvorak HF, Austen KF. The structure of normal skin and the morphology of atopic eczema. J Invest Dermatol 1976; 67: 305–312.

164. Soter NA, Mihm MC Jr. Morphology of atopic eczema. Acta Derm Venereol (Suppl) 1980; 92: 11–15.
165. White CR Jr. Histopathology of atopic dermatitis. Semin Dermatol 1983; 2: 34–38.
166. Hurwitz RM, Detrana C. The cutaneous pathology of atopic dermatitis. J Cutan Pathol 1989; 16: 309 (abstract).
167. Uno H, Hanifin JM. Langerhans cells in acute and chronic epidermal lesions of atopic dermatitis, observed by L-dopa histofluorescence, glycol methacrylate thin section, and electron microscopy. J Invest Dermatol 1980; 75: 52–60.
168. Uehara M. Clinical and histological features of dry skin in atopic dermatitis. Acta Derm Venereol (Suppl) 1985; 114: 82–86.
169. Beran D, Kossard S, Freeman S et al. Immune mechanisms in atopic dermatitis: studies and hypothesis. Australas J Dermatol 1986; 27: 112–117.
170. Sugiura H, Hirota Y, Uehara M. Heterogeneous distribution of mast cells in lichenified lesions of atopic dermatitis. Acta Derm Venereol (Suppl) 1989; 144: 115–118.
171. Uehara M, Miyauchi H. The morphologic characteristics of dry skin in atopic dermatitis. Arch Dermatol 1984; 120: 1186–1190.
172. Finlay AY, Nicholls S, King CS, Marks R. The 'dry' non-eczematous skin associated with atopic eczema. Br J Dermatol 1980; 103: 249–256.
173. Van Neste D, Douka M, Rahier J, Staquet MJ. Epidermal changes in atopic dermatitis. Acta Derm Venereol (Suppl) 1985; 114: 67–71.
174. Leiferman KM, Ackerman SJ, Sampson HA et al. Dermal deposition of eosinophil-granule major basic protein in atopic dermatitis. N Engl J Med 1985; 313: 282–285.
175. Lever R, Turbitt M, Sanderson A, Mackie R. Immunophenotyping of the cutaneous infiltrate and of the mononuclear cells in the peripheral blood in patients with atopic dermatitis. J Invest Dermatol 1987; 89: 4–7.
176. Bieber T, Dannenberg B, Ring J, Braun-Falco O. Keratinocytes in lesional skin of atopic eczema bear HLA-DR, CDIa and IgE molecules. Clin Exp Dermatol 1989; 14: 35–39.
177. Epstein E. Hand dermatitis: practical management and current concepts. J Am Acad Dermatol 1984; 10: 395–424.
178. Menne T, Hjorth N. Pompholyx — dyshidrotic eczema. Semin Dermatol 1983; 2: 75–80.
179. Kutzner H, Wurzel RM, Wolff HH. Are acrosyringia involved in the pathogenesis of "dyshidrosis"? Am J Dermatopathol 1986; 8: 109–116.
180. Meneghini CL, Angelini G. Contact and microbial allergy in pompholyx. Contact Dermatitis 1979; 5: 46–50.
181. Miller RM, Coger RW. Skin conductance conditioning with dyshidrotic eczema patients. Br J Dermatol 1979; 101: 435–440.
182. Norris PG, Levene GM. Pompholyx occurring during hospital admission for treatment of atopic dermatitis. Clin Exp Dermatol 1987; 12: 189–190.
183. Hersle K, Mobacken H. Hyperkeratotic dermatitis of the palms. Br J Dermatol 1982; 107: 195–202.
184. Mackie RM, Hussain SL. Juvenile plantar dermatosis: a new entity? Clin Exp Dermatol 1976; 1: 253–260.
185. Ashton RE, Russell Jones R, Griffiths A. Juvenile plantar dermatosis. A clinicopathologic study. Arch Dermatol 1985; 121: 225–228.
186. Young E. Forefoot eczema — further studies and a review. Clin Exp Dermatol 1986; 11: 523–528.
187. Ashton RE, Griffiths WAD. Juvenile plantar dermatosis — atopy or footwear? Clin Exp Dermatol 1986; 11: 529–534.
188. Svensson A. Prognosis and atopic background of juvenile plantar dermatosis and gluteo-femoral eczema. Acta Derm Venereol 1988; 68: 336–340.
189. Verbov J. Juvenile plantar dermatosis. Acta Derm Venereol (Suppl) 1989; 144: 153–154.
190. Lim KB, Tan T, Rajan VS. Dermatitis palmaris sicca — a distinctive pattern of hand dermatitis. Clin Exp Dermatol 1986; 11: 553–559.
191. van Diggelen MW, van Dijk E, Hausman R. The enigma of juvenile plantar dermatosis. Am J Dermatopathol 1986; 8: 336–340.
192. Shrank AB. The aetiology of juvenile plantar dermatosis. Br J Dermatol 1979; 100: 641–648.
193. Beninson J, Livingood CS. Stasis dermatitis. In: Demis DJ, ed. Clinical dermatology. Philadelphia: Harper and Row, 1986: unit 7.44; 1–6.
194. Cunningham MJ, Zone JJ, Petersen MJ, Green JA. Circulating activated (DR-positive) T lymphocytes in a patient with autoeczematization. J Am Acad Dermatol 1986; 14: 1039–1041.
195. Weedon D. Unpublished observations.
196. Parsons JM. Pityriasis rosea update: 1986. J Am Acad Dermatol 1986; 15: 159–167.
197. Hendricks AA, Lohr JA. Pityriasis rosea in infancy. Arch Dermatol 1979; 115: 896–897.
198. Chuang T-Y, Ilstrup DM, Perry HO, Kurland LT. Pityriasis rosea in Rochester, Minnesota, 1969 to 1978. A 10-year epidemiologic study. J Am Acad Dermatol 1982; 7: 80–89.
199. Kay MH, Rapini RP, Fritz KA. Oral lesions in pityriasis rosea. Arch Dermatol 1985; 121: 1449–1451.
200. Del Campo DV, Barsky S, Tisocco L, Gruszka RJ. Pityriasis rosea unilateralis. Int J Dermatol 1983; 22: 312–313.
201. Garcia RL. Vesicular pityriasis rosea. Arch Dermatol 1976; 112: 410.
202. Chuang T-Y, Perry HO, Ilstrup DM, Kurland LT. Recent upper respiratory tract infection and pityriasis rosea: a case-control study of 249 matched pairs. Br J Dermatol 1983; 108: 587–591.
203. Messenger AG, Knox EG, Summerly R et al. Case clustering in pityriasis rosea: support for role of an infective agent. Br Med J 1982; 284: 371–373.
204. Aoshima T, Komura J, Ofuji S. Virus-like particles in the herald patch of pityriasis rosea. Dermatologica 1981; 162: 64–65.
205. Hudson LD, Adelman S, Lewis CW. Pityriasis rosea. Viral complement fixation studies. J Am Acad Dermatol 1981; 4: 544–546.
206. Burch PRJ, Rowell NR. Pityriasis rosea — an autoaggressive disease? Br J Dermatol 1970; 82: 549–560.
207. Aiba S, Tagami H. Immunohistologic studies in pityriasis rosea. Evidence for cellular immune reaction in the lesional epidermis. Arch Dermatol 1985; 121: 761–765.
208. Maize JC, Tomecki KJ. Pityriasis rosea-like drug

eruption secondary to metronidazole. Arch Dermatol 1977; 113: 1457–1458.

209. Wilkin JK, Kirkendall WM. Pityriasis rosea-like rash from captopril. Arch Dermatol 1982; 118: 186–187.

210. Panizzon R, Bloch PH. Histopathology of pityriasis rosea Gibert. Qualitative and quantitative light-microscopic study of 62 biopsies of 40 patients. Dermatologica 1982; 165: 551–558.

211. Bunch LW, Tilley JC. Pityriasis rosea. A histologic and serologic study. Arch Dermatol 1961; 84: 79–86.

212. Stern JK, Wolf JE Jr, Rosen T. Focal acantholytic dyskeratosis in pityriasis rosea. Arch Dermatol 1979; 115: 497.

213. El-Shiemy S, Nassar A, Mokhtar M, Mabrouk D. Light and electron microscopic studies of pityriasis rosea. Int J Dermatol 1987; 26: 237–239.

214. Okamoto H, Imamura S, Aoshima T et al. Dyskeratotic degeneration of epidermal cells in pityriasis rosea: light and electron microscopic studies. Br J Dermatol 1982; 107: 189–194.

215. Takaki Y, Miyazaki H. Cytologic degeneration of keratinocytes adjacent to Langerhans cells in pityriasis rosea (Gibert). Acta Derm Venereol 1976; 56: 99–103.

216. Gianotti F. The Gianotti–Crosti syndrome. JCE Dermatol 1979; 18(2): 15–25.

217. Eiloart M. The Gianotti–Crosti syndrome. Report of forty-four cases. Br J Dermatol 1966; 78: 488–492.

218. Schneider JA, Poley JR, Millunchick EW et al. Papular acrodermatitis (Gianotti–Crosti syndrome) in a child with anicteric hepatitis B, virus subtype adw. J Pediatr 1982; 101: 219–222.

219. Lee S, Kim KY, Hahn CS et al. Gianotti–Crosti syndrome associated with hepatitis B surface antigen (subtype adr). J Am Acad Dermatol 1985; 12: 629–633.

220. Ishimaru Y, Ishimaru H, Toda G et al. An epidemic of infantile papular acrodermatitis (Gianotti's disease) in Japan associated with hepatitis-B surface antigen subtype ayw. Lancet 1976; 1: 707–709.

221. Konno M, Kikuta H, Ishikawa N et al. A possible association between hepatitis-B antigen-negative infantile papular acrodermatitis and Epstein–Barr virus infection. J Pediatr 1982; 101: 222–224.

222. Iosub S, Santos C, Gromisch DS. Papular acrodermatitis with Epstein–Barr virus infection. Clin Pediatr 1984; 23: 33–34.

223. James WD, Odom RB, Hatch MH. Gianotti–Crosti-like eruption associated with coxsackievirus A-16 infection. J Am Acad Dermatol 1982; 6: 862–866.

224. Sagi EF, Linder N, Shouval D. Papular acrodermatitis of childhood associated with hepatitis A virus infection. Pediatr Dermatol 1985; 3: 31–33.

225. Liehr H, Seelig R, Seelig HP. Cutaneous papulo-vesicular eruptions in non-A, non-B hepatitis. Hepatogastroenterology 1985; 32: 11–14.

226. Berant M, Naveh Y, Weissman I. Papular acrodermatitis with cytomegalovirus hepatitis. Arch Dis Child 1984; 58: 1024–1025.

227. Spear KL, Winkelmann RK. Gianotti–Crosti syndrome. A review of ten cases not associated with hepatitis B. Arch Dermatol 1984; 120: 891–896.

228. Taieb A, Plantin P, Du Pasquier P et al. Gianotti–Crosti syndrome: a study of 26 cases. Br J Dermatol 1986; 115: 49–59.

229. Gianotti F. Papular acrodermatitis of childhood and other papulo-vesicular acro-located syndromes. Br J Dermatol 1979; 100: 49–59.

230. Winkelmann RK, Bourlond A. Infantile lichenoid acrodermatitis. Report of a case of Gianotti–Crosti syndrome. Arch Dermatol 1965; 92: 398–401.

231. Rubenstein D, Esterly NB, Fretzin D. The Gianotti–Crosti syndrome. Pediatrics 1978; 61: 433–437.

232. Fisher AA. Systemic contact-type dermatitis due to drugs. Clin Dermatol 1986; 4: 58–69.

233. Rosen C. Photo-induced drug eruptions. Semin Dermatol 1989; 8: 149–157.

234. Menne T, Veien NK, Maibach HI. Systemic contact-type dermatitis due to drugs. Semin Dermatol 1989; 8: 144–148.

235. VanArsdel PP Jr. Allergy and adverse drug reactions. J Am Acad Dermatol 1982; 6: 833–845.

236. Swinyer LJ. Determining the cause of drug eruptions. Dermatol Clin 1983; 1: 417–431.

237. Bruynzeel DP, van Ketel WG. Patch testing in drug eruptions. Semin Dermatol 1989; 8: 196–203.

238. Addo HA, Ferguson J, Frain-Bell W. Thiazide-induced photosensitivity: a study of 33 subjects. Br J Dermatol 1987; 116: 749–760.

239. Weedon D. Unpublished observations.

240. Bigby M, Stern R. Cutaneous reactions to nonsteroidal anti-inflammatory drugs. A review. J Am Acad Dermatol 1985; 12: 866–876.

241. Stanley J, Fallon-Pellicci V. Phenytoin hypersensitivity reaction. Arch Dermatol 1978; 114: 1350–1353.

242. Tuneu A, Moreno A, de Moragas JM. Cutaneous reactions secondary to heparin injections. J Am Acad Dermatol 1985; 12: 1072–1077.

243. Klein GF, Kofler H, Wolf H, Fritsch PO. Eczema-like, erythematous, infiltrated plaques: A common side effect of subcutaneous heparin therapy. J Am Acad Dermatol 1989; 21: 703–707.

244. Penneys NS. Gold therapy: dermatologic uses and toxicities. J Am Acad Dermatol 1979; 1: 315–320.

245. Ranki A, Niemi K-M, Kanerva L. Clinical, immunohistochemical, and electron-microscopic findings in gold dermatitis. Am J Dermatopathol 1989; 11: 22–28.

246. Kauppinen K, Stubb S. Drug eruptions: causative agents and clinical types. A series of in-patients during a 10-year period. Acta Derm Venereol 1984; 64: 320–324.

247. Fellner MJ, Prutkin L. Morbilliform eruptions caused by penicillin. A study by electron microscopy and immunologic tests. J Invest Dermatol 1970; 55: 390–395.

248. Bennaman O, Sanchez JL. Comparative clinicopathological study on pityriasis lichenoides chronica and small plaque psoriasis. Am J Dermatopathol 1988; 10: 189–196.

249. Hu C-H, Winkelmann RK. Digitate dermatosis. A new look at symmetrical, small plaque parapsoriasis. Arch Dermatol 1973; 107: 65–69.

250. Calnan CD, Meara RH. Parapsoriasis en plaque and chronic superficial dermatitis. Trans St John's Hosp Dermatol Soc 1956; 37: 12–13.

251. Lambert WC, Everett MA. The nosology of parapsoriasis. J Am Acad Dermatol 1981; 5: 373–395.

252. Bluefarb SM. The clinical implications of parapsoriasis. Int J Dermatol 1980; 19: 556–557.
253. Goldberg LC. Xantho-erythrodermia perstans (Crocker). Arch Dermatol 1963; 88: 901–907.
254. Samman PD. The natural history of parapsorais en plaques (chronic superficial dermatitis) and prereticulotic poikiloderma. Br J Dermatol 1972; 87: 405–411.
255. Everett MA, Headington JT. Parapsoriasis. JCE Dermatology 1978; 17(12): 12–24.
256. Altman J. Parapsoriasis: a histopathologic review and classification. Semin Dermatol 1984; 3: 14–21.
257. Sanchez JL, Ackerman AB. The patch stage of mycosis fungoides. Criteria for histologic diagnosis. Am J Dermatopathol 1979; 1: 5–26.
258. Nickoloff BJ. Light-microscopic assessment of 100 patients with patch/plaque-stage mycosis fungoides. Am J Dermatopathol 1988; 10: 469–477.

The vesiculobullous reaction pattern

INTRODUCTION

The vesiculobullous reaction pattern is characterized by the presence of vesicles or bullae at any level within the epidermis or at the dermo-epidermal junction. Pustules, which are vesicles or bullae containing numerous neutrophils or eosinophils, are included in this reaction pattern.

Classification of vesiculobullous diseases

Early lesions should always be biopsied to ensure that a histopathological diagnosis can be made. Once regeneration of the epidermis commences or secondary changes such as infection or ulceration occur, accurate diagnosis of a vesiculobullous lesion may not always be possible. Furthermore, in some blistering diseases, special techniques such as direct immunofluorescence or electron microscopy may assist in making the diagnosis. These special requirements should be kept in mind when one of the vesiculobullous diseases is to be biopsied.

There are three morphological features that may need to be assessed in the diagnosis of vesiculobullous lesions. They are:

1. the anatomical level of the split
2. the mechanism responsible for the split
3. the inflammatory cell component (in the case of subepidermal blisters).

These various aspects will be considered in greater detail.

Anatomical level of the split. The blister may form at any one of four different anatomical levels. The split may be subcorneal (intracorneal splitting is included in this category), within the spinous or malpighian layers, suprabasilar, or beneath the epidermis (subepidermal). In the case of subepidermal blisters there are several different anatomical levels that may be involved but these are 'submicroscopic' and require the use of electron microscopy or other special techniques (see below) for their elucidation.

The mechanism responsible for the split. There are several mechanisms by which blistering can result — spongiosis, acantholysis and ballooning degeneration of keratinocytes. *Spongiosis* refers to the presence of intercellular oedema. In some of the disorders showing the spongiotic reaction pattern (see Ch. 5, pp. 95–125) the oedema may be so pronounced that there is breakdown of the intercellular connections, leading to vesicle formation. Clinically visible vesicles occur in a small proportion of cases with the spongiotic reaction pattern. *Acantholysis* refers to the loss of attachments between keratinocytes resulting in the formation of rounded, detached cells within the blister. Acantholysis may result from damage to the intercellular substance due to the deposition of immune complexes, as in pemphigus, or from abnormalities of the tonofilament-desmosome complexes, which may be an acquired abnormality or have a heredofamilial basis. Acantholysis may also occur secondary to other processes such as ballooning degeneration. *Ballooning degeneration* of keratinocytes refers to the swelling of these cells which follows their infection with certain viruses. The ballooning results in rupture of desmosomal attachments and vesicle formation. Sometimes a few acantholytic cells are present in vesicles as an incidental phenomenon, resulting from the action of enzymes released by neutrophils in the accompanying inflammatory infiltrate. The presence of a few acantholytic cells in these circumstances should not be misinterpreted as indicating that acantholysis is the pathogenetic mechanism responsible for the blister in such a case. *Junctional separation* is sometimes included as a mechanism of blister formation but it is a heterogeneous process involving different mechanisms and different anatomical levels within the basement membrane zone.

Inflammatory cell component. In the case of subepidermal blisters, it is usual to subclassify them further on the basis of the predominant cell in the inflammatory infiltrate in the underlying dermis. In some subepidermal blisters, the proportion of eosinophils and neutrophils may vary from case to case, and with the age of the lesion. These caveats must always be kept in mind when a subepidermal blister with neutrophils or eosinophils is biopsied. The presence of neutrophils within intraepidermal blisters may also have relevance to the diagnosis, even though this aspect is not used in the subclassification of intraepidermal blisters.

Other morphological features. Although the key features in the assessment of any vesiculobullous lesion are the anatomical level of the split, the mechanism responsible for the split and the nature of the inflammatory cell infiltrate, as discussed above, the presence of changes in keratinocytes may assist in making a diagnosis in several diseases. Examples include the presence of dyskeratotic cells in Darier's disease (see p.

281), the presence of multinucleate giant cells in certain virus-induced blisters (see p. 683), and confluent epidermal necrosis in toxic epidermal necrolysis (see p. 46) and in severe erythema multiforme (see p. 44). Shrunken keratinocytes (Civatte bodies) may be seen in bullous lichen planus (see p. 38), bullous fixed drug eruptions (see p. 42) and erythema multiforme (see p. 44).

INTRACORNEAL AND SUBCORNEAL BLISTERS

In this group of vesiculobullous diseases the split occurs within the stratum corneum or directly beneath it. In addition to the conditions discussed below, subcorneal blisters or pustules have been reported uncommonly as a manifestation of epidermolysis bullosa simplex (see p. 141), acute generalized.pustulosis and other pustular vasculitides (see pp. 231 and 229 respectively), mercury poisoning (see p. 421) and pyoderma gangrenosum (see p. 242).[1] There has been one report of a patient with vegetative plaques resembling pemphigus vegetans and a subcorneal spongiform pustule with marked acanthosis of the epidermis on histological examination.[2]

Other causes of intracorneal or subcorneal blisters are discussed below.

IMPETIGO

Impetigo is an acute superficial pyoderma which occurs predominantly in childhood (see p. 596). *Staphylococcus aureus* is the usual organism isolated from this condition. There are two clinical forms of impetigo — a common vesiculopustular type and a rare bullous type.

Histopathology

In impetigo there are subcorneal collections of neutrophils. A few acantholytic cells are sometimes present, particularly in bullous impetigo, as a result of the action of enzymes released from neutrophils. Acantholysis is never as prominent

in impetigo as it is in pemphigus foliaceus. Gram-positive cocci can usually be demonstrated in impetigo, another distinguishing feature of this condition.

STAPHYLOCOCCAL 'SCALDED SKIN' SYNDROME

The staphylococcal 'scalded skin' syndrome (SSSS) is discussed in detail with the bacterial infections on page 597. It results from the production of an epidermolytic toxin by certain strains of *Staphylococcus aureus*.

Histopathology

It is usually difficult to obtain an intact blister in the staphylococcal 'scalded skin' syndrome, as the stratum corneum may be cast off during the biopsy procedure or the subsequent processing of the specimen. A few acantholytic cells and neutrophils are usually present in intact blisters or on the surface of the epidermis if its roof has been shed (Fig. 6.1). Organisms are not usually present in the affected skin, in contrast to bullous impetigo. There is usually only a sparse inflammatory cell infiltrate in the upper dermis, in contrast to bullous impetigo and pemphigus foliaceus in which the infiltrate is usually heavier.

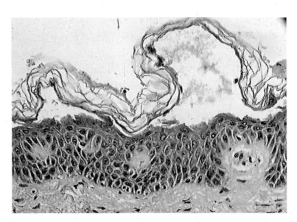

Fig. 6.1 Staphylococcal 'scalded skin' syndrome. A thin layer of normal stratum corneum forms the roof of the blister. There is no inflammation.
Haematoxylin — eosin

DERMATOPHYTOSIS

Subcorneal and intraepidermal blisters are sometimes seen in the dermatophytoses, particularly on the hands and feet. The presence of neutrophils in the stratum corneum or within the epidermis should always prompt consideration of an infectious aetiology, including fungi. Candidosis is another uncommon cause of subcorneal blistering (see p. 645).

PEMPHIGUS FOLIACEUS

Pemphigus foliaceus, which accounts for approximately 10% of all cases of pemphigus, is one of the less severe forms of the disease.[3,4] There are recurrent crops of flaccid bullae that readily rupture, resulting in shallow erosions and crusted erythematous plaques.[5,6] A stinging or burning sensation is sometimes present. Lesions may be localized to the face and trunk initially, but the condition usually spreads to involve large areas of the body. However, mucous membrane involvement is rare.[7,8] No age, including childhood,[9-11] is exempt, although the majority of cases present in late middle life.

Rare clinical presentations have included lesions resembling eruptive seborrhoeic keratoses,[12,13] and in other instances erythematous and vesicular lesions suggestive of dermatitis herpetiformis.[14-19] This latter group often shows transient histological changes of eosinophilic spongiosis (see p. 97).

Pemphigus foliaceus has been reported in association with bullous pemphigoid,[20] lupus erythematosus,[21] rheumatoid arthritis, myasthenia gravis,[7,22,23] lichen planus,[24] Graves' disease[21] and mycosis fungoides.[25] It has also been associated with the use of penicillamine,[26,27] gold, pyritinol, rifampicin,[28] captopril,[29] methimazole (thiamazole) and α-mercaptopropionylglycine (tiopronin).[30-32]

Pemphigus foliaceus is the most common form of pemphigus complicating the use of penicillamine.[26] Pemphigus develops in nearly 10% of those taking penicillamine for prolonged periods, and it may persist for many months after the drug is discontinued.[33,34] Sometimes the eruption that ensues is not typical of a specific type of pemphigus but shares clinical or immunohistological features of different types of the disease.[35-38]

Pemphigus foliaceus results from the formation of autoantibodies of IgG type reactive with antigens in the intercellular spaces or on the surface of epidermal cells.[39] In one subgroup of patients these autoantibodies are directed to desmoglein 1, a desmosomal core glycoprotein.[40,41] Complement, including the terminal complement sequence (membrane-attack complex),[42] and plasmin appear to be important mediators in the detachment of the epidermal cells.[39,43] Antibody levels fluctuate during the course of the disease and have some correlation with disease activity.

Endemic pemphigus foliaceus. This variant is also known by the Portuguese expression *fogo selvagem* ('wild fire') and as Brazilian pemphigus foliaceus.[44,45] It affects mostly children and young adults and it is endemic in certain rural areas of South America, particularly parts of Brazil.[46] The epidemiology strongly suggests an infectious agent, probably a virus, and this is supported by the finding of elevated levels of thymosin alpha 1 in many affected individuals.[47,48] The endemic variant has an abrupt onset and a variable course.[49] Familial cases occur in 10%, in contrast to their rarity in the more usual form of pemphigus foliaceus.[50] The circulating intercellular antibodies have similar antigenic specificity to those found in the non-endemic form of the disease.[51-53] Of interest is the recent finding that the intraperitoneal injection into mice of IgG from patients with endemic pemphigus foliaceus causes acantholysis in the animals.[54]

Histopathology

Established lesions of pemphigus foliaceus of both the endemic and non-endemic forms show a superficial bulla with the split high in the granular layer or directly beneath the stratum corneum.[55] The bulla contains fibrin, some neutrophils and scattered acantholytic keratinocytes. No bacteria are present, unlike bullous impetigo.[55]

The earliest change appears to be the formation of vacuoles in the intercellular spaces in the upper layers of the epidermis.[56] These expand, leading to cleft formation. Uncommonly, eosinophilic spongiosis is seen as a precursor lesion and transitions between this picture and that of pemphigus foliaceus may be seen.

In late lesions of pemphigus foliaceus the epidermis may be hyperplastic, with overlying focal parakeratosis and some orthokeratosis.[57] Dyskeratotic cells with hyperchromatic nuclei and somewhat resembling the 'grains' found in Darier's disease are a distinctive feature of the granular layer (Fig. 6.2).

The superficial dermis is oedematous with a mixed inflammatory cell infiltrate which usually includes both eosinophils and neutrophils. In drug-induced lesions, eosinophils may predominate in the dermal infiltrate.

With direct immunofluorescence, there is intercellular staining for IgG and C3 in both affected and normal skin.[58,59] Sometimes the staining is localized to the upper levels of the epidermis.[60,61] Rarely, these immunoreactants may be present along the basement membrane, even in cases that clinically resemble pemphigus foliaceus rather than pemphigus erythematosus (see below).[62] In a few instances, IgA rather than IgG has been present in the intercellular regions.[63] These cases of IgA pemphigus foliaceus have shown features overlapping with subcorneal pustular dermatosis, with the presence of subcorneal pustules but with prominent acantholysis (see p. 132).[63,64]

Electron microscopy. Acantholysis in pemphigus foliaceus appears to result from separation of the non-specific junctions and subsequent rupture of desmosomal junctions.[57] The tonofilament-desmosomal complexes remain intact, although irregular bundles of tonofilaments are found within the acantholytic cells.[65] Immunoelectronmicroscopy shows immunoglobulins deposited over the plasma membrane of the keratinocytes and permeating the desmosomal junctions.[65]

PEMPHIGUS ERYTHEMATOSUS

Pemphigus erythematosus (Senear–Usher syndrome), which accounts for approximately 10% of all cases of pemphigus,[4,66] is a variant of pemphigus foliaceus which combines some of the immunological features of both pemphigus and lupus erythematosus.[5] It usually develops insidiously with erythematous, scaly and crusted plaques in a butterfly distribution over the nose and malar areas.[67] It may also involve other 'seborrhoeic areas' such as the scalp, pectoral and interscapular regions, as well as intertriginous areas. Usually, there is no visceral involvement. Pemphigus erythematosus may persist almost indefinitely as a localized disease.[16] Sunlight sometimes adversely affects its course.[3]

Pemphigus erythematosus is occasionally found in association with other autoimmune diseases, especially myasthenia gravis with an accompanying thymoma.[68–70] Rare cases of concurrent pemphigus erythematosus and systemic lupus erythematosus have been documented.[71] There are reports of its association with parathyroid adenoma,[72] internal cancers,[73] burns[74]

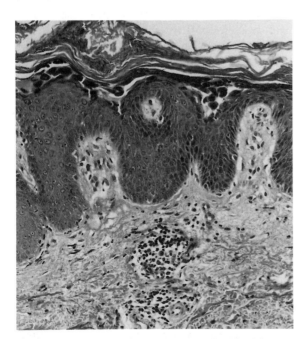

Fig. 6.2 Pemphigus foliaceus. Dyskeratotic cells with hyperchromatic nuclei are a distinctive feature in the granular layer in this older lesion.
Haematoxylin — eosin

and X-radiation. Drugs which may induce pemphigus erythematosus[67] include penicillamine,[27,36,75,76] propranolol,[67] captopril,[77] pyritinol,[67] thiopronine[78] and heroin.[79]

Antinuclear antibodies and circulating antibodies to the intercellular regions are often present. Antibodies to DNA are usually absent.[75]

Histopathology

The appearances are identical to those of pemphigus foliaceus, with a subcorneal blister containing occasional acantholytic cells (see above).[80] Eroded and crusted lesions may develop.

Direct immunofluorescence usually demonstrates IgG and/or complement both in the intercellular spaces and at the dermo–epidermal junction.[81,82] The intercellular staining may be more pronounced in the upper layers of the epidermis. The lupus band test is sometimes positive in uninvolved skin.[75]

SUBCORNEAL PUSTULAR DERMATOSIS

Subcorneal pustular dermatosis is a chronic, relapsing, vesiculopustular dermatosis with a predilection for the trunk, particularly intertriginous areas, and the flexor aspect of the limbs.[83–85] It usually spares the face and mucous membranes, and there are usually no constitutional symptoms.[86] The condition is more common in women, particularly occurring in those in the fourth and fifth decades of life. Cases purporting to be subcorneal pustular dermatosis in children[87] have been disputed.[88]

The pustules are flaccid. They are initially sterile but secondary infection sometimes develops. A transient erythematous flare surrounds the pustules in the early stages.[84]

The aetiology and pathogenesis remain unknown. A small number of patients have had an associated monoclonal gammopathy, most commonly of IgA type.[86,89–91] In two cases, the lesions developed several hours after the performance of echography.[92] Subcorneal pustular dermatosis is regarded by some authorities as a variant of pustular psoriasis.[93,94] This confusion

has arisen, in part, because cases not conforming to the original description in 1956 by Sneddon and Wilkinson have been reported misleadingly as cases of subcorneal pustular dermatosis. Some of these cases have been examples of the annular variant of pustular psoriasis.[85,95] It should be noted that 7 of the 23 purported cases of subcorneal pustular dermatosis seen at the Mayo Clinic subsequently developed generalized pustular psoriasis.[96]

Pustular eruptions with some histological or clinical resemblance to subcorneal pustular dermatosis have been reported following the ingestion of isoniazid,[97] diltiazem,[98] the cephalosporins[99] and amoxycillin.[100] New lesions have been precipitated in a patient with subcorneal pustular dermatosis following the ingestion of dapsone and of quinidine sulphate.[101] Sterile, subcorneal pustules sometimes form in pustular vasculitis (see p. 229).

Histopathology

The subcorneal pustule is filled with neutrophils, with an occasional eosinophil. Neutrophils also migrate through the epidermis, but they do not form spongiform pustules.[85] The pustule appears to 'sit' on the epidermis (Fig. 6.3), and usually it causes no depression of the latter. An occasional acantholytic cell may be present in older lesions, a result of the activity of the proteolytic enzymes released from neutrophils.[85] Mitotic figures are

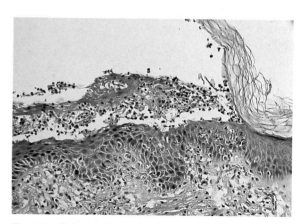

Fig. 6.3 Subcorneal pustular dermatosis. The subcorneal pustule contains fibrin and a modest number of neutrophils. Haematoxylin — eosin

usually absent within the epidermis, unlike pustular psoriasis.[102]

A mixed superficial perivascular inflammatory cell infiltrate is present in the underlying dermis. In early lesions the infiltrate includes quite a few neutrophils.

Direct immunofluorescence is usually negative, although immunoreactants have been described in the epidermis in rare cases.[89] Several cases have been reported of a condition resembling subcorneal pustular dermatosis clinically but in which a biopsy of the lesions showed intercellular IgA. Such cases have recently been classified as IgA pemphigus foliaceus (see p. 131), although a case could be made for the retention of some of them as variants of subcorneal pustular dermatosis.[103] A closely related and, possibly, an identical entity is intraepidermal neutrophilic IgA dermatosis,[103a] in which there are intraepidermal pustules and IgA deposits on or between epidermal cells.

INFANTILE ACROPUSTULOSIS

Infantile acropustulosis is an uncommon pustular dermatosis characterized by recurrent crops of intensely pruritic vesiculopustules on the distal parts of the extremities of infants.[104–113] The lesions measure 1–2 mm in diameter. The condition was first described in 1979.[108,109] Its onset is at birth or in the first few months of life, and resolution occurs at 2–3 years of age.[110] There is a predilection for black males. The aetiology is unknown, although several cases are said to have followed scabies.[113] Peripheral eosinophilia and atopy[111] have been present in several patients.

Because of overlapping clinical and histological features, infantile acropustulosis, erythema neonatorum toxicum and transient neonatal pustular melanosis can be grouped together as the 'pustular dermatoses of infancy' (see below).

Histopathology[112]

In early lesions there is an intraepidermal pustule containing neutrophils and sometimes varying numbers of eosinophils.[113] This progresses to form a subcorneal pustule. There is a sparse

perivascular mixed inflammatory cell infiltrate in the upper dermis.

ERYTHEMA NEONATORUM TOXICUM

Erythema neonatorum toxicum is a common entity which appears within the first week of life as erythematous macules, papules and pustules, mostly located on the trunk.[114–116] The lesions resolve within a few days. The aetiology is unknown.

Histopathology[114,117]

There are subcorneal or intraepidermal pustules, filled with eosinophils, and related to the orifices of the pilosebaceous follicles.[114] An inflammatory infiltrate composed predominantly of eosinophils is present in the upper dermis in the vicinity of the follicles and there is some exocytosis of these cells into the epithelium of the involved follicles.[114]

The histological appearances resemble those of eosinophilic pustular folliculitis but the clinical features of the two conditions differ.[118]

TRANSIENT NEONATAL PUSTULAR MELANOSIS

This uncommon condition presents at birth with pigmented macules, often with a distinct collarette of scale, and vesiculopustules which are clustered beneath the chin, on the forehead, the neck and the back, and sometimes on the extremities.[119–121] The vesiculopustules usually resolve after several days, often transforming into pigmented macules. The pigmented lesions persist for several weeks or more, and then slowly fade.[119] The aetiology of the condition is unknown, but there appears to be a predilection for black races.[119]

Histopathology[119]

The vesiculopustules are intracorneal or subcorneal collections of neutrophils, admixed with fibrin and a few eosinophils. There may be a mild infiltrate of inflammatory cells around vessels in the upper dermis.

The pigmented macules show increased melanin in the basal and suprabasal keratinocytes but, surprisingly, there is no melanin in the dermis.

MILIARIA CRYSTALLINA

The condition known as miliaria crystallina is associated with small 1–2 mm vesicles which rupture easily (see p. 98).

Histopathology

The vesicle forms within, or directly beneath, the stratum corneum. It is centred on the acrosyringium.

INTRAEPIDERMAL BLISTERS

The term 'intraepidermal blister' refers to the formation of lesions within the malpighian layers; it does not include those vesiculobullous diseases in which the split occurs beneath the stratum corneum or in a suprabasilar position. It should be noted, however, that biopsies from some of the diseases listed as forming subcorneal or suprabasilar blisters may sometimes show splitting within the malpighian layers. This is particularly likely in lesions of some days' duration in which regeneration of the epidermis may alter the level of the split.

Intraepidermal blisters usually form as the outcome of spongiosis or ballooning degeneration. The primary acantholytic diseases usually form blisters that are subcorneal or suprabasilar in position, before regeneration occurs. Most of the intraepidermal blistering diseases have been discussed elsewhere, but with the exception of hydroa vacciniforme (see p. 581) they are mentioned below.

SPONGIOTIC BLISTERING DISEASES

Although most of the diseases that produce the

spongiotic reaction pattern (see Ch.5, pp. 95–125) can sometimes be associated with clinically visible vesicles and even bullae, the ones most often associated with blisters are allergic contact dermatitis (see p. 102), nummular dermatitis (see p. 105), pompholyx (see p. 109), polymorphous light eruption (vesicular type — see p. 115), insect bite reactions (see p. 116), incontinentia pigmenti (first stage — see p. 98), and miliaria rubra (see p. 98). The presence of spongiosis adjacent to the vesicle or elsewhere in the biopsy is the clue to this group of blistering diseases. Eosinophils are prominent in the infiltrate in insect bite reactions and incontinentia pigmenti.

Palmoplantar pustulosis commences as a spongiotic vesicle but pustulation rapidly ensues (see below).

PALMOPLANTAR PUSTULOSIS

In palmoplantar pustulosis there are erythematous scaly plaques with recurrent sterile pustules symmetrically distributed on the palms and soles.[122,123] Initially, only a palm or a sole may be involved.[124] Onset of the disease is usually between the ages of 40 and 60 years. Women are predominantly affected.[124] Palmoplantar pustulosis is sometimes associated with a focus of infection somewhere in the body,[125] although elimination of the infectious process has no influence on the course of the disease,[122,126] which is usually protracted and somewhat unpredictable.

Psoriasis is present in at least 6% of cases;[127] some studies have shown a much greater incidence.[128] However, unlike psoriasis, there are no clear associations with any particular HLA type.[129] There is also a difference in the surface receptors on neutrophils in the two conditions.[130] Both psoriasis and palmoplantar pustulosis may be precipitated by lithium.[131] Furthermore, a seronegative spondyloarthropathy is sometimes present.[132]

Other clinical findings in palmoplantar pustulosis include the presence of sternocostoclavicular ossification in 10% of cases,[132] and an increased incidence of autoantibodies to thyroid antigens.[133]

Palmoplantar pustulosis has been regarded as a form of psoriasis, a bacterid (an inflammatory reaction at a site remote from that of a bacterial infection presumed to be of pathogenetic significance), and a distinct clinicopathological entity, probably with an immunological pathogenesis.[134,135] The last of these theories is supported by the finding of increased numbers of Langerhans cells in active lesions.[133] There is some evidence that the very rare acute form of palmoplantar pustulosis, which may progress into the chronic form, is a bacterid with an associated vasculitis.[136]

Histopathology[135,137]

The earliest lesion is a spongiotic vesicle in the lower malpighian layer which contains mononuclear cells and some neutrophils.[122] This progresses to a unilocular, well delimited pustule within the epidermis and extending upwards to the undersurface of the stratum corneum (Fig. 6.4).[122] There may be overlying, focal parakeratosis. In the dermis, a mixed perivascular and diffuse infiltrate of inflammatory cells is present.

Controversy exists as to whether it is possible to differentiate pustular psoriasis and palmoplantar pustulosis on histopathological grounds.[138,139] Spongiform pustulation is often present at the upper margins of the pustule in palmoplantar pustulosis but the focus is usually much smaller than that seen in pustular psoriasis.[139] Sometimes there is spongiosis without associated pustulation; this feature is not present in pustular psoriasis.[139]

Immunoreactants are present in the stratum corneum in some cases of palmoplantar pustulosis.[140,141]

VIRAL BLISTERING DISEASES

Intraepidermal vesicles are seen in herpes simplex (see p. 682), herpes zoster (see p. 685), varicella (see p. 684), hand-foot-and-mouth disease (see p. 692) and some cases of milker's nodule (see p. 680) and orf (see p. 681). In the case of herpes simplex, herpes zoster and varicella there is ballooning degeneration of keratinocytes with secondary acantholysis of cells. Multinucleate keratinocytes, some with intranuclear inclusion bodies, may also be seen. In hand-foot-and-mouth disease there is both spongiosis and intracellular oedema while in milker's nodule and orf there may be pronounced intracellular oedema with pallor and degeneration of keratinocytes in the upper layers of the epidermis.

EPIDERMOLYSIS BULLOSA (WEBER–COCKAYNE TYPE)

In the Weber–Cockayne type of epidermolysis bullosa simplex (see p. 142), the split is usually in the mid or upper layers of the epidermis, although in induced blisters the split develops in the basal layer. An occasional dyskeratotic cell may be present in the epidermis.

FRICTION BLISTER

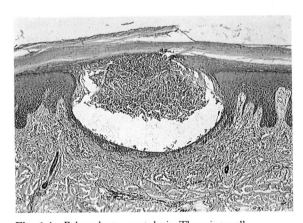

Fig. 6.4 Palmoplantar pustulosis. There is a well-delimited, unilocular pustule extending to the undersurface of the stratum corneum.
Haematoxylin — eosin

Friction blisters are produced at sites where the epidermis is thick and firmly attached to the underlying dermis, as on the palms, soles, heels, and the back of the fingers (see p. 572).

Histopathology

The blister usually forms just beneath the stratum granulosum. The keratinocytes in the base of the blister show variable oedema and pallor and even degenerative changes.

SUPRABASILAR BLISTERS

The suprabasilar blistering diseases — pemphigus vulgaris, pemphigus vegetans, familial benign chronic pemphigus (Hailey–Hailey disease), Darier's disease, Grover's disease (transient acantholytic dermatosis) and acantholytic solar keratosis — all result from acantholysis. In blisters of some days' duration, the split may be present at a higher level within the epidermis as a result of epidermal growth.

PEMPHIGUS VULGARIS

Pemphigus vulgaris is a rare vesiculobullous condition which accounts for approximately 80% of all cases of pemphigus.[142] The initial presentation is often with oral blisters,[143] ulcers and erosions which are followed within weeks to months by the development of cutaneous lesions.[5] These take the form of flaccid blisters on a normal or erythematous base; there is a predilection for the trunk, groins, axillae, scalp, face and pressure points.[5] The blisters break easily, giving eroded and crusted areas. Application of pressure to a blister leads to its extension (Nikolsky's sign).[142] Burning and itching may be present.[143] The lesions generally heal without scarring.[5]

In addition to oral lesions, which eventually develop in 80–90% of cases,[144] other mucosal surfaces may be involved. These include the conjunctiva[145] and larynx[66] and, rarely, the oesophagus,[146–148] urethra, anorectum, vulva and cervix.[149]

Rare clinical presentations include the development of lesions in childhood,[150] the development of transient blisters in a neonate whose mother has pemphigus,[151–153] the development of vegetative[154] or acanthosis-nigricans-like lesions[155] in resolving bullae, and the coexis-

tence of pemphigus vulgaris with bullous pemphigoid.[156] Herpetiform lesions with histological features of eosinophilic spongiosis are more commonly seen in pemphigus foliaceus than in pemphigus vulgaris. Internal cancer,[157] thymoma,[157,158] myasthenia gravis,[159] localized scleroderma,[160] oral submucosal fibrosis[161] and oral herpes simplex infection[162] are rare clinical associations.

The prognosis has improved considerably in recent years, although the mortality is still 5–15%; deaths are due to infections complicating corticosteroid therapy[163] and biochemical abnormalities associated with extensive disease.[164] The titre of circulating antibodies to intercellular cement substance tends to parallel disease activity, although this is of little value in monitoring the clinical management of the patient.[165,166] Recently, it has been found that plasmapheresis reduces the levels of circulating pemphigus antibodies more rapidly than conventional therapy, indicating a likely role for this method of treatment in the future.[167]

Acantholysis is the mechanism by which the bullae form, and it appears that antibodies to intercellular cement substance, and possibly to desmosomes also,[168] induce the acantholysis.[5] This results either from the activation of complement[39,42,169] or by local stimulation of the plasminogen–plasmin system, independent of complement.[170] Various inflammatory mediators have been isolated from blister fluid and these presumably have a role in eliciting the accompanying inflammatory response.[171] What stimulates the formation of antibodies is unknown, although minor trauma[4] and exposure to chemicals[172] have occasionally been documented prior to the onset of the disease. There are also cases in which rifampicin,[173] ampicillin,[174] penicillin[175] and possibly other drugs[32] have precipitated pemphigus vulgaris.

Histopathology

Established lesions of pemphigus vulgaris are suprabasal bullae with acantholysis (Fig. 6.5). The clefting may extend down adnexal structures. The basal cells lose their intercellular bridges but they remain attached to the dermis,

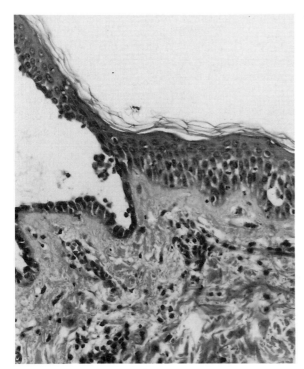

Fig. 6.5 Pemphigus vulgaris. The suprabasal blister contains a few acantholytic cells.
Haematoxylin — eosin

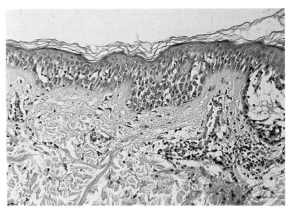

Fig. 6.6 Pemphigus vulgaris. The earliest changes are intercellular oedema and disappearance of the intercellular bridges in the lower epidermis.
Haematoxylin — eosin

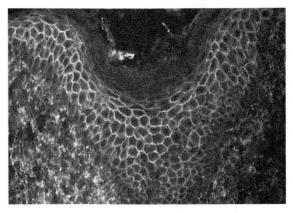

Fig. 6.7 Pemphigus vulgaris. IgG is deposited in the intercellular regions of the epidermis.
Direct immunofluorescence

giving a 'tombstone appearance'.[176] The blister cavity usually contains a few acantholytic cells which often show degenerative changes. Occasionally, a few eosinophils or neutrophils are present in the cavity.[5]

The earliest changes in pemphigus vulgaris consist of oedema and disappearance of the intercellular bridges of keratinocytes in the lower epidermis (Fig. 6.6). This leads to acantholysis and subsequent suprabasal blisters. Eosinophilic spongiosis and subepidermal splitting are two rare presentations of pemphigus vulgaris.[177] Vegetative lesions show epidermal hyperplasia but a paucity of eosinophils, in contrast to pemphigus vegetans.

Dermal changes are of little significance. There is usually a mild, superficial, mixed inflammatory cell infiltrate which usually includes scattered eosinophils.

Direct immunofluorescence usually demonstrates IgG in the intercellular regions of the epidermis in and around the affected parts of the skin (Fig. 6.7);[178] IgG_1 and IgG_4 are the subclasses of IgG found most commonly in patients with active lesions;[179] C3, IgM and IgA are present less frequently.[178,180] Patients in clinical remission, who have positive direct immunofluorescence on a skin biopsy, are more likely to relapse than those with negative immunofluorescence findings.[181] Circulating intercellular antibodies, are present in 80–90% of patients with pemphigus vulgaris, although they may be absent in early cases.[182] Their demonstration depends to some extent on the substrate used; monkey oesophagus gives a higher yield of positive results than guinea-pig oesophagus or human skin.[183] Pemphigus-like antibodies have also been reported in a wide range of inflammatory dermatoses, as well as following burns.[182,184–186]

Electron microscopy.[5] There is dissolution of the intercellular cement substance leading to a widening of the intercellular spaces and eventual separation of the desmosomal attachment plaques. As acantholysis progresses, the desmosomes gradually disappear, followed by retraction of the tonofilaments to the perinuclear area. The keratinocytes often develop numerous, interdigitating processes. Immunoelectron-microscopy shows that the immunoglobulins are deposited on the surface of the epidermal cells in a discontinuous globular pattern.

PEMPHIGUS VEGETANS

Pemphigus vegetans is a rare variant of pemphigus vulgaris[3] which differs from it by the presence of vegetating erosions, primarily affecting flexural areas.[187] Two variants of pemphigus vegetans have been recognized.[187] In the *Neumann type* the initial lesions are vesicular and erosive, resembling pemphigus vulgaris, but the lesions progressively evolve into vegetating plaques. The less common *Hallopeau type* commences with pustular lesions and has a relatively benign course with few, if any, relapses.[188–190]

Oral lesions are almost invariably present in pemphigus vegetans, and these may be the presenting or dominant feature.[191] Sometimes the surface of the tongue assumes a cerebriform pattern.[192] Similar thickening of the epidermis of the scalp may rarely lead to the clinical picture of cutis verticis gyrata.[192] Another clinical feature is the frequent presence of eosinophilia in the peripheral blood.[187]

Recent immunological studies[193] provide further evidence for the close relationship between pemphigus vegetans and pemphigus vulgaris.[194,195] Circulating antibodies have been found in patients with pemphigus vegetans that precipitate with the 130 and 85 kd polypeptides of the pemphigus vulgaris antigen, but there are additional antibodies directed against as yet uncharacterized antigens.[193]

Histopathology[187,192,193]

In the early pustular lesions of the *Hallopeau type*, the appearances resemble those of eosinophilic spongiosis with transmigration of eosinophils into the epidermis and the formation of spongiotic microvesicles and eosinophilic microabscesses.[189] Charcot–Leyden crystals have been seen within these microabscesses.[196] Sporadic acantholytic cells may be present, although they are not usually seen in Tzanck smears prepared from the pustules.[192]

In early lesions of the *Neumann type* there are intraepidermal vesicles with suprabasal acantholysis but no eosinophilic microabscesses.

The vegetative lesions of both types of pemphigus vegetans are similar, with hyperkeratosis, some papillomatosis and prominent acanthosis with downward proliferation of the rete ridges (Fig. 6.8). There are suprabasal lacunae containing some eosinophils. A few acantholytic cells may be present, particularly in the Neumann type.

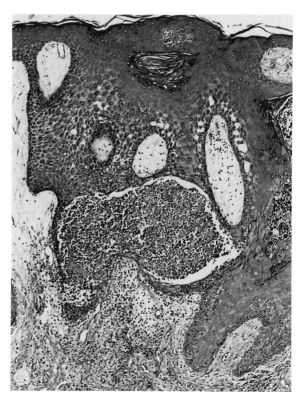

Fig. 6.8 Pemphigus vegetans. Suprabasal clefts containing eosinophils are present in the markedly acanthotic epidermis. Haematoxylin — eosin

In both types of pemphigus vegetans the upper dermis contains a heavy infiltrate of lymphocytes and eosinophils, together with a few neutrophils. There may be oedema of the papillary dermis.

The direct immunofluorescence findings are similar to those in pemphigus vulgaris with the intercellular deposition of IgG and C3.[197] Circulating antibodies to the intercellular region are usually detectable by indirect immunofluorescence.

Electron microscopy.[197,198] There is a reduction in tonofilaments and desmosomes in keratinocytes in skin adjoining the lesion; only rare desmosomes are found in affected skin.[198] Migration of eosinophils into the epidermis through a damaged basement membrane is frequently observed.

FAMILIAL BENIGN CHRONIC PEMPHIGUS

Familial benign chronic pemphigus (Hailey–Hailey disease) is an uncommon genodermatosis with recurrent, erythematous, vesicular plaques which progress to small flaccid bullae with subsequent rupture and crusting. This condition is discussed on page 283.

Histopathology

Early lesions show suprabasilar clefting with acantholytic cells lining and within the clefts. Widespread partial acantholysis at different levels of the epidermis gives rise to the 'dilapidated brick wall' appearance that is so characteristic of the disease. In contrast to Darier's disease, corps ronds are infrequent and grains are rare. Pemphigus vulgaris usually has less acantholysis and more cells showing pronounced dyskeratosis than familial benign chronic pemphigus. Direct immunofluorescence is negative in familial benign chronic pemphigus.

DARIER'S DISEASE

Darier's disease is an autosomal dominant genodermatosis with greasy, crusted papules and papulovesicles, mainly in the seborrhoeic areas of the head, neck and trunk. It is characterized by the minor tissue reaction pattern known as acantholytic dyskeratosis; it is discussed in Chapter 9 (p. 280).

Histopathology

The papulovesicles of Darier's disease show suprabasilar clefting with acantholysis and dyskeratotic cells in the form of corps ronds and grains. There is an overlying keratin plug composed of orthokeratotic and parakeratotic material.

Darier's disease shows more dyskeratosis than pemphigus vulgaris and less acantholysis than familial benign chronic pemphigus.

GROVER'S DISEASE

Grover's disease, also referred to as transient acantholytic dermatosis, is characterized by the sudden onset of small, sometimes crusted, erythematous papules and papulovesicles, particularly on the upper part of the trunk. Like Darier's disease it shows acantholytic dyskeratosis; it is discussed in Chapter 9 (p. 281).

Histopathology

Four histological patterns may be seen in Grover's disease — the so-called Darier-like pattern, the Hailey–Hailey-like pattern, the pemphigus-vulgaris-like pattern and the spongiotic pattern. Subtle histopathological features may allow a lesion of Grover's disease to be distinguished from the three diseases which Grover's disease may resemble microscopically. Lesions of Grover's disease usually have a much thinner keratin plug than Darier's disease. The size of an individual lesion, and the extent of the acantholysis, are usually less in Grover's disease than in either familial benign chronic pemphigus or pemphigus vulgaris. Furthermore, the pemphigus-vulgaris-like lesions of Grover's disease sometimes involve the epidermis adjacent to a hair follicle, in contrast to the random distribution and the more extensive lesions of pemphigus vulgaris itself.

ACANTHOLYTIC SOLAR KERATOSIS

Acantholytic solar keratoses are not always clinically distinct from other types of solar keratosis (see p. 739); they may sometimes resemble a superficial basal cell carcinoma.

Histopathology

Acantholytic solar keratoses are characterized by suprabasilar clefting with acantholytic cells both in the cleft and in its margins. Atypical (dysplastic) keratinocytes are also present. The underlying dermis shows variable solar elastosis. The presence of dysplastic epithelial cells distinguishes acantholytic solar keratosis from the other suprabasilar diseases.

THE CLASSIFICATION OF SUBEPIDERMAL BLISTERS

As stated in the Introduction to this chapter, the subclassification of the subepidermal blistering diseases is usually based on the pattern of inflammation in the underlying dermis.[199] Some overlap occurs between the various categories, particularly with subepidermal vesiculobullous diseases in which neutrophils or eosinophils are the predominant cell in the dermal infiltrate.

The use of special techniques — such as electron microscopy, immuno-electronmicroscopy, direct immunofluorescence using salt-split skin, and immunoperoxidase techniques using monoclonal antibodies directed against various components of the basement membrane zone — has allowed many of the subepidermal blistering diseases to be characterized, in recent times, on the basis of the anatomical level of the split within the basement membrane zone. These techniques have little practical application in most laboratories at present; in routine practice, the nature of the dermal infiltrate is used to distinguish the various subepidermal blistering diseases.

Some knowledge of the basement membrane zone and the various antigens associated with it is required for a proper understanding of the subepidermal blistering diseases.

The epidermal basement membrane

Basement membranes are thin, extracellular matrices which separate epithelia and endothelium from their underlying connective tissue.[200-202] In the skin, basement membranes are found at the dermo–epidermal junction, in the walls of blood vessels and surrounding the various adnexal structures.[200] The discussion which follows relates to the epidermal basement membrane, which has four major structural components: proceeding from the epidermis to the dermis, they are the basal cell plasma membrane, the lamina lucida, the lamina densa, and the sub-lamina-densa zone including the anchoring fibrils.[201,202] In addition to these structural components there are numerous antigenic epitopes within this region.[203] Much of our knowledge about the basement membrane has been gained in recent times; it now appears that the PAS-positive basement membrane, visualized by light microscopists for decades, encompasses more than the true basement membrane.[201]

Plasma membrane. The plasma membrane incorporates the hemidesmosomes, which are studded along the basal surface of the keratinocytes.[201] Tonofilaments insert into the hemidesmosomes. Small anchoring filaments extend between the plasma membrane and the underlying lamina lucida.[202] Little is known of the antigenic structure of this region, although part of the bullous pemphigoid antigen is associated with the attachment plaques of the hemidesmosomes.

Lamina lucida. The lamina lucida is a relatively electron-lucent zone, 20–40 nm in thickness, which is contiguous with the plasma membrane of the overlying basal keratinocytes.[204] The lamina lucida is the weakest link in the dermo–epidermal junction and it represents a plane which is easily severed.[202] At least seven antigens reside in this area: laminin, bullous pemphigoid antigen, cicatricial pemphigoid antigen, fibronectin, AA3, GB3 and 19-DEJ-1.[203,205] This last antigen is localized to the mid-level in the lamina lucida, exclusively in those areas bordered by overlying hemidesmosomes.[205] Laminin and fibronectin are glycoproteins. Fibronectin, which is not confined to a single ultrastructural region, binds to collagen and other components of this zone.

Lamina densa. The lamina densa, which is of epidermal origin, is approximately 30–60 nm in width.[202] It is present just beneath the lamina lucida and it rests on the underlying dermal connective tissue.[204] The lamina densa has been referred to in the past as the basal lamina, but this term has also been applied to the lamina lucida and the lamina densa together.[202] At least eight different antigen structures have been identified in the lamina densa.[203] The main component is type IV collagen which is thought to provide the basement membrane with much of its strength.[200,206] Type IV collagen is resistant to human skin collagenase but it is a substrate for various neutral proteases derived from mast cells, macrophages and granulocytes.[200] Other antigenic components are KF-1, epidermolysis bullosa antigen, nidogen, heparan sulphate proteoglycan, LDA-1, LH 7:2 and chondroitin sulphate proteoglycan.[203]

Sub-lamina-densa. This zone has a variety of components but the major ones are the anchoring fibrils which are the strongest mechanism in securing the epidermis to the dermis.[201] The anchoring fibrils are curved structures with irregularly spaced cross-banding of their central portion.[201] They fan out at either end, inserting into the lamina densa and the papillary dermis. Some fibrils form a sling around islands of type IV collagen and possibly oxytalan fibres, both ends of the sling inserting into the lamina densa.[201] The anchoring fibrils appear to be composed of type VII collagen.[207] The antigens AF-1 and AF-2 are associated with the sub-lamina-densa zone, but the relationship, if any, of these antigens to type VII collagen remains to be elucidated.[203]

Further reference to the basement membrane zone and the antigens within it will be made in the descriptions of the subepidermal blistering diseases that follow.

SUBEPIDERMAL BLISTERS WITH LITTLE INFLAMMATION

This heterogeneous group of vesiculobullous diseases includes variants of epidermolysis bullosa, porphyria cutanea tarda, the cell-poor type of bullous pemphigoid, burns, toxic epidermal necrolysis, suction blisters, the blisters that sometimes form over dermal scar tissue and some bullous drug reactions.

EPIDERMOLYSIS BULLOSA

The term epidermolysis bullosa is applied to a heterogeneous group of non-inflammatory disorders characterized by the development of blisters or erosions following minor trauma to the skin.[208,209] Spontaneous blister formation may occur in some individuals. The clinical presentation may range from minimal involvement of the hands and feet to severe, life-threatening, generalized blistering with dystrophic changes, and extracutaneous involvement.[210]

Epidermolysis bullosa is usually inherited as an autosomal dominant or recessive disorder, although an acquired form (see below) has also been recognized.[209] The incidence of the hereditary forms is 1:50 000 births; the more severe recessive forms have an incidence of 1:200 000 to 1:500 000 births.[210]

These mechanobullous diseases are best classified into three subgroups on the basis of the level at which the skin separates.[211] The three subgroups are:

Epidermolytic (epidermolysis bullosa simplex)
Junctional (junctional epidermolysis bullosa)
Dermolytic (dystrophic epidermolysis bullosa).

For convenience, all forms of epidermolysis bullosa will be considered together because in the majority of cases the appearances on light microscopy are those of a cell-poor subepidermal blister. The epidermolytic group which involves lysis of basal cells will be considered first.

Epidermolysis bullosa simplex

Epidermolysis bullosa simplex, one of the three

major subgroups of epidermolysis bullosa, is a mechanobullous disorder characterized by intraepidermal cleavage, usually through the basal layer of cells.[208,212] There are several distinct clinical variants. Most cases have a mild clinical expression with blisters which heal without scarring and an autosomal dominant inheritance.[213] Rare cases with an autosomal recessive inheritance and a more severe clinical course, sometimes with associated neuromuscular disease, have been reported.[214,215]

The pathogenesis of this group is unknown, although proteases may be the active factor involved in the cell lysis.[216] What triggers the protease cascade is unknown.

Generalized (Koebner) type. This clinical variant is characterized by the development of serous blisters at birth or in early infancy. Blisters may involve the whole body, but they are preferentially distributed on the hands and feet.[208] Cases with oral involvement or with keratoderma of the palms and soles have been reported.[217] The lesions tend to be worse in warmer weather, a feature present in several other variants.

Localized (Weber–Cockayne) type. This form appears to be a localized variant of the Koebner type in which lesions are confined to the hands and feet.[208] Onset is usually within the first two years of life, although it may be delayed into adolescence or beyond.[218] A kindred with autosomal recessive inheritance has been reported.[219]

Epidermolysis bullosa herpetiformis (Dowling—Meara). This is one of the most frequent subtypes and is characterized by the development in the first few months of life of serous or haemorrhagic blisters on the trunk, face and extremities.[220] The blisters may have a herpetiform arrangement. Inflammatory lesions may be present and these sometimes heal with transitory milia or pigmentation.[221] Mucosal lesions and nail involvement may occur, as may keratoderma of the palms and soles.[222] Some improvement occurs with age. This variant has distinct ultrastructural features with clumping of

tonofilaments; the cause of this is unknown.[220,223]

Other variants. Exceedingly rare variants include the *Ogna type* in which there are acral sanguineous blebs and a generalized bruising tendency,[210] the *Fischer and Gedde–Dahl type*[208] in which the blistering tendency is accompanied by mottled pigmentation of the skin,[208,224] and the *superficial type* in which there is subcorneal cleavage mimicking the 'scalded skin' syndrome (see p. 597).[225] Isolated reports claiming new clinical variants appear from time to time.[226–228] The *Bart type*, in which there is congenital localized absence of the skin associated with trauma-induced blisters, is not a specific form of epidermolytic epidermolysis bullosa as sometimes claimed, but probably a mild form of the dermolytic subgroup.[229–232]

Histopathology

In epidermolysis bullosa simplex the cleavage is so low in the epidermis that in routine paraffin sections the blister may appear to be a cell-poor subepidermal blister (Fig. 6.9).[213] With thin plastic-embedded sections, fragments of basal keratinocytes may be observed in the blister base;[213] the PAS-positive basement membrane is also found in that position. Immunofluorescence or immunoperoxidase techniques can also be used to confirm the level of the split. These

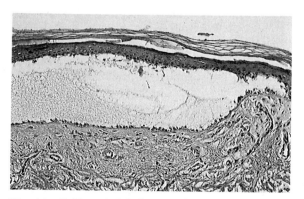

Fig. 6.9 Epidermolysis bullosa simplex with cleavage in the base of the epidermis. Fragments of the basal keratinocytes are present in the floor of the blister. There is no dermal inflammation.
Haematoxylin — eosin

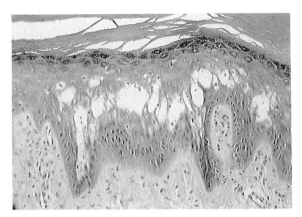

Fig 6.10 Epidermis bullosa (Weber–Cockaybe type). The split is in the mid-epidermis. Haematoxylin — eosin

methods will show that the bullous pemphigoid antigen, laminin, type IV collagen and the LDA-1 antigen (a component of the lamina densa) are all present in the base of the bulla.[233,234]

In the Weber–Cockayne subtype, the level of the split is usually in the mid or upper epidermis (Fig. 6.10), although induced blisters develop in the basal layer.[235] In epidermolysis bullosa herpetiformis a number of eosinophils may be found in the underlying papillary dermis.[221] A rare variant with subcorneal splitting has been reported (see above);[225] a variant with enlarged dyskeratotic basal cells which have eosinophilic clumps in the cytoplasm and show some atypical mitoses is also rare.[236]

Electron microscopy. There is some perinuclear oedema and subnuclear cytolysis of the basal cells[217] but organelles are usually intact. In epidermolysis bullosa herpetiformis the cytolysis is preceded by aggregation and clumping of the tonofilaments which are attached to the hemidesmosomes at the dermo–epidermal junction.[220,222] The basement membrane zone is intact in all variants of epidermolysis bullosa simplex.

Junctional epidermolysis bullosa

Junctional ('lamina lucidolytic') epidermolysis bullosa is an extremely rare group of mechanobullous diseases characterized by autosomal recessive inheritance, lesions which heal without scarring (although in time atrophy may develop), and separation through the lamina lucida.[211] Extracutaneous epithelial involvement may occur.[237] Prenatal diagnosis can be made by fetal skin biopsy.[238,239] Laboratory findings have included reduced natural killer-cell activity[240] and reduced levels of certain trace metals and vitamins.[241] These features are of uncertain significance.

Several antigenic defects have been detected in the lamina lucida in cases of junctional epidermolysis bullosa.[239,242,243] Two such defects are the absence of reactivity using immunofluorescent techniques and either a GB3 monoclonal antibody[244] or a murine monoclonal antibody 19-DEJ-1.[245] These findings may be of diagnostic value, although their pathogenetic significance remains to be elucidated. Reduced adhesion of keratinocytes in culture has also been reported;[246] this appears to result from defective hemidesmosome synthesis.[246a]

There are six clinical variants[247] of junctional epidermolysis bullosa:

Epidermolysis bullosa atrophicans gravis (epidermolysis bullosa letalis). This form has severe generalized involvement with acral accentuation.[248] Erosions and bullae are present at birth.[249] Large non-healing areas of granulation tissue develop on the nape of the neck and in the perioral region. Most affected individuals die in early infancy but a few have survived for longer periods.[208] Clinical associations have included anaemia, pyloric atresia,[250,251] oral lesions, blepharitis and epithelial separation in various internal organs.[252,253]

Epidermolysis bullosa atrophicans mitis (generalized atrophic benign epidermolysis bullosa). In this generalized form lesions heal with atrophy and mild scarring, but there are no milia or contractures.[247,254] There may be some improvement with age. Baldness and absence of pubic and axillary hair are other clinical features.[210]

Epidermolysis bullosa atrophicans inversa. This subtype has truncal blistering with acral sparing.[211] Improvement occurs with age. Chymotrypsin, a proteolytic enzyme thought to digest laminin, was increased in the serum in one reported case.[255]

Epidermolysis bullosa atrophicans localisata. Onset of this form is in early childhood. Lesions are restricted to the soles and pretibial area.[210]

Epidermolysis bullosa progressiva. This rare form presents with nail dystrophy followed some years later by acral blisters.[256] Partial deafness is sometimes present.

Cicatricial junctional epidermolysis bullosa. Clinically, this variant resembles the dystrophic forms with lesions present at birth which heal with scarring.[257] Contractures and scarring of the anterior nares may develop, as also may oral and laryngeal lesions.[257]

Histopathology

The junctional forms appear as subepidermal, cell-poor blisters with the PAS-positive basement membrane in the floor.[252] Laminin, LDA-1 and type IV collagen can also be demonstrated in the base of the blister; the bullous pemphigoid antigen can be detected in the roof.[234,247] If atrophy develops, there is thinning of the epidermis and flattening of the rete ridges. Dermal fibrosis is present in the cicatricial variant.

Electron microscopy. The various junctional forms cannot be distinguished ultrastructurally. They all show separation through the lamina lucida with variable hypoplasia of the hemidesmosomes.[250,258] Disruption of the basement membrane and an increase in dermal fibroblasts are present in the cicatricial variant.[257] Amorphous deposits have been reported in the lamina lucida in epidermolysis

bullosa progressiva but this finding has not been confirmed subsequently.[256]

Dermolytic (dystrophic) epidermolysis bullosa

The dermolytic (dystrophic) forms of epidermolysis bullosa present with trauma-induced blistering which is followed by the formation of scars and milia.[259] There are six clinical subtypes, three of which are inherited in an autosomal dominant fashion. The remainder are recessive in type, and in these cases the lesions tend to be more severe. A transient neonatal variant which does not fit into any of these subtypes has also been reported.[260,260a] Antenatal diagnosis of dermolytic epidermolysis bullosa can be made by fetal skin biopsy.[261]

Other clinical features which may be present include nail dystrophy, and oral[237] and gastrointestinal lesions,[262] particularly oesophageal webs and strictures;[263] congenital localized absence of the skin,[232,264] anaemia, growth retardation and poor nutrition may also be present.[241,265] Squamous cell carcinomas of the skin are an uncommon complication,[266–268] which may be linked to the persistent growth-activated immunophenotype of epidermal keratinocytes that has been found in this disease.[269] Systemic amyloidosis is a rare complication.[270]

The dermolytic variants are all characterized by the development of a split below the basal lamina in the region of the anchoring fibrils. These fibrils are absent in the severe recessive form and diminished in number in many of the other types.[271,272] Abnormal collagenase activity has been demonstrated in the recessive forms and this may be responsible for the destruction of the anchoring fibrils.[216,273,274] Of interest is the finding that drugs which inhibit collagenase and proteases have a favourable therapeutic effect on the course of the disease.[210,275,276] Recent work from several centres suggests that a genetic defect in the synthesis, secretion or molecular assembly of type VII collagen may underlie at least one of the recessive dystrophic forms of epidermolysis bullosa.[277–281] However, type VII collagen was expressed normally in one reported case of dystrophic epidermolysis bullosa inversa (see below), but the anchoring fibrils were defective.[281a] This suggests that different mechanisms may be involved in the pathogenesis of some of the dermolytic types of epidermolysis bullosa.

The various clinical types of dermolytic epidermolysis bullosa are discussed below, commencing with the three dominant forms.

Dermolytic epidermolysis bullosa, hyperplastic variant (Cockayne–Touraine). In this form, blisters commence at birth or in early childhood, but they are usually not debilitating.[282] There is a predilection for acral regions, particularly the extensor surfaces.[211] The scars that develop may be hypertrophic.[210]

Dermolytic epidermolysis bullosa, albopapuloid variant (Pasini). Generalized blistering and erosions commence at birth or in infancy.[211] Pale papules (albopapuloid lesions) develop on the trunk at puberty.[283] Cultured fibroblasts from the skin of affected individuals accumulate excess amounts of glycosaminoglycans; the significance of this is uncertain.[282]

Pretibial epidermolysis bullosa. This rare variant is associated with pretibial blisters which usually develop between the ages of 11 and 24 years.[284–286] Albopapuloid lesions are occasionally present.[208]

Dermolytic epidermolysis bullosa (Hallopeau–Siemens). This autosomal recessive variant is highly debilitating and characterized by large flaccid bullae on any part of the skin from birth.[283] There is a range of severity, with a shortened life span in the severe (gravis) forms.[210,211] The scarring often leads to digital fusion and so-called 'mitten' deformities.[283] The oral, oesophageal, anal and vaginal mucosae are frequently involved with the development of fibrous strictures.[287] Sparse hair, dystrophic teeth, keratitis[288] and growth retardation are common features.[211] A variant with progressive,

symmetrical, centripetal involvement exists.[211,289] Heterozygotes appear to have diminished numbers of anchoring fibrils.[290]

Localized dermolytic epidermolysis bullosa. Blisters develop on the extremities in early childhood.[208] There is some improvement with age.

Dermolytic epidermolysis bullosa inversa. In this variant blisters develop in the skin of the axillae, neck and lower part of the trunk with sparing of the extremities.[291] Milia are usually absent. Mucosal involvement is common and the tongue may be bound to the floor of the mouth.[291]

Histopathology

Routine light microscopy is of little value in the diagnosis of the dermolytic forms of epidermolysis bullosa.[243] There is a cell-poor, subepidermal blister. Superficial dermal scarring and milia are often present. The PAS-positive basement membrane, the bullous pemphigoid antigen, laminin and types IV and V collagen are all found in the roof of the blister.[233] Staining is weak or absent with antibodies to KF-1, AF-1 and AF-2, which are all components of the anchoring fibrils.[210,234,243] If a monoclonal antibody to type VII collagen is used (LH 7:2), staining will occur in the genetically dominant dermolytic forms but only weakly or not at all in the recessive forms.[238,259,279]

Electron microscopy. The anchoring fibrils are totally absent in the generalized recessive form and diminished in number in both the localized recessive and the dominant variants.[211,272] The split occurs beneath the basal lamina.

Epidermolysis bullosa acquisita

Epidermolysis bullosa acquisita (dermolytic pemphigoid) is a rare, non-hereditary, subepidermal bullous disorder with heterogeneous clinical features.[292–294] Typically, there are non-inflammatory bullae which develop in areas subjected to minor trauma such as the extensor surface of the limbs.[295] The lesions eventually heal leaving atrophic scars and milia. In up to 50% of cases the initial presentation is with widespread inflammatory bullae, which are not precipitated by trauma, and which heal without scarring.[292,296] Some such cases, if not all, eventually evolve into the non-inflammatory, scarring type.[292] At times the clinical presentation may mimic bullous pemphigoid or cicatricial pemphigoid.[297-299]

Involvement of the mucous membranes occurs in 30–50% of cases. This usually takes the form of oral erosions and blisters, but ocular involvement can also occur.[300] Vesicular cystitis[301] and scarring alopecia[302] are rarely present.

Onset of the disease is usually in mid-adult life, although a few cases have been reported in children.[303-305] Its course is usually chronic and there is great variability in severity and evolution.[292,306]

Epidermolysis bullosa acquisita has been associated with various systemic diseases, particularly those with a presumed immune pathogenesis.[292,295] They include systemic lupus erythematosus,[307,307a] rheumatoid arthritis, inflammatory bowel disease[302,308] (particularly Crohn's disease),[309] chronic thyroiditis, amyloidosis,[310] mixed cryoglobulinaemia[311] and the multiple endocrinopathy syndrome.[312] Its onset has also been triggered by pregnancy[313] and by penicillamine.[293]

Earlier views[314] that this condition was not a distinct entity but a variant of cicatricial pemphigoid were put to rest by the discovery of the epidermolysis bullosa acquisita (EBA) antigen.[315-318] This antigen has recently been identified as type VII collagen,[319,320] a major component of the anchoring fibrils.[320] It appears to be synthesized by both fibroblasts and keratinocytes.[317] The initiating event in this dermatosis is probably the formation and binding of antibody to the carboxy terminal region of type VII collagen.[319,320a]

Histopathology[292]

There is a subepidermal bulla with fibrin and only a few inflammatory cells in the lumen.[321] The roof of the blister is usually intact and there may be a few dermal fragments attached to the epidermis.[322] In non-inflammatory lesions there is a sparse lymphocytic infiltrate around the vessels of the superficial vascular plexus while in inflammatory lesions there is a heavy dermal inflammatory infiltrate in which neutrophils predominate.[296] Some eosinophils may also be present. The histological heterogeneity presumably results from the heterogeneity of the immune complexes that are deposited, some having greater ability than others to generate complement-derived chemotaxis. In older lesions there will be some dermal scarring and also milia.

With the PAS stain, the basement membrane is split, with most of the PAS-positive material attached to the blister roof.[321] Laminin and type IV collagen can be identified by immunoperoxidase techniques in the roof of the blister.[323] This technique is helpful if facilities are not available for immunoelectronmicroscopy.

Direct immunofluorescence shows linear deposition of immunoglobulins, particularly IgG, and of complement along the basement membrane zone in nearly all lesions;[302,310] cases reported without immunoreactants may form a distinct subgroup.[322,324] Circulating IgG class antibodies to the basement membrane zone are present in up to 50% of cases.[325,326] Using salt-split skin as a substrate these antibodies bind to the dermal floor, in contrast to bullous pemphigoid antibodies which bind to the epidermal roof. A substrate can be prepared in the same way using affected skin and this is then subjected to direct immunofluorescence.[327,328]

Electron microscopy. The split usually occurs in the superficial dermis below the lamina lucida.[329] However, in some of the inflammatory variants splitting may occur within the lamina lucida, possibly as a result of leucocyte-derived proteolytic enzymes acting on the lamina lucida, which appears to be a *locus minoris resistentiae*.[330,331] Electron-dense amorphous deposits are present beneath the lamina densa. On immunoelectronmicroscopy, the immunoreactants which correspond with the electron-dense deposits noted on routine electron microscopy are found within and/or below the lamina densa.[306,331,332]

PORPHYRIA CUTANEA TARDA

Blisters can develop in light-exposed areas, particularly the dorsum of the hands, in porphyria cutanea tarda (see p. 536)

Histopathology

The blisters are subepidermal, with preservation of the dermal papillae in the floor of the lesion ('festooning') (Fig. 6.11). Hyaline material, which is PAS positive and diastase resistant, is present in the walls of the small vessels in the upper dermis and sometimes in the basement membrane of the epidermis. There is usually no inflammatory infiltrate, although patchy haemorrhage is sometimes present in the blister and the underlying dermis.

BULLOUS PEMPHIGOID (CELL-POOR TYPE)

If a biopsy is taken from a bullous lesion in bullous pemphigoid which does not have an erythe-matous base, the lesion will often have few inflammatory cells in the dermis. This is in contrast to lesions with an erythematous base which usually have a heavier dermal infiltrate, including many eosinophils.

BURNS

Subepidermal blisters may develop in second-degree thermal burns and following electrodesiccation therapy. Haemorrhagic blisters may develop after cryotherapy (see p. 577). They are usually cell-poor initially; neutrophils may be present in older lesions, particularly if the lesion becomes infected.

The epidermis is usually necrotic; vertical elongation of keratinocytes is a conspicuous feature after electrodesiccation. The basket-weave pattern of the stratum corneum is usually preserved. A distinctive feature is the fusion of collagen bundles in the upper dermis; they have a refractile eosinophilic appearance.

TOXIC EPIDERMAL NECROLYSIS

Toxic epidermal necrolysis, which is now regarded as a variant of erythema multiforme, presents with generalized tender erythema which rapidly

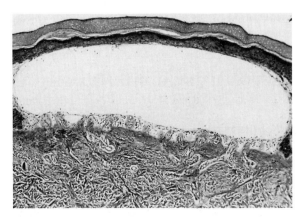

Fig. 6.11 Porphyria cutanea tarda. There is a cell-poor, subepidermal bulla with preservation of the dermal papillae in the floor ('festooning').
Haematoxylin — eosin

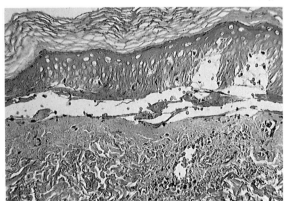

Fig. 6.12 Toxic epidermal necrolysis. This variant of erythema multiforme is characterized by a cell-poor, subepidermal blister with necrosis of the overlying epidermis.
Haematoxylin — eosin

progresses to a blistering phase with extensive shedding of the skin (see p. 45). There is a subepidermal bulla with confluent necrosis of the overlying epidermis (Fig. 6.12). The perivascular infiltrate of lymphocytes, if present at all, is usually sparse, justifying categorization of the condition as a cell-poor blistering disease. Cases with features overlapping those of erythema multiforme are sometimes seen.

Mustard gas, used in chemical warfare, can result in bullae with full-thickness epidermal necrosis resembling toxic epidermal necrolysis.[332a]

SUCTION BLISTERS

Blisters induced by suction are subepidermal in type, in contrast to friction blisters which develop within the epidermis. The dermal papillae are usually preserved in suction blisters ('festooning'). Suction blisters may be a manifestation of dermatitis artefacta (see p . 572).

BLISTERS OVERLYING SCARS

Subepidermal clefting sometimes occurs overlying a dermal scar, particularly if this involves the papillary as well as the reticular dermis. The clefting is usually an incidental histological finding without obvious clinical manifestations. The finding of scar tissue in the base of the blister in association with a clinical history of surgery or some other trauma at the affected site characterizes this entity (Fig. 6.13).

Subepidermal bullae, with a slight lymphocytic infiltrate, have been reported in grafted leg ulcers 4–8 weeks after the operation.[332b] The pathogenetic mechanism is not currently known.

BULLOUS AMYLOIDOSIS

Rarely, bullae may form above the amyloid deposits in the skin in primary systemic amyloidosis (see p. 409). The split is usually in the upper dermis. There are characteristic hyaline deposits of amyloid in the base of the blister. Haemorrhage is often present.

BULLOUS DRUG REACTION

Subepidermal bullae are an uncommon manifestation of a drug reaction. The inflammatory cell infiltrate in the dermis may be variable in intensity and composition. One category is cell-poor and resembles porphyria cutanea tarda (pseudoporphyria). In contrast to porphyria cutanea tarda, drug-induced pseudoporphyria has less PAS-positive material in vessel walls and less obvious 'festooning' (persistence of dermal papillae in the base of the blister). A rare eosinophil may be present in the dermis in the drug-induced cases; this is not a feature of porphyria cutanea tarda.

SUBEPIDERMAL BLISTERS WITH LYMPHOCYTES

All of the conditions in this group have been discussed in other chapters. Accordingly, they will be given only brief mention here.

ERYTHEMA MULTIFORME

The vesiculobullous lesions in erythema multiforme result from damage to the basal cells of the epidermis. Accordingly, this condition is consid-

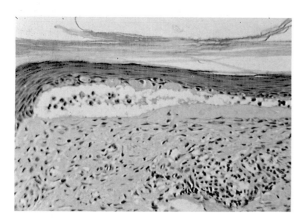

Fig. 6.13 Subepidermal clefting overlying scar tissue. Haematoxylin — eosin

ered among the lichenoid reaction patterns (see Ch. 3, p. 43). Erythema multiforme is characterized by a subepidermal blister with a mild to moderately heavy infiltrate of lymphocytes in the underlying dermis. The infiltrate, which may include a few eosinophils, extends to the level of the mid dermis. The epidermis overlying the blister may show necrosis which may be confluent or involve only small groups of cells. Apoptotic keratinocytes are usually present in the epidermis adjacent to the blister.

FIXED DRUG ERUPTIONS

A bullous variant of fixed drug eruption has been described (see p. 41). The lesions resemble those seen in erythema multiforme; in fixed drug eruptions there is usually deeper extension of the inflammatory cell infiltrate in the dermis, with more eosinophils and sometimes neutrophils in the infiltrate, and melanin in macrophages and lying free in the upper dermis. The inflammatory cell infiltrate tends to obscure the dermo–epidermal interface adjacent to the blister in both erythema multiforme and fixed drug eruptions.

LICHEN SCLEROSUS ET ATROPHICUS

Lichen sclerosus et atrophicus is a chronic dermatosis affecting predominantly the anogenital region of middle-aged and elderly women. Infrequently, haemorrhagic bullae develop. There is a broad zone of oedema or partly sclerotic collagen in the base of the blister with telangiectatic vessels and some haemorrhage. Beneath this oedematous/sclerotic zone there is an infiltrate of lymphocytes which is predominantly perivascular in position (see p. 335).

LICHEN PLANUS PEMPHIGOIDES

Lichen planus pemphigoides is characterized by the development of tense blisters, often located on the extremities, in a patient with lichen planus (see p. 38). There is a mild perivascular infiltrate of lymphocytes, and sometimes there are a few eosinophils beneath the blister. Occasional Civatte bodies are usually present in the basal layer at the margins of the blister. Direct immunofluorescence will usually demonstrate IgG and C3 in the basement membrane zone.

If the bullae develop in papules of lichen planus, as opposed to otherwise uninvolved skin, there is usually a much heavier dermal infiltrate which is superficial and band-like in distribution. There are numerous Civatte bodies in the overlying and adjacent basal keratinocytes. The term *bullous lichen planus* is used in these circumstances.

POLYMORPHOUS LIGHT ERUPTION

Papulovesicular lesions and, rarely, bullae may occur as a clinical subset of polymorphous light eruption (see p. 581). The lesions develop several hours after exposure to the sun. There is pronounced subepidermal oedema leading to blister formation. In early lesions the collagen fibres are separated by the oedema fluid, giving a cobweb-like appearance. Extravasation of red blood cells may be present in this region. A characteristic feature is the presence of a perivascular infiltrate of lymphocytes which involves not only the superficial dermis but also the deep dermis.

FUNGAL INFECTIONS

Pronounced subepidermal oedema leading to vesiculation is a rare manifestation of a fungal infection. It may also be seen in the 'id reaction' to a fungus (see p. 641).

DERMAL ALLERGIC CONTACT DERMATITIS

This is a poorly understood variant of allergic contact dermatitis which may result from contact with various agents, in particular neomycin and zinc and nickel salts (see p. 104). There is pronounced subepidermal oedema leading to vesiculation. The lymphocytes in the infiltrate do not extend as deeply in the dermis as they do in polymorphous light eruption. Epidermal spongiosis is often present and it distinguishes this condition from the other subepidermal blistering diseases.

BULLOUS LEPROSY

Subepidermal bullae are an exceedingly rare manifestation of borderline lepromatous leprosy (see p. 611). Lymphocytes and small collections of macrophages, some with foamy cytoplasm, are present in the dermis; they also surround small cutaneous nerves. Acid-fast bacilli are present within the macrophages.

BULLOUS MYCOSIS FUNGOIDES

Bullae are a very rare manifestation of mycosis fungoides (see p. 1034). They are usually subepidermal in location but intraepidermal splitting has been recorded. The presence of atypical lymphocytes in the underlying dermis and of Pautrier microabscesses in the epidermis characterizes this condition.

SUBEPIDERMAL BLISTERS WITH EOSINOPHILS

Eosinophils are a conspicuous and major component of the inflammatory cell infiltrate in the bullae and in the dermis in bullous pemphigoid and pemphigoid gestationis. They are also found in certain arthropod reactions, particularly in sensitized individuals, and in some bullous drug reactions. Vesiculobullous lesions, resembling insect bites, have been reported in patients with chronic lymphocytic leukaemia.[332c] Eosinophils may be the predominant cell type in some cases of dermatitis herpetiformis (particularly lesions that are more than 48 hours old) and of cicatricial pemphigoid.

BULLOUS PEMPHIGOID

Bullous pemphigoid is a chronic blistering dermatosis in which the split occurs in the lamina lucida.[333] There are multiple, tense bullae of varying size that develop on normal or erythematous skin. Individual lesions may measure several centimetres in diameter. In addition, there may be erythematous macules, urticarial plaques and crusted erosions.[334] Eczematous or urticarial lesions may precede by weeks or months the occurrence of bullous lesions.[335,336] Less common presentations include the development of lesions localized to one area of the body,[337] such as the vulva,[337a] the legs (particularly the pretibial skin),[338,339] a stoma site[340] or the palms and soles,[341] and the development of a haemorrhagic pompholyx.[342,343] The localized variants of bullous pemphigoid must be distinguished from localized cicatricial pemphigoid in which scarring occurs (see p. 160). In established cases of bullous pemphigoid, bullae are found on the lower part of the abdomen, in the groins, and on the flexor surface of the arms and legs. Oral lesions are present in 10–40% of cases,[344] but involvement of other mucosal surfaces is quite rare.[345] Eosinophilia in the blood and elevated serum IgE levels are often present.[334,346] The disease tends to involve older people,[334] but its occurrence in young adults[347] and children has been reported.[348,349]

Several rare clinical variants of bullous pemphigoid have been reported (see below). Immuno-electronmicroscopy of these variants has shown that the immunoreactants deposit in the same position in the basement zone as they do in bullous pemphigoid; this justifies their inclusion as variants of bullous pemphigoid.[350]

Vesicular pemphigoid. There is a chronic eruption of small vesicles which are often pruritic, and occasionally grouped, resembling dermatitis herpetiformis.[351,352] Progression to typical bullous pemphigoid sometimes occurs.[352]

Pemphigoid vegetans. This rare variant resembles pemphigus vegetans clinically with purulent and verrucous, vegetating lesions in intertriginous areas, particularly the groins.[353-356] Inflammatory bowel disease is usually present in patients with this form of bullous pemphigoid.[353]

Polymorphic pemphigoid. This term has been used for cases with features of both dermatitis herpetiformis and bullous pemphigoid.[357] Some of these cases would now be regarded as examples of linear IgA disease.[358] The probable coexistence of bullous pemphigoid and dermatitis herpetiformis has also been reported.[359]

Pemphigoid nodularis. This rare variant combines features of prurigo nodularis with those of bullous pemphigoid, often in the same lesion.[360-363] The verrucous papules or nodules may persist or resolve with scarring. A case with hyperkeratotic islands within areas of denuded blisters, reported as 'pemphigoid en cocarde', is best regarded as a variant of pemphigoid nodularis.[364]

A wide range of diseases, many of presumed autoimmune origin, is reported in association with bullous pemphigoid.[365,366] They include rheumatoid arthritis,[367] systemic lupus erythematosus,[368-370] primary biliary cirrhosis,[371] ulcerative colitis,[372] alopecia areata,[373] diabetes mellitus,[374] thyroid disease,[375,376] multiple sclerosis,[377] acanthosis palmaris,[378] immune complex nephritis,[379,380] pemphigus,[20] psoriasis[381-383] and internal cancer.[384-386] However, it now appears that the association of bullous pemphigoid and internal cancer is not statistically significant.[387]

Bullous pemphigoid runs a chronic course of months to years, with periods of remission and exacerbation.[164] Death is now uncommon in this disease because of improved management.[164]

The initial event in the pathogenesis of bullous pemphigoid appears to be the binding of IgG class antibodies to a transmembrane antigen associated with the lamina lucida and the hemidesmosomes of basal keratinocytes (the bullous pemphigoid antigen).[388-391b] The bullous pemphigoid antigen shows some molecular heterogeneity: the major antigen is a 230 kd basic protein;[392] another antigen (180 kd) has recently been isolated from some patients with bullous pemphigoid.[393] Following the fixation of antibody to the bullous pemphigoid antigen, complement is activated leading to the chemotaxis of neutrophils and eosinophils.[169,394] Mast cells may also be important in the recruitment of eosinophils.[395] The neutrophils and eosinophils release proteolytic enzymes which appear to be responsible for the initial stages of blister formation.[39,396,397]

Although the pathogenetic mechanisms involved in blister formation are reasonably well understood, what triggers the formation of the antibodies to the basement zone is unknown. In a few cases drugs have been incriminated although there is some evidence that the antibodies involved in drug-related cases are, in part, different from those found in usual cases of bullous pemphigoid. The implicated drugs include penicillin derivatives,[398,399] sulphasalazine, ibuprofen,[400] phenacetin,[401] novoscabin, frusemide (furosemide),[402,403] penicillamine[404] and topical fluorouracil.[401] Trauma[405] and radiation[406] have been implicated in a very small number of cases.

Histopathology[199,407]

In bullous pemphigoid there is a unilocular subepidermal blister, eosinophils being the predominant cell in the dermis and blister cavity (Figs 6.14a&b). If the biopsy is taken from a bulla on otherwise normal-appearing skin, there is only a sparse dermal infiltrate; bullae with an erythematous base have a much heavier infiltrate of inflammatory cells in the upper dermis. In addition to eosinophils there are some neutrophils and lymphocytes. Eosinophilic spongiosis may be seen in the clinically erythematous skin bordering the blister.[408]

In lesions of several days' duration, the blister may appear intraepidermal in location at its periphery as a result of regeneration. Sometimes epidermal necrosis occurs in the roof of the blister.[409] There are no isolated, necrotic, basal keratinocytes in the roof of early blisters, as sometimes are seen in pemphigoid gestationis.

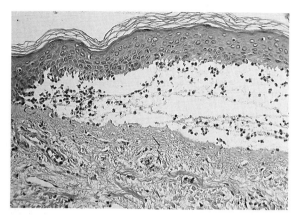

Fig. 6.14a Bullous pemphigoid. There is a subepidermal blister, the lumen of which contains eosinophils. There are relatively few eosinophils in the dermis ('cell-poor' variant). Haematoxylin — eosin

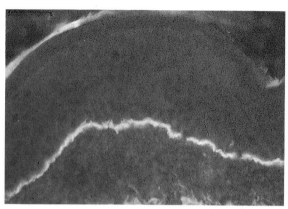

Fig. 6.15 Bullous pemphigoid. The basement membrane zone shows a linear pattern of staining for C3. Direct immunofluorescence

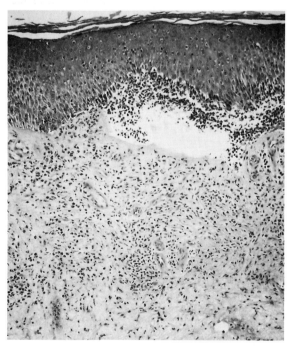

Fig. 6.14b Bullous pemphigoid. This 'cell-rich' variant has numerous eosinophils. Haematoxylin — eosin

The variants of bullous pemphigoid (see above) show some distinguishing histological features reflecting their different clinical appearances. In *vesicular pemphigoid* the lesions are quite small while in *pemphigus vegetans* there is usually prominent acanthosis of the epidermis. Acanthosis is also present in *pemphigoid nodularis*; in addition there is overlying hyperkeratosis and mild papillomatosis.

Prodromal lesions of bullous pemphigoid show oedema of the papillary dermis and a superficial and mid-dermal perivascular infiltrate with numerous eosinophils, occasional lymphocytes and rare neutrophils. Interstitial eosinophils may also be present. A few eosinophils are found within the epidermis.

Direct immunofluorescence almost invariably shows a linear, homogeneous deposition of IgG and/or C3 along the basement membrane zone of the skin around the lesion (Fig. 6.15).[410] In early stages of the disease only C3 may be present. IgM and IgA are present in approximately 20% of cases.[411] The deposition of immunoreactants is probably not influenced by the anatomical site from which the biopsy is taken, as formerly suggested.[412,413] Direct immunofluorescence on suction blisters taken from uninvolved forearm skin of patients with bullous pemphigoid has not shown a consistent pattern of staining.[414] The significance of this finding is uncertain.

Circulating anti-basement-membrane-zone antibodies, usually of IgG class, are present in 60–80% of patients.[415] Their titre does not correlate with disease activity or severity. Antibodies may be absent when circulating immune complexes are formed.[416] Similar antibodies are present in some cases of cicatricial pemphigoid and, rarely, in non-bullous dermatoses.

Electron microscopy.[333,395,417,418] In the cell-poor blisters there is focal thinning and disruption of anchoring filaments with formation of the split in the lamina lucida. In the cell-rich lesions there is more extensive damage in the basement membrane zone following the migration of eosinophils into this region. There is disintegration of the lamina lucida and fragmentation of anchoring fibrils and hemidesmosomes. The basal cells may show some vacuolization.

Immuno-electronmicroscopy shows that the immunoreactants are in the lamina lucida and in the vicinity of the cytoplasmic plaque of the basal cell hemidesmosomes.[391] There are no deposits beneath melanocytes.

PEMPHIGOID GESTATIONIS

Pemphigoid gestationis (formerly known as herpes gestationis) is a rare, pruritic, vesiculobullous dermatosis of pregnancy and the puerperium.[419–424] It occurs in approximately 1 in 10 000 pregnancies, and rarely in association with hydatidiform mole[425] and choriocarcinoma.[426] The onset of the disease is usually in the second or third trimester of pregnancy with the development of papules and urticarial plaques, initially localized to the periumbilical region. Subsequently, the lesions spread to involve the trunk and extremities, becoming vesiculobullous in form.[420] Untreated, the lesions persist through the pregnancy, but they subside within several days or weeks of delivery;[427] persistence for many months or years has been reported.[428,429] Oral contraceptives sometimes cause exacerbations.[430,431]

Pemphigoid gestationis usually recurs in subsequent pregnancies, and at an earlier stage.[432] 'Skipped' pregnancies are more likely to occur following a change in paternity or when the mother and fetus are fully compatible at the HLA-D locus.[426]

Most reports have shown an increased fetal morbidity and mortality, but only rarely does the infant develop transient vesicular lesions resembling those of the mother.[430,432–434]

Pemphigoid gestationis has been reported in association with other autoimmune diseases.[429,435] It also occurs more frequently in patients with the HLA antigens DR3–DR4.[426,436,437] This HLA phenotype is thought to confer a state of heightened immune responsiveness.[426] A major initiating event in pemphigoid gestationis is the aberrant expression of the class II molecules of the major histocompatibility complex in the placenta.[438] Using sensitive techniques it has been found that all patients with pemphigoid gestationis possess a circulating autoantibody of IgG_1 class (the pemphigoid gestationis factor) which has complement-binding activity.[439–441] This antibody is directed against a placental matrix antigen which cross-reacts with an antigen in the basement membrane of skin.[426] The antigen has been further characterized as a basement zone glycoprotein of 180 kd which is antigenically distinct from the bullous pemphigoid antigen.[442] A cytotoxic anti-HLA antibody has also been demonstrated.[443–445] Activation of complement and the release of toxic cationic proteins from eosinophils have an effector role in the formation of the cutaneous lesions.[446]

Histopathology[431,432,447]

In early urticarial lesions there is marked oedema of the papillary dermis and a superficial and mid-dermal infiltrate of lymphocytes, histiocytes and eosinophils. The infiltrate is predominantly perivascular in location. Overlying the tips of the dermal papillae there is often focal spongiosis and, sometimes, necrosis of basal keratinocytes. The vesiculobullous lesions which form are subepidermal. They contain eosinophils, lymphocytes and histiocytes, and a similar infiltrate is present in the superficial dermis (Fig. 6.16). The eosinophils usually form microabscesses in the dermal papillae. A small number of neutrophils may also be present.

Direct immunofluorescence shows C3 and, sometimes, IgG in a linear pattern along the basement membrane zone.[432,448] These im-

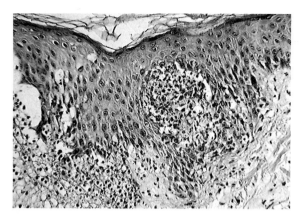

Fig. 6.16 Pemphigoid gestationis. There is subepidermal clefting with both neutrophils and eosinophils in the dermal infiltrate.
Haematoxylin — eosin

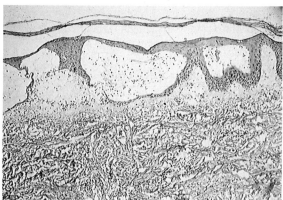

Fig. 6.17 Arthropod bite reaction in a sensitized person. Thin columns of surviving keratinocytes produce a characteristic multilocular blister which is both intraepidermal and subepidermal. There are many eosinophils in the inflammatory infiltrate.
Haematoxylin — eosin

munoreactants are found in the lamina lucida, as in bullous pemphigoid.[449,450] Eosinophil major basic protein can also be detected in the upper dermis by immunofluorescent techniques.[446] Circulating anti-basement-membrane-zone antibodies are uncommon.[451] As mentioned above, a circulating factor (the pemphigoid gestationis factor), which fixes complement at the dermo–epidermal junction of normal human skin, is found in 80% of cases;[452,453] this figure increases to 100% if sensitive techniques are used.[426]

Electron microscopy. The lamina densa is usually located in the floor of the blister, which appears to form as a result of disintegration of basal cells and an accumulation of fluid between the basal cells and the lamina densa.[447] Degenerative changes are present in some of the basal cells.[448]

ARTHROPOD BITES

The bite of certain arthropods will result in a bullous lesion in susceptible individuals.[453a] There may be a subepidermal blister or a mixed intraepidermal and subepidermal lesion with thin strands of keratinocytes bridging the bulla (Fig. 6.17). Eosinophils are usually present in the blister. The dermal infiltrate consists of lymphocytes and eosinophils around vessels in the superficial and deep dermis; interstitial eosinophils are also present.

DRUG REACTIONS

Certain drugs may produce a vesiculobullous eruption which resembles bullous pemphigoid both clinically and histologically (see p. 564). At other times the resemblance is less complete.

SUBEPIDERMAL BLISTERS WITH NEUTROPHILS

Neutrophils are a major component of the inflammatory cell infiltrate in the dermis in early lesions of dermatitis herpetiformis and in linear IgA bullous dermatosis, cicatricial pemphigoid and localized cicatricial pemphigoid. Bullae are an uncommon manifestation of urticaria, acute vasculitis, lupus erythematosus, erysipelas and Sweet's syndrome. Neutrophils may be abundant in some inflammatory forms of epidermolysis bullosa acquisita.

DERMATITIS HERPETIFORMIS

Dermatitis herpetiformis is a rare, chronic, subepidermal blistering disorder characterized by the presence of intensely pruritic papules and vesicles, granular deposition of IgA in the dermal papillae, and a high incidence of gluten-sensitive enteropathy.[454,455] It is of uncertain pathogenesis.

The cutaneous papulovesicles have a characteristic herpetiform grouping and a predilection for extensor surfaces, usually in symmetrical distribution.[455] Sites of involvement include the elbows, the knees, the shoulders, the nape of the neck, the sacral area and the scalp; mucous membranes are infrequently involved.[456,457] In addition to papulovesicles, excoriations are almost invariably present. Bullae are quite uncommon.[455] Onset of the disease is most frequent in early adult life, but it may occur at any age, including childhood.[458] There is a male preponderance; in women with the disease, perimenstrual exacerbations sometimes occur.[459] The HLA antigens B8, DR3 and DQW2 are increased in frequency in those with the disease.[460–462]

A gluten-sensitive enteropathy is present in approximately 90% of cases, although clinical symptoms of this are quite uncommon. A gluten-free diet usually leads to a reversal of the intestinal villous atrophy and improved control of the skin lesions.[463] There is also a high incidence of gluten-sensitive enteropathy in relatives although very few of the relatives with an enteropathy have dermatitis herpetiformis.[460]

Circulating antibodies to reticulin,[464,465] gliadin,[466,467] nuclear components,[464] human jejunum,[468] gastric parietal cells[469] and thyroid antigens[470] have been reported in variable percentages. Only the presence of IgA-class endomysial antibodies is of diagnostic importance.[465,471–473] They are present in 70% of patients with dermatitis herpetiformis on a normal diet and in 100% of those with villous atrophy.[474] Gluten challenge usually converts seronegative cases to seropositive while a gluten-free diet results in a rapid decrease in the titre of various antibodies.[474–476] Demonstration of this antibody may assist in making a diagnosis of dermatitis herpetiformis when clinical and histological features are equivocal.[477]

Dermatitis herpetiformis has been associated sporadically with autoimmune thyroid disease,[365] ulcerative colitis,[478] systemic lupus erythematosus,[479] rheumatoid arthritis,[365] Sjögren's syndrome,[480] Addison's disease,[481] primary biliary cirrhosis,[482] atopic disorders[483] and immune complex nephritis.[484] Although there are reports of its association with internal cancers, only the development of intestinal lymphomas appears to be of statistical significance.[386,485]

If untreated, dermatitis herpetiformis has a protracted course although there may be long periods of remission.[485a,486] Individual lesions persist for days to weeks. Iodine[487] and nonsteroidal anti-inflammatory drugs may provoke or exacerbate the disease in susceptible individuals.[488]

The pathogenesis of dermatitis herpetiformis is unknown, but it has been suggested that IgA antibodies formed in the gut somehow fix to the skin.[485a,489,490] There is some evidence to suggest that these antibodies are not directed against dietary antigens such as gluten.[485a,491] The recent isolation of the IgA deposits from the dermal papillae is likely to lead to their characterization before long.[492] They are localized to the microfibrillar bundles in the dermal papillae, possibly to fibrillin-reactive fibrils.[492a] The IgA deposited in the skin was originally thought to be of A_1 class only,[493] but IgA_2 has also been detected in these deposits.[494] Whatever the mechanism involved in the formation and deposition of IgA deposits, it appears that the final common pathway involves activation of the complement system followed by chemotaxis of neutrophils into the papillary dermis.[490] Enzymes released from these neutrophils alter or destroy at least two basement membrane components (laminin and type IV collagen), contributing to the formation of blisters.[495]

Histopathology[455]

Early lesions are characterized by collections of neutrophils and a varying number of eosinophils at the tips of oedematous dermal papillae, resulting in the so-called papillary microabscesses (Fig. 6.18). Fibrin is also present near the tips of the dermal papillae, imparting a 'necrotic' appearance. An occasional acantholytic basal cell may also be found above the tips of the papillae.

In lesions of 36–48 hours' duration, the number of eosinophils in the infiltrate is propor-

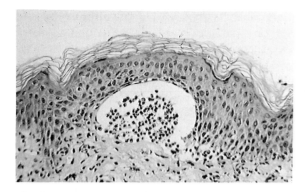

Fig. 6.18 Dermatitis herpetiformis. A microabscess is present in a dermal papilla.
Haematoxylin — eosin

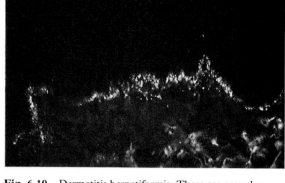

Fig. 6.19 Dermatitis herpetiformis. There are granular deposits of IgA in the dermal papillae.
Direct immunofluorescence

tionately increased. Some fragmentation of neutrophils is also present. Very occasionally, intraepidermal collections of neutrophils appear to be present, such cases requiring distinction from the very rare condition known as *intra-epidermal neutrophilic IgA dermatosis*[496] and IgA pemphigus foliaceus (see p. 131).

In older lesions, subepidermal vesiculation occurs, although initially the interpapillary ridges remain attached leading to multilocularity of the vesicle:[497] after a few days the attachments break down with the formation of a unilocular blister. The vesicles contain fibrin, neutrophils, eosinophils, and very occasional 'shadow' epidermal cells.[469]

Blood vessels in the upper and mid dermis are surrounded by an infiltrate of lymphocytes and histiocytes with a variable admixture of neutrophils and eosinophils. A vasculitis is rarely present. In urticarial lesions there is also marked oedema of the upper dermis. Neutrophils may not be prominent in such lesions.

The histological distinction between dermatitis herpetiformis and linear IgA disease is almost impossible,[498] although subtle distinguishing features have been reported[497,499] (see p. 158). Older lesions of dermatitis herpetiformis may resemble bullous pemphigoid although eosinophils are usually more prominent in the latter condition. [497] Rare cases with overlap features between dermatitis herpetiformis and other bullous diseases have been reported.[500–502] It should be remembered that dermal papillary microabscesses can be seen not only in dermatitis herpetiformis but also in cicatricial pemphigoid, localized cicatricial pemphigoid, and linear IgA bullous dermatosis. Papillary microabscesses also form in pemphigoid gestationis but they are composed of eosinophils in most cases. Neutrophils are also found in some cases of epidermolysis bullosa acquisita.

Direct immunofluorescence shows granular deposits of IgA in the dermal papillae of perilesional and uninvolved skin, although the deposition is not uniform (Fig. 6.19).[503,504] Interestingly, IgA is not found in the skin in coeliac disease without skin lesions.[505] Experience has shown that if IgA is not detected, the disorder usually turns out to be a dermatosis other than dermatitis herpetiformis,[506,507] although very rarely IgA is found on a second biopsy when it was not demonstrated on the initial examination.[508] Other immunoglobulins, particularly IgM, are present in almost 30% of all cases, while C3 is found in approximately 50%.[180,508] Most studies have recorded a diminution in the quantity of IgA and in the incidence of C3 deposition in patients on a gluten-free diet.[509–511]

The exact nosological position of cases with a granular linear pattern of IgA is uncertain,[455] although the presence of J chains coexistent with the IgA is similar to the pattern seen in dermatitis herpetiformis, but different from that in linear IgA bullous dermatosis in which it is absent.[512]

Electron microscopy. The basal lamina remains applied to the basal layer in very early blisters, but is soon disrupted or disappears.[513] The blister forms below this level. Immunoelectronmicroscopy confirms that the IgA is present in clumps in the dermal papillae, closely associated with microfibrillar bundles.[514]

LINEAR IgA BULLOUS DERMATOSIS

Linear IgA bullous dermatosis (linear IgA disease) is a rare, sulphone-responsive, subepidermal blistering disorder of unknown aetiology in which smooth linear deposits of IgA are found in the basement membrane zone.[515,516] There are two clinical variants — chronic bullous dermatosis of childhood and adult linear IgA bullous dermatosis. They are now regarded as different expressions of the same disease[517] as both variants share the same target antigen, which is different to that found in bullous pemphigoid and epidermolysis bullosa acquisita.

Chronic bullous dermatosis of childhood. This variant, known in the past as juvenile dermatitis herpetiformis,[518–520] juvenile pemphigoid[521] and linear IgA disease of childhood, is characterized by the abrupt onset, in the first decade of life, of large, tense bullae on a normal or erythematous base.[516,522,523] They have a predilection for the perioral and genital regions, as well as the lower part of the abdomen and the thighs.[524,525] Often there is a polycyclic grouping, the so-called 'cluster of jewels' sign.[516] The disease usually runs a benign course with remission after several months or years.[526,527] In one series, 12% of the cases persisted beyond puberty.[516] The entity known as childhood cicatricial pemphigoid appears to be a variant of chronic bullous dermatosis of childhood and is characterized by severe scarring lesions of mucosae, particularly the conjunctiva.[516,528]

Adult linear IgA bullous dermatosis. This entity was originally regarded as a subgroup of dermatitis herpetiformis, but it is now known to differ from dermatitis herpetiformis by the absence of gluten-sensitive enteropathy[529,530] and IgA anti-endomysial antibodies,[472,473] although anti-gliadin antibodies are sometimes present.[467] Adult linear IgA bullous dermatosis has a heterogeneous clinical presentation which may clinically resemble dermatitis herpetiformis, bullous pemphigoid or other bullous disorders.[357,531–535] Sometimes the lesions have an annular configuration. Bullae usually involve the trunk and limbs; facial and perineal lesions are not as frequent as in the childhood form.[515] An association with lymphoma,[536] other malignant tumours,[537,538] and immune complex glomerulonephritis[539] has been reported. The disease has also followed the therapeutic use of lithium carbonate,[540] vancomycin,[541] and non-steroidal anti-inflammatory drugs.[515,542] It runs a more chronic course than the childhood form, and lesions may persist indefinitely.[515]

In both the adult and the childhood forms the lesions may be pruritic or burning.[515] Haemorrhagic bullae may form.[523] Mucosal involvement occurs in 80% or more of adults but less frequently in children.[543–545] Scarring conjunctival lesions sometimes develop.[544,546] Other findings have included severe arthralgia,[517] and the presence of organ-specific antibodies and of various histocompatibility antigens, some of which differ from those found in dermatitis herpetiforms.[461] However, the incidence of HLA-B8 is increased in both dermatitis herpetiformis and chronic bullous dermatosis of childhood, and marginally so in the adult form of the latter.[515]

The antigen in linear IgA bullous dermatosis in both childhood and adult forms is found only in stratified squamous epithelium and the amnion of mammalian species.[547] Its localization has varied in different studies, depending on the techniques used.[547,548] Currently, the antigen is thought to be in the sub-lamina-densa region of the basement membrane zone. Circulating IgA antibodies are found in approximately 70% of childhood cases, but in only 20% of adult cases.[515] A higher yield is obtained using split skin as the substrate.[548a] These antibodies are thought to have some pathogenetic significance despite their low incidence in the adult forms of the disease.

Histopathology

Linear IgA bullous dermatosis is a subepidermal blistering disease in which neutrophils are usually the predominant cell in the infiltrate. Accordingly, many cases are indistinguishable on light microscopy from dermatitis herpetiformis, with the presence of dermal papillary micro-abscesses (see p. 155).[533] Some adult cases may mimic bullous pemphigoid by having a predominance of eosinophils in the infiltrate.[515] No attempt has yet been made to ascertain whether the type of the predominant cell in the infiltrate is merely a reflection of the age of the lesion. A scanty infiltrate of lymphocytes usually surrounds the small vessels in the superficial plexus.

Attempts have been made to establish criteria for the distinction of linear IgA bullous dermatosis from dermatitis herpetiformis.[497,499] Fibrin is present at the tips of the dermal papillae with underlying leucocytoclasis in nearly all cases of dermatitis herpetiformis.[497] However, these changes are also present in three-quarters of the cases of linear IgA disease.[497] Furthermore, the neutrophil infiltration in this latter condition tends to be more widespread than that in dermatitis herpetiformis in which there is relative sparing of the rete tips between each dermal papilla (Fig. 6.20).[499] In most cases it is impossible to distinguish between the two conditions.

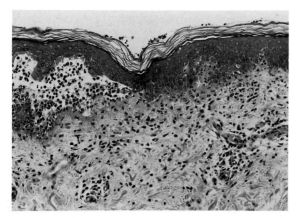

Fig. 6.20   Linear IgA bullous dermatosis. There is a subepidermal blister with neutrophils in the lumen and in the base. They are dispersed in the papillary dermis of the adjacent skin.
Haematoxylin — eosin

Direct immunofluorescence reveals a homogeneous linear pattern of IgA deposition along the basement membrane zone of non-lesional skin.[473] This is the only immunoreactant in nearly 80% of cases.[515] In the remainder, IgG, IgM and/or C3 may be present.[515,549] The IgA is exclusively IgA_1 in contrast to dermatitis herpetiformis in which both IgA_1 and IgA_2 are present.[550] Furthermore, J-chain staining, indicating a mucosal origin for the IgA, is found only in dermatitis herpetiformis.[512] J-chain staining is also found in those few cases that have a granular-linear IgA pattern, suggesting that these cases should be classified with dermatitis herpetiformis.[512] As already mentioned, circulating IgA antibodies are found more often in childhood than adult cases. The deposition of IgA in a linear fashion along the basement membrane is not specific for linear IgA bullous dermatosis, as it may also be found in several bullous dermatoses and cutaneous diseases.[551]

Electron microscopy. Most of the ultrastructural studies have been directed at ascertaining the site of deposition of the IgA, rather than the anatomical level of the split within the basement membrane zone.[552] In some studies the split has been within the lamina lucida,[552,553] while in others it has been below the basal lamina, as in dermatitis herpetiformis.[554] Most recent immuno-electron-microscopical studies have shown that the deposits are below the lamina densa, as in epidermolysis bullosa acquisita,[555,556] or on either side of the lamina densa in a mirror image pattern.[557] A few studies, involving small numbers of cases, have demonstrated deposits within the lamina lucida.[540,558] Split-skin studies have shown that the IgA is above the lamina densa,[548,558] but this is likely to be artefactual and related to the mechanical disruption in this region during the preparation of the specimen.[554]

CICATRICIAL PEMPHIGOID

Cicatricial pemphigoid (benign mucous membrane pemphigoid) is an uncommon, chronic, vesiculobullous disease that is distinguished clinically by its predilection for oral and ocular mucous membranes, and a tendency for the lesions to scar.[559–561] It occurs predominantly in older age groups, but there are several reports of the disease in children and adolescents.[562–564] There is a female predominance.[561]

The mouth is the most frequent site of onset, and it is eventually involved in 85% of cases.[565] There are erosions, irregular ulcers and vesiculo-bullous lesions. Ocular involvement is also common and corneal and conjunctival scarring may lead to blindness.[546,561] Skin lesions occur in about 25% of cases, but in only 10% is the skin the initial site of involvement.[559,566] There may be scattered tense bullae which heal without scarring, or several areas of erythema with blisters which often heal with scarring.[16] There is a tendency for blisters to recur in the same area. Generalized cutaneous lesions resembling bullous pemphigoid are uncommon.[567] The face, neck, scalp and, to a lesser extent, the axillae and distal parts of the limbs are the usual sites of cutaneous lesions.[559] The external genitalia, larynx,[568] pharynx, anus, oesophagus, middle ear[569] and nail plates[570] may also be involved.[561] Coexistence with rheumatoid arthritis[571] and systemic lupus erythematosus[572] and an association with the ingestion of practolol[573] and clonidine[574] have also been reported.

The relationship of cicatricial pemphigoid to several other subepidermal bullous diseases has been a matter for discussion and some controversy. Although mucosal involvement may occur in bullous pemphigoid, and the two share similar immunofluorescent findings, there is a suggestion that the antigen involved in cicatricial pemphigoid is distinct from the bullous pemphigoid antigen, with the plane of cleavage just below that of bullous pemphigoid.[414,575] However, a recent study using immunoblotting showed that the target antigen in cicatricial pemphigoid is similar to the bullous pemphigoid antigens (230–240 kd and 180 kd).[575a] It has also been suggested that cicatricial pemphigoid and epidermolysis bullosa acquisita (EBA) are the same disease,[314] but this is disputed by those who have found the deposits in cicatricial pemphigoid in the lamina lucida[575] rather than below the lamina densa, as seen in EBA.[297,576] Finally, the existence of a rare, scarring, bullous

eruption with linear IgA at the dermo–epidermal junction raises the question of the relationship of these cases to cicatricial pemphigoid and linear IgA bullous dermatosis,[528,577–579] but as little is known about the target antigens in these two conditions there has as yet been no clarification of this issue.[579a]

Histopathology

In cicatricial pemphigoid there is a subepidermal blister which shows a variable infiltrate of cells in its base, depending on the age of the lesion. In lesions of less than 48 hours' duration there are neutrophil microabscesses in the dermal papillae resembling those seen in dermatitis herpetiformis.[580] With increasing age of the lesion there are increasing numbers of eosinophils and later of lymphocytes, and a reducing number of neutrophils. There are always fewer eosinophils than in bullous pemphigoid.[561]

Scarring may be present even in early lesions if the biopsy site corresponds to an area of previous blister formation and subsequent scarring (Fig. 6.21). The earliest stages of scarring may be detected by examination under polarized light. New collagen bundles are arranged parallel to the surface rather than in the usual haphazard distribution.

Direct immunofluorescence shows linear deposits of IgG and often of C3 along the

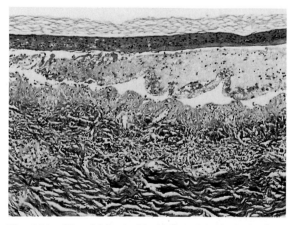

Fig. 6.21 Cicatricial pemphigoid. Scar tissue is present in the dermis beneath the subepidermal blister. Because blisters have a tendency to recur at the site of a previous lesion, scarring may be present in the dermis beneath a 'new' blister. Haematoxylin — eosin

basement membrane zone in approximately 80% of cases.[579,581] The yield is higher in buccal mucosa than in skin.[414,575] A similar band often extends along the basement membrane of the appendages; it has also been reported in a similar position in the mucous glands of the oropharynx.[582] IgA and other immunoglobulins may also be present in approximately 20% of cases,[580] but only rarely (see above) is IgA the only immunoglobulin present.[528,579]

Circulating antibodies to basement membrane zone are found in only 20% of cases, but the use of multiple substrates will increase the number of positives obtained.[583] Circulating pemphigus-like antibodies have been demonstrated in several cases; they are of doubtful significance.[584,585]

Electron microscopy. There is a need for further studies, including immuno-electron-microscopy, to clarify the exact site of the deposits and of the split. Although the lamina lucida is usually quoted as the site of the split,[586] a slightly lower level (the zone below the lamina densa) would be more in keeping with the presence of scarring, which is usually confined to those blistering diseases with splits deeper than the lamina lucida.[587] A recent study (see above) showed that the immunoreactants in cicatricial pemphigoid were mostly localized on the lamina densa, sometimes overflowing on to the anchoring fibrils.[575a] Deposits were occasionally found in the lamina lucida, the site of the split.

LOCALIZED CICATRICIAL PEMPHIGOID

Localized cicatricial pemphigoid (Brunsting–Perry type) is characterized by the occurrence of one or more scarring, plaque-like lesions, usually on the head and neck, but without involvement of mucous membranes, even during prolonged follow-up.[588–592] The temple is the most frequent site,[593–595] but lesions have been reported elsewhere,[596] and also in tissue transplanted to the site of a pre-existing lesion.[591] The exact relationship of this condition to cicatricial pemphigoid is speculative, although they are thought to be closely related diseases.[592]

Localized cicatricial pemphigoid should be

distinguished also from 'localized pemphigoid' which is a variant of bullous pemphigoid in which lesions are localized to one area, such as the vulva,[337a] pretibial region, a stoma site or the palms and soles (see p. 150).[337,340, 597] In contrast to localized cicatricial pemphigoid, the lesions in 'localized pemphigoid' do not scar. It is uncertain whether all cases of 'localized pemphigoid' are variants of bullous pemphigoid: underlying vascular disease and lymphatic obstruction have been present in some cases in the pretibial region.[339] Furthermore, direct immunofluorescence is sometimes negative in these cases.[339] Pretibial epidermolysis bullosa also needs consideration in these circumstances; it usually presents in the first three decades of life (see p. 145).

Histopathology[591]

There is a subepidermal blister with a mixture of neutrophils, eosinophils and lymphocytes, similar to that seen in cicatricial pemphigoid. The proportion of the various cell types in the infiltrate depends on the age of the lesion biopsied. Small papillary microabscesses are present in lesions less than 48 hours old (Fig. 6.22).[593] There is variable fibrosis in the dermis, depending on the presence of a previous blister at the site of biopsy.

In the pretibial form of 'localized pemphigoid'

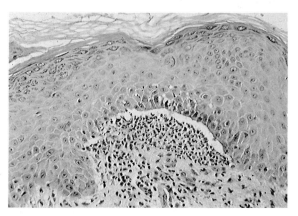

Fig. 6.22 Localized cicatricial pemphigoid. A neutrophil microabscess is present in a dermal papilla, similar to the picture in dermatitis herpetiformis.
Haematoxylin — eosin

there is only a sparse dermal inflammatory cell infiltrate associated with neovascularization of the papillary dermis.[339] There may be some fibrosis of the dermis, but this is rarely a prominent feature.

Immunofluorescence of localized cicatricial pemphigoid usually shows basement membrane zone IgG and/or C3.[591] Indirect immunofluorescence for circulating antibodies is usually negative.[591]

Electron microscopy. Ultrastructural studies have shown that the blister forms below the basal lamina.[592] The basal lamina and anchoring fibrils are well preserved and attached to the intact epidermis which forms the roof of the blister.[592]

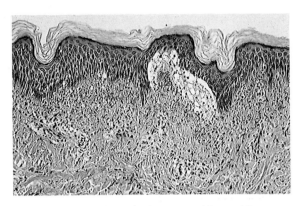

Fig. 6.23   Bullous lupus erythematosus. Neutrophils are present in the superficial dermis in a more dispersed arrangement than in dermatitis herpetiformis. There is a small subepidermal blister.
Haematoxylin — eosin

BULLOUS URTICARIA

Bullae are an uncommon manifestation of urticaria and result from severe oedema of the papillary dermis (see p. 216). Neutrophils and eosinophils are present in the upper dermis; sometimes a mixed infiltrate of lymphocytes and eosinophils is present.

BULLOUS ACUTE VASCULITIS

If bullae form in acute vasculitis they are sometimes haemorrhagic. The vessels in the underlying dermis show the typical features of an acute vasculitis (see p. 220). Leucocytoclasis may be a conspicuous feature. A vasculitis is usually present in the bullous lesions associated with septicaemia caused by *Vibrio vulnificus*[598] and, rarely, by *Escherichia coli*,[599] *Yersinia enterocolitica*[600] and *Morganella morganii*.[600a] Subepidermal bullae have also been reported in the toxic shock syndrome.[600b]

BULLOUS LUPUS ERYTHEMATOSUS

A vesiculobullous eruption is an uncommon manifestation of systemic lupus erythematosus (see p. 50). The lesions vary in appearance from herpetiform vesicles to large haemorrhagic bullae. Sometimes the lesions are limited to sun-exposed areas of the body.

Histopathology[600c]

The appearances closely resemble dermatitis herpetiformis with subepidermal splitting and papillary microabscesses (Fig. 6.23). Nuclear dust is prominent in the papillae and sometimes around superficial blood vessels. The neutrophils tend to extend more deeply in the papillary dermis and around vessels than they do in dermatitis herpetiformis. Vacuolar change is not usually present although occasional Civatte bodies are sometimes seen.

Immuno-electronmicroscopy shows that the deposits (IgG, C3 and often IgA) may be deep to the anchoring fibrils in the upper dermis.

ERYSIPELAS

In erysipelas, subepidermal blisters may form as a result of massive oedema in the upper dermis (see p. 599). Elongated rete ridges may bridge the blister and connect with the underlying dermis. The neutrophilic infiltrate is usually only mild, although there are numerous extravasated erythrocytes.

SWEET'S SYNDROME

Bullae are quite uncommon in Sweet's syndrome (see p. 229). Sometimes there is severe oedema of the upper dermis mimicking early blister formation but the clinical appearances suggest an urticarial plaque, not a blister. There is a heavy infiltrate of neutrophils in the upper and mid dermis, often with leucocytoclasis. There is no fibrinoid change in vessel walls.

EPIDERMOLYSIS BULLOSA ACQUISITA

Neutrophils are present in the dermis in some variants of this disease (see p. 146).

SUBEPIDERMAL BLISTERS WITH MAST CELLS

BULLOUS MASTOCYTOSIS

Bullous lesions are an uncommon manifestation of mastocytosis in neonates and infants (see p. 1007). There are usually numerous mast cells in the dermis beneath the blister.

MISCELLANEOUS BLISTERING DISEASES

The *miscellaneous category* of blistering diseases includes several very rare entities in which the anatomical level of the split is variable, or the disease does not fit appropriately into one of the categories of subepidermal blistering diseases already mentioned. Penicillamine may produce blisters at different anatomical levels in the epidermis, resembling either pemphigus foliaceus or pemphigus vulgaris; this is discussed on pages 130 and 136.

The bullous lesions that develop rarely in diabetes mellitus (see p. 532) may be subepidermal or intraepidermal.

Bullae may be a manifestation of the rare genodermatoses pachyonychia congenita (see p. 276) and Kindler's syndrome (see p. 55). Small, haemorrhagic blisters have been reported in one case of Wilson's disease.[600d]

The following entities are discussed further below:

Drug-overdose-related bullae
Methyl-bromide-induced bullae
Etretinate-induced bullae
PUVA-induced bullae
Cancer-related bullae
Lymphatic bullae.

DRUG-OVERDOSE-RELATED BULLAE

Bullae, tense vesicles, erosions and dusky erythematous plaques may develop at sites of pressure in patients with drug-induced or carbon-monoxide-induced coma, particularly if the coma is deep.[601] Drugs involved have included morphine, heroin, methadone, barbiturates,[602] imipramine, carbamazepine,[602a] amitryp-tyline[603] and diazepam.[604] Rarely, this entity has developed in association with other neurological disorders;[604] it followed treatment with the beta-adrenergic antagonist atenolol, in a patient with phaeochromocytoma.[605]

The lesions are believed to result from tissue ischaemia, which in turn is related to local pressure and to systemic hypoxia.[606]

Histopathology[606,607]

The blisters which form are predominantly subepidermal, but there is also spongiosis in the overlying epidermis which may lead to the formation of intraepidermal vesicles as well. There is focal necrosis of keratinocytes in, and adjacent to, the acrosyringium; sometimes the epithelium in the pilosebaceous follicles also shows focal necrosis. The secretory cells of the sweat glands beneath the bullae are necrotic. The basement membrane of the sweat glands may also be destroyed but the myoepithelial cells usually survive. In the dermis there is only a sparse inflammatory cell infiltrate which includes some neutrophils.

METHYL-BROMIDE-INDUCED BULLAE

A vesiculobullous eruption has been reported

following occupational exposure to high concentrations of methyl bromide used in fumigation.[608]

Histopathology[608]

The bullae induced by methyl bromide are subepidermal in location and associated with marked oedema of the upper dermis. The dermal infiltrate is composed of neutrophils, eosinophils and a few lymphocytes. The infiltrate is distributed around blood vessels in the upper dermis.

Another feature of this entity is the presence of spongiosis of the epidermis and necrosis of epidermal keratinocytes. Neutrophils infiltrate the epidermis.

ETRETINATE-INDUCED BULLAE

Increased skin fragility and subepidermal blistering are a rare complication of therapy with etretinate.[609] The blisters rapidly ulcerate; they are followed by some scarring.

Histopathology[609]

Intact blisters are difficult to obtain. Clefting appears to occur at the dermo–epidermal junction. The overlying epidermis may show spongiosis. The dermal infiltrate includes plasma cells, eosinophils and neutrophils.

PUVA-INDUCED BULLAE

Blisters may develop on the limbs in 10% of patients receiving therapy with psoralens plus long-wave ultraviolet light (PUVA).[610] The lesions appear to result from friction and minor trauma. The mechanism remains to be determined although the blisters apparently develop as a result of damage to the basal and suprabasal layers of the epidermis.[610]

Histopathology[610]

The blistering appears to form in the basal layer of the epidermis as damaged basal cells are sometimes seen in the base of the blisters. There is swelling and destruction of keratinocytes in the overlying epidermis. Apoptotic cells ('sunburn cells') are sometimes present. The dermis contains a very sparse, mixed inflammatory cell infiltrate.

CANCER-RELATED BULLAE

Several patients with cancer have developed bullae in association with gyrate lesions.[611,612] Uncommonly, the bullae are related to trauma.[612] Bullae have been reported in a patient with multiple myeloma, but there were no gyrate lesions.[613]

Not included in this category are the bullous eruptions, resembling bullous pemphigoid (see p. 150) and epidermolysis bullosa acquisita (see p. 146), that sometimes develop in patients with cancer.

Histopathology[612]

The cancer-related bullae with gyrate lesions are usually subepidermal in location and the inflammatory cell infiltrate in the dermis is mild and of mixed type. Direct immunofluorescence may show IgG and C3 in the basement membrane zone.[612]

LYMPHATIC BULLAE

Subepidermal bullae are a very rare complication of lymphoedema or of a lymphatic fistula.[614,615] Uncommonly, vesicular lesions are due to markedly dilated lymphatics in the papillary dermis.[616]

REFERENCES

Intracorneal and subcorneal blisters

1. Wilkinson DS. Pustular dermatoses. Br J Dermatol (Suppl) 1969; 3: 38–45.
2. Tagami H, Iwatsuki K, Shirahama S, Yamada M. Pustulosis vegetans. Arch Dermatol 1984; 120: 1355–1359.
3. Ryan JG. Pemphigus. A 20-year survey of experience with 70 cases. Arch Dermatol 1971; 104: 14–20.
4. Beutner EH, Chorzelski TP. Studies on etiologic factors in pemphigus. J Cutan Pathol 1976; 3: 67–74.
5. Korman N. Pemphigus. J Am Acad Dermatol 1988; 18: 1219–1238.
6. Koulu L, Stanley JR. Clinical, histologic, and immunopathologic comparison of pemphigus vulgaris and pemphigus foliaceus. Semin Dermatol 1988; 7: 82–90.
7. Imamura S, Takigawa M, Ikai K et al. Pemphigus foliaceus, myasthenia gravis, thymoma and red cell aplasia. Clin Exp Dermatol 1978; 3: 285–291.
8. Perry HO, Brunsting LA. Pemphigus foliaceus. Further observations. Arch Dermatol 1965; 91: 10–23.
9. Jones SK, Schwab HP, Norris DA. Childhood pemphigus foliaceus: case report and review of the literature. Pediatr Dermatol 1986; 3: 459–463.
10. Sotiriou L, Herszenson S, Jordon RE. Childhood pemphigus foliaceus. Report of a case. Arch Dermatol 1980; 116: 679–680.
11. Yorav S, Trau H, Schewack-Millet M. Pemphigus foliaceus in an 8-year-old girl. Int J Dermatol 1989; 28: 125–126.
12. Bruckner N, Katz RA, Hood AF. Pemphigus foliaceus resembling eruptive seborrheic keratoses. Arch Dermatol 1980; 8: 815–816.
13. Kahana M, Trau H, Schewach-Millet M, Sofer E. Pemphigus foliaceus presenting as multiple giant seborrheic keratoses. J Am Acad Dermatol 1984; 11: 299–300.
14. Emmerson RW, Wilson Jones E. Eosinophilic spongiosis in pemphigus. Arch Dermatol 1968; 97: 252–257.
15. Knight AG, Black MM, Delaney TJ. Eosinophilic spongiosis. A clinical histological and immunofluorescent correlation. Clin Exp Dermatol 1976; 1: 141–153.
16. Lever WF. Pemphigus and pemphigoid. A review of the advances made since 1964. J Am Acad Dermatol 1979; 1: 2–31.
17. Brodersen I, Frentz G, Thomsen K. Eosinophilic spongiosis in early pemphigus foliaceus. Acta Derm Venereol 1978; 58: 368–369.
18. Osteen FB, Wheeler CE Jr, Briggaman RA, Puritz EM. Pemphigus foliaceus. Early clinical appearance as dermatitis herpetiformis with eosinophilic spongiosis. Arch Dermatol 1976; 112: 1148–1152.
19. Maciejowska E, Jablonska S, Chorzelski T. Is pemphigus herpetiformis an entity? Int J Dermatol 1987; 26: 571–577.
20. Harrington CI, Sneddon IB. Coexistence of bullous pemphigoid and pemphigus foliaceus. Br J Dermatol 1979; 100: 441–445.
21. Levine L, Bernstein JE, Soltani K et al. Coexisting childhood pemphigus foliaceus and Graves' disease. Arch Dermatol 1982; 118: 602–604.
22. Maize JC, Dobson RL, Provost TT. Pemphigus and myasthenia gravis. Arch Dermatol 1975; 111: 1334–1339.
23. Kaufman AJ, Ahmed AR, Kaplan RP. Pemphigus, myasthenia gravis, and pregnancy. J Am Acad Dermatol 1988; 19: 414–418.
24. Neumann-Jensen B, Worsaae N, Dabelsteen E, Ullman S. Pemphigus vulgaris and pemphigus foliaceus coexisting with oral lichen planus. Br J Dermatol 1980; 102: 585–590.
25. Sarnoff DS, DeFeo CP. Coexistence of pemphigus foliaceus and mycosis fungoides. Arch Dermatol 1985; 121: 669–672.
26. Santa Cruz DJ, Prioleau PJ, Marcus MD, Uitto J. Pemphigus-like lesions induced by D-penicillamine. Analysis of clinical, histopathological, and immunofluorescence features in 34 cases. Am J Dermatopathol 1981; 3: 85–92.
27. Kennedy C, Hodge L, Sanderson KV. Skin changes caused by D-penicillamine treatment of arthritis. Clin Exp Dermatol 1978; 3: 107–116.
28. Lee CW, Lim JH, Kang HJ. Pemphigus foliaceus induced by rifampicin. Br J Dermatol 1984; 111: 619–622.
29. Blanken R, Doeglas HMG, De Jong MCJM et al. Pemphigus-like eruption induced by d-penicillamine and captopril in the same patient. Acta Derm Venereol 1988; 68: 456–457.
30. Lucky PA, Skovby F, Thier SO. Pemphigus foliaceus and proteinuria induced by α-mercaptopropionylglycine. J Am Acad Dermatol 1983; 8: 667–672.
31. Pisani M, Ruocco V. Drug-induced pemphigus. Clin Dermatol 1986; 4: 118–132.
32. Anhalt GJ. Drug-induced pemphigus. Semin Dermatol 1989; 8: 166–172.
33. Walton S, Keczkes K, Robinson EA. A case of penicillamine-induced pemphigus, successfully treated by plasma exchange. Clin Exp Dermatol 1987; 12: 275–276.
34. Kristensen JK, Wadskov S. Penicillamine-induced pemphigus foliaceus. Acta Derm Venereol 1977; 57: 69–71.
35. Troy JL, Silvers DN, Grossman ME, Jaffe IA. Penicillamine-associated pemphigus: Is it really pemphigus? J Am Acad Dermatol 1981; 4: 547–555.
36. De Jong MCJM, Doeglas HMG, Dijkstra JWE. Immunohistochemical findings in a patient with penicillamine pemphigus. Br J Dermatol 1980; 102: 333–337.
37. Bahmer FA, Bambauer R, Stenger D. Penicillamine-induced pemphigus foliaceus-like dermatosis. Arch Dermatol 1985; 121: 665–668.
38. Velthuis PJ, Hendrikse JC, Nefkens JJ. Combined features of pemphigus and pemphigoid induced by penicillamine. Br J Dermatol 1985; 112: 615–619.
39. Jordon RE, Kawana S, Fritz KA. Immunopathologic mechanisms in pemphigus and bullous pemphigoid. J Invest Dermatol 1985; 85: 72s–78s.
40. Rubinstein N, Stanley JR. Pemphigus foliaceus antibodies and a monoclonal antibody to desmoglein I

demonstrate stratified squamous epithelial-specific epitopes of desmosomes. Am J Dermatopathol 1987; 9: 510–514.

41. Labib RS, Camargo S, Futamura S et al. Pemphigus foliaceus antigen: Characterization of a keratinocyte envelope associated pool and preparation of a soluble immunoreactive fragment. J Invest Dermatol 1989; 93: 272–279.

42. Kawana S, Geoghegan WD, Jordon RE, Nishiyama S. Deposition of the membrane attack complex of complement in pemphigus vulgaris and pemphigus foliaceus skin. J Invest Dermatol 1989; 92: 588–592.

43. Spillman DH, Magnin PH, Roquel L, Mitsui M. Aprotinin inhibition of experimental pemphigus in Balb-c mice following passive transfer of pemphigus foliaceus serum. Clin Exp Dermatol 1988; 13: 321–327.

44. Diaz LA, Sampaio SA, Rivitti EA. Endemic pemphigus foliaceus (fogo selvagem). I. Clinical features and immunopathology. J Am Acad Dermatol 1989; 20: 657–669.

45. Azulay RD. Brazilian pemphigus foliaceus. Int J Dermatol 1982; 21: 122–124.

46. Diaz LA, Sampaio SAP, Rivitti EA et al. Endemic pemphigus foliaceus (fogo selvagem): II. Current and historic epidemiologic studies. J Invest Dermatol 1989; 92: 4–12.

47. Roscoe JT, Naylor PH, Diaz LA et al. Elevated thymosin alpha 1 levels in Brazilian pemphigus foliaceus. Br J Dermatol 1986; 115: 147–150.

48. Ahmed AR, Rosen GB. Viruses in pemphigus. Int J Dermatol 1989; 28: 209–217.

49. Robledo MA, Prada de C S, Jaramillo D, Leon W. South American pemphigus foliaceus: Study of an epidemic in El Bagre and Nechi, Colombia 1982 to 1986. Br J Dermatol 1988; 118: 737–744.

50. Voelter WW, Newell GB, Schwartz SL et al. Familial occurrence of pemphigus foliaceus. Arch Dermatol 1973; 108: 93–94.

51. Roscoe JT, Diaz L, Sampaio SAP et al. Brazilian pemphigus foliaceus autoantibodies are pathogenic to BALB/c mice by passive transfer. J Invest Dermatol 1985; 85: 538–541.

52. Stanley JR, Klaus-Kovtun V, Sampaio SAP. Antigenic specificity of fogo selvagem autoantibodies is similar to North American pemphigus foliaceus and distinct from pemphigus vulgaris autoantibodies. J Invest Dermatol 1986; 87: 197–201.

53. Kawana S, Diaz LA, Geoghegan WD, Jordon RE. Complement fixation by Brazilian pemphigus foliaceus autoantibodies. J Invest Dermatol 1987; 88: 498 (abstract).

54. Futamura S, Martins C, Rivitti EA. Ultrastructural studies of acantholysis induced in vivo by passive transfer of IgG from endemic pemphigus foliaceus (fogo selvagem). J Invest Dermatol 1989; 93: 480–485.

55. Kouskoukis CE, Ackerman AB. What histologic finding distinguishes superficial pemphigus and bullous impetigo? Am J Dermatopathol 1984; 6: 179–181.

56. Kouskoukis CE, Ackerman AB. Vacuoles in the upper part of the epidermis as a clue to eventuation of superficial pemphigus and bullous impetigo. Am J Dermatopathol 1984; 6: 183–186.

57. Castro RM, Roscoe JT, Sampaio SAP. Brazilian pemphigus foliaceus. Clin Dermatol 1983; 1: 22–41.

58. Bhogal B, Wojnarowska F, Black MM et al. The distribution of immunoglobulins and the C3 component of complement in multiple biopsies from the uninvolved and perilesional skin in pemphigus. Clin Exp Dermatol 1986; 11: 49–53.

59. de Messias IT, von Kuster LC, Santamaria J, Kajdacsy-Balla A. Complement and antibody deposition in Brazilian pemphigus foliaceus and correlation of disease activity with circulating antibodies. Arch Dermatol 1988; 124: 1664–1668.

60. Rodriguez J, Bystryn J-C. Pemphigus foliaceus associated with absence of intercellular antigens in lower layers of epidermis. Arch Dermatol 1977; 113: 1696–1699.

61. Bystryn J-C, Abel E, DeFeo C. Pemphigus foliaceus. Subcorneal intercellular antibodies of unique specificity. Arch Dermatol 1974; 110: 857–861.

62. Maize JC, Green D, Provost TT. Pemphigus foliaceus: A case with serologic features of Senear–Usher syndrome and other autoimmune abnormalities. J Am Acad Dermatol 1982; 7: 736–741.

63. Beutner EH, Chorzelski TP, McDonough Wilson R et al. IgA pemphigus foliaceus. Report of two cases and a review of the literature. J Am Acad Dermatol 1989; 20: 89–97.

64. Hashimoto T, Inamoto N, Nakamura K, Nishikawa T. Intercellular IgA dermatosis with clinical features of subcorneal pustular dermatosis. Arch Dermatol 1987; 123: 1062–1065.

65. Sotto MN, Shimizu SH, Costa JM, De Brito T. South American pemphigus foliaceus: electron microscopy and immunoelectron localization of bound immunoglobulin in the skin and oral mucosa. Br J Dermatol 1980; 102: 521–527.

66. Rosenberg FR, Sanders S, Nelson CT. Pemphigus. A 20-year review of 107 patients treated with corticosteroids. Arch Dermatol 1976; 112: 962–970.

67. Amerian ML, Ahmed AR. Pemphigus erythematosus. Senear–Usher syndrome. Int J Dermatol 1985; 24: 16–25.

68. Lynfield YL, Pertschuk LP, Zimmerman A. Pemphigus erythematosus provoked by allergic contact dermatitis. Occurrence many years after thymoma removal. Arch Dermatol 1973; 108: 690–693.

69. Van Joost T, Stolz E, Blog FB et al. Pemphigus erythematosus: clinical and histo-immunological studies in two unusual cases. Acta Derm Venereol 1984; 64: 257–260.

70. Uhlin SR, Maiocco KJ, Bhatia SG. Pemphigus erythematosus and thymoma. Cutis 1980; 25: 177–182.

71. Ngo AW, Straka C, Fretzin D. Pemphigus erythematosus: A unique association with systemic lupus erythematosus. Cutis 1986; 38: 160–163.

72. Basler RSW. Senear–Usher syndrome with parathyroid adenoma. Br J Dermatol 1974; 91: 465–467.

73. Saikia NK, Macconnell LES. Senear–Usher syndrome and internal malignancy. Br J Dermatol 1972; 87: 1–5.

74. Chorzelski T, Jablonska S, Beutner EH, Kowalska M. Can pemphigus be provoked by a burn? Br J Dermatol 1971; 85: 320–325.

75. Amerian ML, Ahmed AR. Pemphigus erythematosus. Presentation of four cases and review of literature. J Am Acad Dermatol 1984; 10: 215–222.

76. Scherak O, Kolarz G, Holubar K. Pemphigus erythematosus-like rash in a patient on penicillamine. Br Med J 1977; 1: 38.

77. Parfrey PS, Clement M, Vandenburg MJ, Wright P. Captopril-induced pemphigus. Br Med J 1980; 281: 194.

78. Alinovi A, Benoldi D, Manganelli P. Pemphigus erythematosus induced by thioproprine. Acta Derm Venereol 1982; 62: 452–454.

79. Fellner MJ, Wininger J. Pemphigus erythematosus and heroin addiction. Int J Dermatol 1978; 17: 308–311.

80. Ahmed AR. Pemphigus: current concepts. Ann Intern Med 1980; 92: 396–405.

81. Chorzelski T, Jablonska S, Blaszczyk M. Immunopathological investigations in the Senear–Usher syndrome (coexistence of pemphigus and lupus erythematosus). Br J Dermatol 1968; 80: 211–217.

82. Bean SF, Lynch FW. Senear–Usher syndrome (pemphigus erythematosus). Immunofluorescent studies in a patient. Arch Dermatol 1970; 101: 642–645.

83. Sneddon IB, Wilkinson DS. Subcorneal pustular dermatosis. Br J Dermatol 1956; 68: 385–394.

84. Sneddon IB. Subcorneal pustular dermatosis. Int J Dermatol 1977; 16: 640–644.

85. Sneddon IB, Wilkinson DS. Subcorneal pustular dermatosis. Br J Dermatol 1979; 100: 61–68.

86. Dallot A, Decazes JM, Drouault Y et al. Subcorneal pustular dermatosis (Sneddon–Wilkinson disease) with amicrobial lymph node suppuration and aseptic spleen abscesses. Br J Dermatol 1988; 119: 803–807.

87. Johnson SAM, Cripps DJ. Subcorneal pustular dermatosis in children. Arch Dermatol 1974; 109: 73–77.

88. Limmer BL. Subcorneal pustular dermatosis vs pustular psoriasis. Arch Dermatol 1974; 110: 131.

89. Kasha EE Jr, Epinette WW. Subcorneal pustular dermatosis (Sneddon–Wilkinson disease) in association with a monoclonal IgA gammopathy: A report and review of the literature. J Am Acad Dermatol 1988; 19: 854–858.

90. Ryatt KS, Dodman BA, Cotterill JA. Subcorneal pustular dermatosis and IgA gammopathy. Acta Derm Venereol 1981; 61: 560–562.

91. Marsden JR, Millard LG. Pyoderma gangrenosum, subcorneal pustular dermatosis and IgA paraproteinaemia. Br J Dermatol 1986; 114: 125–129.

92. Ingber A, Ideses C, Halevy S, Feuerman EJ. Subcorneal pustular dermatosis (Sneddon–Wilkinson disease) after a diagnostic echogram. Report of two cases. J Am Acad Dermatol 1983; 9: 393–396.

93. Sanchez N, Ackerman AB. Subcorneal pustular dermatosis: a variant of pustular psoriasis. Acta Derm Venereol (Suppl) 1979; 85: 147–151.

94. Chimenti S, Ackerman AB. Is subcorneal pustular dermatosis of Sneddon and Wilkinson an entity *sui generis*? Am J Dermatopathol 1981; 3: 363–376.

95. Wolff K. Subcorneal pustular dermatosis is not pustular psoriasis. Am J Dermatopathol 1981; 3: 381–382.

96. Sanchez NP, Perry HO, Muller SA, Winkelmann RK. Subcorneal pustular dermatosis and pustular psoriasis. A clinicopathologic correlation. Arch Dermatol 1983; 119: 715–721.

97. Yamasaki R, Yamasaki M, Kawasaki Y, Nagasako R. Generalized pustular dermatosis caused by isoniazid. Br J Dermatol 1985; 112: 504–506.

98. Lambert DG, Dalac S, Beer F et al. Acute generalized exanthematous pustular dermatitis induced by diltiazem. Br J Dermatol 1988; 118: 308–309.

99. Stough D, Guin JD, Baker GF, Haynie L. Pustular eruptions following administration of cefazolin: A possible interaction with methyldopa. J Am Acad Dermatol 1987; 16: 1051–1052.

100. Shuttleworth D. A localized recurrent pustular eruption following amoxycillin administration. Clin Exp Dermatol 1989; 14: 367–368.

101. Halevy S, Ingber A, Feuerman J. Subcorneal pustular dermatosis — an unusual course. Acta Derm Venereol 1983; 63: 441–444.

102. Ryan TJ. Sneddon and Wilkinson's pustular dermatosis does exist. Am J Dermatopathol 1981; 3: 383–384.

103. Wallach D, Janssen F, Vignon-Pennamen M-D et al. Atypical neutrophilic dermatosis with subcorneal IgA deposits. Arch Dermatol 1987; 123: 790–795.

103a. Kuan Y-Z, Chiou H-T, Chang H-C et al. Intraepidermal neutrophilic IgA dermatosis. J Am Acad Dermatol 1990; 22: 917–919.

104. Sturman SW. Infantile acropustulosis. Semin Dermatol 1984; 3: 50–52.

105. Kahana M, Schewach-Millet M, Feinstein A. Infantile acropustulosis — report of a case. Clin Exp Dermatol 1987; 12: 291–292.

106. Newton JA, Salisbury J, Marsden A, McGibbon DH. Acropustulosis of infancy. Br J Dermatol 1986; 115: 735–739.

107. Jennings JL, Burrows WM. Infantile acropustulosis. J Am Acad Dermatol 1983; 9: 733–738.

108. Kahn G, Rywlin AM. Acropustulosis of infancy. Arch Dermatol 1979; 115: 831–833.

109. Jarratt M, Ramsdell W. Infantile acropustulosis. Arch Dermatol 1979; 115: 834–836.

110. Findlay RF, Odom RB. Infantile acropustulosis. Am J Dis Child 1983; 137: 455–457.

111. McFadden N, Falk ES. Infantile acropustulosis. Cutis 1985; 36: 49–51.

112. Vignon-Pennamen M-D, Wallach D. Infantile acropustulosis. A clinicopathologic study of six cases. Arch Dermatol 1986; 122: 1155–1160.

113. Bundino S, Zina AM, Ubertalli S. Infantile acropustulosis. Dermatologica 1982; 165: 615–619.

114. Freeman RG, Spiller R, Knox JM. Histopathology of erythema toxicum neonatorum. Arch Dermatol 1960; 82: 586–589.

115. Marino LJ. Toxic erythema present at birth. Arch Dermatol 1965; 92: 402–403.

116. Schachner L, Press S. Vesicular, bullous and pustular disorders in infancy and childhood. Pediatr Clin North Am 1983; 30: 609–629.

117. Luders D. Histologic observations in erythema toxicum neonatorum. Pediatrics 1960; 26: 219–224.

118. Lucky AW, Esterly NB, Heskel N et al. Eosinophilic pustular folliculitis in infancy. Pediatr Dermatol 1984; 1: 202–206.

119. Ramamurthy RS, Reveri M, Esterly NB et al. Transient neonatal pustular melanosis. J Pediatr 1976; 88: 831–835.

120. Auster B. Transient neonatal pustular melanosis. Cutis 1978; 22: 327–328.

121. Barr RJ, Globerman LM, Werber FA. Transient neonatal pustular melanosis. Int J Dermatol 1979; 18: 636–638.

Intraepidermal blisters

122. Uehara M. Pustulosis palmaris et plantaris: Evolutionary sequence from vesicular to pustular lesions. Semin Dermatol 1983; 2: 51–56.
123. Rosen K. Pustulosis palmoplantaris and chronic eczematous hand dermatitis. Acta Derm Venereol (Suppl) 1988; 137: 7–52.
124. Hellgren L, Mobacken H. Pustulosis palmaris et plantaris. Prevalence, clinical observations and prognosis. Acta Derm Venereol 1971; 51: 284–288.
125. Jansen CT, Hollmen A, Pajarre R, Terho P. Antichlamydial antibodies in chronic palmoplantar pustulosis. Acta Derm Venereol 1980; 60: 263–266.
126. Paller AS, Packman L, Rich K et al. Pustulosis palmaris et plantaris: Its association with chronic recurrent multifocal osteomyelitis. J Am Acad Dermatol 1985; 12: 927–930.
127. Enfors W, Molin L. Pustulosis palmaris et plantaris. Acta Derm Venereol 1971; 51: 289–294.
128. Thomsen K, Osterbye P. Pustulosis palmaris et plantaris. Br J Dermatol 1973; 89: 293–296.
129. Ward JM, Barnes RMR. HLA antigens in persistent palmoplantar pustulosis and its relationship to psoriasis. Br J Dermatol 1978; 99: 477–483.
130. Iwatsuki K, Imaizumi S, Tsugiki M et al. Alterations of surface receptors on intralesional neutrophils in pustular psoriasis and palmo-plantar pustulosis. Br J Dermatol 1985; 112: 53–56.
131. White SW. Palmoplantar pustular psoriasis provoked by lithium therapy. J Am Acad Dermatol 1982; 7: 660–662.
132. Jurik AG, Ternowitz T. Frequency of skeletal disease, arthro-osteitis, in patients with pustulosis palmoplantaris. J Am Acad Dermatol 1988; 18: 666–671.
133. Rosen K, Jontell M, Mobacken H, Rosdahl I. Epidermal Langerhans' cells in patients with pustulosis palmoplantaris treated with etretinate or etretinate + methoxsalen photochemotherapy. Acta Derm Venereol 1988; 68: 218–223.
134. Goette DK, Morgan AM, Fox BJ, Horn RT. Treatment of palmoplantar pustulosis with intralesional triamcinolone injections. Arch Dermatol 1984; 120: 319–323.
135. Stevens DM, Ackerman AB. On the concept of bacterids (pustular bacterid, Andrews). Am J Dermatopathol 1984; 6: 281–286.
136. Burge SM, Ryan TJ. Acute palmoplantar pustulosis. Br J Dermatol 1985; 113: 77–83.
137. Uehara M, Ofuji S. The morphogenesis of pustulosis palmaris et plantaris. Arch Dermatol 1974; 109: 518–520.
138. Ashurst PJC. Relapsing pustular eruptions of the hands and feet. Br J Dermatol 1964; 76: 169–180.
139. Thormann J, Heilesen B. Recalcitrant pustular eruptions of the extremities. J Cutan Pathol 1975; 2: 19–24.
140. Danno K, Okamoto H, Imamura S, Ofuji S. Assessment of anti-stratum corneum antibody titres in pustulosis palmaris et plantaris. Br J Dermatol 1982; 107: 183–188.
141. Takematsu H, Ohkohchi K, Tagami H. Demonstration of anaphylatoxins C3a, C4a and C5a in the scales of psoriasis and inflammatory pustular dermatoses. Br J Dermatol 1986; 114: 1–6.

Suprabasilar blisters

142. Ahmed AR. Clinical features of pemphigus. Clin Dermatol 1983; 1: 13–21.
143. Meurer M, Millns JL, Rogers RS III, Jordon RE. Oral pemphigus vulgaris. A report of ten cases. Arch Dermatol 1977; 113: 1520–1524.
144. Shklar G, Cataldo E. Histopathology and cytology of oral lesions of pemphigus. Arch Dermatol 1970; 101: 635–641.
145. Bean SF, Holubar K, Gillett RB. Pemphigus involving the eyes. Arch Dermatol 1975; 111: 1484–1486.
146. Kaneko F, Mori M, Tsukinaga I, Miura Y. Pemphigus vulgaris of esophageal mucosa. Arch Dermatol 1985; 121: 272–273.
147. Raque CJ, Stein KM, Samitz MH. Pemphigus vulgaris involving the esophagus. Arch Dermatol 1970; 102: 371–373.
148. Goldberg NS, Weiss SS. Pemphigus vulgaris of the esophagus in women. J Am Acad Dermatol 1989; 21: 1115–1118.
149. Sagher F, Bercovici B, Romem R. Nikolsky sign on cervix uteri in pemphigus. Br J Dermatol 1974; 90: 407–411.
150. Ahmed AR, Salm M. Juvenile pemphigus. J Am Acad Dermatol 1983; 8: 799–807.
151. Hup JM, Bruinsma RA, Boersma ER, de Jong MCJM. Neonatal pemphigus vulgaris: transplacental transmission of antibodies. Pediatr Dermatol 1986; 3: 468–472.
152. Terpstra H, de Jong MCJM, Klokke AH. In vivo bound pemphigus antibodies in a stillborn infant. Arch Dermatol 1979; 115: 316–319.
153. Moncado B, Sandoval-Cruz JM, Baranda L, Garcia-Reyes J. Neonatal pemphigus. Int J Dermatol 1989; 28: 123–124.
154. Faber WR, Neumann HAM, Flinterman J. Persistent vegetating and keratotic lesions in patients with pemphigus vulgaris during immunosuppressive therapy. Br J Dermatol 1983; 109: 459–463.
155. Coverton RW, Armstrong RB. Acanthosis nigricans developing in resolving lesions of pemphigus vulgaris. Arch Dermatol 1982; 118: 115–116.
156. Leibovici V, Ron N, Goldenhersh M, Holubar K. Coexistence of pemphigus and bullous pemphigoid. Int J Dermatol 1989; 28: 259–260.
157. Krain LS. The association of pemphigus with thymoma or malignancy: a critical review. Br J Dermatol 1974; 90: 397–405.
158. Safai B, Gupta S, Good RA. Pemphigus vulgaris associated with a syndrome of immunodeficiency and thymoma: a case report. Clin Exp Dermatol 1978; 3: 129–134.
159. Vetters JM, Saikia NK, Wood J, Simpson JA. Pemphigus vulgaris and myasthenia gravis. Br J Dermatol 1973; 88: 437–441.
160. Chan LS, Cooper KD. Coexistence of pemphigus vulgaris and progressive localized scleroderma. Arch Dermatol 1989; 125: 1555–1557.
161. Hay RJ, Calnan CD. Oral submucosal fibrosis in a

patient with pemphigus vulgaris. Clin Exp Dermatol 1979; 4: 381–383.

162. Brown P, Taylor B. Herpes simplex infection associated with pemphigus vulgaris. Case report and literature review. J Am Acad Dermatol 1989; 21: 1126–1128.

163. Seidenbaum M, David M, Sandbank M. The course and prognosis of pemphigus. A review of 115 patients. Int J Dermatol 1988; 27: 580–584.

164. Savin JA. The events leading to the death of patients with pemphigus and pemphigoid. Br J Dermatol 1979; 101: 521–534.

165. Creswell SN, Black MM, Bhogal B, Skeete MVH. Correlation of circulating intercellular antibody titers in pemphigus with disease activity. Clin Exp Dermatol 1981; 6: 477–483.

166. Fitzpatrick RE, Newcomer VD. The correlation of disease activity and antibody titers in pemphigus. Arch Dermatol 1980; 116: 285–290.

167. Tan-Lim R, Bystryn J-C. Effect of plasmapheresis therapy on circulating levels of pemphigus antibodies. J Am Acad Dermatol 1990; 22: 35–40.

168. Iwatsuki K, Takigawa M, Imaizumi S, Yamada M. In vivo binding site of pemphigus vulgaris antibodies and their fate during acantholysis. J Am Acad Dermatol 1989; 20: 578–582.

169. Anhalt GJ, Patel H, Diaz LA. Mechanisms of immunologic injury. Pemphigus and bullous pemphigoid. Arch Dermatol 1983; 119: 711–714.

170. Fabbri P, Lotti T, Panconesi E. Pathogenesis of pemphigus. Int J Dermatol 1985; 24: 422–425.

171. Grando SA, Glukhenky BT, Drannik GN et al. Mediators of inflammation in blister fluids from patients with pemphigus vulgaris and bullous pemphigoid. Arch Dermatol 1989; 125: 925–930.

172. Krain LS. Pemphigus. Epidemiologic and survival characteristics of 59 patients, 1955–1973. Arch Dermatol 1974; 110: 862–865.

173. Gange RW, Rhodes EL, Edwards CO, Powell MEA. Pemphigus induced by rifampicin. Br J Dermatol 1976; 95: 445.

174. Brenner S, Livni E. Macrophage migration inhibition factor in pemphigus vulgaris. Arch Dermatol 1986; 14: 453–455.

175. Fellner MJ, Mark AS. Penicillin- and ampicillin-induced pemphigus vulgaris. Int J Dermatol 1980; 19: 392–393.

176. Moy R, Jordon RE. Immunopathology in pemphigus. Clin Dermatol 1983; 1: 72–81.

177. Smolle J, Kerl H. Pitfalls in the diagnosis of pemphigus vulgaris (early pemphigus vulgaris with features of bullous pemphigoid). Am J Dermatopathol 1984; 6: 429–435.

178. Judd KP, Lever WF. Correlation of antibodies in skin and serum with disease severity in pemphigus. Arch Dermatol 1979; 115: 428–432.

179. David M, Katzenelson V, Hazaz B et al. Determination of IgG subclasses in patients with pemphigus with active disease and in remission. Arch Dermatol 1989; 125: 787–790.

180. Maurice PDL, Allen BR, Marriott DW et al. Skin immunofluorescence in the diagnosis of primary bullous diseases — a review of 279 cases. Clin Exp Dermatol 1986; 11: 352–364.

181. David M, Weissman-Katzenelson V, Ben-Chetrit A et al. The usefulness of immunofluorescent tests in pemphigus patients in clinical remission. Br J Dermatol 1989; 120: 391–395.

182. Fellner MJ, Fukuyama K, Moshell A, Klaus MV. Intercellular antibodies in blood and epidermis. Br J Dermatol 1973; 89: 115–126.

183. Feibelman C, Stolzner G, Provost TT. Pemphigus vulgaris. Superior sensitivity of monkey esophagus in the determination of pemphigus antibody. Arch Dermatol 1981; 117: 561–562.

184. Chorzelski TP, Maciejowski E, Jablonska S et al. Coexistence of pemphigus and bullous pemphigoid. Arch Dermatol 1974; 109: 849–853.

185. Anderson HJ, Newcomer VD, Landau JW, Rosenthal LH. Pemphigus and other diseases. Results of indirect intercellular immunofluorescence. Arch Dermatol 1970; 101: 538–546.

186. Ahmed AR, Workman S. Anti-intercellular substance antibodies. Presence in serum samples of 14 patients without pemphigus. Arch Dermatol 1983; 119: 17–21.

187. Ahmed AR, Blose DA. Pemphigus vegetans. Neumann type and Hallopeau type. Int J Dermatol 1984; 23: 135–141.

188. Nelson CG, Apisarnthanarax P, Bean SF, Mullins JF. Pemphigus vegetans of Hallopeau. Immunofluorescent studies. Arch Dermatol 1977; 113: 942–945.

189. Pearson RW, O'Donoghue M, Kaplan SJ. Pemphigus vegetans. Its relationship to eosinophilic spongiosis and favorable response to dapsone. Arch Dermatol 1980; 116: 65–68.

190. Neumann HAM, Faber WR. Pyodermite végétante of Hallopeau. Immunofluorescence studies performed in an early disease stage. Arch Dermatol 1980; 116: 1169–1171.

191. Woo TY, Solomon AR, Fairley JA. Pemphigus vegetans limited to the lips and oral mucosa. Arch Dermatol 1985; 121: 271–272.

192. Premalatha S, Jayakumar S, Yesudian P, Thambiah AS. Cerebriform tongue — a clinical sign in pemphigus vegetans. Br J Dermatol 1981; 104: 587–591.

193. Parodi A, Stanley JR, Ciaccio M, Rebora A. Epidermal antigens in pemphigus vegetans. Report of a case. Br J Dermatol 1988; 119: 799–802.

194. Roenigk HH Jr, Fowler-Bergfeld W. Pemphigus vulgaris-vegetans. Arch Dermatol 1969; 99: 123–124.

195. Matsubara M, Tamaki T, Sato M et al. An unusual form of pemphigus vegetans. Acta Derm Venereol 1981; 61: 259–261.

196. Kuo T-T, Wang CN. Charcot–Leyden crystals in pemphigus vegetans. J Cutan Pathol 1986; 13: 242–245.

197. Guerra-Rodrigo F, Morias Cardoso JP. Pemphigus vegetans. Immunofluorescent and ultrastructural studies in a patient. Arch Dermatol 1971; 104: 412–419.

198. Higashida T, Hino H, Kobayasi T. Desmosomes in pemphigus vegetans. Acta Derm Venereol 1981; 61: 107–113.

The classification of subepidermal blisters

199. Farmer ER. Subepidermal bullous diseases. J Cutan Pathol 1985; 12: 316–321.

200. Sage H. Collagens of basement membranes. J Invest Dermatol 1982; 79: 51s–59s.

201. Eady RAJ. The basement membrane. Interface between the epithelium and the dermis: structural features. Arch Dermatol 1988; 124: 709–712.
202. Katz SI. The epidermal basement membrane zone — structure, ontogeny, and role in disease. J Am Acad Dermatol 1984; 11: 1025–1037.
203. Fine J-D. Antigenic features and structural correlates of basement membranes. Relationship to epidermolysis bullosa. Arch Dermatol 1988; 124: 713–717.
204. Tidman MJ, Eady RAJ. Ultrastructural morphometry of normal human dermal-epidermal junction. The influence of age, sex, and body region on laminar and nonlaminar components. J Invest Dermatol 1984; 83: 448–453.
205. Fine J-D, Horiguchi Y, Couchman JR. 19-DEJ-1, a hemidesmosome-anchoring filament complex-associated monoclonal antibody. Arch Dermatol 1989; 125: 520–523.
206. Stanley JR, Woodley DT, Katz SI, Martin GR. Structure and function of basement membrane. J Invest Dermatol 1982; 79: 69s–72s.
207. Smith LT, Sakai LY, Burgeson RE, Holbrook KA. Ontogeny of structural components at the dermal-epidermal junction in human embryonic and fetal skin: the appearance of anchoring fibrils and type VII collagen. J Invest Dermatol 1988; 90: 480–485.

Subepidermal blisters with little inflammation

208. Haber RM, Hanna W, Ramsay CA, Boxall LBH. Hereditary epidermolysis bullosa. J Am Acad Dermatol 1985; 13: 252–278.
209. Gedde-Dahl T Jr. Sixteen types of epidermolysis bullosa. Acta Derm Venereol (Suppl) 1981; 95: 74–87.
210. Tabas M, Gibbons S, Bauer EA. The mechanobullous diseases. Dermatol Clin 1987; 5: 123–136.
211. Pearson RW. Clinicopathologic types of epidermolysis bullosa and their nondermatological complications. Arch Dermatol 1988; 124: 718–725.
212. Sanchez G, Seltzer JL, Eisen AZ et al. Generalized dominant epidermolysis bullosa simplex: decreased activity of a gelatinolytic protease in cultured fibroblasts as a phenotypic marker. J Invest Dermatol 1983; 81: 576–579.
213. Eady RAJ, Tidman MJ. Diagnosing epidermolysis bullosa. Br J Dermatol 1983; 108: 621–626.
214. Salih MAM, Lake BD, El Hag MA, Atherton DJ. Lethal epidermolytic epidermolysis bullosa: a new autosomal recessive type of epidermolysis bullosa. Br J Dermatol 1985; 113: 135–143.
215. Fine J-D, Stenn J, Johnson L et al. Autosomal recessive epidermolysis bullosa simplex. Arch Dermatol 1989; 125: 931–938.
216. Takamori K, Ikeda S, Naito K, Ogawa H. Proteases are responsible for blister formation in recessive dystrophic epidermolysis bullosa and epidermolysis bullosa simplex. Br J Dermatol 1985; 112: 533–538.
217. Haber RM, Ramsay CA, Boxall LBH. Epidermolysis bullosa simplex with keratoderma of the palms and soles. J Am Acad Dermatol 1985; 12: 1040–1044.
218. DesGroseilliers J-P, Brisson P. Localized epidermolysis bullosa. Report of two cases and evaluation of therapy with glutaraldehyde. Arch Dermatol 1974; 109: 70–72.
219. Fine J-D, Johnson L, Wright T, Horiguchi Y. Epidermolysis bullosa simplex: identification of a kindred with autosomal recessive transmission of the Weber–Cockayne variety. Pediatr Dermatol 1989; 6: 1–5.
220. Hacham-Zadeh S, Rappersberger K, Livshin R, Konrad K. Epidermolysis bullosa herpetiformis Dowling–Meara in a large family. J Am Acad Dermatol 1988; 18: 702–706.
221. Anton-Lamprecht I, Schnyder UW. Epidermolysis bullosa herpetiformis Dowling–Meara. Dermatologica 1982; 164: 221–235.
222. Buchbinder LH, Lucky AW, Ballard E et al. Severe infantile epidermolysis bullosa simplex: Dowling–Meara type. Arch Dermatol 1986; 122: 190–198.
223. Tidman MJ, Eady RAJ, Leigh IM, MacDonald DM. Keratin expression in epidermolysis bullosa simplex (Dowling–Meara). Acta Derm Venereol 1988; 68: 15–20.
224. Bruckner-Tuderman L, Vogel A, Ruegger S et al. Epidermolysis bullosa simplex with mottled pigmentation. J Am Acad Dermatol 1989; 21: 425–432.
225. Fine J-D, Johnson L, Wright T. Epidermolysis bullosa simplex superficialis. Arch Dermatol 1989; 125: 631–638.
226. Medenica-Mojsilovic L, Fenske NA, Espinoza CG. Epidermolysis bullosa herpetiformis with mottled pigmentation and an unusual punctate keratoderma. Arch Dermatol 1986; 122: 900–908.
227. Eisenberg M, Shorey CD, de Chair-Baker W. Epidermolysis bullosa — a new subgroup. Australas J Dermatol 1986; 27: 15–18.
228. Niemi K-M, Sommer H, Kero M et al. Epidermolysis bullosa simplex associated with muscular dystrophy with recessive inheritance. Arch Dermatol 1988; 124: 551–554.
229. Bart BJ, Gorlin RJ, Anderson VE, Lynch FW. Congenital localized absence of skin and associated abnormalities resembling epidermolysis bullosa. Arch Dermatol 1966; 93: 296–304.
230. Bart BJ. Epidermolysis bullosa and congenital localized absence of skin. Arch Dermatol 1970; 101: 78–81.
231. Smith SZ, Cram DL. A mechanobullous disease of the newborn. Bart's syndrome. Arch Dermatol 1978; 114: 81–84.
232. Fisher GB Jr, Greer KE, Cooper PH. Congenital self-healing (transient) mechanobullous dermatosis. Arch Dermatol 1988; 124: 240–243.
233. Kero M, Peltonen L, Foidart JM, Savolainen E-R. Immunohistological localization of three basement membrane components in various forms of epidermolysis bullosa. J Cutan Pathol 1982; 9: 316–328.
234. Fine J-D, Gay S. LDA-1 monoclonal antibody. An excellent reagent for immunofluorescence mapping studies in patients with epidermolysis bullosa. Arch Dermatol 1986; 122: 48–51.
235. Haneke E, Anton-Lamprecht I. Ultrastructure of blister formation in epidermolysis bullosa hereditaria: V. Epidermolysis bullosa simplex localisata type Weber–Cockayne. J Invest Dermatol 1982; 78: 219–223.
236. Niemi K-M, Kero M, Kanerva L, Mattila R.

Epidermolysis bullosa simplex. A new histologic subgroup. Arch Dermatol 1983; 119: 138–141.

237. Holbrook KA. Extracutaneous epithelial involvement n inherited epidermolysis bullosa. Arch Dermatol 1988; 124: 726–731.

238. Eady RAJ. Fetoscopy and fetal skin biopsy for prenatal diagnosis of genetic skin disorders. Semin Dermatol 1988; 7: 2–8.

239. Heagerty AHM, Eady RAJ, Kennedy AR et al. Rapid prenatal diagnosis of epidermolysis bullosa letalis using GB3 monoclonal antibody. Br J Dermatol 1987; 117: 271–275.

240. Tyring SK, Chopra V, Johnson L, Fine J-D. Natural killer cell activity is reduced in patients with severe forms of inherited epidermolysis bullosa. Arch Dermatol 1989; 125: 797–800.

241. Fine J-D, Tamura T, Johnson L. Blood vitamin and trace metal levels in epidermolysis bullosa. Arch Dermatol 1989; 125: 374–379.

242. Kennedy AR, Heagerty AHM, Ortonne J-P et al. Abnormal binding of an anti-amnion antibody to epidermal basement membrane provides a novel diagnostic probe for junctional epidermolysis bullosa. Br J Dermatol 1985; 113: 651–659.

243. Fine J-D. Changing clinical and laboratory concepts in inherited epidermolysis bullosa. Arch Dermatol 1988; 124: 523–526.

244. Thomas L, Faure M, Cambazard F et al. Cultured epithelia from junctional epidermolysis bullosa letalis keratinocytes express the main phenotypic characteristics of the disease. Br J Dermatol 1990; 122: 137–145.

245. Fine J-D, Horiguchi Y, Couchman JR. 19-DEJ-1, a hemidesmosome-anchoring filament complex-associated monoclonal antibody. Definition of a new skin basement membrane antigenic defect in junctional and dystrophic epidermolysis bullosa. Arch Dermatol 1989; 125: 520–523.

246. Leigh IM, Tidman MJ, Eady RAJ. Epidermolysis bullosa: preliminary observations of blister formation in keratinocyte culture. Br J Dermatol 1984; 111: 527–532.

246a. Chapman SJ, Leigh IM, Tidman MJ, Eady RAJ. Abnormal expression of hemidesmosome-like structures by junctional epidermolysis bullosa keratinocytes in vitro. Br J Dermatol 1990; 123: 137–144.

247. Paller AS, Fine J-D, Kaplan S, Pearson RW. The generalized atrophic benign form of junctional epidermolysis bullosa. Arch Dermatol 1986; 122: 704–710.

248. Turner TW. Two cases of junctional epidermolysis bullosa (Herlitz–Pearson). Br J Dermatol 1980; 102: 97–107.

249. Skoven I, Drzewiecki KT. Congenital localized skin defect and epidermolysis bullosa hereditaria letalis. Acta Derm Venereol 1979; 59: 533–537.

250. Peltier FA, Tschen EH, Raimer SS, Kuo T-t. Epidermolysis bullosa letalis associated with congenital pyloric atresia. Arch Dermatol 1981; 117: 728–731.

251. Berger TG, Detlefs RL, Donatucci CF. Junctional epidermolysis bullosa, pyloric atresia, and genitourinary disease. Pediatr Dermatol 1986; 3: 130–134.

252. Pearson RW, Potter B, Strauss F. Epidermolysis bullosa hereditaria letalis. Arch Dermatol 1974; 109: 349–355.

253. Schachner L, Lazarus GS, Dembitzer H. Epidermolysis bullosa hereditaria letalis. Br J Dermatol 1977; 96: 51–58.

254. Hintner H, Wolff K. Generalized atrophic benign epidermolysis bullosa. Arch Dermatol 1982; 118: 375–384.

255. Heng MCY, Barrascout CE, Rasmus W et al. Elevated serum chymotrypsin levels in a patient with junctional epidermolysis bullosa. Int J Dermatol 1987; 26: 385–388.

256. Haber RM, Hanna W. Epidermolysis bullosa progressiva. J Am Acad Dermatol 1987; 16: 195–200.

257. Haber RM, Hanna W, Ramsay CA, Boxall LBH. Cicatricial junctional epidermolysis bullosa. J Am Acad Dermatol 1985; 12: 836–844.

258. Oakley CA, Wilson N, Ross JA, Barnetson R St C. Junctional epidermolysis bullosa in two siblings: clinical observations, collagen studies and electron microscopy. Br J Dermatol 1984; 111: 533–543.

259. Heagerty AHM, Kennedy AR, Leigh IM et al. Identification of an epidermal basement membrane defect in recessive forms of dystrophic epidermolysis bullosa by LH 7:2 monoclonal antibody: use in diagnosis. Br J Dermatol 1986; 115: 125–131.

260. Hashimoto K, Matsumoto M, Iacobelli D. Transient bullous dermolysis of the newborn. Arch Dermatol 1985; 121: 1429–1438.

260a. Hashimoto K, Burk JD, Bale GF et al. Transient bullous dermolysis of the newborn: Two additional cases. J Am Acad Dermatol 1989; 21: 708–713.

261. Bauer EA, Ludman MD, Goldberg JD et al. Antenatal diagnosis of recessive dystrophic epidermolysis bullosa: collagenase expression in cultured fibroblasts as a biochemical marker. J Invest Dermatol 1986; 87: 597–601.

262. Sehgal VN, Rege VL, Ghosh SK, Kamat SM. Dystrophic epidermolysis bullosa. Interesting gastro-intestinal manifestations. Br J Dermatol 1977; 96: 389–392.

263. Tidman MJ, Martin IR, Wells RS et al. Oesophageal web formation in dystrophic epidermolysis bullosa. Clin Exp Dermatol 1988; 13: 279–281.

264. Wojnarowska FT, Eady RAJ, Wells RS. Dystrophic epidermolysis bullosa presenting with congenital localized absence of skin: report of four cases. Br J Dermatol 1983; 108: 477–483.

265. Lechner-Gruskay D, Honig PJ, Pereira G, McKinney S. Nutritional and metabolic profile of children with epidermolysis bullosa. Pediatr Dermatol 1988; 5: 22–27.

266. Reed WB, College J Jr, Francis MJO et al. Epidermolysis bullosa dystrophica with epidermal neoplasms. Arch Dermatol 1974; 110: 894–902.

267. Monk BE, Pembroke AC. Epidermolysis bullosa with squamous-cell carcinoma. Clin Exp Dermatol 1987; 12: 373–374.

268. Carapeto FJ, Pastor JA, Martin J, Agurruza J. Recessive dystrophic epidermolysis bullosa and multiple squamous cell carcinomas. Dermatologica 1982; 165: 39–46.

269. Smoller BA, McNutt NS, Carter DM et al. Recessive dystrophic epidermolysis bullosa skin displays a

chronic growth-activated immunophenotype. Implications for carcinogenesis. Arch Dermatol 1990; 126: 78–83.

270. Yi S, Naito M, Takahashi K et al. Complicating systemic amyloidosis in dystrophic epidermolysis bullosa, recessive type. Pathology 1988; 20: 184–187.

271. Briggaman RA. Is there any specificity to defects of anchoring fibrils in epidermolysis bullosa dystrophica, and what does this mean in terms of pathogenesis? J Invest Dermatol 1985; 84: 371–373.

272. Tidman MJ, Eady RAJ. Evaluation of anchoring fibrils and other components of the dermal-epidermal junction in dystrophic epidermolysis bullosa by a quantitative ultrastructural technique. J Invest Dermatol 1985; 84: 374–377.

273. Takamori K, Naito K, Taneda A, Ogawa H. Increased neutral protease and collagenase activity in recessive dystrophic epidermolysis bullosa. Br J Dermatol 1983; 108: 687–694.

274. Kero M, Palotie A, Peltonen L. Collagen metabolism in two rare forms of epidermolysis bullosa. Br J Dermatol 1984; 110: 177–184.

275. Ikeda S, Manabe M, Muramatsu T et al. Protease inhibitor therapy for recessive dystrophic epidermolysis bullosa. J Am Acad Dermatol 1988; 18: 1246–1252.

276. Bauer EA, Tabas M. A perspective on the role of collagenase in recessive dystrophic epidermolysis bullosa. Arch Dermatol 1988; 124: 734–736.

277. Leigh IM, Eady RAJ, Heagerty AHM et al. Type VII collagen is a normal component of epidermal basement membrane, which shows altered expression in recessive dystrophic epidermolysis bullosa. J Invest Dermatol 1988; 90: 639–642.

278. Smith LT, Sybert VP. Intra-epidermal retention of type VII collagen in a patient with recessive dystrophic epidermolysis bullosa. J Invest Dermatol 1990; 94: 261–264.

279. Bruckner-Tuderman L, Mitsuhashi Y, Schnyder UW, Bruckner P. Anchoring fibrils and type VII collagen are absent from skin in severe recessive dystrophic epidermolysis bullosa. J Invest Dermatol 1989; 93: 3–9.

280. Rusenko KW, Gammon WR, Fine J-D, Briggaman RA. The carboxyl-terminal domain of type VII collagen is present at the basement membrane in recessive dystrophic epidermolysis bullosa. J Invest Dermatol 1989; 92: 623–627.

281. Fine J-D, Horiguchi Y, Stein DH et al. Intraepidermal type VII collagen. Evidence for abnormal intracytoplasmic processing of a major basement membrane protein in rare patients with dominant and possibly localized recessive forms of dystrophic epidermolysis bullosa. J Am Acad Dermatol 1990; 22: 188–195.

281a. Bruckner-Tuderman L, Niemi K-M, Kero M et al. Type VII collagen is expressed but anchoring fibrils are defective in dystrophic epidermolysis bullosa inversa. Br J Dermatol 1990; 122: 383–390.

282. Fine J-D. Epidermolysis bullosa. Clinical aspects, pathology, and recent advances in research. Int J Dermatol 1986; 25: 143–157.

283. Kero M, Niemi K-M. Epidermolysis bullosa. Int J Dermatol 1986; 25: 75–82.

284. Garcia-Perez A, Carapeto FJ. Pretibial epidermolysis bullosa: report of two families and review of the literature. Dermatologica 1975; 150: 122–128.

285. Furue M, Ando I, Inoue Y et al. Pretibial epidermolysis bullosa. Arch Dermatol 1986; 122: 310–313.

286. Lichtenwald DJ, Hanna W, Sauder DN et al. Pretibial epidermolysis bullosa: Report of a case. J Am Acad Dermatol 1990; 22: 346–350.

287. Gryboski JD, Touloukian R, Campanella RA. Gastrointestinal manifestations of epidermolysis bullosa in children. Arch Dermatol 1988; 124: 746–752.

288. Gans LA. Eye lesions of epidermolysis bullosa. Arch Dermatol 1988; 124: 762–764.

289. Fine J-D, Osment LS, Gay S. Dystrophic epidermolysis bullosa. A new variant characterized by progressive symmetrical centripetal involvement with scarring. Arch Dermatol 1985; 121: 1014–1017.

290. Tidman MJ, Eady RAJ. Structural and functional properties of the dermoepidermal junction in obligate heterozygotes for recessive forms of epidermolysis bullosa. Arch Dermatol 1986; 122: 278–281.

291. Pearson RW, Paller AS. Dermolytic (dystrophic) epidermolysis bullosa inversa. Arch Dermatol 1988; 124: 544–547.

292. Woodley DT, Briggaman RA, Gammon WT. Review and update of epidermolysis bullosa acquisita. Semin Dermatol 1988; 7: 111–122.

293. Roenigk HH Jr, Pearson RW. Epidermolysis bullosa acquisita. Arch Dermatol 1981; 117: 383.

294. Gammon WR. Epidermolysis bullosa acquisita. Semin Dermatol 1988; 7: 218–224.

295. Roenigk HH Jr, Ryan JG, Bergfeld WF. Epidermolysis bullosa acquisita. Report of three cases and review of all published cases. Arch Dermatol 1971; 103: 1–10.

296. Gammon WR, Briggaman RA, Wheeler CE Jr. Epidermolysis bullosa acquisita presenting as an inflammatory bullous disease. J Am Acad Dermatol 1982; 7: 382–387.

297. Dahl MGC. Epidermolysis bullosa acquisita — a sign of cicatricial pemphigoid? Br J Dermatol 1979; 101: 475–484.

298. Gammon WR, Briggaman RA, Woodley DT et al. Epidermolysis bullosa acquisita — a pemphigoid-like disease. J Am Acad Dermatol 1984; 11: 820–832.

299. Richter BJ, McNutt S. The spectrum of epidermolysis bullosa acquisita. Arch Dermatol 1979; 115: 1325–1328.

300. Lang PG Jr, Tapert MJ. Severe ocular involvement in a patient with epidermolysis bullosa acquisita. J Am Acad Dermatol 1987; 16: 439–443.

301. Lee CW. Epidermolysis bullosa acquisita associated with vesicular cystitis. Br J Dermatol 1988; 119: 101–105.

302. Medenica-Mojsilovic L, Fenske NA, Espinoza CG. Epidermolysis bullosa acquisita. Direct immunofluorescence and ultrastructural studies. Am J Dermatopathol 1987; 9: 324–333.

303. Rubenstein R, Esterly NB, Fine J-D. Childhood epidermolysis bullosa acquisita. Detection in a 5-year-old girl. Arch Dermatol 1987; 123: 772–776.

304. Borok M, Heng MCY, Ahmed AR. Epidermolysis bullosa acquisita in an 8-year-old girl. Pediatr Dermatol 1986; 3: 315–322.

305. McCuaig CC, Chan LS, Woodley DT et al.

Epidermolysis bullosa acquisita in childhood. Differentiation from hereditary epidermolysis bullosa. Arch Dermatol 1989; 125: 944–949.

306. Briggaman RA, Gammon WR, Woodley DT. Epidermolysis bullosa acquisita of the immunopathological type (dermolytic pemphigoid). J Invest Dermatol 1985; 85: 79s–84s.

307. Dotson AD, Raimer SS, Pursley TV, Tschen J. Systemic lupus erythematosus occurring in a patient with epidermolysis bullosa acquisita. Arch Dermatol 1981; 117: 422–426.

307a. Boh E, Roberts LJ, Lieu T-S et al. Epidermolysis bullosa acquisita preceding the development of systemic lupus erythematosus. J Am Acad Dermatol 1990; 22: 587–593.

308. Ray TL, Levine JB, Weiss W, Ward PA. Epidermolysis bullosa acquisita and inflammatory bowel disease. J Am Acad Dermatol 1982; 6: 242–252.

309. Livden JK, Nilsen R, Thunold S, Schjonsby H. Epidermolysis bullosa acquisita and Crohn's disease. Acta Derm Venereol 1978; 58: 241–244.

310. Palestine RF, Kossard S, Dicken CH. Epidermolysis bullosa acquisita: A heterogeneous disease. J Am Acad Dermatol 1981; 5: 43–53.

311. Krivo JM, Miller F. Immunopathology of epidermolysis bullosa acquisita. Association with mixed cryoglobulinemia. Arch Dermatol 1978; 114: 1218–1220.

312. Burke WA, Briggaman RA, Gammon WR. Epidermolysis bullosa acquisita in a patient with multiple endocrinopathies syndrome. Arch Dermatol 1986; 122: 187–189.

313. Kero M, Niemi K-M, Kanerva L. Pregnancy as a trigger of epidermolysis bullosa acquisita. Acta Derm Venereol 1983; 63: 353–356.

314. Reed RJ. The relationship of epidermolysis bullosa acquisita to cicatricial pemphigoid. Am J Dermatopathol 1981; 3: 69–72.

315. Caughman SW. Epidermolysis bullosa acquisita. The search for identity. Arch Dermatol 1986; 122: 159–161.

316. Furue M, Iwata M, Tamaki K, Ishibashi Y. Anatomical distribution and immunological characteristics of epidermolysis bullosa acquisita antigen and bullous pemphigoid antigen. Br J Dermatol 1986; 114: 651–659.

317. Woodley DT, Briggaman RA, Gammon WR et al. Epidermolysis bullosa acquisita antigen, a major cutaneous basement membrane component is synthesized by human dermal fibroblasts and other cutaneous tissues. J Invest Dermatol 1986; 87: 227–231.

318. Woodley DT, O'Keefe EJ, Reese MJ et al. Epidermolysis bullosa acquisita antigen, a new major component of cutaneous basement membrane, is a glycoprotein with collagenous domains. J Invest Dermatol 1986; 86: 668–672.

319. Gammon WR, Briggaman RA. Functional heterogeneity of immune complexes in epidermolysis bullosa acquisita. J Invest Dermatol 1987; 89: 478–483.

320. Tatnall FM, Whitehead PC, Black MM et al. Identification of the epidermolysis bullosa acquisita antigen by LH 7.2 monoclonal antibody: use in diagnosis. Br J Dermatol 1989; 120: 533–539.

320a. Shimizu H, McDonald JN, Gunner DB et al. Epidermolysis bullosa acquisita antigen and the carboxy terminus of type VII collagen have a common immunolocalization to anchoring fibrils and lamina densa of basement membrane. Br J Dermatol 1990; 122: 577–585.

321. Wilson BD, Birnkrant AF, Beutner EH, Maize JC. Epidermolysis bullosa acquisita: A clinical disorder of varied etiologies. J Am Acad Dermatol 1980; 3: 280–291.

322. Lacour J-P, Juhlin L, El Baze P, Ortonne J-P. Epidermolysis bullosa acquisita with negative direct immunofluorescence. Arch Dermatol 1985; 121: 1183–1185.

323. Barthelemy H, Kanitakis J, Cambazard F et al. Epidermolysis bullosa acquisita — mapping of antigenic determinants by an immunofluorescent technique. Clin Exp Dermatol 1986; 11: 378–386.

324. Unis ME, Pfau RG, Patel H et al. An acquired form of epidermolysis bullosa with immunoreactants. Report of a case. J Am Acad Dermatol 1985; 13: 377–380.

325. Nieboer C, Boorsma DM, Woerdeman MJ, Kalsbeek GL. Epidermolysis bullosa acquisita. Br J Dermatol 1980; 102: 383–392.

326. Zhu X, Niimi Y, Bystryn J-C. Epidermolysis bullosa acquisita. Incidence in patients with basement membrane zone antibodies. Arch Dermatol 1990; 126: 171–174.

327. Woodley DT. Immunofluorescence on salt-split skin for the diagnosis of epidermolysis bullosa acquisita. Arch Dermatol 1990; 126: 229–231.

328. Gammon WR, Kowalewski C, Chorzelski TP et al. Direct immunofluorescence studies of sodium chloride-separated skin in the differential diagnosis of bullous pemphigoid and epidermolysis bullosa acquisita. J Am Acad Dermatol 1990; 22: 664–670.

329. Gibbs RB, Minus HR. Epidermolysis bullosa acquisita with electron microscopical studies. Arch Dermatol 1975; 111: 215–220.

330. Klein GF, Hintner H, Schuler G, Fritsch P. Junctional blisters in acquired bullous disorders of the dermal-epidermal junction zone: role of the lamina lucida as the mechanical locus minoris resistentiae. Br J Dermatol 1983; 109: 499–508.

331. Fine J-D, Tyring S, Gammon WR. The presence of intra-lamina lucida blister formation in epidermolysis bullosa acquisita: possible role of leukocytes. J Invest Dermatol 1989; 92: 27–32.

332. Yaoita H, Briggaman RA, Lawley TJ et al. Epidermolysis bullosa acquisita: ultrastructural and immunological studies. J Invest Dermatol 1981; 76: 288–292.

332a. Requena L, Requena C, Sanchez M et al. Chemical warfare. Cutaneous lesions from mustard gas. J Am Acad Dermatol 1988; 19: 529–536.

332b. Baran R, Juhlin L, Brun P. Bullae in skin grafts. Br J Dermatol 1984; 111: 221–225.

Subepidermal blisters with eosinophils

332c. Rosen LB, Frank BL, Rywlin AM. A characteristic vesiculobullous eruption in patients with chronic lymphocytic leukemia. J Am Acad Dermatol 1986; 15: 943–950.

333. Thivolet J, Barthelemy H. Bullous pemphigoid. Semin Dermatol 1988; 7: 91–103.
334. Korman N. Bullous pemphigoid. J Am Acad Dermatol 1987; 16: 907–924.
335. Asbrink E, Hovmark A. Clinical variants in bullous pemphigoid with respect to early symptoms. Acta Derm Venereol 1981; 61: 417–421.
336. Amato DA, Silverstein J, Zitelli J. The prodrome of bullous pemphigoid. Int J Dermatol 1988; 27: 560–563.
337. van Joost T, Vuzevski VD, ten Kate F, Tank B. Localized bullous pemphigoid, a T cell-mediated disease? Electron microscopic and immunologic studies. Acta Derm Venereol 1989; 69: 341–344.
337a. Guenther LC, Shum D. Localized childhood vulvar pemphigoid. J Am Acad Dermatol 1990; 22: 762–764.
338. Provost TT, Maize JC, Ahmed AR et al. Unusual subepidermal bullous diseases with immunologic features of bullous pemphigoid. Arch Dermatol 1979; 115: 156–160.
339. Person JR. Hydrostatic bullae and pretibial pemphigoid. Int J Dermatol 1983; 22: 237–238.
340. Salomon RJ, Briggaman RA, Wernikoff SY, Kayne AL. Localized bullous pemphigoid. A mimic of acute contact dermatitis. Arch Dermatol 1987; 123: 389–392.
341. Liu H-NH, Su WPD, Rogers RS III. Clinical variants of pemphigoid. Int J Dermatol 1986; 25: 17–27.
342. Duhra P, Ryatt KS. Haemorrhagic pompholyx in bullous pemphigoid. Clin Exp Dermatol 1988; 13: 342–343.
343. Barth JH, Fairris GM, Wojnarowska F, White JE. Haemorrhagic pompholyx is a sign of bullous pemphigoid and an indication for low-dose prednisolone therapy. Clin Exp Dermatol 1986; 11: 409–412.
344. Shklar G, Meyer I, Zacarian SA. Oral lesions in bullous pemphigoid. Arch Dermatol 1969; 99: 663–670.
345. Eng TY, Hogan WJ, Jordon RE. Oesophageal involvement in bullous pemphigoid. Br J Dermatol 1978; 99: 207–210.
346. Bushkell LL, Jordon RE. Bullous pemphigoid: A cause of peripheral blood eosinophilia. J Am Acad Dermatol 1983; 8: 648–651.
347. Miyagawa S, Ishii H, Kitamura W, Sakamoto K. Bullous pemphigoid in a man and his nephew. Arch Dermatol 1983; 119: 605–606.
348. Robison JW, Odom RB. Bullous pemphigoid in children. Arch Dermatol 1978; 114: 899–902.
349. Oranje AP, van Joost T. Pemphigoid in children. Pediatr Dermatol 1989; 6: 267–274.
350. Shimizu H, Hayakawa K, Nishikawa T. A comparative immunoelectron microscopic study of typical and atypical cases of pemphigoid. Br J Dermatol 1988; 119: 717–722.
351. Bean SF, Michel B, Furey N et al. Vesicular pemphigoid. Arch Dermatol 1976; 112: 1402–1404.
352. Gruber GG, Owen LG, Callen JP. Vesicular pemphigoid. J Am Acad Dermatol 1980; 3: 619–622.
353. Winkelmann RK, Su WPD. Pemphigoid vegetans. Arch Dermatol 1979; 115: 446–448.
354. Al-Najjar A, Reilly GD, Bleehen SS. Pemphigoid vegetans: a case report. Acta Derm Venereol 1984; 64: 450–452.
355. Kuokkanen K, Helin H. Pemphigoid vegetans. Report of a case. Arch Dermatol 1981; 117: 56–57.
356. Ueda Y, Nashiro K, Seki Y et al. Pemphigoid vegetans. Br J Dermatol 1989; 120: 449–453.
357. Honeyman JF, Honeyman AR, De la Parra MA et al. Polymorphic pemphigoid. Arch Dermatol 1979; 115: 423–427.
358. Jablonska S, Chorzelski TP, Beutner EH et al. Dermatitis herpetiformis and bullous pemphigoid. Intermediate and mixed forms. Arch Dermatol 1976; 112: 45–48.
359. Sander HM, Utz MMP, Peters MS. Bullous pemphigoid and dermatitis herpetiformis: mixed bullous disease or coexistence of two separate entities? J Cutan Pathol 1989; 16: 370–374.
360. Massa MC, Connolly SM. Bullous pemphigoid with features of prurigo nodularis. Arch Dermatol 1982; 118: 937–939.
361. Yung CW, Soltani K, Lorincz AL. Pemphigoid nodularis. J Am Acad Dermatol 1981; 5: 54–60.
362. Roenigk RK, Dahl MV. Bullous pemphigoid and prurigo nodularis. J Am Acad Dermatol 1986; 14: 944–947.
363. Tani M, Murata Y, Masaki H. Pemphigoid nodularis. J Am Acad Dermatol 1989; 21: 1099–1104.
364. Gawkrodger DJ, O'Doherty C St J. Pemphigoid en cocarde. J Am Acad Dermatol 1989; 20: 1125.
365. Callen JP. Internal disorders associated with bullous disease of the skin. J Am Acad Dermatol 1980; 3: 107–119.
366. Ahmed AR, Hardy D. Bullous pemphigoid family of autoimmune diseases. Int J Dermatol 1981; 20: 541–543.
367. Giannini JM, Callen JP, Gruber GG. Bullous pemphigoid and rheumatoid arthritis. J Am Acad Dermatol 1981; 4: 695–697.
368. Szabo E, Husz S, Kovacs L. Coexistent atypical bullous pemphigoid and systemic lupus erythematosus. Br J Dermatol 1981; 104: 71–75.
369. Kumar V, Binder WL, Schotland E et al. Coexistence of bullous pemphigoid and systemic lupus erythematosus. Arch Dermatol 1978; 114: 1187–1190.
370. Jacoby RA, Abraham AA. Bullous dermatosis and systemic lupus erythematosus in a 15-year-old boy. Arch Dermatol 1979; 115: 1094–1097.
371. Hamilton DV, McKenzie AW. Bullous pemphigoid and primary biliary cirrhosis. Br J Dermatol 1978; 99: 447–450.
372. Barth JH, Kelly SE, Wojnarowska F et al. Pemphigoid and ulcerative colitis. J Am Acad Dermatol 1988; 19: 303–308.
373. Lynfield YL, Green K, Gopal R. Bullous pemphigoid and multiple autoimmune diseases. J Am Acad Dermatol 1983; 9: 257–261.
374. Chuang T-Y, Korkij W, Soltani K et al. Increased frequency of diabetes mellitus in patients with bullous pemphigoid: A case-control study. J Am Acad Dermatol 1984; 11: 1099–1102.
375. Callen JP, McCall MW. Bullous pemphigoid and Hashimoto's thyroiditis. J Am Acad Dermatol 1981; 5: 558–560.
376. How J, Bewsher PD, Stankler L. Bullous pemphigoid,

polymyalgia rheumatica and thyroid disease. Br J Dermatol 1980; 103: 201–204.

377. Masouye I, Schmied E, Didierjean L et al. Bullous pemphigoid and multiple sclerosis: More than a coincidence? Report of three cases. J Am Acad Dermatol 1989; 21: 63–68.

378. Razack EM, Premalatha S, Rao NR, Zahra A. Acanthosis palmaris in a patient with bullous pemphigoid. J Am Acad Dermatol 1987; 16: 217–219.

379. van Joost T, Muntendam J, Heule F et al. Subepidermal bullous autoimmune disease associated with immune nephritis. Immunomorphologic studies. J Am Acad Dermatol 1986; 14: 214–220.

380. Simon CA, Winkelmann RK. Bullous pemphigoid and glomerulonephritis. J Am Acad Dermatol 1986; 14: 456–463.

381. Abel EA, Bennett A. Bullous pemphigoid. Occurrence in psoriasis treated with psoralens plus long-wave ultraviolet radiation. Arch Dermatol 1979; 115: 988–989.

382. Grattan CEH. Evidence of an association between bullous pemphigoid and psoriasis. Br J Dermatol 1985; 113: 281–283.

383. Robinson JK, Baughman RD, Provost TT. Bullous pemphigoid induced by PUVA therapy. Br J Dermatol 1978; 99: 709–713.

384. Stone SP, Schroeter AL. Bullous pemphigoid and associated malignant neoplasms. Arch Dermatol 1975; 111: 991–994.

385. Graham-Brown RAC. Bullous pemphigoid with figurate erythema associated with carcinoma of the bronchus. Br J Dermatol 1987; 117: 385–388.

386. Jablonska S, Chorzelski TP, Blaszczyk M, Maciejowska E. Bullous diseases and malignancy. Semin Dermatol 1984; 3: 316–326.

387. Lindelof B, Islam N, Eklund G, Arfors L. Pemphigoid and cancer. Arch Dermatol 1990; 126: 66–68.

388. Westgate GE, Weaver AC, Couchman JR. Bullous pemphigoid antigen localization suggests an intracellular association with hemidesmosomes. J Invest Dermatol 1985; 84: 218–224.

389. Bernard P, Didierjean L, Denis F et al. Heterogeneous bullous pemphigoid antibodies: detection and characterization by immunoblotting when absent by indirect immunofluorescence. J Invest Dermatol 1989; 92: 171–174.

390. Logan RA, Bhogal B, Das AK et al. Localization of bullous pemphigoid antibody — an indirect immunofluorescence study of 228 cases using a split-skin technique. Br J Dermatol 1987; 117: 471–478.

391. Mutasim DF, Morrison LH, Takahashi Y et al. Definition of bullous pemphigoid antibody binding to intracellular and extracellular antigen associated with hemidesmosomes. J Invest Dermatol 1989; 92: 225–230.

391a. Meyer LJ, Taylor TB, Kadunce DP, Zone JJ. Two groups of bullous pemphigoid antigens are identified by affinity-purified antibodies. J Invest Dermatol 1990; 94: 611–616.

391b. Robledo MA, Kim S-C, Korman NJ et al. Studies of the relationship of the 230-kD and 180-kD bullous pemphigoid antigens. J Invest Dermatol 1990; 94: 793–797.

392. Mueller S, Klaus-Kovtun V, Stanley JR. A 230-kD basic protein is the major bullous pemphigoid antigen. J Invest Dermatol 1989; 92: 33–38.

393. Cook AL, Hanahoe THP, Mallett RB, Pye RJ. Recognition of two distinct major antigens by bullous pemphigoid sera. Br J Dermatol 1990; 122: 435–444.

394. Naito K, Morioka S, Ogawa H. The pathogenic mechanisms of blister formation in bullous pemphigoid. J Invest Dermatol 1982; 79: 303–306.

395. Sams WM Jr, Gammon WR. Mechanism of lesion production in pemphigus and pemphigoid. J Am Acad Dermatol 1982; 6: 431–449.

396. Dubertret L, Bertaux B, Fosse M, Touraine R. Cellular events leading to blister formation in bulloupemphigoid. Br J Dermatol 1980; 104: 615–624.

397. Takamori K, Yoshiike T, Morioka S, Ogawa H. The role of proteases in the pathogenesis of bullous dermatoses. Int J Dermatol 1988; 27: 533–539.

398. Alcalay J, David M, Ingber A et al. Bullous pemphigoid mimicking bullous erythema multiforme: An untoward side effect of penicillins. J Am Acad Dermatol 1988; 18: 345–349.

399. Hodak E, Ben-Shetrit A, Ingber A, Sandbank M. Bullous pemphigoid — an adverse effect of ampicillin. Clin Exp Dermatol 1990; 15: 50–52.

400. Laing VB, Sherertz EF, Flowers FP. Pemphigoid-like eruption related to ibuprofen. J Am Acad Dermatol 1988; 19: 91–94.

401. Kashihara M, Danno K, Miyachi Y et al. Bullous pemphigoid-like lesions induced by phenacetin. Arch Dermatol 1984; 120: 1196–1199.

402. Castel T, Gratacos R, Castro J et al. Bullous pemphigoid induced by Frusemide. Clin Exp Dermatol 1981; 6: 635–638.

403. Fellner MJ, Katz JM. Occurrence of bullous pemphigoid after furosemide therapy. Arch Dermatol 1976; 112: 75–77.

404. Rasmussen HB, Jepsen LV, Brandrup F. Penicillamine-induced bullous pemphigoid with pemphigus-like antibodies. J Cutan Pathol 1989; 16: 154–157.

405. Macfarlane AW, Verbov JL. Trauma-induced bullous pemphigoid. Clin Exp Dermatol 1989; 14: 245–249.

406. Duschet P, Schwarz T, Gschnait F. Bullous pemphigoid after radiation therapy. J Am Acad Dermatol 1988; 18: 441–444.

407. Ahmed AR. Diagnosis of bullous disease and studies in the pathogenesis of blister formation using immunopathological techniques. J Cutan Pathol 1984; 11: 237–248.

408. Nishioka K, Hashimoto K, Katayama I et al. Eosinophilic spongiosis in bullous pemphigoid. Arch Dermatol 1984; 120: 1166–1168.

409. Saxe N, Kahn LB. Subepidermal bullous disease. A correlated clinico-pathologic study of 51 cases. J Cutan Pathol 1976; 3: 88–94.

410. Ahmed AR, Maize JC, Provost TT. Bullous pemphigoid. Clinical and immunological follow-up after successful therapy. Arch Dermatol 1977; 113: 1043–1046.

411. Peters MS, Rogers RS III. Clinical correlations of linear IgA deposition at the cutaneous basement membrane zone. J Am Acad Dermatol 1989; 20: 761–770.

412. Weigand DA. Effect of anatomic region on immunofluorescence diagnosis of bullous pemphigoid. J Am Acad Dermatol 1985; 12: 274–278.
413. Weigand DA, Clements MK. Direct immunofluorescence in bullous pemphigoid: Effects of extent and location of lesions. J Am Acad Dermatol 1989; 20: 437–440.
414. Venning VA, Allen J, Millard PR, Wojnarowska F. The localization of the bullous pemphigoid and cicatricial pemphigoid antigens: direct and indirect immunofluorescence of suction blisters. Br J Dermatol 1989; 120: 305–315.
415. Hodge L, Black MM, Ramnarain N, Bhogal B. Indirect complement immunofluorescence in the immunopathological assessment of bullous pemphigoid, cicatricial pemphigoid, and herpes gestationis. Clin Exp Dermatol 1978; 3: 61–67.
416. Gomes MA, Dambuyant C, Thivolet J, Bussy R. Bullous pemphigoid: a correlative study of autoantibodies, circulating immune complexes and dermo-epidermal deposits. Br J Dermatol 1982; 107: 43–52.
417. Giannotti B, Fabbri P, Panconesi E. Ultrastructural findings in bullous pemphigoid. J Cutan Pathol 1975; 2: 103–108.
418. Schaumburg-Lever G, Orfanos CE, Lever WF. Electron microscopic study of bullous pemphigoid. Arch Dermatol 1972; 106: 662–667.
419. Carruthers JA. Herpes gestationis: a reappraisal. Clin Exp Dermatol 1978; 3: 199–202.
420. Holmes RC, Black MM. The specific dermatoses of pregnancy. J Am Acad Dermatol 1983; 8: 405–412.
421. Winton GB, Lewis CW. Dermatoses of pregnancy. J Am Acad Dermatol 1982; 6: 977–998.
422. Shornick JK. Herpes gestationis. J Am Acad Dermatol 1987; 17: 539–556.
423. Sasseville D, Wilkinson RD, Schnader JY. Dermatoses of pregnancy. Int J Dermatol 1981; 20: 223–241.
424. Mayou SE, Black MM, Holmes RC. Pemphigoid 'herpes' gestationis. Semin Dermatol 1988; 7: 104–110.
425. Tindall JG, Rea TH, Shulman I, Quismorio FP. Herpes gestationis in association with a hydatidiform mole. Immunopathologic studies. Arch Dermatol 1981; 117: 510–512.
426. Kelly SE, Black MM. Pemphigoid gestationis: placental interactions. Semin Dermatol 1989; 8: 12–17.
427. Jurecka W, Holmes RC, Black MM et al. An immunoelectron microscopy study of the relationship between herpes gestationis and polymorphic eruption of pregnancy. Br J Dermatol 1983; 108: 147–151.
428. Fine J-D, Omura EF. Herpes gestationis. Persistent disease activity 11 years post partum. Arch Dermatol 1985; 121: 924–926.
429. Holmes R, Black MM, Williamson DM, Scutt RWB. Herpes gestationis and bullous pemphigoid: a disease spectrum. Br J Dermatol 1980; 103: 535–541.
430. Lawley TJ, Stingl G, Katz SI. Fetal and maternal risk factors in herpes gestationis. Arch Dermatol 1978; 114: 552–555.
431. Hertz KC, Katz SI, Maize J, Ackerman AB. Herpes gestationis. A clinicopathologic study. Arch Dermatol 1976; 112: 1543–1548.

432. Shornick JK, Bangert JL, Freeman RG, Gilliam JN. Herpes gestationis: Clinical and histologic features of twenty-eight cases. J Am Acad Dermatol 1983; 8: 214–224.
433. Katz A, Minta JO, Toole JWP, Medwidsky W. Immunopathologic study of herpes gestationis in mother and infant. Arch Dermatol 1977; 113: 1069–1072.
434. Holmes RC, Black MM. The fetal prognosis in pemphigoid gestationis (herpes gestationis). Br J Dermatol 1984; 110: 67–72.
435. Holmes RC, Black MM. Herpes gestationis. A possible association with autoimmune thyrotoxicosis (Graves' disease). J Am Acad Dermatol 1980; 3: 474–477.
436. Holmes RC, Black MM, Jurecka W et al. Clues to the aetiology and pathogenesis of herpes gestationis. Br J Dermatol 1983; 109: 131–139.
437. Holmes RC, Black MM, Dann J et al. A comparative study of toxic erythema of pregnancy and herpes gestationis. Br J Dermatol 1982; 106: 499–510.
438. Kelly SE, Black MM, Fleming S. Antigen-presenting cells in the skin and placenta in pemphigoid gestationis. Br J Dermatol 1990; 122: 593–599.
439. Kelly SE, Cerio R, Bhogal BS, Black MM. The distribution of IgG subclasses in pemphigoid gestationis: PG factor is an IgG1 autoantibody. J Invest Dermatol 1989; 92: 695–698.
440. Kelly SE, Bhogal BS, Wojnarowska F, Black MM. Expression of a pemphigoid gestationis-related antigen by human placenta. Br J Dermatol 1988; 118: 605–611.
441. Ortonne J-P, Hsi B-L, Verrando P et al. Herpes gestationis factor reacts with the amniotic epithelial basement membrane. Br J Dermatol 1987; 117: 147–154.
442. Kelly SE, Bhogal BS, Wojnarowska F et al. Western blot analysis of the antigen in pemphigoid gestationis. Br J Dermatol 1990; 122: 445–449.
443. Karvonen J, Ilonen J, Reunala T, Tiilikainen A. Immunity in herpes gestationis: inhibition of mixed lymphocyte culture by patients' sera. Br J Dermatol 1984; 111: 183–189.
444. Eberst E, Tongio MM, Eberst B et al. Herpes gestationis and anti-HLA immunization. Br J Dermatol 1981; 104: 543–559.
445. Reunala T, Karvonen J, Tiilikainen A, Salo OP. Herpes gestationis. A high titre of anti-HLA-B8 antibody in the mother and pemphigoid-like immunohistological findings in the mother and the child. Br J Dermatol 1977; 96: 563–571.
446. Scheman AJ, Hordinsky MD, Groth DW et al. Evidence for eosinophil degranulation in the pathogenesis of herpes gestationis. Arch Dermatol 1989; 125: 1079–1083.
447. Schaumburg-Lever G, Saffold OE, Orfanos CE, Lever WF. Herpes gestationis. Histology and ultrastructure. Arch Dermatol 1973; 107: 888–892.
448. Harrington CI, Bleehen SS. Herpes gestationis: immunopathological and ultrastructural studies. Br J Dermatol 1979; 100: 389–399.
449. Cutler TP. Herpes gestationis. Clin Exp Dermatol 1982; 7: 201–207.
450. Holubar K, Konrad K, Stingl G. Detection by immunoelectron microscopy of immunoglobulin G

deposits in skin of immunofluorescence negative herpes gestationis. Br J Dermatol 1977; 96: 569–571.

451. Quimby SR, Xenias SJ, Perry HO. Herpes gestationis. Mayo Clin Proc 1982; 57: 520–526.

452. Carruthers JA, Black MM, Ramnarain N. Immunopathological studies in herpes gestationis. Br J Dermatol 1977; 96: 35–43.

453. Katz SI, Hertz KC, Yaoita H. Herpes gestationis. Immunopathology and characterization of the HG factor. J Clin Invest 1976; 57: 1434–1441.

453a. Walker GB, Harrison PV. Seasonal bullous eruption due to mosquitoes. Clin Exp Dermatol 1985; 10: 127–132.

Subepidermal blisters with neutrophils

454. Thiers BH. Dermatitis herpetiformis. J Am Acad Dermatol 1981; 5: 114–117.

455. Faure M. Dermatitis herpetiformis. Semin Dermatol 1988; 7: 123–129.

456. Greenberg RD. Laryngeal involvement in dermatitis herpetiformis: Case report. J Am Acad Dermatol 1989; 20: 690–691.

457. Fraser NG, Kerr NW, Donald D. Oral lesions in dermatitis herpetiformis. Br J Dermatol 1973; 89: 439–450.

458. Ermacora E, Prampolini L, Tribbia G et al. Long-term follow-up of dermatitis herpetiformis in children. J Am Acad Dermatol 1986; 15: 24–30.

459. Leitao EA, Bernhard JD. Perimenstrual nonvesicular dermatitis herpetiformis. J Am Acad Dermatol 1990; 22: 331–334.

460. Meyer LJ, Zone JJ. Familial incidence of dermatitis herpetiformis. J Am Acad Dermatol 1987; 17: 643–647.

461. Sachs JA, Leonard J, Awad J et al. A comparative serological and molecular study of linear IgA disease and dermatitis herpetiformis. Br J Dermatol 1988; 118: 759–764.

462. Hall RP, Clark RE, Ward FE. Dermatitis herpetiformis in two American blacks: HLA type and clinical characteristics. J Am Acad Dermatol 1990; 22: 436–439.

463. Fry L, Leonard JN, Swain F et al. Long term follow-up of dermatitis herpetiformis with and without dietary gluten withdrawal. Br J Dermatol 1982; 107: 631–640.

464. Ljunghall K, Scheynius A, Forsum U. Circulating reticulin autoantibodies of IgA class in dermatitis herpetiformis. Br J Dermatol 1979; 100: 173–176.

465. Kumar V, Hemedinger E, Chorzelski TP et al. Reticulin and endomysial antibodies in bullous diseases. Comparison of specificity and sensitivity. Arch Dermatol 1987; 123: 1179–1182.

466. Kieffer M, Barnetson R St C. Increased gliadin antibodies in dermatitis herpetiformis and pemphigoid. Br J Dermatol 1983; 108: 673–678.

467. Ciclitira PJ, Ellis HJ, Venning VA et al. Circulating antibodies to gliadin subfractions in dermatitis herpetiformis and linear IgA dermatosis of adults and children. Clin Exp Dermatol 1986; 11: 502–509.

468. Karpati S, Torok E, Kosnai I. IgA class antibody against human jejunum in sera of children with dermatitis herpetiformis. J Invest Dermatol 1986; 87: 703–706.

469. Buckley DB, English J, Molloy W et al. Dermatitis herpetiformis: a review of 119 cases. Clin Exp Dermatol 1983; 8: 477–487.

470. Weetman AP, Burrin JM, Mackay D et al. The prevalence of thyroid autoantibodies in dermatitis herpetiformis. Br J Dermatol 1988; 118: 377–383.

471. Chorzelski TP, Jablonska S, Chadzynska M et al. IgA endomysium antibody in children with dermatitis herpetiformis treated with gluten-free diet. Pediatr Dermatol 1986; 3: 291–294.

472. Beutner EH, Chorzelski TP, Kumar V et al. Sensitivity and specificity of IgA-class antiendomysial antibodies for dermatitis herpetiformis and findings relevant to their pathogenic significance. J Am Acad Dermatol 1986; 15: 464–473.

473. Peters MS, McEvoy MT. IgA antiendomysial antibodies in dermatitis herpetiformis. J Am Acad Dermatol 1989; 21: 1225–1231.

474. Reunala T, Chorzelski TP, Viander M et al. IgA anti-endomysial antibodies in dermatitis herpetiformis: correlation with jejunal morphology, gluten-free diet and anti-gliadin antibodies. Br J Dermatol 1987; 117: 185–191.

475. Ljunghall K, Scheynius A, Jonsson J et al. Gluten-free diet in patients with dermatitis herpetiformis. Effect on the occurrence of antibodies to reticulin and gluten. Arch Dermatol 1983; 119: 970–974.

476. Chorzelski TP, Rosinska D, Beutner EH et al. Aggressive gluten challenge of dermatitis herpetiformis cases converts them from seronegative to seropositive for IgA-class endomysial antibodies. J Am Acad Dermatol 1988; 18: 672–678.

477. Accetta P, Kumar V, Beutner EH et al. Anti-endomysial antibodies. A serologic marker of dermatitis herpetiformis. Arch Dermatol 1986; 122: 459–462.

478. Dodd HJ. Dermatitis herpetiformis and ulcerative colitis: report of a case. Clin Exp Dermatol 1984; 9: 99–101.

479. Fligiel A, Aronson PJ, Kitajima J, Payne RR. Dermatitis herpetiformis — bullous lupus erythematosus overlap syndrome of 27 years pre- and postdating discoid lupus and septal panniculitis. J Cutan Pathol 1988; 15: 307 (abstract).

480. Fraser NG, Rennie AGR, Donald D. Dermatitis herpetiformis and Sjogren's syndrome. Br J Dermatol 1979; 100: 213–215.

481. Reunala T, Salmi J, Karvonen J. Dermatitis herpetiformis and celiac disease associated with Addison's disease. Arch Dermatol 1987; 123: 930–932.

482. Walton C, Walton S. Primary biliary cirrhosis in a diabetic male with dermatitis herpetiformis. Clin Exp Dermatol 1987; 12: 46–47.

483. Davies MG, Fifield R, Marks R. Atopic disease and dermatitis herpetiformis. Br J Dermatol 1979; 101: 429–434.

484. Reunala T, Helin H, Pasternack A et al. Renal involvement and circulating immune complexes in dermatitis herpetiformis. J Am Acad Dermatol 1983; 9: 219–223.

485. Jenkins D, Lynde CW, Stewart WD. Histiocytic lymphoma occurring in a patient with dermatitis herpetiformis. J Am Acad Dermatol 1983; 9: 252–256.

485a. Katz SI, Strober W. The pathogenesis of dermatitis

herpetiformis. J Invest Dermatol 1978; 70: 63–75.

486. Mobacken H, Andersson H, Dahlberg E et al. Spontaneous remission of dermatitis herpetiformis: dietary and gastrointestinal studies. Acta Derm Venereol 1986; 66: 245–250.

487. From E, Thomsen K. Dermatitis herpetiformis. A case provoked by iodine. Br J Dermatol 1974; 91: 221–224.

488. Griffiths CEM, Leonard JN, Fry L. Dermatitis herpetiformis exacerbated by indomethacin. Br J Dermatol 1985; 112: 443–445.

489. Burnie J. A possible immunological mechanism for the pathogenesis of dermatitis herpetiformis with reference to coeliac disease. Clin Exp Dermatol 1980; 5: 451–463.

490. Hall RP. The pathogenesis of dermatitis herpetiformis: Recent advances. J Am Acad Dermatol 1987; 16: 1129–1144.

491. Hall RP, Waldbauer GV. Characterization of the mucosal immune response to dietary antigens in patients with dermatitis herpetiformis. J Invest Dermatol 1988; 90: 658–663.

492. Meyer LJ, Carioto L, Zone JJ. Dermatitis herpetiformis: extraction of intact IgA from granular deposits in dermal papillae. J Invest Dermatol 1987; 88: 559–563.

492a. Dahlback K, Sakai L. IgA immunoreactive deposits collocal with fibrillin immunoreactive fibers in dermatitis herpetiformis skin. Acta Derm Venereol 1990; 70: 194–198.

493. Olbricht SM, Flotte TJ, Collins AB et al. Dermatitis herpetiformis. Cutaneous deposition of polyclonal IgA1. Arch Dermatol 1986; 122: 418–421.

494. Wojnarowska F, Delacroix D, Gengoux P. Cutaneous IgA subclasses in dermatitis herpetiformis and linear IgA disease. J Cutan Pathol 1988; 15: 272–275.

495. Karttunen T, Autio-Harmainen H, Rasanen O et al. Immunohistochemical localization of epidermal basement membrane laminin and type IV collagen in bullous lesions of dermatitis herpetiformis. Br J Dermatol 1984; 111: 389–394.

496. Huff JC, Golitz LE, Kunke KS. Intraepidermal neutrophilic IgA dermatosis. N Engl J Med 1985; 313: 1643–1645.

497. Blenkinsopp WK, Fry L, Haffenden GP, Leonard JN. Histology of linear IgA disease, dermatitis herpetiformis, and bullous pemphigoid. Am J Dermatopathol 1983; 5: 547–554.

498. Marsden RA, McKee PH, Bhogal B et al. A study of benign chronic bullous dermatosis of childhood and comparison with dermatitis herpetiformis and bullous pemphigoid occurring in childhood. Clin Exp Dermatol 1980; 5: 159–172.

499. Smith SB, Harrist TJ, Murphy GF et al. Linear IgA bullous dermatosis v dermatitis herpetiformis. Quantitative measurements of dermoepidermal alterations. Arch Dermatol 1984; 120: 324–328.

500. De Mento FJ, Grover RW. Acantholytic herpetiform dermatitis. Arch Dermatol 1973; 107: 883–887.

501. de Jong MCJM, van der Meer JB, de Nijs JAM, van der Putte SCJ. Concomitant immunohistochemical characteristics of pemphigoid and dermatitis herpetiformis in a patient with atypical bullous dermatosis. Acta Derm Venereol 1983; 63: 476–482.

502. Jawitz J, Kumar V, Nigra TP, Beutner EH. Vesicular pemphigoid vs dermatitis herpetiformis. J Am Acad Dermatol 1984; 10: 892–896.

503. Haffenden G, Wojnarowska F, Fry L. Comparison of immunoglobulin and complement deposition in multiple biopsies from the uninvolved skin in dermatitis herpetiformis. Br J Dermatol 1979; 101: 39–45.

504. Beutner EH, Chorzelski TP, Jablonska S. Immunofluorescence tests. Clinical significance of sera and skin in bullous diseases. Int J Dermatol 1985; 24: 405–421.

505. Karlsson IJ, Dahl MGC, Marks JM. Absence of cutaneous IgA in coeliac disease without dermatitis herpetiformis. Br J Dermatol 1978; 99: 621–625.

506. Fry L, Seah PP. Dermatitis herpetiformis: an evaluation of diagnostic criteria. Br J Dermatol 1974; 90: 137–146.

507. Fry L, Walkden V, Wojnarowska F et al. A comparison of IgA positive and IgA negative dapsone responsive dermatoses. Br J Dermatol 1980; 102: 371–382.

508. Seah PP, Fry L. Immunoglobulins in the skin in dermatitis herpetiformis and their relevance in diagnosis. Br J Dermatol 1975; 92: 157–166.

509. Fry L, Haffenden G, Wojnarowska F et al. IgA and C3 complement in the uninvolved skin in dermatitis herpetiformis after gluten withdrawal. Br J Dermatol 1978; 99: 31–37.

510. Ljunghall K, Tjernlund U. Dermatitis herpetiformis: effect of gluten-restricted and gluten free diet on dapsone requirement and on IgA and C3 deposits in uninvolved skin. Acta Derm Venereol 1983; 63: 129–136.

511. Reunala T. Gluten-free diet in dermatitis herpetiformis. Br J Dermatol 1978; 98: 69–78.

512. Leonard JN, Haffenden GP, Unsworth DJ et al. Evidence that the IgA in patients with linear IgA disease is qualitatively different from that of patients with dermatitis herpetiformis. Br J Dermatol 1984; 110: 315–321.

513. Riches DJ, Martin BGH, Seah PP, Fry L. Ultrastructural observations on uninvolved skin in dermatitis herpetiformis. Br J Dermatol 1973; 88: 323–330.

514. Pehamberger H, Konrad K, Holubar K. Juvenile dermatitis herpetiformis: an immunoelectron microscopic study. Br J Dermatol 1979; 101: 271–277.

515. Wojnarowska F, Marsden RA, Bhogal B, Black MM. Chronic bullous disease of childhood, childhood cicatricial pemphigoid, and linear IgA disease of adults. A comparative study demonstrating clinical and immunopathologic overlap. J Am Acad Dermatol 1988; 19: 792–805.

516. Wojnarowska F. Chronic bullous disease of childhood. Semin Dermatol 1988; 7: 58–65.

517. Leigh G, Marsden RA, Wojnarowska F. Linear IgA dermatosis with severe arthralgia. Br J Dermatol 1988; 119: 789–792.

518. Kim R, Winkelmann RK. Dermatitis herpetiformis in children. Relationship to bullous pemphigoid. Arch Dermatol 1961; 83: 895–902.

519. Jordon RE, Bean SF, Triftshauser CT, Winkelmann RK. Childhood bullous dermatitis herpetiformis. Arch Dermatol 1970; 101: 629–634.

520. Bean SF, Jordon RE. Chronic nonhereditary blistering

disease in children. Arch Dermatol 1974; 110: 941–944.

521. Faber WR, Van Joost T. Juvenile pemphigoid. Br J Dermatol 1973; 89: 519–522.

522. Marsden RA, Skeete MVH, Black MM. The chronic acquired bullous diseases of childhood. Clin Exp Dermatol 1979; 4: 227–240.

523. Rogers M, Bartlett B, Walder B, Cains J. Chronic bullous disease of childhood — aspects of management. Australas J Dermatol 1982; 23: 62–69.

524. Ratnam KV, Lee CT, Tan T. Chronic bullous dermatosis of childhood in Singapore. Int J Dermatol 1986; 25: 34–37.

525. Chorzelski TP, Jablonska S. IgA linear dermatosis of childhood (chronic bullous disease of childhood). Br J Dermatol 1979; 101: 535–542.

526. Surbrugg SK, Weston WL. The course of chronic bullous disease of childhood. Pediatr Dermatol 1985; 2: 213–215.

527. Burge S, Wojnarowska F, Marsden A. Chronic bullous dermatosis of childhood persisting into adulthood. Pediatr Dermatol 1988; 5: 246–249.

528. Wojnarowska F, Marsden RA, Bhogal B, Black MM. Childhood cicatricial pemphigoid with linear IgA deposits. Clin Exp Dermatol 1984; 9: 407–415.

529. Leonard JN, Haffenden GP, Ring NP et al. Linear IgA disease in adults. Br J Dermatol 1982; 107: 301–316.

530. Leonard JN, Griffiths CEM, Powles AV et al. Experience with a gluten free diet in the treatment of linear IgA disease. Acta Derm Venereol 1987; 67: 145–148.

531. Wilson BD, Beutner EH, Kumar V et al. Linear IgA bullous dermatosis. An immunologically defined disease. Int J Dermatol 1985; 24: 569–574.

532. Argenyi ZB, Bergfeld WF, Valenzuela R et al. Linear IgA bullous dermatosis mimicking erythema multiforme in adult. Int J Dermatol 1987; 26: 513–517.

533. Mobacken H, Kastrup W, Ljunghall K et al. Linear IgA dermatosis: a study of ten adult patients. Acta Derm Venereol 1983; 63: 123–128.

534. Tanita Y, Masu S, Kato T, Tagami H. Linear IgA bullous dermatosis clinically simulating pemphigus vulgaris. Arch Dermatol 1986; 122: 246–248.

535. Ratnam KV. IgA dermatosis in an adult Chinese population. A 10-year study of linear IgA and dermatitis herpetiformis in Singapore. Int J Dermatol 1988; 27: 21–24.

536. Barnadas MA, Moreno A, Brunet S et al. Linear IgA bullous dermatosis associated with Hodgkin's disease. J Am Acad Dermatol 1988; 19: 1122–1124.

537. Russell Jones R, Goolamali SK. IgA bullous pemphigoid: a distinct blistering disorder. Case report and review of the literature. Br J Dermatol 1980; 102: 719–725.

538. McEvoy MT, Connolly SM. Linear IgA dermatosis: Association with malignancy. J Am Acad Dermatol 1990; 22: 59–63.

539. Chappe SG, Esterly NB, Furey NL et al. Subepidermal bullous disease and glomerulonephritis in a child. J Am Acad Dermatol 1981; 5: 280–289.

540. McWhirter JD, Hashimoto K, Fayne S, Ito K. Linear IgA bullous dermatosis related to lithium carbonate. Arch Dermatol 1987; 123: 1120–1122.

541. Baden LA, Apovian C, Imber MJ, Dover JS.

542. Gabrielsen TO, Staerfelt F, Thune PO. Drug-induced bullous dermatosis with linear IgA deposits along the basement membrane. Acta Derm Venereol 1981; 61: 439–441.

543. Verhelst F, Demedts M, Verschakelen J et al. Adult linear IgA bullous dermatosis with bronchial involvement. Br J Dermatol 1987; 116: 587–590.

544. Kelly SE, Frith PA, Millard PR et al. A clinicopathological study of mucosal involvement in linear IgA disease. Br J Dermatol 1988; 119: 161–170.

545. Chan LS, Regezi JA, Cooper KD. Oral manifestations of linear IgA disease. J Am Acad Dermatol 1990; 22: 362–365.

546. Leonard JN, Wright P, Williams DM et al. The relationship between linear IgA disease and benign mucous membrane pemphigoid. Br J Dermatol 1984; 110: 307–314.

547. Pothupitiya GM, Wojnarowska F, Bhogal BS, Black MM. Distribution of the antigen in adult linear IgA disease and chronic bullous dermatosis of childhood suggests that it is a single and unique antigen. Br J Dermatol 1988; 118: 175–182.

548. Aboobaker J, Bhogal B, Wojnarowska F et al. The localization of the binding site of circulating IgA antibodies in linear IgA disease of adults, chronic bullous disease of childhood and childhood cicatricial pemphigoid. Br J Dermatol 1987; 116: 293–302.

548a. Wilsteed E, Bhogal BS, Black MM et al. Use of 1M NaCl split skin in the indirect immunofluorescence of the linear IgA bullous dermatoses. J Cutan Pathol 1990; 17: 144–148.

549. Petersen MJ, Gammon WR, Briggaman RA. A case of linear IgA disease presenting initially with IgG immune deposits. J Am Acad Dermatol 1986; 14: 1014–1019.

550. Flotte TJ, Olbricht SM, Collins AB, Harrist TJ. Immunopathologic studies of adult linear IgA bullous dermatosis. Arch Pathol Lab Med 1985; 109: 457–459.

551. Blickenstaff RD, Perry HO, Peters MS. Linear IgA deposition associated with cutaneous varicella-zoster infection. J Cutan Pathol 1988; 15: 49–52.

552. Horiguchi Y, Toda K, Okamoto H, Imamura S. Immunoelectron microscopic observations in a case of linear IgA bullous dermatosis of childhood. J Am Acad Dermatol 1986; 14: 593–599.

553. Ortonne JP, Schmitt D, Jacquelin L. Chronic bullous dermatosis of childhood. Immunological and ultrastructural studies on the melanocyte-dermal junction. Acta Derm Venereol 1978; 58: 291–296.

554. Chorzelski T, Jablonska S. Evolving concept of IgA linear dermatosis. Semin Dermatol 1988; 7: 225–232.

555. Bhogal B, Wojnarowska F, Marsden RA et al. Linear IgA bullous dermatosis of adults and children: an immunoelectron microscopic study. Br J Dermatol 1987; 117: 289–296.

556. Bhogal BS, Wojnarowska F, Black MM et al. Immunopathology of linear IgA bullous dermatosis. J Cutan Pathol 1988; 15: 298 (abstract).

557. Prost C, Colonna De Leca A, Combemale P et al. Diagnosis of adult linear IgA dermatosis by immunoelectronmicroscopy in 16 patients with linear IgA deposits. J Invest Dermatol 1989; 92: 39–45.

558. Roberts LJ, Sontheimer RD. Chronic bullous dermatosis of childhood: immunopathologic studies. Pediatr Dermatol 1987; 4: 6–10.

559. Hardy KM, Perry HO, Pingree GC et al. Benign mucous membrane pemphigoid. Arch Dermatol 1971; 104: 467–475.

560. Bean SF. Cicatricial pemphigoid. Int J Dermatol 1975; 14: 23–26.

561. Ahmed AR, Hombal SM. Cicatricial pemphigoid. Int J Dermatol 1986; 25: 90–96.

562. Rosenbaum MM, Esterly NB, Greenwald MJ, Gerson CR. Cicatricial pemphigoid in a 6-year-old child: Report of a case and review of the literature. Pediatr Dermatol 1984; 2: 13–22.

563. Jolliffe DS, Sim-Davis D. Cicatricial pemphigoid in a young girl: report of a case. Clin Exp Dermatol 1977; 2: 281–284.

564. Rogers M, Painter D. Cicatricial pemphigoid in a four-year-old child: a case report. Australas J Dermatol 1981; 22: 21–23.

565. Venning VA, Frith PA, Bron AJ et al. Mucosal involvement in bullous and cicatricial pemphigoid. A clinical and immunopathological study. Br J Dermatol 1988; 118: 7–15.

566. Harrington CI, Sneddon IB. An unusual case of benign mucous membrane pemphigoid. Acta Derm Venereol 1977; 57: 459–467.

567. Behlen CH II, Mackey DM. Benign mucous membrane pemphigus with a generalized eruption. Arch Dermatol 1965; 92: 566–567.

568. Fisher I, Dahl MV, Christiansen TA. Cicatricial pemphigoid confined to the larynx. Cutis 1980; 25: 371–373.

569. Thomson J, Lang W, Craig JA. Deafness complicating mucous membrane pemphigoid: a case report. Br J Dermatol 1975; 93: 337–339.

570. Burge SM, Powell SM, Ryan TJ. Cicatricial pemphigoid with nail dystrophy. Clin Exp Dermatol 1985; 10: 472–475.

571. Spigel GT, Winkelmann RK. Cicatricial pemphigoid and rheumatoid arthritis. Arch Dermatol 1978; 114: 415–417.

572. Redman RS, Thorne EG. Cicatricial pemphigoid in a patient with systemic lupus erythematosus. Arch Dermatol 1981; 117: 109–110.

573. Van Joost TH, Crone RA, Overdijk AD. Ocular cicatricial pemphigoid associated with practolol therapy. Br J Dermatol 1976; 94: 447–450.

574. Van Joost TH, Faber WR, Manuel HR. Drug-induced anogenital cicatricial pemphigoid. Br J Dermatol 1980; 102: 715–718.

575. Fine J-D, Neises GR, Katz SI. Immunofluorescence and immunoelectron microscopic studies in cicatricial pemphigoid. J Invest Dermatol 1984; 82: 39–43.

575a. Bernard P, Prost C, Lecerf V et al. Studies of cicatricial pemphigoid autoantibodies using direct immunoelectron microscopy and immunoblot analysis. J Invest Dermatol 1990; 94: 630–635.

576. Nieboer C, Boorsma DM, Woerdeman MJ. Immunoelectron microscopic findings in cicatricial pemphigoid: their significance in relation to epidermolysis bullosa acquisita. Br J Dermatol 1982; 106: 419–422.

577. Langeland T. Childhood cicatricial pemphigoid with linear IgA deposits: a case report. Acta Derm Venereol 1985; 65: 354–355.

578. Kumar V, Rogozinski T, Yarbrough C et al. A case of cicatricial pemphigoid or cicatricial linear IgA bullous dermatosis. J Am Acad Dermatol 1980; 2: 327–331.

579. Leonard JN, Hobday CM, Haffenden GP et al. Immunofluorescent studies in ocular cicatricial pemphigoid. Br J Dermatol 1988; 118: 209–217.

579a. Petit A, Perrin P, Bernard P et al. A case of cicatricial pemphigoid with circulating IgA and IgG antibodies directed against 280 kD, 165 kD and 120–130 kD epidermal antigens. Acta Derm Venereol 1990; 70: 236–238.

580. Person JR, Rogers RS III. Bullous and cicatricial pemphigoid. Clinical, histopathologic, and immunopathologic correlations. Mayo Clin Proc 1977; 52: 54–66.

581. Griffith MR, Fukuyama K, Tuffanelli D, Silverman S Jr. Immunofluorescent studies in mucous membrane pemphigoid. Arch Dermatol 1974; 109: 195–199.

582. Fleming MG, Valenzuela R, Bergfeld WF, Tuthill RJ. Mucous gland basement membrane immunofluorescence in cicatricial pemphigoid. Arch Dermatol 1988; 124: 1407–1410.

583. Bean SF. Cicatricial pemphigoid. Immunofluorescent studies. Arch Dermatol 1974; 110: 552–555.

584. Cram DL, Griffith MR, Fukuyama K. Pemphigus-like antibodies in cicatricial pemphigoid. Arch Dermatol 1974; 109: 235–238.

585. Kumar V, Yarbrough C, Beutner EH. Complement-fixing intercellular antibodies in a case of cicatricial pemphigoid. Arch Dermatol 1980; 116: 812–814.

586. Brauner GJ, Jimbow K. Benign mucous membrane pemphigoid. An unusual case with electron microscopic findings. Arch Dermatol 1972; 106: 535–540.

587. Prost C, Labeille B, Chaussade V et al. Immunoelectron microscopy in subepidermal autoimmune bullous diseases. J Invest Dermatol 1987; 89: 567–573.

588. Brunsting LA, Perry HO. Benign pemphigoid? A report of seven cases with chronic, scarring, herpetiform plaques about the head and neck. Arch Dermatol 1957; 75: 489–501.

589. Michel B, Bean SF, Chorzelski T, Fedele CF. Cicatricial pemphigoid of Brunsting-Perry. Arch Dermatol 1977; 113: 1403–1405.

590. MacVicar DN, Graham JH. Localized chronic pemphigoid: A clinicopathologic and histochemical study. Am J Pathol 1966; 48: 52a.

591. Ahmed AR, Salm M, Larson R, Kaplan R. Localized cicatricial pemphigoid (Brunsting-Perry). A transplantation experiment. Arch Dermatol 1984; 120: 932–935.

592. Leenutaphong V, von Kries R, Plewig G. Localized cicatricial pemphigoid (Brunsting-Perry): Electron microscopic study. J Am Acad Dermatol 1989; 21: 1089–1093.

593. Weedon D, Robertson I. Localized chronic pemphigoid. J Cutan Pathol 1976; 3: 41–44.

594. Niboer C, Roeleveld CG, Kalsbeek GL. Localized chronic pemphigoid. Dermatologica 1978; 156: 24–33.

595. Monihan JM, Nguyen TH, Guill MA. Brunsting-Perry pemphigoid simulating basal cell carcinoma. J Am Acad Dermatol 1989; 21: 331–334.

596. Hanno R, Foster DR, Bean SF. Brunsting–Perry cicatricial pemphigoid associated with bullous pemphigoid. J Am Acad Dermatol 1980; 3: 470–473.

597. Person JR, Rogers RS III, Perry HO. Localized pemphigoid. Br J Dermatol 1976; 95: 531–534.

598. Tyring SK, Lee PC. Hemorrhagic bullae associated with *Vibrio vulnificus* septicemia. Report of two cases. Arch Dermatol 1986; 122: 818–820.

599. Fisher K, Berger BW, Keusch GT. Subepidermal bullae secondary to *Escherichia coli* septicemia. Arch Dermatol 1974; 110: 105–106.

600. Olbrych TG, Zarconi J, File TM Jr. Bullous skin lesions associated with *Yersinia enterocolitica* septicemia. Am J Med Sci 1984; 287: 38–39.

600a. Bagel J, Grossman ME. Hemorrhagic bullae associated with *Morganella morganii* septicemia. J Am Acad Dermatol 1985; 12: 575–576.

600b. Elbaum DJ, Wood C, Abuabara F, Morhenn VB. Bullae in a patient with toxic shock syndrome. J Am Acad Dermatol 1984; 10: 267–272.

600c. Tani M, Shimizu R, Ban M et al. Systemic lupus erythematosus with vesiculobullous lesions. Arch Dermatol 1984; 120: 1497–1501.

Miscellaneous blistering diseases

600d. Feldman SR, Jones RS, Lesesne HR et al. A blistering eruption associated with Wilson's disease. J Am Acad Dermatol 1989; 21: 1030–1032.

601. Leavell UW, Farley CH, McIntyre JS. Cutaneous changes in a patient with carbon monoxide poisoning. Arch Dermatol 1969; 99: 429–433.

602. Leavell UW. Sweat gland necrosis in barbiturate poisoning. Arch Dermatol 1969; 100: 218–221.

602a. Godden DJ, McPhie JL. Bullous skin eruption associated with carbamazepine overdosage. Postgrad Med J 1983; 59: 336–337.

603. Herschthal D, Robinson MJ. Blisters of the skin in coma induced by amitryptyline and clorazepate dipotassium. Arch Dermatol 1979; 115: 499.

604. Arndt KA, Mihm MC Jr, Parrish JA. Bullae: a cutaneous sign of a variety of neurologic diseases. J Invest Dermatol 1973; 60: 312–320.

605. Naeyaert JM, Derom E, Santosa S, Rubens R. Sweat-gland necrosis after beta-adrenergic antagonist treatment in a patient with pheochromocytoma. Br J Dermatol 1987; 117: 371–376.

606. Mandy S, Ackerman AB. Characteristic traumatic skin lesions in drug-induced coma. JAMA 1970; 213: 253–256.

607. Brehmer-Andersson E, Pedersen NB. Sweat gland necrosis and bullous skin changes in acute drug intoxication. Acta Derm Venereol 1969; 49: 157–162.

608. Henzemans-Boer M, Toonstra J, Meulenbelt J et al. Skin lesions due to exposure to methyl bromide. Arch Dermatol 1988; 124: 917–921.

609. Ramsay B, Bloxham C, Eldred A et al. Blistering, erosions and scarring in a patient on etretinate. Br J Dermatol 1989; 121: 397–400.

610. Friedmann PS, Coburn P, Dahl MGC et al. PUVA-induced blisters, complement deposition, and damage to the dermoepidermal junction. Arch Dermatol 1987; 123: 1471–1477.

611. Saikia NK, Mackie RM, McQueen A. A case of bullous pemphigoid and figurate erythema in association with metastatic spread of carcinoma. Br J Dermatol 1973; 88: 331–334.

612. Watsky KL, Orlow SJ, Bolognia JL. Figurate and bullous eruption in association with breast carcinoma. Arch Dermatol 1990; 126: 649–652.

613. Vincendeau P, Claudy A, Thivolet J et al. Bullous dermatosis and myeloma. Arch Dermatol 1980; 116: 681–682.

614. Moranz JF, Siegle RJ, Barrett JL. Lymphatic bullae arising as a complication of second-intention healing. J Dermatol Surg Oncol 1989; 15: 874–877.

615. Groff JW, White JW. Vesiculobullous cutaneous lymphatic reflux. Cutis 1988; 42: 31–32.

616. Johnson WT. Cutaneous chylous reflux. "The weeping scrotum". Arch Dermatol 1979; 115: 464–466.

The granulomatous reaction pattern

INTRODUCTION

There are many ways of defining a granulomatous dermatitis. Here, the granulomatous reaction pattern (granulomatous tissue reaction) is defined as a predominantly dermal, chronic inflammatory reaction in which formed granulomas are present: that is, there are organized relatively discrete collections of histiocytes or epithelioid histiocytes within the inflammatory reaction. Multinucleate giant cells of varying types may be present. Conditions in which there is a diffuse infiltrate of histiocytes within the dermis, such as lepromatous leprosy, are not included in this reaction pattern. The group is subdivided by way of :

a. the arrangement of granulomas,
b. the presence of accessory features such as central necrosis, suppuration or necrobiosis, and
c. the presence of foreign material or organisms.

It is difficult to present a completely satisfactory classification of the granulomatous reactions. As Hirsh and Johnson remark in their review of the subject, 'Sometimes a perfect fit can be achieved only with the help of an enlightened shove'.[1] Many conditions described within this group may show only non-specific changes in the early evolution of the inflammatory process and in a late or resolving stage show fibrosis and non-specific changes without granulomas. Occasionally a variety of granuloma types may be seen in one area, e.g. in reactions to foreign bodies or around ruptured hair follicles.

It is necessary in any granulomatous dermatitis to exclude an infectious cause. Culture of fresh tissue as well as histological search increases the chances of identifying a specific infectious agent. The time-consuming examination of multiple sections may be necessary to exclude such a cause. Special stains for organisms may be indicated. Occasionally fungi are shown only by silver stains, such as Grocott methenamine silver, and not by PAS staining. All granulomas should be examined under polarized light to detect or exclude the presence of birefringent foreign material.

Many of the conditions exhibiting a granulomatous tissue reaction have been discussed in other chapters; they will be mentioned only briefly. It is not intended to discuss the general pathogenesis of granulomas here. This has been reviewed elsewhere.[2]

The following classification is based on the structural features of granulomas.

SARCOIDAL GRANULOMAS

Sarcoidal granulomas are found in sarcoidosis and in certain types of reaction to foreign materials and squames.

The prototypic condition in this group is sarcoidosis. Sarcoidal granulomas are discrete, round to oval, and composed of epithelioid histiocytes and multinucleate giant cells which may be of either Langhans or foreign body type. Generally, the type of multinucleate histiocyte present in a granuloma is not helpful in arriving at a specific histological diagnosis. Giant cells may contain asteroid bodies, conchoidal bodies (Schaumann bodies) or crystalline particles. Typical granulomas are surrounded by a sparse rim of lymphocytes and plasma cells and only occasional lymphocytes are present within them. Consequently, they have been described as having a 'naked' appearance. Although the granulomas may be in close proximity to one another, their confluence is not commonly found. With reticulin stains, a network of reticulin fibres is seen surrounding and permeating the histiocytic cluster.

SARCOIDOSIS

This is a multisystem disease which may involve any organ of the body but most commonly affects the lungs, lymph nodes, skin and eyes.[3,4] It is characterized by non-caseating granulomas in the involved organs which may resolve without residua or undergo fibrosis. Despite much investigation sarcoidosis is still a disease of uncertain cause although it is known to be associated with several immunological abnormalities.[4]

Between 10 and 35% of patients with systemic sarcoidosis have cutaneous lesions.[5] Although sarcoidosis is usually a multi-organ disease, chronic cutaneous lesions may be the only manifestation.[6] The skin lesions may be specific, showing a granulomatous histology, or non-specific. The most common non-specific skin lesion is erythema nodosum, which is said to occur in from 3–25% of cases.[5] Sarcoidosis predominantly affects adults; skin lesions are rarely seen in children.[7]

A diversity of clinical forms of cutaneous sarcoidosis occurs. These forms include:

1. papules, plaques and nodules, which may be arranged in an annular or serpiginous pattern;
2. a maculopapular eruption associated with acute lymphadenopathy, uveitis or pulmonary involvement;
3. plaques with marked telangiectasia (angiolupoid sarcoidosis);
4. lupus pernio, consisting of violaceous nodules, particularly on the nose, cheeks and ears;[8]
5. nodular subcutaneous sarcoidosis;[9] and
6. a miscellaneous group which includes cicatricial alopecia,[10] ichthyosiform sarcoidosis,[11] ulcerative, necrotizing and mutilating forms,[12,13] verrucous lesions[14] and erythroderma.[15]

This sixth group represents rare cutaneous manifestations of sarcoidosis. Lupus pernio may resolve with fibrosis and scarring and is often associated with involvement of the upper respiratory tract and lungs.[16] Oral lesions may also occur.[17] The majority of skin lesions resolve without scarring.

It is generally considered that the presence of cutaneous lesions in association with systemic involvement is an indicator of more severe disease. Skin lesions may occur in scars[18] following trauma (including surgery and venipuncture[19]), radiation and chronic infection. In some cases these lesions may be the first manifestation of sarcoidosis. Other cases do not appear to be related to systemic sarcoidosis and may be a sarcoidal reaction to a foreign body. Lesions may also develop in tattoo sites.[20]

Histopathology

There is a dermal infiltrate of granulomas of the type already described (Fig. 7.1). Granulomas may be present only in the superficial dermis or they may extend through the whole thickness of the dermis or subcutis, depending on the type of cutaneous lesion. There is no particular localization to skin appendages or nerves. Necrosis is not usually seen in granulomas but has been reported.[21] Small amounts of fibrinous or granular material may be seen in some granulomas.[3] Slight perigranulomatous fibrosis may be present but marked dermal scarring is unusual except in lupus pernio or necrotizing and ulcerating lesions.

Overlying epidermal hyperplasia occurs in verrucous lesions,[14] and hyperkeratosis occurs in the rare ichthyosiform variant.[11] Otherwise, in most cases, the overlying epidermis is normal or atrophic.

Transepidermal elimination has been reported in sarcoidosis and the histology shows characteristic elimination channels.[22] In some cases the round cell infiltrate surrounding the granulomas is more intense and the granulomas less discrete. The diagnosis of sarcoidosis may then become one of exclusion.

Asteroid bodies and conchoidal bodies (Schaumann bodies) may be seen in multinucleate giant cells but are not specific for sarcoidosis and may occur in other granulomatous reactions including tuberculosis (Fig. 7.2). Schaumann bodies, which are shell-like calcium-impregnated protein complexes, are much more common in the granulomas of sarcoidosis than in those of tuberculosis.[23] Birefringent crystals

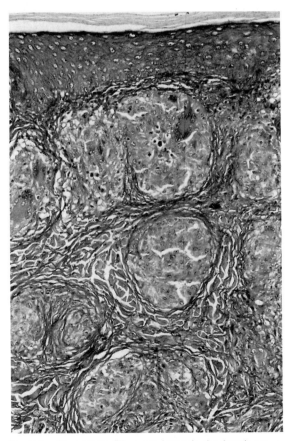

Fig. 7.1   Sarcoidosis. The granulomas in the dermis are composed of epithelioid histiocytes and multinucleate giant cells with only a sparse infiltrate of lymphocytes at the periphery ('naked' granulomas).
Haematoxylin — eosin

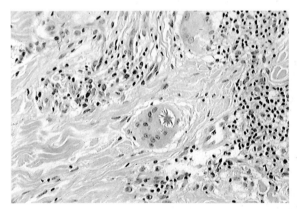

Fig. 7.2   Sarcoidosis. An asteroid body is present in the cytoplasm of a multinucleate giant cell.
Haematoxylin — eosin

of endogenous origin may be present in the granulomas and should not be confused with foreign bodies. These crystals are thought to consist predominantly of calcite (calcium carbonate) and are probably the precursors of Schaumann bodies. Asteroid bodies are said by some to be formed from trapped collagen bundles,[24] or from components of the cytoskeleton, predominantly vimentin intermediate filaments.[25]

Biopsies taken from Kveim–Siltzbach skin test sites, sometimes used in the diagnosis of sarcoidosis, show a variety of changes ranging from poorly formed granulomas with a heavy mononuclear cell infiltrate to small granulomas with few mononuclear cells. The changes seen appear to parallel the changes in the lung.[26]

Immunohistochemical marker studies have shown that the T lymphocytes expressing the suppressor/cytotoxic phenotype are found predominantly in the perigranulomatous mantle whereas those expressing the helper/inducer phenotype are present throughout the granuloma.[27] B lymphocytes are also present in the mantle zone.

Immunofluorescence studies in some cases have shown IgM at the dermo–epidermal junction, IgM within blood vessel walls and IgG within and around the granuloma. A fibrin network is present within granulomas.[28]

REACTIONS TO FOREIGN MATERIALS

A number of foreign substances and materials when introduced into the skin may induce a granulomatous dermatitis which histologically resembles sarcoidosis. These include silica, tattoo pigments, zirconium, beryllium and certain man-made fibres.

Following some kind of trauma, silica may contaminate a wound in the form of dirt, sand, rock or glass (including windshield glass from motor vehicles). Papules and nodules arise in the area of trauma. The granulomas seen in the dermal reaction contain varying numbers of Langhans or foreign body giant cells, some of which may contain clear colourless particles.

These may be difficult to see with routine microscopy but are birefringent in polarized light. The differentiation from true sarcoidosis may be difficult, since granulomas sometimes develop in scars in sarcoidosis and the granulomas can contain birefringent calcite crystals. If there is any doubt, energy-dispersive X-ray analysis techniques using scanning electron microscopy can be used to identify elements present in the crystalline material.[29] The granulomas are thought to develop as a response to colloidal silica particles and not as a result of a hypersensitivity reaction.[30]

A granulomatous dermatitis may occur in response to pigments used in tattooing (see p. 418). The skin lesions are sometimes limited to certain areas of a tattoo where a particular pigment has been used. Two patterns are seen, a foreign body type and a sarcoid type.[31] In the latter form there are aggregates of epithelioid histiocytes and giant cells with a sparse perigranulomatous round cell infiltrate. The histiocytes and giant cells contain pigment particles. True sarcoidosis has also been reported in tattoos, in some cases associated with pulmonary hilar lymphadenopathy. Some of these cases may represent a generalized sarcoid-like reaction to tattoo pigments rather than true sarcoidosis.[32,33] Other granulomatous complications of tattoos include tuberculosis cutis and leprosy.[34]

Zirconium compounds used in underarm deodorants and other skin preparations have been associated with a granulomatous skin reaction in sensitized individuals.[35,36] Histologically the lesions are identical to sarcoidosis. No birefringent material is seen in polarized light.

In the past, cutaneous granulomatous lesions with histology similar to sarcoidosis have been reported in persons exposed to beryllium compounds in industry.[37,38] Other foreign bodies capable of inducing sarcoidal granulomas include acrylic and nylon fibres, wheat stubble and sea urchin spines.[39–41]

Occasionally keratin from ruptured cysts or hair follicles can induce sarcoidal granulomas rather than the more usual foreign-body type of reaction.

TUBERCULOID GRANULOMAS

While the granulomas in this group consist of collections of epithelioid histiocytes, including multinucleate forms, they tend to be less circumscribed than those in the sarcoidal group, have a greater tendency to confluence and are surrounded by a substantial rim of lymphocytes and plasma cells. Langhans giant cells tend to be more characteristic of this group but the foreign body type of giant cell is also seen. There may be areas of caseation in the lesions of tuberculosis.

Tuberculoid granulomas are seen in the following conditions:

Tuberculosis
Tuberculids
Leprosy
Late syphilis
Leishmaniasis
Papular rosacea
Perioral dermatitis
Lupus miliaris disseminatus faciei
Crohn's disease.

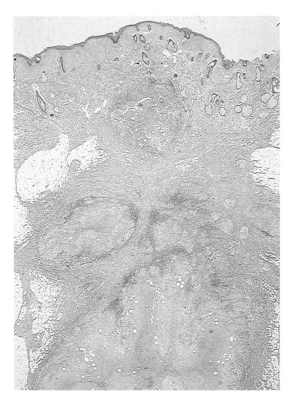

Fig. 7.3 Tuberculosis. The caseating granulomas show some confluence. They extend into the subcutis. Haematoxylin — eosin

TUBERCULOSIS

Typical tuberculoid granulomas can be seen in the dermal inflammatory reaction of late primary inoculation tuberculosis, late miliary tuberculosis, tuberculosis cutis orificialis, tuberculosis verrucosa cutis ('prosector's wart'), scrofuloderma and lupus vulgaris.[42] Cutaneous tuberculosis is discussed in detail with the bacterial infections (see p. 604). A similar pattern of inflammation can be seen after bacille Calmette–Guérin (BCG) vaccination and immunotherapy.[43]

Histopathology

Santa Cruz and Strayer have stressed the variety of histological changes seen in cutaneous tuberculosis.[44] In many forms, particularly in early lesions, there is a mixture of inflammatory cells within the dermis which includes histiocytes and multinucleate cells without well formed epithelioid granulomas. The changes seen in the overlying epidermis are variable. In some forms inflammatory changes extend into the subcutis (Fig. 7.3). Areas of caseation may or may not be present within granulomas. In some cases this may be difficult to distinguish from the necrobiosis seen in rheumatoid nodules (see p. 195). The number of acid-fast organisms varies in different lesions. In lesions with caseation, organisms are most frequently found in the centres of necrotic foci.[45] Generally, where there are well formed granulomas without caseation necrosis, organisms are absent or difficult to find. Neutrophils may be a component of the inflammatory infiltrate and abscesses form in some clinical subtypes. Both Schaumann bodies and asteroid bodies can occasionally be present in multinucleate giant cells.

In lesions with caseation and demonstrable acid-fast organisms, the histological diagnosis may be straightforward. In lupus vulgaris, however, caseation necrosis, if present, is minimal and organisms are rarely found.

Histological differential diagnosis. There is usually a heavier round cell infiltrate about tuberculous granulomas than is seen in sarcoidosis. It is to be remembered that the small foci of fibrinous material sometimes seen in the granulomas of sarcoidosis may mimic, and be mistaken for, caseation. Epidermal changes and dermal fibrosis are not commonly part of the histopathology of sarcoidosis.

Lesions of other non-tuberculous mycobacterial infections of the skin, such as those due to *Mycobacterium marinum*, may be histologically indistinguishable from cutaneous tuberculosis. Organisms are usually difficult to find in *M. marinum* infections; they are described as being longer and broader than typical *M. tuberculosis*. Culture is required for species identification.

The combination of marked irregular epidermal hyperplasia, epidermal and dermal abscesses and dermal tuberculoid granulomas may be seen in tuberculosis verrucosa cutis, caused by *M. tuberculosis*, and in swimming pool granuloma due to *M. marinum* infection. This reaction pattern is also seen in cutaneous fungal infections such as sporotrichosis, chromomycosis and blastomycosis. Diagnosis depends on identification of the appropriate organism.

The lesions of tuberculosis cutis orificialis must be distinguished from those of oral or anal Crohn's disease and from cheilitis granulomatosa (see p. 200). This is not always possible on histological grounds and may depend on clinical history and associated lesions. Foci of caseation and acid-fast organisms may be seen in tuberculous lesions. Marked oedema and granulomas related to or in the lumen of dilated lymphatic channels are present in granulomatous cheilitis.

TUBERCULIDS

The tuberculids are a heterogeneous group of cutaneous disorders associated with tuberculous infections elsewhere in the body, or in other parts of the skin (see p. 607). They include lichen scrofulosorum, papulonecrotic tuberculid and erythema induratum.

In *lichen scrofulosorum* there is a superficial inflammatory reaction about hair follicles and sweat ducts which may include tuberculoid granulomas. Acid-fast organisms are not usually seen or cultured from the lesions.[46] Caseation is rare.[47]

Histopathological studies of *papulonecrotic tuberculid* have shown a subacute or granulomatous vasculitis and dermal coagulative necrosis with, in some cases, a surrounding palisading histiocytic reaction resembling granuloma annulare. Acid-fast bacilli are not found in the lesions. Tuberculoid granulomas were not described in a recent study[48] but have been recorded in others.[42]

In *erythema induratum* (Bazin's disease) there is a lobular panniculitis, although tuberculoid granulomas usually extend into the deep dermis (see p. 503).

LEPROSY

Tuberculoid granulomas are seen in the tuberculoid (TT), borderline tuberculoid (BT) and borderline (BB) groups of the classification of leprosy introduced by Ridley and Jopling.[49] Leprosy is considered further on page 610.

Histopathology[50]

In tuberculoid leprosy (TT), single or grouped epithelioid granulomas with a peripheral rim of lymphocytes are distributed throughout the dermis and subcutis. Unlike lepromatous leprosy this infiltrate does not spare the upper papillary dermis (grenz zone) and it may extend into and destroy the basal layer and part of the stratum malpighii. The granulomas are characteristically arranged in and around neurovascular bundles and arrectores pilorum muscles. Granulomas, particularly in the deeper parts of the infiltrate, tend to be oval and elongated along the course of the nerves and vessels. Small cutaneous nerve bundles are infiltrated and enlarged by the inflammatory cells. There may be destruction of nerves, sometimes with caseation necrosis which may mimic cutaneous tuberculosis. In contrast, the infiltrate in tuberculosis is not particularly related to nerves. The granulomas in tuberculoid leprosy may contain well formed Langhans-type giant cells and less well formed multinucleate foreign body giant cells. The causative organism, *Mycobacterium leprae*, which is best demonstrated by modifications of the Ziehl–Neelsen stain such as the Wade–Fite method, is usually not found in the lesions of tuberculoid leprosy. Rare organisms may be present in nerve fibres.

Granulomas in the *borderline tuberculoid form* (BT) are surrounded by fewer lymphocytes, contain more foreign body giant cells than Langhans cells and may or may not extend up to the epidermis. Organisms may be found in small numbers or not at all. Nerve bundle enlargement is not so prominent and there is no caseation necrosis or destruction of the epidermis.

In the *borderline form* (BB) the granulomas are poorly formed and the epithelioid cells separated by oedema. Scant lymphocytes are present about the granulomas and there are no giant cells. Nerve involvement is slight. Organisms are found, usually only in small numbers.

LATE SYPHILIS

Some lesions of late secondary syphilis and nodular lesions of tertiary syphilis show a superficial and deep dermal inflammatory reaction in which there are tuberculoid granulomas (see p. 634).[51] Plasma cells are generally but not always prominent in the inflammatory infiltrate and there may be swelling of endothelial cells.[52,53] Organisms are rarely demonstrable in these lesions.

LEISHMANIASIS

In chronic cutaneous leishmaniasis (see p. 704) and leishmaniasis recidivans, tuberculoid granulomas are present in the upper and lower dermis.[54] The overlying epidermal changes are variable. Occasionally the granulomas extend to the basal layer of the epidermis as in tuberculoid leprosy.[55] Leishmaniae are usually scarce but

may be found in histiocytes or, rarely, free in the dermis. The organisms have sometimes been mistaken for *Histoplasma capsulatum* but differ from the latter in having a kinetoplast.

PAPULAR ROSACEA

Rosacea is characterized by persistent erythema and telangiectasia, predominantly of the cheeks but also affecting the chin, nose and forehead (see p. 468). In the papular form, papules and papulopustules are superimposed on this background.

Histopathology[56]

The changes seen in biopsies of the papules are variable and relate to the age of the lesion. Early lesions may show only a mild perivascular lymphocytic infiltrate in the dermis. In older lesions there is a mixed inflammatory infiltrate related to the vessels or to vessels and pilosebaceous units. The infiltrate consists of lymphocytes and histiocytes with variable numbers of plasma cells and multinucleate giant cells of Langhans or foreign body type. In some lesions epithelioid histiocytes and giant cells are organized into tuberculoid granulomas (granulomatous rosacea) (Fig. 7.4).[57] An acute folliculitis with follicular and perifollicular

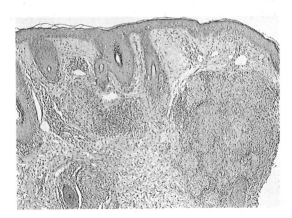

Fig. 7.4 Granulomatous rosacea. Tuberculoid granulomas are present in the dermis. There is some telangiectasia of vessels in the superficial dermis.
Haematoxylin — eosin

pustules and destruction of the hair follicle is sometimes seen. Granulomatous inflammation may be centred on identifiable ruptured hair follicles. There is dermal oedema and vascular dilatation. Epidermal changes, if present, are mild and non-specific.

In granulomatous rosacea, the granulomas are usually of tuberculoid type and not the 'naked' granulomas of sarcoidosis (see p. 182). Differentiation from lupus vulgaris may be difficult. In some cases of rosacea the inflammatory changes may be related to damaged hair follicles. The presence of marked vascular dilatation is suggestive of rosacea.

PERIORAL DERMATITIS

This condition is regarded by some as a distinct entity[58] and by others as a variant of rosacea.[59]

Red papules, papulovesicles or papulopustules on a background of erythema are arranged symmetrically on the chin and nasolabial folds with a characteristic clear zone around the lips. Lesions may occur less commonly on the lower aspect of the cheeks and on the forehead.[60] A periocular variant has also been described.[61] Perioral dermatitis chiefly affects young women, but it has also been reported in children.[62] In many cases the eruption appears to be related to the application of strong topical corticosteroids, particularly fluorinated ones, to the face.[63] Various types of toothpaste have also been implicated.[63a] Perioral dermatitis has also been reported in renal transplant recipients maintained on oral corticosteroids and azathioprine.[64]

Histopathology

The histological changes in perioral dermatitis have been described as identical to those seen in rosacea.[59,62] Others have found the epidermal changes to be more prominent than in rosacea, consisting of parakeratosis, often related to hair follicle ostia, spongiosis which sometimes involves the hair follicle, and slight acanthosis.[65] The changes in the dermis are similar to those in papular rosacea and consist of perivascular or perifollicular infiltrates of lymphocytes and

histiocytes and vascular ectasia. Uncommonly, an acute folliculitis is present. Granulomatous changes are not described.[65]

LUPUS MILIARIS DISSEMINATUS FACIEI

Although the cause of this condition is unknown, it may be related to rosacea.[66] It has also been called acne agminata and acnitis. It is characterized by yellowish brown papules distributed over the central part of the face, including the eyebrows and eyelids. Occasionally lesions occur elsewhere.[67] The lesions last for months and heal with scarring.[68]

Histopathology

Within the dermis are one or more areas of necrosis, sometimes described as caseation necrosis, surrounded by epithelioid histiocytes, multinucleate giant cells and lymphocytes. In many cases granulomas appear to be related to pilosebaceous units.[69] Nuclear fragments may be seen in the necrotic foci. Some lesions show tuberculoid granulomas without necrosis. In one study small vessel changes were also seen, with necrosis of blood vessel walls, thrombi and extravasated red blood cells.[67] Acid-fast bacilli are not found in the areas of necrosis and there is no evidence that this condition is related to tuberculosis.

A recent study of lysozyme in these lesions suggests that there is an immunological mechanism involved in the pathogenesis of this condition rather than a foreign body reaction to an unidentified dermal agent.[70] Conversely, it has been suggested that the lesions represent a granulomatous reaction to damaged pilosebaceous units.[71]

CROHN'S DISEASE

Non-caseating granulomas of tuberculoid type may be found, rarely, in the dermis and subcutis in Crohn's disease (see p. 529). However, they are not uncommon in the wall of perianal sinuses and fistulas. A granulomatous cheilitis has also been reported (see p. 200).

NECROBIOTIC GRANULOMAS

The term 'necrobiosis' has been retained here because of common usage and refers to areas of altered dermal connective tissue in which, by light microscopy, there is blurring and loss of definition of collagen bundles, sometimes separation of fibres, a decrease in connective tissue nuclei and an alteration in staining by routine histological stains, often with increased basophilia or eosinophilia. Granular stringy mucin is sometimes seen in such areas in granuloma annulare and fibrin may be seen in rheumatoid nodules. Necrobiotic areas are partially or completely surrounded by a histiocytic rim which may include multinucleate giant cells. In some cases histiocytes become more spindle-shaped and form a 'palisade'.

Necrobiotic granulomas[72] are found in the following conditions:

Granuloma annulare and its variants
Necrobiosis lipoidica
Rheumatoid nodules
Rheumatic fever nodules.

GRANULOMA ANNULARE

Granuloma annulare is a dermatosis of unknown aetiology in which characteristic necrobiotic granulomas are seen in typical examples.[73] Both localized and generalized forms occur. There is a tendency for the lesions to resolve spontaneously. In one series approximately 50% of lesions cleared within two years.[74] Either the skin or the subcutis, or both, may be involved. There has been one case of cutaneous granuloma annulare associated with histologically similar intra-abdominal visceral lesions in a male with insulin-dependent diabetes.[75]

The clinical variants of granuloma annulare include localized, generalized, perforating[76] and subcutaneous or deep forms.[77,78] A rare linear variant has also been reported.[79]

In the *localized form*, one or more erythematous or skin-coloured papules are found. Grouped papules tend to form annular or arciform plaques. The hands, feet, arms and legs are the sites of predilection in some 80% of cases.[74]

The *generalized form* accounts for approximately 15% of cases.[73] Multiple macules, papules or nodules are distributed over the trunk and limbs.[80] Lesions in *perforating granuloma annulare* are grouped papules, some of which have a central umbilication with scale. The extremities are the most common site. The generalized form may also have perforating lesions.[81] In *subcutaneous (or deep) granuloma annulare*, deep dermal or subcutaneous nodules are found on the lower legs, hands, head and buttocks. These lesions are associated with superficial papules in 25% of cases.[82] This group also includes those lesions described in the past as pseudo-rheumatoid nodules and benign rheumatoid nodules.[83,84] Although arthritis does not occur in children with these nodular lesions, IgM rheumatoid factor has been found in serum in some cases.[85]

Lesions of granuloma annulare have a tendency to regress spontaneously; however, about 40% of cases recur.[74] In the generalized form, the clinical course is chronic with infrequent spontaneous resolution and poor response to therapy.[80]

Females are affected more than twice as commonly as males. The localized and deep forms are more common in children and young adults. Generalized granuloma annulare occurs most frequently in middle-aged to elderly adults. Most cases of granuloma annulare are sporadic but familial cases have occasionally been reported.[86] Patients with the generalized form of the disease show a significantly higher frequency of HLA-BW35 compared with controls and with those who have the localized form of the disease.[87]

Although the aetiology and pathogenesis of the skin lesions in granuloma annulare remain uncertain, possible triggering events include insect bites, trauma, the presence of viral warts and exposure to sunlight. Lesions have occurred in the scars of herpes zoster[88] and at the sites of tuberculin skin tests.[89] The possible link between both the localized and generalized forms and diabetes mellitus remains controversial. There is more convincing evidence of this association with the generalized form than with the localized form.[90,91] Localized, generalized and perforating forms of granuloma annulare have been reported in patients with AIDS.[92–95]

It has been suggested that the underlying

cause of the necrobiotic granulomas is an immunoglobulin-mediated vasculitis.[96] Other studies have stressed the importance of cell-mediated immune mechanisms.[97]

Histopathology

Three histological patterns may be seen in granuloma annulare — necrobiotic granulomas, an interstitial or 'incomplete' form, and granulomas of sarcoidal or tuberculoid type. The third of these patterns is uncommon.[98] In most histopathological studies, the interstitial form is most common.[99]

In the form with *necrobiotic granulomas*, one or more areas of necrobiosis, surrounded by histiocytes and lymphocytes, are present in the superficial and mid dermis (Fig. 7.5). The peripheral rim of histiocytes may form a palisaded pattern (Fig. 7.6). Variable numbers of multinucleate giant cells are found in this zone. Some histiocytes have an epithelioid appearance. The intervening areas of the dermis between the necrobiotic granulomas are relatively normal compared with necrobiosis lipoidica and there is no fibrosis. A perivascular infiltrate of lymphocytes and histiocytes is also present; eosinophils are found in 40% of cases but plasma cells are rare.[100] The central necrobiotic areas contain increased amounts of connective tissue mucins which may appear as basophilic stringy material between collagen bundles. Special stains such as colloidal iron and alcian blue aid in the demonstration of mucin. Elastic fibres may be reduced, absent or unchanged in the involved skin.[101,102]

Occasionally, neutrophils or nuclear fragments are present in necrobiotic areas. An acute or subacute vasculitis has been described in or near foci of necrobiosis, associated with varying

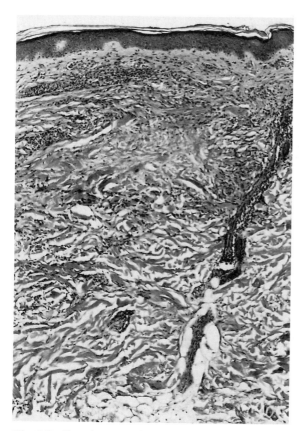

Fig. 7.5 Granuloma annulare. The inflammatory cell infiltrate surrounds the area of 'necrobiosis' on all sides. It is not 'open ended' as in necrobiosis lipoidica. Haematoxylin — eosin

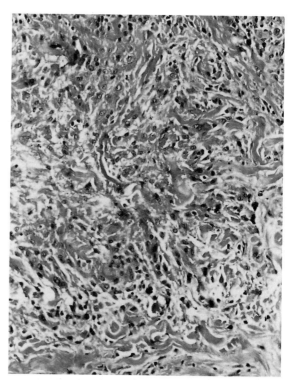

Fig. 7.6 Granuloma annulare. A palisade of inflammatory cells surrounds the central zone of 'necrobiosis'. Haematoxylin — eosin

degrees of endothelial swelling, necrosis of vessel walls, fibrin exudation and nuclear dust.[96]

The lesions of subcutaneous or deep granuloma annulare have areas of necrobiosis which are often larger than in the superficial type (Fig. 7.7). These are distributed in the deep dermis, subcutis and, rarely, muscle.[103] There may be overlying superficial dermal lesions. Eosinophils are more common in this variant than in the superficial lesions.

In the disseminated form of granuloma annulare, the granulomatous foci are often situated in the papillary dermis (Fig. 7.8). Necrobiosis may be inconspicuous. There is some superficial resemblance to lichen nitidus (see p. 39), although in disseminated granuloma annulare there are no acanthotic downgrowths of the epidermis at the periphery of the lesions.

In the *interstitial or 'incomplete' form* of granuloma annulare, the histological changes are subtle and best assessed at lower power. The dermis has a 'busy' look due to increased numbers of inflammatory cells, mainly of histiocytes and lymphocytes (Fig. 7.9). They are arranged about vessels and between collagen bundles which are separated by increased connective tissue mucin. There are no formed areas of necrobiosis. In some cases the interstitial component is minimal.

Cases of the non-necrobiotic *sarcoidal or tuberculoid type* of granuloma annulare are

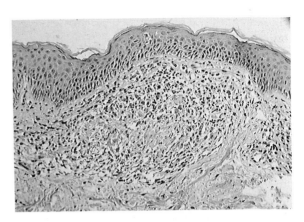

Fig. 7.8 Disseminated granuloma annulare with involvement of the papillary dermis. There are no acanthotic downgrowths of rete pegs at the margins of the inflammatory focus, as seen in lichen nitidus (Fig. 3.10, p. 39). 'Necrobiosis' may be subtle in this form of granuloma annulare.
Haematoxylin — eosin

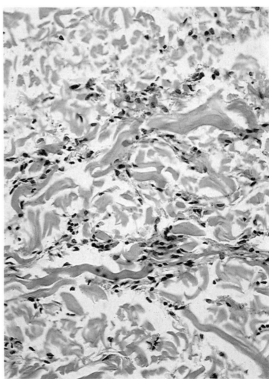

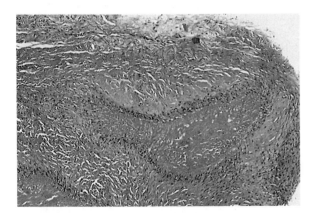

Fig. 7.7 Subcutaneous granuloma annulare. There are large areas of 'necrobiosis' surrounded by a palisade of lymphocytes and histiocytes.
Haematoxylin — eosin

Fig. 7.9 Granuloma annulare of 'incomplete' type. The dermis is hypercellular (a so-called 'busy dermis') and there is an increased amount of interstitial mucin.
Haematoxylin — eosin

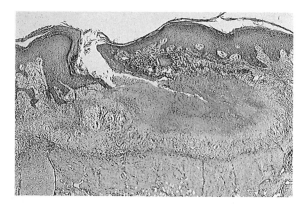

Fig. 7.10   Perforating granuloma annulare.
Haematoxylin — eosin

uncommon and pose a diagnostic problem. The presence of increased dermal mucin or eosinophils may be helpful distinguishing features. Eosinophils and obvious mucin are not seen in sarcoidosis.[100] However, granuloma annulare and sarcoidosis have been reported in the same patient.[104]

In most cases of granuloma annulare, the epidermal changes are minimal. Perforating lesions have a central epidermal perforation which communicates with an underlying necrobiotic granuloma (Fig. 7.10). At the edges of the perforation there are varying degrees of downward epidermal hyperplasia to form a channel. The channel contains necrobiotic material and cellular debris. There is surface hyperkeratosis.[76] The lesions sometimes perforate by way of a hair follicle.[105]

Immunofluorescence studies have shown fibrin in areas of necrobiosis.[104] IgM and C3 were present in blood vessel walls in one series.[96] Immunoperoxidase techniques have demonstrated activated T lymphocytes with an excess of helper/inducer phenotype and CDI-positive dendritic cells related to Langerhans cells in the perivascular and granulomatous infiltrates.[97] A study of the staining pattern of lysozyme in the inflammatory cell infiltrate suggests that this may be useful in distinguishing granuloma annulare from other necrobiotic granulomas.[106]

Electron microscopy. Ultrastructural studies have confirmed the presence of histiocytes in the dermal infiltrate together with cellular debris and fibroblasts. Degenerative changes in collagen in areas of necrobiosis include swelling, loss of periodic banding and fragmentation of fibres. Elastic fibres also show degenerative changes. Fibrin and other amorphous material are present in interstitial areas.[107]

NECROBIOSIS LIPOIDICA

This dermatosis was originally called necrobiosis lipoidica diabeticorum but although many cases are associated with diabetes mellitus (65% in one series),[108,109] it is not peculiar to diabetes. The incidence in diabetics is low — approximately 3 cases per 1000.[108] Although the histology of the lesions varies, areas of necrobiosis with a peripheral histiocytic response are seen at some stage.

The legs, particularly the shins, are overwhelmingly the commonest site of involvement, but lesions may also occur on the forearms, hands and trunk. Three-quarters of cases are bilateral at presentation and many more become bilateral later. Lesions may be single but are more often multiple. Females are affected more than males in a ratio of 3 to 1. The average age of onset in one series was 34 years, but the condition may be seen in children.[110]

The earliest lesions are red papules which enlarge radially to become patches or plaques with an atrophic, slightly depressed, shiny yellow brown centre, and a well-defined raised red to purplish edge. Some lesions resolve spontaneously but many are persistent and chronic and may ulcerate. Rarely, squamous cell carcinoma may arise in longstanding lesions.[111] The simultaneous occurrence of necrobiosis lipoidica with granuloma annulare[112] and with sarcoidosis has been reported.[113]

The strong association of these lesions with diabetes has already been referred to but the role of this metabolic disorder in the development of the cutaneous lesions is not understood. Diabetic vascular changes may be important: in some early lesions a necrotizing vasculitis has been described.[114]

Histopathology

The histopathological changes in necrobiosis lipoidica involve the full thickness of the dermis and often the subcutis (Fig. 7.11). Early lesions are not often biopsied. They are said to show a superficial and deep perivascular and interstitial mixed inflammatory cell infiltrate in the dermis. Similar changes are present in septa of adipose tissue. A necrotizing vasculitis with adjacent areas of necrobiosis and necrosis of adnexal structures is also seen.[114]

In active chronic lesions there is some variability between cases. The characteristic changes are seen at the edge of the lesions. These changes involve most of the dermis but particularly its lower two-thirds. Areas of necrobiosis may be extensive or slight: they are often more extensive and less well defined than in granuloma annulare (Fig. 7.12). The intervening areas of the dermis are also abnormal. Histiocytes, including variable numbers of multinucleate Langhans or foreign body giant cells, outline the areas of necrobiosis. The necrobiosis tends to be irregular and less complete than in granuloma annulare. There is a variable amount of dermal fibrosis and a superficial and deep perivascular inflammatory reaction which, in contrast to the usual picture in granuloma annulare, includes plasma cells (Fig. 7.13). Occasional eosinophils may be present.[100] In some cases necrobiotic areas are less frequent and there are collections of epithelioid histiocytes and multinucleate cells,

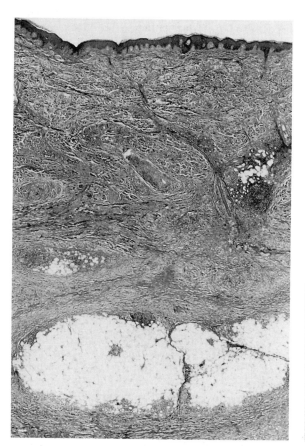

Fig. 7.11 Necrobiosis lipoidica. There is involvement of the full thickness of the dermis with extension into the subcutis. Haematoxylin — eosin

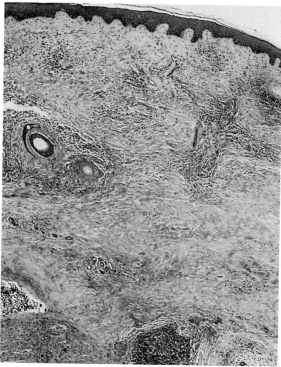

Fig. 7.12 Necrobiosis lipoidica. There are several layers of 'necrobiosis' within the dermis. Haematoxylin — eosin

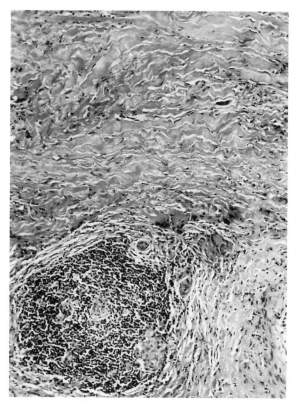

Fig. 7.13 Necrobiosis lipoidica. A perivascular inflammatory cell infiltrate is present in the deep dermis. There is 'necrobiosis' of the adjacent collagen. Haematoxylin — eosin

particularly about dermal vessels. The dermal changes extend into the underlying septa of the subcutis and into the periphery of fat lobules. This septal panniculitis may resemble erythema nodosum but in that condition there are no significant dermal changes. Lymphoid cell aggregates, containing germinal centres, are present in the deep dermis or subcutis in approximately 10% of cases of necrobiosis lipoidica.[115]

In old atrophic lesions and in the centre of plaques there is little necrobiosis and much dermal fibrosis. The underlying subcutis is also fibrotic. Elastic tissue stains demonstrate considerable loss of elastic tissue. Scattered histiocytes may be present.

The presence of lipid in necrobiotic areas (demonstrated by Sudan stains) has been used in the past to distinguish necrobiosis lipoidica from granuloma annulare but recent studies have also shown lipid droplets in granuloma annulare.[102] Fibrin can also be demonstrated in necrobiotic areas.[109] There may be small amounts of mucin in the affected dermis but the presence of large amounts in areas of necrobiosis favours a diagnosis of granuloma annulare.

Vascular changes are more prominent in necrobiosis lipoidica, particularly in the deeper vessels.[72] These range from endothelial swelling to a lymphocytic vasculitis and perivasculitis. Epithelioid granulomas may be present in the vessel wall or adjacent to it. In old lesions the wall may show fibrous thickening. The smaller, more superficial vessels are increased in number and telangiectatic. Apart from atrophy and ulceration, epidermal changes are unremarkable in necrobiosis lipoidica. Transepidermal elimination of degenerate collagen has been reported;[116] it may be associated with focal acanthosis or pseudoepitheliomatous hyperplasia.

Although in most cases it is possible to distinguish necrobiosis lipoidica from granuloma annulare, there are cases in which it is difficult to distinguish between them both clinically and histologically.[109]

Immunofluorescence studies have demonstrated IgM and C3 in the walls of blood vessels in the involved skin. Fibrin is seen in necrobiotic areas. IgM, C3 and fibrinogen may be present at the dermo–epidermal junction.[117]

Ultrastructural studies have shown degeneration of collagen and elastin in the lesions.[118] A recent study has shown a decreased number of S100-positive nerves in plaques, in conformity with the cutaneous anaesthesia that may be a feature of these lesions.[119]

RHEUMATOID NODULES

These nodules occur in approximately 20% of patients with rheumatoid arthritis, usually in the vicinity of joints. Sited primarily in the subcutaneous tissue, they may involve the deep and even the superficial dermis. They vary from millimetres to centimetres in size and consist of fibrous white masses in which there are creamy yellow irregular areas of necrobiosis. Old lesions may have clefts and cystic spaces in these regions. It is most probable that rheumatoid nodules result from a vasculitic process; however, even in very early lesions such a change may be difficult to demonstrate.[120] Nodules usually persist for months to years. Rarely, similar lesions occur in systemic lupus erythematosus.[121]

A papular eruption showing features of a vasculitis and palisading granulomas (rheumatoid papules) has recently been described in a patient with rheumatoid arthritis.[122]

Histopathology

There are one or more irregular areas of necrobiosis in the subcutis and dermis. These are surrounded by a well-developed palisade of elongated histiocytes, with occasional lymphocytes, neutrophils, mast cells and foreign body giant cells (Fig. 7.14). The central necrobiotic focus is usually homogeneous and eosinophilic.[123] There is sometimes obvious fibrin. In contrast, the areas of necrobiosis in the subcutaneous or deep variant of granuloma annulare are often pale and mucinous with a tendency to basophilia. Old rheumatoid nodules may show areas of dense fibrosis, clefts and 'cystic' degeneration of the necrobiotic foci. The dermis and subcutis surrounding the necrobiotic granulomas show a perivascular round cell infiltrate which includes plasma cells. Eosinophils may be present. Uncommonly, an acute vasculitis is seen in the surrounding vessels and sometimes a necrotic blood vessel associated with nuclear fragments or sparse neutrophils may be seen in the centre of areas of necrobiosis. Occasionally, a superficial nodule may perforate the epidermis.[124]

Fibrin is present in the centre of the necrobiotic areas.[125] Rarely, immunoglobulins and complement have been demonstrated in vessels exhibiting a vasculitis. It is unusual to find mucin in necrobiotic foci in rheumatoid nodules and this is the single most useful feature in dis-

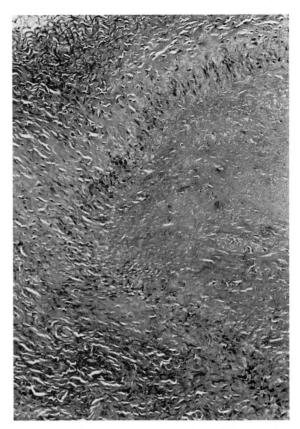

Fig. 7.14 Rheumatoid nodule. A palisade of elongate histiocytes surrounds a zone of 'necrobiosis'. Haematoxylin — eosin

tinguishing these lesions from the deep variant of granuloma annulare.[123]

RHEUMATIC FEVER NODULES

With the decline in the prevalence of rheumatic fever in developed countries, rheumatic nodules are now rarely seen or biopsied. Consequently, most histological studies are found in the older literature.[126] Nodules are more common in children than adults and are usually associated with acute rheumatic carditis. They are usually asymptomatic and are distributed symmetrically over bony prominences, particularly at the elbows.[127] Their size ranges from a few millimetres to 2 to 3 centimetres in diameter. The lesions, unlike rheumatoid nodules, last for only a short time and eventually involute.[126]

Histopathology

Rheumatic nodules form in the subcutis or in the tissue deep to it. They include one or more foci of altered collagen (fibrinoid necrosis, or fibrinoid change): this change is characterized by separation and swelling of the collagen bundles and increased eosinophilia. These foci may contain scattered inflammatory cells[127] or cell debris[126] and are surrounded by histiocytes, sometimes arranged in palisaded array.[126] Multinucleate histiocytes may be seen. A mixed inflammatory cell infiltrate is present at the periphery of these areas and around the vessels. Lipid may be seen in histiocytes about the altered collagen.[126] Apparent differences in the published histological descriptions of these lesions may reflect differences in their age, early lesions being more exudative.

REACTIONS TO FOREIGN MATERIALS

Purified bovine collagen is currently being used, in the form of intracutaneous injections, to treat certain forms of superficial scarring (see p. 425). In some persons this results in a granulomatous reaction resembling granuloma annulare. There are irregular foci of eosinophilic necrobiosis surrounded by a palisading rim of multinucleate and mononuclear histiocytes, with lymphocytes and plasma cells.[128]

Areas of necrobiosis associated with a granulomatous reaction have also been described, rarely, in association with *Trichophyton rubrum* and with the presence of splinters of wood.[129] Necrobiotic areas are also seen in cutaneous berylliosis. Changes which superficially resemble necrobiotic granulomas are also seen in sites of injection of aluminium-adsorbed vaccines[130] and drugs of abuse.[131]

SUPPURATIVE GRANULOMAS

The suppurative granulomas consist of collec-

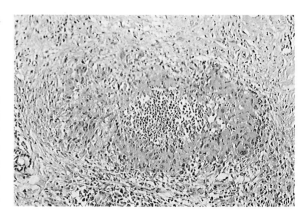

Fig. 7.15 Sporotrichosis. A suppurative granuloma is present.
Haematoxylin — eosin

tions of epithelioid histiocytes, with or without multinucleate giant cells, in the centres of which are collections of neutrophils (Fig. 7.15). Most of the conditions included in this group are discussed in other chapters and only the major differential histological features will be noted here.

Suppurative granulomas are seen in the following conditions:

Chromomycosis and phaeohyphomycosis
Sporotrichosis
Mycobacterium marinum infection
Blastomycosis
Paracoccidioidomycosis
Coccidioidomycosis
Blastomycosis-like pyoderma
Mycetoma, nocardiosis and actinomycosis
Cat-scratch disease
Lymphogranuloma venereum
Pyoderma gangrenosum.
Ruptured cysts and follicles

Histopathology

The first seven conditions listed above show very similar histological changes. These include marked irregular epidermal hyperplasia ('pseudoepitheliomatous' hyperplasia), intra-epidermal and dermal microabscesses, suppurative granulomas and a mixed inflammatory cell infiltrate which includes scattered multinucleate giant cells. Specific diagnosis depends on identification of the causative agent in tissue sections or by culture. Similar changes are seen in halogenodermas but granulomas and giant cells are not seen, except in relation to ruptured hair follicles. It is necessary to cut multiple sections and carefully examine them for microorganisms when such a histopathological pattern is seen. Most organisms can be seen in routine histological sections if care is taken but stains for fungi (for example, the PAS and Grocott methenamine silver methods) and mycobacteria may reveal organisms that escape detection in haematoxylin and eosin preparations.

CHROMOMYCOSIS AND PHAEOHYPHOMYCOSIS

In chromomycosis the characteristic organisms are round to oval thick-walled brown cells about 6–12 μm in diameter (sclerotic bodies, Medlar bodies). Intracellular septation may be seen. Single organisms or small groups are found within multinucleate giant cells, within micro-abscesses, suppurative granulomas or surface crust. Tuberculoid granulomas are occasionally seen in the dermal infiltrate.[132] In phaeo-hyphomycosis, which is clinically distinct from chromomycosis, there are hyphal and yeast forms in suppurative granulomas. Species identification requires culture of the organism. Chromomycosis and phaeohyphomycosis are discussed further in Chapter 25, pages 654–655.

SPOROTRICHOSIS

The causative organism, *Sporothrix schenckii*, is present in the lesions of primary cutaneous sporotrichosis (see p. 655) in the yeast form; it is only rarely found in its hyphal form. The formation of sporothrix asteroids by the encasement of individual yeast cells by a deposit of immune complexes and fibrin is an occasional finding. These asteroids are seen infrequently in sporotrichotic lesions in some parts of the world, but are comparatively common in those seen in Australia and South Africa.[133] The yeast cells are small, round to oval structures, some of which show budding. They may be found within giant cells or in suppurative granulomas. They are difficult to see and may require PAS stains for recognition. The asteroids are found only in microabscesses and the centres of suppurative granulomas. They can be recognized in these locations on careful study of haematoxylin and eosin preparations. Generally, organisms are few in sporotrichosis.

MYCOBACTERIUM MARINUM INFECTION

Tuberculoid or suppurative granulomas may be seen in infections due to this organism (see p. 609). Caseation is not usually seen. The acid-fast organisms are sparse; when found they are usually within histiocytes.[134]

BLASTOMYCOSIS

In the disseminated form of blastomycosis the organisms are scarce and are found either within giant cells or free in the dermis (see p. 651). The organism (*Blastomyces dermatitidis*) is a thick-walled round cell, 8–15 μm in diameter. Multiple nuclei may be seen in the cell. Single broad-based buds are occasionally present on the surface. PAS or Grocott methenamine silver stains make demonstration of the organism easier.

PARACOCCIDIOIDOMYCOSIS

Most cutaneous lesions in paracoccidioidomycosis ('South American blastomycosis') are secondary lesions seen in the course of the disseminated form of the disease (see p. 652). The causative agent, *Paracoccidioides brasiliensis*, is usually found in giant cells. The organisms vary more in size than *Blastomyces dermatitidis* and can be larger. Also, *P. brasiliensis* is thin-walled, lacks multiple nuclei and often has multiple buds arranged round the mother cell.

COCCIDIOIDOMYCOSIS

The cutaneous lesions of coccidioidomycosis are almost always secondary to pulmonary disease (see p. 651). Areas of necrosis are sometimes present in the dermis. Sporangia of *Coccidioides immitis* are rounded structures, 10–80 μm in diameter, which contain multiple sporangiospores, 1–5 μm in diameter. Sporangia are usually easily identified in sections stained with haematoxylin and eosin. Spherules and sporangiospores stain with silver stains. Sporangiospores are PAS-positive whereas spherules may be negative or only weakly positive.[135]

BLASTOMYCOSIS-LIKE PYODERMA

Marked epidermal hyperplasia and epidermal, follicular and dermal abscesses are seen in this condition (see p. 601). In some cases a palisading rim of histiocytes is seen surrounding the suppurative foci in the dermis. Multinucleate giant cells are occasionally present in this zone but they are not as common as in the mycoses discussed above. Bacteria, particularly Gram-positive cocci, may be seen in suppurative foci. *Staphylococcus aureus* is often isolated from tissue samples but not from the skin surface.

MYCETOMAS, NOCARDIOSIS AND ACTINOMYCOSIS

Foci of suppuration in these conditions may become surrounded by a histiocytic rim to form suppurative granulomas. Organisms are present within the suppurative foci. These conditions are discussed in Chapter 25, pages 658–660.

CAT-SCRATCH DISEASE

Suppurative granulomas and zones of necrosis surrounded by a palisade of epithelioid cells may be seen in the skin, at the site of injury, in cat-scratch disease (see p. 618). A variable number of lymphocytes, plasma cells, histiocytes and eosinophils is present in the adjacent tissues.[136]

LYMPHOGRANULOMA VENEREUM

The cutaneous lesions of this disease do not have a specific histopathological appearance (see p. 620). The characteristic suppurative and centrally-necrotic granulomas are found in the regional lymph nodes.[136]

PYODERMA GANGRENOSUM

Superficial granulomatous pyoderma is a recently described variant of pyoderma gangrenosum (see p. 242) in which suppurative granulomas are present in the papillary dermis.[137] Other features of this variant include epidermal hyperplasia, sinus formation, granulation tissue and fibrosis within the dermis and a heavy inflammatory infiltrate in which plasma cells and eosinophils are particularly numerous.

RUPTURED CYSTS AND FOLLICLES

Occasionally suppurative granulomas are seen adjacent to ruptured cysts (epidermal and dermoid cysts, in particular) and to inflamed hair follicles which rupture, liberating their contents into the dermis.

FOREIGN BODY GRANULOMAS

The essential feature in this category of granulomas is the presence either of identifiable *exogenous* (foreign) material or of *endogenous* material which has become altered in some way so that it acts as a foreign body. Around this material are arranged histiocytes (including epithelioid histiocytes), multinucleate giant cells derived from histiocytes and variable numbers of other inflammatory cells. Multinucleate giant cells are often of foreign body type, with nuclei scattered irregularly throughout the cytoplasm but Langhans-type giant cells are also seen. In some cases the reaction consists almost entirely of multinucleate cells. Where there are moderate to large amounts of foreign material, histiocytes are sometimes arranged in an irregular palisade. Some foreign materials, e.g. tattoo pigment, induce granulomas of different types. The causative agent may or may not be birefringent when sections are examined in polarized light.

EXOGENOUS MATERIAL

Foreign body granulomas are formed around such disparate substances as starch,[138] talc,[139] tattoo material (Fig. 7.16),[31] cactus bristles,[140] wood splinters, suture material and insect mouth parts.[141] Some foreign materials such as glass, zirconium, beryllium, acrylic fibres and tattoo pigments may induce local sarcoidal granulomas (see p. 184). Tuberculoid granulomas have been reported in one patient at the site of injection of zinc-containing insulin.[142]

Talc particles are birefringent, as are starch granules; the latter exhibit a characteristic Maltese cross birefringence in polarized light. Incidentally, it is not well known that cryptococci may also be birefringent in polarized light. Materials used to 'cut' heroin and other addictive drugs and the filler materials in crushed tablets may produce cutaneous foreign body granulomas in intravenous drug abusers.[143] The elemental nature of unknown inorganic material can be determined using energy-dispersive X-ray analysis techniques if necessary.

Plant material may be readily identified by its characteristic structure and may be PAS positive.[140] It is prudent to perform stains for bacteria and fungi to exclude contaminating organisms when foreign bodies such as wood splinters or bone fragments are found.

A granulomatous reaction at the site of an arthropod bite may be a reaction to insect fragments or introduced epidermal elements.[141]

A granulomatous reaction is sometimes seen about certain types of suture material, including nylon, silk and dacron.[144] Each type of suture material has a characteristic appearance and birefringence pattern in tissue sections.

ENDOGENOUS MATERIAL

Materials included in this group include calcium deposits, urates, oxalate,[145] keratin and hair.

Both metastatic and dystrophic calcification may be associated with a granulomatous foreign body reaction. This is also seen in idiopathic calcinosis of the scrotum and subepidermal calcified nodules.

A granulomatous reaction to keratin and hair shafts occurs adjacent to ruptured epidermal, pilar and dermoid cysts, pilomatrixomas and any condition associated with rupture or destruction of a hair follicle. Granulomas have been reported as a reaction to autologous hairs incarcerated during hair transplantation.[146] A similar reaction is seen in the interdigital web spaces of barbers from implanted hair.[147] It is not uncommon for enlargement of a banal naevocellular naevus to be due to a granulomatous reaction following damage to a hair follicle. Fragments of keratin may or may not be found in these reactions. Occasional fine wavy eosinophilic squames may be identifiable within spaces in the dermis or within giant cells. Hair shafts are oval or rounded structures when cut in section and sometimes exhibit cortical and medullary layers: they are variably birefringent in polarized light and acid fast when stained by the Ziehl–Neelsen technique.

Cutaneous amyloid is usually inert but in

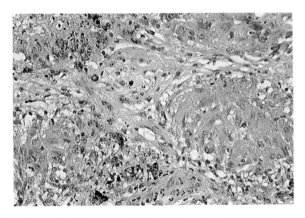

Fig. 7.16 Foreign body granuloma. There is tattoo pigment present.
Haematoxylin — eosin

nodular amyloidosis it may occasionally provoke a foreign body giant cell reaction.

MISCELLANEOUS GRANULOMAS

OROFACIAL GRANULOMATOSIS

This is a rare condition characterized by a syndrome of chronic facial oedema and swelling, particularly of the lips, which is variably associated with gingival overgrowth, oral mucosal tags, fissured tongue and facial nerve paralysis. A granulomatous inflammatory reaction is seen within the swollen tissues of established cases. This syndrome includes the conditions granulomatous cheilitis and Miescher–Melkersson–Rosenthal syndrome.[148–150]

The median age at onset was 20 years in one series and there was an equal sex incidence.[148] Initially, facial swelling may be soft and fluctuating but it becomes firm and persistent with time.[151] The swelling is often asymmetrical and affects predominantly the lower half of the face. The lips are most commonly involved. Unilateral facial nerve palsy occurs in 13–50% of cases.[148,152]

The cause of this condition is unknown but it has been considered to be a manifestation of sarcoidosis, or a reaction to infection or to foreign material such as silicates. In most cases there is a negative Kveim test[153] but occasional cases have been reported in which this is positive.[154] The specificity of this test is doubtful, however.[155] Occasional cases have been associated with other granulomatous skin lesions[148] or granulomatous lymphadenopathy[156] but not generalized sarcoidosis. Eyelid swelling has been reported as a manifestation of systemic sarcoidosis.[157] More important, granulomatous cheilitis with swelling of the lip may be a manifestation of Crohn's disease. In one series, 10% of cases had evidence of Crohn's disease involving the small or large intestine.[148] The lip signs may predate gastrointestinal tract symptoms by years.[158]

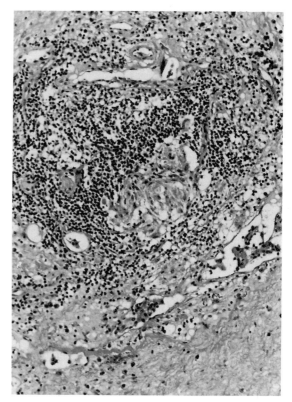

Fig. 7.17   Orofacial granulomatosis. A granulomatous reaction is present adjacent to a vessel containing inflammatory cells.
Haematoxylin — eosin

Histopathology

There is marked oedema in the dermis together with a perivascular inflammatory cell infiltrate consisting of lymphocytes, plasma cells, histiocytes and occasional eosinophils; the infiltrate may extend into underlying muscle. Small 'naked' collections of epithelioid cells, loose tuberculoid granulomas with a peripheral round cell infiltrate or isolated multinucleate giant cells are usually present. The inflammatory infiltrate is more consistently related to vessels than that in sarcoidosis (Fig. 7.17). Schaumann bodies and birefringent fragments may occasionally be seen in histiocytes and giant cells. Lymphatics are usually widely dilated and may contain collections of inflammatory cells. Alternatively, inflammatory cell collections may bulge into the

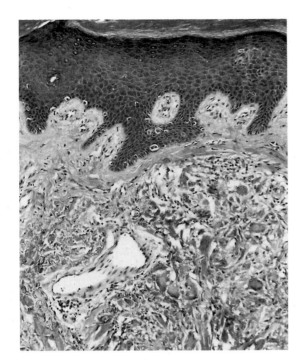

Fig. 7.18 Actinic granuloma. There are many foreign body giant cells arranged around elastotic fibres. Some fibres have been phagocytosed.
Haematoxylin — eosin

lumen of vessels.[159] Older lesions may show dermal fibrosis. Collagenous nodules which represent fibrosed granulomas may be found after treatment with steroids.[160] Overlying epithelial changes are non-specific. There are no reliable features which allow distinction of those cases which represent a manifestation of Crohn's disease.

Similar histological changes are seen in association with chronic oedema and swelling of the vulva and penis in some cases of recurrent infections of this region.[161]

ELASTOLYTIC GRANULOMAS

This group of granulomatous conditions predominantly affects the exposed skin of the head, neck and limbs. It includes actinic granuloma,[162] atypical necrobiosis lipoidica of the face and scalp[163] and Miescher's granuloma.[164]

They are all characterized by annular lesions exhibiting a zonal histological pattern that includes a granulomatous response with giant cells at the annular rim and centrally a loss of elastic fibres or the presence of solar elastotic material. These conditions may represent a single diagnostic entity and have been grouped under the title 'annular elastolytic giant cell granuloma'.[165] The relationship, if any, of this group to the necrobiotic granulomas is controversial. Another lesion, granuloma multiforme, is also very similar clinically and histologically to these conditions and is discussed here.

Actinic granuloma

In 1975, O'Brien described annular skin lesions which occurred in sun-damaged skin and were characterized histologically by disappearance of solar-elastotic fibres and, at the edge of the lesion, by a histiocytic and giant cell inflammatory reaction.[162] His concept of a granulomatous response to solar elastosis was challenged by some,[166] and supported by others.[167,168] Some felt that this lesion was granuloma annulare in sun-damaged skin.[166] Others proposed the term 'annular elastotic giant cell granuloma' because of the absence of solar elastosis in some of their cases.[165] Lesions have also been reported in covered areas of the body.[169] In support of O'Brien, similar changes have been described in association with solar elastosis in pinguecula of the bulbar conjunctiva.[170]

As initially described, actinic granuloma begins as single or grouped pink papules which evolve to annular lesions in sun-exposed regions of the neck, face, chest and arms. Both sexes are affected equally and most of the patients are 40 years of age or older. One case has been reported in association with relapsing polychondritis[171] and another with cutaneous amyloidosis.[172]

Histopathology

In annular lesions, the changes seen at the rim of the lesion differ from those in the centre (Fig. 7.18). The dermis in the region of the rim is

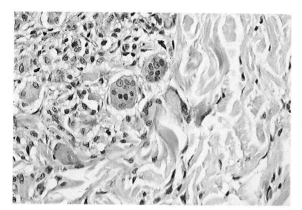

Fig. 7.19 Actinic granuloma. Multinucleate giant cells are engulfing elastotic fibres.
Haematoxylin — eosin

infiltrated by histiocytes and there are many foreign body giant cells. The latter are applied to, and engulf, elastotic fibres (elastoclasis) (Fig. 7.19). There is also a variable component of lymphocytes, plasma cells and eosinophils. Within the central zone, there is complete or almost complete loss of both elastotic fibres and normal elastic fibres. The dermal collagen in this region is relatively normal or slightly increased. Unlike granuloma annulare and necrobiosis lipoidica, necrobiosis is not usually seen. The absence of increased dermal mucin also distinguishes most cases from granuloma annulare. Asteroid bodies are sometimes present in giant cells. In some cases mononuclear histiocytes may be more prominent than multinucleate giant cells, and occasionally tuberculoid granulomas form.[173]

A similar granulomatous response can occur in relation to some basal cell carcinomas and keratoacanthomas.[168] Elastoclasis has also been described in granuloma annulare,[174] elastosis perforans serpiginosa and other lesions occurring in sun-damaged skin.[166] In these cases, elastoclasis may represent a secondary response to elastotic fibres which have been altered in some as yet unknown way by the primary process, whereas in actinic granuloma there is no obvious provoking cause. It has been suggested that there is a cell-mediated immune response to antigenic determinants on actinically altered elastotic fibres.[175] Elastophagocytosis may also be seen in sun-protected skin in association with a variety of inflammatory conditions.[176]

In a recent study comparing actinic granuloma and granuloma annulare, absence of elastotic material in the centre of the lesions and the presence of scarring and giant cells with up to 12 nuclei were characteristic of actinic granuloma. By comparison, granuloma annulare was characterized by moderate amounts of elastotic material within granulomas, scarring was absent and giant cells contained fewer nuclei.[177]

Immunohistochemical studies have shown the presence of lysozyme in giant cells and a predominance of helper T cells in the lymphocytic infiltrate.[175] One ultrastructural study has demonstrated both extracellular and intracellular digestion of elastotic fibres.[178]

Atypical necrobiosis lipoidica

A condition characterized by annular lesions of the upper face and scalp has been called 'atypical necrobiosis lipoidica'.[163] It occurs predominantly in females. The average age of onset is about 35 years. The lesions resolve spontaneously or persist for many years. Unlike necrobiosis lipoidica, they heal without scarring or alopecia. Some patients have necrobiosis lipoidica at other sites.

Lesions with similar clinical and histological features to those seen in atypical necrobiosis lipoidica have been described as Miescher's granuloma of the face.[164] It has been suggested that both conditions represent actinic granulomas although solar elastosis has not been a conspicuous feature in either.[162] The issue is further confused by reports of actinic granuloma with areas of necrobiosis.[173,179]

Histopathology

These lesions are characterized by a central healing zone, in which there is loss of elastic tissue, and a peripheral raised edge. In the latter region there is a lymphocytic and histiocytic dermal infiltrate which is distributed between collagen bundles. The infiltrate includes multinucleate giant cells, some of which contain asteroid bodies. Necrobiotic areas and increased dermal mucin have not been described.

Granuloma multiforme

This granulomatous dermatitis was originally recognized because of its potential importance in the differential diagnosis of tuberculoid leprosy, which it resembles clinically and, to some extent, histologically.[180,181] First reported in Nigeria, granuloma multiforme has also been reported in other central African countries and in Indonesia.[180] Papular and annular lesions occur on exposed regions of the trunk and arms. Both sexes are affected and most of the patients are aged 40 years or more. There was a marked female predominance in one series.[182] It has been suggested that this is a variant of granuloma annulare or necrobiosis lipoidica.[182] Others consider it to be related to actinic granuloma.[162]

Histopathology

The zonal histology described in actinic granuloma is also seen in this condition (see above). There is destruction of dermal elastic tissue, with mild fibrosis in the centre of annular lesions. In the raised active edge of the lesion there is a granulomatous reaction which includes histiocytes, multinucleate giant cells, lymphocytes, eosinophils and plasma cells. Elastoclasis (elastic fibre phagocytosis by histiocytes) is seen in this region. Areas of necrobiosis have been described, surrounded by a palisaded rim of histiocytes, in the middle and upper dermis in the annular rim.[182] Solar elastosis may occur in black-skinned people but it is not clear whether it is present in the lesions of granuloma multiforme in black patients.[183]

In one series of cases there was no evidence of fat within these lesions on special staining; mucin stains were inconclusive.[182]

GRANULOMATOUS T-CELL LYMPHOMA

Rare cases of mycosis fungoides have a granulomatous infiltrate in the dermis (see p. 1036). Granulomas are also present in granulomatous slack skin, a variant of T-cell lymphoma (see p. 1042). In both conditions phagocytosis of elastic fibres and lymphocytes may occur.

REFERENCES

Introduction

1. Hirsh BC, Johnson WC. Concepts of granulomatous inflammation. Int J Dermatol 1984; 23: 90–100.
2. Williams GT, Williams WJ. Granulomatous inflammation — a review. J Clin Pathol 1983; 36: 723–733.

Sarcoidal granulomas

3. Mitchell DN, Scadding JG, Heard BE, Hinson KFW. Sarcoidosis: histopathological definition and clinical diagnosis. J Clin Pathol 1977; 30: 395–408.
4. Kerdel FA, Moschella SL. Sarcoidosis. An updated review. J Am Acad Dermatol 1984; 11: 1–19.
5. Hanno R, Callen JP. Sarcoidosis. A disorder with prominent cutaneous features and their interrelationship with systemic disease. Med Clin North Am 1980; 64: 847–866.
6. Veien NK, Stahl D, Brodthagen H. Cutaneous sarcoidosis in Caucasians. J Am Acad Dermatol 1987; 16: 534–540.
7. O'Driscoll JB, Beck MH, Lendon M et al. Cutaneous presentation of sarcoidosis in an infant. Clin Exp Dermatol 1990; 15: 60–62.
8. Spiteri MA, Matthey F, Gordon T et al. Lupus pernio: a clinico-radiological study of thirty-five cases. Br J Dermatol 1985; 112: 315–322.
9. Vainsencher D, Winkelmann RK. Subcutaneous sarcoidosis. Arch Dermatol 1984; 120: 1028–1031.
10. Golitz LE, Shapiro L, Hurwitz E, Stritzler R. Cicatricial alopecia of sarcoidosis. Arch Dermatol 1973; 107: 758–760.
11. Kauh YC, Goody HE, Luscombe HA. Ichthyosiform sarcoidosis. Arch Dermatol 1978; 114: 100–101.
12. Neill SM, Smith NP, Eady RAJ. Ulcerative sarcoidosis: a rare manifestation of a common disease. Clin Exp Dermatol 1984; 9: 277–279.
13. Verdegem TD, Sharma OP. Cutaneous ulcers in sarcoidosis. Arch Dermatol 1987; 123: 1531–1534.
14. Herzlinger DC, Marland AM, Barr RJ. Verrucous ulcerative skin lesions in sarcoidosis. An unusual clinical presentation. Cutis 1979; 23: 569–572.
15. Greer KE, Harman LE, Kayne AL. Unusual cutaneous

manifestations of sarcoidosis. South Med J 1977; 70: 666–668.

16. Neville E, Mills RGS, Jash DK et al. Sarcoidosis of the upper respiratory tract and its association with lupus pernio. Thorax 1976; 31: 660–664.

17. Gold RS, Sager E. Oral sarcoidosis: review of the literature. J Oral Surg 1976; 34: 237–244.

18. James DG. Dermatological aspects of sarcoidosis. Q J Med 1959; 28: 109–124.

19. Burgdorf WHC, Hoxtell EO, Bart BJ. Sarcoid granulomas in venipuncture sites. Cutis 1979; 24: 52–53.

20. Weidman AI, Andrade R, Franks AG. Sarcoidosis. Report of a case of sarcoid lesions in a tattoo and subsequent discovery of pulmonary sarcoidosis. Arch Dermatol 1966; 94: 320–325.

21. Kuramoto Y, Shindo Y, Tagami H. Subcutaneous sarcoidosis with extensive caseation necrosis. J Cutan Pathol 1988; 15: 188–190.

22. Batres E, Klima M, Tschen J. Transepithelial elimination in cutaneous sarcoidosis. J Cutan Pathol 1982; 9: 50–54.

23. Jones Williams W. The nature and origin of Schaumann bodies. J Path Bact 1960; 79: 193–201.

24. Azar HA, Lunardelli C. Collagen nature of asteroid bodies of giant cells in sarcoidosis. Am J Pathol 1969; 57: 81–92.

25. Cain H, Kraus B. Immunofluorescence microscopic demonstration of vimentin filaments in asteroid bodies of sarcoidosis. Virchows Arch [B] 1983; 42: 213–226.

26. Pierard GE, Pierre S, Damseaux M et al. The histological structure of Kveim tests parallels the evolution of pulmonary sarcoidosis. Am J Dermatopathol 1982; 4: 17–23.

27. Modlin RL, Gottlieb B, Hofman FM et al. Demonstration in situ of subsets of T-lymphocytes in sarcoidosis. Am J Dermatopathol 1984; 6: 423–427.

28. Quismorio FP, Sharma OP, Chandor S. Immunopathological studies on the cutaneous lesions in sarcoidosis. Br J Dermatol 1977; 97: 635–642.

29. Schewach-Millet M, Ziv R, Trau H et al. Sarcoidosis versus foreign-body granulomas. Int J Dermatol 1987; 26: 582–583.

30. Shelley WB, Hurley HJ. The pathogenesis of silica granulomas in man: A non-allergic colloidal phenomenon. J Invest Dermatol 1960; 34: 107–123.

31. Goldstein AP. VII. Histologic reactions in tattoos. J Dermatol Surg Oncol 1979; 5: 896–900.

32. Dickinson JA. Sarcoidal reactions in tattoos. Arch Dermatol 1969; 100: 315–319.

33. Hanada K, Chiyoya S, Katabira Y. Systemic sarcoidal reaction in tattoo. Clin Exp Dermatol 1985; 10: 479–484.

34. Goldstein N. IV. Complications from tattoos. J Dermatol Surg Oncol 1979; 5: 869–878.

35. Shelley WB, Hurley HJ. Allergic origin of zirconium deodorant granuloma. Br J Dermatol 1958; 70: 75–101.

36. LoPresti PJ, Hambrick GW Jr. Zirconium granuloma following treatment of Rhus dermatitis. Arch Dermatol 1965; 92: 188–191.

37. Dutra FR. Beryllium granulomas of the skin. Arch Dermatol Syph 1949; 60: 1140–1147.

38. Helwig EB. Chemical (beryllium) granulomas of skin. Mil Surgeon 1951; 109: 540–558.

39. Pimentel JC. Sarcoid granulomas of the skin produced by acrylic and nylon fibres. Br J Dermatol 1977; 96: 673–677.

40. Pimentel JC. The "wheat–stubble sarcoid granuloma": a new epithelioid granuloma of the skin. Br J Dermatol 1972; 87: 444–449.

41. Kinmont PDC. Sea-urchin sarcoidal granuloma. Br J Dermatol 1965; 77: 335–343.

Tuberculoid granulomas

42. Hirsh BC, Johnson WC. Pathology of granulomatous diseases. Epithelioid granulomas, Part 1. Int J Dermatol 1984; 23: 237–246.

43. Shea C, Imber MJ, Cropley TG et al. Granulomatous eruption after BCG vaccine immunotherapy for malignant melanoma. J Am Acad Dermatol 1989; 21: 1119–1122.

44. Santa Cruz DJ, Strayer DS. The histologic spectrum of the cutaneous mycobacterioses. Hum Pathol 1982; 13: 485–495.

45. Ulbright TM, Katzenstein A-LA. Solitary necrotizing granulomas of the lung. Am J Surg Pathol 1980; 4: 13–28.

46. Smith NP, Ryan TJ, Sanderson KV, Sarkany I. Lichen scrofulosorum. A report of four cases. Br J Dermatol 1976; 94: 319–325.

47. Hudson PM. Tuberculide (lichen scrofulosorum) secondary to osseous tuberculosis. Clin Exp Dermatol 1976; 1: 391–394.

48. Wilson Jones E, Winkelmann RK. The histopathology of papulonecrotic tuberculid (PNT). J Cutan Pathol 1986; 13: 81 (abstract).

49. Ridley DS, Jopling WH. Classification of leprosy according to immunity. A five-group system. Int J Lep 1966; 34: 255–273.

50. Ridley DS. Histological classification and the immunological spectrum of leprosy. Bull WHO 1974; 51: 451–465.

51. Lantis LR, Petrozzi JW, Hurley HJ. Sarcoid granuloma in secondary syphilis. Arch Dermatol 1969; 99: 748–752.

52. Abell E, Marks R, Wilson Jones E. Secondary syphilis: a clinico-pathological review. Br J Dermatol 1975; 93: 53–61.

53. Hirsh BC, Johnson WC. Pathology of granulomatous diseases. Epithelioid granulomas, Part II. Int J Dermatol 1984; 23: 306–313.

54. Farah FS, Malak JA. Cutaneous leishmaniasis. Arch Dermatol 1971; 103: 467–474.

55. Hart M, Livingood CS, Goltz RW, Totonchy M. Late cutaneous leishmaniasis. Arch Dermatol 1969; 99: 455–458.

56. Marks R, Harcourt-Webster JN. Histopathology of rosacea. Arch Dermatol 1969; 100: 683–691.

57. Mullanax MG, Kierland RR. Granulomatous rosacea. Arch Dermatol 1970; 101: 206–211.

58. Marks R, Wilkinson DS. Rosacea and perioral dermatitis. In: Rook A, Wilkinson DS, Ebling FJG et al, eds. Textbook of Dermatology, 4th ed. Oxford: Blackwell Scientific Publications, 1986; 1605–1617.

59. Ackerman AB. Histologic diagnosis of inflammatory skin diseases. Philadelphia: Lea & Febiger 1978; 658.

60. Hjorth N, Osmundsen P, Rook AJ et al. Perioral

dermatitis. Br J Dermatol 1968; 80: 307–313.

61. Fisher AA. Periocular dermatitis akin to the perioral variety. J Am Acad Dermatol 1986; 15: 642–644.

62. Frieden IJ, Prose NS, Fletcher V, Turner ML. Granulomatous perioral dermatitis in children. Arch Dermatol 1989; 125: 369–373.

63. Sneddon I. Perioral dermatitis. Br J Dermatol 1972; 87: 430–434.

63a. Beacham BE, Kurgansky D, Gould WM. Circumoral dermatitis and cheilitis caused by tartar control dentifrices. J Am Acad Dermatol 1990; 22: 1029–1032.

64. Adams SJ, Davison AM, Cunliffe WJ, Giles GR. Perioral dermatitis in renal transplant recipients maintained on corticosteroids and immunosuppressive therapy. Br J Dermatol 1982; 106: 589–592.

65. Marks R, Black MM. Perioral dermatitis — a histopathological study of 26 cases. Br J Dermatol 1971; 84: 242–247.

66. Ackerman AB. Histologic diagnosis of inflammatory skin diseases. Philadelphia: Lea and Febiger 1978; 407.

67. Russell Jones R, Wilson Jones E. Disseminated acne agminata. Br J Dermatol (Suppl) 1981; 19: 76.

68. Kumano K, Tani M, Murata Y. Dapsone in the treatment of miliary lupus of the face. Br J Dermatol 1983; 109: 57–62.

69. Shitara A. Clinicopathological and immunological studies of lupus miliaris disseminatus faciei. J Dermatol 1982; 9: 383–395.

70. Mihara K, Isoda M. Immunohistochemical study of lysozyme in lupus miliaris disseminatus faciei. Br J Dermatol 1986; 115: 187–192.

71. Shitara A. Lupus miliaris disseminatus faciei. Int J Dermatol 1984; 23: 542–544.

Necrobiotic granulomas

72. Johnson WC. Necrobiotic granulomas. J Cutan Pathol 1984; 12: 289–299.

73. Muhlbauer JE. Granuloma annulare. J Am Acad Dermatol 1980; 3: 217–230.

74. Wells RS, Smith MA. The natural history of granuloma annulare. Br J Dermatol 1963; 75: 199–205.

75. Thomas DJB, Rademaker M, Munro DD et al. Visceral and skin granuloma annulare, diabetes, and polyendocrine disease. Br Med J 1986; 293: 977–978.

76. Owens DW, Freeman RG. Perforating granuloma annulare. Arch Dermatol 1971; 103: 64–67.

77. Salomon RJ, Gardepe SF, Woodley DT. Deep granuloma annulare in adults. Int J Dermatol 1986; 25: 109–112.

78. Rubin M, Lynch FW. Subcutaneous granuloma annulare. Comment on familial granuloma annulare. Arch Dermatol 1966; 93: 416–420.

79. Harpster EF, Mauro T, Barr RJ. Linear granuloma annulare. J Am Acad Dermatol 1989; 21: 1138–1141.

80. Dabski K, Winkelmann RK. Generalized granuloma annulare: Clinical and laboratory findings in 100 patients. J Am Acad Dermatol 1989; 20: 39–47.

81. Delaney TJ, Gold SC, Leppard B. Disseminated perforating granuloma annulare. Br J Dermatol 1973; 89: 523–526.

82. Draheim JH, Johnson LC, Helwig EB. A clinico-pathologic analysis of "rheumatoid" nodules occurring in 54 children. Am J Pathol 1959; 35: 678.

83. Burrington JD. "Pseudorheumatoid" nodules in children. Report of 10 cases. Pediatrics 1970; 45: 473–478.

84. Simons FER, Schaller JG. Benign rheumatoid nodules. Pediatrics 1975; 56: 29–33.

85. Berardinelli JL, Hyman CJ, Campbell EE, Fireman P. Presence of rheumatoid factor in ten children with isolated rheumatoid-like nodules. J Pediatr 1972; 81: 751–757.

86. Friedman SJ, Winkelmann RK. Familial granuloma annulare. Report of two cases and review of the literature. J Am Acad Dermatol 1987; 16: 600–605.

87. Friedman-Birnbaum R, Haim S, Gideone O, Barzilai A. Histocompatibility antigens in granuloma annulare. Comparative study of the generalized and localized types. Br J Dermatol 1978; 98: 425–428.

88. Friedman SJ, Fox BJ, Albert HL. Granuloma annulare arising in herpes zoster scars. Report of two cases and review of the literature. J Am Acad Dermatol 1986; 14: 764–770.

89. Beer WE, Wilson Jones E. Granuloma annulare following tuberculin Heaf tests. Trans St John's Hosp Dermatol Soc 1966; 52: 68.

90. Friedman-Birnbaum R. Generalized and localized granuloma annulare. Int J Dermatol 1986; 25: 364–366.

91. Muhlemann MF, Williams DRR. Localized granuloma annulare is associated with insulin-dependent diabetes mellitus. Br J Dermatol 1984; 111: 325–329.

92. Ghadially R, Sibbald RG, Walter JB, Haberman HF. Granuloma annulare in patients with human immunodeficiency virus infections. J Am Acad Dermatol 1989; 20: 232–235.

93. Smith NP. AIDS, Kaposi's sarcoma and the dermatologist. J R Soc Med 1985; 78: 97–99.

94. Penneys NS, Hicks B. Unusual cutaneous lesions associated with acquired immunodeficiency syndrome. J Am Acad Dermatol 1985; 13: 845–852.

95. Huerter CJ, Bass J, Bergfeld WF, Tubbs RR. Perforating granuloma annulare in a patient with acquired immunodeficiency syndrome. Arch Dermatol 1987; 123: 1217–1220.

96. Dahl MV, Ullman S, Goltz RW. Vasculitis in granuloma annulare: histopathology and direct immunofluorescence. Arch Dermatol 1977; 113: 463–467.

97. Modlin RL, Vaccaro SA, Gottlieb B et al. Granuloma annulare. Identification of cells in the cutaneous infiltrate by immunoperoxidase techniques. Arch Pathol Lab Med 1984; 108: 379–382.

98. Umbert P, Winkelmann RK. Histologic, ultrastructural and histochemical studies of granuloma annulare. Arch Dermatol 1977; 113: 1681–1686.

99. Friedman-Birnbaum R, Weltfriend S, Munichor M, Lichtig C. A comparative histopathologic study of generalized and localized granuloma annulare. Am J Dermatopathol 1989; 11: 144–148.

100. Silverman RA, Rabinowitz AD. Eosinophils in the cellular infiltrate of granuloma annulare. J Cutan Pathol 1985; 12: 13–17.

101. Friedman-Birnbaum R, Weltfriend S, Kerner H, Lichtig C. Elastic tissue changes in generalized granuloma annulare. Am J Dermatopathol 1989; 11: 429–433.

102. Dabski K, Winkelmann RK. Generalized granuloma annulare: Histopathology and immunopathology. Systematic review of 100 cases and comparison with localized granuloma annulare. J Am Acad Dermatol 1989; 20: 28–39.

103. Kossard S, Goellner JR, Su WPD. Subcutaneous necrobiotic granulomas of the scalp. J Am Acad Dermatol 1980; 3: 180–185.

104. Umbert P, Winkelmann RK. Granuloma annulare: direct immunofluorescence study. Br J Dermatol 1977; 97: 481–486.

105. Bardach HG. Granuloma annulare with transfollicular perforation. J Cutan Pathol 1977; 4: 99–104.

106. Padilla RS, Mukai K, Dahl MV et al. Differential staining pattern of lysozyme in palisading granulomas: An immunoperoxidase study. J Am Acad Dermatol 1983; 8: 634–638.

107. Friedman-Birnbaum R, Ludatscher RM. Comparative ultrastructural study of generalized and localized granuloma annulare. Am J Dermatopathol 1986; 8: 302–308.

108. Muller SA, Winkelmann RK. Necrobiosis lipoidica diabeticorum. A clinical and pathological investigation of 171 cases. Arch Dermatol 1966; 93: 272–281.

109. Muller SA, Winkelmann RK. Necrobiosis lipoidica diabeticorum. Histopathologic study of 98 cases. Arch Dermatol 1966; 94: 1–10.

110. Muller SA. Dermatologic disorders associated with diabetes mellitus. Mayo Clin Proc 1966; 41: 689–703.

111. Kossard S, Collins E, Wargon O, Downie D. Squamous carcinomas developing in bilateral lesions of necrobiosis lipoidica. Australas J Dermatol 1987; 28: 14–17.

112. Schwartz ME. Necrobiosis lipoidica and granuloma annulare. Simultaneous occurrence in a patient. Arch Dermatol 1982; 118: 192–193.

113. Monk BE, Du Vivier AWP. Necrobiosis lipoidica and sarcoidosis. Clin Exp Dermatol 1987; 12: 294–295.

114. Ackerman AB. Histologic diagnosis of inflammatory skin diseases. Philadelphia: Lea & Febiger 1978; 424.

115. Alegre VA, Winkelmann RK. A new histopathologic feature of necrobiosis lipoidica diabeticorum: lymphoid nodules. J Cutan Pathol 1988; 15: 75–77.

116. Parra CA. Transepithelial elimination in necrobiosis lipoidica. Br J Dermatol 1977; 96: 83–86.

117. Ullman S, Dahl MV. Necrobiosis lipoidica. An immunofluorescence study. Arch Dermatol 1977; 113: 1671–1673.

118. Oikarinen A, Mortenhumer M, Kallioinen M, Savolainen E-R. Necrobiosis lipoidica: ultrastructural and biochemical demonstration of a collagen defect. J Invest Dermatol 1987; 88: 227–232.

119. Boulton AJM, Cutfield RG, Abouganem D et al. Necrobiosis lipoidica diabeticorum: A clinicopathologic study. J Am Acad Dermatol 1988; 18: 530–537.

120. Rasker JJ, Kuipers FC. Are rheumatoid nodules caused by vasculitis? A study of 13 early cases. Ann Rheum Dis 1983; 42: 384–388.

121. Hahn BH, Yardley JH, Stevens MB. "Rheumatoid" nodules in systemic lupus erythematosus. Ann Intern Med 1970; 72: 49–58.

122. Smith ML, Jorizzo JL, Semble E et al. Rheumatoid papules: Lesions showing features of vasculitis and palisading granuloma. J Am Acad Dermatol 1989; 20: 348–352.

123. Patterson JW. Rheumatoid nodule and subcutaneous granuloma annulare. A comparative histologic study. Am J Dermatopathol 1988; 10: 1–8.

124. Patterson JW, Demos PT. Superficial ulcerating rheumatoid necrobiosis: a perforating rheumatoid nodule. Cutis 1985; 36: 323–328.

125. Aherne MJ, Bacon PA, Blake DR et al. Immunohistochemical findings in rheumatoid nodules. Virchows Arch [A] 1985; 407: 191–202.

126. Allen AC. The skin. St. Louis: The C.V. Mosby Company 1954; 146.

127. Bennett GA, Zeller JW, Bauer W. Subcutaneous nodules of rheumatoid arthritis and rheumatic fever. Arch Pathol 1940; 30: 70–89.

128. Barr RJ, King DF, McDonald RM, Bartlow GA. Necrobiotic granulomas associated with bovine collagen test site injections. J Am Acad Dermatol 1982; 6: 867–869.

129. Graham JH. Superficial fungus infections. In: Graham JH, Johnson WC, Helwig EB. Dermal pathology. Hagerstown, Maryland: Harper & Row, 1972; 176.

130. Fawcett HA, Smith NP. Injection-site granuloma due to aluminum. Arch Dermatol 1984; 120: 1318–1322.

131. Rosen VJ. Cutaneous manifestations of drug abuse by parenteral injections. Am J Dermatopathol 1985; 7: 79–83.

Suppurative granulomas

132. Leslie DF, Beardmore GL. Chromoblastomycosis in Queensland: a retrospective study of 13 cases at the Royal Brisbane Hospital. Australas J Dermatol 1979; 20: 23–30.

133. Bullpitt P, Weedon D. Sporotrichosis: a review of 39 cases. Pathology 1978; 10: 249–256.

134. Philpott JA, Woodburne AR, Philpott OS et al. Swimming pool granuloma. A study of 290 cases. Arch Dermatol 1963; 88: 158–162.

135. Hirsh BC, Johnson WC. Pathology of granulomatous diseases. Mixed inflammatory granulomas. Int J Dermatol 1984; 23: 585–597.

136. Reyes-Flores O. Granulomas induced by living agents. Int J Dermatol 1986; 25: 158–165.

137. Wilson-Jones E, Winkelmann RK. Superficial granulomatous pyoderma: A localized vegetative form of pyoderma gangrenosum. J Am Acad Dermatol 1988; 18: 511–521.

Foreign body granulomas

138. Leonard DD. Starch granulomas. Arch Dermatol 1973; 107: 101–103.

139. Tye MJ, Hashimoto K, Fox F. Talc granulomas of the skin. JAMA 1966; 198: 1370–1372.

140. Snyder RA, Schwartz RA. Cactus bristle implantation. Report of an unusual case initially seen with rows of yellow hairs. Arch Dermatol 1983; 119: 152–154.

141. Allen AC. Persistent "insect bites" (dermal eosinophilic granulomas) simulating lymphoblastomas, histiocytoses, and squamous cell carcinomas. Am J Pathol 1948; 24: 367–375.

142. Jordaan HF, Sandler M. Zinc-induced granuloma — a

unique complication of insulin therapy. Clin Exp Dermatol 1989; 14: 227–229.

143. Posner DI, Guill MA III. Cutaneous foreign body granulomas associated with intravenous drug abuse. J Am Acad Dermatol 1985; 13: 869–872.

144. Postlethwait RW, Willigan DA, Ulin AW. Human tissue reaction to sutures. Ann Surg 1975; 181: 144–150.

145. Sina B, Lutz LL. Cutaneous oxalate granuloma. J Am Acad Dermatol 1990; 22: 316–318.

146. Altchek DD, Pearlstein HH. Granulomatous reaction to autologous hairs incarcerated during hair transplantation. J Dermatol Surg Oncol 1978; 4: 928–929.

147. Joseph HL, Gifford H. Barber's interdigital pilonidal sinus. Arch Dermatol 1954; 70: 616–624.

Miscellaneous granulomas

148. Wiesenfeld D, Ferguson MM, Mitchell DN et al. Oro-facial granulomatosis — a clinical and pathological analysis. Q J Med 1985; 54: 101–113.

149. Greene RM, Rogers RS III. Melkersson–Rosenthal syndrome: A review of 36 patients. J Am Acad Dermatol 1989; 21: 1263–1270.

150. Meisel–Stosiek M, Hornstein OP, Stosiek N. Family study on Melkersson–Rosenthal syndrome. Acta Derm Venereol 1990; 70: 221–226.

151. Levenson MJ, Ingerman M, Grimes C, Anand KV. Melkersson–Rosenthal syndrome. Arch Otolaryngol 1984; 110: 540–542.

152. Vistnes LM, Kernahan DA. The Melkersson–Rosenthal syndrome. Plast Reconstr Surg 1971; 48: 126–132.

153. Lindelof B, Eklund A, Liden S. Kveim test reactivity in Melkersson–Rosenthal syndrome (cheilitis granulomatosa). Acta Derm Venereol 1985; 65: 443–445.

154. Shehade SA, Foulds IS. Granulomatous cheilitis and a positive Kveim test. Br J Dermatol 1986; 115: 619–622.

155. Israel HL, Goldstein RA. Relation of Kveim-antigen reaction to lymphadenopathy. Study of sarcoidosis and other diseases. N Engl J Med 1971; 284: 345–349.

156. Nelson HM, Stevenson AG. Melkerssohn–Rosenthal syndrome with positive Kveim test. Clin Exp Dermatol 1988; 13: 49–50.

157. Diestelmeier MR, Sausker WF, Pierson DL, Rodman OG. Sarcoidosis manifesting as eyelid swelling. Arch Dermatol 1982; 118: 356–357.

158. Carr D. Granulomatous cheilitis in Crohn's disease. Br Med J 1974; 4: 636.

159. Rhodes EL, Stirling GA. Granulomatous cheilitis. Arch Dermatol 1965; 92: 40–44.

160. Krutchkoff D, James R. Cheilitis granulomatosa. Successful treatment with combined local triamcinolone injections and surgery. Arch Dermatol 1978; 114: 1203–1206.

161. Westermark P, Henriksson T-G. Granulomatous inflammation of the vulva and penis, a genital counterpart to cheilitis granulomatosa. Dermatologica 1979; 158: 269–274.

162. O'Brien JP. Actinic granuloma. An annular connective tissue disorder affecting sun- and heat-damaged

(elastotic) skin. Arch Dermatol 1975; 111: 460–466.

163. Wilson Jones E. Necrobiosis lipoidica presenting on the face and scalp. An account of 29 patients and a detailed consideration of recent histochemical findings. Trans St. John's Hosp Dermatol Soc 1971; 57: 202–220.

164. Mehregan AH, Altman J. Miescher's granuloma of the face. A variant of the necrobiosis lipoidica-granuloma annulare spectrum. Arch Dermatol 1973; 107: 62–64.

165. Hanke CW, Bailin PL, Roenigk HH. Annular elastolytic giant cell granuloma. A clinicopathologic study of five cases and a review of similar entities. J Am Acad Dermatol 1979; 1: 413–421.

166. Ragaz A, Ackerman AB. Is actinic granuloma a specific condition? Am J Dermatopathol 1979; 1: 43–50.

167. Wilson Jones E. Actinic granuloma. Am J Dermatopathol 1980; 2: 89–90.

168. Weedon D. Actinic granuloma: the controversy continues. Am J Dermatopathol 1980; 2: 90–91.

169. Ishibashi A, Yokoyama A, Hirano K. Annular elastolytic giant cell granuloma occurring in covered areas. Dermatologica 1987; 174: 293–297.

170. Proia AD, Browning DJ, Klintworth GK. Actinic granuloma of the conjunctiva. Am J Ophthalmol 1983; 96: 116–118.

171. Pierard GE, Henrijean A, Foidart JM, Lapiere CM. Actinic granulomas and relapsing polychondritis. Acta Derm Venereol 1982; 62: 531–533.

172. Lee Y-S, Vijayasingam S, Chan H-L. Photosensitive annular elastolytic giant cell granuloma with cutaneous amyloidosis. Am J Dermatopathol 1989; 11: 443–450.

173. O'Brien JP. Actinic granuloma: the expanding significance. Int J Dermatol 1985; 24: 473–490.

174. Burket JM, Zelickson AS. Intracellular elastin in generalized granuloma annulare. J Am Acad Dermatol 1986; 14: 975–981.

175. McGrae JD Jr. Actinic granuloma. A clinical, histopathologic, and immunocytochemical study. Arch Dermatol 1986; 122: 43–47.

176. Barnhill RL, Goldenhersh MA. Elastophagocytosis: a non-specific reaction pattern associated with inflammatory processes in sun-protected skin. J Cutan Pathol 1989; 16: 199–202.

177. Steffen C. Actinic granuloma (O'Brien). J Cutan Pathol 1988; 15: 66–74.

178. Yanagihara M, Kato F, Mori S. Extra- and intra-cellular digestion of elastic fibers by macrophages in annular elastolytic giant cell granuloma. J Cutan Pathol 1987; 14: 303–308.

179. Prendiville J, Griffiths WAD, Russell Jones R. O'Brien's actinic granuloma. Br J Dermatol 1985; 113: 353–358.

180. Meyers WM, Connor DH. In: Binford CH, Connor DH, eds. Pathology of tropical and extraordinary diseases, Volume 2. Washington, D.C.: Armed Forces Institute of Pathology, 1976; 676.

181. Leiker DL, Koh SH, Spaas JAJ. Granuloma multiforme. A new skin disease resembling leprosy. Int J Lepr 1964; 32: 368–376.

182. Allenby CF, Wilson Jones E. Granuloma multiforme. Trans St. John's Hosp Dermatol Soc 1969; 55: 88–98.

183. Kligman AM. Early destructive effect of sunlight on human skin. JAMA 1969; 210: 2377–2380.

The vasculopathic reaction pattern

INTRODUCTION

Diseases of cutaneous blood vessels are an important cause of morbidity. In the case of the vasculitides, mortality may occasionally result. Because blood vessels have a limited number of ways in which they can react to insults of various kinds, considerable morphological overlap exists between the various clinical syndromes that have been described.

The broad classifications used in this chapter are morphologically rather than aetiologically based, as this is the most practical scheme to follow when confronted with a biopsy.

Excluding tumours and telangiectases, which are discussed in Chapter 38, there are five major groups of vascular diseases:

Non-inflammatory purpuras
Vascular occlusive diseases
Urticarias
Vasculitis
Neutrophilic dermatoses.

The *non-inflammatory purpuras* are characterized by the extravasation of erythrocytes into the dermis. There is no inflammation or occlusion of blood vessels.

The *vascular occlusive diseases* exhibit narrowing or obliteration of the lumina of small vessels by fibrin or platelet thrombi, cryoglobulins, cholesterol or other material. Purpura is sometimes a clinical symptom of this group.

The *urticarias* involve the leakage of plasma and some cells from dermal vessels. Some of the urticarias have overlapping features with the vasculitides, further justification for their inclusion in this chapter.

In *vasculitis* there is inflammation of the walls of blood vessels. In subsiding lesions there may only be an inflammatory infiltrate in close contact with vessel walls. The vasculitides are subclassified on the basis of the inflammatory process into acute, chronic lymphocytic and granulomatous forms. Fibrin-platelet thrombi may sometimes form, particularly in acute vasculitis, leading to some overlap with the vascular occlusive diseases.

The *neutrophilic dermatoses* are a recently delineated group of conditions in which there is a prominent dermal infiltrate of neutrophils, but usually without the fibrinoid necrosis of vessel walls that typifies acute allergic (leucocytoclastic) vasculitis. The term 'pustular vasculitis' has been used for some entities in this group. There is increasing evidence that many of these conditions exhibit significant vascular damage, including fibrin extravasation at some stage in their evolution. Their distinctive morphological features justify their separate consideration, despite their close relationship to acute vasculitis.

NON-INFLAMMATORY PURPURAS

Purpura is haemorrhage into the skin. Clinically this may take the form of small lesions less than 3 mm in diameter (petechiae), or larger areas known as ecchymoses. There is a predilection for the limbs. The numerous causes of purpura may be broadly grouped into defects of blood vessels, platelets or coagulation factors. These aspects are considered in Volume 2.

At the histopathological level, purpuras are characterized by an extravasation of red blood cells into the dermis from small cutaneous vessels. If the purpura is chronic or recurrent, haemosiderin or haematoidin pigment may be present.[1,2] Purpuras have traditionally been divided into an inflammatory group (vasculitis), and a non-inflammatory group when there is no inflammation of vessel walls.

The non-inflammatory purpuras include idiopathic thrombocytopenic purpura, senile purpura, the autoerythrocyte sensitization syndrome (psychogenic purpura), traumatic purpura and drug purpuras.[1,3,4] Only senile purpura will be considered in further detail in this volume.

SENILE PURPURA

This common form of non-inflammatory purpura occurs on the extensor surfaces of the forearms and hands of elderly individuals.[5–8] Usually large ecchymoses are present. It has been suggested that the bleeding results from minor shearing injuries to poorly supported cutaneous vessels. Senile purpura tends to persist longer than other forms of purpura, indicating slower removal or breakdown of the erythrocytes. Furthermore, senile purpura does not usually show the colour changes of bruising, as seen in purpura of other causes.

Histopathology

Senile purpura is characterized by extravasation of red blood cells into the dermis. This is most marked in the upper dermis and in a perivascular location. There is also marked solar elastosis and often some thinning of the dermis with atrophy of collagen bundles.[5,6]

VASCULAR OCCLUSIVE DISEASES

Occlusion of cutaneous blood vessels is quite uncommon. The clinical picture that results is varied. It may include purpura, livedo reticularis,[9–11] ulceration or infarction. Cutaneous infarction only occurs when numerous vessels in the lower dermis and subcutis are occluded.

Complete or partial occlusion of cutaneous vessels usually results from the lodgement of fibrin-platelet thrombi. Other causes include platelet-rich thrombi in thrombocythaemia and thrombotic thrombocytopenic purpura, cryoglobulins in cryoglobulinaemia, cholesterol in atheromatous emboli, swollen endothelial cells containing numerous acid-fast bacilli in Lucio's phenomenon of leprosy, fungi in mucormycosis,[12] and fibrous tissue producing intimal thickening in endarteritis obliterans.[13]

Excluding vasculitis, which is considered later, vascular occlusion may be seen in the following circumstances:

Warfarin necrosis
Atrophie blanche
Disseminated intravascular coagulation
Purpura fulminans
Thrombotic thrombocytopenic purpura
Cryoglobulinaemia
Cholesterol embolism
Miscellaneous conditions.

WARFARIN NECROSIS

Cutaneous infarction is a rare, unpredictable complication of anticoagulant therapy with the coumarin derivative warfarin sodium. It has a predilection for fatty areas such as the thighs, buttocks and breasts of obese, middle-aged women.[14,15] Lesions usually develop several days after the commencement of therapy. There are well defined, ecchymotic changes that rapidly progress to blistering and necrosis.[16] Purpuric[17] and linear lesions[18] have been reported.

Warfarin necrosis is related to low levels of protein C, a vitamin-K-dependent plasma protein with potent anticoagulant properties.[19] This deficiency in protein C may be induced by the anticoagulant therapy,[20] or be pre-existing in those who are heterozygous for protein C deficiency.[21] Homozygotes with absent protein C present with neonatal purpura fulminans (see below). Rarely, widespread disseminated intravascular coagulation is associated with warfarin therapy.[22]

Histopathology

Fibrin-platelet thrombi are present in venules and arterioles in the deep dermis and subcutis. There is variable haemorrhage, and subsequently the development of infarction. Large areas of the skin may be involved.[23]

ATROPHIE BLANCHE

Although previously considered to be due to a vasculitis, atrophie blanche (white atrophy) is best regarded as a manifestation of a vasculopathy in which occlusion of small dermal vessels by fibrin thrombi is the primary event.[24] It appears to result from decreased fibrinolytic activity of the blood with defective release of tissue plasminogen activator from vessel walls.[25] The platelets usually show an increased tendency to aggregate.[26] Several cases with a lupus-type anticoagulant and an increased level of anticardiolipin antibodies have been reported.[27] This abnormality can alter fibrinolytic activity.

Atrophie blanche (synonyms — livedo vasculitis, segmental hyalinizing vasculitis) is characterized by the development of telangiectatic, purpuric papules and plaques leading to the formation of small crusted ulcers, which heal after many months to leave white atrophic stellate scars.[28–31] The ulcers are painful and recurrent. Sometimes they are large and slow to heal. The lower parts of the legs, especially the ankles and the dorsum of the feet, are usually involved, although rarely the extensor surfaces of the arms below the elbows can be affected.[28] Many patients also have livedo reticularis, while some may have systemic diseases such as scleroderma, systemic lupus erythematosus and cryoglobulinaemia.[28,32,33] The disorder has a predilection for middle-aged females, but all ages may be affected.[31]

Histopathology[30,34,35]

The changes will depend on the age of the lesion which is biopsied. The primary event is the formation of hyaline thrombi in the lumen of

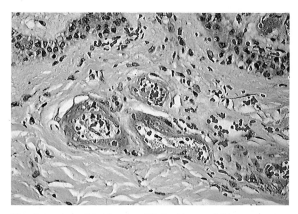

Fig. 8.1 Atrophie blanche. Fibrinoid material is present in the walls of small blood vessels in the upper dermis. Haematoxylin — eosin

small vessels in the upper and mid dermis.[32] Rarely deeper vessels are involved.[31] Fibrinoid material is also present in the walls of these blood vessels and in perivascular stroma (Fig. 8.1). This material is PAS positive and diastase resistant. There is usually infarction of the superficial dermis, often with a small area of ulceration. Sometimes a thin parakeratotic layer is present overlying infarcted or atrophic epidermis. The epidermis adjacent to the ulceration may be spongiotic. A sparse perivascular lymphocytic infiltrate may be present, but there is no vasculitis. Neutrophils, if present, are usually sparse and confined to the infarcted upper dermis and ulcer base. There are often extravasated red cells in the upper dermis. Small blood vessels are often increased in the adjacent papillary dermis, but this is a common feature in biopsies from the lower parts of the legs, and is therefore of no diagnostic value.

In older lesions there is thickening and hyalinization of vessels in the dermis with some endothelial cell oedema and proliferation. Fibrinoid material may also be present in vessel walls. It should be pointed out that fibrinoid material is almost invariably present in blood vessels in the base of ulcers, of many different causes, on the lower legs. In atrophie blanche the involved vessels are not only in the base of any ulcer, but also may be found at a distance beyond this.

In even later lesions, there is dermal sclerosis

and scarring with some dilated lymphatics, and epidermal atrophy. There may be a small amount of haemosiderin in the upper dermis. As these areas may become involved again, it is possible to find dermal sclerosis in some early lesions.

Immunofluorescence will demonstrate fibrin in vessel walls in early lesions, while in later stages there are also immunoglobulins and complement components in broad bands about vessel walls.[24,36]

Electron microscopy. This has confirmed the presence of luminal fibrin deposition with subsequent endothelial damage.[24]

DISSEMINATED INTRAVASCULAR COAGULATION

Disseminated intravascular coagulation (DIC) is an acquired disorder in which activation of the coagulation system leads to the formation of thrombi in the microcirculation of many tissues and organs.[37] As a consequence of the consumption of platelets and of fibrin and other factors during the coagulation process, haemorrhagic manifestations also occur. DIC may complicate infections, various neoplasms, certain obstetrical incidents, massive tissue injury such as burns, and miscellaneous conditions such as liver disease, snake bite and vasculitis.[37,38]

Cutaneous changes are present in approximately 70% of cases, and these may be the initial manifestations of DIC.[39–41] Petechiae, ecchymoses, haemorrhagic bullae, purpura fulminans, bleeding from wounds, acral cyanosis and frank gangrene have all been recorded.[39,41]

The formation of thrombi appears to be a consequence of the release of thromboplastins into the circulation and/or widespread injury to endothelial cells. Decreased levels of protein C have been reported; the level returns to normal with clinical recovery.[42]

Histopathology[38,40,41]

In early lesions, fibrin thrombi are present in capillaries and venules of the papillary dermis, and occasionally in vessels in the reticular dermis

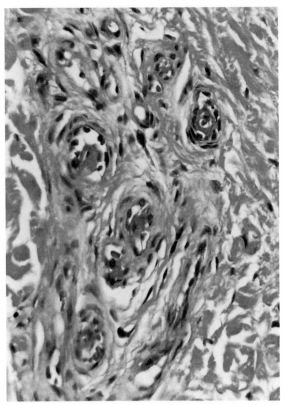

Fig. 8.2 Disseminated intravascular coagulation. Small vessels in the upper dermis contain fibrin-platelet thrombi. Haematoxylin — eosin

and subcutis (Fig. 8.2). Haemorrhage is also present, but there is no vasculitis or inflammation.

In older lesions, of 2–3 days' duration, there may be epidermal necrosis, subepidermal bullae, extensive haemorrhage and patchy necrosis of eccrine glands, the pilosebaceous apparatus and the papillary dermis. Nearby blood vessels are thrombosed but there is only mild inflammation in the dermis. In chronic states, some vascular proliferation and ectasia may occur.

PURPURA FULMINANS

Purpura fulminans is a rare clinical manifestation of disseminated intravascular coagulation (DIC) in which there are large cutaneous ecchymoses and haemorrhagic necrosis of the skin resulting from thrombosis of the cutaneous micro-vasculature.[21,43] Hypotension and fever are also present, but visceral manifestations are uncommon.[44] Only a few cases have been reported in adults,[44,45] the majority arising in infancy and early childhood some days after an infectious illness,[45a] usually of streptococcal, meningococcal,[46] pneumococcal[47] or viral[48] aetiology. Rarely purpura fulminans occurs in the neonatal period associated with severe congenital deficiency of protein C.[21,49–51]

The cutaneous lesions can commence as erythematous macules which rapidly enlarge and develop central purpura. The central zone becomes necrotic and the eventual removal of the resulting eschar leads to an area of ulceration.[21] There is a predilection for the lower extremities and the lateral aspect of the buttocks and thighs. Peripheral gangrene may sometimes develop. The use of fresh frozen plasma has improved considerably the prognosis of this disease.

The rare neonatal cases have been associated with homozygous protein C deficiency.[21] Recent studies suggest that an acquired deficiency of this protein, probably related to the primary infectious process, may be responsible for purpura fulminans in later life.[46] It is not known why only certain patients with DIC develop the full picture of purpura fulminans.[21]

Histopathology[21,44]

Fibrin thrombi fill most of the venules and capillaries in the skin. There is a mild perivascular infiltrate in some areas, but no vasculitis. Extensive haemorrhage is present with the subsequent development of epidermal necrosis. Occasionally a subepidermal bulla develops.

THROMBOTIC THROMBOCYTOPENIC PURPURA

This rare syndrome is characterized by the clinical picture of microangiopathic haemolytic anaemia, thrombocytopenia, neurological symptoms, renal disease and fever.[52,53] Cutaneous haemorrhages in the form of petechiae and ecchymoses are quite common.[52] Prior to the introduction of plasmapheresis and antiplatelet agents, the disease was almost invariably fatal.[54]

It appears to result from prostacyclin inhibition and impaired fibrinolysis. While drugs, infectious agents and obstetrical incidents have been implicated in triggering this syndrome, in the majority of individuals there is no apparent causal event or underlying disease process.[52,55] Coagulation studies fail to show evidence of disseminated intravascular coagulation.

Histopathology

Platelet-rich thrombi admixed with a small amount of fibrin deposit in vessels at the level of the arteriolocapillary junction.[52] There may be slight dilatation of vessels proximal to the thrombi. The material is PAS-positive. There is no evidence of any associated vasculitis. Extravasation of red blood cells also occurs. In severe cases, necrosis of the epidermis may ensue.

CRYOGLOBULINAEMIA

Cryoglobulins are immunoglobulins that reversibly precipitate from the serum or plasma on cooling.[56,57] There are two distinct types of cryoglobulinaemia, monoclonal and mixed, which reflect the composition of the cryoglobulins involved. In the monoclonal type intravascular deposits of cryoglobulins can be seen in biopsy specimens, while the mixed variant is a vasculitis. They are considered together for convenience.

Monoclonal cryoglobulinaemia. This variant, which accounts for approximately 25% of cases of cryoglobulinaemia, is associated with the presence of IgG or IgM cryoglobulin, or rarely of a cryoprecipitable light chain.[56] Monoclonal cryoglobulins, also known as type 1 cryoglobulins, are usually seen in association with multiple myeloma, Waldenström's macroglobulinaemia, and chronic lymphatic leukaemia.[56] Sometimes, no underlying disease is present (essential cryoglobulinaemia). The condition may be asymptomatic or result in pur-

pura, acral cyanosis or focal ulceration, which is usually limited to the lower extremities.[58,59]

Mixed cryoglobulinaemia. In this variant, the cryoglobulins are composed either of a monoclonal immunoglobulin which possesses antibody activity towards, and is attached to, polyclonal IgG (type 2), or of two or more polyclonal immunoglobulins (type 3).[60] Mixed cryoglobulins usually take the form of immune complexes and interreact with complement. They are seen in autoimmune diseases such as rheumatoid arthritis, systemic lupus erythematosus and Sjögren's syndrome, as well as in various chronic infections resulting from the hepatitis and Epstein–Barr viruses.[60,61] In approximately 50% of cases, there is no detectable autoimmune, lymphoproliferative or active infective disease present.[62] These cases of *essential mixed cryoglobulinaemia* are characterized by a chronic course with intermittent palpable purpura, polyarthralgia, Raynaud's phenomenon, and occasionally glomerulonephritis.[61,63] Other cutaneous manifestations that may be present include ulcers, urticaria, digital necrosis and, rarely, pustular purpura.[64,65] A history of preceding hepatitis B infection is sometimes obtained in essential mixed cryoglobulinaemia.[61,62]

Histopathology

Monoclonal cryoglobulinaemia. Purpuric lesions will show extravasation of red blood cells into the dermis. Small vessels in the upper dermis may be filled with homogeneous, eosinophilic material which is also PAS positive.[58,66,67] These intravascular deposits are seen more commonly beneath areas of ulceration.[58] Although there is no vasculitis, there may be a perivascular infiltrate of predominantly mononuclear cells.[66]

Mixed cryoglobulinaemia. The histological features are those of an acute vasculitis.[68] There may be some variation from case to case in the extent of the infiltrate and the degree of leucocytoclasis, probably reflecting the stage of the lesion.[62] There are usually some extravasated red blood cells, and in cases of long standing haemosiderin may be present. Intravascular hyaline deposits are the exception, but they may be found beneath areas of ulceration.[60,64] Immunoglobulins and complement are often found in vessel walls by immunofluorescence.[62]

Electron microscopy. The ultrastructural features depend on the involved immunoglobulins, and on their respective quantities. There may be tubular microcrystals, filaments, or cylindrical and annular bodies.[64,69]

CUTANEOUS CHOLESTEROL EMBOLISM

Cutaneous involvement occurs in 35% of patients with cholesterol crystal embolization.[70] The source of the emboli is atheromatous plaques in major blood vessels, particularly the abdominal aorta. This material may dislodge spontaneously, or following vascular procedures or anticoagulant therapy.[70] There is a high mortality. Cutaneous lesions are found particularly on the lower limbs, and include livedo reticularis, gangrene, ulceration, cyanosis, purpura and cutaneous nodules.[70–72] Rare manifestations have included a haemorrhagic panniculitis on the chest[73] and an eschar on the ear.[74]

Histopathology[70,71]

Multiple sections are sometimes required to find the diagnostic acicular clefts indicating the site of cholesterol crystals in arterioles and small arteries in the lower dermis or subcutis. A fibrin thrombus often surrounds the cholesterol material. Foreign body giant cells and a few inflammatory cells may also be present. Cutaneous infarction and associated inflammatory changes sometimes develop.

MISCELLANEOUS CONDITIONS CAUSING VASCULAR OCCLUSION

Rare causes of cutaneous microthrombi include the hypereosinophilic syndrome,[75,76] the presence of the lupus anticoagulant (cardiolipin antibodies),[77–81] Sneddon's syndrome (livedo reticularis and cerebrovascular thromboses in early adulthood),[82–87] renal failure with hyperparathyroidism,[88] thrombocythaemia, protein C deficiency,[89,90] heparin therapy,[91] the intravascular injection of large amounts of cocaine,[92] ulcerative colitis[93] and embolic processes, including bacterial endocarditis. The eschar found in some rickettsial infections is a cutaneous infarct with fibrin-platelet thrombi in marginal vessels (see p. 621). A lymphocytic vasculitis is usually present as well.

Vascular occlusion, either partial or complete, may occur in endarteritis obliterans as a result of fibrous thickening of the intima. It may be seen in a range of clinicopathological settings which include peripheral atherosclerosis, Raynaud's phenomenon, scleroderma, diabetes, hypertension and healed vasculitis.[13]

URTICARIAS

Urticaria is a cutaneous reaction pattern characterized clinically by transient, often pruritic, oedematous, erythematous papules or wheals which may show central clearing.[94,95] Angio-oedema is a related process in which the oedema involves the subcutaneous tissues and/or mucous membranes. It may coexist with urticaria.[96]

Urticaria is a common affliction, affecting 15% or more of the population on at least one occasion in their life. Most cases are transient (acute) and the aetiology is usually detected.[97] On the other hand, chronic urticaria, which is arbitrarily defined as urticaria persisting for longer than six weeks, is idiopathic in approximately 75% of cases.[95] It tends to involve middle-aged people, in contrast to acute urticaria which occurs more commonly in children and young adults. Chronic urticaria may be aggravated by aspirin, food additives and the like.[98] This has led to the suggestion that chronic urticaria results from an occult allergy to some everyday substance.

Papular urticaria is a clinical variant of urticaria in which the lesions are more persistent than the usual urticarial wheal.[99] It may result from a hypersensitivity reaction to the bites of arthropods such as fleas, lice, mites and bed bugs.[99-101] Rare clinical variants of urticaria include bullous and purpuric forms,[97] urticaria with anaphylaxis[97] and recurrent urticaria with fever and eosinophilia.[102]

Most of the literature on urticaria refers to the chronic form of the disease because this is often an important clinical problem. The remainder of this discussion will refer to chronic urticaria.

CHRONIC URTICARIA

Chronic urticaria is urticaria persisting longer than six weeks. There are many variants of chronic urticaria, although they share in common the presence of erythematous papules or wheals. These variants are usually classified aetiopathogenetically, as follows:[103]

Physical urticarias
Cholinergic urticaria
Angio-oedema
Urticarias due to histamine-releasing agents
IgE-mediated urticarias
Immune-complex-mediated urticarias
Idiopathic urticarias.

Some overlap exists between these various categories. For example, drugs and foodstuffs may produce chronic urticaria through more than one of the above mechanisms.

Variants of urticaria

Physical urticarias.   Physical stimuli such as heat, cold, pressure, light, water and vibration are the most commonly identified causes of chronic urticaria, accounting for approximately 15% of all cases.[104-106] The wheals are usually of short duration and limited to the area of the physical stimulus.[104] Accordingly, the physical urticarias tend to occur on exposed areas. Angio-oedema may coexist.[107] More than one of the physical agents listed above may induce urticaria in some individuals.[105] Some of the physical urticarias can be transferred passively.[107-109] *Cold urticaria,* which is produced at sites of localized cooling of the skin, is usually acquired,

although a rare familial form has been reported.[110,111] It may follow a viral illness[112] or the use of drugs such as penicillin and griseofulvin, although in most cases no underlying cause is found.[113] *Heat urticaria,* by contrast, is exceedingly rare.[114] *Solar urticaria* is another rare physical urticaria which results from exposure to sun and light.[115-118] It has a faster onset and shorter duration than polymorphous light eruption (see p. 581).[119] *Aquagenic urticaria* follows contact with water.[120] Much more common is aquagenic pruritus in which prickly discomfort occurs in the absence of any cutaneous lesion.[121-124] It appears to be an entity distinct from aquagenic urticaria and may follow increased degranulation of a normal number of mast cells.[125] In *pressure urticaria,* deep wheals develop after a delay of several hours following the application of pressure.[126-130] Systemic symptoms, which include an influenza-like illness, may also develop.[131] *Vibratory urticaria* is a related disorder resulting from vibratory stimuli.[105] *Dermographism,* which is the production of a linear wheal in response to a scratch, is an accentuation of the physiological whealing of the Lewis triple response.[132,133] Minor forms are quite common, but only a small percentage of affected persons are symptomatic with pruritus. A delayed form, which is an entity similar to delayed pressure urticaria, also occurs.[129,134]

The physical urticaria which is least well understood is *contact urticaria.*[135-137b] In this variant a wheal and flare response is usually elicited 30-60 minutes after skin contact with various chemicals in medicaments, cosmetics, foods and industrial agents.[135] Distinction from an irritant contact dermatitis may sometimes be difficult (see p. 101).[138] An IgE-mediated form and a non-immunological form have been delineated.[136,138] Contact urticaria may be superimposed on an 'eczematous dermatitis' of different types.[135]

Cholinergic urticaria.   This form of chronic urticaria is produced by exercise, heat and emotion, with general overheating of the body as the final common pathway.[106,139,140] Accordingly, it is sometimes included with the physical urticarias, with which it may coexist.[141,142] Lesions are distinctive and consist of 2–3 mm wheals surrounded by large erythematous flares.[106] There is a predilection for blush areas. Increased sympathetic activity may result in the release of acetylcholine at nerve endings causing mast cells to degranulate.[143]

Angio-oedema.[144]   There is a special form of angio-oedema (hereditary angio-oedema) which may be associated with swelling of the face and limbs or involve the larynx with potentially life-threatening consequences.[145] It results from an absolute or functional deficiency of C1 esterase inhibitor.[146] Non-familial angio-oedema may occur in association with various urticarias.[107]

Urticaria due to histamine-releasing agents.   Histamine may be released by mast cells in response to certain drugs, such as opiates, and some foodstuffs, including strawberries, egg white and lobster.[95]

IgE-mediated urticarias.   Antigen-specific IgE may be responsible for some of the urticarias due to certain foods,[136] drugs,[147] and pollens in addition to the urticaria related to parasitic infestations and stings. Over 300 causes have been identified. Mast cell degranulation is the final common pathway.[97]

Immune-complex-mediated urticarias.   Immune complexes may be involved in the pathogenesis of the chronic urticaria seen in infectious hepatitis, infectious mononucleosis, systemic lupus erythematosus and serum-sickness-like illnesses.[148] They have also been implicated in the urticarial reactions that are an uncommon manifestation of various internal cancers. In some instances, fever, purpura and joint pains are also present. The urticaria is usually more persistent, particularly in those cases with an accompanying vasculitis.

Idiopathic urticaria.   Approximately 75% of all chronic urticarias fall into this category.[103]

Miscellaneous urticarias.   An urticarial reaction is sometimes seen in individuals who are infected with *Candida albicans*;[103] the role of this organism in the causation of urticarias has been overstated in the past. Urticaria may be a manifestation of autoimmune progesterone dermatitis, a disorder which is usually manifest 7–10 days before the menses.[149,150]

Pathogenesis of urticaria

Urticaria results from vasodilatation and increased vascular permeability associated with the extravasation of protein and fluids into the dermis.[146] Angio-oedema results when a similar process occurs in the deep dermis and subcutis. Histamine has generally been regarded as the mediator of these changes although other mediators such as prostaglandins and interleukin 1[151] are possibly involved in some circumstances.[128] Both immunological[152] (type I and type III) and non-immunological mechanisms can cause mast cells and basophils to degranulate, liberating histamine and other substances.[146,153] Eosinophil degranulation also occurs in some urticarias.

Histopathology[154]

The cell type and the intensity of the inflammatory response in urticaria are quite variable.[128] There is increasing evidence to suggest that the age of the lesion biopsied and the nature of the evoking stimulus may influence the type and the intensity of the inflammatory response.

Dermal oedema, which is recognized by separation of the collagen bundles, is an important feature of urticaria. Mild degrees may be difficult to detect. Urticarial oedema differs from the mucinoses by the absence of granular, stringy, basophilic material in the widened interstitium. There is also dilatation of small blood vessels and lymphatics, and swelling of their endothelium is often present (Fig. 8.3). The histopathological changes in urticaria are most marked in the upper dermis, but involvement of the deep dermis may be present, particularly in those with coexisting angio-oedema.

The cellular infiltrate in urticaria is usually mild and perivascular in location. It consists of

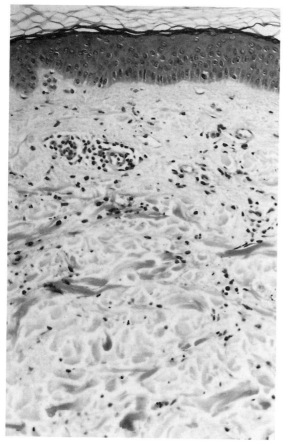

Fig. 8.3 Urticaria. There is mild dermal oedema and a perivascular infiltrate of lymphocytes, mast cells and eosinophils. Occasional interstitial eosinophils are also present.
Haematoxylin — eosin

lymphocytes and, in most cases, a few eosinophils. Occasional interstitial eosinophils and mast cells are also present. Eosinophil granule major basic protein has been identified in the dermis in several types of urticaria.[155,156] Neutrophils are usually noted in early lesions and there is some evidence to suggest that they are more prominent in the physical urticarias.[157–159] An important diagnostic feature of many early urticarias is the presence of neutrophils and sometimes eosinophils in the lumen of small vessels in the upper dermis.[158] Further mention will be made below of the presence of neutrophils in other circumstances. Although mast cells are often increased in early lesions, and even in non-stimulated skin of patients with chronic urticaria,[116] they appear to be decreased in late lesions, apparently due to the failure of histochemical methods to detect degranulated mast cells.[131,143]

Neutrophils have been described in urticaria in several different circumstances.[160–162] As already noted, a few intravascular and perivascular neutrophils are a common feature in early urticaria.[160] At times, there may be sufficient transmigration of neutrophils through vessel walls to give a superficial resemblance to 'vasculitis', but there is no fibrinoid change, haemorrhage or leucocytoclasis. A more diffuse dermal neutrophilia has also been described in nearly 10% of urticarias.[161] In these cases, neutrophils are scattered among the collagen bundles, usually in the upper dermis but sometimes throughout its thickness. The infiltrate is usually mild in intensity.[161] Rare nuclear 'dusting' may also be present. Interstitial eosinophils and perivascular eosinophils and lymphocytes are usually noted as well.[161] Neutrophils are also present in the leucocytoclastic vasculitis that sometimes accompanies chronic urticaria. The term *urticarial vasculitis* has been applied to cases of this type in which the clinical picture is that of an urticaria and the histopathology is a vasculitis.[163–168] In urticarial vasculitis (see also p. 222) the urticarial lesions are usually of longer duration than in the 'usual' chronic urticaria and systemic symptoms may accompany them.[169–172] The incidence of vasculitis in chronic urticaria varies with the strictness of the criteria used for defining vasculitis.[173–174] There appears to be a continuum of changes with a few intravascular and perivascular neutrophils at one end of the spectrum and an established leucocytoclastic vasculitis at the other.

Other histopathological features have been described in several of the specific types of urticaria. In dermographism, perivascular mononuclear cells are increased, even prior to the initiation of a wheal.[175] In contact urticaria, subcorneal vesiculation and spongiosis have been reported, but this may simply reflect a concomitant allergic or irritant contact dermatitis.[135] The inflammatory cell infiltrate in papular urticaria is usually heavier than in other chronic urticarias and consists of lymphocytes and eosinophils in a perivascular location.[99] Interstitial eosinophils may also be present, and in lesions of less than 24 hours' duration there are also some neutrophils.[99] In angio-oedema, the oedema and vascular dilatation involve the deep dermis and/or subcutis, although in the hereditary form there is usually no infiltrate of inflammatory cells.[107]

ACUTE VASCULITIS

The term vasculitis refers to a heterogeneous group of disorders in which there is inflammation and damage of blood vessel walls.[176–178] It may be limited to the skin or some other organ, or be a multisystem disorder with protean manifestations. Numerous classifications of vasculitis have been proposed but there is still no universally acceptable one.[176,179,180]

Vasculitis can be classified on an aetiological basis, although in approximately 50% of cases there is no discernible cause.[181] Furthermore, a single aetiological agent can result in several clinical expressions of vasculitis. Another approach to the classification of the vasculitides has been on the basis of the size and type of blood vessel involved, as this correlates to some extent with the cutaneous manifestations. For example, small or medium-sized arteries are involved in polyarteritis nodosa, Kawasaki disease and nodular vasculitis, while large veins are involved in thrombophlebitis. Both small and large vessels are involved in rheumatoid arthritis and certain 'collagen diseases'. However, most cases of cutaneous vasculitis involve small vessels, particularly venules. The classification to be adopted here is based on the nature of the inflammatory response, with three major categories: acute (neutrophilic) vasculitis, chronic lymphocytic vasculitis and vasculitis with granulomatosis. A fourth category, the neutrophilic dermatoses, is included although most of the diseases in this group have been regarded at various times as instances of acute (neutrophilic) vasculitis. There is an infiltration of neutrophils in the dermis but there is usually no fibrinoid

necrosis of the vessel wall, a cardinal feature of acute vasculitis.[182]

The classification below has some shortcomings because vasculitis is a dynamic process, with the evolution of some acute lesions into a chronic stage.[183,184] Furthermore, lesions are sometimes seen in which there are features of both acute and chronic vasculitis. Whether this represents a stage in the evolution of the disease or a change *de novo* is debatable. Each category of vasculitis can be further subdivided into a number of clinicopathological entities.[185,186] In the case of acute vasculitis, they are as follows:

Hypersensitivity vasculitis
Henoch–Schönlein purpura
Rheumatoid vasculitis
Urticarial vasculitis
Mixed cryoglobulinaemia
Hypergammaglobulinaemic purpura
Septic vasculitis
Erythema elevatum diutinum
Granuloma faciale
Polyarteritis nodosa
Kawasaki disease
Superficial thrombophlebitis
Miscellaneous associations.

HYPERSENSITIVITY VASCULITIS

Hypersensitivity vasculitis is the preferred designation for a clearly defined clinicopathological entity which predominantly affects small vessels of the skin, particularly the post-capillary venules.[186] The term leucocytoclastic vasculitis is often used,[181] but as leucocytoclasis (degeneration of neutrophils) is not invariably present, it is best avoided. Other diagnoses that have been applied to this condition include allergic vasculitis,[187] hypersensitivity angiitis[188] and necrotizing vasculitis.[189]

Hypersensitivity vasculitis usually presents with erythematous macules or palpable purpura, with a predilection for dependent parts, particularly the lower parts of the legs.[190,191] Other lesions which may be present include haemorrhagic vesicles and bullae, nodules,[192] crusted ulcers and, less commonly, livedo reticularis, pustules[193] or annular lesions.[194] Cases with urticarial lesions are classified separately as urticarial vasculitis (see below). Individual lesions vary from 1 mm to several cm in diameter. Large lesions are sometimes painful.[186] There may be a single crop of lesions which subside spontaneously after a few weeks or crops of lesions at different stages of evolution which may recur intermittently.[177,195]

Extracutaneous manifestations occur in approximately 50% of affected individuals and include arthralgia, myositis, low grade fever and malaise.[190] Less commonly, there are renal, gastrointestinal, pulmonary or neurological manifestations.[187,190] There is a low mortality in hypersensitivity vasculitis; death, when due to the vasculitis, is related to involvement of systemic vessels.

There are several different aetiological groups, although in approximately 50% of cases there is no apparent cause. The recognized groups include infections, drugs and chemicals, cancers and systemic diseases.[186,190,196] Miscellaneous causes include certain arthropod bites, severe atherosclerosis[197] and some coral ulcers.[198] Streptococcal infections, particularly of the upper respiratory tract, are the most commonly implicated infections.[186] Others include influenza, hepatitis B, herpes simplex,[199] herpes zoster/varicella,[199] cytomegalic inclusion disease,[200] parvovirus infection,[180] AIDS,[201] and malaria.[186] Drug causes of hypersensitivity vasculitis include penicillin,[181] ampicillin,[202] erythromycin,[203] clindamycin,[204] the cephalosporins,[190] sulphonamides,[202] griseofulvin,[202] frusemide (furosemide),[205] thiouracil,[206] allopurinol,[202] aspirin,[190] phenylbutazone,[202] cimetidine,[188] procainamide,[188] potassium iodide,[202] gold,[207] phenothiazines,[208] thiazides,[190] quinidine,[202] disulfiram[207] and phenytoin (diphenylhydantoin).[202] Chemicals used in industry, hyposensitizing antigens and intravenous drug abuse can be included in this aetiological category [208] The cancers associated with hypersensitivity vasculitis include lymphomas,[209] mycosis fungoides,[210] hairy cell leukaemia,[211,212] and very rarely a visceral tumour.[189] The systemic diseases include systemic lupus erythematosus, Behçet's disease,[213] coeliac disease,[209] inflammatory bowel disease,[214] cystic fibrosis,[215] Sjögren's disease,[216] pyoderma gangrenosum,[217] sarcoidosis,[194] the Wiskott–Aldrich syndrome[215] and α_1-antitrypsin deficiency.[218]

The pathogenesis of hypersensitivity vasculitis involves the deposition of immune complexes in vessel walls with activation of the complement system, particularly the terminal components.[219] Chemotaxis of neutrophils and injury to vessel walls with exudation of serum, erythrocytes and fibrin result. Mast cells may also play a role.[220] The size of the immune complexes, which depends on the valence of the respective antigen and antibody and their relative concentrations (which is in part determined by the number of binding sites on the antigen), determines the likelihood of their deposition.[186] The complexes most likely to precipitate are those with antigens bearing 2–4 binding sites and in a concentration approximately equivalent with antibody.[186] These are the largest immune complexes that ordinarily remain soluble.[186]

Various haemodynamic factors, such as turbulence and increased venous pressure, as well as the reduced fibrinolytic activity that occurs in the legs may explain why localization of lesions to this site commonly occurs.[221] Rarely, lesions may develop in areas of previously traumatized skin — the Koebner phenomenon.[221a] The size and configuration of the complexes may also determine the class of vessel affected. The size of the affected vessels correlates with the clinical features. For example, involvement of small dermal vessels results in erythema or palpable purpura while lesions in larger arteries may lead to nodules, ulcers or livedo reticularis.[215] Deep venous involvement results in nodules without ulceration.[215]

Histopathology[222]

Acute vasculitis is a dynamic process. Accordingly, not all the features described below will necessarily be present at a particular stage in the evolution of the disease.[186] It is best to biopsy a lesion of 18–24 hours' duration as this will show the most diagnostic features (Fig. 8.4).[188] The

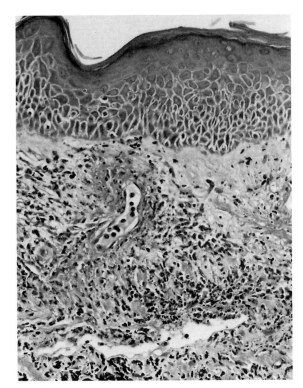

Fig. 8.4 Hypersensitivity vasculitis. Fibrin is present in the walls of small vessels and there is a neutrophilic infiltrate in their vicinity.
Haematoxylin — eosin

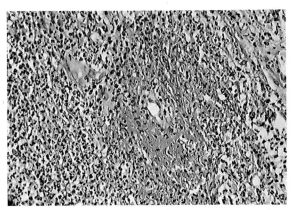

Fig. 8.5 Hypersensitivity vasculitis with extensive extravasation of fibrin around a small blood vessel. There is also a heavy infiltrate of neutrophils and some leucocytoclasis.
Haematoxylin — eosin

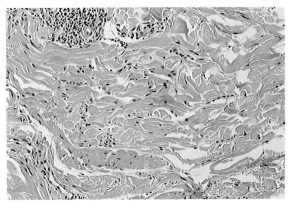

Fig. 8.6 Subsiding vasculitis. It is characterized by a perivascular infiltrate of lymphocytes, a hypercellular ('busy') dermis and some interstitial mucin.
Haematoxylin — eosin

changes to be described usually involve the small venules in the dermis, although in severe cases arterioles may also be affected.[195] There is infiltration of vessel walls with neutrophils which also extend into the perivascular zone and beyond. These neutrophils undergo degeneration (leucocytoclasis) with the formation of nuclear dust. The vessel walls are thickened by the exudate of inflammatory cells and oedema fluid. There is also exudation of fibrin (fibrinoid necrosis) which often extends into the adjacent perivascular connective tissue (Fig. 8.5).[195] Endothelial cells are usually swollen and some are degenerate. Thrombosis of vessels is sometimes present. The dermis shows variable oedema and extravasation of red blood cells.

In some lesions, particularly those of longer duration, eosinophils and lymphocytes are also present, particularly in a perivascular location. In vasculitis due to drugs, a mixed inflammatory cell infiltrate of eosinophils, lymphocytes and occasional neutrophils is commonly seen.[202] In resolving lesions, there is usually only a mild perivascular infiltrate of lymphocytes and some eosinophils. A rare plasma cell may also be present. A striking feature of late resolving lesions is hypercellularity of the dermis with an increased number of interstitial fibroblasts and histiocytes, giving the appearance of a 'busy dermis' (Fig. 8.6). There is sometimes a mild increase in acid mucopolysaccharides, imparting a vague 'necrobiotic' appearance.

Uncommonly, the subepidermal oedema is so pronounced that vesiculobullous lesions result. Cutaneous infarction, usually involving only the epidermis and upper third of the dermis, may follow thrombosis of affected vessels. Rare changes reported in hypersensitivity vasculitis include subepidermal microabscess formation resembling dermatitis herpetiformis[223] and intraepidermal vesiculation with acantholytic cells containing vacuolated nuclei.[224]

Immunofluorescence examination of the affected skin is not particularly useful.[176] It must be performed on lesions less than six hours old. If this is done, immunoglobulins, particularly IgM, C3 and fibrin can be demonstrated in vessel walls and the perivascular space.[181] Immunoreactants are usually undetectable after 24 hours.

HENOCH–SCHÖNLEIN PURPURA

This clinical variant of hypersensitivy vasculitis is characterized by a purpuric rash, usually on the lower parts of the legs, which is often accompanied by one or more of the following: arthritis, abdominal pain, haematuria and, rarely, cardiac or neurological manifestations.[225,226] It is usually preceded by an upper respiratory tract infection or the ingestion of certain drugs or foods, with the formation of IgA-containing complexes, which may precipitate in vessels in the skin and certain other organs.[227,228] The alternate complement pathway is thereby activated. It has a predilection for children, although occurrence in adults is known.[228]

The disease usually runs a self-limited course, although in a small percentage of patients persistent renal involvement occurs.

Histopathology

The appearances are usually indistinguishable from those seen in hypersensitivity vasculitis. IgA is demonstrable in vessel walls in both involved and uninvolved skin in most cases, provided that the biopsy is taken early in the course of the disease.[227,228]

RHEUMATOID VASCULITIS

Rheumatoid vasculitis typically occurs in patients with seropositive, erosive rheumatoid arthritis of long standing.[229,230] A similar vasculitis may occur in some cases of systemic lupus erythematosus, mixed connective tissue disease, Sjögren's syndrome and, rarely, dermatomyositis and scleroderma. Rheumatoid vasculitis is an acute vasculitis which differs from hypersensitivity vasculitis in its involvement of large as well as small blood vessels. This leads to varied clinical presentations which may include digital gangrene, cutaneous ulcers and digital nail fold infarction as well as palpable purpura.[231] Involvement of the vasa nervorum can result in a neuropathy.[231]

In rheumatoid vasculitis, lesions are often recurrent.[181] The overall mortality may approach 30%.[229] Immune complexes appear to be involved in the pathogenesis.[231]

Histopathology[229,231]

As already mentioned, rheumatoid vasculitis is an acute vasculitis with involvement of several sizes of blood vessels. The involvement of medium-sized muscular arteries may be indistinguishable from that seen in polyarteritis nodosa. In the skin, vessels in the lower dermis are sometimes involved, while superficial vessels may be spared. Intimal proliferation and thrombosis of vessels also occur.

Rheumatoid vasculitis should be distinguished from rheumatoid neutrophilic dermatosis, which is one of the neutrophilic dermatoses, and as such has no fibrinoid necrosis of vessels (see p. 231).

URTICARIAL VASCULITIS

Urticarial vasculitis is another clinical variant of hypersensitivity vasculitis in which the cutaneous lesions comprise urticarial wheals and/or angio-oedema, rather than palpable purpura.[163,172] Erythematous papules and plaques may also occur. The wheals usually persist longer than is usual for chronic urticaria without vasculitis, and they may resolve leaving an ecchymotic stain. The lesions are often generalized without any predilection for the lower legs. Systemic involvement, including renal failure, may occur, and this is more likely in those with concurrent hypocomplementaemia.[164,165] A lupus-erythematosus-like syndrome is sometimes present.[232,233] Urticarial vasculitis has been reported in association with hepatitis B infection, Sjögren's syndrome, IgA myeloma, an IgM gammopathy (Schnitzler's syndrome),[233a] systemic lupus erythematosus, and solar and cold urticaria,[170] and following the ingestion of certain drugs.[234]

Histopathology[166]

The changes are similar to those seen in hypersensitivity vasculitis, although there is usually prominent oedema of the upper dermis. The inflammatory infiltrate is sometimes quite mild. A variant with a lymphocytic vasculitis has been reported.[171]

MIXED CRYOGLOBULINAEMIA

Mixed cryoglobulinaemia has been discussed earlier in this chapter along with the monoclonal form (see p. 214). The histopathological changes are those of an acute vasculitis resembling hypersensitivity vasculitis. In contrast to the monoclonal form, intravascular hyaline deposits are the exception, although they are sometimes found beneath areas of ulceration.[235]

HYPERGAMMAGLOBULINAEMIC PURPURA

Hypergammaglobulinaemic purpura (Waldenström) is characterized by recurrent purpura, anaemia, an elevated erythrocyte sedimentation rate and polyclonal hypergammaglobulinamae.[176,186]

Histopathology

The changes are similar to those occurring in hypersensitivity vasculitis.

SEPTIC VASCULITIS

Septic vasculitis, also referred to (somewhat erroneously) as non-leucocytoclastic vasculitis,[236] is a variant of acute vasculitis seen in association with various septicaemic states. These include meningococcal septicaemia, gonococcal septicaemia, *Pseudomonas* septicaemia, infective endocarditis, particularly that due to *Staphylococcus aureus*,[237] and some cases of secondary syphilis. Certain rickettsial infections can produce similar lesions (see p. 620). The condition known as acute generalized pustulosis (see p. 231) is closely related.

Cutaneous lesions occur in 80% or more of cases of acute meningococcal infections.[238] There are erythematous macules, nodules and petechiae which may be surmounted with small pustules.[238] There is a predilection for the extremities and pressure sites. Features of disseminated intravascular coagulation are invariably present (see p. 212).[239] Acute gonococcaemia is exceedingly rare in comparison, although localized pustular lesions have been reported on the digits.[240-242] In *Pseudomonas* infections, haemorrhagic bullae, ulcers and eschars are seen.[243-245] These changes are discussed elsewhere as ecthyma gangrenosum (see p. 598). Acute pustular lesions also occur in infective endocarditis as Osler nodes and Janeway lesions.

Chronic infections with *Neisseria meningitidis* and *N. gonorrhoeae* are characterized by the triad of intermittent fever, arthralgia and vesiculopustular or haemorrhagic lesions.[246-249] In chronic gonococcal septicaemia there is a marked female preponderance and lesions are fewer in number than in chronic meningococcal septicaemia.[250,251] Positive blood cultures have been obtained during febrile episodes.

Histopathology

In *acute meningococcal septicaemia* there is widespread vascular damage characterized by endothelial swelling and focal necrosis, fibrinoid change in vessel walls and occlusive thrombi composed of platelets, fibrin, red blood cells and neutrophils (Fig. 8.7).[252,253] There are neutrophils in and around vessel walls, as well as in the

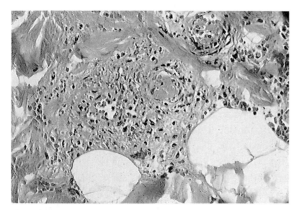

Fig. 8.7 Meningococcal septicaemia. A vessel is occluded by a fibrin thrombus. There are some neutrophils in the surrounding dermis.
Haematoxylin — eosin

interstitium. Leucocytoclasis is often present, although it is usually quite mild.[238] There is also some perivascular haemorrhage. The adnexa may show degenerative changes.[252] Sub-epidermal oedema and pustulation occur as well as intraepidermal pustules.[252] Large numbers of Gram-negative diplococci are seen in endothelial cells and neutrophils.[252,253]

In *chronic meningococcal septicaemia* and *chronic gonococcal septicaemia* there is a vasculitis which differs from hypersensitivity vasculitis in subtle ways. Arterioles are often affected in addition to venules, and deep vessels may show changes just as conspicuous as those in the super-ficial dermis. Extravasation of erythrocytes is often conspicuous. There is also an admixture of mononuclear cells in chronic septic vasculitis and vascular thrombi are more regularly seen.[246,248] Leucocytoclasis is often present, but it is not a prominent feature.[250] Another distinguishing feature is the regular presence of subepidermal and intraepidermal pustules with partial destruction of the epidermis.[246,254] Organisms are usually not found with a Gram stain of tissue sections, although bacterial antigens are commonly identified using immunofluorescence techniques.[246,254–256]

There are conflicting reports on the histo-pathological findings in the Osler nodes and Janeway lesions of infective endocarditis. Osler nodes appear to be a septic vasculitis, involving in part the glomus apparatus,[257] while Janeway lesions have variously been regarded as a similar process,[258,259] or as an embolic suppurative process with or without vasculitis.[260,260a]

ERYTHEMA ELEVATUM DIUTINUM

This is a rare dermatosis in which there are persistent red, violaceous and yellowish papules, plaques and nodules that are usually distributed acrally and symmetrically on extensor surfaces, including the buttocks.[261,262] Pedunculated lesions[263,264] and nodules surmounted by vesi-cles and bullae have also been described.[265,266] Arthralgia is sometimes present,[262] and an association with multiple myeloma[261] and cryoglobulinaemia[267] has been documented. Onset is usually in middle life. Lesions may involute after 5–10 years, but persistence for 20 years has been reported.[268]

The aetiology is unknown but it is thought to be a variant of leucocytoclastic vasculitis resulting from an Arthus-type reaction to bacterial[269] and even viral antigens.[270] The formation of granulation tissue in lesions results in a local perpetuation of the process as newly formed vessels are more vulnerable to injury.

Histopathology[261,262,271]

Erythema elevatum diutinum is typically charac-terized by acute histological features which contrast with the chronic clinical course.[261,272] Nevertheless, the histological appearances vary somewhat according to the age of the lesion.

In early lesions there is a moderately dense perivascular infiltrate of neutrophils, with deposits of fibrin ('toxic hyalin') within and around the walls of small dermal blood vessels.[262,264] These may also show endothelial swelling. Leucocytoclasis is also present. There are lesser numbers of histiocytes and lymphocytes, and only a few eosinophils. Extravasation of red cells is uncommon.

In more established lesions the infiltrate of neutrophils involves the entire dermis. The epidermis is usually uninvolved, but there may be focal spongiosis. In vesiculobullous lesions there is subepidermal vesiculation and pustulation.[266] Focal epidermal necrosis is sometimes present.[266] Basophilic nuclear dust may encrust collagen bundles in some cases.[271] Capillary proliferation is usually present in established lesions.

In late lesions there is variable fibrosis, and in some instances a fascicled proliferation of spindle cells.[271] The low-power picture resembles a dermatofibroma. Small foci of neutrophilic vasculitis are scattered through the fibrotic areas.[264] Capillary proliferation is also present. *Extracellular cholesterosis* of the older literature[272] is now regarded as a variant in which lipids are secondarily deposited between the collagen.[261] Since the introduction of dapsone in the treatment of this entity, cholesterol deposits no longer seem to be recorded.

Although immunoglobulins and complement have been reported in the vicinity of small vessels in the dermis, this has not been an invariable finding.[262,273]

Although the clinical features are quite distinct, the histological features of early lesions may be indistinguishable from the neutrophilic dermatoses (see p. 228) — Sweet's syndrome, rheumatoid neutrophilic dermatosis, the bowel-associated dermatosis-arthritis syndrome and Behçet's disease. Erythema elevatum diutinum differs from granuloma faciale in the predominance of neutrophils rather than eosinophils, and the involvement of the adventitial dermis which is spared in granuloma faciale (see below).[271]

Electron microscopy. In addition to the fibrin deposition and neutrophil fragmentation, there are histiocytes present which contain fat droplets and myelin figures.[271] Cholesterol crystals have been present in some cases, both intracellular and extracellular in position.[271,274] Langerhans cells are increased in the dermis in both early and late lesions.[275]

GRANULOMA FACIALE

Granuloma faciale is a rare dermatosis which manifests as one or several, brown-red plaques, nodules or sometimes papules on the face.[276,277]

There is a predilection for white males of middle age.[278] Extrafacial involvement is quite uncommon.[279,280] The lesions are usually persistent, and essentially asymptomatic.

The aetiology is unknown, but a form of vasculitis, mediated by a localized Arthus-like process has been postulated.[281]

Histopathology[276,277,282]

There is usually a dense, polymorphous, inflammatory cell infiltrate in the upper two-thirds of the dermis, with a narrow, uninvolved grenz zone beneath the epidermis, and often around pilosebaceous follicles (Fig. 8.8). Occasionally the entire dermis, and even the upper

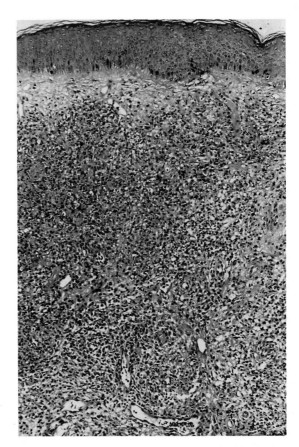

Fig. 8.8 Granuloma faciale. A grenz zone of uninvolved dermis overlies a mixed inflammatory cell infiltrate. A small amount of fibrin is present in vessel walls. The dermal infiltrate is more widespread than in most cases of hypersensitivity vasculitis.
Haematoxylin — eosin

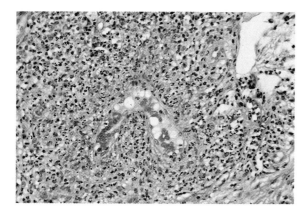

Fig. 8.9 Granuloma faciale. A mixed infiltrate, which includes neutrophils, eosinophils and lymphocytes, surrounds a dermal blood vessel. Haematoxylin — eosin

subcutis are involved.[283] Sometimes the infiltrate is less dense and then tends to show perivascular accentuation. The infiltrate consists of eosinophils, usually quite numerous, together with neutrophils, lymphocytes, histiocytes and a few mast cells and plasma cells (Fig. 8.9). Neutrophils are usually localized around the blood vessels, and there may be mild leucocytoclasis.[284] There is controversy as to whether neutrophils are related to the intensity of the inflammation or the stage of the disease.[276,282] A few foam cells and foreign body giant cells may be present.[281] In lesions of long standing there is usually some fibrosis.

Blood vessels in the upper dermis are usually dilated, often with some endothelial swelling. Eosinophilic fibrinoid material, so-called 'toxic hyalin', may be deposited around some vessels, but many cases do not show this feature. The material is PAS-positive and diastase-resistant. Extravasated red blood cells are often present, and haemosiderin is present in over one-half of all biopsies. A true vasculitis may be present, but this presumably depends on the timing of the biopsy with respect to the course of the disease process.[283]

Immunoglobulins, particularly IgG, and complement are often present along the basement membrane and around blood vessels.[285,286] Fibrin is usually present around the vessels, even when toxic hyalin is not present on light microscopy.[285]

Erythema elevatum diutinum (see above) has many histological similarities, but in this condition the proportion of neutrophils to eosinophils is higher than in granuloma faciale, and there is usually no well defined grenz zone.[282] Toxic hyalin is more abundant and often intimately related to the vessel wall in erythema elevatum diutinum.[277]

Electron microscopy. This has shown abundant eosinophils, often with cytoplasmic degenerative changes.[287]

POLYARTERITIS NODOSA

Polyarteritis nodosa is a rare inflammatory disease of small and medium-sized muscular arteries; it usually involves multiple organs.[288] These include the kidneys, liver, gastrointestinal tract and nervous system.[289] The skin is involved in approximately 10–15% of cases, resulting in palpable purpura and sometimes ulceration of the lower extremities.[290] There are usually constitutional symptoms such as fever, weight loss, fatigue, arthralgia and myalgia.[288] No age is exempt, but there is a predilection for adult males.[291]

The course is variable, but it is not possible to predict those likely to develop progressive disease.[288] The 5-year survival rate is approximately 50%; death is usually the result of involvement of the kidneys or gastrointestinal tract.[288]

A *cutaneous form* of polyarteritis nodosa, with a chronic relapsing course but no evidence of systemic disease, has been reported.[292–294] This variant usually presents with nodules, livedo reticularis or ulceration involving the lower limbs. There may be mild constitutional symptoms but the prognosis is nevertheless good. An unusual complication has been the formation of periosteal new bone beneath the cutaneous lesions.[295]

There are probably many causes of polyarteritis nodosa. Immune complexes appear to play an important role in the pathogenesis. Hepatitis B surface antigen has been detected in up to 50% of systemic cases[296] but this figure is much higher than has been recorded in most series.[297] The antigen has also been reported in the localized cutaneous form.[298,299]

Polyarteritis-nodosa-like lesions have been reported in association with Crohn's disease,[300,301] Kawasaki's disease (see below), rheumatoid arthritis, angioimmunoblastic lymphadenopathy, and following the repair of coarctation of the aorta.[302,303] They have also been noted following the intravenous injection of methylamphetamine (metamphetamine, 'speed').[304]

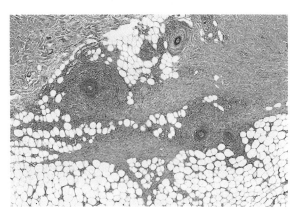

Fig. 8.10 Cutaneous polyarteritis nodosa. The affected small arteries in the upper subcutis show marked fibrin extravasation into their walls. Haematoxylin — eosin

Histopathology[291,305]

In the early stages there is marked thickening of the wall of the vessel, particularly the intima, as a result of oedema and a fibrinous and cellular exudate. The infiltrate is composed of neutrophils, with some eosinophils and lymphocytes. Leucocytoclasis is sometimes present.[294] In older lesions there is a greater proportion of mononuclear cells, particularly lymphocytes. Luminal thrombi and aneurysms may form. Initially the lesions are segmental but the infiltrate expands to involve the full circumference of the artery. The changes are often localized to the region of a bifurcation of the vessel. At a still later stage there is intimal and mural fibrosis leading to obliteration of the vessel. A characteristic feature of polyarteritis nodosa is the presence of lesions at all stages of development.

In the *cutaneous form* small and medium-sized arteries in the subcutis, and occasionally the deep dermis, are involved. The inflammation is localized to the vessel and its immediate vicinity, allowing a distinction to be made from the various panniculitides (Fig. 8.10). There may be a mild perivascular lymphocytic infiltrate in the overlying dermis.

Immunofluorescence of the cutaneous form has shown IgM and sometimes C3 in the vessel walls.[293]

KAWASAKI SYNDROME

Kawasaki syndrome (Kawasaki disease, mucocutaneous lymph node syndrome) is an acute, multisystem, febrile illness of unknown cause that occurs predominantly in infancy and early childhood.[306,307] Adult cases have been reported, but some of these may represent erythema multiforme or the toxic shock syndrome.[308] In addition to the prolonged fever, clinical features include non-exudative conjunctivitis, cervical lymphadenopathy, oropharyngeal inflammation, thrombocytosis and a vasculitis which predominantly involves the coronary arteries, leading to coronary artery aneurysms or ectasias in 20% or more of cases.[307,309,310] The disease is usually self-limited although 1% may end fatally, almost exclusively from the cardiac involvement.[311]

Cutaneous manifestations include a polymorphous, exanthematous rash, accompanied by brawny oedema and erythema of the palms and soles.[307,309] This is followed by desquamation which particularly involves the tips of the fingers and toes. An erythematous, desquamating perineal eruption is a distinctive feature in many cases.[312] A pustular rash resembling miliaria pustulosa also occurs in some of the patients.[313]

Although the aetiology is unknown, a microbial cause is suggested by the clinical features, by the occurrence of epidemic outbreaks and by the amelioration of coronary artery abnormalities by the use of gamma globulin.[314] A retrovirus and *Propionibacterium acnes* have been incriminated but no agent has been consistently demonstrable.[315]

Histopathology

Biopsies of the skin lesions are infrequently performed. They have shown non-specific features which include oedema of the papillary dermis and a mild perivascular infiltrate of lymphocytes and mononuclear cells.[309,316] Subtle vascular changes, including subendothelial oedema, focal endothelial cell necrosis and vascular deposition of small amounts of fibrinoid material, were noted in one report.[316] The pustular lesions are small intraepidermal and subcorneal abscesses; they are not related to eccrine ducts.[313]

Although autopsies on fatal cases have shown a polyarteritis-nodosa-like involvement of the coronary and some other visceral arteries, no cutaneous vasculitis has been reported.[306]

SUPERFICIAL THROMBOPHLEBITIS

Superficial thrombophlebitis presents with tender, erythematous swellings or cord-like thickenings of the subcutis, usually on the lower parts of the legs. Multiple segments of a vein may be involved over time, hence the use of the term 'migratory' in the older literature to describe this process. Superficial thrombophlebitis may occur in association with Behçet's disease (see p. 232), Buerger's disease (thromboangiitis obliterans) or an underlying cancer, most often a carcinoma of the pancreas or of the stomach.[317,317a] It may be associated with various hypercoagulable states.[317b,317c]

Mondor's disease is a variant of superficial thrombophlebitis occurring in relation to the breast or anterolateral chest wall.[318,319] A history of preceding trauma, including breast surgery, is obtained in a number of cases.

Histopathology

Superficial thrombophlebitis involves veins in the upper subcutis. In early lesions, the inflammatory cell infiltrate is composed of numerous neutrophils, although at a later stage there are lymphocytes and occasional multinucleate giant cells. Intramural microabscesses are commonly present in the vein in the thrombophlebitis which accompanies Buerger's disease; there is some controversy whether this finding is specific for this disease. The inflammatory cell infiltrate extends only a short distance into the surrounding fat, in contrast to the more extensive panniculitis seen in nodular vasculitis (see p. 502).

Thrombus is often present in the lumen of the affected veins and this eventually undergoes recanalization.

MISCELLANEOUS ASSOCIATIONS

An acute vasculitis is a feature of erythema nodosum leprosum (see p. 614). It has also been reported in the rose spots of paratyphoid fever,[320] and in the Jarisch–Herxheimer reaction which may follow therapy for syphilis.[321] In this latter condition, the acute inflammatory changes are superimposed on a background of chronic inflammation in which plasma cells are usually prominent.[321]

The condition known as nodular vasculitis is also an acute vasculitis. It results in a panniculitis and accordingly is discussed with the panniculitides on page 502.

NEUTROPHILIC DERMATOSES

The neutrophilic dermatoses are a clinically heterogeneous group of entities characterized histopathologically by the presence of a heavy dermal infiltrate of neutrophils and variable leucocytoclasis.[322] On casual examination of tissue sections the appearances suggest an acute vasculitis, although on closer inspection there is no significant fibrinoid necrosis of vessel walls. Limited vascular damage in the form of endothelial swelling may be present, and in some biopsies fibrinoid necrosis of some vessel walls may be found. The term *pustular vasculitis* has been proposed as an alternative designation, further evidence of the confusion which surrounds the nosological classification of this group.[323,324]

Circulating immune complexes with heightened chemotaxis of neutrophils are thought to have an important pathogenetic role.[324,325] The immune complexes appear to be of diverse origin.

The following diseases will be considered in this category, although it should be noted that the lesions in some stages of Behçet's syndrome do not qualify for inclusion:

Sweet's syndrome
Bowel-associated dermatosis-arthritis syndrome
Rheumatoid neutrophilic dermatosis
Acute generalized pustulosis
Behçet's syndrome.

Although having many histopathological features in common with this group, erythema elevatum diutinum has prominent fibrinoid change in vessel walls and is best included with the acute vasculities (see p. 224). Pyoderma gangrenosum has also been included in this group by some authorities (see p. 242).[182]

SWEET'S SYNDROME

Sweet's syndrome (acute febrile neutrophilic dermatosis) is a rare dermatosis characterized by the abrupt onset of tender or painful, erythematous plaques and nodules on the face[326] and extremities, and less commonly on the trunk, in association with fever, malaise and a neutrophil leucocytosis.[327-330] A variant with raised annular lesions has been reported.[331] The skin lesions are sometimes studded with small vesicles or pustules,[332] but ulceration is unusual and true bullae are uncommon. Lesions usually heal without scarring although there may be residual pigmentation attributed to haemosiderin.[332] There is a predilection for females; the patients may be of any age.[333] Other clinical features may

include polyarthritis, conjunctivitis and episcleritis.[330,334]

In 10–15% of cases an associated leukaemia, usually of acute myelomonocytic type, is present.[335-341] In some of these cases, features of atypical pyoderma gangrenosum may be present and it has been suggested that Sweet's syndrome and pyoderma gangrenosum may be at opposite ends of the spectrum of one process.[342-345] Other associations have included polycythaemia vera,[346,347] lymphoma,[348,349] myeloma,[350] solid cancers,[330,351,352] Behçet's syndrome,[353,354] rheumatoid arthritis, lupus erythematosus,[355,356] ulcerative colitis,[327] Crohn's disease,[357] BCG vaccination,[358] and treatment with frusemide (furosemide).[359]

The aetiology is unknown, but the syndrome is assumed to represent a hypersensitivity reaction triggered by some antecedent process.[339] There is sometimes a history of a preceding upper respiratory tract infection.[334] Enhanced chemotaxis for neutrophils has been reported in several cases.[360-362]

Histopathology[330,363]

There is a dense infiltrate of mature neutrophils in the upper half of the dermis. Neutrophils may extend throughout the dermis and even into the subcutis. The epidermis is usually spared, although it may be pale staining. Neutrophils may be so dense in the centre of the lesion that the appearances simulate an incipient abscess. Leucocytoclasis with the formation of nuclear dust is usually present but there is no true vasculitis or fibrinoid extravasation (Fig. 8.11). However, the vessels often show endothelial swelling. Lymphocytes are present in older lesions but are usually perivascular and few in number. A few eosinophils may be present in the infiltrate. In later lesions, macrophages containing phagocytosed neutrophils are sometimes prominent in the upper dermis.

There is often marked oedema of the papillary dermis which may lead to the appearance of subepidermal vesiculation (Fig. 8.12). Delicate strands of dermal collagen usually stretch across this pseudobullous space.[330] Dilated vessels and

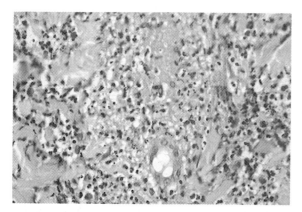

Fig. 8.11 Sweet's syndrome. There are numerous neutrophils surrounding a dermal blood vessel which is devoid of fibrin in its wall.
Haematoxylin — eosin

extravasated red blood cells may be found in this zone.

The appearances resemble erythema elevatum diutinum (see p. 224), except for the absence of fibrinoid material in Sweet's syndrome.[332] In granuloma faciale (see p. 225) there are more eosinophils, even in early lesions, and there is a well-defined grenz zone.[332]

BOWEL-ASSOCIATED DERMATOSIS-ARTHRITIS SYNDROME

The use of intestinal bypass surgery for the treatment of morbid obesity is complicated in from 10–20% of patients by an influenza-like illness with malaise, fever, polyarthritis, and the development of small pustular lesions in the skin of the upper extremities and trunk.[364,365] Erythema nodosum-like lesions are sometimes present.[366] A similar clinicopathological syndrome has been reported rarely in patients with other bowel conditions,[367] such as ulcerative colitis, Crohn's disease and intestinal diverticula, and following partial gastrectomy.[368–370] This has prompted the new designation used above, in place of the previous term, the *bowel bypass syndrome*.[370]

The deposition of immune complexes containing the bacterial antigen peptidoglycan, derived from an overgrowth of bacteria in a blind

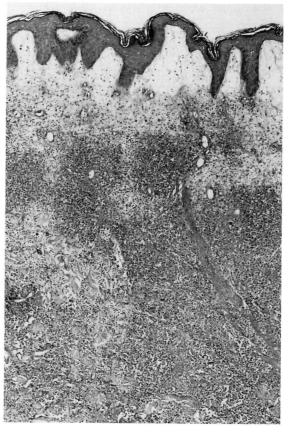

Fig. 8.12 Sweet's syndrome with marked subepidermal oedema. The underlying dermis contains a heavy infiltrate of neutrophils.
Haematoxylin — eosin

loop or abnormal segment of bowel, may be responsible for this syndrome.[365,371] Cryoglobulins are also often present.[371]

Histopathology

The changes resemble those of Sweet's syndrome, with subepidermal oedema and a heavy infiltrate of neutrophils in the upper and mid dermis which is both perivascular and diffuse in distribution.[369] There is variable leucocytoclasis. In older lesions, lymphocytes, eosinophils and macrophages containing neutrophil debris are also present. Although signs of vascular damage are usually limited to some endothelial swelling, fibrin deposition around vessels can be present.[372,373] A purulent folliculitis has also been reported, but this is more common in the pustular lesions, particularly on the face, in patients with ulcerative colitis.[374] Septal and lower dermal inflammation is present in the erythema nodosum-like lesions.[366]

Immunofluorescence findings have not been consistent. Immunoglobulins and complement have been noted at the dermo–epidermal junction and even in vessel walls.[366,371]

RHEUMATOID NEUTROPHILIC DERMATOSIS

Rheumatoid neutrophilic dermatosis is a rare cutaneous manifestation of severe rheumatoid arthritis. It has received scant attention in the literature.[375–377a] Clinically, it presents with plaques and nodules overlying joints of the extremities, particularly the hands, and resembling erythema elevatum diutinum.[375] At other times the lesions are flat, erythematous plaques, more widely distributed on the extremities and sometimes on the trunk.[376,378]

Histopathology

There is a dense neutrophilic infiltrate throughout the dermis, but particularly in the upper and middle levels. There is variable leucocytoclasis. In late lesions lymphocytes, plasma cells and macrophages containing neutrophilic debris are also present (Fig. 8.13). There is no vasculitis. Sometimes the neutrophils collect in the papillary dermis, forming microabscesses similar to those seen in dermatitis herpetiformis.[375,378]

ACUTE GENERALIZED PUSTULOSIS

There have been several reports of the occurrence of a widespread pustular purpura following an infection or occurring as an idiopathic phenomenon (Fig. 8.14).[379–381] The terms 'acute generalized pustular bacterid'[379] and 'primary idiopathic cutaneous pustular vasculitis'[381] refer to the same condition. This condition should probably be incorporated into the

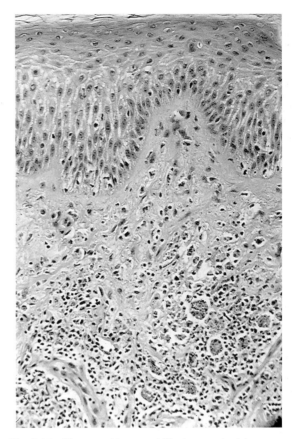

Fig. 8.13 Rheumatoid neutrophilic dermatosis. A late lesion is shown. Macrophages have neutrophil debris in their cytoplasm.
Haematoxylin — eosin

concept known as pustular vasculitis (see p. 229). There are circulating immune complexes and enhancement of neutrophil migration.[380,381]

Histopathology[379–381a]

There is a large subcorneal or intraepidermal pustule overlying a massive perivascular and interstitial infiltrate of neutrophils in the upper and mid dermis. There is some exocytosis of neutrophils through the epidermis. Leucocytoclasis is variable. Vessel walls may show fibrinoid necrosis. In older lesions there are perivascular collections of lymphocytes and some eosinophils in addition to the neutrophils.

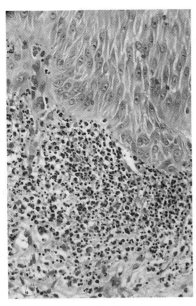

Fig. 8.14 Generalized pustulosis. A subepidermal pustule is present. There is leucocytoclasis but no vasculitis. Haematoxylin — eosin

BEHÇET'S DISEASE

Behçet's disease is a multisystem disorder in which the presence of recurrent aphthous ulcers in the oral cavity is an almost universal feature.[382] These are painful, measure 2–10 mm in diameter, and heal within 7–14 days, only to recur subsequently.[383] Other characteristic signs include genital ulceration, ocular abnormalities such as uveitis, hypopyon and iridocyclitis, and cutaneous lesions.[384,385] Less frequent manifestations include synovitis, neurological lesions including meningoencephalitis, and epididymitis.[385] The clinical course is variable; death may result from central nervous system involvement or arterial aneurysms.

The most characteristic cutaneous lesions are erythema nodosum-like nodules on the legs,[386] superficial and/or deep thrombophlebitis[387] and the development of self-healing, sterile pustules at sites of trauma ('pathergy').[388,389] Pathergic lesions, which may be induced by a needle prick, are commonly seen in cases reported from Turkey, but are less common in the United Kingdom.[390] Lesions resembling those seen in Sweet's syndrome have also been a presenting feature.[391]

Behçet's disease occurs most often in young adult males.[392] There are different prevalence rates in different geographical areas: the highest incidence has been reported in Japan, Korea, China, and Eastern Mediterranean countries.[393] A strong association with certain HLA types, particularly Bw51 and B12, has been reported.[385] Familial cases occur.[394]

Numerous causes have been proposed, and these may be grouped into viral, bacterial, immunological and environmental.[385,393] An immunological basis is most favoured because of the wide variety of immunological disturbances that have been identified. These include the presence of circulating immune complexes,[395] enhanced chemotactic activity of neutrophils,[395] alteration of T-cell subsets,[396,397] lymphocytotoxicity to oral epithelial cells[398] and evidence of delayed hypersensitivity to certain streptococcal antigens.[399] The common denominator in all systems appears to be a vasculitis with early infiltration by mononuclear cells and the later presence of neutrophils in some sites.[382]

Histopathology

In aphthous ulcers there is a variable infiltrate of lymphocytes, macrophages and neutrophils in the base of the ulcer.[396] The infiltrate is accentuated around small vessels, and also extends into the epithelium at the margins of the ulcer.[399,400] Some of the intraepithelial lymphocytes appear activated with large indented nuclei.[401] Degenerating prickle cells may be present in the marginal epithelium. There is a virtual absence of plasma cells in early lesions, but these may be quite prominent in older lesions.[400]

The erythema-nodosum-like lesions show a perivascular infiltrate of lymphocytes and other mononuclear cells in the deep dermis and the septa of the subcutaneous fat.[402] Lymphocytes may extend into vessel walls in the manner of a lymphocytic vasculitis, but fibrin is not present. Endothelial cells are often enlarged, and sometimes these show degenerative features, particularly on ultrastructural examination.[402]

Subsequently neutrophils are found in the perivascular collections, and in some cases are quite numerous.[402] The lesions lack the histiocytic granulomas of the usual type of erythema nodosum (see p. 500).[385] A lobular panniculitis has also been described in lesions of Behçet's disease.[386]

In pathergic lesions there is a heavy neutrophil infiltrate, without fibrinoid changes, in the vessel walls.[403] This has been called pustular vasculitis or 'Sweet's-like vasculitis' to distinguish it from leucocytoclastic vasculitis in which fibrinoid change and leucocytoclasis are prominent features (see p. 229).[404] Subsequently there is an influx of chronic inflammatory cells and large numbers of mast cells in the pathergic lesions.[405]

The thrombophlebitic lesions are rarely biopsied. Folliculitis, acneiform lesions, dermal abscesses and a necrotizing vasculitis[213] have all been described in Behçet's disease.[406]

Immunofluorescence studies have shown IgM and C3 in aphthous lesions, often diffusely distributed.[399] Immunoreactants are a less constant feature in the erythema-nodosum-like lesions.

CHRONIC LYMPHOCYTIC VASCULITIS

Lymphocytic vasculitis is not a disease *sui generis*, but rather a group term for a number of clinically heterogeneous diseases which on histopathological examination have evidence of a lymphocytic vasculitis; that is, there is a predominantly lymphocytic infiltrate involving and surrounding the walls of small vessels in the dermis.[407] Often there is associated endothelial cell swelling and some extravasation of erythrocytes, but nuclear dusting is uncommon. While there may be an extravasation of fibrin into vessel walls, this feature should *not* be a requirement for the diagnosis of lymphocytic vasculitis. After all, exudative phenomena are not usually a feature of chronic inflammation.

The following clinical conditions may be regarded as lymphocytic vasculitides:

Toxic erythema
Toxic erythema of pregnancy
Prurigo of pregnancy
Gyrate erythemas
Pityriasis lichenoides
Pigmented purpuric dermatoses
Malignant atrophic papulosis (Degos)
Perniosis
Rickettsial and viral infections
Pyoderma gangrenosum
Polymorphous light eruption (one variant)
Sclerosing lymphangitis of the penis.

It should be noted at the outset that the inclusion of the last three entities is controversial; this will be considered further in the discussion of these entities. A lymphocytic vasculitis has also been reported in the toxic shock syndrome, which results from a toxin produced by *Staphylococcus aureus*,[408] but it is not an invariable finding in this condition.

TOXIC ERYTHEMA

Toxic erythema is a poorly defined clinical entity in which there is a macular or blotchy erythema, sometimes with a small purpuric component. It is usually present on the trunk and proximal extremities. The histopathological term lymphocytic vasculitis is sometimes given clinical connotations and used in place of toxic erythema: this usage should be avoided because the histological picture that this term describes is common to several clinically distinct conditions.

Toxic erythema may result from the ingestion of various drugs, including antibiotics, oral contraceptives,[409] aspirin and, rarely, paracetamol, as well as from various preservatives and dyes added to foods. Viral infections are sometimes implicated. On many occasions the aetiology of toxic erythema is unknown, or at best presumptive.

Histopathology

The appearances are those of a lymphocytic vasculitis, as described above (Fig. 8.15). A small amount of nuclear dust is sometimes present, although fibrin extravasation is quite uncommon.

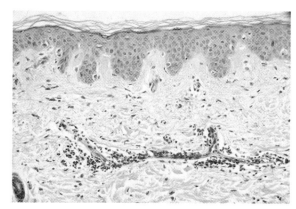

Fig. 8.15   Toxic erythema with a lymphocytic vasculitis. There is no fibrin in vessel walls. Fibrin is often absent in the lymphocytic vasculitides.
Haematoxylin — eosin

TOXIC ERYTHEMA OF PREGNANCY

Toxic erythema of pregnancy,[410] which occurs in approximately 1 in 200 pregnancies, has many synonyms, such as polymorphic eruption of pregnancy,[411,412] late onset prurigo of pregnancy[413–415] and pruritic urticarial papules and plaques of pregnancy (PUPPP).[416–418] It presents as an intensely pruritic eruption of papules and urticarial plaques, sometimes studded with small vesicles. The lesions develop in and around the abdominal striae in the last few weeks of pregnancy.[410] Subsequently they may become widespread on the trunk and limbs, but in contrast to pemphigoid gestationis (herpes gestationis) there is usually sparing of the periumbilical region.[410] The rash usually resolves spontaneously, or with delivery. Only occasionally does it recur in subsequent pregnancies.[417] The finding of increased maternal weight gain, increased neonatal birth weight, and increased twin rate suggests that abdominal distension or a reaction to it may play a role in the development of this condition.[419,419a]

Histopathology[410]

There is a lymphocytic vasculitis with a varying admixture of eosinophils and variable oedema of the papillary dermis.[414,420] The infiltrate may only involve the superficial plexus, although at

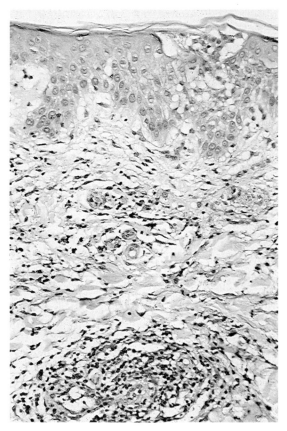

Fig. 8.16   Toxic erythema of pregnancy. Focal spongiosis overlies a lymphocytic vasculitis.
Haematoxylin — eosin

other times it extends to a deeper level. There is sometimes perivascular oedema in the dermis. Nuclear dust has been present in a few cases,[421] but there is no fibrin extravasation. Epidermal changes are present in about one-third of cases and include focal spongiosis and parakeratosis (Fig. 8.16).[422] Exocytosis of inflammatory cells is sometimes present.

Immunofluorescence studies are consistently negative, in contrast to the finding of C3 in the basement membrane zone in pemphigoid gestationis.[411,423]

PRURIGO OF PREGNANCY

This term has been proposed for another pruritic eruption of pregnancy characterized by widely scattered papules, usually arising earlier in pregnancy than toxic erythema.[424-426] It is possibly a heterogeneous entity, which includes prurigo gestationis of Besnier, early onset prurigo of Nurse,[413] pruritic papules of pregnancy[427] and papular dermatitis of pregnancy.[422,428] This last condition is controversial, because in one report the fetal mortality was high, a feature not described in the other pruritic eruptions of pregnancy and not confirmed in subsequent reports.[422]

Histopathology

There are few descriptions of the histopathological changes. A lymphocytic vasculitis similar to that of toxic erythema of pregnancy is present, with the additional features of focal parakeratosis, acanthosis and sometimes excoriations.[427] In some cases the infiltrate is only loosely arranged around vessels and there is then no evidence of vasculitis.

GYRATE ERYTHEMAS

The gyrate erythemas are a heterogeneous group of dermatoses which are akin to toxic erythema[429] in having a tight perivascular lymphohistiocytic infiltrate, which at times involves the vessel walls in the manner of a lymphocytic vasculitis. Clinically, there are one or more circinate, arcuate or polycyclic lesions which may be fixed or migratory.[429-432]

Histopathologically, the gyrate erythemas have been divided on the basis of the distribution of the perivascular infiltrate into a superficial type and a deep type.[433] The superficial gyrate erythemas are usually accompanied by slight spongiosis and focal parakeratosis, which corresponds to the peripheral scale noted clinically; in the deep type there is no spongiosis or parakeratosis and clinically the lesions have a firm cord-like border but no scale. Both types have been included within the entity known as erythema annulare centrifugum, suggesting that it is a heterogeneous entity.[434] The various clinical forms of gyrate erythema fall into one or other of these pathological groups.

The following gyrate erythemas will be considered:

Erythema annulare centrifugum
Erythema gyratum repens
Erythema marginatum
Annular erythemas of infancy
Erythema chronicum migrans.

Erythema annulare centrifugum

This condition is characterized by the presence of one or more annular, erythematous lesions which may spread outwards or remain stationary.[429,430] A fine scale is sometimes present inside the advancing edge. The lesions may be pruritic. They are found most commonly on the trunk and proximal parts of the limbs.

A variety of agents have been implicated in the aetiology of erythema annulare centrifugum,[435] but in a significant number of cases no aetiological agent can be found.[430] The condition has been associated with infections by bacteria,[436] viruses,[437] and fungi, and with infestation by parasites.[438] Malignant tumours,[439-441] foods[430] and drugs[442] have also been blamed. The drugs have included penicillin, cimetidine,[443] salicylates, thiazides,[444] oestrogen-progesterone in oil, and antimalarials.[445] The annular erythema which is occasionally seen in association with Sjögren's syndrome has a wide, elevated border.[446]

The pathogenetic mechanism is unknown; a hypersensitivity reaction to one or other of the agents mentioned above has been suggested.[444]

Histopathology[430,434]

As mentioned above, two distinct patterns — a superficial type and a deep type — may be found. In the superficial variant there is a moderately dense infiltrate of lymphocytes, histiocytes, and, rarely, eosinophils around vessels of the superficial vascular plexus. The infiltrate is well demarcated and has a 'coat-sleeve' distribution. Cells may extend into the walls of the small vessels, but there is never any fibrin extravasation. There may be slight oedema of the papillary dermis. At the advancing edge there is slight spongiosis and focal parakeratosis.

In the deep type a similar infiltrate involves both the superficial and deep vascular plexuses. The epidermis is normal.

Erythema gyratum repens

This rare dermatosis is the most distinctive of the gyrate erythemas.[430,431] There are broad erythematous bands arranged in an arcuate or polycyclic pattern, often accompanied by a trailing scale, and likened to wood grain or marble.[447] The eruption, which is often pruritic,[448] may migrate up to 1 cm per day. It is usually confined to the trunk and proximal parts of the limbs; the face is not affected.[429]

Erythema gyratum repens is usually associated with an internal cancer, particularly of pulmonary origin.[449-451] It has been reported in association with pulmonary tuberculosis,[452] ichthyosis[453] and in the resolving stage of pityriasis rubra pilaris.[454] It also occurs in otherwise healthy individuals.[455,456]

Histopathology[430]

There is usually mild spongiosis with focal parakeratosis and mild acanthosis. A sparse to moderately heavy lymphohistiocytic infiltrate is present around vessels of the superficial plexus, often associated with mild oedema of the papillary dermis.[457] Sometimes the infiltrate includes variable numbers of eosinophils.[458] Its extension to involve the deep vascular plexus has also been reported.[434]

Erythema marginatum

Erythema marginatum is a diagnostic manifestation of rheumatic fever, seen in less than 10% of cases.[449,459] It may develop at any time during the course of the disease, and is more likely to occur in children than adults. The annular eruption is macular or slightly raised, with a pink or red border and a paler centre.[460] Lesions are asymptomatic, transient and migratory.

Histopathology[449,460]

Erythema marginatum is included here because of its clinical appearances. The histopathological changes are not usually those of a lymphocytic vasculitis.[461] Rather, there is a perivascular infiltrate in the upper dermis which includes many neutrophils in addition to a few lymphocytes and eosinophils. It is often said that there is no vasculitis, although mild leucocytoclasis was noted in earlier accounts of the disease.

Annular erythemas of infancy

This term refers to a rare, heterogeneous group of annular erythemas reported under various titles, including familial annular erythema,[462] annular erythema of infancy,[463-465] persistent annular erythema of infancy,[466] erythema gyratum atrophicans transiens neonatale,[467] and infantile epidermodysplastic erythema gyratum.[468] Clinical differences exist between all these entities. Several cases have been associated with maternal lupus erythematosus.[469,470]

Histopathology

Most annular erythemas of infancy show a superficial and deep lymphohistiocytic infiltrate in a perivascular distribution, as seen in the so-called deep gyrate erythemas (see p. 235).[466] They differ by the presence usually of eosinophils and sometimes of neutrophils in the infiltrate. Epidermal atrophy was present in one variant,[467] while bowenoid features were recorded in the epidermis in another.[468]

Erythema chronicum migrans

This annular erythema, caused by *Borrelia burgdorferi*, has been discussed in detail with the spirochaetal infections (see p. 635). The histopathological changes are those of a deep gyrate erythema.

PITYRIASIS LICHENOIDES

Pityriasis lichenoides is an uncommon, self-limiting dermatosis of disputed histogenesis with a spectrum of clinical changes. At one end is a relatively acute disorder with haemorrhagic papules which resolve, leaving varioliform scars — pityriasis lichenoides et varioliformis acuta (PLEVA); at the other end of the spectrum is a less severe disease with small, scaly, red-brown maculopapules, known as pityriasis lichenoides chronica.[471] The distinction between the acute and chronic forms is not always clear-cut.[472] Pityriasis lichenoides may develop at all ages, but there is a predilection for males in the second and third decades of life.[473] Lesions, which vary in number from 20 or so to several hundred, are most common on the anterior aspect of the trunk and the flexor surfaces of the proximal parts of the extremities.

PLEVA. The acute form of pityriasis lichenoides is a papular eruption in which the lesions may become haemorrhagic or crusted before healing to leave a superficial varioliform scar. The lesions appear in crops which heal in several weeks; new lesions may continue to appear for many months or even years, with varying periods of remission. A severe form with ulceronecrotic lesions and constitutional symptoms has been described.[474,475] Fortunately it is quite rare.

Pityriasis lichenoides chronica. The chronic form is more scaly and less haemorrhagic and consists of red-brown inflammatory papules and macules with a characteristic, centrally adherent, 'mica' scale which is easily detached. Post-inflammatory hypopigmentation is quite common in dark-skinned individuals.[476,477]

The pathogenesis of pityriasis lichenoides is unknown: cell-mediated immune mechanisms, possibly related to viral[475] or other infections,[478] may be important.[479] It is usually regarded as a lymphocytic vasculitis. Its relationship to lymphomatoid papulosis is controversial, although a favoured view is that the two diseases are pathogenetically distinct.[480]

Histopathology[480–482]

Pityriasis lichenoides is essentially a lymphocytic vasculitis in which the associated inflammatory cell infiltrate shows exocytosis into the epidermis with obscuration of the dermo–epidermal interface.[483] There is variable death of epidermal keratinocytes which may involve scattered single cells or sheets of cells, resulting in confluent necrosis of the epidermis.[484] Some of the keratinocytes undergo apoptosis. The inflammatory infiltrate and the degree of epidermal changes are more prominent in PLEVA than in pityriasis lichenoides chronica.

In *PLEVA* there is a sharply delimited, sparse to moderately dense inflammatory cell infiltrate involving the superficial vascular plexus. Sometimes this extends in a wedge-shaped pattern to involve also the lower dermis. The infiltrate is composed of lymphocytes and some macrophages; in florid cases there may be some perivascular neutrophils as well. A few atypical lymphoid cells may be found in a small number of cases. There is endothelial swelling involving small vessels and extravasation of red blood cells. Only occasionally do the vessels show fibrinoid necrosis.[474,485] The papillary dermis is variably oedematous.

Lymphocytes and some erythrocytes extend into the epidermis (Fig. 8.17). This is associated with some basal vacuolar change and spongiosis.[482] Degenerate keratinocytes are not restricted to the basal layer, and they are often more prominent in the upper layers of the epidermis. In advanced lesions there is often extensive epidermal necrosis. Overlying parakeratosis is quite common and there may be some neutrophils forming a parakeratotic crust.[481]

In *pityriasis lichenoides chronica*[486] the infiltrate is less dense and more superficial than in PLEVA and the epidermal changes are much less pronounced.[487] There is a relatively sparse perivascular infiltrate with only subtle features of a lymphocytic vasculitis. A few extravasated erythrocytes may be present. There are small areas of basal vacuolar change associated with minimal exocytosis of lymphocytes and occasional degenerate keratinocytes.

The epidermis shows variable acanthosis and is sometimes vaguely psoriasiform. Pallor of the upper epidermis may be noted, with overlying parakeratosis. Late lesions may show mild

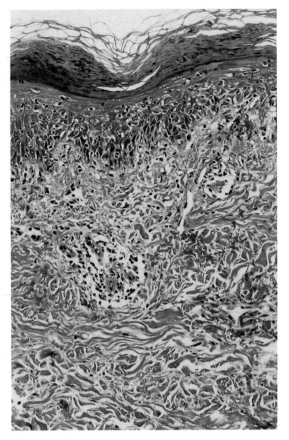

Fig. 8.17 Pityriasis lichenoides. In this acute variant there is a lichenoid reaction pattern with 'interface obscuring'. The lymphocytic vasculitis is not well shown in this field. Haematoxylin — eosin

fibrosis of the papillary dermis and the presence of some melanophages, changes which are also found in late lesions of PLEVA.

Immunofluorescence reveals the presence of immunoreactants, particularly IgM and C3, along the basement membrane zone and in vessels of the papillary dermis in a small number of cases.[488–490] Immunoperoxidase studies have shown that the lymphocytes in the dermal infiltrate are T cells, particularly of cytotoxic/suppressor type.[479] Approximately 5% of the perivascular cells are Langerhans or indeterminate cells.[479] The epidermis in the lesions is HLA-DR positive.[487]

PIGMENTED PURPURIC DERMATOSES

The pigmented purpuric dermatoses are a group of chronic skin disorders with overlapping clinical and histopathological features.[491–493] The lesions are purpuric, with variable pigmentation resulting from the deposition of haemosiderin, which is, in turn, a consequence of the extravasation of red blood cells from capillaries in the papillary dermis. There is a predilection for the lower extremities of young adults. Cases have been reported also in children.[494] Four clinical variants have been recognized.

Progressive pigmentary dermatosis (Schamberg's disease) is the most common type.[495] There are numerous punctate purpuric macules forming confluent patches. These are usually symmetrically distributed in the pretibial region. Familial cases have been described.[496] The eczematid-like purpura of Doucas and Kapetanakis,[497] the itching purpura of Loewenthal[498–500] and disseminated pruriginous angiodermatitis[501] are now regarded as variants of Schamberg's disease. These pruritic forms usually have an acute onset and a self-limited course.

Purpura annularis telangiectodes of Majocchi has annular patches with perifollicular, red punctate lesions and telangiectasias.[492]

Pigmented purpuric lichenoid dermatosis of Gougerot and Blum consists of lichenoid papules which may coalesce to give plaque-like lesions. They are often symmetrically distributed on the lower legs.[492] If unilateral, the plaque may mimic Kaposi's sarcoma.[502]

Lichen aureus consists of grouped macules or lichenoid papules having a rusty, golden or even purplish colour.[503–505] Lesions may occur on the trunk or upper extremity, although the lower parts of the legs are the site of predilection.[506,507] Involvement of the glans penis has been reported.[508] Lichen aureus is usually unilateral.[505]

Three different pathogenetic mechanisms have been proposed for the pigmented purpuric dermatoses.[509] These include disturbed humoral immunity, cellular immune reactions related to the dermal infiltrate of lymphocytes, macrophages and Langerhans cells,[509,510] and weakness of blood vessels with increased capillary fragility.[511] Perforator vein incompetence was present in one series of cases of lichen aureus.[512] There are isolated reports implicating sensitivity to oils used in wool processing,[513] exposure to dyes,[514] and treatment with thiamine,[514] carbromal and meprobamate.[515]

Histopathology

There is a variable infiltrate of lymphocytes and macrophages in the upper dermis. This is band-like and heavy in lichen aureus, and less dense and with perivascular accentuation in the other variants (Figs 8.18 and 8.19). A lymphocytic vasculitis involving vessels in the papillary dermis may be present in active cases (Fig. 8.20). The infiltrate is composed predominantly of helper/inducer T lymphocytes with some OKT–6 (CDI) reactive Langerhans cells.[509] Plasma cells are sometimes present in lichen aureus, while a few neutrophils are usually seen in the infiltrate in the lesions of itching purpura (Fig. 8.21). There is often exocytosis of lymphocytes, and associated spongiosis of the epidermis in all

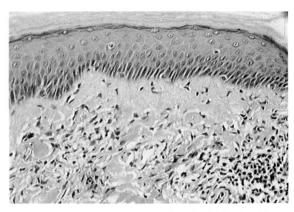

Fig. 8.19   Pigmented purpuric eruption. The infiltrate is less heavy in this case and it fills the papillary dermis. Haemosiderin is present in macrophages. Haematoxylin — eosin

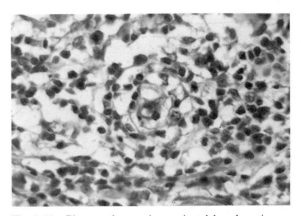

Fig. 8.20   Pigmented purpuric eruption. A lymphocytic vasculitis is present. It is not always as obvious as in this case. Haematoxylin — eosin

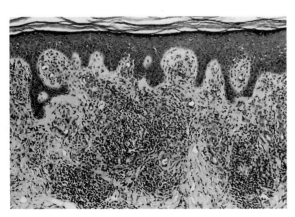

Fig. 8.18   Pigmented purpuric eruption. This condition is characterized by an infiltrate which involves the papillary dermis. Tight lymphocytic cuffing of vessels in the papillary dermis is often present. Haematoxylin — eosin

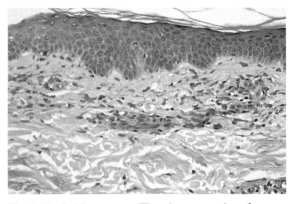

Fig. 8.21   Itching purpura. There is extravasation of erythrocytes and mild cuffing of small vessels in the papillary dermis by lymphocytes. Haematoxylin — eosin

variants except lichen aureus; in the latter a thin layer of uninvolved collagen separates the undersurface of the epidermis from the inflammatory infiltrate below.[516,517] When spongiosis is present, there is often focal parakeratosis as well.

There is variable extravasation of red blood cells into the papillary dermis. Haemosiderin is present, predominantly in macrophages, although small amounts are sometimes found lying free in the papillary dermis, and even in the epidermis. Sometimes the macrophages containing the haemosiderin are at or below the lower margin of the inflammatory infiltrate, but the haemosiderin is never as deep in the dermis as in stasis dermatitis.[491] Haemosiderin is usually absent in early lesions of itching purpura. Blood vessels in the papillary dermis may be dilated, but more often there is endothelial swelling causing luminal narrowing. Occasionally, there is hyaline thickening of blood vessel walls or pericapillary fibrosis.

An eruption which resembles pigmented purpuric dermatosis both clinically and histologically is an uncommon presentation of mycosis fungoides.[518] At this early stage of the latter there may be no distinguishing features.

Immunofluorescence studies have usually been negative, except for the presence of perivascular fibrin. In one study C3, and sometimes immunoglobulins, were present in vessel walls.[519]

Electron microscopy. Ultrastructural studies have not contributed in any way to our understanding of these dermatoses.[520] Langerhans cells have been identified in the inflammatory infiltrate.

MALIGNANT ATROPHIC PAPULOSIS

Malignant atrophic papulosis (Degos' disease) is a rare, often fatal, multisystem disorder in which pathognomonic skin lesions are frequently associated with infarctive lesions of other viscera, particularly the gastrointestinal tract.[521–523] Patients develop crops of papules, approximately 0.5–1 cm in diameter, which evolve slowly to become umbilicated, with a porcelain white centre and a telangiectatic rim, and finally leave an atrophic scar.[522] There are approximately 10 to 40 lesions at any time, in different stages of evolution. In 60% of cases, gastrointestinal involvement supervenes, usually within a year, but sometimes after a long interval.[523] This takes the form of infarction with perforation, leading to fatal peritonitis. Some patients have only cutaneous lesions and a relatively benign course.[524,525] Involvement of the central nervous system may also occur;[526,527] less commonly, other viscera also develop infarcts.[528] There are several reports of familial involvement,[529,530] including one in which the mother and five children were affected.[531]

Malignant atrophic papulosis has been regarded as an 'endovasculitis', or primary endothelial defect,[532] with secondary thrombosis leading to infarctive lesions.[533] Impaired fibrinolytic activity has been detected in cutaneous lesions,[524,534] but there are no circulating immune complexes.[532] Most authors agree that the condition is not a vasculitis in the sense that allergic vasculitis and polyarteritis nodosa are;[532] however a study of ultrathin sections led to the conclusion that it is a lymphocyte-mediated necrotizing vasculitis.[535] Malignant atrophic papulosis has also been regarded as a mucinosis (see p. 393).[521]

Histopathology[523,535]

A well-developed lesion shows epidermal atrophy with overlying hyperkeratosis, and an underlying wedge-shaped area of cutaneous ischaemia, the apex of which extends into the deep dermis (Fig. 8.22). This dermal area is uniformly hypereosinophilic and relatively acellular. A mild to moderately dense lymphocytic infiltrate is present at the edge of the ischaemic wedge, particularly in the mid and lower dermis.[525,535] The infiltrate has a perivenular and intervenular distribution. There is marked endothelial swelling of venules, and to a lesser extent arterioles, sometimes with obliteration of the lumen. There are fibrin-platelet thrombi in some small vessels and there is some perivenular distribution of fibrin in the

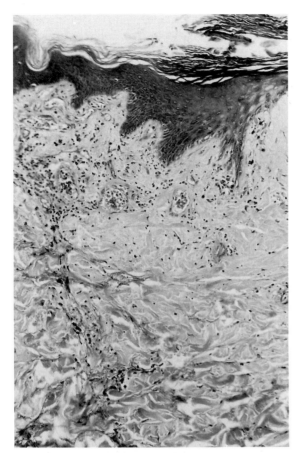

Fig. 8.22 Malignant atrophic papulosis. There is central epidermal parakeratosis, mild lymphocytic cuffing of vessels in the deep dermis and separation of collagen bundles at the periphery resulting from an increase in interstitial mucin. Haematoxylin — eosin

dermis.[535] A study using thin sections has also shown ghost-like infarcted small vessels and demyelination of cutaneous nerves.[535] Red cells fill the lumen of some small vessels.

Sometimes the epidermis shows focal infarction or scattered necrotic keratinocytes in addition to the atrophy. There may also be some basal vacuolar change.

A prominent feature is the presence of abundant acid mucopolysaccharides in the dermis.[521,536] Initially these are localized to the ischaemic zone, but in older lesions the material is confined to the margins of this zone.[537] They stain with the colloidal iron or alcian blue methods.

Immunofluorescence studies have given conflicting results. Fibrin is always demonstrated, and sometimes immunoglobulins and complement may be found around small dermal vessels, or near the basement membrane.[535]

Electron microscopy. There is swelling of endothelial cells with various degenerative changes,[535] and sometimes luminal occlusion by endothelial cells and cell fragments. Tubular aggregates are often seen in the endothelial cells.[538,539]

PERNIOSIS

Perniosis is a localized inflammatory lesion which develops in certain individuals exposed to cold temperatures.[540,541] Classic perniosis (chilblains) occurs on the fingers and toes, but plaques have also been described on the thighs.[541] Lupus erythematosus is uncommonly complicated by perniosis (chilblain lupus erythematosus).[542] A possible occasional association with chronic myelomonocytic leukaemia has also been suggested.[543]

Histopathology[541]

Perniosis is a lymphocytic vasculitis in which there is oedema and thickening of vessel walls associated with a mural and perivascular infiltrate of lymphocytes. A few neutrophils and eosinophils may be present in early lesions. The term 'fluffy oedema' has been used to describe the vessel wall changes.[541] Sometimes vessels at all levels of the dermis are involved, while at other times the process is confined to the more superficial vessels. There is variable oedema of the papillary dermis which is sometimes quite intense.[541] Basal vacuolar change is present in lupus pernio.[542]

RICKETTSIAL AND VIRAL INFECTIONS

A lymphocytic vasculitis, often associated with fibrin extravasation, is characteristic of the maculopapular rash of the various rickettsial infections (see p. 620). If an eschar is present, necrosis of the epidermis and upper dermis will be found, with a vasculitis at the periphery of the lesion. Fibrin thrombi are often present in these vessels.

Herpes virus, and possibly other viral infections, may be associated with a lymphocytic vasculitis. In the case of herpes virus this has been reported in association with a lichenoid inflammatory infiltrate.[544]

PYODERMA GANGRENOSUM

Pyoderma gangrenosum is a clinically distinctive disorder characterized by the development of an erythematous pustule or nodule which rapidly progresses to become a necrotic ulcer with a ragged, undermined, violaceous edge.[545,546] Lesions may be single or multiple.[547] Although most ulcers are less than 3 cm in diameter, large lesions up to 20 cm or more in diameter may result from coalescence of smaller ulcers.[547] Not infrequently minor trauma may initiate the onset of a lesion, a process known as pathergy.[548]

Pyoderma gangrenosum has a predilection for the lower extremities,[546] although sometimes the trunk, and rarely the head and neck,[549] may also be involved. Onset is usually in mid-adult life, but onset in childhood has been recorded.[550,551] Familial occurrence is exceedingly rare.[552]

In cases associated with haematological malignancies, the lesions may develop bullae at the advancing edge.[553–556] This clinical variant is histogenetically similar to Sweet's syndrome and cases with overlap features have been recorded (see p. 229). Another clinical variant is *malignant pyoderma*, a rare, ulcerating, destructive condition of the skin of the head, neck and upper part of the trunk, but which has a predilection for the preauricular region.[548,557–559] Individual lesions lack the undermined, violaceous border of pyoderma gangrenosum, and there is usually no associated systemic disease.[558,560] Another clinicopathological variant has been reported as *superficial granulomatous pyoderma*.[561,562] It is characterized by a superficial ulcer, usually solitary and on the trunk. It may arise at sites of surgical incision or

other pathergic stimuli. Draining sinuses may be present.[561] It runs a chronic course, although it usually responds to topical therapy.[562]

In more than half of the cases of pyoderma gangrenosum there is an associated systemic illness such as ulcerative colitis,[563] Crohn's disease,[564–566] rheumatoid arthritis,[546] seronegative polyarthritis, or a monoclonal gammopathy, particularly of IgA type.[567] Rare clinical associations[568] have included chronic active hepatitis,[569,570] chronic persistent hepatitis,[571] thyroid disease,[546] sarcoidosis, hidradenitis suppurativa,[546] Behçet's disease,[572] subcorneal pustular dermatosis,[573] internal cancer,[574,575] diabetes mellitus,[576] polycythaemia rubra vera,[577] and an immunosuppressed state.[578,579]

Pyoderma gangrenosum may run an acute progressive course with rapidly expanding lesions which require systemic treatment to arrest their growth.[580,581] Other cases pursue a more chronic course with slow extension, and sometimes spontaneous regression after weeks or months.[580] Lesions eventually heal leaving a parchment or cribriform scar.

Multiple abnormalities of humoral immunity, cell-mediated immunity and neutrophil function have been reported, although the pathogenetic significance of these findings remains an enigma.[545,582–585] Some of these abnormalities may be nothing more than epiphenomena. The role, if any, of a vasculitis in the pathogenesis of pyoderma gangrenosum is debatable (see below).[586]

Histopathology[545,546,587]

The findings are quite variable and depend on the age of the lesion and the site biopsied. The most controversial aspect of the histopathology relates to the presence (or not) of a vasculitis.[571] A lymphocytic vasculitis has been reported at the advancing erythematous border,[546] although Ackerman has written, 'I now believe that all cases of pyoderma gangrenosum begin as folliculitides and that vasculitis is not a primary event in pyoderma gangrenosum'.[588]

The earliest lesion shows follicular and perifollicular inflammation with intradermal abscess formation.[551,588] In later lesions there is

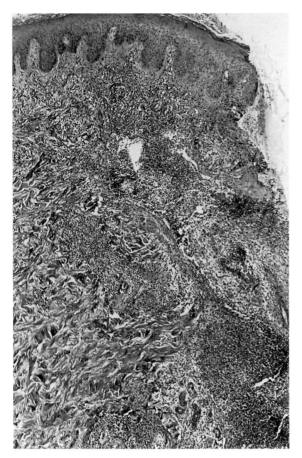

Fig. 8.23 Pyoderma gangrenosum. A deep ulcer is present. Tight lymphocytic cuffing of vessels in the margin of the ulcer is present.
Haematoxylin — eosin

necrosis of the superficial dermis and epidermis forming an ulcer, the base of which shows a mixed inflammatory cell infiltrate with abscess formation.[587] The process may extend into the underlying subcutis (Fig. 8.23).

At the advancing edge there is a tight perivascular infiltrate of lymphocytes and plasma cells with endothelial swelling and fibrinoid extravasation representing a lymphocytic vasculitis.[587] This finding has been disputed by some authors.[581] A leucocytoclastic vasculitis is rarely present.[589,590]

There is often subepidermal oedema at the advancing edge. This is prominent and associated with intraepidermal bullae with pustulation in those variants with bullous changes at the advancing edge.[556] Acanthosis is a prominent change in the perilesional erythematous zone.

In the variant known as *superficial granulomatous pyoderma*, there are superficial dermal abscesses surrounded by a narrow zone of histiocytes and some giant cells of foreign body type.[561,562] Beyond this there is a mixed inflammatory cell infiltrate which often includes plasma cells and eosinophils. There is often pseudoepitheliomatous hyperplasia. The follicular infundibula may be enlarged, possibly in association with transepidermal elimination of inflammatory debris. There is some resemblance to the changes seen in blastomycosis-like pyoderma, although in this latter condition the inflammatory process is usually much deeper in the dermis and palisading histiocytes are not usually prominent; furthermore, the two processes usually occur at different sites (see p. 601).

Immunoreactants have been reported around blood vessels in the dermis in over 50% of cases of pyoderma gangrenosum in one series.[591] They have not been detected by others.[581]

POLYMORPHOUS LIGHT ERUPTION

In some cases of polymorphous light eruption, particularly the papulovesicular variant, the tight perivascular lymphocytic infiltrate mimics closely the picture seen in lymphocytic vasculitis, although there is never any fibrinoid change in the vessels. Red cell extravasation is invariably present in the papulovesicular variant. Polymorphous light eruption is discussed further on page 581.

SCLEROSING LYMPHANGITIS OF THE PENIS

This condition is characterized by the sudden appearance of a firm, cord-like, nodular lesion in the coronal sulcus or on the dorsum of the shaft of the penis.[592] It is usually asymptomatic and subsides after several weeks. Recurrences are documented. The aetiology is unknown, but sexual intercourse,[593,594] herpes infection[595]

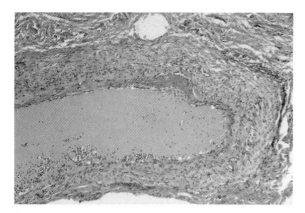

Fig. 8.24   Sclerosing lymphangitis of the penis. Condensed eosinophilic material fills the lumen of a vessel, most likely a vein.
Haematoxylin — eosin

and secondary syphilis[596] have been incriminated in some cases.

Histopathology[597–599]

Established lesions show a dilated vessel, the lumen of which contains condensed eosinophilic material or a fibrin thrombus in the process of recanalization (Fig. 8.24). Lymphocytes and macrophages are often present within the thrombus. The wall of the vessel shows prominent fibrous thickening.[592] There is usually a mild inflammatory cell infiltrate and some oedema around the involved channel. The vessel is usually said to be a lymphatic but the suggestion has been made that it is in fact a vein and that the condition may be likened to Mondor's phlebitis (see p. 228).[600]

Electron microscopy.   Small lymphatic capillaries containing lymphocytes form within the luminal thrombus.[597] Newly formed collagen fibrils are present in the vessel walls.

VASCULITIS WITH GRANULOMATOSIS

The term 'vasculitis with granulomatosis' is the preferred designation for those diseases which show varying degrees of granulomatosis, both angiocentric and unrelated to vessels, in combination with a vasculitis which may be necrotizing.[601,602] The term 'granulomatous vasculitis', although often used interchangeably, is more limited in its meaning[603,604] and, strictly interpreted, refers to granulomatous involvement of vessel walls[605] without the formation of extravascular granulomas.

The important clinical entities showing vasculitis with granulomatosis include Wegener's granulomatosis, lymphomatoid granulomatosis, allergic granulomatosis (Churg–Strauss syndrome) and midline granuloma.[601] Temporal arteritis and Takayasu's arteritis are usually considered with this group, although the granulomatous inflammation is restricted to the vessel walls. Granulomatous involvement of vessel walls and/or perivascular granulomas may also be seen in a wide range of clinical settings which include lymphoma, angioimmunoblastic lymphadenopathy, sarcoidosis, Crohn's disease,[606] drug reactions,[607] rheumatoid arthritis, infectious granulomatous diseases such as tuberculosis and tertiary syphilis, and less well defined circumstances.[608] The important entities will be considered below.

WEGENER'S GRANULOMATOSIS

Wegener's granulomatosis is a rare systemic disease with necrotizing vasculitis and granulomas involving the upper and lower respiratory tracts, accompanied usually by a focal necrotizing glomerulitis. A vasculitis involving both arteries and veins may involve other organs, including the skin.[609] The disease usually presents in the fourth and fifth decades of life with symptoms related to the upper respiratory tract such as persistent rhinorrhoea and sinus pain.[609,610] Other clinical features may include a cough, haemoptysis, otitis media, ocular signs, arthralgia and constitutional symptoms.[604]

Cutaneous manifestations occur in 40–50% of cases and may occasionally be the presenting complaint.[611,612] They often take the form of papulonecrotic lesions distributed symmetrically over the elbows, knees, and sometimes the buttocks. Other reported clinical lesions[613] include purpura,[610] vesicular and urticarial eruptions, subcutaneous nodules, necrotizing granulomas in scars, and, in one case,[614] breast involvement.

An important clinical variant is the so-called *limited form* in which pulmonary lesions predominate and a glomerulitis is absent.[615,616] Cutaneous lesions are less frequent and may take the form of subcutaneous nodules. The limited form has a better prognosis. Another clinical variant is characterized by protracted mucosal and cutaneous lesions, even in untreated cases.[605]

Wegener's granulomatosis is almost uniformly fatal if not treated; deaths may occur despite treatment.[617,618]

The aetiology and pathogenesis are unknown, but it appears to result from an immunological disturbance in which both immune complexes and delayed hypersensitivity reactions may be implicated.[619] Of interest is the recent finding in the serum of IgG antibodies which react against cytoplasmic components of neutrophils. While these have diagnostic implication their pathogenetic significance awaits further elucidation.[620,621]

A clinical response to antibiotics has been demonstrated, but it should be stressed that this does not necessarily imply an infective aetiology.[622]

Histopathology[605,612,623,623a]

The full picture of a necrotizing vasculitis with granulomatosis is seen in the skin in 20% or less of cases of Wegener's granulomatosis.[601] Sometimes the findings are quite non-specific, with only a chronic inflammatory cell infiltrate in the dermis. In specifically diagnostic lesions, vascular and extravascular changes are present in varying proportions.

Extravascular changes include small foci of necrosis and fibrinoid degeneration, usually without vascular participation. There may be some neutrophil infiltration and nuclear dusting in these foci. Palisading, which varies from minimal to well-defined, may develop in older lesions. Poorly formed granulomas, unrelated to necrotic areas, may also be present. Giant cells are almost invariably present in the palisading margins of the granulomas, in granulation tissue lining ulcerated surfaces, or scattered irregularly in the chronic inflammation which forms a background to the entire process.[605] Rarely, eosinophils are prominent in the infiltrate.[624] No atypical mononuclear cells are present. Granulomas resembling those seen in allergic granulomatosis (Churg–Strauss syndrome) have been reported in several cases (see p. 246).[625]

Vascular changes may take the form of a necrotizing angiitis involving small and medium-sized dermal vessels. Fibrin extends around the vessel walls and sometimes there is a fibrin thrombus in the lumen. Red cell extravasation accompanies the vasculitis. Less commonly, a granulomatous vasculitis with angiocentric granulomas is present.[612]

Special stains are non-contributory, although specific infective causes of granulomas should always be kept in mind in the differential diagnosis. Immunofluorescence microscopy will sometimes show C3 and immunoglobulins related to vessels in early lesions.

LYMPHOMATOID GRANULOMATOSIS

Lymphomatoid granulomatosis, first described in 1972,[626] is a unique form of pulmonary angiitis and granulomatosis which frequently has extrapulmonary manifestations.[627] Skin lesions have been noted in 40–60% of cases, and these may be the presenting complaint.[628–631] They take the form of erythematous or violaceous nodules and plaques which may be widely distributed on the trunk and lower extremities.[630,632] Rarely, paranasal or ulcerated palatal lesions are present.[633] Any of the lesions may become ulcerated, with surface eschar formation, but this is more common with nodules on the leg.

Other clinical features include fever, cough, malaise, weight loss, dyspnoea and pulmonary infiltrates.[627] Onset is usually in early middle age; the illness runs a rapid course with a median survival of 14 months.[627] Death is usually from respiratory failure. In an increasing number of cases (up to 40%), a widespread lymphoma has developed:[627,634,635] this has been described as resembling immunoblastic lymphoma; recent cases have shown T-cell markers.[636-638]

Although the aetiology is unknown, it appears that the atypical proliferative cells are of T-cell origin,[639-642] like those in the lymphomas that sometimes develop in this condition (see above). Lymphomatoid granulomatosis has some features that overlap with those seen in angiocentric T-cell lymphoma (see p. 1042).

Histopathology[630]

There is a polymorphous infiltrate in the dermis, with perivascular, periappendageal and perineural accentuation.[629,634] Sweat glands are particularly involved.[639] The infiltrate often

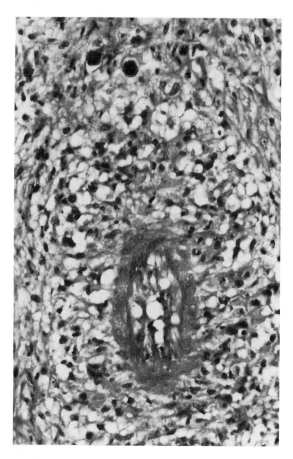

Fig. 8.25 Lymphomatoid granulomatosis. An atypical infiltrate involves the wall of a small artery in the deep dermis.
Haematoxylin — eosin

extends into the subcutis, although the epidermis and papillary dermis are usually spared.[643]

The infiltrate is composed of a mixture of lymphocytes, histiocytes and 'lymphohistiocytoid' cells, some of which may show plasmacytoid features.[629] Occasional giant cells impart a vague granulomatous aura. However, granulomas are less conspicuous and much less distinct than in Wegener's granulomatosis.[601] Occasional eosinophils may be present in the infiltrate, but neutrophils are rare, except beneath ulcerated surfaces. There may be atypical cells and scattered mitoses, but the degree of atypia, which is never as great in the skin as in other organs, varies from case to case.[644]

As well as being angiocentric, the infiltrate is frequently angioinvasive (Fig. 8.25). Sometimes an endothelium-lined lumen in the centre of a lymphohistiocytic aggregate is the only sign of a residual vessel.[643] Both arteries and veins may be affected. Fibrinoid necrosis of vessel walls and infarction are not usually prominent features in the skin. Marked fibroblastic proliferation may be present in some lesions.[645]

Sometimes the histology of the skin lesions is not diagnostic, despite the presence of typical changes in other organs of the body.

ALLERGIC GRANULOMATOSIS

Allergic granulomatosis (Churg–Strauss syndrome) is a clinically distinctive, idiopathic disease in which systemic vasculitis and hypereosinophilia develop in individuals with pre-existing asthma and allergic rhinitis.[646-648] Tissue eosinophilia, peripheral neuropathy, cardiac lesions and mild renal disease may also be present. A limited form of the disease, in which not all of the above features are present, has been described.[649]

Cutaneous lesions are common and include purpura, erythema or urticarial lesions, and distinctive nodules.[650] These nodules, which are often tender, arise on the scalp or symmetrically on the extremities.

The prognosis is variable, but most patients

appear to have a good response to corticosteroid therapy.

The aetiology of allergic granulomatosis is unknown. Of interest is the report of its occurrence in a patient with antibodies to hepatitis B virus and to the human immunodeficiency virus.[651]

Histopathology

The three major histological features are a necrotizing vasculitis, tissue infiltration by eosinophils and extravascular granulomas.[647] The vasculitis involves small arteries and veins, but it may also affect larger arteries and resemble polyarteritis nodosa.[652] Older lesions show healing with scarring. The tissue infiltration with eosinophils is accompanied by destruction of some of these cells, leading to release of their granules and increased eosinophilia of the collagen.[647] The extravascular granulomas, which result in the cutaneous nodules found in some patients, show central necrosis which may be fibrinoid or partly basophilic, with interspersed neutrophils, eosinophils and debris.[650] This area is surrounded by a granulomatous proliferation of histiocytes, lymphocytes and giant cells, often in palisaded array.[650] Granulomas were present in less than half the autopsy cases included in one review.[647] Non-necrotizing granulomas were present in a case of limited allergic granulomatosis.[649]

It should be noted that the three components mentioned above do not always coexist temporally or spatially.[647] Furthermore, similar extravascular granulomas, sometimes referred to as Churg–Strauss granulomas, have been described in association with systemic vasculitis and autoimmune or immunoreactive disorders:[653] these include Wegener's granulomatosis, polyarteritis nodosa, Takayasu's aortitis,[654] systemic lupus erythematosus, rheumatoid arthritis, various lymphoproliferative disorders[655] and some other conditions.[652] In the granulomas found in these diseases, the central necrotic area is invariably basophilic.[656] Furthermore, there is an absence of the tissue eosinophilia within and around the granulomas that is seen in allergic granulomatosis.

LETHAL MIDLINE GRANULOMA

Lethal midline granuloma (Stewart type of non-healing necrotizing granuloma) is a controversial disease category which has been regarded by some as a distinct clinicopathological entity,[657,658] and by others as merely a clinical term to describe any rapidly evolving, destructive lesion of the nose and deep facial tissues.[659–661] Those ascribing to the latter view believe that this clinical picture is an expression of either Wegener's granulomatosis or malignant lymphoma derived from peripheral T cells.[659] Further controversy revolves around its relationship to lymphomatoid granulomatosis, which may also present with this clinical picture. An account of this difficult and challenging subject is included in Volume 1 of this book.[661a] It would seem that the final words on this controversy have not yet been written.[662]

Based on several reports of patients in whom neither malignant lymphoma nor Wegener's granulomatosis is a sustainable diagnosis, it appears that a group of patients exists who present with indurated swelling of the cheek and nose with relentless destruction of midline facial structures.[601,658] There is often a preceding history of non-specific sinusitis and rhinitis. The process does not involve lungs or kidneys.[663] Although progression to lymphoma has been reported, some of these cases may represent malignancy de novo.[658] There is a good response to radiotherapy in lethal midline granuloma with survival exceeding 7–10 years.[663]

Histopathology[658]

Lethal midline granuloma is included here because granulomas and vasculitis may occur.[601] The usual picture is a dense polymorphic infiltrate composed of lymphocytes, plasma cells and some polygonal and spindle-shaped histiocytes in a background of granulation and fibrous tissue. Necrosis is usually prominent. Vasculitis is uncommon but endarteritis obliterans may be seen. Clear-cut granulomas were present in 4 of the 10 cases in one series.[658] Atypical cells are uncommon, although those who equate the diagnosis of 'midline malignant reticulosis' with the Stewart type of lethal midline granuloma report atypical lymphoid cells in all cases.[660] In my view these are examples of peripheral T-cell lymphoma.

GIANT CELL (TEMPORAL) ARTERITIS

Giant cell arteritis is a granulomatous vasculitis involving large or medium-sized elastic arteries, with a predilection for the superficial temporal and ophthalmic arteries, and to a lesser extent other extracranial branches of the carotid arteries.[664,665] The onset is usually late in life. The protean clinical manifestations include severe headache, jaw claudication, and visual and neurological disturbances.[666,667] Its relationship to polymyalgia rheumatica is controversial.[668]

Cutaneous manifestations are uncommon, the most frequent being necrosis of the scalp with ulceration.[668-671] This may be localized to one side, or it may be bitemporal with large areas of necrosis.[672,673] Alopecia, hyperpigmentation and scalp tenderness may occur.[674]

The aetiology is unknown. It has been suggested that the condition results from inflammation and elastolysis (with resorption), involving actinically damaged fibres of the internal elastic lamina of the temporal artery.[675,676] Another suggestion is that cell-mediated immunity, especially a T-cell-regulated granulomatous reaction, may play a role in the pathogenesis of temporal arteritis.[677]

Histopathology [678]

It has been suggested that as a significant number of patients with clinical temporal arteritis have negative biopsies, a trial of steroid therapy would be a better indicator of this diagnosis than temporal artery biopsy.[679] The percentage of positive biopsies depends on the number of sections examined, as skip lesions do occur.[680] The histological changes will also reflect the stage of the disease process.

The classic findings are a granulomatous arteritis involving the inner media, with prominent giant cells of both Langhans and 'foreign

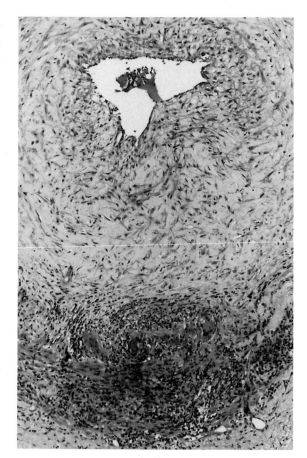

Fig. 8.26 Temporal arteritis. An inflammatory cell infiltrate is present in relation to the elastic lamina. Haematoxylin — eosin

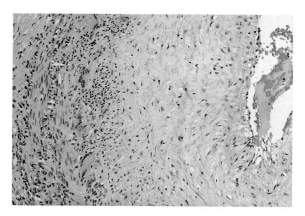

Fig. 8.27 Temporal arteritis. A few multinucleate giant cells and some lymphocytes are present in the wall of the temporal artery adjacent to the internal elastic lamina. Haematoxylin — eosin

body' type (Figs 8.26 and 8.27). This is associated with fragmentation and focal destruction of the internal elastic lamina. A non-specific inflammatory cell infiltrate which includes variable numbers of lymphocytes, histiocytes and even eosinophils is often present. Giant cells are not mandatory for the diagnosis,[681] and their absence may not indicate a worse prognosis,[682] as suggested in one report.[683]

Some biopsies show intimal thickening with a proliferation of fibroblasts and myointimal cells, but little or no change in the media.[678] There is usually an abundant myxomatoid stroma, and a scattering of inflammatory cells. The internal elastic lamina is fragmented or thickened, with some loss of staining with elastic stains. The lumen is narrowed. These changes appear to represent an active process, and not a healed stage, as once thought.[678] In old lesions, there

may be evidence of recanalization of the lumen.

A much more florid inflammatory reaction is present in the exceedingly rare cases of Buerger's disease (thromboangiitis obliterans) of the temporal artery.[684]

TAKAYASU'S ARTERITIS

Takayasu's arteritis (aortic arch syndrome, pulseless disease) is an uncommon large vessel granulomatous vasculitis, with a predilection for young females.[685] It results in fibrosis leading to constriction or occlusion of the aorta and its main branches. Associated skin lesions include erythema nodosum, pyodermatous ulcers, non-specific erythematous rashes, urticaria and necrotizing vasculitis.[654,685] Takayasu's arteritis does not involve cutaneous vessels.

REFERENCES

Non-inflammatory purpuras

1. Rasmussen JE. Puzzling purpuras in children and young adults. J Am Acad Dermatol 1982; 6: 67–72.
2. Ackerman Z, Michaeli J, Gorodetsky R. Skin discoloration in chronic idiopathic thrombocytopenic purpura: detection of local iron deposition by X-ray spectrometry. Dermatologica 1986; 172: 222–224.
3. Pearson B, Mazza JJ. Gardner–Diamond syndrome with multiple glomus tumors. Arch Dermatol 1975; 111: 893–895.
4. Stocker WW, McIntyre R, Clendenning WE. Psychogenic purpura. Arch Dermatol 1977: 113: 606–609.
5. Tattersall RN, Seville R. Senile purpura. Q J Med 1950; 19: 151–159.
6. Shuster S, Scarborough H. Senile purpura. Q J Med 1961; 30: 33–40.
7. Feinstein RJ, Halprin KM, Penneys NS et al. Senile purpura. Arch Dermatol 1973; 108: 229–232.
8. Haboubi NY, Haboubi NAA, Gyde O et al. Zinc deficiency in senile purpura. J Clin Pathol 1985; 38: 1189–1191.

Vascular occlusive diseases

9. Copeman PWM. Livedo reticularis. Signs in the skin of disturbance of blood viscosity and of blood flow. Br J Dermatol 1975; 93: 519–529.
10. Champion RH. Livedo reticularis. A review. Br J Dermatol 1965; 77: 167–179.
11. Bruce S, Wolf JE Jr. Quinidine-induced photosensitive

livedo reticularis-like eruption. J Am Acad Dermatol 1985; 12: 332–336.
12. Kramer BS, Hernandez AD, Reddick RL, Levine AS. Cutaneous infarction. Manifestation of disseminated mucormycosis. Arch Dermatol 1977; 113: 1075–1076.
13. Kossard S, Spigel GT, Winkelmann RK. Cutaneous and subcutaneous endarteritis obliterans. Arch Dermatol 1978; 114: 1652–1658.
14. Schleicher SM, Fricker MP. Coumarin necrosis. Arch Dermatol 1980; 116: 444–445.
15. Kirby JD, Marriott PJ. Skin necrosis following warfarin therapy. Br J Dermatol 1976; 94: 97–99.
16. Schiff BL, Kern AB. Cutaneous reactions to anticoagulants. Arch Dermatol 1968; 98: 136–137.
17. Stone MS, Rosen T. Acral purpura: An unusual sign of coumarin necrosis. J Am Acad Dermatol 1986; 14: 797–802.
18. Schwartz RA, Moore C III, Lambert WC. Linear localized coumarin necrosis. Dermatologica 1984; 168: 31–34.
19. Rose VL, Kwaan HC, Williamson K et al. Protein C antigen deficiency and warfarin necrosis. Am J Clin Pathol 1986; 86: 653–655.
20. Teepe RGC, Broekmans AW, Vermeer BJ et al. Recurrent coumarin-induced skin necrosis in a patient with an acquired functional protein C deficiency. Arch Dermatol 1986; 122: 1408–1412.
21. Auletta MJ, Headington JT. Purpura fulminans. A cutaneous manifestation of severe protein C deficiency. Arch Dermatol 1988; 124: 1387–1391.

22. Norris PG. Warfarin skin necrosis treated with prostacyclin. Clin Exp Dermatol 1987; 12: 370–372.
23. Jones RR, Cunningham J. Warfarin skin necrosis. The role of factor VII. Br J Dermatol 1979; 100: 561–565.
24. Shornick JK, Nicholas BK, Bergstresser PR, Gilliam JN. Idiopathic atrophie blanche. J Am Acad Dermatol 1983; 8: 792–798.
25. Pizzo SV, Murray JC, Gonias SL. Atrophie blanche. A disorder associated with defective release of tissue plasminogen activator. Arch Pathol Lab Med 1986; 110: 517–519.
26. Drucker CR, Duncan WC. Antiplatelet therapy in atrophie blanche and livedo vasculitis. J Am Acad Dermatol 1982; 7: 359–363.
27. Grob JJ, Bonerandi JJ. Thrombotic skin disease as a marker of the anticardiolipin syndrome. J Am Acad Dermatol 1989; 20: 1063–1069.
28. Stevanovic DV. Atrophie blanche. A sign of dermal blood occlusion. Arch Dermatol 1974; 109: 858–862.
29. Kern AB. Atrophie blanche. Report of two patients treated with aspirin and dipyridamole. J Am Acad Dermatol 1982; 6: 1048–1053.
30. Stieffer RE, Bergfeld WF. Atrophie blanche. Int J Dermatol 1982; 21: 1–7.
31. Suster S, Ronnen M, Bubis JJ, Schewach-Millet M. Familial atrophie blanche-like lesions with subcutaneous fibrinoid vasculitis. The Georgian ulcers. Am J Dermatopathol 1986; 8: 386–391.
32. Milstone LM, Braverman IM, Lucky P, Fleckman P. Classification and therapy of atrophie blanche. Arch Dermatol 1983; 119: 963–969.
33. Winkelmann RK, Schroeter AL, Kierland RR, Ryan TM. Clinical studies of livedo vasculitis (segmental hyalinizing vasculitis). Mayo Clin Proc 1974; 49: 746–750.
34. Gray HR, Graham JH, Johnson W, Burgoon CF. Atrophie blanche: periodic painful ulcers of lower extremities. Arch Dermatol 1966; 93: 187–193.
35. Bard JW, Winkelmann RK. Livedo vasculitis. Segmental hyalinizing vasculitis of the dermis. Arch Dermatol 1967; 96: 489–499.
36. Schroeter AL, Diaz-Perez JL, Winkelmann RK, Jordon RE. Livedo vasculitis (the vasculitis of atrophie blanche). Immunohistopathologic study. Arch Dermatol 1975; 111: 188–193.
37. Bell WR. Disseminated intravascular coagulation. Johns Hopkins Med J 1980; 146: 289–299.
38. Kim H-S, Suzuki M, Lie JT, Titus JL. Clinically unsuspected disseminated intravascular coagulation (DIC). An autopsy survey. Am J Clin Pathol 1976; 66: 31–39.
39. Colman RW, Minna JD, Robboy SJ. Disseminated intravascular coagulation: A dermatologic disease. Int J Dermatol 1977; 16: 47–51.
40. Robboy SJ, Colman RW, Minna JD. Pathology of disseminated intravascular coagulation (DIC). Analysis of 26 cases. Hum Pathol 1972; 3: 327–343.
41. Robboy SJ, Mihm MC, Colman RW, Minna JD. The skin in disseminated intravascular coagulation. Br J Dermatol 1973; 88: 221–229.
42. Marlar RA, Endres-Brooks J, Miller C. Serial studies of protein C and its plasma inhibitor in patients with disseminated intravascular coagulation. Blood 1985; 66: 59–63.
43. Cram DL, Soley RL. Purpura fulminans. Br J Dermatol 1968; 80: 323–327.
44. Spicer TE, Rau JM. Purpura fulminans. Am J Med 1976; 61: 566–571.
45. Silverman RA, Rhodes AR, Dennehy PH. Disseminated intravascular coagulation and purpura fulminans in a patient with candida sepsis. Am J Med 1986; 80: 679–684.
45a. Herbst JS, Raffanti S, Pathy A, Zaiac MN. Dysgonic fermenter type 2 septicemia with purpura fulminans. Dermatologic features of a zoonosis acquired from household pets. Arch Dermatol 1989; 125: 1380–1382.
46. Powars DR, Rogers ZR, Patch MJ et al. Purpura fulminans in meningococcemia: Association with acquired deficiencies of proteins C and S. N Engl J Med 1987; 317: 571–572.
47. Hautekeete ML, Berneman ZN, Bieger R et al. Purpura fulminans in pneumococcal sepsis. Arch Intern Med 1986; 146: 497–499.
48. Becker FT, Buckley RP. Purpura fulminans associated with varicella. Arch Dermatol 1966; 94: 613–618.
49. Marciniak E, Wilson HD, Marlar RA. Neonatal purpura fulminans: A genetic disorder related to the absence of protein C in blood. Blood 1985; 65: 15–20.
50. Yuen P, Cheung A, Lin HJ et al. Purpura fulminans in a Chinese boy with congenital protein C deficiency. Pediatrics 1986; 77: 670–676.
51. Sills RH, Marlar RA, Montgomery RR et al. Severe homozygous protein C deficiency. J Pediatr 1984; 105: 409–413.
52. Ridolfi RL, Bell WR. Thrombotic thrombocytopenic purpura. Report of 25 cases and review of the literature. Medicine (Baltimore) 1981; 60: 413–428.
53. Amorosi EL, Ultmann JE. Thrombotic thrombocytopenic purpura: Report of 16 cases and review of the literature. Medicine (Baltimore) 1966; 45: 139–159.
54 Myers TJ, Wakem CJ, Ball ED, Tremont SJ. Thrombotic thrombocytopenic purpura: combined treatment with plasmapheresis and antiplatelet agents. Ann Intern Med 1980; 92: 149–155.
55. Bone RC, Henry JE, Petterson J, Amare M. Respiratory dysfunction in thrombotic thrombocytopenic purpura. Am J Med 1978; 65: 262–270.
56. Heim LR. Cryoglobulins: Characterization and classification. Cutis 1979; 23: 259–266.
57. Meltzer M, Franklin EC. Cryoglobulinemia — a study of twenty-nine patients. Am J Med 1966; 40: 828–836.
58. Baughman RD, Sommer RG. Cryoglobulinemia presenting as "factitial ulceration". Arch Dermatol 1966; 94: 725–731.
59. McKenzie AW, Earle JHO, Lockey E, Mitchell-Heggs GB. Essential cryoglobulinaemia. Br J Dermatol 1961; 73: 22–29.
60. Brouet J-C, Clauvel J-P, Danon F et al. Biologic and clinical significance of cryoglobulins. Am J Med 1974; 57: 775–788.
61. Boom BW, Brand A, Bavinck J-NB et al. Severe leukocytoclastic vasculitis of the skin in a patient with essential mixed cryoglobulinemia treated with high-dose gamma-globulin intravenously. Arch Dermatol 1988; 124: 1550–1553.
62. Gorevic PD, Kassab HJ, Levo Y et al. Mixed

cryoglobulinemia: Clinical aspects and long-term follow-up of 40 patients. Am J Med 1980; 69: 287–308.

63. Solinas A, Cottoni F, Tanda F, Tocco A. Toxic epidermal necrolysis in a patient affected by mixed essential cryoglobulinemia. J Am Acad Dermatol 1988; 18: 1165–1169.

64. Berliner S, Weinberger A, Ben-Bassat M et al. Small skin blood vessel occlusions by cryoglobulin aggregates in ulcerative lesions in IgM-IgG cryoglobulinemia. J Cutan Pathol 1982; 9: 96–103.

65. Nir MA, Pick AI, Schreibman S, Feuerman EJ. Mixed IgG-IgM cryoglobulinemia with follicular pustular purpura. Arch Dermatol 1974; 109: 539–542.

66. Koda H, Kanaide A, Asahi M, Urabe H. Essential IgG cryoglobulinemia with purpura and cold urticaria. Arch Dermatol 1978; 114: 784–786.

67. Ellis FA. The cutaneous manifestations of cryoglobulinemia. Arch Dermatol 1964; 89: 690–697.

68. Cream JJ. Cryoglobulins in vasculitis. Clin Exp Immunol 1972; 10: 117–126.

69. Stoebner P, Renversez JC, Groulade J et al. Ultrastructural study of human IgG and IgG-IgM crystal cryoglobulins. Am J Clin Pathol 1979; 71: 404–410.

70. Falanga V, Fine MJ, Kapoor WN. The cutaneous manifestations of cholesterol crystal embolization. Arch Dermatol 1986; 122: 1194–1198.

71. Kalter DC, Rudolph A, McGavran M. Livedo reticularis due to multiple cholesterol emboli. J Am Acad Dermatol 1985; 13: 235–242.

72. Deschamps P, Leroy D, Mandard JC et al. Livedo reticularis and nodules due to cholesterol embolism in the lower extremities. Br J Dermatol 1977; 97: 93–97.

73. Day LL, Aterman K. Haemorrhagic panniculitis caused by atheromatous embolization. A case report and brief review. Am J Dermatopathol 1984; 6: 471–478.

74. Chesney TMcC. Atheromatous embolization to the skin. Am J Dermatopathol 1982; 4: 271–273.

75. Sanchez JL, Padilla MA. Hypereosinophilic syndrome. Cutis 1982; 29: 490–494.

76. Fitzpatrick JE, Johnson C, Simon P, Owenby J. Cutaneous microthrombi: A histologic clue to the diagnosis of hypereosinophilic syndrome. Am J Dermatopathol 1987; 9: 419–422.

77. Dodd HJ, Sarkany I, O'Shaughnessy D. Widespread cutaneous necrosis associated with the lupus anticoagulant. Clin Exp Dermatol 1985; 10: 581–586.

78. Grob J-J, Bonerandi J-J. Cutaneous manifestations associated with the presence of the lupus anticoagulant. J Am Acad Dermatol 1986; 15: 211–219.

79. Alegre VA, Winkelmann RK. Histopathologic and immunofluorescence study of skin lesions associated with circulating lupus anticoagulant. J Am Acad Dermatol 1988; 19: 117–124.

79a. O'Neill A, Gatenby PA, McGaw B et al. Widespread cutaneous necrosis associated with cardiolipin antibodies. J Am Acad Dermatol 1990; 22: 356–359.

80. Weinstein C, Miller MH, Axtens R et al. Livedo reticularis associated with increased titers of anticardiolipin antibodies in systemic lupus erythematosus. Arch Dermatol 1987; 123: 596–600.

81. Alegre VA, Gastineau DA, Winkelmann RK. Skin lesions associated with circulating lupus anticoagulant. Br J Dermatol 1989; 120: 419–429.

82. Sneddon IB. Cerebro-vascular lesions and livedo reticularis. Br J Dermatol 1965; 77: 180–185.

83. Deffer TA, Berger TG, Gelinas-Sorell D. Sneddon's syndrome. A case report. J Am Acad Dermatol 1987; 16: 1084–1087.

84. Quimby SR, Perry HO. Livedo reticularis and cerebrovascular accidents. J Am Acad Dermatol 1980; 3: 377–383.

85. Thomas DJ, Kirby JDT, Britton KE, Galton DJ. Livedo reticularis and neurological lesions. Br J Dermatol 1982; 106: 711–712.

86. Marsch WC, Muckelmann R. Generalized racemose livedo with cerebrovascular lesions (Sneddon syndrome): an occlusive arteriolopathy due to proliferation and migration of medial smooth muscle cells. Br J Dermatol 1985; 112: 703–708.

86a. Alegre VA, Winkelmann RK, Gastineau DA. Cutaneous thrombosis, cerebrovascular thrombosis, and lupus anticoagulant — the Sneddon syndrome. Report of 10 cases. Int J Dermatol 1990; 29: 45–49.

87. Grattan CEH, Burton JL, Boon AP. Sneddon's syndrome (livedo reticularis and cerebral thrombosis) with livedo vasculitis and anticardiolipin antibodies. Br J Dermatol 1989; 120: 441–447.

88. Miller JA, Machin SJ, Dowd PM. Cutaneous gangrene with hyperparathyroidism. Clin Exp Dermatol 1988; 13: 204–206.

89. Miller SJ. The dermatologist and protein C. J Am Acad Dermatol 1988; 19: 904–907.

90. Marlar RA, Adcock DM. Clinical evaluation of protein C: a comparative review of antigenic and functional assays. Hum Pathol 1989; 20: 1040–1047.

91. Levine LE, Bernstein JE, Soltani K et al. Heparin-induced cutaneous necrosis unrelated to injection sites. Arch Dermatol 1983; 119: 400–403.

92. Heng MCY, Haberfeld G. Thrombotic phenomena associated with intravenous cocaine. J Am Acad Dermatol 1987; 16: 462–468.

93. Stapleton SR, Curley RK, Simpson WA. Cutaneous gangrene secondary to focal thrombosis — an important cutaneous manifestation of ulcerative colitis. Clin Exp Dermatol 1989; 14: 387–389.

Urticarias

94. Synkowski D, Dore N, Provost TT. Urticaria and urticaria-like lesions. Clin Rheum Dis 1982; 8: 383–395.

95. Monroe EW. Urticaria. Int J Dermatol 1981; 20: 32–41.

96. Juhlin L. Recurrent urticaria: clinical investigation of 330 patients. Br J Dermatol 1981; 104: 369–381.

97. Champion RH. Acute and chronic urticaria. Semin Dermatol 1987; 6: 286–291.

98. Michaelsson G, Juhlin L. Urticaria induced by preservatives and dye additives in food and drugs. Br J Dermatol 1973; 88: 525–532.

99. Heng MCY, Kloss SG, Haberfelde GC. Pathogenesis of papular urticaria. J Am Acad Dermatol 1984; 10: 1030–1034.

100. Hannuksela M. Urticaria in children. Semin Dermatol 1987; 6: 321–325.

101. Monroe EW. Urticaria and urticarial vasculitis. Med Clin North Am 1980; 64: 867–883.
102. Gleich GJ, Schroeter AL, Marcoux JP et al. Episodic angioedema associated with eosinophilia. N Engl J Med 1984; 310: 1621–1626.
103. Champion RH. Urticaria: then and now. Br J Dermatol 1988; 119: 427–436.
104. Gorevic PD, Kaplan AP. The physical urticarias. Int J Dermatol 1980; 19: 417–435.
105. Sibbald RG. Physical urticaria. Dermatol Clin 1984; 3: 57–69.
106. Jorizzo JL, Smith EB. The physical urticarias. An update and review. Arch Dermatol 1982; 118: 194–201.
107. Soter NA. Physical urticaria/angioedema. Semin Dermatol 1987; 6: 302–312.
108. Duschet P, Leyen P, Schwarz T et al. Solar urticaria — effective treatment by plasmapheresis. Clin Exp Dermatol 1987; 12: 185–188.
109. Kojima M, Horiko T, Nakamura Y, Aoki T. Solar urticaria. The relationship of photoallergen and action spectrum. Arch Dermatol 1986; 122: 550–555.
110. Neittaanmaki H. Cold urticaria. Clinical findings in 220 patients. J Am Acad Dermatol 1985; 13: 636–644.
111. Lawlor F, Kobza Black A, Breathnach AS et al. A timed study of the histopathology, direct immunofluorescence and ultrastructural findings in idiopathic cold-contact urticaria over a 24-h period. Clin Exp Dermatol 1989; 14: 416–420.
112. Doeglas HMG, Rijnten WJ, Schroder FP, Schirm J. Cold urticaria and virus infections: a clinical and serological study in 39 patients. Br J Dermatol 1986; 114: 311–318.
113. Black AK. Cold urticaria. Semin Dermatol 1987; 6: 292–301.
114. Freeman PA, Watt GC. Localized heat urticaria (heat contact urticaria). Australas J Dermatol 1988; 29: 43–46.
115. Armstrong RB, Horan DB, Silvers DN. Leukocytoclastic vasculitis in urticaria induced by ultraviolet irradiation. Arch Dermatol 1985; 121: 1145–1148.
116. Rantanen T, Suhonen R. Solar urticaria: a case with increased skin mast cells and good therapeutic response to an antihistamine. Acta Derm Venereol 1980; 60: 363–365.
117. Armstrong RB. Solar urticaria. Dermatol Clin 1986; 4: 253–259.
118. Horio T, Fujigaki K. Augmentation spectrum in solar urticaria. J Am Acad Dermatol 1988; 18: 1189–1193.
119. Ramsay CA. Solar urticaria. Int J Dermatol 1980; 19: 233–236.
120. Bonnetblanc JM, Andrieu-Pfahl F, Meraud JP, Roux J. Familial aquagenic urticaria. Dermatologica 1979; 158: 468–470.
121. Archer CB, Greaves MG. Aquagenic pruritus. Semin Dermatol 1988; 7: 301–303.
122. Kligman AM, Greaves MW, Steinman H. Water-induced itching without cutaneous signs. Aquagenic pruritus. Arch Dermatol 1986; 122: 183–186.
123. Bircher AJ, Meier-Ruge W. Aquagenic pruritus. Water-induced activation of acetylcholinesterase. Arch Dermatol 1988; 124: 84–89.
124. Wolf R, Krakowski A. Variations in aquagenic pruritus and treatment alternatives. J Am Acad Dermatol 1988; 18: 1081–1083.
125. Steinman HK, Greaves MW. Aquagenic pruritus. J Am Acad Dermatol 1985; 13: 91–96.
126. Estes SA, Yung CW. Delayed pressure urticaria: An investigation of some parameters of lesion induction. J Am Acad Dermatol 1981; 5: 25–31.
127. Lawlor F, Black AK, Ward AM et al. Delayed pressure urticaria, objective evaluation of a variable disease using a dermographometer and assessment of treatment using colchicine. Br J Dermatol 1989; 120: 403–408.
128. Lawlor F, Barr R, Kobza-Black A et al. Arachidonic acid transformation is not stimulated in delayed pressure urticaria. Br J Dermatol 1989; 121: 317–321.
129. Dover JS, Black AK, Ward AM, Greaves MW. Delayed pressure urticaria. Clinical features, laboratory investigations, and response to therapy of 44 patients. J Am Acad Dermatol 1988; 18: 1289–1298.
130. Warin RP. Clinical observations on delayed pressure urticaria. Br J Dermatol 1989; 121: 225–228.
131. Czarnetzki BM, Meentken J, Kolde G, Brocker E-B. Morphology of the cellular infiltrate in delayed pressure urticaria. J Am Acad Dermatol 1985; 12: 253–259.
132. Breathnach SM, Allen R, Milford Ward A, Greaves MW. Symptomatic dermographism: natural history, clinical features, laboratory investigations and response to therapy. Clin Exp Dermatol 1983; 8: 463–476.
133. Lawlor F, Kobza Black A, Murdoch RD, Greaves MW. Symptomatic dermographism: wealing, mast cells and histamine are decreased in the skin following long-term application of a potent topical corticosteroid. Br J Dermatol 1989; 121: 629–634.
134. Ryan TJ, Shim-Young N, Turk JL. Delayed pressure urticaria. Br J Dermatol 1968; 80: 485–490.
135. Burdick AE, Mathias CGT. The contact urticaria syndrome. Dermatol Clin 1985; 3: 71–84.
136. von Krogh G, Maibach HI. The contact urticaria syndrome — an updated review. J Am Acad Dermatol 1981; 5: 328–342.
137. Turjanmaa K, Reunala T, Rasanen L. Comparison of diagnostic methods in latex surgical glove contact urticaria. Contact Dermatitis 1988; 19: 241–247.
137a. Kligman AM. The spectrum of contact urticaria. Wheals, erythema, and pruritus. Dermatol Clin 1990; 8: 57–60.
137b. Pecquet C, Leynadier F, Dry J. Contact urticaria and anaphylaxis to natural latex. J Am Acad Dermatol 1990; 22: 631–633.
138. Lahti A, Maibach HI. Immediate contact reactions: contact urticaria syndrome. Semin Dermatol 1987; 6: 313–320.
139. Jorizzo JL. Cholinergic urticaria. Arch Dermatol 1987; 123: 455–457.
140. Berth-Jones J, Graham-Brown RAC. Cholinergic pruritus, erythema and urticaria: a disease spectrum responding to danazol. Br J Dermatol 1989; 121: 235–237.
141. Mayou SC, Kobza Black A, Eady RAJ, Greaves MW. Cholinergic dermographism. Br J Dermatol 1986; 115: 371–377.

142. Ormerod AD, Kobza-Black A, Milford-Ward A, Greaves MW. Combined cold urticaria and cholinergic urticaria — clinical characterization and laboratory findings. Br J Dermatol 1988; 118: 621–627.
143. Hirschmann JV, Lawlor F, English JSC et al. Cholinergic urticaria. A clinical and histological study. Arch Dermatol 1987; 123: 462–467.
144. Warin RP, Cunliffe WJ, Greaves MW, Wallington TB. Recurrent angioedema: familial and oestrogen-induced. Br J Dermatol 1986; 115: 731–734.
145. Tappeiner G, Hintner H, Glatzl J, Wolff K. Hereditary angio-oedema: treatment with danazol. Br J Dermatol 1979; 100: 207–212.
146. Jorizzo JL. Classification of urticaria and the reactive inflammatory vascular dermatoses. Dermatol Clin 1985; 3: 3–28.
147. Gammon WR. Manifestations of drug reactions: urticaria and cutaneous necrotizing venulitis. Clin Dermatol 1986; 4: 50–57.
148. Bielory L, Yancey KB, Young NS et al. Cutaneous manifestations of serum sickness in patients receiving antithymocyte globulin. J Am Acad Dermatol 1985; 13: 411–417.
149. Stephens CJM, Black MM. Perimenstrual eruptions: autoimmune progesterone dermatitis. Semin Dermatol 1989; 8: 26–29.
150. Miura T, Matsuda M, Yanbe H, Sugiyama S. Two cases of autoimmune progesterone dermatitis. Immunohistochemical and serological studies. Acta Derm Venereol 1989; 69: 308–310.
151. Shelley WB, Shelley ED. Delayed pressure urticaria syndrome: a clinical expression of interleukin 1. Acta Derm Venereol 1987; 67: 438–441.
152. Leenutaphong V, Holzle E, Plewig G. Pathogenesis and classification of solar urticaria: A new concept. J Am Acad Dermatol 1989; 21: 237–240.
153. Czarnetzki BM. Mechanisms and mediators in urticaria. Semin Dermatol 1987; 6: 272–285.
154. Synkowski DR, Levine MI, Rabin BS, Yunis EJ. Urticaria. An immunofluorescence and histopathology study. Arch Dermatol 1979; 115: 1192–1194.
155. McEvoy MT, Winkelmann RK, Kobza-Black A et al. Eosinophil degranulation in delayed pressure urticaria. J Cutan Pathol 1988; 15: 328 (abstract).
156. Leiferman KM, Norris PG, Murphy GM et al. Evidence for eosinophil degranulation with deposition of granule major basic protein in solar urticaria. J Am Acad Dermatol 1989; 21: 75–80.
157. Winkelmann RK, Black AK, Dover J, Greaves MW. Pressure urticaria — histopathological study. Clin Exp Dermatol 1986; 11: 139–147.
158. Norris PG, Murphy GM, Hawk JLM, Winkelmann RK. A histological study of the evolution of solar urticaria. Arch Dermatol 1988; 124: 80–83.
159. Winkelmann RK. The histology and immunopathology of dermographism. J Cutan Pathol 1985; 12: 486–492.
160. Peters MS, Winkelmann RK. Neutrophilic urticaria. Br J Dermatol 1985; 113: 25–30.
161. Winkelmann RK, Reizner GT. Diffuse dermal neutrophilia in urticaria. Hum Pathol 1988; 19: 389–393.
162. Winkelmann RK, Wilson-Jones E, Smith NP et al. Neutrophilic urticaria. Acta Derm Venereol 1988; 68: 129–133.
163. Gammon WR, Wheeler CE Jr. Urticarial vasculitis. Report of a case and review of the literature. Arch Dermatol 1979; 115: 76–80.
164. Callen JP, Kalbfleisch S. Urticarial vasculitis: a report of nine cases and review of the literature. Br J Dermatol 1982; 107: 87–94.
165. Sanchez NP, Winkelmann RK, Schroeter AL, Dicken CH. The clinical and histopathologic spectrums of urticarial vasculitis: Study of forty cases. J Am Acad Dermatol 1982; 7: 599–605.
166. Russell Jones R, Bhogal B, Dash A, Schifferli J. Urticaria and vasculitis: a continuum of histological and immunopathological changes. Br J Dermatol 1983; 108: 695–703.
167. Russell Jones R, Eady RAJ. Endothelial cell pathology as a marker for urticarial vasculitis: a light microscopic study. Br J Dermatol 1984; 110: 139–149.
168. Monroe EW. Urticarial vasculitis. Semin Dermatol 1987; 6: 328–333.
169. Wanderer AA, Nuss DD, Tormey AD, Giclas PC. Urticarial leukocytoclastic vasculitis with cold urticaria. Arch Dermatol 1983; 119: 145–151.
170. Eady RAJ, Keahey TM, Sibbald RG, Black AK. Cold urticaria with vasculitis: report of a case with light and electron microscopic, immunofluorescence and pharmacological studies. Clin Exp Dermatol 1981; 6: 355–366.
171. Aboobaker J, Greaves MW. Urticarial vasculitis. Clin Exp Dermatol 1986; 11: 436–444.
172. Monroe EW. Urticarial vasculitis: An updated review. J Am Acad Dermatol 1981; 5: 88–95.
173. Monroe EW, Schulz CI, Maize JC, Jordon RE. Vasculitis in chronic urticaria: an immunopathologic study. J Invest Dermatol 1981; 76: 103–107.
174. Peteiro C, Toribio J. Incidence of leukocytoclastic vasculitis in chronic idiopathic urticaria. Study of 100 cases. Am J Dermatopathol 1989; 11: 528–533.
175. English JSC, Murphy GM, Winkelmann RK, Bhogal B. A sequential histopathological study of dermographism. Clin Exp Dermatol 1988; 13: 314–317.

Acute vasculitis

176. Sams WM Jr. Necrotizing vasculitis. J Am Acad Dermatol 1980; 3: 1–13.
177. Fauci AS. The spectrum of vasculitis. Clinical, pathologic, immunologic, and therapeutic considerations. Ann Intern Med 1978; 89: 660–676.
178. Ryan TJ. Cutaneous vasculitis. J Cutan Pathol 1985; 12: 381–387.
179. Callen JP, Chandra JJ, Voorhees JJ. Cutaneous angiitis (vasculitis). Int J Dermatol 1978; 17: 105–113.
180. Conn DL. Update on systemic necrotizing vasculitis. Mayo Clin Proc 1989; 64: 535–543.
181. Mackel SE, Jordon RE. Leukocytoclastic vasculitis. A cutaneous expression of immune complex disease. Arch Dermatol 1982; 118: 296–301.
182. Jorizzo JL, Solomon AR, Zanolli MD, Leshin B. Neutrophilic vascular reactions. J Am Acad Dermatol 1988; 19: 983–1005.
183. Zax RH, Hodge SJ, Callen JP. Cutaneous leukocytoclastic vasculitis. Serial histopathologic evaluation demonstrates the dynamic nature of the

infiltrate. Arch Dermatol 1990; 126: 69–72.

184. Smoller BR, McNutt NS, Contreras F. The natural history of vasculitis. What the histology tells us about pathogenesis. Arch Dermatol 1990; 126: 84–89.

185. Sams WM Jr, Thorne EG, Small P et al. Leukocytoclastic vasculitis. Arch Dermatol 1976; 112: 219–226.

186. Sams WM Jr. Immunologic aspects of cutaneous vasculitis. Semin Dermatol 1988; 7: 140–148.

187. Ramsay C, Fry L. Allergic vasculitis: clinical and histological features and incidence of renal involvement. Br J Dermatol 1969; 81: 96–102.

188. Sams WM Jr. Hypersensitivity angiitis. J Invest Dermatol 1989; 93: 78s–81s.

189. Handel DW, Roenigk HH Jr, Shainoff J, Deodhar S. Necrotizing vasculitis. Etiologic aspects of immunology and coagulopathy. Arch Dermatol 1975; 111: 847–852.

190. Ekenstam EA, Callen JP. Cutaneous leukocytoclastic vasculitis. Clinical and laboratory features of 82 patients seen in private practice. Arch Dermatol 1984; 120: 484–489.

191. Hodge SJ, Callen JP, Ekenstam E. Cutaneous leukocytoclastic vasculitis: correlation of histopathological changes with clinical severity and course. J Cutan Pathol 1987; 14: 279–284.

192. Gougerot H, Duperrat B. The nodular allergides of Gougerot. Br J Dermatol 1954; 66: 283–286.

193. Diaz LA, Provost TT, Tomasi TB Jr. Pustular necrotizing angiitis. Arch Dermatol 1973; 108: 114–118.

194. Branford WA, Farr PM, Porter DI. Annular vasculitis of the head and neck in a patient with sarcoidosis. Br J Dermatol 1982; 106: 713–716.

195. Gammon R. Leucocytoclastic vasculitis. Clin Rheum Dis 1982; 8: 397–413.

196. Callen JP. Cutaneous vasculitis and its relationship to systemic disease. Australas J Dermatol 1987; 28: 49–55.

197. Alegre VA, Winkelmann RK. Necrotizing vasculitis and atherosclerosis. Br J Dermatol 1988; 119: 381–384.

198. Bianchini G, Lotti T, Campolmi P et al. Coral ulcer as a vasculitis. Int J Dermatol 1988; 27: 506–507.

199. Cohen C, Trapuckd S. Leukocytoclastic vasculitis associated with cutaneous infection by herpesvirus. Am J Dermatopathol 1984; 6: 561–565.

200. Curtis JL, Egbert BM. Cutaneous cytomegalovirus vasculitis: an unusual clinical presentation of a common opportunistic pathogen. Hum Pathol 1982; 13: 1138–1141.

201. Chren M-M, Silverman RA, Sorensen RU, Elmets CA. Leukocytoclastic vasculitis in a patient infected with human immunodeficiency virus. J Am Acad Dermatol 1989; 21: 1161–1164.

202. Mullick FG, McAllister HA Jr, Wagner BM, Fenoglio JJ Jr. Drug related vasculitis. Clinicopathologic correlations in 30 patients. Hum Pathol 1979; 10: 313–325.

203. Roenigk HH Jr. Vasculitis. Int J Dermatol 1976; 15: 395–404.

204. Lambert WC, Kolber LR, Proper SA. Leukocytoclastic angiitis induced by clindamycin. Cutis 1982; 30: 615–619.

205. Hendricks WM, Ader RS. Furosemide-induced cutaneous necrotizing vasculitis. Arch Dermatol 1977; 113: 375.

206. Cox NH, Dunn LK, Williams J. Cutaneous vasculitis associated with long-term thiouracil therapy. Clin Exp Dermatol 1985; 10: 292–295.

207. Sanchez NP, Van Hale HM, Su WPD. Clinical and histopathologic spectrum of necrotizing vasculitis. Report of findings in 101 cases. Arch Dermatol 1985; 121: 220–224.

208. Bickley LK, Schwartz RA, Lambert WC. Localized cutaneous leukocytoclastic vasculitis in an intravenous drug abuser. Int J Dermatol 1988; 27: 512–513.

209. Alegre VA, Winkelmann RK, Diez-Martin JL, Banks PM. Adult celiac disease, small and medium vessel cutaneous necrotizing vasculitis, and T cell lymphoma. J Am Acad Dermatol 1988; 19: 973–978.

210. Granstein RD, Soter NA, Haynes HA. Necrotizing vasculitis with cutaneous lesions of mycosis fungoides. J Am Acad Dermatol 1983; 9: 128–133.

211. Kenny PGW, Shum DT, Smout MS. Leukocytoclastic vasculitis in hairy cell leukemia (leukemic reticuloendotheliosis). Arch Dermatol 1983; 119: 1018–1019.

212. Spann CR, Callen JP, Yam LT, Apgar JT. Cutaneous leukocytoclastic vasculitis complicating hairy cell leukemia (leukemic reticuloendotheliosis). Arch Dermatol 1986; 122: 1057–1059.

213. Lee SH, Chung KY, Lee WS, Lee S. Behçet's syndrome associated with bullous necrotizing vasculitis. J Am Acad Dermatol 1989; 21: 327–330.

214. Newton JA, McGibbon DH, Marsden RA. Leucocytoclastic vasculitis and angio-oedema associated with inflammatory bowel disease. Clin Exp Dermatol 1984; 9: 618–623.

215. Resnick AH, Esterly NB. Vasculitis in children. Int J Dermatol 1985; 24: 139–146.

216. Alexander E, Provost TT. Sjögren's syndrome. Association of cutaneous vasculitis with central nervous system disease. Arch Dermatol 1987; 123: 801–810.

217. Thompson DM, Main RA, Beck JS, Albert-Recht F. Studies on a patient with leucocytoclastic vasculitis 'pyoderma gangrenosum' and paraproteinaemia. Br J Dermatol 1973; 88: 117–125.

218. Brandrup F, Ostergaard PA. α1-antitrypsin deficiency associated with persistent cutaneous vasculitis. Occurrence in a child with liver disease. Arch Dermatol 1978; 114: 921–924.

219. Boom BW, Out-Luiting CJ, Baldwin WM et al. Membrane attack complex of complement in leukocytoclastic vasculitis of the skin. Arch Dermatol 1987; 123: 1192–1195.

220. Tosca N, Stratigos JD. Possible pathogenetic mechanisms in allergic cutaneous vasculitis. Int J Dermatol 1988; 27: 291–296.

221. Cunliffe WJ. Fibrinolysis and vasculitis. Clin Exp Dermatol 1976; 1: 1–16.

221a. Chan LS, Cooper KD, Rasmussen JE. Koebnerization as a cutaneous manifestation of immune complex-mediated vasculitis. J Am Acad Dermatol 1990; 22: 775–781.

222. Jones RE Jr (Editor). Questions to the Editorial Board and other authorities. Am J Dermatopathol 1985; 7: 181–187.

223. Russell Jones R, Bhogal B. Dermatitis herpetiformis-like changes in cutaneous leucocytoclastic vasculitis with IgA deposition. Clin Exp Dermatol 1981; 6: 495–501.

224. Minkowitz S, Adler M, Alderete MN. Nuclear vacuolar acantholytic vesicular dermatitis associated with leukocytoclastic vasculitis. J Am Acad Dermatol 1986; 15: 1083–1089.

225. Ansell BM. Henoch–Schönlein purpura with particular reference to the prognosis of the renal lesion. Br J Dermatol 1970; 82: 211–215.

226. Heng MCY. Henoch–Schönlein purpura. Br J Dermatol 1985; 112: 235–240.

227. Van Hale HM, Gibson LE, Schroeter AL. Henoch–Schönlein vasculitis: Direct immunofluorescence study of uninvolved skin. J Am Acad Dermatol 1986; 15: 665–670.

228. Piette WW, Stone MS. A cutaneous sign of IgA-associated small dermal vessel leukocytoclastic vasculitis in adults (Henoch–Schönlein purpura). Arch Dermatol 1989; 125: 53–56.

229. Scott DGI, Bacon PA, Tribe CR. Systemic rheumatoid vasculitis: a clinical and laboratory study of 50 cases. Medicine (Baltimore) 1981; 60: 288–297.

230. Upchurch KS, Heller K, Brass NM. Low-dose methotrexate therapy for cutaneous vasculitis of rheumatoid arthritis. J Am Acad Dermatol 1987; 17: 355–359.

231. Gordon GV. Rheumatoid vasculitis. Int J Dermatol 1981; 20: 546–547.

232. Gammon WR. Urticarial vasculitis. Dermatol Clin 1985; 3: 97–105.

233. Bisaccia E, Adamo V, Rozan SW. Urticarial vasculitis progressing to systemic lupus erythematosus. Arch Dermatol 1988; 124: 1088–1090.

233a. Borradori L, Rybojad M, Puissant A et al. Urticarial vasculitis associated with a monoclonal IgM gammopathy: Schnitzler's syndrome. Br J Dermatol 1990; 123: 113–118.

234. Berg RE, Kantor GR, Bergfeld WF. Urticarial vasculitis. Int J Dermatol 1988; 27: 468–472.

235. Cohen SJ, Pittelkow MR, Su WPD. Cryoglobulinemia: a cutaneous clinical and pathologic study. J Cutan Pathol 1989; 16: 300 (abstract).

236. Ackerman AB. Histologic diagnosis of inflammatory skin diseases. Philadelphia: Lea & Febiger, 1978; 356–362.

237. Plaut ME. Staphylococcal septicemia and pustular purpura. Arch Dermatol 1969; 99: 82–85.

238. Hill WR, Kinney TD. The cutaneous lesions in acute meningococcemia. A clinical and pathologic study. JAMA 1947; 134: 513–518.

239. Winkelstein A, Songster CL, Caras TS et al. Fulminant meningococcemia and disseminated intravascular coagulation. Arch Intern Med 1969; 124: 55–59.

240. Scott MJ Jr, Scott MJ Sr. Primary cutaneous Neisseria gonorrhoeae infections. Arch Dermatol 1982; 118: 351–352.

241. Prager KM. Primary extragenital cutaneous gonorrhea. Arch Dermatol 1973; 107: 112.

242. Rosen T. Unusual presentations of gonorrhea. J Am Acad Dermatol 1982; 6: 369–372.

243. Hurwitz RM, Leaming RD, Horine RK. Necrotic cellulitis. A localized form of septic vasculitis. Arch Dermatol 1984; 120: 87–92.

244. Hall JH, Callaway JL, Tindall JP, Smith JG Jr. Pseudomonas aeruginosa in dermatology. Arch Dermatol 1968; 97: 312–324.

245. Mandell IN, Feiner HD, Price NM, Simberkoff M. Pseudomonas cepacia endocarditis and ecthyma gangrenosum. Arch Dermatol 1977; 113: 199–202.

246. Shapiro L, Teisch JA, Brownstein MH. Dermatohistopathology of chronic gonococcal sepsis. Arch Dermatol 1973; 107: 403–406.

247. Ognibene AJ, Dito WR. Chronic meningococcemia. Arch Intern Med 1964; 114: 29–32.

248. Nielsen LT. Chronic meningococcemia. Arch Dermatol 1970; 102: 97–101.

249. Ackerman AB. Haemorrhagic bullae in gonococcemia. N Engl J Med 1970; 282: 793–794.

250. Scherer R, Braun-Falco O. Alternative pathway complement activation: a possible mechanism inducing skin lesions in benign gonococcal sepsis. Br J Dermatol 1976; 95: 303–309.

251. Bjornberg A. Benign gonococcal sepsis. Acta Derm Venereol 1970; 50: 313–316.

252. Sotto MN, Langer B, Hoshino-Shimizu S, de Brito T. Pathogenesis of cutaneous lesions in acute meningococcemia in humans: light, immunofluorescent, and electron microscopic studies of skin biopsy specimens. J Infect Dis 1976; 133: 506–514.

253. Dalldorf FG, Jennette JC. Fatal meningococcal septicemia. Arch Pathol Lab Med 1977; 101: 6–9.

254. Ackerman AB, Miller RC, Shapiro L. Gonococcemia and its cutaneous manifestations. Arch Dermatol 1965; 91: 227–232.

255. Kahn G, Danielsson D. Septic gonococcal dermatitis. Arch Dermatol 1969; 99: 421–425.

256. Abu-Nassar H, Hill N, Fred HL, Yow EM. Cutaneous manifestations of gonococcemia. A review of 14 cases. Arch Intern Med 1963; 112: 731–737.

257. Von Gemmingen GR, Winkelmann RK. Osler's node of subacute bacterial endocarditis. Focal necrotizing vasculitis of the glomus body. Arch Dermatol 1967; 95: 91–94.

258. Alpert JS, Krous HF, Dalen JE et al. Pathogenesis of Osler's nodes. Ann Intern Med 1976; 85: 471–473.

259. Rubenfeld S, Min K-W. Leukocytoclastic angiitis in subacute bacterial endocarditis. Arch Dermatol 1977; 113: 1073–1074.

260. Kerr A Jr, Tan JS. Biopsies of the Janeway lesion of infective endocarditis. J Cutan Pathol 1979; 6: 124–129.

260a. Cardullo AC, Silvers DN, Grossman ME. Janeway lesions and Osler's nodes: A review of histopathologic findings. J Am Acad Dermatol 1990; 22: 1088–1090.

261. Mrez JP, Newcomer VD. Erythema elevatum diutinum. Arch Dermatol 1967; 96: 235–246.

262. Katz SI, Gallin JI, Hertz KC et al. Erythema elevatum diutinum: skin and systemic manifestations, immunologic studies, and successful treatment with dapsone. Medicine (Baltimore) 1977; 56: 443–455.

263. English JSC, Smith NP, Kersy PJW, Levene GM. Erythema elevatum diutinum — an unusual case. Clin Exp Dermatol 1985; 10: 577–580.

264. Caputo R, Alessi E. Unique aspects of a lesion of erythema elevatum diutinum. Am J Dermatopathol 1984; 6: 465–469.

265. Kohler IK, Lorincz AL. Erythema elevatum diutinum treated with niacinamide and tetracycline. Arch Dermatol 1980; 116: 693–695.

266. Vollum DI. Erythema elevatum diutinum — vesicular lesions and sulphone response. Br J Dermatol 1968; 80: 178–183.

267. Morrison JGL, Hull PR, Fourie E. Erythema
elevatum diutinum, cryoglobulinaemia, and fixed
urticaria on cooling. Br J Dermatol 1977; 97: 99–104.

268. Fort SL, Rodman OG. Erythema elevatum diutinum.
Response to dapsone. Arch Dermatol 1977; 113:
819–822.

269. Cream JJ, Levene GM, Calnan CD. Erythema
elevatum diutinum. An unusual reaction to
streptococcal antigen and response to dapsone. Br J
Dermatol 1971; 84: 393–399.

270. da Cunha Bang F, Weismann K, Ralfkiaer E et al.
Erythema elevatum diutinum and pre-AIDS. Acta
Derm Venereol 1986; 66: 272–274.

271. LeBoit PE, Yen TSB, Wintroub B. The evolution of
lesions in erythema elevatum diutinum. Am J
Dermatopathol 1986; 8: 392–402.

272. Haber H. Erythema elevatum diutinum. Br J Dermatol
1955; 67: 121–145.

273. Ramsey ML, Gibson B, Tschen JA, Wolf JE Jr.
Erythema elevatum diutinum. Cutis 1984; 34: 41–43.

274. Wolff HH, Maciejewski W, Scherer R. Erythema
elevatum diutinum. Electron microscopy of a case with
extracellular cholesterosis. Arch Dermatol Res 1978;
261: 7–16.

275. Lee AY, Nakagawa H, Nogita T, Ishibashi Y. Erythema
elevatum diutinum: an ultrastructural case study. J
Cutan Pathol 1989; 16: 211–217.

276. Pedace FJ, Perry HO. Granuloma faciale. A clinical
and histopathologic review. Arch Dermatol 1966; 94:
387–395.

277. Johnson WC, Higdon RS, Helwig EB. Granuloma
faciale. Arch Dermatol 1959; 79: 42–52.

278. Jacyk WK. Facial granuloma in a patient treated with
clofazimine. Arch Dermatol 1981; 117: 597–598.

279. Rusin LJ, Dubin HV, Taylor WB. Disseminated
granuloma faciale. Arch Dermatol 1976; 112:
1575–1577.

280. Okun MR, Bauman L, Minor D. Granuloma faciale
with lesions on the face and hand. Arch Dermatol
1965; 92: 78–80.

281. Guill MA, Aton JK. Facial granuloma responsive to
dapsone therapy. Arch Dermatol 1982; 118: 332–335.

282. Lever WF, Leeper RW. Eosinophilic granuloma of the
skin. Arch Dermatol 1950; 62: 85–96.

283. Frost FA, Heenan PJ. Facial granuloma. Australas J
Dermatol 1984; 25: 121–124.

284. Cobane JH, Straith CL, Pinkus H. Facial granulomas
with eosinophilia. Arch Dermatol 1950; 61: 442–454.

285. Nieboer C, Kalsbeek GL. Immunofluorescence studies
in granuloma eosinophilicum faciale. J Cutan Pathol
1978; 5: 68–75.

286. Schroeter AL, Copeman PWM, Jordon RE et al.
Immunofluorescence of cutaneous vasculitis associated
with systemic disease. Arch Dermatol 1971; 104:
254–259.

287. Schnitzler L, Verret JL, Schubert B. Granuloma
faciale. Ultrastructural study of three cases. J Cutan
Pathol 1977; 4: 123–133.

288. Cohen RD, Conn DL, Ilstrup DM. Clinical features,
prognosis, and response to treatment in polyarteritis.
Mayo Clin Proc 1980; 55: 146–155.

289. Patalano VJ, Sommers SC. Biopsy diagnosis of
periarteritis nodosa. Arch Pathol 1961; 72: 1–21.

290. Vertzman L. Polyarteritis nodosa. Clin Rheum Dis
1980; 6: 297–317.

291. Alarcón-Segovia D, Brown AL Jr. Classification and
etiologic aspects of necrotizing angiitides: an analytic
approach to a confused subject with a critical review of
the evidence for hypersensitivity in polyarteritis
nodosa. Mayo Clin Proc 1964; 39: 205–222.

292. Diaz-Perez JL, Winkelmann RK. Cutaneous
periarteritis nodosa. Arch Dermatol 1974; 110:
407–414.

293. Diaz-Perez JL, Schroeter AL, Winkelmann RK.
Cutaneous periarteritis nodosa. Immunofluorescence
studies. Arch Dermatol 1980; 116: 56–58.

294. Borrie P. Cutaneous polyarteritis nodosa. Br J
Dermatol 1972; 87: 87–95.

295. Brandrup F, Petersen EM, Hansen BF. Localized
polyarteritis nodosa in the lower limb with new bone
formation. Acta Derm Venereol 1980; 60: 182–184.

296. Trepo CG, Zuckerman AJ, Bird RC, Prince AM. The
role of circulating hepatitis B antigen/antibody immune
complexes in the pathogenesis of vascular and hepatic
manifestations in polyarteritis nodosa. J Clin Pathol
1974; 27: 863–868.

297. Gocke DJ, Hsu K, Morgan C et al. Association
between polyarteritis and Australia antigen. Lancet
1970; 2: 1149–1153.

298. Whittaker SJ, Dover JS, Greaves MW. Cutaneous
polyarteritis nodosa associated with hepatitis B surface
antigen. J Am Acad Dermatol 1986; 15: 1142–1145.

299. Van de Pette JEW, Jarvis JM, Wilton JMA, MacDonald
DM. Cutaneous periarteritis nodosa. Arch Dermatol
1984; 120: 109–111.

300. Dyer NH, Verbov JL, Dawson AM et al. Cutaneous
polyarteritis nodosa associated with Crohn's disease.
Lancet 1970; 1: 648–650.

301. Goslen JB, Graham W, Lazarus GS. Cutaneous
polyarteritis nodosa. Report of a case associated with
Crohn's disease. Arch Dermatol 1983; 119: 326–329.

302. Fernandez-Diaz J. General pathology of necrotizing
vasculitis. Clin Rheum Dis 1980; 6: 279–295.

303. Alarcón-Segovia D. The necrotizing vasculitides. A
new pathogenetic classification. Med Clin North Am
1977; 61: 241–260.

304. Citron BP, Halpern M, McCarron M et al. Necrotizing
angiitis associated with drug abuse. N Engl J Med
1970; 283: 1003–1011.

305. Rose GA, Spencer H. Polyarteritis nodosa. Q J Med
1957; 26: 43–81.

306. Kawasaki T, Kosaki F, Okawa S et al. A new infantile
acute febrile mucocutaneous lymph node syndrome
(MLNS) prevailing in Japan. Pediatrics 1974; 54:
271–276.

307. Hicks RV, Melish ME. Kawasaki syndrome. Pediatr
Clin North Am 1986; 33: 1151–1175.

308. Butler DF, Hough DR, Friedman SJ, Davis HE. Adult
Kawasaki syndrome. Arch Dermatol 1987; 123:
1356–1361.

309. Weston WL, Huff JC. The mucocutaneous lymph node
syndrome: a critical re-examination. Clin Exp
Dermatol 1981; 6: 167–178.

310. Bell DM, Brink EW, Nitzkin JL et al. Kawasaki
syndrome: description of two outbreaks in the United
States. N Engl J Med 1981; 304: 1568–1575.

311. Everett ED. Acute febrile mucocutaneous lymph node
syndrome — Kawasaki syndrome. Int J Dermatol
1982; 21: 506–509.

312. Friter BS, Lucky AW. The perineal eruption of

Kawasaki syndrome. Arch Dermatol 1988; 124: 1805–1810.

313. Kimura T, Miyazawa H, Watanabe K, Moriya T. Small pustules in Kawasaki disease. A clinicopathological study of four patients. Am J Dermatopathol 1988; 10: 218–223.

314. Newburger JW, Takahashi M, Burns JC et al. The treatment of Kawasaki syndrome with intravenous gamma globulin. N Engl J Med 1986; 315: 341–347.

315. Rauch AM. Kawasaki syndrome: review of new epidemiologic and laboratory developments. Pediatr Infect Dis 1987; 6: 1016–1021.

316. Hirose S, Hamashima Y. Morphological observations on the vasculitis in the mucocutaneous lymph node syndrome. A skin biopsy study of 27 cases. Eur J Pediatr 1978; 129: 17–27.

317. Giblin WJ, James WD, Benson PM. Buerger's disease. Int J Dermatol 1989; 28: 638–642.

317a. Abdullah AN, Keczkes K. Thromboangiitis obliterans (Bürger's disease) in a woman — a case report and review of the literature. Clin Exp Dermatol 1990; 15: 46–49.

317b. Samlaska CP, James WD. Superficial thrombophlebitis I. Primary hypercoagulable states. J Am Acad Dermatol 1990; 22: 975–989.

317c. Samlaska CP, James WD. Superficial thrombophlebitis II. Secondary hypercoagulable states. J Am Acad Dermatol 1990; 23: 1–18.

318. Skipworth GB, Morris JB, Goldstein N. Bilateral Mondor's disease. Arch Dermatol 1967; 95: 95–97.

319. Aloi FG, Tomasini CF, Moliners A. Railway track-like dermatitis: An atypical Mondor's disease? J Am Acad Dermatol 1989; 20: 920–923.

320. Fine JD, Harrist TJ. Cutaneous leukocytoclastic vasculitis in the rose spot of paratyphoid fever. Int J Dermatol 1982; 21: 216–217.

321. Rosen T, Rubin H, Ellner K et al. Vesicular Jarisch–Herxheimer reaction. Arch Dermatol 1989; 125: 77–81.

Neutrophilic dermatoses

322. Hunt SJ, Santa Cruz DJ. Neutrophilic dermatoses. Semin Dermatol 1989; 8: 266–275.

323. Jorizzo JL. Pustular vasculitis: An emerging disease concept. J Am Acad Dermatol 1983; 9: 160–162.

324. Jorizzo JL, Schmalstieg FC, Dinehart SM et al. Bowel-associated dermatosis-arthritis syndrome. Immune complex-mediated vessel damage and increased neutrophil migration. Arch Intern Med 1984; 144: 738–740.

325. Ely PH, Utsinger PD. Clinical observations and immunologic abnormalities following bowel bypass surgery. J Am Acad Dermatol 1980; 2: 529–530.

326. Whittle CH, Beck GA, Champion RH. Recurrent neutrophilic dermatosis of the face — a variant of Sweet's syndrome. Br J Dermatol 1968; 80: 806–810.

327. Sweet RD. An acute febrile neutrophilic dermatosis. Br J Dermatol 1964; 76: 349–356.

328. Sweet RD. Further observations on acute febrile neutrophilic dermatosis. Br J Dermatol 1968; 80: 800–805.

329. Sweet RD. Acute febrile neutrophilic dermatosis — 1978. Br J Dermatol 1979; 100: 93–99.

330. Greer KE, Cooper PH. Sweet's syndrome (acute febrile neutrophilic dermatosis). Clin Rheum Dis 1982; 8: 427–441.

331. Christensen OB, Holst R, Svensson A. Chronic recurrent annular neutrophilic dermatosis. An entity? Acta Derm Venereol 1989; 69: 415–418.

332. Goldman GC, Moschella SL. Acute febrile neutrophilic dermatosis (Sweet's syndrome). Arch Dermatol 1971; 103: 654–660.

333. Itami S, Nishioka K. Sweet's syndrome in infancy. Br J Dermatol 1980; 103: 449–451.

334. Gunawardena DA, Gunawardena KA, Ratnayaka RMRS, Vasanthanathan NS. The clinical spectrum of Sweet's syndrome (acute febrile neutrophilic dermatosis) — a report of eighteen cases. Br J Dermatol 1975; 92: 363–373.

335. Raimer SS, Duncan WC. Febrile neutrophilic dermatosis in acute myelogenous leukemia. Arch Dermatol 1978; 114: 413–414.

336. Behm FG, Kay S, Aportela R. Febrile neutrophilic dermatosis associated with acute leukemia. Am J Clin Pathol 1981; 76: 344–347.

337. Gisser SD. Acute febrile neutrophilic dermatosis (Sweet's syndrome) in a patient with hairy-cell leukemia. Am J Dermatopathol 1983; 5: 283–288.

338. Ilchyshyn A, Smith AG, Phaure TAJ. Sweet's syndrome associated with chronic lymphatic leukaemia. Clin Exp Dermatol 1987; 12: 277–279.

339. Soderstrom RM. Acute febrile neutrophilic dermatosis (Sweet's syndrome) and internal malignancy. Semin Dermatol 1984; 3: 337–339.

340. Cooper PH, Innes DJ, Greer KE. Acute febrile neutrophilic dermatosis (Sweet's syndrome) and myeloproliferative disorders. Cancer 1983; 51: 1518–1526.

341. Clemmensen OJ, Menne T, Brandrup F et al. Acute febrile neutrophilic dermatosis — a marker of malignancy? Acta Derm Venereol 1989; 69: 52–58.

342. Burton JL. Sweet's syndrome, pyoderma gangrenosum and acute leukaemia. Br J Dermatol 1980; 102: 239.

343. Gibson LE, Dicken CH, Flach DB. Neutrophilic dermatoses and myeloproliferative disease: Report of two cases. Mayo Clin Proc 1985; 60: 735–740.

344. Caughman W, Stern R, Haynes H. Neutrophilic dermatosis of myeloproliferative disorders. J Am Acad Dermatol 1983; 9: 751–758.

345. Callen JP. Acute febrile neutrophilic dermatosis (Sweet's syndrome) and the related conditions of "bowel bypass" syndrome and bullous pyoderma gangrenosum. Dermatol Clin 1985; 3: 153–163.

346. Grob JJ, Mege JL, Prax AM, Bonerandi JJ. Disseminated pustular dermatosis in polycythemia vera. J Am Acad Dermatol 1988; 1 febrile neutrophilic dermatosis (Sweet's syndrome) associated with lymphoma. Hum Pathol 1985; 16: 520–522.

347. Horan MP, Redmond J, Gehle D et al. Postpolycythemic myeloid metaplasia, Sweet's syndrome, and acute myeloid leukemia. J Am Acad Dermatol 1987; 16: 458–462.

348. Krolikowski FJ, Reuter K, Shultis EW. Acute febrile neutrophilic dermatosis (Sweet's syndrome) associated with lymphoma. Hum Pathol 1985; 16: 520–522.

349. Schwartz RA, French SW, Rubenstein DJ, Lambert WC. Acute neutrophilic dermatosis with diffuse histiocytic lymphoma. J Am Acad Dermatol 1984; 10: 350–354.

350. Berth-Jones J, Hutchinson PE. Sweet's syndrome and malignancy: a case associated with multiple myeloma and review of the literature. Br J Dermatol 1989; 121: 123–127.
351. Mali-Gerrits MGH, Rampen FHJ. Acute febrile neutrophilic dermatosis (Sweet's syndrome) and adenocarcinoma of the rectum. Clin Exp Dermatol 1988; 13: 105–106.
352. Dyall-Smith D, Billson V. Sweet's syndrome associated with adenocarcinoma of the prostate. Australas J Dermatol 1988; 29: 25–27.
353. Mizoguchi M, Chikakane K, Goh K et al. Acute febrile neutrophilic dermatosis (Sweet's syndrome) in Behçet's disease. Br J Dermatol 1987; 116: 727–734.
354. Mizoguchi M, Matsuki K, Mochizuki M et al. Human leukocyte antigen in Sweet's syndrome and its relationship to Behçet's disease. Arch Dermatol 1988; 124: 1069–1073.
355. Goette DK. Sweet's syndrome in subacute cutaneous lupus erythematosus. Arch Dermatol 1985; 121: 789–791.
356. Servitje O, Ribera M, Juanola X, Rodriguez-Moreno J. Acute neutrophilic dermatosis associated with hydralazine-induced lupus. Arch Dermatol 1987; 123: 1435–1436.
357. Becuwe C, Delaporte E, Colombel JF et al. Sweet's syndrome associated with Crohn's disease. Acta Derm Venereol 1989; 69: 444–445.
358. Radeff B, Harms M. Acute febrile neutrophilic dermatosis (Sweet's syndrome) following BCG vaccination. Acta Derm Venereol 1986; 66: 357–358.
359. Cobb MW. Furosemide-induced eruption simulating Sweet's syndrome. J Am Acad Dermatol 1989; 21: 339–343.
360. Aram H. Acute febrile neutrophilic dermatosis (Sweet's syndrome). Response to dapsone. Arch Dermatol 1984; 120: 245–247.
361. Kaplan SS, Wechsler HL, Basford RE et al. Increased plasma chemoattractant in Sweet's syndrome. J Am Acad Dermatol 1985; 12: 1013–1021.
362. Keefe M, Wakeel RA, Kerr REI. Sweet's syndrome, plantar pustulosis and vulval pustules. Clin Exp Dermatol 1988; 13: 344–346.
363. Jordaan HF. Acute febrile neutrophilic dermatosis. A histopathological study of 37 patients and a review of the literature. Am J Dermatopathol 1989; 11: 99–111.
364. Dicken CH, Seehafer JR. Bowel bypass syndrome. Arch Dermatol 1979; 115: 837–839.
365. Ely PH. The bowel bypass syndrome: A response to bacterial peptidoglycans. J Am Acad Dermatol 1980; 2: 473–487.
366. Kennedy C. The spectrum of inflammatory skin disease following jejuno-ileal bypass for morbid obesity. Br J Dermatol 1981; 105: 425–436.
367. Kemp DR, Gin D. Bowel-associated dermatosis-arthritis syndrome. Med J Aust 1990; 152: 43–45.
368. Dicken CH. Bowel-associated dermatosis-arthritis syndrome: bowel bypass syndrome without bowel bypass. Mayo Clin Proc 1984; 59: 43–46.
369. Dicken CH. Bowel-associated dermatosis-arthritis syndrome: bowel bypass syndrome without bowel bypass. J Am Acad Dermatol 1986; 14: 792–796.
370. Jorizzo JL, Apisarnthanarax P, Subrt P et al. Bowel-bypass syndrome without bowel bypass. Bowel-associated dermatosis-arthritis syndrome. Arch Intern Med 1983; 143: 457–461.
371. Utsinger PD. Systemic immune complex disease following intestinal bypass surgery: Bypass disease. J Am Acad Dermatol 1980; 2: 488–495.
372. Morrison JGL, Fourie ED. A distinctive skin eruption following small-bowel by-pass surgery. Br J Dermatol 1980; 102: 467–471.
373. Goldman JA, Casey HL, Davidson ED et al. Vasculitis associated with intestinal bypass surgery. Arch Dermatol 1979; 115: 725–727.
374. O'Loughlin S, Perry HO. A diffuse pustular eruption associated with ulcerative colitis. Arch Dermatol 1978; 114: 1061–1064.
375. Ackerman AB. Histologic diagnosis of inflammatory skin diseases. Philadelphia: Lea & Febiger, 1978; 449–451.
376. Scherbenske JM, Benson PM, Lupton GP, Samlaska CP. Rheumatoid neutrophilic dermatitis. Arch Dermatol 1989; 125: 1105–1108.
377. Delaporte E, Graveau DJ, Piette FA, Bergoend HA. Acute febrile neutrophilic dermatosis (Sweet's syndrome). Association with rheumatoid vasculitis. Arch Dermatol 1989; 125: 1101–1104.
377a. Sanchez JL, Cruz A. Rheumatoid neutrophilic dermatitis. J Am Acad Dermatol 1990; 22: 922–925.
378. Weedon D. Unpublished observations.
379. Tan RS-H. Acute generalized pustular bacterid. An unusual manifestation of leukocytoclastic vasculitis. Br J Dermatol 1974; 91: 209–215.
380. Miyachi Y, Danno K, Yanase K, Imamura S. Acute generalized pustular bacterid and immune complexes. Acta Derm Venereol 1980; 60: 66–69.
381. McNeely MC, Jorizzo JL, Solomon AR Jr et al. Primary idiopathic cutaneous pustular vasculitis. J Am Acad Dermatol 1986; 14: 939–944.
381a. Rustin MHA, Robinson TWE, Dowd PM. Toxic pustuloderma: a self-limiting eruption. Br J Dermatol 1990; 123: 119–124.
382. James DG. Behçet's syndrome. N Engl J Med 1979; 301: 431–432.
383. Jorizzo JL, Taylor RS, Schmalstieg FC et al. Complex aphthosis: A forme fruste of Behçet's syndrome? J Am Acad Dermatol 1985; 13: 80–84.
384. Haim S. Contribution of ocular symptoms in the diagnosis of Behçet's disease. Study of 23 cases. Arch Dermatol 1968; 98: 478–480.
385. Arbesfeld SJ, Kurban AK. Behçet's disease. New perspectives on an enigmatic syndrome. J Am Acad Dermatol 1988; 19: 767–779.
386. Chun SI, Su WPD, Lee S, Rogers RS III. Erythema nodosum-like lesions in Behçet's syndrome: a histopathologic study of 30 cases. J Cutan Pathol 1989; 16: 259–265.
387. Haim S, Sobel JD, Friedman-Birnbaum R. Thrombophlebitis. A cardinal symptom of Behçet's syndrome. Acta Derm Venereol 1974; 54: 299–301.
388. Chajek T, Fainaru M. Behçet's disease. Report of 41 cases and a review of the literature. Medicine (Baltimore) 1975; 54: 179–196.
389. Gilhar A, Winterstein G, Turani H et al. Skin hyperreactivity response (pathergy) in Behçet's disease. J Am Acad Dermatol 1989; 21: 547–552.
390. Wong RC, Ellis CN, Diaz LA. Behçet's disease. Int J Dermatol 1984; 23: 25–32.
391. Cho KH, Shin KS, Sohn SJ et al. Behçet's disease with Sweet's syndrome-like presentation — a report of six cases. Clin Exp Dermatol 1989; 14: 20–24.

392. Rakover Y, Adar H, Tal I et al. Behcet disease: long-term follow-up of three children and review of the literature. Pediatrics 1989; 83: 986–992.

393. Jorizzo JL. Behçet's disease. An update based on the 1985 international conference in London. Arch Dermatol 1986; 122: 556–558.

394. Dundar SV, Gencalp U, Simsek H. Familial cases of Behcet's disease. Br J Dermatol 1985; 113: 319–321.

395. Jorizzo JL, Hudson RD, Schmalstieg FC et al. Behçet's syndrome: Immune regulation, circulating immune complexes, neutrophil migration, and colchicine therapy. J Am Acad Dermatol 1984; 10: 205–214.

396. Kaneko F, Takahashi Y, Muramatsu R et al. Natural killer cell numbers and function in peripheral lymphoid cells in Behcet's disease. Br J Dermatol 1985; 113: 313–318.

397. Lim SD, Haw CR, Kim NI, Fusaro RM. Abnormalities of T-cell subsets in Behçet's syndrome. Arch Dermatol 1983; 119: 307–310.

398. Rogers RS III, Sams WM Jr, Shorter RG. Lymphocytotoxicity in recurrent aphthous stomatitis. Lymphocytotoxicity for oral epithelial cells in recurrent aphthous stomatitis and Behcet syndrome. Arch Dermatol 1974; 109: 361–366.

399. Kaneko F, Takahashi Y, Muramatsu Y, Miura Y. Immunological studies on aphthous ulcer and erythema nodosum-like eruptions in Behξet's disease. Br J Dermatol 1985; 113: 303–312.

400. Muller W, Lehner T. Quantitative electron microscopical analysis of leukocyte infiltrate in oral ulcers of Behcet's syndrome. Br J Dermatol 1982; 106: 535–544.

401. Honma T, Saito T, Fujioka Y. Intraepithelial atypical lymphocytes in oral lesions of Behcet's syndrome. Arch Dermatol 1981; 117: 83–85.

402. Bang D, Honma T, Saito T et al. The pathogenesis of vascular changes in erythema nodosum-like lesions of Behçet's syndrome: an electron microscopic study. Hum Pathol 1987; 18: 1172–1179.

403. Haim S, Sobel JD, Friedman-Birnbaum R, Lichtig C. Histological and direct immunofluorescence study of cutaneous hyperreactivity in Behçet's disease. Br J Dermatol 1976; 95: 631–636.

404. Jorizzo JL, Solomon AR, Cavallo T. Behçet's syndrome. Arch Pathol Lab Med 1985; 109: 747–751.

405. Lichtig C, Haim S, Hammel I, Friedman-Birnbaum R. The quantification and significance of mast cells in lesions of Behcet's disease. Br J Dermatol 1980; 102: 255–259.

406. Toroko Y, Seto T, Abe Y et al. Skin lesions in Behçet's disease. Int J Dermatol 1977; 16: 227–244.

Chronic lymphocytic vasculitis

407. Massa MC, Su WPD. Lymphocytic vasculitis: is it a special clinicopathologic entity? J Cutan Pathol 1984; 11: 132–139.

408. Vuzevski VD, van Joost T, Wagenvoort JHT, Day JJM. Cutaneous pathology in toxic shock syndrome. Int J Dermatol 1989; 28: 94–97.

409. Coskey RJ. Eruptions due to oral contraceptives. Arch Dermatol 1977; 113: 333–334.

410. Holmes RC, Black MM, Dann J et al. A comparative study of toxic erythema of pregnancy and herpes gestationis. Br J Dermatol 1982; 106: 499–510.

411. Jurecka W, Holmes RC, Black MM et al. An immunoelectron microscopy study of the relationship between herpes gestationis and polymorphic eruption of pregnancy. Br J Dermatol 1983; 108: 147–151.

412. Charles-Holmes R. Polymorphic eruption of pregnancy. Semin Dermatol 1989; 8: 18–22.

413. Nurse DS. Prurigo of pregnancy. Australas J Dermatol 1968; 9: 258–267.

414. Faber WR, Van Joost T, Hausman R, Weenink GH. Late prurigo of pregnancy. Br J Dermatol 1982; 106: 511–516.

415. Cooper AJ, Fryer JA. Prurigo of late pregnancy. Australas J Dermatol 1980; 21: 79–84.

416. Lawley TJ, Hertz KC, Wade TR et al. Pruritic urticarial papules and plaques of pregnancy. JAMA 1979; 241: 1696–1699.

417. Yancey KB, Hall RP, Lawley TJ. Pruritic urticarial papules and plaques of pregnancy. Clinical experience in twenty-five patients. J Am Acad Dermatol 1984; 10: 473–480.

418. Uhlin SR. Pruritic urticarial papules and plaques of pregnancy. Involvement in mother and infant. Arch Dermatol 1981; 117: 238–239.

419. Cohen LM, Capeless EL, Krusinski PA, Maloney ME. Pruritic urticarial papules and plaques of pregnancy and its relationship to maternal-fetal weight gain and twin pregnancy. Arch Dermatol 1989; 125: 1534–1536.

419a. Bunker CB, Erskine K, Rustin MHA, Gilkes JJH. Severe polymorphic eruption of pregnancy occurring in twin pregnancies. Clin Exp Dermatol 1990; 15: 228–231.

420. Sasseville D, Wilkinson RD, Schnader JY. Dermatoses of pregnancy. Int J Dermatol 1981; 20: 223–241.

421. Callen JP, Hanno R. Pruritic urticarial papules and plaques of pregnancy (PUPPP). A clinicopathologic study. J Am Acad Dermatol 1981; 5: 401–405.

422. Winton GB, Lewis CW. Dermatoses of pregnancy. J Am Acad Dermatol 1982; 6: 977–998.

423. Ahmed AR, Kaplan R. Pruritic urticarial papules and plaques of pregnancy. J Am Acad Dermatol 1981; 4: 679–681.

424. Holmes RC, Black MM. The specific dermatoses of pregnancy: a reappraisal with specific emphasis on a proposed simplified clinical classification. Clin Exp Dermatol 1982; 7: 65–73.

425. Holmes RC, Black MM. The specific dermatoses of pregnancy. J Am Acad Dermatol 1983; 8: 405–412.

426. Black MM. Prurigo of pregnancy, papular dermatitis of pregnancy, and pruritic folliculitis of pregnancy. Semin Dermatol 1989; 8: 23–25.

427. Rahbari H. Pruritic papules of pregnancy. J Cutan Pathol 1978; 5: 347–352.

428. Spangler AS, Reddy W, Bardawil WA et al. Papular dermatitis of pregnancy: A new clinical entity? JAMA 1962; 181: 577–581.

429. Harrison PV. The annular erythemas. Int J Dermatol 1979; 18: 282–290.

430. Hurley HJ, Hurley JP. The gyrate erythemas. Semin Dermatol 1984; 3: 327–336.

431. White JW Jr. Gyrate erythema. Dermatol Clin 1985; 3: 129–139.

432. White JW, Perry HO. Erythema perstans. Br J Dermatol 1969; 81: 641–651.

433. Ackerman AB. Histologic diagnosis of inflammatory

skin diseases. Philadelphia: Lea & Febiger, 1978; 231–233.

434. Bressler GS, Jones RE Jr. Erythema annulare centrifugum. J Am Acad Dermatol 1981; 4: 597–602.

435. Braunstein BL. Erythema annulare centrifugum and Graves' disease. Arch Dermatol 1982; 118: 623.

436. Burkhart CG. Erythema annulare centrifugum. A case due to tuberculosis. Int J Dermatol 1982; 21: 538–539.

437. Vasily DB, Bhatia SG. Erythema annulare centrifugum and molluscum contagiosum. Arch Report of two further cases associated with carcinoma. Br J Dermatol 1970; 82: 406–411.

438. Hendricks AA, Lu C, Elfenbein GJ, Hussain R. Erythema annulare centrifugum associated with ascariasis. Arch Dermatol 1981; 117: 582–585.

439. Stillians A. Erythema annulare centrifugum. Its relation to internal disease. Arch Dermatol 1953; 67: 590–593.

440. Everall JD, Dowd PM, Ardalan B. Unusual cutaneous associations of a malignant carcinoid tumour of the bronchus — erythema annulare centrifugum and white banding of the toe nails. Br J Dermatol 1975; 93: 341–345.

441. Dodd HJ, Kirby JDT, Chambers TJ, Stansfeld AG. Erythema annulare centrifugum and malignant histiocytosis — report of a case. Clin Exp Dermatol 1984; 9: 608–613.

442. Mahood JM. Erythema annulare centrifugum: a review of 24 cases with special reference to its association with underlying disease. Clin Exp Dermatol 1983; 8: 383–387.

443. Merrett AC, Marks R, Dudley FJ. Cimetidine-induced erythema annulare centrifugum: no cross-sensitivity with ranitidine. Br Med J 1981; 283: 698.

444. Goette DK, Beatrice E. Erythema annulare centrifugum caused by hydrochlorothiazide-induced interstitial nephritis. Int J Dermatol 1988; 27: 129–130.

445. Ashurst PJ. Erythema annulare centrifugum; due to hydroxychloroquine sulfate and chloroquine sulfate. Arch Dermatol 1967; 95: 37–39.

446. Teramoto N, Katayama I, Arai H et al. Annular erythema: A possible association with primary Sjögren's syndrome. J Am Acad Dermatol 1989; 20: 596–601.

447. Olsen TG, Milroy SK, Jones-Olsen S. Erythema gyratum repens with associated squamous cell carcinoma of the lung. Cutis 1984; 34: 351–355.

448. Skolnick M, Mainman ER. Erythema gyratum repens with metastatic adenocarcinoma. Arch Dermatol 1975; 111: 227–229.

449. Willis WF. The gyrate erythemas. Int J Dermatol 1978; 17: 698–702.

450. Appell ML, Ward WQ, Tyring SK. Erythema gyratum repens. A cutaneous marker of malignancy. Cancer 1988; 62: 548–550.

451. Holt PJA, Davies MG. Erythema gyratum repens — an immunologically mediated dermatosis? Br J Dermatol 1977; 96: 343–347.

452. Barber PV, Doyle L, Vickers DM, Hubbard H. Erythema gyratum repens with pulmonary tuberculosis. Br J Dermatol 1978; 98: 465–468.

453. Juhlin L, Lacour JP, Larrouy JC et al. Episodic erythema gyratum repens with ichthyosis and

palmoplantar hyperkeratosis without signs of internal malignancy. Clin Exp Dermatol 1989; 14: 223–226.

454. Cheesbrough MJ, Williamson DM. Erythema gyratum repens, a stage in the resolution of pityriasis rubra pilaris? Clin Exp Dermatol 1985; 10: 466–471.

455. Stankler L. Erythema gyratum repens: spontaneous resolution in a healthy man. Br J Dermatol 1978; 99: 461.

456. Langlois JC, Shaw JM, Odland GF. Erythema gyratum repens unassociated with internal malignancy. J Am Acad Dermatol 1985; 12: 911–913.

457. Thomson J, Stankler L. Erythema gyratum repens. 114–116.

458. Leavell UW Jr, Winternitz WW, Black JH. Erythema gyratum repens and undifferentiated carcinoma. Arch Dermatol 1967; 95: 69–72.

459. Okoroma OE, Ihenacho HNC, Anyanwu CH. Rheumatic fever in Nigerian children. A prospective study of 66 patients. Am J Dis Child 1981; 135: 236–238.

460. Troyer C, Grossman M, Silvers DN. Erythema marginatum in rheumatic fever: Early diagnosis by skin biopsy. J Am Acad Dermatol 1983; 8: 724–728.

461. Sahn EE, Maize JC, Silver RM. Erythema marginatum: an unusual histopathologic manifestation. J Am Acad Dermatol 1989; 21: 145–147.

462. Beare JM, Froggatt P, Jones JH, Neill DW. Familial annular erythema. An apparently new dominant mutation. Br J Dermatol 1966; 78: 59–68.

463. Peterson AO Jr, Jarratt M. Annular erythema of infancy. Arch Dermatol 1981; 117: 145–148.

464. Cox NH, McQueen A, Evans TJ, Morley WN. An annular erythema of infancy. Arch Dermatol 1987; 123: 510–513.

465. Hebert AA, Esterly NB. Annular erythema of infancy. J Am Acad Dermatol 1986; 14: 339–343.

466. Toonstra J, de Wit RFE. 'Persistent' annular erythema of infancy. Arch Dermatol 1984; 120: 1069–1072.

467. Gianotti F, Ermacora E. Erythema gyratum atrophicans transiens neonatale. Arch Dermatol 1975; 111: 615–616.

468. Saurat JH, Janin-Mercier A. Infantile epidermodysplastic erythema gyratum responsive to imidazoles. A new entity? Arch Dermatol 1984; 120: 1601–1603.

469. Hammar H, Ronnerfalt L. Annular erythemas in infants associated with autoimmune disorders in their mothers. Dermatologica 1977; 154: 115–127.

470. Miyagawa S, Kitamura W, Yoshioka J, Sakamoto K. Placental transfer of anticytoplasmic antibodies in annular erythema of newborns. Arch Dermatol 1981; 117: 569–572.

471. Marks R, Black M, Wilson Jones E. Pityriasis lichenoides: a reappraisal. Br J Dermatol 1972; 86: 215–225.

472. Truhan AP, Hebert AA, Esterly NB. Pityriasis lichenoides in children: Therapeutic response to erythromycin. J Am Acad Dermatol 1986; 15: 66–70.

473. Shavin JS, Jones TM, Aton JK et al. Mucha–Habermann's disease in children. Treatment with erythromycin. Arch Dermatol 1978; 114: 1679–1680.

474. Burke DP, Adams RM, Arundell FD. Febrile ulceronecrotic Mucha–Habermann's disease. Arch Dermatol 1969; 100: 200–206.

475. Auster BI, Santa Cruz DJ, Eisen AZ. Febrile ulceronecrotic Mucha–Habermann's disease with interstitial pneumonitis. J Cutan Pathol 1979; 6: 66–76.

476. Clayton R, Warin A. Pityriasis lichenoides chronica presenting as hypopigmentation. Br J Dermatol 1979; 100: 297–302.

477. Warin AP. Hypochromic variant of pityriasis lichenoides chronica. Clin Exp Dermatol 1978; 3: 85–88.

478. Zlatkov NB, Andreev VC. Toxoplasmosis and pityriasis lichenoides. Br J Dermatol 1972; 87: Dermatol 1978; 114: 1853.

479. Muhlbauer JE, Bhan AK, Harrist TJ et al. Immunopathology of pityriasis lichenoides acuta. J Am Acad Dermatol 1984; 10: 783–795.

480. Willemze R, Scheffer E. Clinical and histologic differentiation between lymphomatoid papulosis and pityriasis lichenoides. J Am Acad Dermatol 1985; 13: 418–428.

481. Marks R, Black MM. The epidermal component of pityriasis lichenoides. Br J Dermatol 1972; 87: 106–113.

482. Hood AF, Mark EJ. Histopathologic diagnosis of pityriasis lichenoides et varioliformis acuta and its clinical correlation. Arch Dermatol 1982; 118: 478–482.

483. Szymanski FJ. Pityriasis lichenoides et varioliformis acuta: Histopathological evidence that it is an entity distinct from parapsoriasis. Arch Dermatol 1959; 79: 7–16.

484. Longley J, Demar L, Feinstein RP et al. Clinical and histologic features of pityriasis lichenoides et varioliformis acuta in children. Arch Dermatol 1987; 123: 1335–1339.

485. Black MM, Marks R. The inflammatory reaction in pityriasis lichenoides. Br J Dermatol 1972; 87: 533–539.

486. Benmaman O, Sanchez JL. Comparative clinicopathological study on pityriasis lichenoides chronica and small plaque parapsoriasis. Am J Dermatopathol 1988; 10: 189–196.

487. Wood GS, Strickler JG, Abel EA et al. Immunohistology of pityriasis lichenoides et varioliformis acuta and pityriasis lichenoides chronica. Evidence for their interrelationship with lymphomatoid papulosis. J Am Acad Dermatol 1987; 16: 559–570.

488. Thivolet J, Faure M, Chouvet B. Immunofluorescence study of pityriasis lichenoides. Br J Dermatol 1979; 101: 237.

489. Clayton R, Haffenden G. An immunofluorescence study of pityriasis lichenoides. Br J Dermatol 1978; 99: 491–493.

490. Faber WR, van Joost T. Pityriasis lichenoides, an immune complex disease? Acta Derm Venereol 1980; 60: 259–261.

491. Graham RM, English JS, Emmerson RW. Lichen aureus — a study of twelve cases. Clin Exp Dermatol 1984; 9: 393–401.

492. Newton RC, Raimer SS. Pigmented purpuric eruptions. Dermatol Clin 1985; 3: 165–169.

493. Jorizzo JL, Gonzalez EB, Apisarnthanarax P, Daniels JC. Pigmented purpuric eruption in a patient with rheumatoid arthritis. Arch Intern Med 1982; 142: 2184–2185.

494. Stell JS, Moyer DG. Schamberg's disease. Arch Dermatol 1966; 94: 626–627.

495. Randall SJ, Kierland RR, Montgomery H. Pigmented purpuric eruptions. Arch Dermatol 1951; 64: 177–191.

496. Baden HP. Familial Schamberg's disease. Arch Dermatol 1964; 90: 400.

497. Doucas C, Kapetanakis J. Eczematid-like purpura. Dermatologica 1953; 106: 86–95.

498. Loewenthal LJA. Itching purpura. Br J Dermatol 1954; 66: 95–103.

499. Osment LS, Noojin RO, Lewis RA, Lupton CH. Transitory pigmented purpuric eruption of the lower extremities. Arch Dermatol 1960; 81: 591–598.

500. Pravda DJ, Moynihan GD. Itching purpura. Cutis 1980; 25: 147–151.

501. Mosto SJ, Casala AM. Disseminated pruriginous angiodermatitis (itching purpura). Arch Dermatol 1965; 91: 351–356.

502. Wong RC, Solomon AR, Field SI, Anderson TF. Pigmented purpuric lichenoid dermatitis of Gougerot–Blum mimicking Kaposi's sarcoma. Cutis 1983; 31: 406–410.

503. Ayala F, Donofrio P. Lichen aureus vel purpuricus: report of a case. Clin Exp Dermatol 1984; 9: 205–208.

504. Abramovits W, Landau JW, Lowe NJ. A report of two patients with lichen aureus. Arch Dermatol 1980; 116: 1183–1184.

505. Price ML, Wilson Jones E, Calnan CD, MacDonald DM. Lichen aureus: A localized persistent form of pigmented purpuric dermatitis. Br J Dermatol 1985; 112: 307–314.

506. English J. Lichen aureus. J Am Acad Dermatol 1985; 12: 377–378.

507. Rudolph RI. Lichen aureus. J Am Acad Dermatol 1983; 8: 722–724.

508. Kossard S, Shumack S. Lichen aureus of the glans penis as an expression of Zoon's balanitis. J Am Acad Dermatol 1989; 21: 804–806.

509. Aiba S, Tagami H. Immunohistologic studies in Schamberg's disease. Evidence for cellular immune reaction in lesional skin. Arch Dermatol 1988; 124: 1058–1062.

510. Simon M Jr, Heese A, Gotz A. Immunopathological investigations in purpura pigmentosa chronica. Acta Derm Venereol 1989; 69: 101–104.

511. Reinhardt L, Wilkin JK, Tausend R. Vascular abnormalities in lichen aureus. J Am Acad Dermatol 1983; 8: 417–420.

512. Shelley WB, Swaminathan R, Shelley ED. Lichen aureus: A haemosiderin tattoo associated with perforator vein incompetence. J Am Acad Dermatol 1984; 11: 260–264.

513. Greenwood K. Dermatitis with capillary fragility. Arch Dermatol 1960; 81: 947–952.

514. Nishioka K, Sarashi C, Katayama I. Chronic pigmented purpura induced by chemical substances. Clin Exp Dermatol 1980; 5: 213–218.

515. Peterson WC Jr, Manick KP. Purpuric eruptions associated with use of carbromal and meprobamate. Arch Dermatol 1967; 95: 40–42.

516. Waisman M, Waisman M. Lichen aureus. Arch Dermatol 1976; 112: 696–697.

517. Waisman M. Lichen aureus. Int J Dermatol 1985; 24: 645–646.

518. Barnhill RL, Braverman IM. Progression of pigmented purpura-like eruptions to mycosis fungoides: Report of

three cases. J Am Acad Dermatol 1988; 19: 25–31.

519. Iwatsuki K, Aoshima T, Tagami H et al. Immunofluorescence study in purpura pigmentosa chronica. Acta Derm Venereol 1980; 60: 341–345.

520. Geiger JM, Grosshans E, Hanau D. Lichen aureus: Ultrastructural study. J Cutan Pathol 1981; 8: 150.

521. Magrinat G, Kerwin KS, Gabriel DA. The clinical manifestations of Degos' syndrome. Arch Pathol Lab Med 1989; 113: 354–362.

522. Black MM. Malignant atrophic papulosis (Degos' disease). Int J Dermatol 1976; 15: 405–411.

523. Degos R. Malignant atrophic papulosis. Br J Dermatol 1979; 100: 21–35.

524. Muller SA, Landry M. Malignant atrophic papulosis (Degos disease). Arch Dermatol 1976; 112: 357–363.

525. Roenigk HH, Farmer RG. Degos' disease (malignant papulosis). Report of three cases with clues to etiology. JAMA 1968; 206: 1508–1514.

526. Howsden SM, Hodge SJ, Herndon JH, Freeman RG. Malignant atrophic papulosis of Degos. Report of a patient who failed to respond to fibrinolytic therapy. Arch Dermatol 1976; 112: 1582–1588.

527. Barlow RJ, Heyl T, Simson IW, Schulz EJ. Malignant atrophic papulosis (Degos' disease) — diffuse involvement of brain and bowel in an African patient. Br J Dermatol 1988; 118: 117–123.

528. Nomland R, Layton JM. Malignant papulosis with atrophy (Degos). Fatal cutaneointestinal syndrome. Arch Dermatol 1960; 81: 181–197.

529. Hall-Smith P. Malignant atrophic papulosis (Degos' disease). Two cases occurring in the same family. Br J Dermatol 1969; 81: 817–822.

530. Newton JA, Black MM. Familial malignant atrophic papulosis. Clin Exp Dermatol 1984; 9: 298–299.

531. Kisch LS, Bruynzeel DP. Six cases of malignant atrophic papulosis (Degos' disease) occurring in one family. Br J Dermatol 1984; 111: 469–471.

532. Tribble K, Archer ME, Jorizzo JL et al. Malignant atrophic papulosis: Absence of circulating immune complexes or vasculitis. J Am Acad Dermatol 1986; 15: 365–369.

533. Muller SA, Landry M. Exchange autografts in malignant atrophic papulosis (Degos' disease). Mayo Clin Proc 1974; 49: 884–888.

534. Black MM, Nishioka K, Levene GM. The role of dermal blood vessels in the pathogenesis of malignant atrophic papulosis (Degos' disease). Br J Dermatol 1973; 88: 213–219.

535. Soter NA, Murphy GF, Mihm MC. Lymphocytes and necrosis of the cutaneous microvasculature in malignant atrophic papulosis: A refined light microscope study. J Am Acad Dermatol 1982; 7: 620–630.

536. Feuerman EJ, Dollberg L, Salvador O. Malignant atrophic papulosis with mucin in the dermis. Arch Pathol 1970; 90: 310–315.

537. Black MM. Malignant atrophic papulosis (Degos' syndrome). Br J Dermatol 1971; 85: 290–292.

538. Bleehen SS. Intra-endothelial tubular aggregates in malignant atrophic papulosis (Degos' disease). Clin Exp Dermatol 1977; 2: 73–74.

539. Stahl D, Thomsen K, Hou-Jensen K. Malignant atrophic papulosis. Treatment with aspirin and dipyridamole. Arch Dermatol 1978; 114: 1687–1689.

540. Coskey RJ, Mehregan AH. Shoe boot pernio. Arch Dermatol 1974; 109: 56–57.

541. Wall LM, Smith NP. Perniosis: a histopathological review. Clin Exp Dermatol 1981; 6: 263–271.

542. Millard LG, Rowell NR. Chilblain lupus erythematosus (Hutchinson). Br J Dermatol 1978; 98: 497–506.

543. Kelly JW, Dowling JP. Pernio. A possible association with chronic myelomonocytic leukemia. Arch Dermatol 1985; 121: 1048–1052.

544. Ferguson DL, Hawk RJ, Covington NM, Reed RJ. Lichenoid lymphocytic vasculitis with a high component of histiocytes. Am J Dermatopathol 1989; 11: 259–269.

545. Schwaegerle SM, Bergfeld WF, Senitzer D, Tidrick RT. Pyoderma gangrenosum: A review. J Am Acad Dermatol 1988; 18: 559–568.

546. Powell FC, Schroeter AL, Su WPD, Perry HO. Pyoderma gangrenosum: a review of 86 patients. Q J Med 1985; 55: 173–186.

547. Prystowsky JH, Kahn SN, Lazarus GS. Present status of pyoderma gangrenosum. Review of 21 cases. Arch Dermatol 1989; 125: 57–64.

548. Malkinson FD. Pyoderma gangrenosum vs malignant pyoderma. Arch Dermatol 1987; 123: 333–337.

549. Snyder RA. Pyoderma gangrenosum involving the head and neck. Arch Dermatol 1986; 122: 295–302.

550. Powell FC, Perry HO. Pyoderma gangrenosum in childhood. Arch Dermatol 1984; 120: 757–761.

551. Barnes L, Lucky AW, Bucuvalas JC, Suchy FJ. Pustular pyoderma gangrenosum associated with ulcerative colitis in childhood. J Am Acad Dermatol 1986; 15: 608–614.

552. Shands JW Jr, Flowers FP, Hill HM, Smith JO. Pyoderma gangrenosum in a kindred. J Am Acad Dermatol 1987; 16: 931–934.

553. Callen JP, Dubin HV, Gehrke CF. Recurrent pyoderma gangrenosum and agnogenic myeloid metaplasia. Arch Dermatol 1977; 113: 1585–1586.

554. Horton JJ, Trounce JR, MacDonald DM. Bullous pyoderma gangrenosum and multiple myeloma. Br J Dermatol 1984; 110: 227–230.

555. Sheps M, Shapero H, Ramsay C. Bullous pyoderma gangrenosum and acute leukemia. Arch Dermatol 1978; 114: 1842–1843.

556. Pye RJ, Choudhury C. Bullous pyoderma as a presentation of acute leukaemia. Clin Exp Dermatol 1977; 2: 33–38.

557. Perry HO, Winkelmann RK, Muller SA, Kierland RR. Malignant pyodermas. Arch Dermatol 1968; 98: 561–576.

558. Dicken CH. Malignant pyoderma. J Am Acad Dermatol 1985; 13: 1021–1025.

559. Wernikoff S, Merritt C, Briggaman RA, Woodley DT. Malignant pyoderma or pyoderma gangrenosum of the head and neck? Arch Dermatol 1987; 123: 371–375.

560. Novice FM, Hacker P, Unger WP, Keystone EC. Malignant pyoderma. Int J Dermatol 1987; 26: 42–44.

561. Wilson-Jones E, Winkelmann RK. Superficial granulomatous pyoderma: A localized vegetative form of pyoderma gangrenosum. J Am Acad Dermatol 1988; 18: 511–521.

562. Quimby SR, Gibson LE, Winkelmann RK. Superficial granulomatous pyoderma: clinicopathologic spectrum. Mayo Clin Proc 1989; 64: 37–43.

563. Basler RSW. Ulcerative colitis and the skin. Med Clin North Am 1980; 64: 941–954.

564. Burgdorf W. Cutaneous manifestations of Crohn's

disease. J Am Acad Dermatol 1981; 5: 689–695.

565. Schoetz DJ Jr, Coller JA, Veidenheimer MC. Pyoderma gangrenosum and Crohn's disease. Dis Colon Rectum 1983; 26: 155–158.

566. Gellert A, Green ES, Beck ER, Ridley CM. Erythema nodosum progressing to pyoderma gangrenosum as a complication of Crohn's disease. Postgrad Med J 1983; 59: 791–793.

567. Powell FC, Schroeter AL, Su WPD, Perry HO. Pyoderma gangrenosum and monoclonal gammopathy. Arch Dermatol 1983; 119: 468–472.

568. Hickman JG, Lazarus GS. Pyoderma gangrenosum: a reappraisal of associated systemic diseases. Br J Dermatol 1980; 102: 235–237.

569. Norris DA, Weston WL, Thorne EG, Humbert JR. Pyoderma gangrenosum. Abnormal monocyte function corrected in vitro with hydrocortisone. Arch Dermatol 1978; 114: 906–911.

570. Burns DA, Sarkany I. Active chronic hepatitis and pyoderma gangrenosum: report of a case. Clin Exp Dermatol 1979; 4: 465–469.

571. Green LK, Hebert AA, Jorizzo JL et al. Pyoderma gangrenosum and chronic persistent hepatitis. J Am Acad Dermatol 1985; 13: 892–897.

572. Munro CS, Cox NH. Pyoderma gangrenosum associated with Behçet's syndrome — response to thalidomide. Clin Exp Dermatol 1988; 13: 408–410.

573. Venning VA, Ryan TJ. Subcorneal pustular dermatosis followed by pyoderma gangrenosum. Br J Dermatol 1986; 115: 117–118.

574. Mahood JM, Sneddon IB. Pyoderma gangrenosum complicating non-Hodgkin's lymphoma. Br J Dermatol 1980; 102: 223–225.

575. Cartwright PH, Rowell NR. Hairy-cell leukaemia presenting with pyoderma gangrenosum. Clin Exp Dermatol 1987; 12: 451–452.

576. Philpott JA Jr, Goltz RW, Park RK. Pyoderma gangrenosum, rheumatoid arthritis, and diabetes mellitus. Arch Dermatol 1966; 94: 732–738.

577. Cox NH, White SI, Walton S et al. Pyoderma gangrenosum associated with polycythaemia rubra vera. Clin Exp Dermatol 1987; 12: 375–377.

578. Haim S, Friedman-Birnbaum R. Pyoderma gangrenosum in immunosuppressed patients. Dermatologica 1976; 153: 44–48.

579. van de Kerkhof PCM, de Vaan GAM, Holland R. Pyoderma gangrenosum in acute myeloid leukaemia during immunosuppression. Eur J Pediatr 1988; 148: 34–36.

580. Holt PJA. The current status of pyoderma gangrenosum. Clin Exp Dermatol 1979; 4: 509–516.

581. Holt PJA, Davies MG, Saunders KC, Nuki G. Pyoderma gangrenosum. Clinical and laboratory findings in 15 patients with special reference to polyarthritis. Medicine (Baltimore) 1980; 59: 114–133.

582. Breathnach SM, Wells GC, Valdimarsson H. Idiopathic pyoderma gangrenosum and impaired lymphocyte function: failure of azathioprine and corticosteroid therapy. Br J Dermatol 1981; 104: 567–573.

583. Asghar SS, Bos JD, Kammeijer A, Cormane RH. Immunologic and biochemical studies on a patient with pyoderma gangrenosum. Int J Dermatol 1984; 23: 112–116.

584. Greenberg SJ, Jegasothy BV, Johnson RB, Lazarus GS.

585. Berbis P, Mege JL, Capo C et al. Hyperimmunoglobulin E and impaired neutrophil functions in a case of pyoderma gangrenosum: Effect of clofazimine. J Am Acad Dermatol 1988; 18: 574–576.

Pyoderma gangrenosum. Occurrence with altered cellular immunity and a circulating serum factor. Arch Dermatol 1982; 118: 498–502.

586. Perry HO. Pyoderma gangrenosum. Australas J Dermatol 1982; 23: 53–61.

587. Su WPD, Schroeter AL, Perry HO, Powell FC. Histopathologic and immunopathologic study of pyoderma gangrenosum. J Cutan Pathol 1986; 13: 323–330.

588. Ackerman AB. Questions to the Editorial Board. Am J Dermatopathol 1983; 5: 409–410.

589. English JSC, Fenton DA, Barth J et al. Pyoderma gangrenosum and leucocytoclastic vasculitis in association with rheumatoid arthritis — report of two cases. Clin Exp Dermatol 1984; 9: 270–276.

590. Wong E, Greaves MW. Pyoderma gangrenosum and leucocytoclastic vasculitis. Clin Exp Dermatol 1985; 10: 68–72.

591. Powell FC, Schroeter AL, Perry HO, Su WPD. Direct immunofluorescence in pyoderma gangrenosum. Br J Dermatol 1983; 108: 287–293.

592. Nickel WR, Plumb RT. Nonvenereal sclerosing lymphangitis of penis. Arch Dermatol 1962; 86: 761–763.

593. Fiumara NJ. Nonvenereal sclerosing lymphangitis of the penis. Arch Dermatol 1975; 111: 902–903.

594. Greenberg RD, Perry TL. Nonvenereal sclerosing lymphangitis of the penis. Arch Dermatol 1972; 105: 728–729.

595. Van Der Staak WJBM. Non-venereal sclerosing lymphangitis of the penis following herpes progenitalis. Br J Dermatol 1977; 96: 679–680.

596. Baden HP, Provan J, Tanenbaum L. Circular indurated lymphangitis of the penis. Arch Dermatol 1976; 112: 1146.

597. Marsch WC, Stuttgen G. Sclerosing lymphangitis of the penis: a lymphangiofibrosis thrombotica occlusiva. Br J Dermatol 1981; 104: 687–695.

598. Lassus A, Niemi KM, Valle SL, Kiistala U. Sclerosing lymphangitis of the penis. Br J Vener Dis 1972; 48: 545–548.

599. Kandil E, Al-Kashlan IM. Non-venereal sclerosing lymphangitis of the penis. A clinicopathologic treatise. Acta Derm Venereol 1970; 50: 309–312.

600. Findlay GH, Whiting DA. Mondor's phlebitis of the penis. A condition miscalled 'non-venereal sclerosing lymphangitis'. Clin Exp Dermatol 1977; 2: 65–67.

Vasculitis with granulomatosis

601. Chanda JJ, Callen JP. Necrotizing vasculitis (angiitis) with granulomatosis. Int J Dermatol 1984; 23: 101–107.

602. Yevich I. Necrotizing vasculitis with granulomatosis. Int J Dermatol 1988; 27: 540–546.

603. Hoekstra JA, Fauci AS. The granulomatous vasculitides. Clin Rheum Dis 1980; 6: 373–388.

604. Fauci AS, Wolff SM. Wegener's granulomatosis: Studies in eighteen patients and a review of the literature. Medicine (Baltimore) 1973; 52: 535–561.

605. Fienberg R. The protracted superficial phenomenon in

pathergic (Wegener's) granulomatosis. Hum Pathol 1981; 12: 458–467.

606. Chalvardjian A, Nethercott JR. Cutaneous granulomatous vasculitis associated with Crohn's disease. Cutis 1982; 30: 645–648.

607. Eeckhout E, Willemsen M, Deconinck A, Somers G. Granulomatous vasculitis as a complication of potassium iodide treatment for Sweet's syndrome. Acta Derm Venereol 1987; 67: 362–364.

608. Gibson LE, Winkelmann RK. Cutaneous granulomatous vasculitis. Its relationship to systemic disease. J Am Acad Dermatol 1986; 14: 492–501.

609. Godman GC, Churg J. Wegener's granulomatosis. Pathology and review of the literature. Arch Pathol 1954; 58: 533–553.

610. Chyu JYH, Hagstrom WJ, Soltani K et al. Wegener's granulomatosis in childhood: Cutaneous manifestations as the presenting signs. J Am Acad Dermatol 1984; 10: 341–346.

611. Cupps TR, Fauci AS. Wegener's granulomatosis. Int J Dermatol 1980; 19: 76–80.

612. Hu C-H, O'Loughlin S, Winkelmann RK. Cutaneous manifestations of Wegener granulomatosis. Arch Dermatol 1977; 113: 175–182.

613. Kesseler ME. Wegener's granulomatosis. Clin Exp Dermatol 1982; 7: 103–108.

614. Elsner B, Harper FB. Disseminated Wegener's granulomatosis with breast involvement. Arch Pathol 1969; 87: 544–547.

615. Carrington CB, Liebow AA. Limited forms of angiitis and granulomatosis of Wegener's type. Am J Med 1966; 41: 497–527.

616. Cassan SM, Coles DT, Harrison EG Jr. The concept of limited forms of Wegener's granulomatosis. Am J Med 1970; 49: 366–379.

617. Keczkes K. Wegener's granulomatosis. Br J Dermatol 1976; 94: 391–399.

618. De Remee RA, McDonald TJ, Harrison EG Jr, Coles DT. Wegener's granulomatosis. Anatomic correlates, a proposed classification. Mayo Clin Proc 1976; 51: 777–781.

619. Kornblut AD, Fauci AS. Wegener's granulomatosis. Cutis 1985; 35: 27–35.

620. Specks U, Wheatley CL, McDonald TJ et al. Anticytoplasmic autoantibodies in the diagnosis and follow-up of Wegener's granulomatosis. Mayo Clin Proc 1989; 64: 28–36.

621. Cross CE, Lillington GA. Serodiagnosis of Wegener's granulomatosis: pathobiologic and clinical implications. Mayo Clin Proc 1989; 64: 119–122.

622. De Remee RA, McDonald TJ, Weiland LH. Wegener's granulomatosis: Observations on treatment with antimicrobial agents. Mayo Clin Proc 1985; 60: 27–32.

623. Le T, Pierard GE, Lapiere CM. Granulomatous vasculitis of Wegener. J Cutan Pathol 1981; 8: 34–39.

623a. Devaney KO, Travis WD, Hoffman G et al. Interpretation of head and neck biopsies in Wegener's granulomatosis. A pathologic study of 126 biopsies in 70 patients. Am J Surg Pathol 1990; 14: 555–564.

624. Yousem SA, Lombard CM. The eosinophilic variant of Wegener's granulomatosis. Hum Pathol 1988; 19: 682–688.

625. Finan MC, Winkelmann RK. The cutaneous extravascular necrotizing granuloma (Churg–Strauss granuloma) and systemic disease: A review of 27 cases. Medicine (Baltimore) 1983; 62: 142–158.

626. Liebow AA, Carrington CRB, Friedman PJ. Lymphomatoid granulomatosis. Hum Pathol 1972; 3: 457–533.

627. Katzenstein A-LA, Carrington CB, Liebow AA. Lymphomatoid granulomatosis. A clinicopathologic study of 152 cases. Cancer 1979; 43: 360–373.

628. Holden CA, Wells RS, MacDonald DM. Cutaneous lymphomatoid granulomatosis. Clin Exp Dermatol 1982; 7: 449–454.

629. Jambrosic J, From L, Assaad DA et al. Lymphomatoid granulomatosis. J Am Acad Dermatol 1987; 17: 621–631.

630. James WD, Odom RB, Katzenstein A-LA. Cutaneous manifestations of lymphomatoid granulomatosis. Report of 44 cases and a review of the literature. Arch Dermatol 1981; 117: 196–202.

631. Camisa C. Lymphomatoid granulomatosis: Two cases with skin involvement. J Am Acad Dermatol 1989; 20: 571–578.

632. MacDonald DM, Sarkany I. Lymphomatoid granulomatosis. Clin Exp Dermatol 1976; 1: 163–173.

633. Crissman JD. Midline malignant reticulosis and lymphomatoid granulomatosis. A case report. Arch Pathol Lab Med 1979; 103: 561–564.

634. Brodell RT, Miller CW, Eisen AZ. Cutaneous lesions of lymphomatoid granulomatosis. Arch Dermatol 1986; 122: 303–306.

635. Fauci AS, Haynes BF, Costa J et al. Lymphomatoid granulomatosis. Prospective clinical and therapeutic experience over 10 years. N Engl J Med 1982; 306: 68–74.

636. Chan JKC, Ng CS, Ngan KC et al. Angiocentric T-cell lymphoma of the skin. An aggressive lymphoma distinct from mycosis fungoides. Am J Surg Pathol 1988; 12: 861–876.

637. Foley JF, Linder J, Koh J et al. Cutaneous necrotizing granulomatous vasculitis with evolution to T cell lymphoma. Am J Med 1987; 82: 839–844.

638. Carlson KC, Gibson LE. The cutaneous signs of lymphomatoid granulomatosis. J Cutan Pathol 1989; 16: 298.

639. Wood ML, Harrington CI, Slater DN et al. Cutaneous lymphomatoid granulomatosis: a rare cause of recurrent skin ulceration. Br J Dermatol 1984; 110: 619–625.

640. Sordillo PP, Epremian B, Koziner B et al. Lymphomatoid granulomatosis. An analysis of clinical and immunologic characteristics. Cancer 1982; 49: 2070–2076.

641. Jauregui HO. Lymphomatoid granulomatosis after immunosuppression for pemphigus. Arch Dermatol 1978; 114: 1052–1055.

642. Minars N, Kay S, Escobar MR. Lymphomatoid granulomatosis of the skin. A new clinicopathologic entity. Arch Dermatol 1975; 111: 493–496.

643. Kessler S, Lund HZ, Leonard DD. Cutaneous lesions of lymphomatoid granulomatosis. Comparison with lymphomatoid papulosis. Am J Dermatopathol 1981; 3: 115–127.

644. Kay S, Fu Y-S, Minars N, Brady JW. Lymphomatoid granulomatosis of the skin: light microscopic and ultrastructural studies. Cancer 1974; 34: 1675–1682.

645. Patton WF, Lynch JP III. Lymphomatoid granulomatosis. Clinicopathologic study of four cases and literature review. Medicine (Baltimore) 1982; 61: 1–12.

646. Churg J, Strauss L. Allergic granulomatosis, allergic angiitis, and periarteritis nodosa. Am J Pathol 1951; 27: 277–301.

647. Lanham JG, Elkon KB, Pusey CD, Hughes GR. Systemic vasculitis with asthma and eosinophilia: A clinical approach to the Churg–Strauss syndrome. Medicine (Baltimore) 1984; 63: 65–81.

648. Lie JT. The classification of vasculitis and a reappraisal of allergic granulomatosis and angiitis (Churg–Strauss syndrome). Mt Sinai J Med (NY) 1986; 53: 429–439.

649. Nissim F, Von der Valde J, Czernobilsky B. A limited form of Churg-Strauss syndrome. Ocular and cutaneous manifestations. Arch Pathol Lab Med 1982; 106: 305–307.

650. Crotty CP, De Remee RA, Winkelmann RK. Cutaneous clinicopathologic correlation of allergic granulomatosis. J Am Acad Dermatol 1981; 5: 571–581.

651. Cooper LM, Patterson JAK. Allergic granulomatosis and angiitis of Churg–Strauss. Case report in a patient with antibodies to human immunodeficiency virus and hepatitis B virus. Int J Dermatol 1989; 28: 597–599.

652. Chumbley LC, Harrison EG Jr, De Remee RA. Allergic granulomatosis and angiitis (Churg–Strauss syndrome). Report and analysis of 30 cases. Mayo Clin Proc 1977; 52: 477–484.

653. Finan MC, Winkelmann RK. The cutaneous extravascular necrotizing granuloma (Churg–Strauss granuloma) and systemic disease: a review of 27 cases. Medicine (Baltimore) 1983; 62: 142–158.

654. Perniciaro C, Winkelmann RK. Cutaneous extravascular necrotizing granuloma in a patient with Takayasu's aortitis. Arch Dermatol 1986; 122: 201–204.

655. Finan MC, Winkelmann RK. Cutaneous extravascular necrotizing granuloma and lymphocytic lymphoma. Arch Dermatol 1983; 119: 419–422.

656. Dicken CH, Winkelmann RK. The Churg–Strauss granuloma. Cutaneous necrotizing, palisading granuloma in vasculitis syndromes. Arch Pathol Lab Med 1978; 102: 576–580.

657. Schlechter SL, Bole GG, Walker SE. Midline granuloma and Wegener's granulomatosis: clinical and therapeutic considerations. J Rheumatol 1976; 3: 241–250.

658. Fauci AS, Johnson RE, Wolff SM. Radiation therapy of midline granuloma. Ann Intern Med 1976; 84: 140–147.

659. Ishii Y, Yamanaka N, Ogawa K et al. Nasal T-cell lymphoma as a type of so-called "lethal midline granuloma". Cancer 1982; 50: 2336–2344.

660. Wetmore SJ, Platz CE. Idiopathic midface lesions. Ann Otol 1978; 87: 60–69.

661. Kassel SH, Echevarria RA, Guzzo FP. Midline malignant reticulosis (so-called lethal midline granuloma). Cancer 1969; 23: 920–935.

661a. Friedmann I. Non-healing nasal granulomas of unknown cause. In: Friedmann I, ed. Nose, throat and ears. Systemic pathology, 3rd ed. Edinburgh: Churchill Livingstone, 1986; 1: 48–62.

662. Friedmann I. Midline granuloma. Proc R Soc Med 1964; 57: 289–297.

663. Lober CW, Kaplan RJ, West WH. Midline granuloma. Stewart type. Arch Dermatol 1982; 118: 52–54.

664. Russell RWR. Giant-cell arteritis. A review of 35 cases. Q J Med 1959; 28: 471–489.

665. Bunker CB, Dowd PM. Giant cell arteritis and systemic lupus erythematosus. Br J Dermatol 1988; 119: 115–120.

666. Hamilton CR Jr, Shelley WM, Tumulty PA. Giant cell arteritis and polymyalgia rheumatica. Medicine (Baltimore) 1971; 50: 1–27.

667. Healey LA, Wilske KR. Manifestations of giant cell arteritis. Med Clin North Am 1977; 61: 261–270.

668. Soderstrom CW, Seehafer JR. Bilateral scalp necrosis in temporal arteritis. A rare complication of Horton's disease. Am J Med 1976; 61: 541–546.

669. Barefoot SW, Lund HZ. Temporal (giant-cell) arteritis associated with ulcerations of scalp. Arch Dermatol 1966; 93: 79–83.

670. Berth-Jones J, Holt PJA. Temporal arteritis presenting with scalp necrosis and a normal erythrocyte sedimentation rate. Clin Exp Dermatol 1988; 13: 200–201.

671. Abdullah AN, Keczkes K, Wyatt EH. Skin necrosis in giant cell (temporal) arteritis: report of three cases. Br J Dermatol 1989; 120: 843–846.

672. Hitch JM. Dermatologic manifestations of giant-cell (temporal, cranial) arteritis. Arch Dermatol 1970; 101: 409–415.

673. Kinmont PDC, McCallum DI. Skin manifestations of giant-cell arteritis. Br J Dermatol 1964; 76: 299–308.

674. Baum EW, Sams WM Jr, Payne RR. Giant cell arteritis: A systemic disease with rare cutaneous manifestations. J Am Acad Dermatol 1982; 6: 1081–1088.

675. O'Brien JP. A concept of diffuse actinic arteritis. Br J Dermatol 1978; 98: 1–13.

676. O'Brien JP. Vascular accidents after actinic (solar) exposure. An aspect of the temporal arteritis/polymyalgia rheumatica syndrome. Int J Dermatol 1987; 26: 366–370.

677. Shiki H, Shimokama T, Watanabe T. Temporal arteritis: cell composition and the possible pathogenetic role of cell-mediated immunity. Hum Pathol 1989; 20: 1057–1064.

678. Mambo NC. Temporal (granulomatous) arteritis: a histopathological study of 32 cases. Histopathology 1979; 3: 209–221.

679. Allsop CJ, Gallagher PJ. Temporal artery biopsy in giant-cell arteritis. A reappraisal. Am J Surg Pathol 1981; 5: 317–323.

680. Klein RG, Campbell RJ, Hunder GG, Carney JA. Skip lesions in temporal arteritis. Mayo Clin Proc 1976; 51: 504–510.

681. Goodman BW Jr. Temporal arteritis. Am J Med 1979; 67: 839–852.

682. Huston KA, Hunder GG, Lie JT et al. Temporal arteritis. A 25-year epidemiologic, clinical and pathologic study. Ann Intern Med 1978; 88: 162–167.

683. Morgan GJ Jr, Harris EJ Jr. Prognostic implications of non-giant cell temporal arteritis. Arthritis Rheum 1976; 19: 812 (abstract).

684. Lie JT, Michet CJ Jr. Thromboangiitis obliterans with eosinophilia (Buerger's disease) of the temporal arteries. Hum Pathol 1988; 19: 598–602.

685. Hall S, Barr W, Lie JT et al. Takayasu arteritis. A study of 32 North American patients. Medicine (Baltimore) 1985; 64: 89–99.

Disorders of epidermal maturation and keratinization

INTRODUCTION

This chapter deals with a heterogeneous group of diseases in which an abnormality of maturation, of keratinization or of structural integrity of the epidermis is present. Most of these conditions are genetically determined, although a few are acquired diseases of adult life. The process of normal keratinization has been considered in Chapter 1 (p. 3).

ICHTHYOSES

The ichthyoses are a heterogeneous group of hereditary and acquired disorders of keratinization characterized by the presence of visible scales on the skin surface.[1-2a] The name is derived from the Greek word for fish — *ichthys*. There are four major types of ichthyosis: ichthyosis vulgaris, X-linked ichthyosis, lamellar ichthyosis and epidermolytic hyperkeratosis (bullous ichthyosiform erythroderma). In addition, there are several rare syndromes in which ichthyosis is a major feature.

Kinetic studies have shown that lamellar ichthyosis and epidermolytic hyperkeratosis are characterized by hyperproliferation of the epidermis with transit times of 4 to 5 days, whereas the scale in ichthyosis vulgaris and X-linked ichthyosis is related to prolonged retention of the stratum corneum.[1,2]

Although the mode of inheritance was originally used as a major criterion in the delineation of the various forms of ichthyosis, recent studies have shown some evidence of genetic heterogeneity in the various groups.[3,4]

ICHTHYOSIS VULGARIS

This is the most common type of ichthyosis (incidence 1:250), with an onset in early childhood and an autosomal dominant inheritance.[1] It may have only very mild expression and be misdiagnosed as dry skin. The disorder is lifelong. It is characterized by fine, whitish scales involving particularly the extensor surfaces of the arms and legs, as well as the scalp. Flexures are spared. There may be accentuation of palmar and plantar markings, keratosis pilaris and features of atopy.

Recent studies have demonstrated an abnormality in filaggrin generation.[5]

Histopathology

The epidermis may be of normal thickness or slightly thinned with some loss of the rete ridges. There is mild to moderate hyperkeratosis, associated paradoxically with diminution or absence of the granular layer (Fig. 9.1). The thickened stratum corneum is often laminated in appearance. The hyperkeratosis may extend into the hair follicles.[6] The sebaceous and sweat glands are often reduced in size and number.

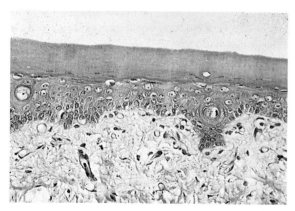

Fig. 9.1 Ichthyosis vulgaris. There is a thickened layer of compact orthokeratosis overlying a diminished granular layer.
Haematoxylin — eosin

Electron microscopy. This shows defective keratohyaline synthesis with small granules having a crumbled or spongy appearance.[5,7]

X-LINKED ICHTHYOSIS

This form, which is inherited as an X-linked recessive trait, is present at birth or develops in the first few months of life.[8-9] It is characterized by large polygonal scales which are dirty brown in colour and adherent. X-linked ichthyosis may involve the entire body in varying degree, although there is sparing of the palms and soles. The pre-auricular region is characteristically involved in this variant of ichthyosis; in contrast, this site is usually spared in ichthyosis vulgaris.[9a] Corneal opacities also occur in X-linked ichthyosis.[10]

Its incidence is approximately 1 in 6000 males, but occasionally female heterozygotes have mild scaling of the legs.

This condition is characterized by a deficiency of steroid sulphatase in a wide range of tissues, including leucocytes and fibroblasts, and as a result there is an accumulation of cholesterol sulphate in the pathological scales, and in serum and leucocytes.[11-14] The deficiency in placental sulphatase which is also present results in decreased maternal urinary oestrogens and a failure to initiate labour in some cases.[10]

Histopathology

There is usually conspicuous acanthosis with thickening of the stratum corneum and a normal to thickened granular layer. Thinning of the granular layer is sometimes present.[14a] There is often hyperkeratosis of follicular and sweat duct orifices.[9] There may be a few lymphocytes around the vessels in the superficial dermis.

LAMELLAR ICHTHYOSIS

This is a rare, severe, autosomal recessive form of ichthyosis which is usually manifest at birth. It may present with the infant encased in a tight membrane — the so-called 'collodion baby'.[2,15,16] Lamellar ichthyosis appears to be a heterogeneous entity[17–17b] with a classic form characterized by large plate-like scales and an erythrodermic form (*non-bullous congenital ichthyosiform erythroderma*) in which there is erythroderma with finer, pale scales and a high content of n-alkanes in the scale.[12,18,19]

In lamellar ichthyosis there is generalized involvement of the skin, including the palms and soles.[2] Ectropion is often present.

Histopathology

There is hyperkeratosis, focal parakeratosis and a normal or thickened granular layer.[6] The hyperkeratosis is more marked in lamellar ichthyosis than other variants and there is easily discernible parakeratosis in the erythrodermic form.[18] There is often some acanthosis and occasionally there is irregular psoriasiform epidermal hyperplasia (Fig. 9.2).[4] Vacuolation of cells in the granular layer is a rare finding.[19a] Keratotic plugging of follicular orifices may also be present. The dermis often shows a mild superficial perivascular infiltrate of lymphocytes.

Electron microscopy. There is a reduced cellular content of tonofibrils and keratohyaline in the granular layer and prominent lipid vacuoles in the horny layer.[17,20] The marginal band of the cornified layer may be absent.[20] The morphological features of this condition are also expressed in cultured keratinocytes that have been grafted on to athymic mice.[20a]

BULLOUS ICHTHYOSIS

The term bullous ichthyosis is preferred to bullous congenital ichthyosiform erythroderma and to epidermolytic hyperkeratosis (which merely describes a histological reaction pattern). Bullous ichthyosis is a rare, autosomal dominant condition which is usually severe and characterized at birth by widespread erythema and some blistering.[2] Coarse, verrucous scales, particularly in the flexures, develop as the disposition to blistering subsides during childhood.

The fundamental defect is unknown, although a structural abnormality in keratins has been suggested.[2] Prenatal diagnosis can be made at approximately 19 weeks by fetal skin biopsy examined by light and electron microscopy; this shows abnormal aggregation of keratin filaments.[21]

The rare ichthyosis bullosa of Siemens is histologically similar but clinically lacks the erythroderma.[22,22a]

Histopathology

The histological pattern is that of epidermolytic hyperkeratosis, characterized by marked hyperkeratosis and granular and vacuolar change in the upper spinous and granular layers (Fig. 9.3).[23] The keratohyaline granules appear coarse and basophilic with clumping. There is moderate acanthosis. The histological features of blistering can sometimes be subtle, with only slight separation of the markedly vacuolar cells in the mid and upper dermis. There is usually a mild perivascular inflammatory cell infiltrate in the upper dermis.

Electron microscopy. There is aggregation of tonofilaments at the cell periphery with perinuclear areas free of tonofilaments and containing endoplasmic reticulum.[24] In the upper granular layer there are numerous keratohyaline granules, sometimes embedded in clumped tonofilaments. Although desmosomes

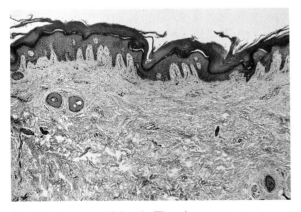

Fig. 9.2 Lamellar ichthyosis. There is compact orthokeratosis and psoriasiform hyperplasia of the epidermis. Haematoxylin — eosin

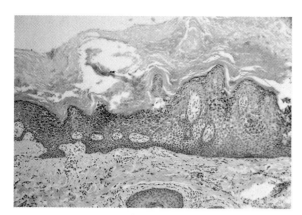

Fig. 9.3 Bullous ichthyosis with hyperkeratosis and granular and vacuolar change of the keratinocytes in the upper layers of the epidermis. Blistering is not shown in this field.
Haematoxylin — eosin

appear normal, there is often an abnormality in the association of tonofilaments and desmosomes.

ICHTHYOSIS LINEARIS CIRCUMFLEXA

This is a rare autosomal recessive condition characterized by migratory annular and polycyclic erythema with scaling borders distributed on the trunk and extremities. Some patients have hair shaft abnormalities.[25] Netherton's syndrome is the term used for the triad of ichthyosis linearis circumflexa, trichorrhexis invaginata and an atopic diathesis.[26] Intermittent aminoaciduria and mental retardation may also be present.[27] Other hair shaft abnormalities such as pili torti, trichorrhexis nodosa and monilethrix have also been reported in Netherton's syndrome;[28,28a] the ichthyosiform component may, rarely, be of another type.[26]

Recent studies have shown that the keratin filaments from the scales in this condition are composed of reduced amounts of high molecular subunits and increased amounts of low molecular subunits.[25]

Histopathology

The skin lesions show hyperkeratosis, a well developed granular layer and acanthosis. The margin shows focal parakeratosis with absence of the granular layer and more obvious psoriasiform epidermal hyperplasia.[25,29] Epidermal mitoses are increased. In some cases PAS-positive, diastase-resistant granules can be found in the prickle cells. There is often a mild perivascular inflammatory cell infiltrate in the superficial dermis.

Electron microscopy. This shows an increase in mitochondria and numerous round or oval opaque (lipoid) bodies in the stratum corneum.[25,30]

ERYTHROKERATODERMIA VARIABILIS

This rare, autosomal dominant form of ichthyosis develops in infancy. There are transient erythematous patches and erythematous hyperkeratotic plaques which are often polycyclic or circinate.[1,31] There is retention hyperkeratosis associated with a basal cell type of keratin.[32]

Histopathology

The findings are not distinctive. There is hyperkeratosis, irregular acanthosis, very mild papillomatosis in some biopsies and a mild superficial perivascular infiltrate of lymphocytes. Dyskeratotic, grain-like cells may be seen in the lower stratum corneum.[33]

Electron microscopy. There is a reduction in keratinosomes in the stratum granulosum.[33] The dyskeratotic cells have clumped tonofilaments.[33]

HARLEQUIN FETUS

This severe disorder of cornification, which is usually incompatible with extrauterine life, is of autosomal recessive inheritance.[2,33a] There appears to be genetic heterogeneity.[34,34a] It is characterized by thick, plate-like scales with deep fissures.[35] Prenatal diagnosis can be made by skin biopsy of the intrauterine fetus at about 20 weeks.[36] Harlequin ichthyosis is a disorder of epidermal keratinization in which there are altered lamellar granules and a variation in the expression of keratin and filaggrin.[34a] Lipid levels may be increased in the stratum corneum.[37]

Histopathology

There is massive hyperkeratosis in all biopsies. Some cases have parakeratosis with a thin or absent granular layer while others have had persistence of the granular layer.[37]

Electron microscopy. The stratum corneum is thickened and contains lipid and vacuolar inclusions.[37a] Lamellar granules are abnormal or absent.[34a]

FOLLICULAR ICHTHYOSIS

This is a rare, distinctive form of ichthyosis in which the abnormal epidermal differentiation occurs mainly in hair follicles.[38] Its onset is at birth or early in childhood. The hyperkeratosis is more prominent on the head and neck. Photophobia and alopecia are often present.[38a] Three of the patients reported have also had acanthosis-nigricans-like lesions.[38]

Histopathology

There is marked follicular hyperkeratosis which is compact and extends deep within the follicle. There is a prominent granular layer.[38] In keratosis pilaris the hyperkeratosis has a more open basket-weave pattern and is confined to the infundibular region of the follicle (see p. 467).

ACQUIRED ICHTHYOSIS

This variant of ichthyosis, which occurs in adult life, is similar to ichthyosis vulgaris both clinically and histologically.[39] It is usually associated with an underlying malignant disease, particularly a lymphoma,[40] but it usually appears some time after other manifestations of the malignant process. Ichthyosis has also been associated with malnutrition, hypothyroidism, leprosy, sarcoidosis,[41,42] and drugs such as clofazimine and nafoxidine.[43] Acquired ichthyosis must be distinguished from asteatosis (dry skin). It may be related to an essential fatty acid deficiency in some cases.[42]

Pityriasis rotunda, which is manifested by sharply demarcated, circular, scaly patches of variable diameter and number, is probably a variant of acquired ichthyosis. It is more common in black and oriental patients than in whites. An underlying malignant neoplasm or systemic illness is often present.[43a-43f]

REFSUM'S SYNDROME

This rare autosomal recessive disorder is characterized by ichthyosis, cerebellar ataxia, peripheral neuropathy and retinitis pigmentosa.[2] The skin most resembles ichthyosis vulgaris but the onset of scale is often delayed until adulthood. There is an inability to oxidize phytanic acid, and improvement occurs when the patient adheres to a diet free from chlorophyll, which contains phytol, the precursor of this fatty acid.[2]

Histopathology

A biopsy will show hyperkeratosis, a granular layer that may be increased or decreased in amount, and some acanthosis. Basal keratinocytes are vacuolated, and these stain for neutral lipid.[44] Lipid vacuoles are also present in keratinocytes in the rare Dorfman–Chanarin syndrome in which congenital ichthyosis is present.[45]

Electron microscopy. There are non-membrane-bound vacuoles in the basal and suprabasal keratinocytes.[44]

OTHER ICHTHYOSIS-RELATED SYNDROMES

There are a number of rare syndromes in which ichthyosis is a feature. As histologically they resemble the already described forms of ichthyosis, they will be discussed only briefly. The *Sjögren–Larsson syndrome* is an autosomal recessive disorder characterized by the triad of congenital ichthyosis (most resembling lamellar ichthyosis), spastic paralysis and mental retardation.[46] A prenatal diagnosis can be made by fetal skin biopsy.[47] The thickened keratin layer may still retain its basket-weave appearance.[48] The *'KID' syndrome* comprises *k*eratitis, *i*chthyosis and *d*eafness.[49–51b] *Conradi's syndrome* combines chondrodysplasia with ichthyosis and palmar and plantar hyperkeratosis.[1,52,52a] The *'CHILD' syndrome* includes *c*ongenital *h*emidysplasia, *i*chthyosiform erythroderma and *l*imb *d*efects.[1,53] *Tay's syndrome* is associated with close-set eyes, a beaked nose and sunken cheeks.[1] *'IBIDS'* combines *i*chthyosis with *b*rittle hair, *i*mpaired intelligence, *d*ecreased fertility and *s*hort stature.[54,55] *Multiple sulphatase deficiency* includes severe neurodegenerative disease, ichthyosis and signs of mucopolysaccharidosis.[2] *Neutral lipid storage disease*, in which neutral lipid accumulates in the cytoplasm of many cells of the body, combines fatty liver with muscular dystrophy and ichthyosis.[2] Other unnamed associations have been described.[1,56]

PALMOPLANTAR KERATODERMAS AND RELATED CONDITIONS

In addition to the group of disorders usually categorized as the palmoplantar keratodermas, there are several rare genodermatoses that are usually regarded as discrete entities, in which palmoplantar keratoderma is a major clinicopathological feature. These disorders include hidrotic ectodermal dysplasia (see p. 275), acrokeratoelastoidosis (see p. 275), pachyonychia congenita (see p. 276), tyrosinosis (see p. 274) and pachydermoperiostosis (see p. 333).

PALMOPLANTAR KERATODERMAS

The palmoplantar keratodermas are a heterogeneous group of congenital and acquired disorders of keratinization, characterized by diffuse or localized hyperkeratosis of the palms and soles, sometimes accompanied by other ectodermal abnormalities.[57] At least 10 different hereditary variants, most with eponymous designations, have been distinguished on the basis of their mode of inheritance, sites of involvement, and associated abnormalities.[58] The autosomal recessive types are usually the most severe and include mal de Meleda, Papillon–Lefèvre syndrome, some mutilating variants and a recently described variant associated with generalized ichthyosis.[58a] The other hereditary forms are autosomal dominant, although sporadic cases of most syndromes occur.[59]

Another feature used to distinguish the various subtypes of keratoderma is the presence of hyperkeratosis beyond the palms and soles. These 'transgrediens' lesions occur in the Olmstead, Greither, Vohwinkel and mal de Meleda types.[60] Onset of most keratodermas is at birth or early infancy, but later onset is seen in the punctate and acquired forms.

Brief mention will be made of the important clinical features of the various keratodermas:

Unna–Thost syndrome. This is the most common diffuse form. Deafness is sometimes present,[61] while acrocyanosis is a rare association.[61a]

Greither's syndrome. In this 'transgrediens' form (hyperkeratosis beyond the palms and soles), the elbows and knees may be more involved than the palms and soles.[57,62,63]

Olmsted's syndrome. Periorificial keratoderma and oral leucokeratosis accompany the palmoplantar keratoderma.[60,63a]

Vohwinkel's syndrome. There is a honeycombing pattern of keratoderma with starfish-shaped keratoses on the dorsa of the digits and linear keratoses on the knees and elbows.[64–66] Ainhum-like constriction bands develop, leading to gangrene of the digits in adolescence.[65,67–69] A recessive variant is associated with ectodermal dysplasia.[70]

Epidermolytic keratoderma. This variant is clinically indistinguishable from the Unna–Thost type, although the histology is unique, with epidermolytic hyperkeratosis.[71–76] A kindred with associated internal malignancies has been reported.[77]

Howel–Evans syndrome. The palmoplantar keratoderma begins early in life and affected family members develop a squamous cell carcinoma of the oesophagus in middle adult life.[78] Squamous cell carcinoma sometimes develops in the thickened skin of the palms.[79] Interestingly, palmoplantar keratoderma has been reported in one patient with post-corrosive stricture of the oesophagus.[80]

Papillon–Lefèvre syndrome. In this condition, there is periodontosis accompanied by premature loss of the deciduous and permanent teeth.[81–83] Involvement of the elbows and knees and calcification of the choroid plexus may occur.[84]

Mal de Meleda. This rare, autosomal recessive variant was first described in families living on the small island of Meleda in the Adriatic sea.[85] Onset is at birth, or in infancy. Lesions may extend from the palms and soles on to the dorsum of the hands and feet respectively, although there is a sharp 'cut-off' at the wrists and ankles.[85–87] Hyperhidrosis leads to severe maceration.[58]

Punctate keratoderma. This localized variant is characterized by discrete, hard, keratotic plugs arising in normal skin.[88–89] A variant with verrucoid lesions has been reported.[90] The plugs form again if removed. Onset is usually in adolescence, but it may be much later.[91] Sometimes the lesions are confined to the palmar creases, particularly in blacks.[92–94] An underlying malignancy has been present in a few cases.[95] Punctate lesions, which are characterized histologically by a cornoid lamella, are best classified as punctate porokeratotic keratoderma;[88] they are clinically indistinguishable from the other punctate forms.[89–95a]

Circumscribed keratoderma. Focal areas of thickening, sometimes tender, may develop on the palms and soles.[96] Some have an autosomal recessive inheritance. This is a clinically heterogeneous group,[96] which includes the conditions of hereditary painful callosities[97,98] and keratoderma palmoplantaris striata.[98a] Corneal dystrophy has been present in some circumscribed variants.[96] Localized hypertrophy of the skin of the soles and palms can occur in the Proteus syndrome, a rare disorder in which the major manifestations are skeletal overgrowth, digital hypertrophy, exostoses of the skull, subcutaneous lipomas and, sometimes, epidermal naevi.[98b]

Acquired keratoderma. Palmoplantar keratoderma or discrete keratotic lesions may rarely develop in cases of myxoedema,[99,100] mycosis fungoides,[101] and internal cancers,[102–105] following exposure to arsenic, and after the menopause or following bilateral oophorectomy (keratoderma climactericum).[106] Rugose lesions of the palms may occur in association with acanthosis nigricans, so-called 'tripe palms' (pachydermatoglyphy);[107] in a few instances, this condition has been reported in association with a cancer, without concurrent acanthosis nigricans.[107a] Recently, keratoderma has been described in patients with AIDS, following the infusion of glucan, which was used as an immunostimulant.[108] Keratoderma can also occur in patients with papulosquamous conditions such as lichen planus and pityriasis rubra pilaris.[109]

Histopathology

The *diffuse forms* show prominent orthokeratotic hyperkeratosis, with variable amounts of focal parakeratosis. The granular layer is often thickened. There is also some acanthosis of the epidermis and a sparse, superficial, perivascular infiltrate of chronic inflammatory cells.

The *epidermolytic form* shows epidermolytic hyperkeratosis. This tissue reaction is described on page 278.

The *punctate forms* show a dense, homogeneous keratin plug which often results in an undulating appearance in the epidermis.[89,91]

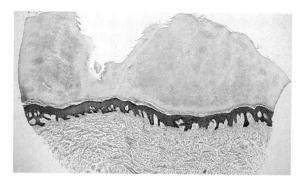

Fig. 9.4 Punctate keratoderma. There is slight depression of the epidermis beneath a keratin plug. There is a pit in the adjacent stratum corneum.
Haematoxylin — eosin

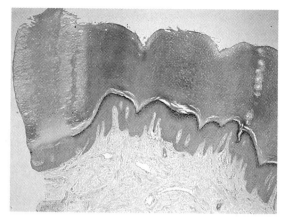

Fig. 9.5 Punctate porokeratotic keratoderma. A wide cornoid lamella is present towards one edge of the field.
Haematoxylin — eosin
Provided by Dr J J Sullivan.

There is usually a slight depression in the epidermis beneath the plug (Fig. 9.4).[89] Those punctate cases with a parakeratotic plug are best classified as punctate porokeratotic keratoderma (Figs 9.5 and 9.6).[110] Focal acantholytic dyskeratosis was present in the punctate lesions in one reported case.[110a]

In *hereditary callosities with blisters*, there is intraepidermal vesiculation with cytolysis of keratinocytes and clumping of tonofilaments.[97] The changes resemble those seen in pachyonychia congenita (see p. 276).

Electron microscopy. Ultrastructural studies have not shown consistent abnormalities. A recent report of a new clinical variant found that the keratohyaline granules were abnormal in distribution and structure.[57] They did not show normal association with keratin filaments. Based on other evidence as well, it seems that the normal association of filaggrin and keratin filaments does not occur in the stratum corneum.[57] Nucleolar hypertrophy has been noted in the punctate form.[89] Ultrastructural studies of the Papillon–Lefèvre syndrome have shown lipid-like vacuoles in corneocytes, abnormally shaped keratohyaline granules, and a reduction in tonofilaments.[111]

OCULOCUTANEOUS TYROSINOSIS

This condition, also known as tyrosinaemia II and the Richner–Hanhart syndrome, is an ex-

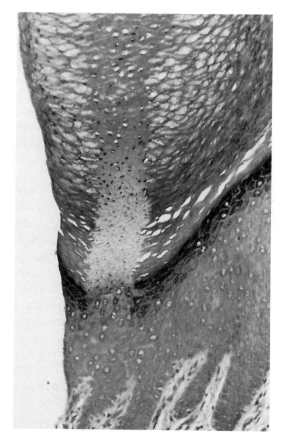

Fig. 9.6 Punctate porokeratotic keratoderma. The granular layer is absent beneath the parakeratotic zone.
Haematoxylin — eosin
Provided by Dr J J Sullivan.

tremely rare, autosomal recessive genodermatosis caused by a deficiency of hepatic tyrosine aminotransferase.[112–116] It is usually characterized by corneal ulcerations and painful keratotic lesions on the palms and soles, but ocular lesions have been absent in some kindreds.[117–118] The palmoplantar lesions vary from fine 1–2 mm keratoses, to linear or diffuse keratotic thickenings.[116] Erosions and blisters have also been reported.[119] Mental retardation is often present. The condition is treated by a dietary restriction of tyrosine and phenylalanine.[120]

Histopathology[113]

The palmoplantar lesions show prominent hyperkeratosis and parakeratosis with variable epidermal hyperplasia. Scattered mitoses and multinucleate keratinocytes may be present.[121] Epidermolytic hyperkeratosis and intraepidermal bulla formation have been present in some families.[119]

Electron microscopy. Lipid-like granules have been noted in the upper epidermis.[120] An increase in tonofibrils and keratohyalin has also been seen in affected skin.[121]

HIDROTIC ECTODERMAL DYSPLASIA

This autosomal dominant variant of ectodermal dysplasia (see p. 289 for a discussion of the ectodermal dysplasias) is characterized by the triad of alopecia, dystrophic nails and palmoplantar keratoderma.[122–124] Dental abnormalities may also be present, but sweating is normal in contrast to many other ectodermal dysplasias.

Histopathology

The palms and soles show prominent hyperkeratosis of orthokeratotic type. There is some acanthosis. The granular layer is of normal thickness.

ACROKERATOELASTOIDOSIS

Acrokeratoelastoidosis (Costa's papular acrokeratosis)[125] is a variant of palmoplantar keratoderma which occurs both sporadically and as an autosomal dominant genodermatosis.[126,127] There appears to be some variability in the morphological expression of the disease.[128] Its onset is in childhood or early adult life, and there is a female predominance. There are multiple, small (2–5 mm in diameter), firm, translucent papules which are most numerous along the junction of the dorsal and palmar or plantar surfaces of the hands and feet respectively.[128a] They may be localized to the sides of the fingers, particularly the inner side of the thumb and the adjoining index finger. In this situation, they resemble clinically the lesions seen in collagenous and elastotic plaques of the hands, an entity which is found predominantly in males over the age of 50, and which results from trauma and actinic damage.[125] In acrokeratoelastoidosis there may also be a mild diffuse hyperkeratosis of the palms and soles; this was a prominent feature in one report.[129] There may also be isolated lesions over interphalangeal joints and elsewhere on the dorsum of the hands and feet.[130]

Histopathology

There may be slight hyperkeratosis with a shallow depression in the underlying epidermis, which shows a prominent granular layer and mild acanthosis. The dermis may be normal or slightly thickened. The elastic fibres are decreased in number, thin and somewhat fragmented in the mid and deep reticular dermis.[131] In some cases the elastic fibres are coarse and fragmented.[130] Cases have been reported with no light microscopic changes in the dermis.[126] The group which lacks elastorrhexis has been designated 'focal acral hyperkeratosis'.[132,133]

Electron microscopy. In acrokeratoelastoidosis there is disaggregation of elastic fibres with fragmentation of the microfibrils.[126] In one report the fibroblasts contained dense granules in the cytoplasm and there was an absence of extracellular fibres, leading to the hypothesis that there was a block in the synthesis of elastic fibres by the fibroblasts.[134]

PACHYONYCHIA CONGENITA

Pachyonychia congenita is a rare genodermatosis in which symmetrical, hard thickening of the nails of the fingers and toes is the most striking and consistent feature.[135,135a] Various other abnormalities of keratinization are usually present.[136] These include palmar and plantar keratoderma, follicular keratoses on the extensor surfaces of the knees and elbows, keratosis pilaris, blister formation on the feet and sometimes on the palms, callosities of the feet, leucokeratosis of the oral mucosa (often complicated by candidosis),[137] hair abnormalities, and hyperhidrosis of the palms and soles. These clinical features typify the so-called Type I cases.[136] Patients with the Type II variant have the addition of natal teeth (teeth erupted prior to birth) and multiple cutaneous cysts, either epidermal cysts or steatocystomas,[138] but no oral leucokeratosis.[139] In Type III, there are the features of Type I, together with leucokeratosis of the cornea. Type IV combines the clinical features of the other types with laryngeal lesions, mental retardation and alopecia.[140]

There is some variability in the age of onset of the various manifestations, but nail changes are usually present at birth or soon afterwards and become progressively more disfiguring over the first year of life.

Pachyonychia congenita is usually inherited as an autosomal dominant trait with incomplete penetrance, although several cases with autosomal recessive inheritance have been reported.[135]

Histopathology

The involved mucous membranes and skin, including the nail bed, show marked intracellular oedema involving cells in the upper malpighian layer and in the thickened stratum corneum.[135,136,141–144] There is sometimes rupture of cell walls, particularly with lesions on plantar surfaces, with the formation of intraepidermal vesicles. The epidermis is markedly thickened as a consequence of the oedema and of the accompanying hyperkeratosis and focal parakeratosis.

The hyperkeratotic papules on the knees and elbows show hyperkeratosis, a prominent granular layer and acanthosis.[135,145] There is usually a thick horny plug extending above the infundibulum of the hair follicle. In one case, the plug resembled a cornoid lamella (see below);[146] in another, the plug, which was not related to a follicle, penetrated into the dermis in the manner seen in Kyrle's disease (see p. 286).[147] Horny plugs have also been described in sweat pores.[145]

The plantar callosities show hyperkeratosis, focal parakeratosis and sometimes mild papillomatosis and acanthosis. The granular layer is thick except for the area overlying any papillomatous foci.[136]

Two kindreds have been reported with pigment incontinence and amyloid in the papillary dermis.[148]

CORNOID LAMELLATION

The cornoid lamella is a thin column of parakeratotic cells with an absent or decreased underlying granular zone and vacuolated or dyskeratotic cells in the spinous layer. It is the key histological feature of porokeratosis and its clinical variants, but like some of the other minor 'tissue reaction patterns' (see Ch. 2, p. 25) can be found as an incidental phenomenon in a range of inflammatory, hyperplastic and neoplastic conditions of the skin. The cornoid lamella represents a localized area of faulty keratinization and is manifest clinically as a raised keratotic or thin thread-like border to an annular, gyrate or linear lesion.

Cornoid lamellation has been regarded as a clonal disease[149] and as a morphological expression of disordered epithelial metabolism.[150] Abnormal DNA ploidy has been demonstrated in the epidermis in some lesions of porokeratosis.[151,152]

POROKERATOSIS AND VARIANTS

Porokeratosis is a genodermatosis with many different clinical expressions.[153] Lesions may be solitary or numerous, inconspicuous or prominent, small or large, atrophic or hyperkeratotic, and asymptomatic or pruritic.[154] The lip,[155] mouth and glans penis are sites that are rarely involved. Although originally regarded as a familial disease with autosomal dominant inheritance,[156] numerous non-familial cases have now been reported. The most important clinical forms are porokeratosis of Mibelli (characterized by one or more round, oval or gyrate plaques with an atrophic centre and a thin, elevated, guttered, keratotic rim which may show peripheral expansion), and disseminated superficial actinic porokeratosis[157,158] — DSAP — consisting of multiple, annular, keratotic lesions less than 1 cm in diameter, with a hyperkeratotic, thread-like border and occurring particularly on the exposed extremities. Rare clinical variants include a linear[159–161] or systematized[162,163] variant, a reticulate form,[164] porokeratosis plantaris discreta[165,166] (painful plantar lesions), punctate porokeratotic keratoderma, also known as punctate porokeratosis[167–169] and porokeratosis punctata palmaris et plantaris[170] (asymptomatic pits or plugs, usually on the palms, digits or soles), porokeratosis plantaris, palmaris et disseminata[171–175] (annular and serpiginous lesions on the palms and soles with later involvement of other areas), and the related superficial disseminated eruptive form.[176] Other rare variants of porokeratosis are a hyperkeratotic verrucous type,[177] and a facial variant.[178] Closely related are the cases with cornoid lamellae in eccrine and hair follicle ostia, described as 'porokeratotic eccrine ostial and dermal duct naevus',[179–181] 'porokeratotic eccrine duct and hair follicle naevus'[182] and 'reticular erythema with ostial porokeratosis'.[183]

The disseminated superficial actinic variant coexists rarely with other types of porokeratosis.[161,184] Lesions in this type may be exacerbated by exposure to ultraviolet light.[185] Both DSAP and porokeratosis of Mibelli have developed in immunosuppressed patients.[186–188]

The development of squamous cell carcinoma[189–192] or intraepidermal carcinoma[193] is a rare clinical complication of several of the variants of porokeratosis. The term malignant disseminated porokeratosis has been applied to several cases in which the porokeratotic lesions had a significant potential to undergo malignant degeneration.[194,195]

Histopathology

It is important that the biopsy is taken across the edge of the peripheral rim in order to show the typical cornoid lamella, the features of which have been described above. Multiple cornoid lamellae will usually be seen in biopsies from the linear and reticulate form. There may be two cornoid lamellae, one on each side of a keratotic plug, at either edge of a lesion of DSAP.[196] In porokeratosis of Mibelli there is invagination of the epidermis at the site of the cornoid lamella with adjacent mild papillomatosis. Beneath the lamella there is absence or diminution of the granular layer, sometimes only several cells in width (Fig. 9.7). However, in the solitary palmar

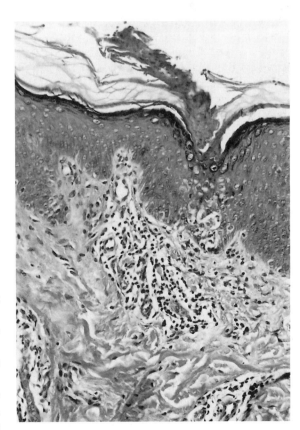

Fig. 9.7 Porokeratosis. The thin parakeratotic column (cornoid lamella) overlies an area several cells in width, in which the granular layer is absent.
Haematoxylin — eosin

or plantar lesions the cornoid lamella is quite broad with a corresponding wide zone where the underlying granular zone is absent or markedly reduced. Sometimes one or more dyskeratotic cells are present in the spinous layer.

Beneath the lamella there are often dilated capillaries in the papillary dermis, associated with a lymphocytic infiltrate. The most prominent inflammatory changes are seen in DSAP in which a superficial band-like infiltrate with lichenoid qualities (including Civatte bodies) is usually present. In addition, the epidermis between the lamellae is often atrophic in this form, with overlying hyperkeratosis, and the dermis may show solar elastotic changes. Focal epidermal necrosis has been reported at the periphery of a lesion of porokeratosis.[197] Amyloid has been found in the papillary dermis in several cases.[198,199]

Electron microscopy. Scanning electron microscopy has shown bud-like spreading of the active edge,[200] while transmission electron microscopy has demonstrated that the basophilic granular material in the cornoid lamella consists of degenerate cells with pyknotic nuclei.[201] The granular layer is inconspicuous with only small amounts of keratohyalin. Vacuolated cells and others showing filamentous degeneration ('dyskeratotic' cells) are often present. Apoptotic bodies may be seen in the basal layer and in the dermal papillae.[202]

EPIDERMOLYTIC HYPERKERATOSIS

This abnormality of epidermal maturation is characterized by compact hyperkeratosis, accompanied by granular and vacuolar degeneration of the cells of the spinous and granular layers (Fig. 9.8). It may be a congenital or an acquired defect. This histological pattern may be seen in a number of different clinical settings, some of which will be considered in other sections of this chapter. It may be:

Generalized: bullous ichthyosis (see p. 269)
Systematized or linear: epidermal naevus variant (see below and p. 729)

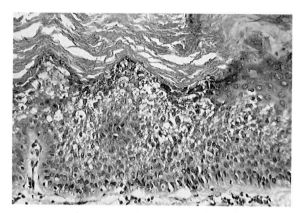

Fig. 9.8   Epidermolytic hyperkeratosis. Compact orthokeratosis overlies an epidermis showing granular and vacuolar change in its upper layers.
Haematoxylin — eosin

Palmoplantar: palmoplantar keratoderma variant (see p. 272)
Solitary: epidermolytic acanthoma (see below)
Multiple discrete: disseminated epidermolytic acanthoma (see below)
Incidental: focal epidermolytic hyperkeratosis (see below)
Solar keratosis-related: a rare variant of solar keratosis (see p. 739)
Follicular: naevoid follicular epidermolytic hyperkeratosis (see below)
Mucosal: epidermolytic leucoplakia.

Epidermolytic hyperkeratosis is a relatively uncommon histological pattern in epidermal naevi, being present in only 8 of 160 cases reported from the Mayo Clinic (the clinical appearance of the lesions in this series is not described).[203] There are reports of cases with a systematized pattern[204,205] (ichthyosis hystrix), and with a linear pattern (naevus unius lateris).[205] Bullous ichthyosis (generalized epidermolytic hyperkeratosis) has been reported in the offspring of two patients with the linear form of the disease.[206]

Focal epidermolytic hyperkeratosis has been found incidentally in a range of circumstances, including the wall of a pilar cyst, in a seborrhoeic keratosis, in a cutaneous horn and a skin tag, overlying an intradermal naevus and even in association with dermatoses.[23] It may be found adjacent to any lesion as an incidental phenomenon. It may also involve the intraepidermal eccrine sweat duct[207,208] and oral mucosa.[209]

The naevoid follicular variant[210] presents as comedo-like follicular papules that may have the appearance of naevus comedonicus.[211,212]

Epidermolytic hyperkeratosis has also been found rarely in solar keratoses[213] and in leucoplakic lesions of the lips[213,214] and prepuce.[215]

Electron microscopy. There are similar ultrastructural changes in the different variants of epidermolytic hyperkeratosis.[216] There is clumping of tonofilaments and cytoplasmic vacuolation.[217] Keratohyaline granules are of variable size.

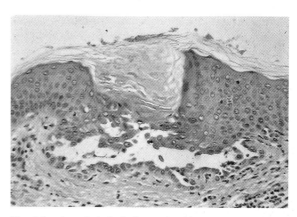

Fig. 9.9 Acantholytic dyskeratosis with suprabasal clefting and occasional acantholytic and dyskeratotic cells. The patient had an eruption with a zosteriform distribution. Haematoxylin — eosin

EPIDERMOLYTIC ACANTHOMA

This is an uncommon lesion which presents clinically as a wart, in patients of all ages.[218] A disseminated form has also been reported.[219,220]

Histopathology

The lesions show the typical features of epidermolytic hyperkeratosis. The entire thickness of the epidermis may be involved, or only the upper part of the nucleated epidermis.

ACANTHOLYTIC DYSKERATOSIS

Acantholytic dyskeratosis is a histological reaction pattern characterized by suprabasilar clefting with acantholytic and dyskeratotic cells at all levels of the epidermis (Fig. 9.9).[221] It may also be regarded as a special subdivision of the vesiculobullous tissue reaction, but it is considered in this chapter because the vesiculation is not usually apparent clinically and the primary abnormality involves the tonofilament-desmosome complex with disordered epidermal maturation.

Like epidermolytic hyperkeratosis, acantholytic dyskeratosis may be found in a number of different clinical settings.[221] The two histological

patterns have even been found in the same biopsy.[222] Acantholytic dyskeratosis may be:

Generalized: Darier's disease (see p. 280)
Systematized or linear: zosteriform Darier's disease or linear naevus (see below and p. 729)
Transient: Grover's disease (see p. 281)
Palmoplantar: a very rare form of keratoderma (see p. 274)
Solitary: warty dyskeratoma (see p. 284)
Incidental: focal acantholytic dyskeratosis (see below)
Solar keratosis-related: acantholytic solar keratosis (see p. 739)
Mucosal: vulval and anal acantholytic dyskeratosis (see below).

Of the various clinical settings listed above, focal acantholytic dyskeratosis, Darier's disease, Grover's disease and warty dyskeratoma will be considered separately. Familial benign chronic pemphigus (Hailey–Hailey disease) is also included in this section because of some overlap features with Darier's disease. However, in Hailey–Hailey disease the acantholysis is more extensive and dyskeratosis is not a prominent feature. Only brief mention will be made of the other clinical settings because of their rarity, or because they belong more appropriately to another section of this volume.

The occurrence of acantholytic dyskeratosis in lesions with a linear or systematized distribution is now regarded as a variant of epidermal naevus, rather than as a forme fruste of Darier's disease.[223,224] Acantholytic dyskeratosis was present in only 2 of a series of 167 epidermal naevi reported from the Mayo Clinic.[203] Acantholytic dyskeratosis has also been reported as a rare pattern in familial dyskeratotic comedones, a condition with some features in common with naevus comedonicus (see p. 731).[225]

Acantholytic dyskeratosis appears to affect cells within the germinative cellular pool of the epidermis.[226] The dyskeratosis that occurs within the acantholytic cells is probably a secondary phenomenon as the acantholytic cells are metabolically inert.[226]

FOCAL ACANTHOLYTIC DYSKERATOSIS

Although the term focal acantholytic dyskeratosis is often used both for clinically inapparent incidental foci and for clinically apparent solitary lesions with the histological pattern of acantholytic dyskeratosis, some authors restrict its use to its incidental finding in histological sections. This is not an uncommon event.[227] The term papular acantholytic dyskeratoma has recently been applied to the clinically apparent solitary lesions,[228] and papular acantholytic dyskeratosis to the exceedingly rare cases in which multiple lesions have developed on the vulva,[229–231] perianal area[232] or penis.[233]

Histopathology

There is acantholytic dyskeratosis, as already defined (see above). Hyperkeratosis is less prominent in incidental lesions than in Darier's disease. Warty dyskeratomas differ from focal acantholytic dyskeratomas by having more prominent villi, clefting and corps ronds. Some of the vulval cases (see above) have a histological resemblance to Hailey–Hailey disease (familial benign chronic pemphigus — see p. 283) ,[231,234] with marked acantholysis and little dyskeratosis.

Acantholysis, with little or no dyskeratosis, is a feature of acantholytic acanthoma,[235] a solitary lesion of the skin (see p. 734). It was also a feature in a patient with multiple cutaneous papules[236] and in another with a variant of epidermal naevus with horn-like processes. The latter case was reported as 'naevus corniculatus'.[237]

DARIER'S DISEASE

Darier's disease is an autosomal dominant genodermatosis in which greasy, yellow to brown, crusted papular lesions develop, mainly in the seborrhoeic areas of the head, neck and trunk.[238] The coalescence of papules gives plaques which may at times become papillomatous. Onset is usually in adolescence and the disease runs a chronic course. Verrucous lesions resembling acrokeratosis verruciformis may be present on the dorsum of the hands and feet.[239] Punctate keratoses are sometimes found on the palms and soles.[239] Longitudinal striations are usually present in the nails.[240] Rare clinical variants include a bullous[241–243] and a hypertrophic form.[244,245] Cutaneous depigmentation,[246] mucosal lesions,[247,248] ocular disorders,[249] bone cysts[250] and mental deficiency[251] have also been recorded.

There is a predisposition to bacterial, fungal and viral infections, although no consistent and specific immunological abnormality has been demonstrated.[238,252,253] Infection with herpes simplex virus, vaccinia[254] and even coxsackievirus A16[255] may produce the features of Kaposi's varicelliform eruption[256,257] (see Ch. 26, p. 684).

The mechanism of acantholysis in Darier's disease is still the subject of controversy.[238] It is usually ascribed to a defect in the synthesis, organization, or maturation of the tonofilament-desmosome complexes.[258] It is possible that the primary defect is in the formation or maintenance of the intercellular contact layer.[259] The pathogenetic significance of the recent finding that there is a delay in the expression of the suprabasal skin-specific keratins is uncertain.[260] Another study has found plasminogen in the suprabasal cells in Darier's disease;[261] plasminogen is confined to the basal layer in normal skin.

Histopathology

An individual papule of Darier's disease shows suprabasal acantholysis with the formation of a small cleft (lacuna). Irregular projections of the papillary dermis covered by a layer of basal cells, the so-called villi, extend into the lacunae (Fig. 9.10).[238] A thick orthokeratotic plug, often showing focal parakeratosis, overlies each lesion. Mild papillomatosis is often present.

Two characteristic types of dyskeratotic cell are present — *corps ronds* and *grains*. The *corps ronds* are found as solitary cells, or sometimes small groups of separated cells, in the upper malpighian layer and stratum corneum.[262] They have a small pyknotic nucleus, a clear perinuclear halo, and brightly eosinophilic cytoplasm. The *grains* are small cells with elongated nuclei and scant cytoplasm in the upper layers of the epidermis. They resemble parakeratotic cells but are somewhat larger.

The keratotic papules on the dorsum of the hands resemble those seen in acrokeratosis

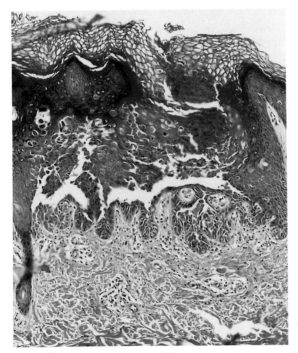

Fig. 9.10 Darier's disease. There is suprabasal clefting with a thickened stratum corneum and some dyskeratotic cells in the epidermis.
Haematoxylin — eosin

verruciformis, but small foci of suprabasal acantholytic dyskeratosis may be seen if serial sections are examined.

Immunoglobulins and C3 have been found in the intercellular areas of affected skin by direct immunofluorescence;[263] this finding has not been confirmed in other studies.[242]

Electron microscopy. The *corps ronds* have a vacuolated perinuclear halo surrounded by a ring of tonofilaments aggregated with keratohyaline granules.[264–266] The *grains* show premature aggregation of tonofilaments.[266] The synthesis of keratohyalin in association with clumped tonofilaments is peculiar to Darier's disease.[266] It is not seen in Hailey–Hailey disease. As already mentioned, there is controversy whether the withdrawal of the tonofilaments from the attachment plate of the desmosomes is the primary event in the acantholytic process, or merely secondary to the splitting of the desmosomes.[259] Another ultrastructural finding in Darier's disease is the presence of cytoplasmic processes projecting from the basal keratinocytes into the underlying dermis through small defects in the basal lamina.[267]

GROVER'S DISEASE

The eponymous designation Grover's disease is the preferred title for several closely related dermatoses characterized by the sudden onset of small, discrete, sometimes crusted, erythematous papules and papulovesicles.[268,269] They usually develop on the upper trunk of older men. Lesions may be transient, lasting for weeks or several months[268] (transient acantholytic dermatosis) or they may persist for several years[270] (persistent acantholytic dermatosis,[271–273] or papular acantholytic dermatosis[274]). Intense pruritus is often present. Oral involvement has been reported,[275] as has the coexistence of other dermatoses such as asteatotic eczema,[276,277] allergic contact dermatitis,[277] atopic eczema,[277] psoriasis[276] and pemphigus foliaceus.[278]

Some cases of Grover's disease have followed, or been exacerbated by, exposure to ultraviolet light.[272,274] Recently, the role of heat, persistent fever and sweating has been postulated in the aetiology of this condition.[279–281]

Histopathology

Four histological patterns may be seen[276] — Darier-like, Hailey–Hailey-like, pemphigus-vulgaris-like and spongiotic (Figs 9.11 and 9.12). The Darier pattern is most common.[270] In the spongiotic type there are a few acantholytic cells within and contiguous with spongiotic foci.[271,276] More than one of these histological patterns may be present. In some reports, the persistent cases have tended to have either a Darier-like[272] or pemphigus pattern.[274] In addition to the epidermal changes, there is usually a superficial dermal infiltrate of lymphocytes and sometimes eosinophils.[270,271]

Older lesions may have considerable acanthosis and only subtle clefting and acantholysis (Fig. 9.13). They may be misdiagnosed as a solar keratosis or non-specific lesion. Small, non-pigmented seborrhoeic keratoses seem to be increased in number[282] and are sometimes biopsied instead of the lesions of Grover's disease. The transient, vesiculobullous variant with a pemphigus foliaceus pattern on histology is best regarded as a variant of pemphigus foliaceus and not of Grover's disease.[283]

Direct immunofluorescence is usually negative,[279] although there are several reports describing variable patterns of immunoglobulin and complement deposition.[271,284,285]

Electron microscopy. Ultrastructural changes reflect the light microscopic features with variable degrees of acantholysis, dyskeratosis and cytoplasmic vacuolization.[286,287] The dyskeratosis is represented by an increase in tonofilaments with some clumping.[287] There is some loss of desmosomes in the affected area, but the hemidesmosomes of the basal layer are preserved.[282]

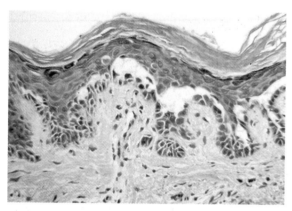

Fig. 9.11 Grover's disease. A few acantholytic cells are present within the suprabasal cleft. There is a mild inflammatory infiltrate in the dermis.
Haematoxylin — eosin

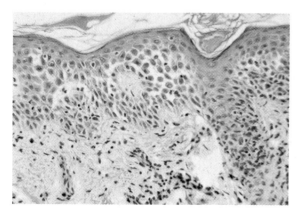

Fig. 9.12 Grover's disease. There is prominent acantholysis resembling Hailey-Hailey disease.
Haematoxylin — eosin

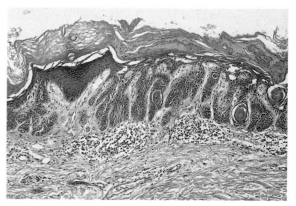

Fig. 9.13 Grover's disease. This lesion was of some duration and accordingly there is conspicuous acanthosis. Clefting is just visible in the upper layers of the epidermis. Biopsies of lesions such as this are often misdiagnosed as a solar keratosis.
Haematoxylin — eosin

FAMILIAL BENIGN CHRONIC PEMPHIGUS

Familial benign chronic pemphigus (Hailey–Hailey disease) is an uncommon genodermatosis with recurrent, erythematous, vesicular plaques, which progress to small flaccid bullae with subsequent rupture and crusting.[288,289] The plaques are well demarcated and spread peripherally, often with a circinate border. Rare clinical forms include papular,[290] verrucous,[291] annular and vesiculopustular variants.[292] Nikolsky's sign may be positive. There is a predilection for the neck, axillae and intertriginous areas such as the genitocrural, perianal and inframammary region. Occasionally large areas of the skin are involved.[293] There are rare reports of involvement of oral, ocular, oesophageal,[294] and vaginal[295] mucous membranes, or of lesions limited to the vulva[230,296,297] or perianal[298] region.

The disease is inherited as an autosomal dominant condition with incomplete gene penetrance. Nearly one-third of cases are sporadic. Onset is usually in the late teens and there is a tendency for the disease to improve in late adulthood.

The chronic course is punctuated by periods of spontaneous remission with subsequent exacerbations. Lesions may be induced in genetically predisposed tissues by trauma,[299,300] heat, ultraviolet light,[301] perspiration, and infection with bacteria,[302] herpes virus,[303] or yeasts. Lesions are often mildly pruritic or burning. They are also malodorous.

Rare associations have included psoriasis,[299,304,305] Darier's disease,[306,307] localized bullous pemphigoid,[308] syringomas of the vulva[309] and basal cell carcinoma.[310] Selected cases, which have been refractory to other forms of treatment, have benefited by excision of affected skin and split-skin grafting using uninvolved skin.[311–315] Conversely, if suspensions of keratinocytes from affected skin are placed on to healthy heterologous dermis, devoid of its epidermis, the morphological features of the disease are reproduced in vitro.[316]

Histopathology

In early lesions, there are lacunae formed by suprabasilar clefting, with acantholytic cells either singly or in clumps lining the clefts and lying free within them. The lacunae progress to broad, acantholytic vesicles and bullae (Fig. 9.14). Intercellular oedema leading to partial acantholysis gives rise to areas with a characteristic 'dilapidated brick wall' appearance (Fig. 9.15).[317]

Epidermal hyperplasia is commonly seen, and this is formed, in part, by downward elongation of the rete ridges. Elongated papillae covered by one or several layers of keratinocytes ('villi') may protrude up into the bullae.

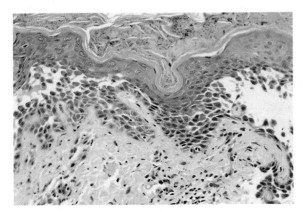

Fig. 9.14 Hailey-Hailey disease. There is suprabasal clefting with pronounced acantholysis.
Haematoxylin — eosin

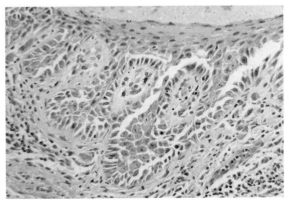

Fig. 9.15 Hailey-Hailey disease with many acantholytic keratinocytes.
Haematoxylin — eosin

Some acantholytic cells are dyskeratotic but they have a well defined nucleus and preserved cytoplasm in contrast to the degenerating dyskeratotic cells of pemphigus. Corps ronds are infrequent and grains are rare.

Neutrophils are sometimes numerous within the vesicles or in the surface parakeratotic crust. Bacteria may also be present in the crust.[288] The dermis shows a variable, superficial chronic inflammatory cell infiltrate.

The Hailey–Hailey variant of Grover's disease (see p. 282) has only a narrow vesicle involving no more than a few rete ridges, in contrast to the broad lesions of familial benign chronic pemphigus.[317] Although pemphigus vulgaris usually has less acantholysis and some of its cells show more pronounced dyskeratosis, it can be difficult sometimes to distinguish between it and familial benign pemphigus without recourse to immunofluorescence.

Electron microscopy.   Although earlier ultrastructural studies reported that detachment of tonofilaments from desmosomes with the subsequent disruption and disappearance of the latter was the primary event leading to acantholysis,[318] subsequent studies have shown that the initial event is a series of changes in the microvilli leading to loss of cellular adhesions.[319,320] Desmosomes are then separated and invaginated into cells. Thickened bundles of tonofilaments, sometimes in whorls, are found in cells of the prickle cell and granular layers.[319]

WARTY DYSKERATOMA

Warty dyskeratomas are rare, usually solitary, papules or nodules with an umbilicated or porelike centre.[321,322] They have a predilection for the head and neck of middle-aged and elderly individuals.[323] Oral lesions have also been reported, but some of these appear to be examples of isolated focal acantholytic dyskeratosis (see p. 280).[324,325] Warty dyskeratomas average 5 mm in diameter, although an unusually large example, 3 cm in diameter, has been described.[326]

They occasionally bleed or intermittently discharge cheesy material.[322]

Histopathology[322,323]

There is a circumscribed, cup-shaped, invaginating lesion extending into the underlying dermis (Fig. 9.16). The central depression is filled with a plug of keratinous material containing some grains. These keratin plugs have sometimes been dislodged, particularly in oral lesions.[325] The epidermal component shows suprabasilar clefting with numerous acantholytic and dyskeratotic cells within the lacuna. Protruding into the lacuna are villi which are dermal papillae covered by a layer of basal cells. The papillae contain dilated vessels, occasional melanophages and a few inflammatory cells; inflammatory cells are

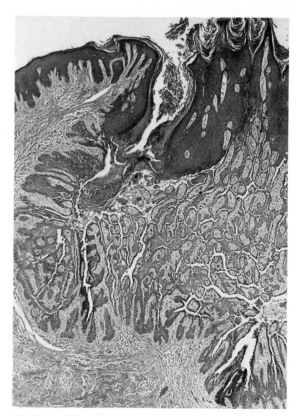

Fig. 9.16   Warty dyskeratoma. There is suprabasal clefting and conspicuous basal proliferation.   There is not the usual keratin plug.
Haematoxylin — eosin

also present in the underlying dermis. Pilo-sebaceous follicles may open into the lesion.

Corps ronds and grains are better developed in the skin lesions than in those in the mouth.[325]

COLLOID KERATOSIS

Colloid keratosis is characterized by the presence of homogeneous eosinophilic masses of variable size and number within the upper layers of squamous epithelia.[327] It has been seen as an incidental finding in neoplastic and non-neoplastic lesions in the skin and respiratory tract,[328] as well as in pachyonychia congenita and other onychoses.[327] Reports have appeared mainly in the non-English and dental literature.

It appears to result from a defect in keratinization with the accumulation of cytokeratin precursors or related protein products. Colloid keratosis has no clinical significance and it is a reaction pattern rather than a disease entity.

Histopathology[327]

Homogeneous and rounded pools of eosinophilic material are found in the upper layers of the epidermis (Fig. 9.17). The material is PAS positive and diastase resistant. Ultrastructurally it is amorphous and devoid of any filaments.

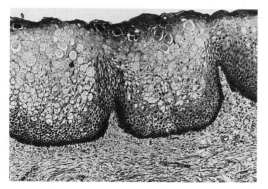

Fig. 9.17 Colloid keratosis characterized by pools of homogeneous eosinophilic material in the upper layers of the epidermis.
Haematoxylin — eosin
Photomicrograph provided by Dr Sergio Gonzalez, Catholic University, Santiago, Chile.

Colloid keratosis must be distinguished from pagetoid dyskeratosis, which is another incidental histological finding. It is characterized by cells with a pyknotic nucleus with a clear halo and a rim of pale cytoplasm.[329] Both entities must be distinguished from clear cell papulosis in which clear cells, containing mucin and keratin, are present in the epidermis.[330] It has been suggested that the clear cells might be precursor cells for cutaneous Paget's disease.[330]

DISCRETE KERATOTIC LESIONS

There is a group of rare genodermatoses of late onset in which multiple, discrete, keratotic lesions develop as a result of abnormal keratinization. This group includes hyperkeratosis lenticularis perstans, Kyrle's disease and disseminated spiked hyperkeratosis. Discrete keratotic lesions associated with palmar-plantar involvement (see p. 273) or cornoid lamellation (see p. 277) are considered elsewhere in this chapter. Certain acquired lesions such as warts, cutaneous horns, callosities, corns, stucco keratoses, solar keratoses, seborrhoeic keratoses and lesions produced by tar may present as discrete keratotic lesions. They are not included in this section which is concerned essentially with keratotic genodermatoses.

HYPERKERATOSIS LENTICULARIS PERSTANS

Hyperkeratosis lenticularis perstans (Flegel's disease)[331] is a rare genodermatosis of late onset in which an abnormality in keratinization results in the development of multiple, discrete, 1–5 mm keratoses.[332,333] An autosomal dominant inheritance is sometimes present.[334–336] The lesions are most prominent on the dorsum of the feet and the anterior aspect of the lower legs, but they may also develop on the thighs, upper limbs and pinnae.[333,337] The keratoses develop in mid to late adult life and persist. Removal of the spiny scale causes slight bleeding.[338]

Several reports, but not all,[337,339] have documented a decrease in or qualitative defects of the membrane-coating granules (lamellar or Odland bodies) in affected areas of epidermis.[340–343] It has been suggested that these abnormalities are the basis for the defect in keratinization.[341]

Histopathology[333,337,341]

There is a discrete zone of compact, deeply eosinophilic hyperkeratosis, with patchy areas of parakeratosis.[336] There is some acanthosis at the margins of the lesions, but the epidermis at the base of the plaque of keratin is thinned with effacement of the rete ridge pattern.[333] The malpighian layer may eventually be only three cells thick. The granular layer is usually less prominent in this area. There may be some basal vacuolar change[344] and occasional apoptotic cells.[333] They were prominent in a case reported by Hunter and Donald.[345] The superficial dermis has a dense band-like infiltrate of lymphocytes, some of which appear activated.[342] Capillary proliferation is sometimes present.

It is tempting to speculate that the inflammatory infiltrate is an immunological reaction directed against emerging clones of abnormal epidermal cells, in much the same way that this occurs in some cases of porokeratosis.[346]

Electron microscopy.   Studies have shown a reduction in keratohyaline granules and some persistence of desmosomal components in the stratum corneum.[339] The disparate findings with regard to membrane-coating granules (lamellar bodies) have been referred to above.[339]

KYRLE'S DISEASE

The eponymous designation Kyrle's disease is preferable to the original designation of hyperkeratosis follicularis et parafollicularis in cutem penetrans.[347] This controversial entity is regarded by some as a late onset genodermatosis in which abnormal clones of epidermal cells lead to premature keratinization at the expense of epidermal thickness, with the subsequent introduction of keratinous material into the dermis.[348,349] Others regard it as a variant of perforating folliculitis, a view which is supported by the finding of perforating lesions in patients with chronic renal failure on dialysis, with clinical and histological overlap features between Kyrle's disease, perforating folliculitis and even reactive perforating collagenosis.[350–352] It has also been suggested that Kyrle's disease and Flegel's disease (hyperkeratosis lenticularis perstans — see above) may be different manifestations of the same disease process.[353,354]

Kyrle's disease, as traditionally described, consists of hyperkeratotic papules 2–8 mm in diameter, containing a central, cone-shaped plug.[347,355] The papules may be follicular or extrafollicular in location and they may coalesce to form a verrucous plaque. There is a predilection for the lower limbs, but lesions may also occur on the upper limbs and less often on the head and neck.[355,356] Palmar and plantar surfaces are rarely involved.[357] A female preponderance has been noted in some series.[349] Onset is usually in the fourth decade. A family history has been present in a few cases.[349] Kyrle's disease has been associated with chronic renal failure[358–360] and with diabetes mellitus,[359] and more rarely with hepatic dysfunction.[355,361]

Histopathology[362,363]

There is a keratotic plug overlying an invaginated atrophic epidermis. Focal parakeratosis is present in part of the plug; often there is some basophilic cellular debris, which does not stain for elastin. If serial sections are studied, a focus where the epidermal cells are absent and the keratotic plug is in contact with the dermis will often be seen. An inflammatory infiltrate which includes lymphocytes, occasional neutrophils and sometimes a few foreign body giant cells will be present in these areas. Follicular involvement may be present, particularly in those with chronic renal failure where overlap with perforating folliculitis occurs. Eccrine duct involvement was present in one atypical case reported in the literature.[357]

In Flegel's disease (see p. 285), in contrast, there is massive orthokeratosis and only focal parakeratosis, but no basophilic debris in the keratin layer.[349] Also, the inflammatory infiltrate is more conspicuous and usually band-like in distribution.

DISSEMINATED SPIKED HYPERKERATOSIS

This is a rare disorder of keratinization, sometimes with an autosomal dominant inheritance,[364,365] in which hundreds of minute keratotic spikes develop in early adult life. There is a predilection for the upper parts of the trunk and for the proximal parts of the limbs.[366,367]

A closely related entity, *minute aggregate keratoses*,[368] has dome-shaped papules and crateriform or annular lesions in addition to the spicular lesions seen in disseminated spiked hyperkeratosis.

Minute keratotic spikes resembling those seen in disseminated spiked hyperkeratosis have been reported as an acquired phenomenon following X-irradiation (see below), and in Crohn's disease.[369] They have also developed transiently following inflammatory skin disease.[370] In another case, the lesions were localized to the palms and soles.[371]

Histopathology

The spicules are composed of densely compacted, thin stacks of orthokeratotic material, often arising from a finely pointed epidermal elevation. The keratinous spicules are 1–3 mm in height. They are not related to hair follicles. There may be mild underlying epidermal hyperplasia. The dermis is normal. The digitate keratoses that developed in a patient following irradiation to the area were characterized by parakeratotic plugs and underlying epidermal invaginations.[372] Parakeratotic horns were also present in the patient with Crohn's disease, referred to above.

Electron microscopy. This shows a thickened stratum corneum and a reduced keratohyaline content in the superficial epidermis.[373] Odland bodies are present.[364,373]

MISCELLANEOUS EPIDERMAL GENODERMATOSES

This group includes such disparate conditions as acrokeratosis verruciformis, xeroderma pigmentosum, the ectodermal dysplasias and aplasia cutis congenita.

ACROKERATOSIS VERRUCIFORMIS

Acrokeratosis verruciformis is an autosomal dominant genodermatosis in which multiple papules, resembling plane warts, develop on the dorsum of the hands and fingers, and to a lesser extent on the feet, forearms and legs.[374–378] Onset is usually before puberty, but late onset has been recorded.[374–377] It is more common in males.[377]

Lesions identical to those of acrokeratosis verruciformis develop in a significant number of patients with Darier's disease (see p. 280). Such lesions may precede, follow or develop concurrently with the onset of the more usual lesions of Darier's disease.[379] Acrokeratosis verruciformis has been reported in the relatives of individuals with Darier's disease.[380] There is considerable controversy as to the nature of the relationship of these two conditions, and also about their relationship to the palmar and plantar keratoses which may accompany either disease. One view is that the acral lesions of Darier's disease and acrokeratosis verruciformis are separate entities.[377] This is based on the finding of small foci of acantholytic dyskeratosis in some acral lesions of Darier's disease if multiple sections are examined. The contrary view is that both diseases result from a single autosomal dominant genetic defect with variable expressivity of the gene.[379,381,382]

Histopathology[374,377]

Sections show hyperkeratosis, regular acanthosis and low papillomatosis imparting a regular undulating appearance to the surface (Fig. 9.18). These changes have been likened to 'church spires'. There is no parakeratosis, no epidermal

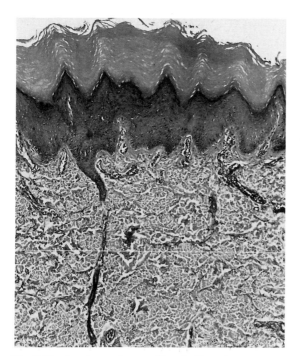

Fig. 9.18 Acrokeratosis verruciformis. There is compact orthokeratosis and low papillomatosis imparting an undulating appearance to the epidermis. Haematoxylin — eosin

vacuolation and no significant dermal inflammatory infiltrate.

Squamous cell carcinomas have been reported in two cases of long standing.[377]

XERODERMA PIGMENTOSUM

Xeroderma pigmentosum is a rare, autosomal recessive genodermatosis characterized by photophobia, severe solar sensitivity, cutaneous pigmentary changes, xerosis, and the early development of mucocutaneous and ocular cancers, particularly in sun-exposed areas.[383–386] Neurological abnormalities are present in up to 20%,[387] and these are most severe in the De Sanctis–Cacchione syndrome (microcephaly, dwarfism, choreoathetosis and mental deficiency).[383,385,388] The earliest changes usually develop before the age of 2 with a severe sunburn reaction and the development of multiple freckles with variable intensity of melanin pigmentation and interspersed hypopigmented macules.[389,390] Pigmentation often develops on the palms and soles and mucous membranes. Later there is dry, scaly skin (xerosis) with poikilodermatous features. Skin tumours which include solar keratoses, cutaneous horns, keratoacanthomas, squamous and basal cell carcinomas, malignant melanomas and angiomas may develop in late childhood; patients may ultimately die from the consequences of their tumours.[387] The development of the cutaneous lesions can be retarded by protection from the sun from birth.[391] Immunological abnormalities have been present in some patients.[392]

Xeroderma pigmentosum involves both sexes and all races with an incidence of 1:250 000 and a gene frequency of 1:200.[383] There is a high incidence of consanguinity.[393] Heterozygotes cannot be reliably demonstrated in the laboratory. They are asymptomatic, although there is one report of an increased incidence of malignant skin tumours in these individuals.[383] Prenatal diagnosis of xeroderma pigmentosum can be made by an analysis of DNA repair in cells cultured from the amniotic fluid of women at risk.[394]

There is genetic heterogeneity with at least ten different groups recognized by somatic cell fusion studies — so-called complementation groups.[383] Nine of these groups (labelled A to I) have deficient excision repair of ultraviolet radiation-induced DNA damage, while in one (the so-called XP variant) there is defective ability to convert newly synthesized DNA from low to high molecular weight after UV irradiation (post-replication repair).[383,395,396] These different complementation groups have different clinical correlations, including different susceptibility to the various cutaneous tumours.[397] For example, XP-A is the most severe form, and some of this group have the De Sanctis–Cacchione syndrome (see above). XP-E is the mildest form, with late onset and a higher residual capacity to repair UV-induced DNA damage in in-vitro studies.[398] XP-F,[399,400] XP-G,[401] XP-B and XP-H are extremely rare and the latter two groups have been associated with the Cockayne syndrome (short stature, photosensitivity, deafness, mental deficiency, large ears and nose and sunken eyes).[383,386,402] Squamous cell carcinomas are commonly found in groups A and H, basal cell carcinomas in groups C and E and in the variant form, and malignant melanomas in groups C and D and also in the variant form.[383,403]

Recently, a skin fibroblast cell strain from a patient with xeroderma pigmentosum was reported to have shown spontaneous morphological transformation to an anchorage-independent form after serial passage.[404] This presumably has some significance in the development of tumours in vivo; the finding of reduced natural killer cell activity may have a similar significance.[405]

It is now well established that cultured fibroblasts from patients with xeroderma pigmentosum show defective DNA repair following ultraviolet radiation. This abnormality is also present in keratinocytes and melanocytes cultured from affected patients.[406]

Histopathology[384]

In the initial stages there are no diagnostically specific features. There may be variability in epidermal melanin concentration, telangiectasia of superficial vessels and a mild perivascular inflammatory cell reaction. With time, the pigmentary changes are more marked, with areas of prominent melanin pigmentation of the basal, malpighian and spinous layers, and pigmentary incontinence. Areas of hypopigmentation, sometimes with epidermal atrophy, may be seen. There is eventually prominent solar elastosis and the development of areas of hyperkeratosis. Keratoses and the other tumours already mentioned eventually develop. Tumours of the anterior part of the tongue have also been reported.[407,408]

Electron microscopy. Various changes have been noted. They include irregular nuclear morphology, melanosomes with a high degree of polymorphism, and dilated rough endoplasmic reticulum, vacuoles and disrupted desmosomes in basal keratinocytes.[409] Fibroblast-like cells may show melanophagic activity.[409] Structures resembling anchoring fibrils and the basal lamina

have been noted in the dilated endoplasmic reticulum of these cells.[410]

ECTODERMAL DYSPLASIAS

The ectodermal dysplasias are an expanding, but nevertheless rare, group of genodermatoses characterized by a diffuse, non-progressive disorder of the epidermis and at least one of its appendages.[122,411] The epidermal component may involve keratinocytes, melanocytes[412] or Langerhans cells, or any combination thereof; the 'appendageal' component may affect the hair, sebaceous or eccrine glands, the nails or the teeth.[413] The ectodermal dysplasias comprise nearly 100 clinically distinct syndromes and the limits of this entity are not clearly defined.[414] Abnormalities of non-ectodermal structures may also be present.

The traditional classification of the ectodermal dysplasias into hidrotic and anhidrotic types is not appropriate for the broad range of abnormalities that may occur in this group.[415] They are now classified on the basis of the presence or absence of trichodysplasia, dental abnormalities, onychodysplasia and dyshidrosis. Most of the syndromes are extremely rare and of little dermatopathological importance. Three of them merit further discussion.

Anhidrotic ectodermal dysplasia. In this X-linked recessive disorder, also known as the Christ–Siemens–Touraine syndrome, there is anhidrosis or marked hypohidrosis, complete or partial anodontia, hypotrichosis and a characteristic facies.[122,416,417] Less frequent manifestations include nail dystrophy, genital anomalies, absence of mammary glands, impaired immunity[418] and mental retardation.[419,420] A prenatal diagnosis can be made by an examination of fetal skin.[421] Female carriers may show reduced sweating and faulty dentition.[422]

Hidrotic ectodermal dysplasia. In this variant, also known as Clouston's syndrome, there is a normal ability to perspire.[122–124] Palmar-plantar keratoderma is usually a prominent feature (see p. 275). The recent finding of an increased number of desmosomal discs in the thickened stratum corneum suggests that the hyperkeratosis in this disorder is due to delayed desquamation of the stratum corneum.[423]

Orofaciodigital syndrome. This is an X-linked dominant disorder which is usually lethal in males.[122,424] There is a marked reduction in sebaceous glands on the scalp or face, dental dysplasia, evanescent facial milia, cleft lip and palate, and malformation of the digits. Mental retardation may be present.

Histopathology

The histological features will obviously vary according to which epidermal and appendageal components are involved.

In *anhidrotic ectodermal dysplasia* the epidermis is thinned. Eccrine glands are absent or rudimentary, although poorly formed intraepidermal eccrine ducts may be present.[425] Apocrine glands may also be hypotrophic. There is a reduction in pilosebaceous follicles although, paradoxically, foci of sebaceous hyperplasia have sometimes been noted on the upper cheeks.[426] Other reported features include a reduction in seromucous glands in the respiratory tract,[427] a reduction in epidermal Langerhans cells and fragmentation of dermal elastic fibres. As eccrine glands do not develop until 20–24 weeks of gestation, whereas hair follicles should be present at this time, it is the absence of pilar units which is used to make the diagnosis on fetal skin biopsies taken at this period of gestation.[421]

In *hidrotic ectodermal dysplasia* there is pronounced hyperkeratosis, particularly of the palms and soles, and a normal number of sweat glands. The sweat glands are also normal in number in the *orofaciodigital syndrome*, but sebaceous glands are diminished or absent.[424] The epidermis may be somewhat atrophic.

CUTANEOUS AND MUCOSAL DYSKERATOSIS

There has been a report describing a father and son with brownish papules with central keratotic plugs.[428] Single cell keratinization (dyskeratosis) was present in the epidermis, as well as in the epithelium of the mouth and the conjunctiva.[428] In another case, numerous dyskeratotic cells were present in epithelium of the lips, palate and gums and on the labial surfaces of the genitalia, as an acquired phenomenon: this condition was referred to as acquired dyskeratotic leucoplakia.[429] Dyskeratotic cells were also a feature of the cases reported as hereditary muco-epithelial dysplasia.[430]

REFERENCES

Ichthyoses

1. Rand RE, Baden HP. The ichthyoses — a review. J Am Acad Dermatol 1983; 8: 285–305.
2. Williams ML. The ichthyoses — pathogenesis and prenatal diagnosis: a review of recent advances. Pediatr Dermatol 1983; 1: 1–24.
2a. Williams ML, Elias PM. Genetically transmitted, generalized disorders of cornification. The ichthyoses. Dermatol Clin 1987; 5: 155–178.
3. Williams ML, Elias PM. Ichthyosis. Genetic heterogeneity, genodermatoses, and genetic counseling. Arch Dermatol 1986; 122: 529–531.
4. Bernhardt M, Baden HP. Report of a family with an unusual expression of recessive ichthyosis. Report of 42 cases. Arch Dermatol 1986; 122: 428–433.
5. Sybert VP, Dale BA, Holbrook KA. Ichthyosis vulgaris: identification of a defect in synthesis of filaggrin correlated with an absence of keratohyaline granules. J Invest Dermatol 1985; 84: 191–194.
6. Schnyder UW. Inherited ichthyosis. Arch Dermatol 1970; 102: 240–251.
7. Anton-Lamprecht I. Electron microscopy in the early diagnosis of genetic disorders of the skin. Dermatologica 1978; 157: 65–85.
8. Shapiro LJ. X-linked ichthyosis. Int J Dermatol 1981; 20: 26–31.
8a. Elliott ST. X-linked ichthyosis: A metabolic disease. J Am Acad Dermatol 1979; 1: 139–143.
9. De Unamuno P, Martin-Pascual A, Garcia-Perez A. X-linked ichthyosis. Br J Dermatol 1977; 97: 53–58.
9a. Okano M, Kitano Y, Yoshikawa K et al. X-linked ichthyosis and ichthyosis vulgaris: comparison of their clinical features based on biochemical analysis. Br J Dermatol 1988; 119: 777–783.

10. Honour JW, Goolamali SK, Taylor NF. Prenatal diagnosis and variable presentation of recessive X-linked ichthyosis. Br J Dermatol 1985; 112: 423–430.

11. Yoshiike T, Matsui T, Ogawa H. Steroid sulphatase deficiency in patients initially diagnosed as ichthyosis vulgaris or recessive X-linked ichthyosis. Br J Dermatol 1985; 112: 431–433.

12. Brown BE, Williams ML, Elias PM. Stratum corneum lipid abnormalities in ichthyosis. Detection by a new lipid microanalytical method. Arch Dermatol 1984; 120: 204–209.

13. Jobsis AC, De Groot WP, Meijer AEFH, Van Der Loos CM. A new method for the determination of steroid sulphatase activity in leukocytes in X-linked ichthyosis. Br J Dermatol 1983; 108: 567–572.

14. Dijkstra AC, Vermeesch-Markslag AMG, Vromans EWM et al. Substrate specific sulfatase activity from hair follicles in recessive X-linked ichthyosis. Acta Derm Venereol 1987; 67: 369–376.

14a. Piccirillo A, Auricchio L, Fabbrocini G et al. Ocular findings and skin histology in a group of patients with X-linked ichthyosis. Br J Dermatol 1988; 119: 185–188.

15. Lentz CL, Altman J. Lamellar ichthyosis. The natural clinical course of collodion baby. Arch Dermatol 1968; 97: 3–13.

16. Frenk E, Mevorah B. The keratinization disorder in collodion babies evolving into lamellar ichthyosis. J Cutan Pathol 1977; 4: 329–337.

17. Rossmann-Ringdahl I, Anton-Lamprecht I, Swanbeck G. A mother and two children with nonbullous congenital ichthyosiform erythroderma. Arch Dermatol 1986; 122: 559–564.

17a. Finlay AY. Major autosomal recessive ichthyoses. Semin Dermatol 1988; 7: 26–36.

17b. Bergers M, Traupe H, Dunnwald SC et al. Enzymatic distinction between two subgroups of autosomal recessive lamellar ichthyosis. J Invest Dermatol 1990; 94: 407–412.

18. Hazell M, Marks R. Clinical, histologic, and cell kinetic discriminants between lamellar ichthyosis and nonbullous congenital ichthyosiform erythroderma. Arch Dermatol 1985; 121: 489–493.

19. Dover R, Burge S, Ralfs I, Ryan TJ. Congenital non-bullous ichthyosiform erythroderma — cell kinetics before and after treatment with etretinate. Clin Exp Dermatol 1986; 11: 431–435.

19a. Niemi K-M, Kanerva L. Ichthyosis with laminated membrane structures. Am J Dermatopathol 1989; 11: 149–156.

20. Kanerva L, Niemi K-M, Lauharanta J, Lassus A. New observations on the fine structure of lamellar ichthyosis and the effect of treatment with etretinate. Am J Dermatopathol 1983; 5: 555–568.

20a. Haftek M, Thivolet J, Thomas L et al. Re-expression of disease — characteristic features of non-bullous congenital ichthyosiform erythroderma (CIE) after grafting of the pathological keratinocyte cultures to athymic mice. J Cutan Pathol 1989; 16: 1–6.

21. Holbrook KA. Progress in prenatal diagnosis of bullous congenital ichthyosiform erythroderma (epidermolytic hyperkeratosis). Semin Dermatol 1984; 3: 216–220.

22. Traupe H, Kolde G, Hamm H, Happle R. Ichthyosis bullosa of Siemens: a unique type of epidermolytic hyperkeratosis. J Am Acad Dermatol 1986; 14: 1000–1005.

22a. Murdoch ME, Leigh IM. Ichthyosis bullosa of Siemens and bullous ichthyosiform erythroderma — variants of the same disease? Clin Exp Dermatol 1990; 15: 53–56.

23. Ackerman AB. Histopathologic concept of epidermolytic hyperkeratosis. Arch Dermatol 1970; 102: 253–259.

24. Wilgram GF, Caulfield JB. An electron microscopic study of epidermolytic hyperkeratosis. Arch Dermatol 1966; 94: 127–143.

25. Yoshiike T, Manabe M, Negi M, Ogawa H. Ichthyosis linearis circumflexa: morphological and biochemical studies. Br J Dermatol 1985; 112: 277–283.

26. Greene SL, Muller SA. Netherton's syndrome. Report of a case and review of the literature. J Am Acad Dermatol 1985; 13: 329–337.

27. Yesudian P, Srinivas K. Ichthyosis with unusual hair shaft abnormalities in siblings. Br J Dermatol 1977; 96: 199–203.

28. Caputo R, Vanotti P, Bertani E. Netherton's syndrome in two adult brothers. Arch Dermatol 1984; 120: 220–222.

28a. Stevanovic DV. Multiple defects of the hair shaft in Netherton's disease. Association with ichthyosis linearis circumflexa. Br J Dermatol 1969; 81: 851–857.

29. Altman J, Stroud J. Netherton's syndrome and ichthyosis linearis circumflexa. Arch Dermatol 1969; 100: 550–558.

30. Zina AM, Bundino S. Ichthyosis linearis circumflexa Comel and Netherton's syndrome; an ultrastructural study. Dermatologica 1979; 158: 404–412.

31. Gewirtzman GB, Winkler NW, Dobson RL. Erythrokeratodermia variabilis. A family study. Arch Dermatol 1978; 114: 259–261.

32. McFadden N, Oppedal BR, Ree K, Brandtzaeg P. Erythrokeratodermia variabilis: immunohistochemical and ultrastructural studies of the epidermis. Acta Derm Venereol 1987; 67: 284–288.

33. Rappaport IP, Goldes JA, Goltz RW. Erythrokeratodermia variabilis treated with isotretinoin. A clinical, histologic, and ultrastructural study. Arch Dermatol 1986; 122: 441–445.

33a. Roberts LJ. Long-term survival of a harlequin fetus. J Am Acad Dermatol 1989; 21: 335–339.

34. Baden HP, Kubilus J, Rosenbaum K, Fletcher A. Keratinization in the harlequin fetus. Arch Dermatol 1982; 118: 14–18.

34a. Dale BA, Holbrook KA, Fleckman P et al. Heterogeneity in harlequin ichthyosis, an inborn error of epidermal keratinization: variable morphology and structural protein expression and a defect in lamellar granules. J Invest Dermatol 1990; 94: 6–18.

35. Unamuno P, Pierola JM, Fernandez E et al. Harlequin foetus in four siblings. Br J Dermatol 1987; 116: 569–572.

36. Blanchet-Bardon C, Dumez Y. Prenatal diagnosis of a harlequin fetus. Semin Dermatol 1984; 3: 225–228.

37. Buxman MM, Goodkin PE, Fahrenbach WH, Dimond RL. Harlequin ichthyosis with epidermal lipid abnormality. Arch Dermatol 1979; 115: 189–193.

37a. Fleck RM, Barnadas M, Schulz WW et al. Harlequin ichthyosis: An ultrastructural study. J Am Acad Dermatol 1989; 21: 999–1006.

38. Hazell M, Marks R. Follicular ichthyosis. Br J Dermatol 1984; 111: 101–109.

38a. Eramo LR, Esterly NB, Zieserl EJ et al. Ichthyosis

follicularis with alopecia and photophobia. Arch Dermatol 1985; 121: 1167–1174.

39. Dykes PJ, Marks R. Acquired ichthyosis: multiple causes for an acquired generalized disturbance in desquamation. Br J Dermatol 1977; 97: 327–334.

40. Flint GL, Flam M, Soter NA. Acquired ichthyosis. A sign of nonlymphoproliferative malignant disorders. Arch Dermatol 1975; 111: 1446–1447.

41. Kauh YC, Goody HE, Luscombe HA. Ichthyosiform sarcoidosis. Arch Dermatol 1978; 114: 100–101.

42. Banse-Kupin L, Pelachyk JM. Ichthyosiform sarcoidosis. Report of two cases and a review of the literature. J Am Acad Dermatol 1987; 17: 616–620.

43. Aram H. Acquired ichthyosis and related conditions. Int J Dermatol 1984; 23: 458–461.

43a. El-Hefnawi H, Rasheed A. Pityriasis rotunda. Arch Dermatol 1966; 93: 84–86.

43b. Kahana M, Levy A, Ronnen M et al. Pityriasis rotunda in a white patient. Report of the second case and review of the literature. J Am Acad Dermatol 1986; 15: 362–365.

43c. Rubin MG, Mathes B. Pityriasis rotunda: Two cases in black Americans. J Am Acad Dermatol 1986; 14: 74–78.

43d. DiBisceglie AM, Hodkinson HJ, Berkowitz I, Kew MC. Pityriasis rotunda. A cutaneous marker of hepatocellular carcinoma in South African blacks. Arch Dermatol 1986; 122: 802–804.

43e. Berkowitz I, Hodkinson HJ, Kew MC, DiBisceglie AM. Pityriasis rotunda as a cutaneous marker of hepatocellular carcinoma: a comparison with its prevalence in other diseases. Br J Dermatol 1989; 120: 545–549.

43f. Segal R, Hodak E, Sandbank M. Pityriasis rotunda in a Caucasian woman from the Mediterranean area. Clin Exp Dermatol 1989; 14: 325–327.

44. Davies MG, Marks R, Dykes PJ, Reynolds D. Epidermal abnormalities in Refsum's disease. Br J Dermatol 1977; 97: 401–406.

45. Srebrnik A, Tur E, Perluk C et al. Dorfman-Chanarin syndrome. A case report and a review. J Am Acad Dermatol 1987; 17: 801–808.

46. Liden S, Jagell S. The Sjögren-Larsson syndrome. Int J Dermatol 1984; 23: 247–253.

47. Trepeta R, Stenn KS, Mahoney MJ. Prenatal diagnosis of Sjögren-Larsson syndrome. Semin Dermatol 1984; 3: 221–224.

48. Hofer PA, Jagell S. Sjögren-Larsson syndrome: a dermato-histopathological study. J Cutan Pathol 1982; 9: 360–376.

49. Harms M, Gilardi S, Levy PM, Saurat JH. KID syndrome (keratitis, ichthyosis, and deafness) and chronic mucocutaneous candidiasis: case report and review of the literature. Pediatr Dermatol 1984; 2: 1–7.

50. Grob JJ, Breton A, Bonafe JL et al. Keratitis, ichthyosis, and deafness (KID) syndrome. Vertical transmission and death from multiple squamous cell carcinomas. Arch Dermatol 1987; 123: 777–782.

50a. Mallory SB, Haynie LS, Williams ML, Hall W. Ichthyosis, deafness, and Hirschsprung's disease. Pediatr Dermatol 1989; 6: 24–27.

51. Singh K. Keratitis, ichthyosis and deafness (KID syndrome). Australas J Dermatol 1987; 28: 38–41.

51a. McGrae JD Jr. Keratitis, ichthyosis, and deafness (KID) syndrome with adult onset of keratitis component. Int J Dermatol 1990; 29: 145–146.

51b. McGrae JD Jr. Keratitis, ichthyosis and deafness (KID) syndrome. Int J Dermatol 1990; 29: 89–93.

52. Bodian EL. Skin manifestations of Conradi's disease. Chondrodystrophia congenita punctata. Arch Dermatol 1966; 94: 743–748.

52a. Kalter DC, Atherton DJ, Clayton PT. X-linked dominant Conradi-Hünermann syndrome presenting as congenital erythroderma. J Am Acad Dermatol 1989; 21: 248–256.

53. Hebert AA, Esterly NB, Holbrook KA, Hall JC. The CHILD syndrome. Histologic and ultrastructural studies. Arch Dermatol 1987; 123: 503–509.

54. Jorizzo JL, Atherton DJ, Crounse RG, Wells RS. Ichthyosis, brittle hair, impaired intelligence, decreased fertility and short stature (IBIDS syndrome). Br J Dermatol 1982; 106: 705–710.

55. Rebora A, Crovato F. PIBI(D)S syndrome — trichothiodystrophy with xeroderma pigmentosum (group D) mutation. J Am Acad Dermatol 1987; 16: 940–947.

56. Baden HP, Bronstein BR. Ichthyosiform dermatosis and deafness. Report of a case and review of the literature. Arch Dermatol 1988; 124: 102–106.

Palmoplantar keratodermas and related conditions

57. Sybert VP, Dale BA, Holbrook KA. Palmar-plantar keratoderma. A clinical, ultrastructural, and biochemical study. J Am Acad Dermatol 1988; 18: 75–86.

58. Bergfeld WF, Derbes VJ, Elias PM et al. The treatment of keratosis palmaris et plantaris with isotretinoin. J Am Acad Dermatol 1982; 6: 727–731.

58a. Pujol RM, Moreno A, Alomar A, de Moragas JM. Congenital ichthyosiform dermatosis with linear keratotic flexural papules and sclerosing palmoplantar keratoderma. Arch Dermatol 1989; 125: 103–106.

59. Thomas JR III, Greene SL, Su WPD. Epidermolytic palmo-plantar keratoderma. Int J Dermatol 1984; 23: 652–655.

60. Poulin Y, Perry HO, Muller SA. Olmsted syndrome — congenital palmoplantar and periorificial keratoderma. J Am Acad Dermatol 1984; 10: 600–610.

61. Hatamochi A, Nakagawa S, Ueki H et al. Diffuse palmoplantar keratoderma with deafness. Arch Dermatol 1982; 118: 605–607.

61a. Gamborg Nielsen P. Diffuse palmoplantar keratoderma associated with acrocyanosis. A family study. Acta Derm Venereol 1989; 69: 156–161.

62. Kansky A, Arzensek J. Is palmoplantar keratoderma of Greither's type a separate nosologic entity? Dermatologica 1979; 158: 244–248.

63. Rook AJ. Progressive palmo-plantar keratoderma — Greither's syndrome. Br J Dermatol 1967; 79: 302.

63a. Atherton DJ, Sutton C, Jones BM. Mutilating palmoplantar keratoderma with periorificial keratotic plaques (Olmsted's syndrome). Br J Dermatol 1990; 122: 245–252.

64. Camisa C, Rossana C. Variant of keratoderma hereditaria mutilans (Vohwinkel's syndrome). Arch Dermatol 1984; 120: 1323–1328.

65. Goldfarb MT, Woo TY, Rasmussen JE. Keratoderma hereditaria mutilans (Vohwinkel's syndrome): a trial of isotretinoin. Pediatr Dermatol 1985; 2: 216–218.

66. Gibbs RC, Frank SB. Keratoderma hereditaria mutilans (Vohwinkel). Differentiating features of conditions with constriction of digits. Arch Dermatol 1966; 94: 619–625.

67. Chang Sing Pang AFI, Oranje AP, Vuzevki VD, Stolz E. Successful treatment of keratoderma hereditaria mutilans with an aromatic retinoid. Arch Dermatol 1981; 117: 225–228.

68. Reddy BSN, Gupta SK. Mutilating keratoderma of Vohwinkel. Int J Dermatol 1983; 22: 530–533.

69. Singh K. Mutilating palmo-plantar keratoderma. Int J Dermatol 1986; 25: 436–439.

70. Gamborg Nielsen P. Mutilating palmo-plantar keratoderma. Acta Derm Venereol 1983; 63: 365–367.

71. Fritsch P, Honigsman H, Jaschke E. Epidermolytic hereditary palmoplantar keratoderma. Br J Dermatol 1978; 99: 561–568.

72. Blasik LG, Dimond RL, Baughman RD. Hereditary epidermolytic palmoplantar keratoderma. Arch Dermatol 1981; 117: 229–231.

73. Camisa C, Williams H. Epidermolytic variant of hereditary palmoplantar keratoderma. Br J Dermatol 1985; 112: 221–225.

74. Klaus S, Weinstein GD, Frost P. Localized epidermolytic hyperkeratosis. A form of keratoderma of the palms and soles. Arch Dermatol 1970; 101: 272–275.

75. Kanitakis J, Tsoitis G, Kanitakis C. Hereditary epidermolytic palmoplantar keratoderma (Vörner type). J Am Acad Dermatol 1987; 17: 414–422.

76. Moriwaki S, Tanaka T, Horiguchi Y et al. Epidermolytic hereditary palmoplantar keratoderma. Arch Dermatol 1988; 124: 555–559.

77. Blanchet-Bardon C, Nazzaro V, Chevrant-Breton J et al. Hereditary epidermolytic palmoplantar keratoderma associated with breast and ovarian cancer in a large kindred. Br J Dermatol 1987; 117: 363–370.

78. Howel-Evans W, McConnell RB, Clarke CA, Sheppard PM. Carcinoma of the oesophagus with keratosis palmaris et plantaris (tylosis). A study of two families. Q J Med 1958; 27: 413–429.

79. Yesudian P, Premalatha S, Thambiah AS. Genetic tylosis with malignancy: a study of a South Indian pedigree. Br J Dermatol 1980; 102: 597–600.

80. Thambiah AS, Yesudian P, Augustine SM et al. Tylosis following post-corrosive stricture of the oesophagus. Br J Dermatol 1975; 92: 219–221.

81. Nguyen TQ, Greer KE, Fisher GB Jr, Cooper PH. Papillon-Lefèvre syndrome. Report of two patients treated successfully with isotretinoin. J Am Acad Dermatol 1986; 15: 46–49.

82. Puliyel JM, Iyer KSS. A syndrome of keratosis palmo-plantaris congenita, pes planus, onychogryphosis, periodontosis, arachnodactyly and a peculiar acro-osteolysis. Br J Dermatol 1986; 115: 243–248.

83. El Darouti MA, Al Raubaie SM, Eiada MA. Papillon-Lefèvre syndrome. Successful treatment with oral retinoids in three patients. Int J Dermatol 1988; 27: 63–66.

84. Bach JN, Levan NE. Papillon-Lefèvre syndrome. Arch Dermatol 1968; 97: 154–158.

85. Reed ML, Stanley J, Stengel F et al. Mal de Meleda treated with 13-cis retinoic acid. Arch Dermatol 1979; 115: 605–608.

86. Jee S-H, Lee Y-Y, Wu Y-C et al. Report of a family with mal de Meleda in Taiwan: a clinical,

histopathological and immunological study. Dermatologica 1985; 171: 30–37.

87. Salamon T, Plavsic B, Nikulin A. Electron microscopic study of fingernails in the disease of Mljet (Mal de Meleda). Acta Derm Venereol 1984; 64: 302–307.

88. Stone OJ, Mullins JF. Nail changes in keratosis punctata. Arch Dermatol 1965; 92: 557–558.

88a. Rustad OJ, Corwin Vance J. Punctate keratoses of the palms and soles and keratotic pits of the palmar creases. J Am Acad Dermatol 1990; 22: 468–476.

89. Rubenstein DJ, Schwartz RA, Hansen RC, Payne CM. Punctate hyperkeratosis of the palms and soles. An ultrastructural study. J Am Acad Dermatol 1980; 3: 43–49.

90. Baran R, Juhlin L. Keratodermia palmoplantare papuloverrucoides progressiva: successful treatment with etretinate. J Am Acad Dermatol 1983; 8: 700–702.

91. Buchanan RN Jr. Keratosis punctata palmaris et plantaris. Arch Dermatol 1963; 88: 644–650.

92. Anderson WA, Elam MD, Lambert WC. Keratosis punctata and atopy. Report of 31 cases with a prospective study of prevalence. Arch Dermatol 1984; 120: 884–890.

93. Kalter DC, Stone MS, Kettler A et al. Keratosis punctata of the palmar creases: Extremely uncommon? J Am Acad Dermatol 1986; 14: 510–511.

94. Ortega M, Quintana J, Camacho F. Keratosis punctata of the palmar creases. J Am Acad Dermatol 1985; 13: 381–382.

95. Bennion SD, Patterson JW. Keratosis punctata palmaris et plantaris and adenocarcinoma of the colon. J Am Acad Dermatol 1984; 10: 587–591.

95a. Friedman SJ, Herman PS, Pittelkow MR, Su WPD. Punctate porokeratotic keratoderma. Arch Dermatol 1988; 124: 1678–1682.

96. Callan NJ. Circumscribed palmoplantar keratoderma. Aust J Dermatol 1970; 11: 76–81.

97. Baden HP, Bronstein BR, Rand RE. Hereditary callosities with blisters. Report of a family and review. J Am Acad Dermatol 1984; 11: 409–415.

98. Wachters DHJ, Frensdorf EL, Hausman R, van Dijk E. Keratosis palmoplantaris nummularis ("hereditary painful callosities"). Clinical and histopathologic aspects. J Am Acad Dermatol 1983; 9: 204–209.

98a. Casado M, Jimenez-Acosta F, Borbujo J et al. Keratoderma palmoplantaris striata. Clin Exp Dermatol 1989; 14: 240–242.

98b. Viljoen DL, Saxe N, Temple-Camp C. Cutaneous manifestations of the Proteus syndrome. Pediatr Dermatol 1988; 5: 14–21.

99. Tan OT, Sarkany I. Severe palmar keratoderma in myxoedema. Clin Exp Dermatol 1977; 2: 287–288.

99a. Fartasch M, Vigneswaran N, Diepgen TL, Hornstein OP. Abnormalities of keratinocyte maturation and differentiation in keratosis palmoplantaris striata. Immunohistochemical and ultrastructural study before and during etretinate therapy. Am J Dermatopathol 1990; 12: 275–282.

100. Hodak E, David M, Feuerman EJ. Palmoplantar keratoderma in association with myxedema. Acta Derm Venereol 1986; 66: 354–357.

101. Aram H, Zeidenbaum M. Palmoplantar hyperkeratosis in mycosis fungoides. J Am Acad Dermatol 1985; 13: 897–899.

102. Parnell DD, Johnson SAM. Tylosis palmaris et

plantaris. Its occurrence with internal malignancy. Arch Dermatol 1969; 100: 7–9.

103. Millard LG, Gould DJ. Hyperkeratosis of the palms and soles associated with internal malignancy and elevated levels of immunoreactive human growth hormone. Clin Exp Dermatol 1976; 1: 363–367.

104. Murata Y, Kumano K, Tani M et al. Acquired diffuse keratoderma of the palms and soles with bronchial carcinoma: report of a case and review of the literature. J Am Acad Dermatol 1988; 124: 497–498.

105. Kerdel FA, MacDonald DM. Palmo-plantar keratoderma associated with carcinoma of the bronchus. Acta Derm Venereol 1982; 62: 178–180.

106. Wachtel TJ. Plantar and palmar hyperkeratosis in young castrated women. Int J Dermatol 1981; 20: 270–271.

107. Breathnach SM, Wells GC. Acanthosis palmaris: tripe palms. A distinctive pattern of palmar keratoderma frequently associated with internal malignancy. Clin Exp Dermatol 1980; 5: 181–189.

107a. Pujol RM, Puig L, Garcia-Marques JM, de Moragas JM. Acquired pachydermatoglyphy. A cutaneous sign of internal malignancy. Int J Dermatol 1988; 27: 688–689.

108. Duvic M, Reisman M, Finley V et al. Glucan-induced keratoderma in acquired immunodeficiency syndrome. Arch Dermatol 1987; 123: 751–756.

109. Reed WB, Porter PS. Keratosis. Arch Dermatol 1971; 104: 99–100.

110. Herman PS. Punctate porokeratotic keratoderma. Dermatologica 1973; 147: 206–213.

110a. Caputo R, Carminati G, Ermacora E, Menni S. Keratosis punctata palmaris et plantaris as an expression of focal acantholytic dyskeratosis. Am J Dermatopathol 1989; 11: 574–576.

111. Nazzaro V, Blanchet-Bardon C, Mimoz C et al. Papillon-Lefèvre syndrome. Ultrastructural study and successful treatment with acitretin. Arch Dermatol 1988; 124: 533–539.

112. Goldsmith LA. Tyrosinemia II. Arch Intern Med 1985; 145: 1697–1700.

113. Goldsmith LA. Tyrosinemia II: Lesions in molecular pathophysiology. Pediatr Dermatol 1983; 1: 25–34.

114. Hunziker N. Richner-Hanhart syndrome and tyrosinemia type II. Dermatologica 1980; 160: 180–189.

115. Fraser NG, MacDonald J, Griffiths WAD, McPhie JL. Tyrosinaemia type II (Richner-Hanhart syndrome) — report of two cases treated with etretinate. Clin Exp Dermatol 1987; 12: 440–443.

116. Goldsmith LA. Tyrosine-induced skin disease. Br J Dermatol 1978; 98: 119–123.

117. Rehak A, Selim MM, Yadav G. Richner-Hanhart syndrome (tyrosinaemia-II): (report of four cases without ocular involvement). Br J Dermatol 1981; 104: 469–475.

118. Lestringant GG. Tyrosinemia II with incomplete Richner-Hanhart's syndrome. Int J Dermatol 1988; 27: 43–44.

119. Zaleski WA, Hill A, Kushniruk W. Skin lesions in tyrosinosis: response to dietary treatment. Br J Dermatol 1973; 88: 335–340.

120. Goldsmith LA, Kang E, Bienfang DC et al. Tyrosinemia with plantar and palmar keratosis and keratitis. J Pediatr 1973; 83: 798–805.

121. Machino H, Miki Y, Kawatsu T et al. Successful dietary control of tyrosinemia II. J Am Acad Dermatol 1983; 9: 533–539.

122. Solomon LM, Cook B, Klipfel W. The ectodermal dysplasias. Dermatol Clin 1987; 5: 231–237.

123. McNaughton PZ, Pierson DL, Rodman OG. Hidrotic ectodermal dysplasia in a black mother and daughter. Arch Dermatol 1976; 112: 1448–1450.

124. Rajagopalan K, Tay CH. Hidrotic ectodermal dysplasia. Study of a large Chinese pedigree. Arch Dermatol 1977; 113: 481–485.

125. Rahbari H. Acrokeratoelastoidosis and keratoelastoidosis marginalis — any relation? J Am Acad Dermatol 1981; 5: 348–350.

126. Johansson EA, Kariniemi AL, Niemi KM. Palmoplantar keratoderma of punctate type: acrokeratoelastoidosis Costa. Acta Derm Venereol 1980; 60: 149–153.

127. Costa OG. Akrokerato-elastoidosis (a hitherto undescribed skin disease). Dermatologica 1953; 107: 164–168.

128. Highet AS, Rook A, Anderson JR. Acrokeratoelastoidosis. Br J Dermatol 1982; 106: 337–344.

128a. Shbaklo Z, Jamaleddine NF, Kibbi A-G et al. Acrokeratoelastoidosis. Int J Dermatol 1990; 29: 333–336.

129. Matthews CNA, Harman RRM. Acrokerato-elastoidosis in a Somerset mother and her two sons. Br J Dermatol (Suppl) 1977; 15: 42–43.

130. Korc A, Hansen RC, Lynch PJ. Acrokeratoelastoidosis of Costa in North America. A report of two cases. J Am Acad Dermatol 1985; 12: 832–836.

131. Jung EG, Beil FU, Anton-Lamprecht I et al. Akrokeratoelastoidosis. Hautarzt 1974; 25: 127–133.

132. Dowd PM, Harman RRM, Black MM. Focal acral hyperkeratosis. Br J Dermatol 1983; 109: 97–103.

133. Handfield-Jones S, Kennedy CTC. Acrokeratoelastoidosis treated with etretinate. J Am Acad Dermatol 1987; 17: 881–882.

134. Masse R, Quillard A, Hery B et al. Acrokerato-elastoidose de Costa. Ann Dermatol Venereol 1977; 104: 441–445.

135. Haber RM, Rose TH. Autosomal recessive pachyonychia congenita. Arch Dermatol 1986; 122: 919–923.

135a. Su WPD, Chun SI, Hammond DE, Gordon H. Pachyonychia congenita: a clinical study of 12 cases and review of the literature. Pediatr Dermatol 1990; 7: 33–38.

136. Schönfeld PHIR. The pachyonychia congenita syndrome. Acta Derm Venereol 1980; 60: 45–49.

137. Mawhinney H, Creswell S, Beare JM. Pachyonychia congenita with candidiasis. Clin Exp Dermatol 1981; 6: 145–149.

138. Vineyard WR, Scott RA. Steatocystoma multiplex with pachyonychia congenita. Arch Dermatol 1961; 84: 824–827.

139. Soderquist NA, Reed WB. Pachyonychia congenita with epidermal cysts and other congenital dyskeratoses. Arch Dermatol 1968; 97: 31–33.

140. Feinstein A, Friedman J, Schewach-Millet M. Pachyonychia congenita. J Am Acad Dermatol 1988; 19: 705–711.

141. Forslind B, Nylén B, Swanbeck G et al. Pachyonychia congenita. A histologic and microradiographic study. Acta Derm Venereol 1973; 53: 211–216.
142. Anneroth G, Isacsson G, Lagerholm B et al. Pachyonychia congenita. Acta Derm Venereol 1975; 55: 387–394.
143. Kelly EW Jr, Pinkus H. Report of a case of pachyonychia congenita. Arch Dermatol 1958; 77: 724–726.
144. Witkop CJ, Gorlin RJ. Four hereditary mucosal syndromes. Arch Dermatol 1961; 84: 762–771.
145. Thormann J, Kobayasi T. Pachyonychia congenita Jadassohn-Lewandowsky: a disorder of keratinization. Acta Derm Venereol 1977; 57: 63–67.
146. Wilkin JK, Rosenberg EW, Kanzaki T. Cornoid lamella in pachyonychia congenita. Arch Dermatol 1978; 114: 1795–1796.
147. Ruiz-Maldonado R, Tamayo L. Pachyonychia congenita (Jadassohn-Lewandowsky) and Kyrle's disease in the same patient. Int J Dermatol 1977; 16: 675–678.
148. Tidman MJ, Wells RS, MacDonald DM. Pachyonychia congenita with cutaneous amyloidosis and hyperpigmentation — a distinct variant. J Am Acad Dermatol 1987; 16: 935–940.

Cornoid lamellation

149. Reed RJ, Leone P. Porokeratosis — a mutant clonal keratosis of the epidermis. I. Histogenesis. Arch Dermatol 1970; 101: 340–347.
150. Wade TR, Ackerman AB. Cornoid lamellation. A histologic reaction pattern. Am J Dermatopathol 1980; 2: 5–15.
151. Otsuka F, Shima A, Ishibashi Y. Porokeratosis as a premalignant condition of the skin. Cytologic demonstration of abnormal DNA ploidy in cells of the epidermis. Cancer 1989; 63: 891–896.
152. Otsuka F, Shima A, Ishibashi Y. Porokeratosis has neoplastic clones in the epidermis: microfluorometric analysis of DNA content of epidermal cell nuclei. J Invest Dermatol 1989; 92: 231s–233s.
153. Chernosky ME. Porokeratosis. Arch Dermatol 1986; 122: 869–870.
154. Mikhail GR, Wertheimer FW. Clinical variants of porokeratosis (Mibelli). Arch Dermatol 1968; 98: 124–131.
155. Dupré A, Christol B. Mibelli's porokeratosis of the lips. Arch Dermatol 1978; 114: 1841–1842.
156. Pirozzi DJ, Rosenthal A. Disseminated superficial actinic porokeratosis. Analysis of an affected family. Br J Dermatol 1976; 95: 429–432.
157. Schwarz T, Seiser A, Gschnait F. Disseminated superficial "actinic" porokeratosis. J Am Acad Dermatol 1984; 11: 724–730.
158. Shumack SP, Commens CA. Disseminated superficial actinic porokeratosis: A clinical study. J Am Acad Dermatol 1989; 20: 1015–1022.
159. McMillan GL, Krull EA, Mikhail GR. Linear porokeratosis with giant cornoid lamella. Arch Dermatol 1976; 112: 515–516.
160. Rahbari H, Cordero AA, Mehregan AH. Linear porokeratosis. A distinctive clinical variant of porokeratosis of Mibelli. Arch Dermatol 1974; 109: 526–528.
161. Commens CA, Shumack SP. Linear porokeratosis in two families with disseminated superficial actinic porokeratosis. Pediatr Dermatol 1987; 4: 209–214.
162. Razack EMA, Natarajan M. Ulcerative systematized porokeratosis (Mibelli). Arch Dermatol 1977; 113: 1583–1584.
163. Karadaglic DL, Berger S, Jankovic D, Stefanovic Z. Zosteriform porokeratosis of Mibelli. Int J Dermatol 1988; 27: 589–590.
164. Helfman RJ, Poulos EG. Reticulated porokeratosis. A unique variant of porokeratosis. Arch Dermatol 1985; 121: 1542–1543.
165. Mandojana RM, Katz R, Rodman OG. Porokeratosis plantaris discreta. J Am Acad Dermatol 1984; 10: 679–682.
166. Kang WH, Chun SI. Porokeratosis plantaris discreta. A case showing transepidermal elimination. Am J Dermatopathol 1988; 10: 229–233.
167. Sakas EL, Gentry RH. Porokeratosis punctata palmaris et plantaris (punctate porokeratosis). Case report and literature review. J Am Acad Dermatol 1985; 13: 908–912.
168. Rahbari H, Cordero AA, Mehregan AH. Punctate porokeratosis. A clinical variant of porokeratosis of Mibelli. J Cutan Pathol 1977; 4: 338–341.
169. Roberts LC, De Villez RL. Congenital unilateral punctate porokeratosis. Am J Dermatopathol 1984; 6: 57–61.
170. Lestringant GG, Berge T. Porokeratosis punctata palmaris et plantaris. A new entity? Arch Dermatol 1989; 125: 816–819.
171. McCallister RE, Estes SA, Yarbrough CL. Porokeratosis plantaris, palmaris, et disseminata. Report of a case and treatment with isotretinoin. J Am Acad Dermatol 1985; 13: 598–603.
172. Shaw JC, White CR Jr. Porokeratosis plantaris palmaris et disseminata. J Am Acad Dermatol 1984; 11: 454–460.
173. Marschalko M, Somlai B. Porokeratosis plantaris, palmaris, et disseminata. Arch Dermatol 1986; 122: 890–891.
174. Neumann RA, Knobler RM, Gebhart W. Unusual presentation of porokeratosis palmaris, plantaris et disseminata. J Am Acad Dermatol 1989; 21: 1131–1133.
175. Patrizi A, Passarini B, Minghetti G, Masina M. Porokeratosis palmaris et plantaris disseminata: An unusual clinical presentation. J Am Acad Dermatol 1989; 21: 415–418.
176. Eng AM, Kolton B. Generalized eruptive porokeratosis of Mibelli with associated psoriasis. J Cutan Pathol 1975; 2: 203–213.
177. Sato A, Bohm W, Bersch A. Hyperkeratotic form of porokeratosis Mibelli. Dermatologica 1977; 155: 340–349.
178. Mehregan AH, Khalili H, Fazel Z. Mibelli's porokeratosis of the face. A report of seven cases. J Am Acad Dermatol 1980; 3: 394–396.
179. Abell E, Read SI. Porokeratotic eccrine ostial and dermal duct naevus. Br J Dermatol 1980; 103: 435–441.
180. Aloi FG, Pippione M. Porokeratotic eccrine ostial and dermal duct nevus. Arch Dermatol 1986; 122: 892–895.
181. Driban NE, Cavicchia JC. Porokeratotic eccrine ostial

and dermal duct nevus. J Cutan Pathol 1987; 14: 118–121.

182. Coskey RJ, Mehregan AH, Hashimoto K. Porokeratotic eccrine duct and hair follicle nevus. J Am Acad Dermatol 1982; 6: 940–943.

183. Kossard S, Freeman S. Reticular erythema with ostial porokeratosis. J Am Acad Dermatol 1990; 22: 913–916.

184. Dover JS, Phillips TJ, Burns DA, Krafchik BR. Disseminated superficial actinic porokeratosis. Coexistence with other porokeratotic variants. Arch Dermatol 1986; 122: 887–889.

185. Neumann RA, Knobler RM, Jurecka W, Gebhart W. Disseminated superficial actinic porokeratosis: Experimental induction and exacerbation of skin lesions. J Am Acad Dermatol 1989; 21: 1182–1188.

186. Bencini PL, Crosti C, Sala F. Porokeratosis: immunosuppression and exposure to sunlight. Br J Dermatol 1987; 116: 113–116.

187. Neumann RA, Knobler RM, Metze D, Jurecka W. Disseminated superficial porokeratosis and immunosuppression. Br J Dermatol 1988; 119: 375–380.

188. Komorowski RA, Clowry LJ. Porokeratosis of Mibelli in transplant recipients. Am J Clin Pathol 1989; 91: 71–74.

189. Shrum JR, Cooper PH, Greer KE, Landes HB. Squamous cell carcinoma in disseminated superficial actinic porokeratosis. J Am Acad Dermatol 1982; 6: 58–62.

190. Chernosky ME, Rapini RP. Squamous cell carcinoma in lesions of disseminated superficial actinic porokeratosis: a report of two cases. Arch Dermatol 1986; 122: 853–855.

191. James WD, Rodman OG. Squamous cell carcinoma arising in porokeratosis of Mibelli. Int J Dermatol 1986; 25: 389–391.

192. Lozinski AZ, Fisher BK, Walter JB, Fitzpatrick PJ. Metastatic squamous cell carcinoma in linear porokeratosis of Mibelli. J Am Acad Dermatol 1987; 16: 448–451.

193. Coskey RJ, Mehregan A. Bowen disease associated with porokeratosis of Mibelli. Arch Dermatol 1975; 111: 1480–1481.

194. Brodkin RH, Rickert RR, Fuller FW, Saporito C. Malignant disseminated porokeratosis. Arch Dermatol 1987; 123: 1521–1526.

195. Waldman JS, Barr RJ. Familial disseminated malignant porokeratosis. J Cutan Pathol 1988; 15: 349 (abstract).

196. Rapini RP, Chernosky ME. Histologic changes in early lesions of disseminated superficial actinic porokeratosis. J Cutan Pathol 1988; 15: 340 (abstract).

197. Burge SM, Ryan TJ. Punched-out porokeratosis. A histological variant of disseminated superficial actinic porokeratosis. Am J Dermatopathol 1987; 9: 240–242.

198. Piamphongsant T, Sittapairoachana D. Localized cutaneous amyloidosis in disseminated superficial actinic porokeratosis. J Cutan Pathol 1974; 1: 207–210.

199. Lee JYY, Lally M, Abell E. Disseminated superficial porokeratosis with amyloid deposits in a Chinese man. J Cutan Pathol 1988; 15: 323 (abstract).

200. Menter MA, Fourie PB. A surface impression and scanning electron microscopy study of porokeratosis of Mibelli. Br J Dermatol 1977; 96: 393–397.

201. Mann PR, Cort DF, Fairburn EA, Abdel-Aziz A. Ultrastructural studies on two cases of porokeratosis of Mibelli. Br J Dermatol 1974; 90: 607–617.

202. Sato A, Masu S, Seiji M. Electron microscopic studies of porokeratosis Mibelli — Civatte bodies and amyloid deposits in the dermis. J Dermatol 1980; 7: 323–333.

Epidermolytic hyperkeratosis

203. Su WPD. Histopathologic varieties of epidermal nevus. A study of 160 cases. Am J Dermatopathol 1982; 4: 161–170.

204. Adam JE, Richards R. Ichthyosis hystrix. Epidermolytic hyperkeratosis; discordant in monozygotic twins. Arch Dermatol 1973; 107: 278–282.

205. Zeligman I, Pomeranz J. Variations of congenital ichthyosiform erythroderma. Arch Dermatol 1965; 91: 120–125.

206. Nazzaro V, Ermacora E, Santucci B, Caputo R. Epidermolytic hyperkeratosis: generalized form in children from parents with systematized linear form. Br J Dermatol 1990; 122: 417–422.

207. Mehregan AH. Epidermolytic hyperkeratosis. Incidental findings in the epidermis and in the intraepidermal eccrine sweat duct units. J Cutan Pathol 1978; 5: 76–80.

208. Zina AM, Bundino S, Pippione MG. Acrosyringial epidermolytic papulosis neviformis. Dermatologica 1985; 171: 122–125.

209. Goette DK, Lapins NA. Epidermolytic hyperkeratosis as an incidental finding in normal oral mucosa. Report of two cases. J Am Acad Dermatol 1984; 10: 246–249.

210. Plewig G, Christophers E. Nevoid follicular epidermolytic hyperkeratosis. Arch Dermatol 1975; 111: 223–226.

211. Barsky S, Doyle JA, Winkelmann RK. Nevus comedonicus with epidermolytic hyperkeratosis. A report of four cases. Arch Dermatol 1981; 117: 86–88.

212. Lookingbill DP, Ladda RL, Cohen C. Generalized epidermolytic hyperkeratosis in the child of a parent with nevus comedonicus. Arch Dermatol 1984; 120: 223–226.

213. Ackerman AB, Reed RJ. Epidermolytic variant of solar keratosis. Arch Dermatol 1973; 107: 104–106.

214. Vakilzadeh F, Happle R. Epidermolytic leukoplakia. J Cutan Pathol 1982; 9: 267–270.

215. Kolde G, Vakilzadeh F. Leukoplakia of the prepuce with epidermolytic hyperkeratosis: a case report. Acta Derm Venereol 1983; 63: 571–573.

216. Haneke E. Epidermolytic hyperkeratosis. J Cutan Pathol 1983; 10: 289–290.

217. Wilgram GF, Caulfield JB. An electron microscopic study of epidermolytic hyperkeratosis. Arch Dermatol 1966; 94: 127–143.

218. Shapiro L, Baraf CS. Isolated epidermolytic acanthoma. A solitary tumor showing granular degeneration. Arch Dermatol 1970; 101: 220–223.

219. Miyamoto Y, Ueda K, Sato M, Yasuno H. Disseminated epidermolytic acanthoma. J Cutan Pathol 1979; 6: 272–279.

220. Hirone T, Fukushiro R. Disseminated epidermolytic acanthoma. Acta Derm Venereol 1973; 53: 393–402.

Acantholytic dyskeratosis

221. Ackerman AB. Focal acantholytic dyskeratosis. Arch Dermatol 1972; 106: 702–706.
222. Ackerman AB, Goldman G. Combined epidermolytic hyperkeratosis and focal acantholytic dyskeratosis. Arch Dermatol 1974; 109: 385–386.
223. Starink TM, Woerdeman MJ. Unilateral systematized keratosis follicularis. A variant of Darier's disease or an epidermal naevus (acantholytic dyskeratotic epidermal naevus)? Br J Dermatol 1981; 105: 207–214.
224. Demetree JW, Lang PG, St Clair JT. Unilateral, linear, zosteriform epidermal nevus with acantholytic dyskeratosis. Arch Dermatol 1979; 115: 875–877.
225. Hall JR, Holder W, Knox JM et al. Familial dyskeratotic comedones. Report of three cases and review of the literature. J Am Acad Dermatol 1987; 17: 808–814.
226. Pierard-Franchimont C, Pierard GE. Suprabasal acantholysis. A common biological feature of distinct inflammatory diseases. Am J Dermatopathol 1983; 5: 421–426.
227. Kolbusz RV, Fretzin DF. Focal acantholytic dyskeratosis in condyloma acuminata. J Cutan Pathol 1989; 16: 44–47.
228. O'Connell BM, Nickoloff BJ. Solitary labial papular acantholytic dyskeratoma in an immunocompromised host. Am J Dermatopathol 1987; 9: 339–342.
229. Coppola G, Muscardin LM, Piazza P. Papular acantholytic dyskeratosis. Am J Dermatopathol 1986; 8: 364.
230. Chorzelski TP, Kudejko J, Jablonska S. Is papular acantholytic dyskeratosis of the vulva a new entity? Am J Dermatopathol 1984; 6: 557–560.
231. Cooper PH. Acantholytic dermatosis localized to the vulvocrural area. J Cutan Pathol 1989; 16: 81–84.
232. Warkel RL, Jager RM. Focal acantholytic dyskeratosis of the anal canal. Am J Dermatopathol 1986; 8: 362–363.
233. van der Putte SCJ, Oey HB, Storm I. Papular acantholytic dyskeratosis of the penis. Am J Dermatopathol 1986; 8: 365–366.
234. Weedon D. Papular acantholytic dyskeratosis of vulva. Am J Dermatopathol 1986; 8: 363.
235. Brownstein MH. Acantholytic acanthoma. J Am Acad Dermatol 1988; 19: 783–786.
236. van Joost T, Vuzevski VD, Menke HE. Benign papular acantholytic non-dyskeratotic eruption: a new paraneoplastic syndrome? Br J Dermatol 1989; 121: 147–148.
237. Happle R, Steijlen PM, Kolde G. Naevus corniculatus: a new acantholytic disorder. Br J Dermatol 1990; 122: 107–112.
238. Rand R, Baden HP. Commentary: Darier-White disease. Arch Dermatol 1983; 119: 81–83.
239. Beck AL Jr, Finocchio AF, White JP. Darier's disease: a kindred with a large number of cases. Br J Dermatol 1977; 97: 335–339.
240. Zaias N, Ackerman AB. The nail in Darier-White disease. Arch Dermatol 1973; 107: 193–199.
241. Reed WB. Bullous Darier's disease. Arch Dermatol 1969; 100: 508–509.
242. Hori Y, Tsuru N, Niimura M. Bullous Darier's disease. Arch Dermatol 1982; 118: 278–279.
243. Telfer NR, Burge SM, Ryan TJ. Vesiculo-bullous Darier's disease. Br J Dermatol 1990; 122: 831–834.
244. Dolezal JF. An unusual variant of Darier disease. Arch Dermatol 1977; 113: 374.
245. Peck GL, Kraemer KH, Wetzel B et al. Cornifying Darier disease — a unique variant. Arch Dermatol 1976; 112: 495–503.
246. Berth-Jones J, Hutchinson PE. Darier's disease with peri-follicular depigmentation. Br J Dermatol 1989; 120: 827–830.
247. Klein A, Burns L, Leyden JJ. Rectal mucosa involvement in keratosis follicularis. Arch Dermatol 1974; 109: 560–561.
248. Weathers DR, Olansky S, Sharpe LO. Darier's disease with mucous membrane involvement. A case report. Arch Dermatol 1969; 100: 50–53.
249. Itin P, Buchner SA, Gloor B. Darier's disease and retinitis pigmentosa; is there a pathogenetic relationship? Br J Dermatol 1988; 119: 397–402.
250. Crisp AJ, Rowland Payne CME, Adams J et al. The prevalence of bone cysts in Darier's disease: a survey of 31 cases. Clin Exp Dermatol 1984; 9: 78–83.
251. Getzler NA, Flint A. Keratosis follicularis. A study of one family. Arch Dermatol 1966; 93: 545–549.
252. Henry JC, Padilla RS, Becker LE, Bankhurst AD. Cell-mediated immunity in Darier's disease. J Am Acad Dermatol 1979; 1: 348–351.
253. Halevy S, Weltfriend S, Pick AI et al. Immunologic studies in Darier's disease. Int J Dermatol 1988; 27: 101–105.
254. Salo OP, Valle MJ. Eczema vaccinatum in a family with Darier's disease. Br J Dermatol 1973; 89: 417–422.
255. Higgins PG, Crow KD. Recurrent Kaposi's varicelliform eruption in Darier's disease. Br J Dermatol 1973; 88: 391–394.
256. Toole JWP, Hofstader SL, Ramsay CA. Darier's disease and Kaposi's varicelliform eruption. J Am Acad Dermatol 1979; 1: 321–324.
257. Carney JF, Caroline NL, Nankervis GA, Pomeranz JR. Eczema vaccinatum and eczema herpeticum in Darier disease. Arch Dermatol 1973; 107: 613–614.
258. Caulfield JB, Wilgram GF. An electron-microscopic study of dyskeratosis and acantholysis in Darier's disease. J Invest Dermatol 1963; 41: 57–65.
259. Mann PR, Haye KR. An electron microscope study on the acantholytic and dyskeratotic processes in Darier's disease. Br J Dermatol 1970; 82: 561–566.
260. Burge SM, Fenton DA, Dawber RPR, Leigh IM. Darier's disease: an immunohistochemical study using monoclonal antibodies to human cytokeratins. Br J Dermatol 1988; 118: 629–640.
261. Burge SM, Ryan TJ, Cederholm-Williams SA. Darier's disease: an immunohistochemical study using antibodies to proteases. Br J Dermatol 1989; 121: 613–621.
262. Steffen C. Dyskeratosis and the dyskeratoses. Am J Dermatopathol 1988; 10: 356–363.
263. Vedtofte P, Joensen HD, Dabelsteen E, Veien N. Intercellular and circulating antibodies in patients with dyskeratosis follicularis, Darier's disease. Acta Derm Venereol 1978; 58: 51–55.
264. De Panfilis G, Manara GC, Ferrari C et al. Darier's keratosis follicularis: an ultrastructural study during and after topical treatment with retinoic acid alone or in combination with 5-fluorouracil. J Cutan Pathol 1981; 8: 214–218.

265. Gottlieb SK, Lutzner MA. Darier's disease. An electron microscopic study. Arch Dermatol 1973; 107: 225–230.
266. Sato A, Anton-Lamprecht I, Schnyder UW. Ultrastructure of dyskeratosis in morbus Darier. J Cutan Pathol 1977; 4: 173–184.
267. El-Gothamy Z, Kamel MM. Ultrastructural observations in Darier's disease. Am J Dermatopathol 1988; 10: 306–310.
268. Grover RW. Transient acantholytic dermatosis. Arch Dermatol 1970; 101: 426–434.
269. Helfman RJ. Grover's disease treated with isotretinoin. Report of four cases. J Am Acad Dermatol 1985; 12: 981–984.
270. Heenan PJ, Quirk CJ. Transient acantholytic dermatosis. Br J Dermatol 1980; 102: 515–520.
271. Simon RS, Bloom D, Ackerman AB. Persistent acantholytic dermatosis. A variant of transient acantholytic dermatosis (Grover disease). Arch Dermatol 1976; 112: 1429–1431.
272. Fawcett HA, Miller JA. Persistent acantholytic dermatosis related to actinic damage. Br J Dermatol 1983; 109: 349–354.
273. Dodd HJ, Sarkany I. Persistent acantholytic dermatosis. Clin Exp Dermatol 1984; 9: 431–434.
274. Heaphy MR, Tucker SB, Winkelmann RK. Benign papular acantholytic dermatosis. Arch Dermatol 1976; 112: 814–821.
275. Kanzaki T, Hashimoto K. Transient acantholytic dermatosis with involvement of oral mucosa. J Cutan Pathol 1978; 5: 23–30.
276. Chalet M, Grover R, Ackerman AB. Transient acantholytic dermatosis. A reevaluation. Arch Dermatol 1977; 113: 431–435.
277. Grover RW, Rosenblaum R. The association of transient acantholytic dermatosis with other skin diseases. J Am Acad Dermatol 1984; 11: 253–256.
278. Fleckman P, Stenn K. Transient acantholytic dermatosis associated with pemphigus foliaceus. Coexistence of two acantholytic diseases. Arch Dermatol 1983; 119: 155–156.
279. Hu C-H, Michel B, Farber EM. Transient acantholytic dermatosis (Grover's disease). A skin disorder related to heat and sweating. Arch Dermatol 1985; 121: 1439–1441.
280. Horn TD, Groleau GE. Transient acantholytic dermatosis in immunocompromised febrile patients with cancer. Arch Dermatol 1987; 123: 238–240.
281. Zelickson BD, Tefferi A, Gertz MA et al. Transient acantholytic dermatosis associated with lymphomatous angioimmunoblastic lymphadenopathy. Acta Derm Venereol 1989; 69: 445–448.
282. Kennedy C, Moss R. Transient acantholytic dermatosis. Br J Dermatol (Suppl) 1979; 17: 67–69.
283. Waisman M, Stewart JJ, Walker AE. Bullous transient acantholytic dermatosis. Arch Dermatol 1976; 112: 1440–1441.
284. Bystryn J-C. Immunofluorescence studies in transient acantholytic dermatosis (Grover's disease). Am J Dermatopathol 1979; 1: 325–327.
285. Millns JL, Doyle JA, Muller SA. Positive cutaneous immunofluorescence in Grover's disease. Arch Dermatol 1980; 116: 515.
286. Grover RW. Transient acantholytic dermatosis. Electron microscope study. Arch Dermatol 1971; 104: 26–37.
287. Grover RW, Duffy JL. Transient acantholytic dermatosis. Electron microscopic study of the Darier type. J Cutan Pathol 1975; 2: 111–127.
288. Palmer DD, Perry HO. Benign familial chronic pemphigus. Arch Dermatol 1962; 86: 493–502.
289. Michel B. Commentary: Hailey-Hailey disease. Familial benign chronic pemphigus. Arch Dermatol 1982; 118: 781–783.
290. Witkowski JA, Parish LC. Familial benign chronic pemphigus. A papular variant. Arch Dermatol 1973; 108: 842–843.
291. Barron DR, Estes SA. Papuloverrucoid Hailey-Hailey disease: an unusual presentation. J Cutan Pathol 1989; 16: 296 (abstract).
292. Lyles TW, Knox JM, Richardson JB. Atypical features in familial benign chronic pemphigus. Arch Dermatol 1958; 78: 446–453.
293. Marsch WC, Stuttgen G. Generalized Hailey-Hailey disease. Br J Dermatol 1978; 99: 553–560.
294. Kahn D, Hutchinson E. Esophageal involvement in familial benign chronic pemphigus. Arch Dermatol 1974; 109: 718–719.
295. Vaclavinkova V, Neumann E. Vaginal involvement in familial benign chronic pemphigus (morbus Hailey-Hailey). Acta Derm Venereol 1982; 62: 80–81.
296. Evron S, Leviatan A, Okon E. Familial benign chronic pemphigus appearing as leukoplakia of the vulva. Int J Dermatol 1984; 23: 556–557.
297. Hazelrigg DE, Stoller LJ. Isolated familial benign chronic pemphigus. Arch Dermatol 1977; 113: 1302.
298. Cooper DL. Familial benign chronic pemphigus of perianal skin. Arch Dermatol 1971; 103: 219–220.
299. Morales A, Livingood CS, Hu F. Familial benign chronic pemphigus. Arch Dermatol 1966; 93: 324–328.
300. Izumi AK, Shmunes E, Wood MG. Familial benign chronic pemphigus. The role of trauma including contact sensitivity. Arch Dermatol 1971; 104: 177–181.
301. Cram DL, Muller SA, Winkelmann RK. Ultraviolet-induced acantholysis in familial benign chronic pemphigus. Detection of the forme fruste. Arch Dermatol 1967; 96: 636–641.
302. Montes LF, Narkates AJ, Hunt D et al. Microbial flora in familial benign chronic pemphigus. Arch Dermatol 1970; 101: 140–144.
303. Leppard B, Delaney TJ, Sanderson KV. Chronic benign familial pemphigus. Induction of lesions by Herpesvirus hominis. Br J Dermatol 1973; 88: 609–613.
304. Fisher I, Orkin M, Bean S. Familial benign chronic pemphigus and psoriasis vulgaris in the same patient. Acta Derm Venereol 1967; 47: 111–117.
305. Heaphy MR, Winkelmann RK. Coexistence of benign familial pemphigus and psoriasis vulgaris. Arch Dermatol 1976; 112: 1571–1574.
306. Nicolis G, Tosca A, Marouli O, Stratigos J. Keratosis follicularis and familial benign chronic pemphigus in the same patient. Dermatologica 1979; 159: 346–351.
307. Ganor S, Sagher F. Keratosis follicularis (Darier) and familial benign chronic pemphigus (Hailey-Hailey) in the same patient. Br J Dermatol 1965; 77: 24–29.
308. Mehregan DA, Umbert IJ, Peters MS. Histologic findings of Hailey-Hailey disease in a patient with bullous pemphigoid. J Am Acad Dermatol 1989; 21: 1107–1112.
309. King DT, Hirose FM, King LA. Simultaneous

occurrence of familial benign chronic pemphigus (Hailey-Hailey disease) and syringoma of the vulva. Arch Dermatol 1978; 114: 801.

310. Furue M, Seki Y, Oohara K, Ishibashi Y. Basal cell epithelioma arising in a patient with Hailey-Hailey's disease. Int J Dermatol 1987; 26: 461–462.

311. Sonck CE, Rintala A. Treatment of familial benign chronic pemphigus by skin grafting. Acta Derm Venereol 1975; 55: 395–397.

312. Bitar A, Giroux J-M. Treatment of benign familial pemphigus (Hailey-Hailey) by skin grafting. Br J Dermatol 1970; 83: 402–404.

313. Shelley WB, Randall P. Surgical eradication of familial benign chronic pemphigus from the axillae. Report of a case. Arch Dermatol 1969; 100: 275–276.

314. Thorne FL, Hall JH, Mladick RA. Surgical treatment of familial chronic pemphigus (Hailey-Hailey disease). Report of a case. Arch Dermatol 1968; 98: 522–524.

315. Berger RS, Lynch PJ. Familial benign chronic pemphigus. Surgical treatment and pathogenesis. Arch Dermatol 1971; 104: 380–384.

316. De Dobbeleer G, De Graef C, M'Poudi E et al. Reproduction of the characteristic morphologic changes of familial benign chronic pemphigus in cultures of lesional keratinocytes onto dead deepidermized dermis. J Am Acad Dermatol 1989; 21: 961–965.

317. Steffen CG. Familial benign chronic pemphigus. Am J Dermatopathol 1987; 9: 58–73.

318. Wilgram GF, Caulfield JB, Lever WF. An electronmicroscopic study of acantholysis and dyskeratosis in Hailey and Hailey's disease. J Invest Dermatol 1962; 39: 373–381.

319. Gottlieb SK, Lutzner MA. Hailey-Hailey disease — an electron microscopic study. J Invest Dermatol 1970; 54: 368–376.

320. De Dobbeleer G, Achten G. Disrupted desmosomes in induced lesions of familial benign chronic pemphigus. J Cutan Pathol 1979; 6: 418–424.

321. Szymanski FJ. Warty dyskeratoma. A benign cutaneous tumor resembling Darier's disease microscopically. Arch Dermatol 1957; 75: 567–572.

322. Graham JH, Helwig EB. Isolated dyskeratosis follicularis. Arch Dermatol 1958; 77: 377–389.

323. Tanay A, Mehregan AH. Warty dyskeratoma. Dermatologica 1969; 138: 155–164.

324. Gorlin RJ, Peterson WC. Warty dyskeratoma. A note concerning its occurrence on the oral mucosa. Arch Dermatol 1967; 95: 292–293.

325. Harrist TJ, Murphy GF, Mihm MC. Oral warty dyskeratoma. Arch Dermatol 1980; 116: 929–931.

326. Panja RK. Warty dyskeratoma. J Cutan Pathol 1977; 4: 194–200.

Colloid keratosis

327. Gonzalez SB. Colloid keratosis. Morphologic characterization of a nonspecific reaction pattern of squamous epithelium. Am J Dermatopathol 1986; 8: 194–201.

328. Gardner DG, Hyams VJ, Heffner DK. Eosinophilic pooling. Am J Surg Pathol 1983; 7: 502–503.

329. Tschen JA, McGavran MH, Kettler AH. Pagetoid dyskeratosis: A selective keratinocytic response. J Am Acad Dermatol 1988; 19: 891–894.

330. Kuo T-t, Chan H-L, Hsueh S. Clear cell papulosis of

the skin. A new entity with histogenetic implications for cutaneous Paget's disease. Am J Surg Pathol 1987; 11: 827–834.

Discrete keratotic lesions

331. Flegel H. Hyperkeratosis lenticularis perstans. Hautarzt 1958; 9: 362–364.

332. Kocsard E, Bear CL, Constance TJ. Hyperkeratosis lenticularis perstans (Flegel). Dermatologica 1968; 136: 35–42.

333. Price ML, Wilson Jones E, MacDonald DM. A clinicopathological study of Flegel's disease (hyperkeratosis lenticularis perstans). Br J Dermatol 1987; 116: 681–691.

334. Bean SF. Hyperkeratosis lenticularis perstans. A clinical, histopathologic, and genetic study. Arch Dermatol 1969; 99: 705–709.

335. Bean SF. The genetics of hyperkeratosis lenticularis perstans. Arch Dermatol 1972; 106: 72.

336. Beveridge GW, Langlands AO. Familial hyperkeratosis lenticularis perstans associated with tumours of the skin. Br J Dermatol 1973; 88: 453–458.

337. Pearson LH, Smith JG Jr, Chalker DK. Hyperkeratosis lenticularis perstans. J Am Acad Dermatol 1987; 16: 190–195.

338. Raffle EJ, Rogers J. Hyperkeratosis lenticularis perstans. Arch Dermatol 1969; 100: 423–428.

339. Tidman MJ, Price ML, MacDonald DM. Lamellar bodies in hyperkeratosis lenticularis perstans. J Cutan Pathol 1987; 14: 207–211.

340. Ikai K, Murai T, Oguchi M et al. An ultrastructural study of the epidermis in hyperkeratosis lenticularis perstans. Acta Derm Venereol 1978; 58: 363–365.

341. Frenk E, Tapernoux B. Hyperkeratosis lenticularis perstans (Flegel). A biological model for keratinization occurring in the absence of Odland bodies? Dermatologica 1976; 153: 253–262.

342. Kuokkanen K, Alavaikko M, Pitkanen R. Hyperkeratosis lenticularis perstans (Flegel's disease). Acta Derm Venereol 1983; 63: 357–360.

343. van de Staak WJBM, Bergers AMG, Bongaarts P. Hyperkeratosis lenticularis perstans (Flegel). Dermatologica 1980; 161: 340–346.

344. Ikada J. Hyperkeratosis lenticularis perstans. Arch Dermatol 1974; 110: 464–465.

345. Hunter GA, Donald GF. Hyperkeratosis lenticularis perstans (Flegel) or dyskeratotic psoriasiform dermatosis. A single dermatosis or two? Arch Dermatol 1968; 98: 239–247.

346. Büchner SA. Hyperkeratosis lenticularis perstans (Flegel's disease). In situ characterization of T cell subsets and Langerhans' cells. Acta Derm Venereol 1988; 68: 341–345.

347. Holubar K. Hyperkeratosis follicularis et parafollicularis in cutem penetrans. Josef Kyrle and "his" disease. Am J Dermatopathol 1985; 7: 261–263.

348. Woo TY, Rasmussen JE. Disorders of transepidermal elimination. Part 2. Int J Dermatol 1985; 24: 337–348.

349. Cunningham SR, Walsh M, Matthews R et al. Kyrle's disease. J Am Acad Dermatol 1987; 16: 117–123.

350. Patterson JW. The perforating disorders. J Am Acad Dermatol 1984; 10: 561–581.

351. White CR Jr. The dermatopathology of perforating disorders. Semin Dermatol 1986; 5: 359–366.

352. Price ML, Wilson Jones E, MacDonald DM. Flegel's

disease, not Kyrle's disease. J Am Acad Dermatol 1988; 18: 1366.

353. Kocsard E, Palmer G, Constance TJ. Coexistence of hyperkeratosis lenticularis perstans (Flegel) and hyperkeratosis follicularis et parafollicularis in cutem penetrans (Kyrle) in a patient. Acta Derm Venereol 1970; 50: 385–390.

354. Walsh M, Cunningham SR, Burrows D. Flegel's disease, not Kyrle's disease. Reply. J Am Acad Dermatol 1988; 18: 1366–1367.

355. Carter VH, Constantine VS. Kyrle's disease. I. Clinical findings in five cases and review of the literature. Arch Dermatol 1968; 97: 624–632.

356. Baer RL. Kyrle's disease (hyperkeratosis follicularis et parafollicularis in cutem penetrans). Arch Dermatol 1967; 96: 351–352.

357. Schamroth JM, Kellen P, Grieve TP. Atypical Kyrle's disease. Int J Dermatol 1986; 25: 310–313.

358. Gupta AK, Gupta MA, Cardella CJ, Haberman HF. Cutaneous associations of chronic renal failure and dialysis. Int J Dermatol 1986; 25: 498–504.

359. Hood AF, Hardegen GL, Zarate AR et al. Kyrle's disease in patients with chronic renal failure. Arch Dermatol 1982; 118: 85–88.

360. Stone RA. Kyrle-like lesions in two patients with renal failure undergoing dialysis. J Am Acad Dermatol 1981; 5: 707–709.

361. Aram H, Szymanski FJ, Bailey WE. Kyrle's disease. Hyperkeratosis follicularis et parafollicularis in cutem penetrans. Arch Dermatol 1969; 100: 453–456.

362. Constantine VS, Carter VH. Kyrle's disease. II. Histopathologic findings in five cases and review of the literature. Arch Dermatol 1968; 97: 633–639.

363. Moss HV. Kyrle's disease. Cutis 1979; 23: 463–466.

364. Balus L, Donati P, Amantea A, Breathnach AS. Multiple minute digitate hyperkeratosis. J Am Acad Dermatol 1988; 18: 431–436.

365. Nedwich JA, Sullivan JJ. Disseminated spiked hyperkeratosis. Int J Dermatol 1987; 26: 358–361.

366. Goldstein N. Multiple minute digitate hyperkeratoses. Arch Dermatol 1967; 96: 692–693.

367. Yoon SW, Gibbs RB. Multiple minute digitate hyperkeratoses. Arch Dermatol 1975; 111: 1176–1177.

368. Shuttleworth D, Graham-Brown RAC, Hutchinson PE. Minute aggregate keratoses — a report of three cases. Clin Exp Dermatol 1985; 10: 566–571.

369. Aloi FG, Molinero A, Pippione M. Parakeratotic horns in a patient with Crohn's disease. Clin Exp Dermatol 1989; 14: 79–81.

370. Cox NH, Ince P. Transient post-inflammatory digitate keratoses. Clin Exp Dermatol 1989; 14: 170–172.

371. Knobler EH, Grossman ME, Rabinowitz AD. Multiple minute palmar-plantar digitate hyperkeratoses. Br J Dermatol 1989; 121: 239–242.

372. Burns DA. Post-irradiation digitate keratoses. Clin Exp Dermatol 1986; 11: 646–649.

373. Frenk E, Mevorah B, Leu F. Disseminated spiked hyperkeratosis. An unusual discrete nonfollicular keratinization disorder. Arch Dermatol 1981; 117: 412–414.

Miscellaneous epidermal genodermatoses

374. Waisman M. Verruciform manifestations of keratosis follicularis. Arch Dermatol 1960; 81: 1–14.

375. Niedelman ML, McKusick VA. Acrokeratosis verruciformis (Hopf). A follow-up study. Arch Dermatol 1962; 86: 779–782.

376. Rook A, Stevanovic D. Acrokeratosis verruciformis. Br J Dermatol 1957; 69: 450–451.

377. Panja RK. Acrokeratosis verruciformis (Hopf) — a clinical entity? Br J Dermatol 1977; 96: 643–652.

378. Schueller WA. Acrokeratosis verruciformis of Hopf. Arch Dermatol 1972; 106: 81–83.

379. Herndon JH, Wilson JD. Acrokeratosis verruciformis (Hopf) and Darier's disease. Genetic evidence for a unitary origin. Arch Dermatol 1966; 93: 305–310.

380. Niordson AM, Sylvest B. Bullous dyskeratosis follicularis and acrokeratosis verruciformis. Report of a case. Arch Dermatol 1965; 92: 166–168.

381. Verbov J. Acrokeratosis verruciformis of Hopf with steatocystoma multiplex and hypertrophic lichen planus. Br J Dermatol 1972; 86: 91–94.

382. Penrod JN, Everett MA, McCreight WG. Observations on keratosis follicularis. Arch Dermatol 1960; 82: 367–370.

383. Jung EG. Xeroderma pigmentosum. Int J Dermatol 1986; 25: 629–633.

384. Kraemer KH, Slor H. Xeroderma pigmentosum. Clin Dermatol 1985; 3: 33–69.

385. Kraemer KH, Lee MM, Scotto J. Xeroderma pigmentosum. Cutaneous, ocular and neurologic abnormalities in 830 published cases. Arch Dermatol 1987; 123: 241–250.

386. Lambert WC. Genetic diseases associated with DNA and chromosomal instability. Dermatol Clin 1987; 5: 85–108.

387. English JSC, Swerdlow AJ. The risk of malignant melanoma, internal malignancy and mortality in xeroderma pigmentosum patients. Br J Dermatol 1987; 117: 457–461.

388. Reed WB, Sugarman GI, Mathis RA. DeSanctis-Cacchione syndrome. A case report with autopsy findings. Arch Dermatol 1977; 113: 1561–1563.

389. Kraemer KH. Xeroderma pigmentosum. A prototype disease of environmental-genetic interaction. Arch Dermatol 1980; 116: 541–542.

390. Nishigori C, Miyachi Y, Takebe H, Imamura S. A case of xeroderma pigmentosum with clinical appearance of dyschromatosis symmetrica hereditaria. Pediatr Dermatol 1986; 3: 410–413.

391. Lynch HT, Frichot BC, Lynch JF. Cancer control in xeroderma pigmentosum. Arch Dermatol 1977; 113: 193–195.

392. Wysenbeek AJ, Weiss H, Duczyminer-Kahana M et al. Immunologic alterations in xeroderma pigmentosum patients. Cancer 1986; 58: 219–221.

393. Bhutani LK. The photodermatoses as seen in tropical countries. Semin Dermatol 1982; 1: 175–181.

394. Auerbach AD. Diagnosis of diseases of DNA synthesis and repair that affect the skin using cultured amniotic fluid cells. Semin Dermatol 1984; 3: 172–184.

395. Cleaver JE. Xeroderma pigmentosum: genetic and environmental influences in skin carcinogenesis. Int J Dermatol 1978; 17: 435–444.

396. Friedberg EC. Xeroderma pigmentosum. Recent studies on the DNA repair defects. Arch Pathol Lab Med 1978; 102: 3–7.

397. Fischer E, Jung EG. Photosensitivity and the genodermatoses. Semin Dermatol 1982; 1: 169–174.

398. Kondo S, Fukuro S, Mamada A et al. Assignment of three patients with xeroderma pigmentosum to complementation group E and their characteristics. J Invest Dermatol 1988; 90: 152–157.

399. Norris PG, Hawk JLM, Avery JA, Giannelli F. Xeroderma pigmentosum complementation group F in a non-Japanese patient. J Am Acad Dermatol 1988; 18: 1185–1188.

400. Yamamura K, Ichihashi M, Hiramoto T et al. Clinical and photobiological characteristics of xeroderma pigmentosum complementation group F: a review of cases from Japan. Br J Dermatol 1989; 121: 471–480.

401. Norris PG, Hawk JLM, Avery JA, Giannelli F. Xeroderma pigmentosum complementation group G — report of two cases. Br J Dermatol 1987; 116: 861–866.

402. Otsuka F, Robbins JH. The Cockayne syndrome — an inherited multisystem disorder with cutaneous photosensitivity and defective repair of DNA. Comparison with xeroderma pigmentosum. Am J Dermatopathol 1985; 7: 387–392.

403. Lynch HT, Fusaro RM, Johnson JA. Xeroderma pigmentosum. Complementation group C and malignant melanoma. Arch Dermatol 1984; 120: 175–179.

404. Nagasawa H, Zamansky GB, McCone EF et al. Spontaneous transformation to anchorage-independent growth of a xeroderma pigmentosum fibroblast cell strain. J Invest Dermatol 1987; 88: 149–153.

405. Norris PG, Limb GA, Hamblin AS et al. Immune function, mutant frequency, and cancer risk in the DNA repair defective genodermatoses xeroderma pigmentosum, Cockayne's syndrome, and trichothiodystrophy. J Invest Dermatol 1990; 94: 94–100.

406. Kraemer KH, Herlyn M, Yuspa SH et al. Reduced DNA repair in cultured melanocytes and nevus cells from a patient with xeroderma pigmentosum. Arch Dermatol 1989; 125: 263–268.

407. Wade MH, Plotnick H. Xeroderma pigmentosum and squamous cell carcinoma of the tongue. Identification of two black patients as members of complementation group C. J Am Acad Dermatol 1985; 12: 515–521.

408. Harper JI, Copeman PWM. Carcinoma of the tongue in a boy with xeroderma pigmentosum. Clin Exp Dermatol 1981; 6: 601–604.

409. Plotnick H, Lupulescu A. Ultrastructural studies of xeroderma pigmentosum. J Am Acad Dermatol 1983; 9: 876–882.

410. Tsuji T. Electron microscopic studies of xeroderma pigmentosum: unusual changes in the keratinocyte. Br J Dermatol 1974; 91: 657–666.

411. Friere-Maia N, Pinheiro M. Ectodermal dysplasias: a clinical and genetic syndrome. New York: Alan R Liss, 1984.

412. Lucky AW, Esterly NB, Tunnessen WW Jr. Ectodermal dysplasia and abnormal thumbs. J Am Acad Dermatol 1980; 2: 379–384.

413. Solomon LM, Keuer EJ. The ectodermal dysplasias. Problems of classification and some newer syndromes. Arch Dermatol 1980; 116: 1295–1299.

414. Tsakalakos N, Jordaan FH, Taljaard JJF, Hough SF. A previously undescribed ectodermal dysplasia of the tricho-odonto-onychial subgroup in a family. Arch Dermatol 1986; 122: 1047–1053.

415. Freire-Maia N, Pinheiro M. So-called "anhidrotic ectodermal dysplasia". Int J Dermatol 1980; 19: 455–456.

416. Martin-Pascual A, De Unamuno P, Aparicio M, Herreros V. Anhidrotic (or hypohidrotic) ectodermal dysplasia. Dermatologica 1977; 154: 235–243.

417. Sybert VP. Hypohidrotic ectodermal dysplasia: argument against an autosomal recessive form clinically indistinguishable from X-linked hypohidrotic ectodermal dysplasia (Christ-Siemens-Touraine syndrome). Pediatr Dermatol 1989; 6: 76–81.

418. Davis JR, Solomon LM. Cellular immunodeficiency in anhidrotic ectodermal dysplasia. Acta Derm Venereol 1976; 56: 115–120.

419. Reed WB, Lopez DA, Landing B. Clinical spectrum of anhidrotic ectodermal dysplasia. Arch Dermatol 1970; 102: 134–143.

420. Reddy BSN, Chandra S, Jha PK, Singh G. Anhidrotic ectodermal dysplasia. Int J Dermatol 1978; 17: 139–141.

421. Arnold M-L, Rauskolb R, Anton-Lamprecht I et al. Prenatal diagnosis of anhidrotic ectodermal dysplasia. Prenatal Diagnosis 1984; 4: 85–98.

422. Verbov J. Hypohidrotic (or anhidrotic) ectodermal dysplasia — an appraisal of diagnostic methods. Br J Dermatol 1970; 83: 341–348.

423. Ando Y, Tanaka T, Horiguchi Y et al. Hidrotic ectodermal dysplasia: a clinical and ultrastructural observation. Dermatologica 1988; 176: 205–211.

424. Solomon LM, Fretzin D, Pruzansky S. Pilosebaceous dysplasia in the oral-facial-digital syndrome. Arch Dermatol 1970; 102: 598–602.

425. Lambert WC, Bilinski DL. Diagnostic pitfalls in anhidrotic ectodermal dysplasia: indications for palmar skin biopsy. Cutis 1983; 31: 182–187.

426. Katz SI, Penneys NS. Sebaceous gland papules in anhidrotic ectodermal dysplasia. Arch Dermatol 1971; 103: 507–509.

427. Frix CD III, Bronson DM. Acute miliary tuberculosis in a child with anhidrotic ectodermal dysplasia. Pediatr Dermatol 1986; 3: 464–467.

428. From E, Philipsen HP, Thormann J. Dyskeratosis benigna intraepithelialis mucosae et cutis hereditaria. A report of this disorder in father and son. J Cutan Pathol 1978; 5: 105–115.

429. James WD, Lupton GP. Acquired dyskeratotic leukoplakia. Arch Dermatol 1988; 124: 117–120.

430. Scheman AJ, Ray DJ, Witkop CJ Jr, Dahl MV. Hereditary mucoepithelial dysplasia. Case report and review of the literature. J Am Acad Dermatol 1989; 21: 351–357.

10

David Weedon

Disorders of pigmentation

INTRODUCTION

This chapter deals with the various disorders of cutaneous pigmentation, excluding those entities in which there is an obvious lentiginous proliferation of melanocytes in sections stained with haematoxylin and eosin; it also excludes tumours of the naevus-cell–melanocyte system. Both of the excluded categories are discussed in Chapter 32. Cutaneous pigmentation may also result from the deposition of drug complexes in the dermis. This category of pigmentation is discussed among other cutaneous deposits in Chapter 14.

Cutaneous pigmentary disorders can be divided into two major categories: disorders with hypopigmentation and those with hyperpigmentation. The dyschromatoses in which areas both of hypopigmentation and of hyperpigmentation are present have been arbitrarily included with the disorders of hyperpigmentation.

The pigmentary system

The pigmentary system involves a complex set of reactions with numerous potential sites for dysfunction. Melanin is produced in melanosomes in the cytoplasm of melanocytes by the action of tyrosinase on tyrosine. A number of intermediate steps involving the formation of dopa and dopaquinone take place prior to the synthesis of melanin. The melanin synthesized in any one melanocyte is then transferred to an average of 36 keratinocytes by the phagocytosis of the melanin-laden dendritic tips of the melanocytes.[1] This transfer of melanin can be disrupted by any inflammatory process involving the basal layer of the epidermis. Specific enzyme defects and destruction of melanocytes are other theoretical causes of hypopigmentation.

The pathogenesis of hyperpigmentation is not as well understood. Prominent pigment incontinence is an obvious cause of hyperpigmentation. Ultrastructural examination in some disorders of hyperpigmentation has shown an increase in size or melanization of the melanosomes, although in others the reasons for the basal hyperpigmentation have not been determined.

The disorders of hypopigmentation will be discussed first.

DISORDERS CHARACTERIZED BY HYPOPIGMENTATION

There are multiple potential sites for dysfunction in the formation of melanin pigment in basal melanocytes.[1] Attempts have been made to categorize the various diseases with hypopigmentation on the basis of their presumed pathogenesis. The following categories may be considered:

1. *Abnormal migration/differentiation of melanoblasts*: piebaldism, Waardenburg's and Woolf's syndromes.
2. *Destruction of melanocytes*: vitiligo, Vogt–Koyanagi–Harada syndrome, chemical leucoderma.
3. *Reduced tyrosinase activity*: oculocutaneous albinism type IA, phenylketonuria(?).
4. *Abnormal structure of melanosomes*: 'ash leaf spots' of tuberous sclerosis, Chédiak–Higashi syndrome, progressive macular hypomelanosis.
5. *Reduced melanization and/or numbers of melanosomes*: albinism (other tyrosinase-positive variants), idiopathic guttate hypomelanosis, hypomelanosis of Ito, 'ash leaf spots', pityriasis versicolor (tinea versicolor), naevus depigmentosus.
6. *Reduced transfer to keratinocytes*: naevus depigmentosus, pityriasis alba, post-inflammatory leucoderma, pityriasis versicolor (tinea versicolor), Chédiak–Higashi syndrome. Increased degradation of melanosomes within

melanocytes may also apply in some conditions listed in this section.
7. *Abnormal vasculature*: naevus anaemicus.

In addition to the conditions listed above, there are isolated reports of one or more cases in which the hypopigmentation does not correspond neatly to any of the named diseases.[2,3] These cases will not be considered further.

Phenylketonuria, an autosomal recessive disorder with a deficiency of the enzyme L-phenylalanine hydroxylase, is characterized by oculocutaneous pigmentary dilution in addition to neurological abnormalities.[1,4] There are several steps in the biosynthesis of melanin which may be affected by this enzyme deficiency. As biopsies are rarely taken, this condition will not be discussed further.

PIEBALDISM

In piebaldism (partial albinism), an autosomal dominant disorder, there are non-progressive, discrete patches of leucoderma present from birth.[1] The chalk-white areas of hypomelanosis involve the anterior part of the trunk, the mid-region of the extremities, the forehead and the mid-frontal area of the scalp beneath a white forelock.[1] This hair change is present in up to 90% of those with piebaldism, and it is sometimes found as an isolated change in the absence of cutaneous leucoderma.[5] Within the areas of hypomelanosis there are hyperpigmented and normally-pigmented macules of various sizes.[5a]

There are several rare syndromes in which extracutaneous manifestations accompany the piebaldism.[1,6,7] Examples include *Waardenburg's syndrome* in which piebaldism is associated with neurosensory hearing loss and other abnormalities,[8,9] and *Woolf's syndrome* in which the hearing loss is the only associated feature.[1]

It has been suggested that the absence of melanocytes from the depigmented areas results from defective migration of melanoblasts from the neural crest in embryogenesis, or from failure of these cells to differentiate into viable melanocytes once they reach the skin.[5] The successful use of autologous grafts to repigment the affected areas is not inconsistent with these theories.[10]

Histopathology

There are usually no melanocytes and no melanin in the leucodermic areas. Sometimes a small number of morphologically abnormal melanocytes is present, particularly near the margins of hypopigmentation. These melanocytes may have spherical melanosomes. Some clear cells, representing Langerhans cells, are usually present in the epidermis.[11]

The hyperpigmented islands contain normal numbers of melanocytes: there are abundant melanosomes in the melanocytes and in keratinocytes. There are no dopa-positive melanocytes in the hair bulbs of the white forelock.[9]

Recently, some doubt has been cast on these traditional findings by a study which showed some dopa-positive melanocytes in depigmented areas. This awaits confirmation.[12]

VITILIGO

Vitiligo is an acquired, idiopathic disorder in which there are depigmented macules of variable size which enlarge and coalesce to form extensive areas of leucoderma.[13-15] An erythematous border is occasionally present in the initial stages.[1] The incidence in Caucasians is approximately 1%. This condition may develop at any age, although in 50% of affected persons it appears before the age of 20 years.[16] A family history is present in up to 25% of cases; the inheritance appears to be multifactorial.[14]

There is a predilection for the face, backs of the hands, axillae, groins, umbilicus and genitalia and for the skin overlying bony areas such as the knees and elbows.[14] Sometimes the depigmented area is segmental or dermatomal in distribution (type B); oftener it is more generalized (type A).[17,18] Repigmentation seldom occurs in type B, which is also resistant to treatment, and more common in children.[18]

Approximately 20–30% of individuals with vitiligo have an associated autoimmune and/or

endocrine disorder[1] such as Hashimoto's disease, hyperthyroidism, pernicious anaemia, Addison's disease, insulin-dependent diabetes mellitus[19,20] and alopecia areata.[21] Less frequent associations include various lymphoproliferative diseases, morphoea,[22] Crohn's disease[23,24] and chronic mucocutaneous candidosis.[25] The reported association of vitiligo with psoriasis and erythema dyschromicum perstans[26] is probably fortuitous.

Vitiligo may be accompanied by a variety of ocular pigmentary disturbances,[27] the best known of which is the *Vogt–Koyanagi–Harada syndrome* which includes uveitis, poliosis, dysacusis, alopecia, vitiligo and signs of meningeal irritation.[28] Not all these features are present in all cases.

Sometimes there is a history in the patient or the patient's immediate family of premature greying of the hair (poliosis), a halo naevus, or even a malignant melanoma.[29] It is interesting to note that individuals with metastatic melanoma who develop vitiligo-like depigmentation have a better prognosis than those who do not.[30,31]

The onset of vitiligo is usually insidious with no precipitating cause. In approximately 20% of cases it develops after severe sunburn or some severe emotional or physical stress.[14] In generalized forms the depigmentation may eventually involve large areas of skin. Some repigmentation may occur but it is usually incomplete and short lived.[14,28] Eventually the process of depigmentation ceases.

Three hypotheses have been proposed to explain the destruction of melanocytes which results in the depigmentation.[28] These may be summarized as the neural, the self-destructive and the immune theories. The *neural hypothesis* suggests that a neurochemical mediator released at nerve endings results in destruction of melanocytes. It has been proposed that the segmental form (type B) of vitiligo results from dysfunction of sympathetic nerves in the affected areas.[18] The *self-destruction hypothesis* is based on the known toxicity of melanin precursors for melanocytes. It is assumed that affected individuals have an intrinsic inability to eliminate or handle these toxic precursors, which accumulate and result in the destruction of melanocytes.[15] The *immune hypothesis*, which is currently most favoured, particularly for the generalized forms, proposes that antibody-dependent, cell-mediated cytotoxicity utilizing natural killer cells is responsible for the loss of melanocytes. Several abnormalities in the immune system have been recorded in vitiligo.[32] These include a decrease in T-helper cells,[33–34a] an increase in natural killer cells,[34,35] circulating antibodies to melanocytes[36,37] and to certain melanoma cell lines,[38] and possible functional impairment of Langerhans cells.[39,40] Grafting studies have until recently shown variable results;[41,42] localized vitiligo has now been successfully treated using autologous grafts.[43] Further information relating to the pathogenesis of vitiligo is now forthcoming from the animal models that exist in the mouse and in the Smyth chicken.[44,45]

Finally, depigmentation resembling vitiligo has been reported following contact with hydroquinones, certain phenolic agents,[14] cinnamic aldehyde in toothpaste[46] and PUVA therapy.[47,48]

Histopathology

Vitiliginous skin shows a complete loss of melanin pigment from the epidermis and an absence of melanocytes (Fig. 10.1). At the advancing border the melanocytes may be increased in size with an increased number of dendrites.[14] Occasional lymphocytes may be present in this region;[49] these cells are invariably present if there is an inflammatory border clinically. In these instances there is also a perivascular infiltrate of mononuclear cells involving the superficial plexus, as well as some superficial oedema.[50] Ultrathin sections will often show vacuolated keratinocytes and extracellular granular material in the basal layer of the normal skin adjacent to areas of vitiligo.[51] If serial sections are examined a lymphocyte will sometimes be found in close apposition to a melanocyte at the advancing edge (unpublished observation — Fig. 10.2). Degenerative changes have also been reported in nerves and sweat glands.[52]

Electron microscopy. Melanocytes and keratinocytes adjacent to the vitiliginous areas show degenerative changes in the form of intracellular oedema and vacuolar formation.[51,53,54] Extracellular material derived from degenerating keratinocytes is sometimes present.[51] Fibrillar

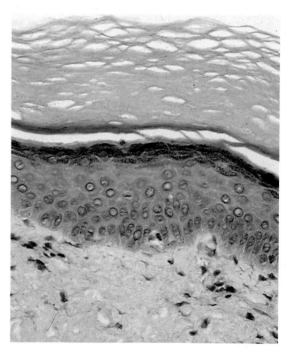

Fig. 10.2 Vitiligo. A lymphocyte is in contact with a melanocyte in the basal layer at the advancing edge of an area of vitiligo. This is support for the theory that some cases of vitiligo result from lymphocyte-mediated destruction of melanocytes.
Haematoxylin — eosin

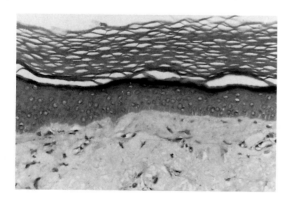

Fig. 10.1 Vitiligo. Melanocytes and melanin are absent from the basal layer.
Haematoxylin — eosin

masses similar to colloid bodies may also be present in the upper dermis and in the basal layer.[51] Numerous nerve endings may be seen in close contact with the basal lamina.[53]

OCULOCUTANEOUS ALBINISM

Oculocutaneous albinism is a genetically heterogeneous group of disorders in which there is a generalized decrease or absence of melanin pigment in the eyes, hair and skin.[55] At least ten forms of this condition have been identified, each presumably resulting from a different biochemical block in the synthesis of melanin.[1] Only in Type IA, the classic type, is the defect known: it is a complete absence of tyrosinase activity in melanocytes.[56] Other types show variable or normal tyrosinase activity and the defect is thought to be at a later stage in the pathway of the synthesis of melanin.[56,57] Inheritance is autosomal recessive in type, except for Type II oculocutaneous albinism, the most prevalent form, in which it is autosomal dominant.

The usual finding at birth is white hair and skin, and blue eyes. In all phenotypes except Type IA, there is some increase in pigment with age, the amount depending on the ethnic background of the individual and the particular subtype of the disorder.[55] Red-yellow phaeomelanin is the first to form; black-brown eumelanin is synthesized only after a long period of phaeomelanin formation.[55]

Ocular disorders include photophobia, nystagmus, strabismus and reduced visual acuity. In the skin there is accelerated photoageing and an increased incidence of keratoses and squamous and basal cell carcinomas.[58] Malignant melanomas develop occasionally. The dysplastic naevus syndrome has also been reported in individuals with oculocutaneous albinism.[59] Lentigines and naevi do not form in Type IA, the tyrosinase-negative phenotype.[1]

Systemic features are present in the Hermansky–Pudlak syndrome, one of the clinical variants of oculocutaneous albinism, in which there is also a defect in platelets.[1] Lipid and ceroid pigment are present in macrophages in various organs, including the skin.[59a] The

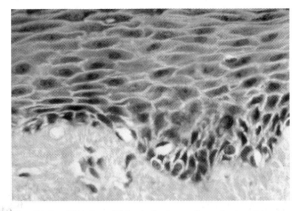

Fig. 10.3 Albinism. Melanin is absent from the basal layer but melanocytes are normal in number and morphology. Haematoxylin — eosin

Chédiak–Higashi syndrome (see below) is sometimes regarded as another clinical variant.[1]

Histopathology

There is a complete or partial reduction in melanin pigment in the skin and hair bulbs. Melanocytes are normal in number and morphology (Fig. 10.3). Tyrosinase activity is lacking in melanocytes in freshly-plucked anagen hair bulbs in Type IA;[60] it is reduced in heterozygotes with this phenotype and variably reduced in some of the other types. Tyrosinase activity is normal in Type II.[56]

Electron microscopy. Melanocytes and melanosomes are normal in configuration. There are no stage III or IV melanosomes in Type IA.

CHEDIAK–HIGASHI SYNDROME

The Chédiak–Higashi syndrome is a rare, autosomal recessive disorder in which there is partial oculocutaneous albinism associated with frequent pyogenic infections and the presence of abnormal, large granules in leucocytes and some other cells.[61] The disease usually enters an accelerated phase in childhood, with pancytopenia, hepatosplenomegaly and lymphohistiocytic infiltrates in various organs.[62] This phase, which resembles the virus-associated haemophagocytic syndrome, is usually followed by death.[62]

The pigmentary dilution involves at least one, and often all three, of the following — skin, hair and eyes.[61,63] There is increased susceptibility to burning. The hair is usually blond or light brown in colour.

The increased susceptibility to infection is related to impaired function of leucocytes and natural killer cells associated with lysosomal defects, while the reduced skin pigmentation is related to similar defects in melanocytes.[62,64] The inclusions found in these and other cells are massive secondary lysosomal structures formed through a combined process of fusion, cytoplasmic injury and phagocytosis.[62,64]

Histopathology

There is a striking reduction or even absence of melanin pigment in the basal layer, and in hair follicles.[61] A few large pigment granules corresponding to giant melanosomes are present.[65] In less affected individuals, and in some heterozygotes, clumps of enlarged pigment granules may also be present in the dermis in macrophages and endothelial cells and lying free in the interstitium.[63]

Staining with toluidine blue demonstrates large cytoplasmic inclusions in cutaneous mast cells.[65]

Electron microscopy. Giant melanosomes and degenerating cytoplasmic residues are found in melanocytes.[66] The pigment granules passed to keratinocytes are bigger than normal.[66] The giant melanosomes appear to arise from defective premelanosomes.[66] Giant cytoplasmic granules have also been found in Langerhans cells.[66a] They are believed to be derived from the fusion of lysosomes or some portion of Birbeck granules.[66a]

PROGRESSIVE MACULAR HYPOMELANOSIS

Progressive macular hypomelanosis of the trunk is an acquired form of hypopigmentation with a predisposition to affect the back of young adult females of Caribbean origin.[67] The hypopigmented macules, which measure 1–3 cm in diameter, coalesce into large patches. The disease remits in 3–4 years.

Histopathology[67]

There is a decrease in melanin pigment within the epidermis. Melanocytes are normal in number.

Electron microscopy. There is a reduction in stage IV (negroid) melanosomes which are replaced by small type I–III melanosomes in an aggregated (caucasoid) pattern.

TUBEROUS SCLEROSIS

Tuberous sclerosis is characterized by the triad of epilepsy, mental retardation and multiple angiofibromas ('adenoma sebaceum'). In addition, circumscribed macules of hypopigmentation known as 'ash leaf spots' can be present at birth on the trunk and lower extremities.[1,68] They vary in diameter from 1 mm to 12 cm. The more common shapes are oval, polygonal or ash-leaf-like. The basic abnormality appears to be an arrest in the maturation of melanosomes.[1]

Histopathology

Epidermal melanin is reduced, but not absent.

Electron microscopy.[1,69] This has shown a normal number of melanocytes and a reduction in the number, size and melanization of the melanosomes.[68] The small melanosomes often form aggregates within the keratinocytes.

IDIOPATHIC GUTTATE HYPOMELANOSIS

This is a common leucodermic dermatosis of unknown aetiology in which multiple achromic or hypochromic macules, 2–5 mm in diameter, develop over many years.[70–73] They are usually found on the sun-exposed extremities of elderly individuals, but scattered lesions may occur on the trunk.[74,75] Repigmentation does not occur.

Histopathology[72,73]

There is a decrease in melanin pigment in the basal layer of the epidermis and a reduction in the number of dopa-positive melanocytes, although these cells are never completely absent. The epidermis usually shows some atrophy, with flattening of the rete pegs. There may be basket-weave hyperkeratosis.

Electron microscopy. Some of the melanocytes remaining in affected areas of skin show a reduction in dendritic processes and melanosomes.[76,77]

HYPOMELANOSIS OF ITO

Hypomelanosis of Ito (incontinentia pigmenti achromians) presents at birth or in infancy with sharply demarcated, hypopigmented macular lesions on the trunk and extremities, with a distinctive linear or whorled pattern.[78–79] The pattern resembles a negative image of the pigmentation seen in incontinentia pigmenti (see p. 317).[80] The coexistence of hypomelanosis of Ito and incontinentia pigmenti in the same family, even though disputed by a subsequent author,[81] and the report of several patients with a preceding erythematous or verrucous stage[82,83] have led several authorities to postulate a link between these two conditions.[79,82]

Other features of hypomelanosis of Ito include a female preponderance, a tendency for lesions to become somewhat pigmented in late childhood, a family history in a few cases,[84] and the coexistence in a high percentage of patients of abnormalities of the central nervous system (particularly seizures and mental retardation), eyes, hair, teeth and musculoskeletal system.[78,79]

Histopathology

The hypopigmented areas show a reduction in melanin pigment in the basal layer, but this is usually not discernible in haematoxylin and eosin stained sections and requires a Masson–Fontana stain for confirmation. Dopa stains show a reduction in staining of melanocytes, and sometimes shortening of their dendrites.[85] A reduction in the number of melanocytes[86] and vacuolization of basal keratinocytes have been mentioned in some reports but specifically excluded in most.[87]

Electron microscopy. This has shown a reduction in melanosomes in melanocytes in the hypopigmented areas and a decrease in the number of melanin granules in keratinocytes.[78] There are isolated reports of aggregation of melanosomes, vacuolization of melanocytes,[53] and an increase in the number of Langerhans cells in the epidermis.[88]

NAEVUS DEPIGMENTOSUS

Naevus depigmentosus (achromic naevus) is a little-studied entity consisting of isolated, circular or rectangular, hypopigmented macules with a predisposition for the trunk and proximal parts of the extremities.[1] It may also occur in a dermatomal or systematized pattern, the latter having some clinical resemblance to the pattern seen in hypomelanosis of Ito.[69,89] However, the lesions in naevus depigmentosus are present at birth, there are usually no associated abnormalities in other organs and they are more localized and stable than the lesions of hypomelanosis of Ito.[1]

Histopathology

Melanocytes are said to be normal or slightly reduced in number, although there is reduced dopa activity.[1]

Electron microscopy.[69] Melanosomes are normal in size but there is some abnormal aggregation of them within melanocytes. Degradation of melanosomes within autophagosomes of melanocytes has been noted. Melanosomes are decreased in number in keratinocytes, suggesting impaired transfer.

PITYRIASIS ALBA

Pityriasis alba consists of variably hypopig-mented, slightly scaly patches with a predilection for the face, neck and shoulders of dark-skinned atopic individuals.[90–92] The aetiology is unknown although it has been regarded as post-inflammatory hypopigmentation following eczema.[90]

A supposed variant with extensive non-scaling macules involving the lower part of the trunk has been reported, but there is no real evidence that this is the same process.[91,92] It is not related to atopy.

Histopathology

There are no detailed studies of the usual facial type of pityriasis alba. In a personally studied case there was mild hyperkeratosis, focal parakeratosis and focal mild spongiosis with prominent exocytosis of lymphocytes.[93] There was also a mild superficial perivascular inflammatory cell infiltrate in the dermis. Melanin pigmentation of the basal layer was markedly reduced, but there was no melanin incontinence.[93] Melanocytes were normal in number. This conforms with one other reported case.[94]

A study of the 'extensive' variant showed reduced basal pigmentation, a decreased number of functional melanocytes on the dopa prepara-tion and a reduction in the number and size of melanosomes.[91]

POST-INFLAMMATORY LEUCODERMA

Hypopigmented areas may develop during the course of a number of inflammatory diseases of the skin, usually during the resolving phases.[1] Examples include the various eczematous der-matitides, psoriasis, discoid lupus erythemato-sus, pityriasis rosea, variants of parapsoriasis, lichen sclerosus et atrophicus, syphilis and the viral exanthems.[1] Uncommonly, hypopigmenta-tion may follow lichen planus and other lichenoid eruptions. Hypomelanotic lesions occur in an early stage of the disease, albeit uncommonly, in some of the following lesions — alopecia muci-nosa, sarcoidosis, mycosis fungoides, pityriasis lichenoides chronica, pityriasis versicolor (tinea versicolor), onchocerciasis, yaws and leprosy.[1]

The mechanism in many of these conditions is thought to be a block in the transfer of melano-somes from melanocytes to keratinocytes; in the lichenoid dermatoses damage to melanocytes may also contribute. In pityriasis versicolor, melanosomes are poorly melanized; impaired transfer is also present.

Various mechanisms have been proposed for the hypopigmentation of lesions in indeterminate and tuberculoid leprosy (see p. 612).

Histopathology

There is a reduction in melanin pigment in the basal layer, although not a complete absence. Melanocytes are usually normal in number. Pigment-containing melanophages are sometimes present in the upper dermis, particularly in black patients. Residual features of the preceding or concurrent inflammatory dermatosis may also be present.

NAEVUS ANAEMICUS

Naevus anaemicus is an uncommon congenital disorder in which there is usually a solitary asymptomatic patch that is paler than the sur-rounding normal skin.[95] Its margin is irregular and there may be islands of sparing within the lesion.[96] The pale area averages 5–10 cm in diameter. There is a predilection for the upper trunk, although involvement of the face and extremities has been reported.[97] Naevus anaemi-cus sometimes occurs in association with neuro-fibromatosis.[98]

Naevus anaemicus is regarded as a pharmaco-logical naevus in which the pallor is attributable to increased sensitivity of the blood vessels in the area to catecholamines.[99] Naevus oligaemicus is a related entity in which there is livid erythema rather than pallor.[100]

Histopathology

No abnormalities have been shown by light or electron microscopy.

DISORDERS CHARACTERIZED BY HYPERPIGMENTATION

This is a heterogeneous group of diseases comprising a bewildering number of rare conditions. Japanese people are predisposed to many of the entities to be discussed below. Several factors are taken into consideration in the clinical categorization of these various disorders, including the distribution, arrangement and morphology of individual lesions as well as the presence or absence of hypopigmented areas.[101,102] Four clinical categories of hyperpigmentation can be recognized.

1. *Diffuse hyperpigmentation:* generalized hyperpigmentary disorders (scleroderma, Addison's disease, myxoedema, Graves' disease, malnutrition including pellagra, chronic liver disease including haemochromatosis and Wilson's disease, porphyria, folate and vitamin B_{12} deficiency, heavy metal toxicity, and the ingestion of certain drugs and chemicals), universal acquired melanosis, and the generalized melanosis that may develop in malignant melanoma.
2. *Localized (patchy) hyperpigmentation:* ephelis (freckle), café-au-lait spots, macules of Albright's syndrome, macules of Peutz–Jeghers syndrome, Becker's naevus, acromelanosis, melasma, fixed drug eruption, frictional melanosis, notalgia paraesthetica, and familial progressive hyperpigmentation.
3. *Punctate, reticulate hyperpigmentation (including whorls and streaks):* Dowling–Degos disease, Kitamura's disease, Naegeli–Franceschetti–Jadassohn syndrome, dermatopathia pigmentosa reticularis, macular amyloidosis, 'ripple neck' in atopic dermatitis, hereditary diffuse hyperpigmentation, incontinentia pigmenti, prurigo pigmentosa, confluent and reticulated papillomatosis, patterned hypermelanosis, and chimerism.

4. *Dyschromatosis (hyperpigmentation and hypopigmentation):* dyskeratosis congenita, dyschromatosis symmetrica hereditaria (Dohi), dyschromatosis universalis, heterochromia extremitarum,[102] and hereditary congenital hypopigmented and hyperpigmented macules.[103]

Theoretically, the hyperpigmentation observed in these various conditions could result from increased basal pigmentation and/or melanin incontinence. Alterations in the epidermal configuration can also produce apparent pigmentation of the skin.

Although there is some variability in the histopathological features reported in some of the disorders of hyperpigmentation, the following subclassification provides a useful approach to a biopsy from such a disease.

Disorders with basal hyperpigmentation (mild melanin incontinence is sometimes present also): generalized hyperpigmentary disorders, universal acquired melanosis, acromelanosis (increased melanocytes were noted in one report), familial progressive hyperpigmentation, dyschromatosis symmetrica hereditaria, dyschromatosis universalis, patterned hypermelanosis, chimerism, melasma, ephelis (freckle), café-au-lait spots, macules of Albright's syndrome, macules of Peutz–Jeghers syndrome, and Becker's naevus (melanosis).

Disorders with epidermal changes: Dowling–Degos disease (the epidermal changes resemble those of solar lentigo), Kitamura's disease (the epidermal changes resembling Dowling–Degos disease but with intervening epidermal atrophy also), and confluent and reticulated papillomatosis of Gougerot–Carteaud (the epidermal changes are those of papillomatosis).

Disorders with striking melanin incontinence: post-inflammatory melanosis, prurigo pigmentosa, generalized melanosis in malignant melanoma, dermatopathia pigmentosa reticularis, Naegeli–Franceschetti–Jadassohn syndrome, incontinentia pigmenti, and late fixed drug eruptions.

Disorders with melanin incontinence and epidermal atrophy or 'dyskeratotic' cells: dyskeratosis congenita, frictional melanosis, notalgia paraesthetica, 'ripple neck' in atopic dermatitis, active fixed drug eruptions, and active prurigo pigmentosa.

Fixed drug eruptions and dyskeratosis congenita are discussed with the lichenoid reaction pattern on page 41 and page 56 respectively. Confluent and reticulated papillomatosis is considered on page 553.

GENERALIZED HYPERPIGMENTARY DISORDERS

As mentioned above, generalized cutaneous hyperpigmentation can be seen in a number of metabolic, endocrine, hepatic and nutritional disorders, as well as following intake of certain drugs and heavy metals. Hyperpigmentation may follow sympathectomy.[104] It may also occur in the Crow–Fukase (POEMS) syndrome[105] (see p. 1002).

Histopathology

Biopsies of the pigmented skin are not often taken from individuals with these conditions. There is an increase in melanin in the lower layers of the epidermis, and sometimes a small amount of pigment in the dermis. Of interest is the finding of large nuclei in the keratinocytes of the pigmented skin in some megaloblastic anaemias.[106,107]

UNIVERSAL ACQUIRED MELANOSIS

This extremely rare condition, also known as the 'carbon baby' syndrome, is characterized by progressive pigmentation of the skin during childhood, resembling that seen in black races.[108]

Histopathology

In the reported case there was hyperpigmentation of the epidermis and an increase in type III and IV (negroid pattern) melanosomes in melanocytes.[108]

ACROMELANOSIS

Acromelanosis refers to the presence of pigmented patches and macules on the dorsal surface of the phalanges, usually in coloured people.[101,102] Several clinical variants have been recognized on the basis of the distribution of the pigment and of the progression of the disorder.[102,109]

Histopathology

Basal hyperpigmentation is the usual finding, although an increase in basal melanocytes with associated acanthosis has also been reported.[109]

FAMILIAL PROGRESSIVE HYPERPIGMENTATION

Patches of hyperpigmentation are present at birth in this rare genodermatosis.[110] They increase in size and number with age. Eventually a large percentage of the skin and mucous membranes becomes hyperpigmented.[110]

Histopathology[110]

The most striking change is an increase in melanin pigment within the epidermis, especially in the basal layer. There is some concentration at the tips of the rete ridges.

DYSCHROMATOSIS SYMMETRICA HEREDITARIA

This disorder, also known as reticulate acropigmentation of Dohi, consists of freckle-like lesions on the dorsum of the hands and feet with scattered depigmented macules in between.[101,102]

Histopathology

The epidermis shows increased pigmentation in the hyperpigmented areas and reduced pigmentation, sometimes accompanied by a reduction in the number of melanocytes, in hypopigmented areas.[102]

DYSCHROMATOSIS UNIVERSALIS

This is the prototype condition for a group of dyschromatoses characterized by areas of hypopigmentation and hyperpigmentation.[101] The absence of atrophy and telangiectasia distinguishes this group from the poikilodermas.[101] Onset is in early childhood, with involvement most prominent on the trunk and extremities. Clinical variants have been described.[111–113]

Histopathology

There is variable epidermal pigmentation which may be accompanied by some pigment incontinence. The number of melanocytes is sometimes reduced in the hypopigmented areas.[111]

PATTERNED HYPERMELANOSIS

This term is proposed for several rare dermatoses with overlapping features which have been reported in the past by different names. They are characterized by linear, whorled or reticulate areas of hyperpigmentation.[102] Although the term 'zosteriform' has been used to describe the pattern of the pigmentation in some of these cases, it has been pointed out that this term has not always been used correctly; the hyperpigmentation usually follows Blaschko's lines (the boundary lines separating areas of the skin subserved by different peripheral nerves) and not the courses of the nerves themselves as in a zosteriform pattern.[114]

Included in the patterned hypermelanoses are cases reported as 'linear and whorled nevoid hypermelanosis,'[114] 'reticulate hyperpigmentation distributed in a zosteriform fashion',[115] 'progressive cribriform and zosteriform hyperpigmentation',[116] 'zebra-like hyperpigmentation',[117] 'progressive zosteriform macular pigmented lesions'[118] and 'infant with abnormal pigmentation'.[119] The term patterned hypermelanosis is not applicable to well-defined entities such as incontinentia pigmenti and the reticulate acral pigmentations of Kitamura and of Dowling and Degos (see p. 315).

Histopathology

In all cases there has been an increase in melanin pigment in the basal layer. Pigment incontinence has been present in several cases.[118] A mild increase in the number of melanocytes, usually demonstrable only when quantitative studies are made, has been reported in a few cases.[114,117,119]

CHIMERISM

Chimerism results from double fertilization of an ovum producing an individual (a chimera) with differing sets of chromosomes.[120] Abnormalities of skin pigmentation, usually in the form of irregular areas of hyperpigmentation, are a rare manifestation of the chimeric state.[120]

Histopathology

Melanin is increased in the basal layers of the epidermis in the hyperpigmented lesions.[120]

MELASMA

Melasma (chloasma) refers to the symmetrical hyperpigmentation of the forehead and cheeks which develops in some women who are pregnant or taking oral contraceptives.[121,122] The hormonal basis for melasma is not understood.

Histopathology

There is increased melanin in the epidermis, particularly in the basal layers. Mild pigment incontinence is sometimes present.

EPHELIS (FRECKLE)

Ephelides (freckles) are small, well-defined pigmented macules 1–2 mm in diameter with a predilection for the face, arms and shoulder regions of fair-skinned individuals. They appear at an early age and may follow an episode of severe sunburn.

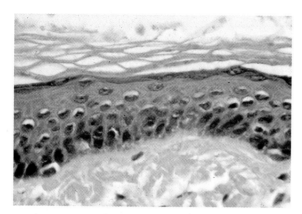

Fig. 10.4 Freckle (ephelis). Melanin is increased in the basal layers of the epidermis but melanocytes are normal in number and morphology. Haematoxylin — eosin

Histopathology

The epidermis appears normal in structure. The basal cells in the affected areas are more heavily pigmented with melanin than those in the surrounding skin, and there is usually sharp delimitation of the abnormal areas from the normal (Fig. 10.4). There are normal numbers of melanocytes.[123]

CAFÉ-AU-LAIT SPOTS

Café-au-lait spots are uniformly pigmented, tan to dark brown macules which vary in size from small, freckle-like lesions to large patches 20 cm or more in diameter. They may be present at birth or develop within the first few years of life.[124] They are found in approximately 15% of individuals.[125] They are not increased in patients with tuberous sclerosis, contrary to common belief.[126] Multiple café-au-lait spots are a feature of neurofibromatosis;[124] axillary freckling is often also present in these cases (see p. 927).

Histopathology

In haematoxylin and eosin preparations, the lesions resemble freckles, with basal hyperpigmentation but no apparent increase in the number of melanocytes. However, quantitative studies have shown a slight increase in melanocytes.[127]

Giant melanin granules (macromelanosomes), measuring up to 6 μm in diameter and recognizable on light microscopy, can be seen in café-au-lait spots in many patients with neurofibromatosis.[128] The diagnostic significance of macromelanosomes is diminished by their absence in some children with neurofibromatosis and their presence in normal skin and other pigmented macular lesions.[129–132]

MACULES OF ALBRIGHT'S SYNDROME

Albright's syndrome is characterized by the triad of polyostotic fibrous dysplasia, sexual precocity, especially in the female, and pigmented macules. These macules are large, often unilateral and related to the side of the bone lesions. The outline of the macules is very irregular in contrast to that of café-au-lait spots.

Histopathology

The lesions resemble freckles, showing hyperpigmentation of the basal layer. Rarely, macromelanosomes can be identified.[130]

PEUTZ–JEGHERS SYNDROME

This syndrome is characterized by the association of gastrointestinal polyposis with the presence of pigmented macules on the buccal mucosa, lips, perioral skin and sometimes the digits.

Histopathology

There is basal hyperpigmentation in the pigmented macules. There are conflicting views as to whether the melanocytes are quantitatively increased.[133,134]

BECKER'S NAEVUS

Becker's naevus (melanosis) is usually found in the region of the shoulder girdle of young men as unilateral, hyperpigmented areas of somewhat thickened skin.[131,135] Hypertrichosis may develop after the pigmentation but is not invariable. A Becker's naevus is usually acquired in adolescence, but a congenital onset has been recorded,[136] as have familial cases.[137] Occasionally, lesions have been said to follow severe sunburn. Lesional tissue has been found to have an increased level of androgen receptors, suggesting that heightened local androgen sensitivity may result in the hypertrichosis.[138] Various skeletal malformations have been reported in individuals with a Becker's naevus.[139,140] Other associations have included a connective tissue naevus[141] and an accessory scrotum.[142]

Histopathology

The epidermal changes are variable but usually there is acanthosis and sometimes mild papillomatous hyperplasia (Fig. 10.5). The changes may resemble those seen in an epidermal naevus (see p. 730).[131] There is variable hyperpigmentation of the basal layer with some melanophages in the dermis. Melanocyte proliferation is usually mild and not always obvious in routine sections; special studies have shown a quantitative increase.[143] There is sometimes an increase in the number and size of hair follicles and sebaceous glands. There may be smooth muscle hypertrophy of the arrectores pilorum as well as smooth muscle bundles in the dermis which are not related to cutaneous adnexa.[144,145] Controversy exists about the relationship of these cases to smooth muscle hamartoma (see p. 917).[146]

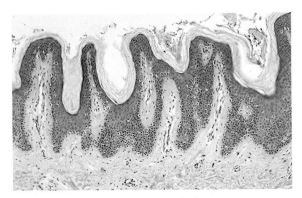

Fig. 10.5 Becker's naevus. The epidermis shows mild papillomatosis and basal hyperpigmentation. Haematoxylin — eosin

Electron microscopy. There is an increase in the number and size of melanosome complexes in the basal and prickle cells of the epidermis with an increase in the number of melanosomes in the complexes.[147] There are also many single collagen fibrils in the dermis.

DOWLING–DEGOS DISEASE

This condition, also known as reticulate pigmented anomaly of the flexures, is a rare autosomal dominant genodermatosis in which there are spotted and reticulate pigmented macules of the flexures.[148,149] Less constant features include pigmented pits in the perioral area, scattered comedo-like lesions and seborrhoeic keratoses.[148,150] The condition usually develops in early adult life, and is slowly progressive.[148]

It is now considered that Haber's disease,[151,152] in which there are rosacea-like facies and seborrhoeic-keratosis-like lesions, and reticulate acropigmentation of Kitamura,[153–156] in which there are reticulate, slightly depressed, pigmented macules on the extensor surface of the hands and feet in association with palmar 'pits', are different phenotypic expressions of the same genodermatosis.[157–160] A further related entity, characterized by reticulate pigmentation on the face and neck and epidermal cysts on the trunk, has been reported.[161]

Histopathology[148]

There are filiform downgrowths of the epidermis, and also of the variably dilated pilosebaceous follicles.[148,162] Small horn cysts and comedo-like lesions are also present. Hyperpigmentation is quite pronounced at the tips of the rete ridges. There is a superficial resemblance to the adenoid form of seborrhoeic keratosis (see p. 735) although the downgrowths are more digitate than in seborrhoeic keratosis, and there is no papillomatosis. In Kitamura's disease the appearances resemble those seen in a solar lentigo, with club-shaped elongations of the rete ridges but with intervening epidermal atrophy.[158,163]

Electron microscopy. Melanosomes are

markedly increased in keratinocytes, and these may be dispersed through the cytoplasm or loosely aggregated.[164,165] They are of normal size. Melanocytes are increased in number in Kitamura's variant.[163]

POST-INFLAMMATORY MELANOSIS

Hyperpigmentation may follow a number of inflammatory dermatoses, particularly those involving damage to the basal layer. Thus, it may follow various disorders that present a lichenoid reaction pattern, such as lichen planus, lichenoid drug eruptions and fixed drug eruptions. Prominent hyperpigmentation is almost invariable in the resolving phases of a phytophotodermatitis (see p. 579).

Histopathology

In addition to prominent melanin incontinence there may be normal or increased amounts of melanin in the basal layer of the epidermis. Basal pigmentation is prominent in phytophotodermatitis. If basal pigmentation is markedly reduced, the clinical appearance will be of hypopigmentation. There may also be occasional lymphocytes around vessels in the papillary dermis and a mild increase in fibroblasts and even collagen in the papillary dermis. There is usually no evidence of the underlying dermatosis which resulted in the area of pigmentation.

PRURIGO PIGMENTOSA

Prurigo pigmentosa is a pruritic dermatosis in which erythematous papules coalesce to form a reticulate pattern. This stage resolves within days, leaving a mottled or reticulate hyperpigmentation.[166–168] Most cases have been reported from Japan, leading to the suggestion that an environmental factor is responsible. Prurigo pigmentosa may be classed as a post-inflammatory melanosis.

Histopathology[166–168]

In the papular stage there is acanthosis, mild spongiosis, and exocytosis of lymphocytes, resulting in the death of isolated keratinocytes. That is, there is a lichenoid reaction pattern although the changes are not confined to the basal layer. The dermal infiltrate is predominantly perivascular and involves the superficial and mid dermis. A few eosinophils are included in the infiltrate. The published descriptions suggest a florid lichenoid drug reaction, but with a bizarre pattern.

In the late stages there is prominent melanin incontinence with numerous melanophages in the dermis.

GENERALIZED MELANOSIS IN MALIGNANT MELANOMA

Cutaneous pigmentation which is slate grey or bluish black in colour may rarely develop in patients with disseminated malignant melanoma (see page 801).[169,170] Although generalized, the pigmentation is often accentuated in areas exposed to the light.

The pathogenesis of the pigmentation is controversial.[170] It has been attributed to epidermal hyperpigmentation, the deposition of melanophages which have circulated in the blood, the presence of scattered melanoma cells within the dermis,[171] and the regression of dermal tumour cells.

Histopathology[170]

The usual finding is the presence of melanin pigment throughout the dermis in perivascular and interstitial melanophages and as free granules. A scant perivascular infiltrate of lymphocytes and sometimes plasma cells may be present. Individual melanoma cells are not usually present.

DERMATOPATHIA PIGMENTOSA RETICULARIS

This condition combines reticulate pigmentation

with nail dystrophy and partial alopecia.[172,172a] Macules of hypopigmentation may develop at a later stage. There are similarities to the Naegeli–Franceschetti–Jadassohn syndrome, although the associated features are different.

Histopathology

The hyperpigmented areas show conspicuous melanin incontinence.[172] The epidermis appears normal.

NAEGELI–FRANCESCHETTI–JADASSOHN SYNDROME

This extremely rare, autosomal dominant disorder combines dark brown, reticulate pigmentation of the trunk and limbs with diffuse or punctate hyperkeratosis of the palms and soles.[173] Hypohidrosis, enamel hypoplasia and nail dystrophy may also be present. Similar pigmentation was present in a case reported as 'hereditary diffuse hyperpigmentation' but there was no anhidrosis and the teeth were normal.[174]

Histopathology

Melanin is increased in the basal layers of the epidermis and there is prominent melanin incontinence.[173]

INCONTINENTIA PIGMENTI

Incontinentia pigmenti is an uncommon, multisystem genodermatosis with cutaneous, skeletal, ocular, neurological and dental abnormalities.[175,176] The cutaneous lesions evolve through vesiculobullous, verrucous and pigmentary stages, but in a small number of individuals pigmentation is the first manifestation. The vesiculobullous lesions, accompanied by erythematous areas, are present at birth or soon after, in a linear arrangement on the extremities and lateral aspects of the trunk. The verrucous lesions evolve some weeks or months later and resolve spontaneously to give atrophy, depigmentation or both. In the third stage, which has a peak onset from 3–6 months, there are streaks and whorls of brown to slate grey pigmentation, often asymmetrically distributed on the trunk and sometimes on the extremities.[176] The pigmentation, which is not necessarily in areas of the earlier lesions, progressively fades at about puberty. Areas of hypopigmentation may remain. Uncommonly, streaks of hypopigmentation are the predominant feature.[177]

Other cutaneous manifestations include alopecia, woolly hair naevus,[178] nail dystrophy, and painful subungual tumours which may involve several fingers and sometimes toes. These keratotic tumours have an onset in late adolescence and may involute spontaneously.[179,180] Several cases of incontinentia pigmenti have been associated with cancer in childhood.[181]

Incontinentia pigmenti is a chromosomal instability disorder which is inherited as an X-linked dominant gene that usually causes the death in utero of affected males.[178,181,182] The small number of males reported with the condition[183] may represent gene mutations.[176]

Several patients have had defects in neutrophil chemotaxis and lymphocyte function.[184–186] Leucotriene B_4 has been demonstrated in extracts of the crusted scales from vesiculobullous lesions, and this may have an important role in the chemotaxis of eosinophils into the epidermis.[187]

It has been postulated that the manifestations of incontinentia pigmenti can be explained as an autoimmune attack on ectodermal clones expressing an abnormal surface antigen,[188] or as premature (programmed) cell death in defective ectodermal clones.[189]

Histopathology

The first stage of incontinentia pigmenti is characterized by eosinophilic spongiosis; that is, spongiosis progressing to intraepidermal vesicle formation with prominent exocytosis of eosinophils into and around them (Fig. 10.6). A few basophils are also present.[190] The erythematous areas show only minimal spongiosis, but there is still prominent exocytosis of eosinophils. There are occasional dyskeratotic cells with eosinophilic hyaline cytoplasm in the epidermis

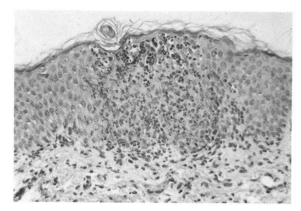

Fig. 10.6 Incontinentia pigmenti (first stage). Numerous eosinophils extend into the epidermis. Spongiosis is mild in this field.
Haematoxylin — eosin

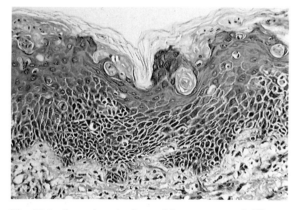

Fig. 10.7 Incontinentia pigmenti (verrucous stage). There are many dyskeratotic cells within the epidermis.
Haematoxylin — eosin

adjacent to the vesicles.[178] The superficial dermis contains an infiltrate of eosinophils and some mononuclear cells.

In the verrucous stage, there are hyperkeratosis, acanthosis, mild irregular papillomatosis and numerous dyskeratotic cells (Fig. 10.7). Some macrophages migrate into the epidermis, and on electron microscopy these have been shown to phagocytose the dyskeratotic cells as well as melanosomes. Inflammatory cells are quite sparse. In the third stage there is pronounced melanin incontinence. Pale scarred areas may be found on the lower part of the legs; these show a

reduction in the number of melanocytes and some increase in dermal collagen.[191]

The subungual lesions show hyperkeratosis, verrucous or pseudoepitheliomatous hyperplasia, and dyskeratotic cells at all levels of the epidermis.[179,180] Neighbouring keratinocytes may form whorls around the dyskeratotic cells.

Electron microscopy. This shows that some of the dyskeratotic cells have masses of loosely arranged tonofilaments, although most have clumped, electron-dense tonofilaments.[192] Pigment incontinence appears to result from phagocytosis of melanosomes by macrophages.[193,194]

FRICTIONAL MELANOSIS

Localized hyperpigmentation may develop at sites of chronic friction.[195] This condition must be distinguished from macular amyloidosis which clinically it resembles.

Histopathology

A prominent feature is the presence in the upper dermis of melanin, most of which is contained in melanophages.[195] Vacuolar change and scattered degenerate keratinocytes have also been noted in some cases.[195]

NOTALGIA PARAESTHETICA

This condition is a sensory neuropathy involving the posterior primary rami of thoracic nerves T2 to T6, and presenting as a localized area of pruritus of the back.[196] The affected region is sometimes lightly pigmented and composed of groups of small tan macules. Similar cases have been reported in the literature as 'peculiar spotty pigmentation'[197] and 'idiopathic pigmentation of the upper back'.[198] Clinically, notalgia paraesthetica resembles macular amyloidosis, a condition which in one report required ultrastructural examination to confirm the presence of amyloid, as histochemical tests were negative.[199]

Histopathology

There is melanin pigment in macrophages in the upper dermis, sometimes accompanied by mild hyperpigmentation of the basal layer.[198] In one reported case, scattered degenerate keratinocytes were present in all layers of the epidermis.[196]

'RIPPLE' PIGMENTATION OF THE NECK

Although 'ripple' pigmentation is usually regard-ed as a feature of macular amyloidosis, it has also been described on the neck in nearly 2% of individuals with atopic dermatitis of long standing.[200,201]

Histopathology

The most prominent feature is the presence of melanin in the upper dermis, both free and in macrophages.[200] An increase in melanocytes with associated mild vacuolar change in the basal layer has been an inconstant feature.[201]

REFERENCES

Introduction

1. Bolognia JL, Pawelek JM. Biology of hypopigmentation. J Am Acad Dermatol 1988; 19: 217–255.

Disorders characterized by hypopigmentation

2. Cole GW, Barr RJ. Hypomelanosis associated with a colonic abnormality. A possible result of defective development of the neural crest. Am J Dermatopathol 1987; 9: 45–50.
3. Cole LA. Hypopigmentation with punctate keratosis of the palms and soles. Arch Dermatol 1976; 112: 998–1000.
4. Jablonska S, Stachow A, Suffczynska M. Skin and muscle indurations in phenylketonuria. Arch Dermatol 1967; 95: 443–450.
5. Mosher DB, Fitzpatrick TB. Piebaldism. Arch Dermatol 1988; 124: 364–365.
5a. Fukai K, Hamada T, Ishii M et al. Acquired pigmented macules in human piebald lesions. Ultrastructure of melanocytes in hypomelanotic skin. Acta Derm Venereol 1989; 69: 524–527.
6. Mahakrishnan A, Srinivasan MS. Piebaldism with Hirschsprung's disease. Arch Dermatol 1980; 116: 1102.
7. Reed WB, Stone VM, Boder E, Ziprkowski L. Pigmentary disorders in association with congenital deafness. Arch Dermatol 1967; 95: 176–186.
8. Perrot H, Ortonne J-P, Thivolet J. Ultrastructural study of leukodermic skin in Waardenburg–Klein syndrome. Acta Derm Venereol 1977; 57: 195–200.
9. Ortonne J-P. Piebaldism, Waardenburg's syndrome, and related disorders. "Neural crest depigmentation syndromes"? Dermatol Clin 1988; 6: 205–216.
10. Selmanowitz VJ. Pigmentary correction of piebaldism by autografts. II. Pathomechanism and pigment spread in piebaldism. Cutis 1979; 24: 66–73.
11. Comings DE, Odland GF. Partial albinism. JAMA 1966; 195: 519–523.
12. Hayashibe K, Mishima Y. Tyrosinase-positive melanocyte distribution and induction of pigmentation in human piebald skin. Arch Dermatol 1988; 124: 381–386.
13. Koranne RV, Sachdeva KG. Vitiligo. Int J Dermatol 1988; 27: 676–681.
14. Nordlund JJ, Lerner AB. Vitiligo. It is important. Arch Dermatol 1982; 118: 5–8.
15. Sharquie KE. Vitiligo. Clin Exp Dermatol 1984; 9: 117–126.
16. Halder RM, Grimes PE, Cowan CA et al. Childhood vitiligo. J Am Acad Dermatol 1987; 16: 948–954.
17. Koga M. Vitiligo: a new classification and therapy. Br J Dermatol 1977; 97: 255–261.
18. Koga M, Tango T. Clinical features and course of type A and type B vitiligo. Br J Dermatol 1988; 118: 223–228.
19. Gould IM, Gray RS, Urbaniak SJ et al. Vitiligo in diabetes mellitus. Br J Dermatol 1985; 113: 153–155.
20. Macaron C, Winter RJ, Traisman HS et al. Vitiligo and juvenile diabetes mellitus. Arch Dermatol 1977; 113: 1515–1517.
21. Grimes PE, Halder RM, Jones C et al. Autoantibodies and their clinical significance in a black vitiligo population. Arch Dermatol 1983; 119: 300–303.
22. Saihan EM, Peachey RDG. Vitiligo and morphoea. Clin Exp Dermatol 1979; 4: 103–106.
23. Monroe EW. Vitiligo associated with regional enteritis. Arch Dermatol 1976; 112: 833–834.
24. McPoland PR, Moss RL. Cutaneous Crohn's disease and progressive vitiligo. J Am Acad Dermatol 1988; 19: 421–425.
25. Howanitz N, Nordlund JL, Lerner AB, Bystryn J-C. Antibodies to melanocytes. Occurrence in patients with vitiligo and chronic mucocutaneous candidiasis. Arch Dermatol 1981; 117: 705–708.
26. Henderson CD, Tschen JA, Schaefer DG. Simultaneously active lesions of vitiligo and erythema dyschromicum perstans. Arch Dermatol 1988; 124: 1258–1260.
27. Cowan CL Jr, Halder RM, Grimes PE et al. Ocular disturbances in vitiligo. J Am Acad Dermatol 1986; 15: 17–24.

28. Barnes L. Vitiligo and the Vogt–Koyanagi–Harada syndrome. Dermatol Clin 1988; 6: 229–239.

29. Lerner AB, Kirkwood JM. Vitiligo and melanoma: Can genetically abnormal melanocytes result in both vitiligo and melanoma within a single family? J Am Acad Dermatol 1984; 11: 696–701.

30. Bystryn J-C, Rigel D, Friedman RJ, Kopf A. Prognostic significance of hypopigmentation in malignant melanoma. Arch Dermatol 1987; 123: 1053–1055.

31. Nordlund JJ. Hypopigmentation, vitiligo, and melanoma. New data, more enigmas. Arch Dermatol 1987; 123: 1005–1008.

32. Ghoneum M, Grimes PE, Gill G, Kelly AP. Natural cell-mediated cytotoxicity in vitiligo. J Am Acad Dermatol 1987; 17: 600–605.

33. Grimes PE, Ghoneum M, Stockton T et al. T cell profiles in vitiligo. J Am Acad Dermatol 1986; 14: 196–201.

34. Halder RM, Walters CS, Johnson BA et al. Aberrations in T lymphocytes and natural killer cells in vitiligo: A flow cytometric study. J Am Acad Dermatol 1986; 14: 733–737.

34a. Mozzanica N, Frigerio U, Finzi AF et al. T cell subpopulations in vitiligo: A chronobiologic study. J Am Acad Dermatol 1990; 22: 223–230.

35. Mozzanica N, Frigerio U, Negri M et al. Circadian rhythm of natural killer cell activity in vitiligo. J Am Acad Dermatol 1989; 20: 591–596.

36. Naughton GK, Eisinger M, Bystryn J-C. Detection of antibodies to melanocytes in vitiligo by specific immunoprecipitation. J Invest Dermatol 1983; 81: 540–542.

37. Naughton GK, Reggiardo D, Bystryn J-C. Correlation between vitiligo antibodies and extent of depigmentation in vitiligo. J Am Acad Dermatol 1986; 15: 978–981.

38. Takei M, Mishima Y, Uda H. Immunopathology of vitiligo vulgaris, Sutton's leukoderma and melanoma-associated vitiligo in relation to steroid effects. I. Circulating antibodies for cultured melanoma cells. J Cutan Pathol 1984; 11: 107–113.

39. Uehara M, Miyauchi H, Tanaka S. Diminished contact sensitivity response in vitiliginous skin. Arch Dermatol 1984; 120: 195–198.

40. Hatchome N, Aiba S, Kato T et al. Possible functional impairment of Langerhans' cells in vitiliginous skin. Arch Dermatol 1987; 123: 51–54.

41. Beck H-I, Schmidt H. Graft exchange in vitiligo. Acta Derm Venereol 1986; 66: 311–315.

42. Falabella R, Escobar C, Borrero I. Transplantation of in vitro-cultured epidermis bearing melanocytes for repigmenting vitiligo. J Am Acad Dermatol 1989; 21: 257–264.

43. Lerner AB. Repopulation of pigment cells in patients with vitiligo. Arch Dermatol 1988; 124: 1701–1702.

44. Lerner AB, Shiohara T, Boissy RE et al. A mouse model for vitiligo. J Invest Dermatol 1986; 87: 299–304.

45. Gilhar A, Pillar T, Eidelman S, Etzioni A. Vitiligo and idiopathic guttate hypomelanosis. Repigmentation of skin following engraftment onto nude mice. Arch Dermatol 1989; 125: 1363–1366.

46. Mathias CGT, Maibach HI, Conant MA. Perioral leukoderma simulating vitiligo from use of a toothpaste containing cinnamic aldehyde. Arch Dermatol 1980; 116: 1172–1173.

47. Todes-Taylor N, Abel EA, Cox AJ. The occurrence of vitiligo after psoralens and ultraviolet A therapy. J Am Acad Dermatol 1983; 9: 526–532.

48. Falabella R, Escobar CE, Carrascal E, Arroyave JA. Leukoderma punctata. J Am Acad Dermatol 1988; 18: 485–494.

49. Gopinathan T. A study of the lesion of vitiligo. Arch Dermatol 1965; 91: 397–404.

50. Kumakiri M, Kimura T, Miura Y, Tagawa Y. Vitiligo with an inflammatory erythema in Vogt–Koyanagi–Harada disease: demonstration of filamentous masses and amyloid deposits. J Cutan Pathol 1982; 9: 258–266.

51. Bhawan J, Bhutani LK. Keratinocyte damage in vitiligo. J Cutan Pathol 1983; 10: 207–212.

52. Gokhale BB, Mehta LN. Histopathology of vitiliginous skin. Int J Dermatol 1983; 22: 477–480.

53. Morohashi M, Hashimoto K, Goodman TF Jr et al. Ultrastructural studies of vitiligo, Vogt–Koyanagi syndrome, and incontinentia pigmenti achromians. Arch Dermatol 1977; 113: 755–766.

54. Moellmann G, Klein-Angerer S, Scollay DA et al. Extracellular granular material and degeneration of keratinocytes in the normally pigmented epidermis of patients with vitiligo. J Invest Dermatol 1982; 79: 321–330.

55. King RA, Summers CG. Albinism. Dermatol Clin 1988; 6: 217–228.

56. King RA, Olds DP. Hairbulb tyrosinase activity in oculocutaneous albinism: suggestions for pathway control and block location. Am J Med Genet 1985; 20: 49–55.

57. King RA, Wirtschafter JD, Olds DP, Brumbaugh J. Minimal pigment: a new type of oculocutaneous albinism. Clin Genet 1986; 29: 42–50.

58. Okoro AN. Albinism in Nigeria. A clinical and social study. Br J Dermatol 1975; 92: 485–492.

59. Levin DL, Roth DE, Muhlbauer JE. Sporadic dysplastic nevus syndrome in a tyrosinase-positive oculocutaneous albino. J Am Acad Dermatol 1988; 19: 393–396.

59a. Schachne JP, Glaser N, Lee S et al. Hermansky–Pudlak syndrome: Case report and clinicopathologic review. J Am Acad Dermatol 1990; 22: 926–932.

60. King RA, Olds DP, Witkop CJ. Characterization of human hair bulb tyrosinase: Properties of normal and albino enzyme. J Invest Dermatol 1978; 71: 136–139.

61. Blume RS, Wolff SM. The Chediak–Higashi syndrome: studies in four patients and a review of the literature. Medicine (Baltimore) 1972; 51: 247–280.

62. Barak Y, Nir E. Chediak–Higashi syndrome. Am J Pediatr Hematol Oncol 1987; 9: 42–55.

63. Bedoya V. Pigmentary changes in Chediak–Higashi syndrome. Microscopic study of 12 homozygous and heterozygous subjects. Br J Dermatol 1971; 85: 336–347.

64. White JG, Clawson CC. The Chediak–Higashi syndrome: The nature of the giant neutrophil granules and their interactions with cytoplasm and foreign particulates. Am J Pathol 1980; 98: 151–196.

65. Moran TJ, Estevez JM. Chediak–Higashi disease. Morphologic studies of a patient and her family. Arch Pathol 1969; 88: 329–339.

66. Zelickson AS, Windhorst DB, White JG, Good RA. The Chediak–Higashi syndrome: Formation of giant melanosomes and the basis of hypopigmentation. J Invest Dermatol 1967; 49: 575–581.

66a. Carrillo-Farga J, Gutierrez-Palomera G, Ruiz-Maldonado R et al. Giant cytoplasmic granules in Langerhans cells in Chediak–Higashi syndrome. Am J Dermatopathol 1990; 12: 81–87.

67. Guillet G, Helenon R, Gauthier Y et al. Progressive macular hypomelanosis of the trunk: primary acquired hypopigmentation. J Cutan Pathol 1988; 15: 286–289.

68. Fitzpatrick TB, Szabo G, Hori Y et al. White leaf-shaped macules. Earliest visible sign of tuberous sclerosis. Arch Dermatol 1968; 98: 1–6.

69. Jimbow K, Fitzpatrick TB, Szabo G, Hori Y. Congenital circumscribed hypomelanosis: a characterization based on electron microscopic study of tuberous sclerosis, nevus depigmentosus, and piebaldism. J Invest Dermatol 1975; 64: 50–62.

70. Whitehead WJ, Moyer DG, Vander Ploeg DE. Idiopathic guttate hypomelanosis. Arch Dermatol 1966; 94: 279–281.

71. Hamada T, Saito T. Senile depigmented spots (idiopathic guttate hypomelanosis). Arch Dermatol 1967; 95: 665.

72. Falabella R, Escobar C, Giraldo N et al. On the pathogenesis of idiopathic guttate hypomelanosis. J Am Acad Dermatol 1987; 16: 35–44.

73. Falabella R. Idiopathic guttate hypomelanosis. Dermatol Clin 1988; 6: 241–247.

74. Wilson PD, Lavker RM, Kligman AM. On the nature of idiopathic guttate hypomelanosis. Acta Derm Venereol 1982; 62: 301–306.

75. Cummings KI, Cottel WI. Idiopathic guttate hypomelanosis. Arch Dermatol 1966; 93: 184–186.

76. Ortonne J-P, Perrot H. Idiopathic guttate hypomelanosis. Arch Dermatol 1980; 116: 664–668.

77. Savall R, Ferrandiz C, Ferrer I, Peyri J. Idiopathic guttate hypomelanosis. Br J Dermatol 1980; 103: 635–642.

78. Buzas JW, Sina B, Burnett JW. Hypomelanosis of Ito. Report of a case and review of the literature. J Am Acad Dermatol 1981; 4: 195–204.

78a. Sybert VP. Hypomelanosis of Ito. Pediatr Dermatol 1990; 7: 74–76.

79. Takematsu H, Sato S, Igarashi M, Seiji M. Incontinentia pigmenti acromians (Ito). Arch Dermatol 1983; 119: 391–395.

80. Hamada T, Saito T, Sugai T, Morita Y. "Incontinentia pigmenti acromians (Ito)". Arch Dermatol 1967; 96: 673–676.

81. Jelinek JE, Bart RS, Schiff GM. Hypomelanosis of Ito ("Incontinentia pigmenti achromians"). Report of three cases and review of the literature. Arch Dermatol 1973; 107: 596–601.

82. Griffiths A, Payne C. Incontinentia pigmenti achromians. Arch Dermatol 1975; 111: 751–752.

83. Mittal R, Handa F, Sharma SC. Incontinentia pigmenti et achromians. Dermatologica 1975; 150: 355–359.

84. Rubin MB. Incontinentia pigmenti achromians. Multiple cases within a family. Arch Dermatol 1972; 105: 424–425.

85. Nordlund JJ, Klaus SN, Gino J. Hypomelanosis of Ito. Acta Derm Venereol 1977; 57: 261–264.

86. Hellgren L. Incontinentia pigmenti achromians (Ito). Acta Derm Venereol 1975; 55: 237–240.

87. Maize JC, Headington JT, Lynch PJ. Systematized hypochromic nevus. Incontinentia pigmenti achromians of Ito. Arch Dermatol 1972; 106: 884–885.

88. Pena L, Ruiz-Maldonado R, Tamayo L et al. Incontinentia pigmenti achromians (Ito's hypomelanosis). Int J Dermatol 1977; 16: 194–202.

89. Coupe RL. Unilateral systematized achromic naevus. Dermatologica 1967; 134: 19–35.

90. Hanifin JM. Clinical and basic aspects of atopic dermatitis. Semin Dermatol 1983; 2: 5–19.

91. Zaynoun ST, Aftimos BG, Tenekjian KK et al. Extensive pityriasis alba: a histological histochemical and ultrastructural study. Br J Dermatol 1983; 108: 83–90.

92. Zaynoun S, Jaber LAA, Kurban AK. Oral methoxsalen photochemotherapy of extensive pityriasis alba. J Am Acad Dermatol 1986; 15: 61–65.

93. Weedon D. Unpublished observations.

94. Wells BT, Whyte HJ, Kierland RR. Pityriasis alba. A ten-year survey and review of the literature. Arch Dermatol 1960; 82: 183–189.

95. Mountcastle EA, Diestelmeier MR, Lupton GP. Nevus anemicus. J Am Acad Dermatol 1986; 14: 628–632.

96. Daniel RH, Hubler WR Jr, Wolf JE Jr, Holder WR. Nevus anemicus. Donor-dominant defect. Arch Dermatol 1977; 113: 53–56.

97. Mandal SB, Dutta AK. Pathophysiology of nevus anemicus. JCE Dermatol 1978; 16(4): 13–18.

98. Fleisher TL. Nevus anemicus. Arch Dermatol 1969; 100: 750–755.

99. Greaves MW, Birkett D, Johnson C. Nevus anemicus: a unique catecholamine-dependent nevus. Arch Dermatol 1970; 102: 172–176.

100. Davies MG, Greaves MW, Coutts A, Black AK. Nevus oligemicus. A variant of nevus anemicus. Arch Dermatol 1981; 117: 111–113.

Disorders characterized by hyperpigmentation

101. Fulk CS. Primary disorders of hyperpigmentation. J Am Acad Dermatol 1984; 10: 1–16.

102. Griffiths WAD. Reticulate pigmentary disorders — a review. Clin Exp Dermatol 1984; 9: 439–450.

103. Westerhof W, Beemer FA, Cormane RH et al. Hereditary congenital hypopigmented and hyperpigmented macules. Arch Dermatol 1978; 114: 931–936.

104. Samuel C, Bird DR, Burton JL. Hyperpigmentation after sympathectomy. Clin Exp Dermatol 1980; 5: 349–350.

105. Shelley WB, Shelley ED. The skin changes in the Crow–Fukase (POEMS) syndrome. Arch Dermatol 1987; 123: 85–87.

106. Marks VJ, Briggaman RA, Wheeler CE Jr. Hyperpigmentation in megaloblastic anaemia. J Am Acad Dermatol 1985; 12: 914–917.

107. Lee SH, Lee WS, Whang KC et al. Hyperpigmentation in megaloblastic anemia. Int J Dermatol 1988; 27: 571–575.

108. Ruiz-Maldonado R, Tamayo L, Fernandez-Diez J.

Universal acquired melanosis. The carbon baby. Arch Dermatol 1978; 114: 775–778.

109. Gonzalez JR, Botet MV. Acromelanosis. A case report. J Am Acad Dermatol 1980; 2: 128–131.

110. Chernosky ME, Anderson DE, Chang JP. Familial progressive hyperpigmentation. Arch Dermatol 1971; 103: 581–598.

111. Foldes C, Wallach D, Launay J-M, Chirio R. Congenital dyschromia with erythrocyte, platelet, and tryptophan metabolism abnormalities. J Am Acad Dermatol 1988; 19: 642–655.

112. Petrozzi JW. Unusual dyschromia in a malnourished infant. Arch Dermatol 1971; 103: 515–519.

113. Rycroft RJG, Calnan CD, Wells RS. Universal dyschromatosis, small stature and high-tone deafness. Clin Exp Dermatol 1977; 2: 45–48.

114. Kalter DC, Griffiths WA, Atherton DJ. Linear and whorled nevoid hypermelanosis. J Am Acad Dermatol 1988; 19: 1037–1044.

115. Iijima S, Naito Y, Naito S, Uyeno K. Reticulate hyperpigmentation distributed in a zosteriform fashion: a new clinical type of hyperpigmentation. Br J Dermatol 1987; 117: 503–510.

116. Rower JM, Carr RD, Lowney ED. Progressive cribriform and zosteriform hyperpigmentation. Arch Dermatol 1978; 114: 98–99.

117. Alimurung FM, Lapenas D, Willis I, Lang P. Zebra-like hyperpigmentation in an infant with multiple congenital defects. Arch Dermatol 1979; 115: 878–881.

118. Simoes GA. Progressive zosteriform macular pigmented lesions. Arch Dermatol 1980; 116: 20.

119. Ment L, Alper J, Sirota RL, Holmes LB. Infant with abnormal pigmentation, malformations, and immune deficiency. Arch Dermatol 1978; 114: 1043–1044.

120. Findlay GH, Moores PP. Pigment anomalies of the skin in the human chimaera: their relation to systematized naevi. Br J Dermatol 1980; 103: 489–498.

121. Kovacs G, Marks R. Contraception and the skin. Australas J Dermatol 1987; 28: 86–92.

122. Jelinek JE. Cutaneous side effects of oral contraceptives. Arch Dermatol 1970; 101: 181–186.

123. Breathnach AS. Melanocyte distribution in forearm epidermis of freckled human subjects. J Invest Dermatol 1957; 29: 253–261.

124. Riccardi VM. Von Recklinghausen neurofibromatosis. N Engl J Med 1981; 305: 1617–1627.

125. Kopf AW, Levine LJ, Rigel DS et al. Prevalence of congenital-nevus-like nevi, nevi spili, and café-au-lait spots. Arch Dermatol 1985; 121: 766–769.

126. Bell SD, MacDonald DM. The prevalence of café-au-lait patches in tuberous sclerosis. Clin Exp Dermatol 1985; 10: 562–565.

127. Johnson BL, Charneco DR. Café au lait spot in neurofibromatosis and in normal individuals. Arch Dermatol 1970; 102: 442–446.

128. Jimbow K, Szabo G, Fitzpatrick TB. Ultrastructure of giant pigment granules (macromelanosomes) in the cutaneous pigmented macules of neurofibromatosis. J Invest Dermatol 1973; 61: 300–309.

129. Silvers DN, Greenwood RS, Helwig EB. Café au lait spots without giant pigment granules. Occurrence in suspected neurofibromatosis. Arch Dermatol 1974; 110: 87–88.

130. Benedict PH, Szabo G, Fitzpatrick TB, Sinesi SJ. Melanotic macules in Albright's syndrome and in neurofibromatosis. JAMA 1968; 205: 618–626.

131. Bhawan J, Chang WH. Becker's melanosis. Dermatologica 1979; 159: 221–230.

132. Bhawan J, Purtilo DT, Riordan JA et al. Giant and "granular melanosomes" in leopard syndrome: an ultrastructural study. J Cutan Pathol 1976; 3: 207–216.

133. Blank AA, Schneider BV, Panizzon R. Pigmentfleckenpolypose (Peutz-Jeghers-Syndrom). Hautarzt 1981; 32: 296–300.

134. Yamada K, Matsukawa A, Hori Y, Kukita A. Ultrastructural studies on pigmented macules of Peutz–Jeghers syndrome. J Dermatol 1981; 8: 367–377.

135. Becker SW. Concurrent melanosis and hypertrichosis in distribution of nevus unius lateris. Arch Dermatol Syph 1949; 60: 155–160.

136. Picascia DD, Esterly NB. Congenital Becker's melanosis. Int J Dermatol 1989; 28: 127–128.

137. Jain HC, Fisher BK. Familial Becker's nevus. Int J Dermatol 1989; 28: 263–264.

138. Person JR, Longcope C. Becker's nevus: An androgen-mediated hyperplasia with increased androgen receptors. J Am Acad Dermatol 1984; 10: 235–238.

139. Glinick SE, Alper JC, Bogaars H, Brown JA. Becker's melanosis: Associated abnormalities. J Am Acad Dermatol 1983; 9: 509–514.

140. Moore JA, Schosser RH. Becker's melanosis and hypoplasia of the breast and pectoralis major muscle. Pediatr Dermatol 1985; 3: 34–37.

141. Fenske NA, Donelan PA. Becker's nevus coexistent with connective-tissue nevus. Arch Dermatol 1984; 120: 1347–1350.

142. Szylit J-A, Grossman ME, Luyando Y et al. Becker's nevus and an accessory scrotum. A unique occurrence. J Am Acad Dermatol 1986; 14: 905–907.

143. Tate PR, Hodge SJ, Owen LG. A quantitative study of melanocytes in Becker's nevus. J Cutan Pathol 1980; 7: 404–409.

144. Urbanek RW, Johnson WC. Smooth muscle hamartoma associated with Becker's nevus. Arch Dermatol 1978; 114: 104–106.

145. Haneke E. The dermal component of melanosis naeviformis Becker. J Cutan Pathol 1979; 6: 53–58.

146. Glinick SE, Alper JA. Spectrum of Becker's melanosis changes is greater than believed. Arch Dermatol 1986; 122: 375.

147. Frenk E, Delacretaz J. Zur Ultrastruktur der Becker schen Melanose. Hautarzt 1970; 21: 397–400.

148. Wilson Jones E, Grice K. Reticulate pigmented anomaly of the flexures. Dowling Degos disease, a new genodermatosis. Arch Dermatol 1978; 114: 1150–1157.

149. Crovato F, Nazzari G, Rebora A. Dowling–Degos disease (reticulate pigmented anomaly of the flexures) is an autosomal dominant condition. Br J Dermatol 1983; 108: 473–476.

150. Boyle J, Burton JL. Reticulate pigmented anomaly of the flexures and seborrhoeic warts. Clin Exp Dermatol 1985; 10: 379–383.

151. Seiji M, Otaki N. Haber's syndrome. Familial rosacea-like dermatosis with keratotic plaques and

pitted scars. Arch Dermatol 1971; 103: 452–455.

152. Kikuchi I, Saita B, Inoue S. Haber's syndrome. Report of a new family. Arch Dermatol 1981; 117: 321–324.

153. Woodley DT, Caro I, Wheeler CE Jr. Reticulate acropigmentation of Kitamura. Arch Dermatol 1979; 115: 760–761.

154. Griffiths WAD. Reticulate acropigmentation of Kitamura. Br J Dermatol 1976; 95: 437–443.

154a. Kanwar AJ, Kaur S, Rajagopalan M. Reticulate acropigmentation of Kitamura. Int J Dermatol 1990; 29: 217–219.

155. Griffiths WAD. Reticulate pigmentary disorders — a review. Clin Exp Dermatol 1984; 9: 439–450.

156. Berth-Jones J, Graham-Brown RAC. A family with Dowling Degos disease showing features of Kitamura's reticulate acropigmentation. Br J Dermatol 1989; 120: 463–466.

157. Crovato F, Desirello G, Rebora A. Is Dowling–Degos disease the same disease as Kitamura's reticulate acropigmentation? Br J Dermatol 1983; 109: 105–110.

158. Rebora A, Crovato F. The spectrum of Dowling–Degos disease. Br J Dermatol 1984; 110: 627–630.

159. Crovato F, Rebora A. Reticulate pigmented anomaly of the flexures associating reticulate acropigmentation: One single entity. J Am Acad Dermatol 1986; 14: 359–361.

160. Kikuchi I, Crovato F, Rebora A. Haber's syndrome and Dowling–Degos disease. Int J Dermatol 1988; 27: 96–97.

161. Hori Y, Kubota Y. Pigmentatio reticularis faciei et colli with multiple epithelial cysts. Arch Dermatol 1985; 121: 109–111.

162. Howell JB, Freeman RG. Reticular pigmented anomaly of the flexures. Arch Dermatol 1978; 114: 400–403.

163. Mizoguchi M, Kukita A. Behavior of melanocytes in reticulate acropigmentation of Kitamura. Arch Dermatol 1985; 121: 659–661.

164. Grosshans E, Geiger JM, Hanau D et al. Ultrastructure of early pigmentary changes in Dowling–Degos' disease. J Cutan Pathol 1980; 7: 77–87.

165. Brown WG. Reticulate pigmented anomaly of the flexures. Case reports and genetic investigation. Arch Dermatol 1982; 118: 490–493.

166. Cox NH. Prurigo pigmentosa. Br J Dermatol 1987; 117: 121–124.

167. Joyce AP, Horn TD, Anhalt GJ. Prurigo pigmentosa. Report of a case and review of the literature. Arch Dermatol 1989; 125: 1551–1554.

168. Shimizu H, Yamasaki Y, Harada T, Nishikawa T. Prurigo pigmentosa. Case report with an electron microscopic observation. J Am Acad Dermatol 1985; 12: 165–169.

169. Silverberg I, Kopf AW, Gumport SL. Diffuse melanosis in malignant melanoma. Arch Dermatol 1968; 97: 671–677.

170. Sexton M, Snyder CR. Generalized melanosis in occult primary melanoma. J Am Acad Dermatol 1989; 20: 261–266.

171. Schuler G, Honigsman H, Wolff K. Diffuse melanosis in metastatic melanoma. Further evidence for disseminated single cell metastases in the skin. J Am Acad Dermatol 1980; 3: 363–369.

172. Rycroft RJG, Calnan CD, Allenby CF. Dermatopathia pigmentosa reticularis. Clin Exp Dermatol 1977; 2: 39–44.

172a. Maso MJ, Schwartz RA, Lambert WC. Dermatopathia pigmentosa reticularis. Arch Dermatol 1990; 126: 935–939.

173. Sparrow GP, Samman PD, Wells RS. Hyperpigmentation and hypohidrosis. (The Naegeli–Franceschetti–Jadassohn syndrome): report of a family and review of the literature. Clin Exp Dermatol 1976; 1: 127–140.

174. Verbov J. Hereditary diffuse hyperpigmentation. Clin Exp Dermatol 1980; 5: 227–234.

175. Carney RG, Carney RG Jr. Incontinentia pigmenti. Arch Dermatol 1970; 102: 157–162.

176. Carney RG Jr. Incontinentia pigmenti. A world statistical analysis. Arch Dermatol 1976; 112: 535–542.

177. Moss C, Ince P. Anhidrotic and achromians lesions in incontinentia pigmenti. Br J Dermatol 1987; 116: 839–849.

178. Wiklund DA, Weston WL. Incontinentia pigmenti. A four-generation study. Arch Dermatol 1980; 116: 701–703.

179. Mascaro JM, Palou J, Vives P. Painful subungual keratotic tumors in incontinentia pigmenti. J Am Acad Dermatol 1985; 13: 913–918.

180. Simmons DA, Kegel MF, Scher RK, Hines YC. Subungual tumors in incontinentia pigmenti. Arch Dermatol 1986; 122: 1431–1434.

181. Roberts WM, Jenkins JJ, Moorhead EL II, Douglass EC. Incontinentia pigmenti, a chromosomal instability syndrome, is associated with childhood malignancy. Cancer 1988; 62: 2370–2372.

182. Bjellerup M. Incontinentia pigmenti with dental anomalies: a three-generation study. Acta Derm Venereol 1982; 62: 262–264.

183. Bargman HB, Wyse C. Incontinentia pigmenti in a 21-year-old man. Arch Dermatol 1975; 111: 1606–1608.

184. Jessen RT, Van Epps DE, Goodwin JS, Bowerman J. Incontinentia pigmenti. Evidence for both neutrophil and lymphocyte dysfunction. Arch Dermatol 1978; 114: 1182–1186.

185. Dahl MV, Matula G, Leonards R, Tuffanelli DL. Incontinentia pigmenti and defective neutrophil chemotaxis. Arch Dermatol 1975; 111: 1603–1605.

186. Menni S, Piccinno R, Biolchini A et al. Incontinentia pigmenti and Behcet's syndrome: an unusual combination. Acta Derm Venereol 1986; 66: 351–354.

187. Takematsu H, Terui T, Torinuki W, Tagami H. Incontinentia pigmenti: eosinophil chemotactic activity of the crusted scales in the vesiculobullous stage. Br J Dermatol 1986; 115: 61–66.

188. Person JR. Incontinentia pigmenti: a failure of immune tolerance? J Am Acad Dermatol 1985; 13: 120–124.

189. Wilkin JK. Response. J Am Acad Dermatol 1985; 13: 123–124.

190. Schmalstieg FC, Jorizzo JL, Tschen J, Subrt P. Basophils in incontinentia pigmenti. J Am Acad Dermatol 1984; 10: 362–364.

191. Ashley JR, Burgdorf WHC. Incontinentia pigmenti: pigmentary changes independent of incontinence. J Cutan Pathol 1987; 14: 248–250.

192. Schamburg-Lever G, Lever WF. Electron microscopy of incontinentia pigmenti. J Invest Dermatol 1973; 61: 151–158.
193. Caputo R, Gianotti F, Innocenti M. Ultrastructural findings in incontinentia pigmenti. Int J Dermatol 1975; 14: 46–55.
194. Guerrier CJW, Wong CK. Ultrastructural evolution of the skin in incontinentia pigmenti (Bloch–Sulzberger). Dermatologica 1974; 149: 10–22.
195. Magana-Garcia M, Carrasco E, Herrera-Goepfert R, Pueblitz-Peredo S. Hyperpigmentation of the clavicular zone: a variant of friction melanosis. Int J Dermatol 1989; 28: 119–122.
196. Weber PJ, Poulos EG. Notalgia paresthetica. Case reports and histologic appraisal. J Am Acad Dermatol 1988; 18: 25–30.
197. Gibbs RC, Frank SB. A peculiar, spotty pigmentation: report of five cases. Dermatol Int 1969; 8: 14–16.
198. El Zawahry M. Idiopathic pigmentation of the upper back. Arch Dermatol 1974; 109: 101–102.
199. Black MM, Maibach HI. Macular amyloidosis simulating naevoid hyperpigmentation. Br J Dermatol 1974; 90: 461–464.
200. Colver GB, Mortimer PS, Millard PR et al. The 'dirty neck' — a reticulate pigmentation in atopics. Clin Exp Dermatol 1987; 12: 1–4.
201. Manabe T, Inagaki Y, Nakagawa S et al. Ripple pigmentation of the neck in atopic dermatitis. Am J Dermatopathol 1987; 9: 301–307.

Disorders of collagen

INTRODUCTION

Collagen is the major structural constituent of mammalian connective tissues.[1] It accounts for well over 70% of the dry weight of the skin.[2] There are at least ten genetically distinct types of collagen and it is the relative content of these different collagen types, as well as the amount of elastic tissue and non-structural constituents such as the proteoglycans, that determines the specific biomechanical properties of the various connective tissues.[3,4]

Normal collagen

Before discussing the disorders of collagen in the skin, a brief account will be given of the composition, types and metabolism of collagen.

Composition of collagen[1]

The structural collagens — types I, II and III — are composed of three polypeptide chains, called alpha chains, each of which contains approximately 1000 amino acid residues, one-third of which are glycine. Proline and hydroxyproline are other important amino acids, constituting up to 20% of the amino acids. The sequence and composition of amino acids differ in the alpha chains of the various collagens.[4] Each of the alpha chains is coiled in a helix, and the three chains which together constitute a collagen molecule are in turn coiled on each other to form a triple helical structure. Short non-helical extensions are found at both ends of the molecule at the time it is secreted into the tissues. These extensions are soon cleaved from the pro-collagen molecules by two different proteases. This produces a shorter molecule which by lateral and longitudinal association with others produces collagen fibrils. At the same time, oxidation of lysyl and hydroxylysine residues results in the formation of stable cross-links which give tensile strength to the collagen.

Types of collagen[3-6]

As mentioned above, at least ten genetically distinct collagens have now been characterized, and at least 20 distinct genes encode the subunits of the various types of collagen.[7] Two of the three structural collagens, types I and III, are important constituents of the skin, while type IV collagen is an important constituent of the basement membrane (see p. 140). Only small amounts of the other collagen types are found in the skin.[3]

Type I collagen is the most abundant collagen in the dermis.[3] It is composed of two identical alpha chains and a third chain of different amino acid composition. The genes for these different chains are thought to be on chromosomes 17 and 7 respectively.

Type III collagen constitutes approximately 50% of fetal skin but less than 20% of adult skin.[2] It is also present in internal organs. This collagen type is composed of three identical alpha chains. Type III collagen is believed to accommodate the expansion and contraction of tissues such as blood vessels and viscera.[8] Reticulin fibres may represent type III collagen.[9]

Type IV collagen has a honeycomb or reticular pattern in contrast to the fibrillar pattern of the other major collagen types.[10,11] It is an important constituent of the lamina densa of the basement membrane.[10,11] Type VII collagen has recently been found in the sub-lamina densa region of the basement membrane zone (see p. 141).

Metabolism of collagen[4]

The metabolism of collagen is a complex process involving a balance between its synthesis and its degradation.[12] There are numerous steps involved in the synthesis of collagen and the regulatory mechanisms are not fully understood. Procollagen is formed in the rough endoplasmic reticulum of fibroblasts. After passing through the Golgi apparatus it is transported to the cell surface and secreted into the interstitium of the connective tissue.[12] Here occur cleavage of the terminal extensions of procollagen and the subsequent cross-linking of molecules to form stable collagen.[13] Collagen appears to be turned over continuously and its degradation is brought about by collagenase. It is remarkably resistant to proteolysis by most tissue proteinases.[12]

Various substances can interfere with the synthesis of collagen: the most important are the corticosteroids, which appear to act at several levels in the biosynthetic pathway.[13]

Categorization of collagen disorders

Although the various disorders of connective tissue have been assigned to a particular chapter of this volume on the basis of which element is most affected, it must be emphasized that an alteration in one component of connective tissue may influence the synthesis, deposition and structure of other components.[14] For instance, alterations in the elastic tissue and proteoglycan composition of the dermis may be found in some of the primary disorders of collagen.

The following categories will be considered, although it is acknowledged that the allocation of some of the disorders to a particular section is somewhat arbitrary:

Scleroderma
Sclerodermoid disorders
Other hypertrophic collagenoses
Atrophic collagenoses
Perforating collagenoses
Variable collagen changes
Syndromes of premature ageing.

It should be noted that diseases such as systemic lupus erythematosus and polyarteritis nodosa, which have been regarded in the past as 'collagen diseases', are not included in this chapter as they are not disorders of collagen in the strict sense. They are discussed with their appropriate tissue reaction pattern (pp. 50 and 226).

SCLERODERMA

The term scleroderma refers to a group of diseases in which there is deposition of collagen in the skin and sometimes other organs as well. It may occur as a localized cutaneous disease in which the disorder of connective tissue is limited to the skin and sometimes structures beneath the affected skin, or it may occur as a systemic disease in which cutaneous lesions are accompanied by Raynaud's phenomenon and variable involvement of other organs.[15–18]

The following classification of scleroderma will be used in the account which follows:

1. *Localized scleroderma*
Morphoea and variants
Linear scleroderma
2. *Systemic scleroderma*
Diffuse form (progressive systemic sclerosis)
Limited form (includes acrosclerosis and the 'CREST' syndrome)
3. *Mixed connective tissue disease*
4. *Eosinophilic fasciitis.*

LOCALIZED SCLERODERMA

Localized scleroderma is the most common form of scleroderma. It generally occurs in children and young adults and there is a female preponderance.[19] There is no visceral involvement or Raynaud's phenomenon, and it usually has a self-limiting course. Progression to the systemic form is rare.[19] Antinuclear antibodies are uncommon except in the linear form,[20] and antibodies to single-stranded DNA are sometimes present, particularly in generalized morphoea.[21]

Morphoea

Morphoea is the commonest form of scleroderma. Usually it presents as one or several indurated plaques on the trunk or extremities with an ivory centre and a violaceous border (the 'lilac ring'). Irregular areas of hyperpigmentation or hypopigmentation may be present within the lesion.[22] Other clinical forms include guttate, generalized, subcutaneous, keloidal and bullous

types.[19,23] Occasionally, more than one type is present in the same individual.

Guttate morphoea consists of small, pale, slightly indurated lesions on the upper part of the trunk which may resemble lichen sclerosus et atrophicus.[24] In the rare *generalized morphoea* there are large plaque-like lesions, often with vague symmetry, involving the trunk and extremities.[25] Atrophy and fibrosis of the deep tissues may lead to crippling deformities. Ulceration and calcification may also develop in some of the lesions.[24] *Disabling pansclerotic morphoea* is an aggressive variant of the generalized type and is of early onset.[26,27] Lesions may extend circumferentially on an extremity leading to massive pansclerosis and atrophy.[24] Peripheral eosinophilia and mild non-progressive visceral changes are sometimes present in this variant.[27] *Subcutaneous morphoea* (morphoea profunda) consists of one or more ill-defined, deep sclerotic plaques on the abdomen, sacral area or extremities; its progression is slow but relentless.[28–29] *Keloidal (nodular) scleroderma* may be part of this spectrum, although the nodules may also be in the dermis, clinically resembling a keloid.[19,29a] Nodules are a rare finding in systemic scleroderma.[30,31] *Bullous lesions* may rarely complicate both localized and systemic scleroderma.[32]

Lesions of morphoea may coexist with lichen sclerosus et atrophicus (see p. 335),[33] and there are isolated reports of localized sclerodermatous lesions occurring in association with elastosis perforans serpiginosa ('perforating morphoea'),[34] discoid lupus erythematosus[35] and the presence of the so-called lupus anticoagulant (see p. 211).[36]

The aetiology of morphoea is controversial. Antibodies to *Borrelia burgdorferi*, the cause of Lyme disease, have been detected in a significant number of patients with morphoea in Austria, and spirochaetes have been demonstrated in tissue sections in some cases using a modified silver stain[36a] or an avidin–biotin immunoperoxidase system.[37,38] However, these findings have not been confirmed in most other countries,[39,40] and this leads to the view that in most instances there is no association between *B. burgdorferi* infection and morphoea.[41–41b]

Morphoea has developed, in a few instances, at the site of previous radiotherapy.[41c] It has also been reported in a patient taking the semisynthetic ergot alkaloid bromocriptine, a drug that has been associated with pulmonary fibrosis.[41d]

Linear scleroderma

Linear scleroderma is a variant of localized scleroderma in which sclerotic areas of skin develop in a linear pattern.[42,43] It may occur on the head, trunk or extremities; on the limbs it may extend the full length, leading to contractures of the joints that it crosses.[44]

Linear scleroderma involving the frontoparietal area is referred to as *en coup de sabre* from its supposed likeness to the scar of a sabre cut.[45,46] This variant, which is more likely to be bilateral than the other forms of linear scleroderma,[47] may be associated with various degrees of facial hemiatrophy (Romberg's disease).[19,48,48a] Rarely, linear scleroderma has been observed overlying the sclerosing bone dystrophy known as melorrheostosis.[49,50]

The onset of linear scleroderma is sometimes abrupt, and occasionally it follows trauma.[42] Its mean duration is longer than for plaque-type morphoea, and it is less likely to resolve as completely.

Histopathology[19]

Localized scleroderma is characterized by three outstanding features — the deposition of collagen in the dermis and subcutis, vascular changes, and an inflammatory cell infiltrate, particularly in early lesions.[51] These changes are now considered in detail.

The epidermis may be normal, somewhat atrophic, or even slightly thicker than usual.[52]

The dermis is increased in thickness and composed of broad sclerotic collagen bundles which stain strongly with the trichrome stain. Collagen also replaces the fat around the sweat glands and extends into the subcutis. In the latter site the collagen is homogenized and less compact than in the dermis and it shows only weak birefringence and trichrome staining;[53]

there is an increased number of fibroblasts. However, the collagen in the subcutis stains strongly with the PAS stain in contrast to the very weak staining of that in the dermis. Mucopolysaccharides are present in the early lesions, particularly in the subcutis.

There is atrophy of adnexal structures, particularly the pilosebaceous units. Eccrine glands are situated at a relatively high level in the dermis as a result of the collagen deposited below them (Fig. 11.1). The arrectores pilorum are often hypertrophied. The mesenchymal elements of peripheral nerves are involved in the sclerotic process.[54]

The vascular changes are thickening of the walls of small blood vessels and narrowing of

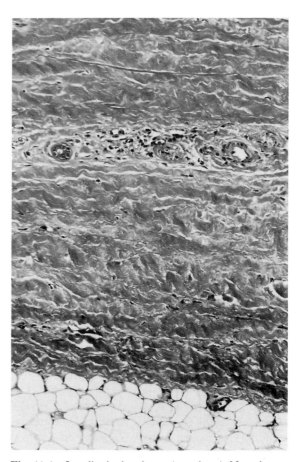

Fig. 11.1 Localized scleroderma (morphoea). Note the swollen collagen bundles, the atrophic sweat glands and the straight edge of the dermal-subcutaneous interface. Haematoxylin — eosin

their lumen. In small arteries there is fibro-mucinous thickening of the intima.

The inflammatory cell infiltrate is composed of lymphocytes with some macrophages and plasma cells. It is distributed around blood vessels or more diffusely through the lower dermis and subcutis, particularly at the border of early lesions. The infiltrate is more marked in localized scleroderma than systemic sclero-derma, and in early rather than late lesions.

In *guttate lesions* the changes are more superficial with less collagen sclerosis but with subepidermal oedema, resembling this feature of lichen sclerosus et atrophicus. *Linear lesions* may show a deeper and more diffuse inflammatory cell infiltrate extending into the underlying muscle. Vascular changes are usually prominent. Ossification of the dermis has been recorded.[55] The inflammation in the subcutis is also marked in the *generalized form*[56] and in subcutaneous morphoea; in both there may be marked fibrosis in the subcutis.[24]

In *subcutaneous morphoea* there is thickening and hyalinization of collagen in the deep dermis and in the septa and fascia.[57,58] Some confusion has arisen because of the variable use of the term subcutaneous morphoea. One group has suggested that the term morphoea profunda be used as an all-embracing one to include cases with dermal, subcutaneous and fascial involvement, while subcutaneous morphoea should be used for cases in which the subcutaneous fat is mainly affected.[57] According to this concept, eosinophilic fasciitis (p. 332) is the fascial component of morphoea profunda.[57] The concept has not yet gained wide acceptance. Markedly thickened fascia has been reported in a few patients with stony-hard induration of the skin and deeper tissues of the lower part of the body.[58a] There were no changes in the deep dermis or subcutaneous fat in these cases of the 'stiff skin syndrome'.[58a]

In *keloidal nodules* there are hyalinized thick collagen bundles associated with an increase in fibroblasts and mucin.[30] *Bullous lesions* show subepidermal oedema with dilated lymphatics in the underlying dermis.[23,57]

Immunofluorescence is usually negative in the lesions of localized scleroderma although a few deposits of IgM may be found in the basement membrane zone and in small dermal blood vessels.[24]

Electron microscopy. There is disarray and variable thickness of collagen at the advancing border.[59] Endothelial cells in blood vessels contain vacuoles and there is widening of the gap between the cells.[51] Collagen fibrils in the subcutis have a reduced diameter.[60]

SYSTEMIC SCLERODERMA

Systemic scleroderma (systemic sclerosis) is an uncommon connective tissue disease charac-terized by symmetrical tightness, thickening and induration of the skin, Raynaud's phenomenon, and sometimes involvement of one or more internal organs.[61,62] The spectrum of systemic scleroderma varies from a relatively mild form with limited acral skin involvement to a more rapidly progressive diffuse form with early and significant involvement of various internal organs.[16,61]

Diffuse systemic scleroderma. This form accounts for 20–40% of cases of systemic scleroderma. There is usually truncal and acral skin involvement of abrupt onset, associated with the appearance of Raynaud's phenomenon and constitutional symptoms.[61] Synovitis is common. Other features include oesophageal hypomotility and strictures, rectal prolapse, sigmoid volvulus, nodular regenerative hyperplasia of the liver, primary biliary cirrhosis, idiopathic pulmonary fibrosis, pulmonary hypertension, Sjögren's disease, thrombosis of major vessels[63,64] and renal failure.[61] Antibodies to Scl-70 (antitopo-isomerase) are present in approximately 30% of patients.[61,65,66]

Limited systemic scleroderma. This variant of systemic scleroderma typically affects older women. Raynaud's phenomenon often precedes the onset of cutaneous thickening, which is usually limited to the digits. Hair loss and anhidrosis are present in affected areas. Facial telangiectasia and cutaneous calcification often develop and there is an increased incidence of late onset pulmonary hypertension. Anticentromere antibodies are present in up to 70–80% of patients.[67–71]

Limited systemic scleroderma includes the condition referred to as the CREST syndrome,[72,73] which derives its name from the clinical features of *c*alcinosis, *R*aynaud's phenomenon, *e*sophageal dysfunction, *s*clerodactyly and *t*elangiectasia.[74] Not all of these features are invariably present, leading to suggestions that the acronym should be dropped in favour of the term 'limited systemic scleroderma'.[18]

Pigmentary changes may be found in both the diffuse and the limited forms of systemic scleroderma.[75] They may take the form of vitiligo-like areas with perifollicular and sometimes supravascular sparing, diffuse hyperpigmentation with accentuation in sun-exposed areas, or pigmentary changes in areas of sclerosis.[76] Livedo reticularis and livedoid vasculitis with ulcers occur uncommonly.[64]

Other clinical features of systemic scleroderma include a weak association with certain HLA antigen types, particularly DR5 and DR1,[77] and rare familial cases.[78,79] Antinuclear antibodies are present in almost all patients, usually with a speckled or nucleolar pattern.[69,80] Further characterization of these antibodies is possible now that specific nuclear macromolecules have been identified.[69] Antibodies to the cytoplasmic antigen Ro/SSA are present in approximately one-third of cases.[80a]

Pathogenesis of scleroderma[61,81–83]

Although the pathogenetic basis for the fibrosis in scleroderma is still not elucidated, theories relate this to changes in the vascular system, immune disturbances or alterations of fibroblast function. It is probable that these three factors will prove to be interdependent and interrelated.[83]

Vascular changes include the formation of gaps between endothelial cells, reduplication of the basal lamina and disruption of endothelial cells.[82] It has been suggested that the endothelial cell is the principal target.[84] Cutaneous hypoxia, which results from the fibromucinous intimal change in larger vessels, may play a role in the modulation of dermal fibroblast activity.[85]

Alterations in the immune system include the presence of autoantibodies and circulating immune complexes[67,86] as well as an increase in the T-helper/T-suppressor cell ratio.[82] There is also an association with other autoimmune diseases and a similarity to chronic graft-versus-host disease. It has been suggested that lymphokines and monokines produced by cells in the inflammatory infiltrate may play a role in fibroblast regulation;[82] histamine released from mast cells may also influence the activity of fibroblasts.[86a]

Numerous studies have attempted to elucidate the mechanisms controlling fibroblast activity in scleroderma.[82] There is an increase in the synthesis, deposition and degradation of collagen, proteoglycans and fibronectin. The increased collagen may result from the accumulation of a distinct subpopulation of fibroblasts capable of increased collagen synthesis.[87] Some of the type III collagen that is initially produced retains the aminopeptide on its surface, resulting in the formation of thin collagen fibrils, 30–40 nm in diameter.[88,89] These fibrils may form bundles in the subcutis or at the advancing edge, or be mixed with larger diameter fibrils.[88] In the later stages, the ratio of type III to type I collagen is normal.[90] Fibroblasts in scleroderma show increased responsiveness to a platelet-release fraction, which is possibly released following the aggregation of platelets in response to endothelial damage in small vessels.[91] Another finding of possible pathogenetic significance is the presence of a glycosaminoglycan in the urine of patients with scleroderma which will induce a sclerodermatous change when injected into mice.[92]

Finally, cell-wall-deficient bacteria have been reported in the affected tissues in cases of scleroderma.[93,94] Their significance is doubtful.

Histopathology[61,95–97]

The histopathological changes in systemic scleroderma are similar to those described above in the localized forms, although minor differ-

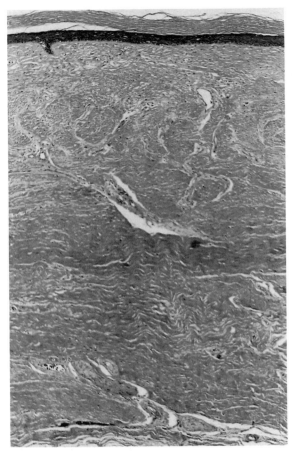

Fig. 11.2 Systemic scleroderma with thick collagen bundles in the dermis. Inflammation is absent. Haematoxylin — eosin

ences exist (Fig. 11.2). The inflammatory changes are less marked in systemic lesions and the deposition of collagen can be quite subtle in the early stages, particularly on the fingers. Vascular changes are sometimes more prominent, particularly severe intimal fibrosis in small arteries and arterioles.[98] These may show evidence of recent or old thrombosis and adventitial fibrosis.[63]

Other changes described include calcification an increase in mast cells in the dermis of early lesions[99] and of clinically uninvolved skin,[99a] and pigmentary changes corresponding to the clinical changes. For example, the vitiligo-like areas show an absence of melanocytes and of melanin in the basal layer.[75,76]

Direct immunofluorescence is usually nega-

tive although a few cases have been described with a speckled nuclear pattern in epidermal cells similar to that seen in mixed connective tissue disease (see below).[100,101]

Electron microscopy. The changes are similar to those described above for the localized form.[102]

MIXED CONNECTIVE TISSUE DISEASE

Mixed connective tissue disease (MCTD) is a distinct clinical syndrome sharing some clinical features of systemic lupus erythematosus, scleroderma and polymyositis. It is associated with the presence of circulating antibody to ribonucleoprotein.[103] Antibodies to the Sm antigen and to native DNA are usually absent.[104] *S*wollen or sclerotic fingers, *R*aynaud's phenomenon and *a*rthritis are important clinical features, leading to a suggestion that the acronym SRA is more appropriate than MCTD.[105] Less constant clinical features include muscle tenderness and proximal weakness, lymphadenopathy, alopecia, oesophageal hypomotility and pigmentary disturbances.[105-107] Approximately 20% develop restrictive lung disease.[105]

MCTD usually runs a chronic and benign course and shows a good response to systemic corticosteroids.

Histopathology

If lupus-like lesions are present clinically, then a biopsy from such an area will show the features of cutaneous lupus erythematosus. In the early stages, a biopsy from a swollen finger reveals marked dermal oedema with separation of collagen bundles.[106] In later lesions, dermal sclerosis resembling that seen in scleroderma may be present. The walls of vessels in the subcutis may be thickened with luminal narrowing.

Direct immunofluorescence of uninvolved skin shows a characteristic pattern of speckled epidermal nuclear staining, with specificity for IgG.[108]

EOSINOPHILIC FASCIITIS

In eosinophilic fasciitis (Shulman syndrome) there is a sudden onset, sometimes following strenuous physical activity, of symmetrical induration of the skin and subcutaneous tissues of the limbs.[109,110] There is usually sparing of the fingers. Localized variants, with involvement of part of a limb, have been reported.[111] The disease usually begins in mid-adult life, but no age is exempt.[112] Other clinical features include peripheral eosinophilia[113,114] and hyper-gammaglobulinaemia,[110] although rare cases with specific immunoglobulin deficiencies have been reported.[115] Visceral involvement and Raynaud's phenomenon are usually absent.[116] The majority of affected patients experience a complete or near complete recovery after 2–4 years, usually following steroid therapy but sometimes occurring spontaneously.[117]

Eosinophilic fasciitis is regarded as a variant of scleroderma.[118–120] Like scleroderma, fibro-blasts in the involved skin of patients with eosinophilic fasciitis exhibit an activated phenotype.[120a] Progression to scleroderma has been documented in several circumstances,[121] including a group of patients with the Spanish toxic oil syndrome (see p. 334). Patchy lesions of morphoea are sometimes present on the trunk, further evidence of the close association between eosinophilic fasciitis and the various scleroderma syndromes.[112,122] Recently, the spirochaete *Borrelia burgdorferi* has been implicated in the aetiology of eosinophilic fasciitis.[123,124] Similar changes have also resulted from the subcutaneous injection of phytomenadione (phytonadione)[125] and from the ingestion of products containing L-tryptophan.[125a]

Histopathology[112,126]

The earliest changes occur in the interlobular fibrous septa of the subcutis and the deep fascia. There is oedema and an infiltration of lymphocytes, histiocytes, plasma cells and eosinophils.[126] Eosinophils are sometimes quite prominent, but in most instances there are only focal collections of these cells.[127] Lymphoid nodules may also be present.

Eventually, there is striking thickening of the deep fascia and septa of the subcutis with fibrosis and hyalinization of the collagen.[126,128] This process extends into the deep dermis where there is atrophy of appendages associated with the sclerosis of the lower dermis. Inflammatory changes may also extend into the fibrous septa of the underlying muscle.[129]

Immunoglobulins and C3 have been present in the walls of vessels in the fascia and subcutis in some cases.

Thickening and fibrosis of the fascia may also be seen in scleroderma but there is usually a notable lack of inflammatory cells in the fascia in contrast to the more conspicuous inflammation found in eosinophilic fasciitis.[130,131]

SCLERODERMOID DISORDERS

The sclerodermoid disorders are a hetero-geneous group of diseases in which lesions develop that may mimic clinically and/or histopathologically the changes found in scleroderma.[15,132,132a] The sclerodermoid disorders, some of which are discussed elsewhere, as indicated below, include:

Winchester's syndrome
Pachydermoperiostosis
Acro-osteolysis
Chemical- and drug-related disorders
Lichen sclerosus et atrophicus
Scleroedema (p. 389)
Scleromyxoedema (p. 387)
Porphyria cutanea tarda (p. 536)
Chronic graft-versus-host disease (p. 46)
Chronic radiation dermatitis (p. 574)
Werner's syndrome (p. 349)
Progeria (p. 349).

No detailed mention need be made of the carcinoid syndrome and of phenylketonuria,[133] both of which are exceedingly rare causes of sclerodermatous skin lesions.

It should be noted that squeezing the skin with forceps, during a biopsy procedure, can produce an artefactual change locally in the dermis which resembles scleroderma somewhat on histopathological examination. Separation of the collagen bundles at the margins of this zone, or artefactual changes in the overlying epidermis may also be present.

WINCHESTER'S SYNDROME

The Winchester syndrome is an exceedingly rare inherited disorder of connective tissue which consists of dwarfism, carpal-tarsal osteolysis, rheumatoid-like small joint destruction and corneal opacities.[134,135] Cutaneous manifestations include a thick, leathery skin with areas of hypertrichosis and hyperpigmentation.[136]

Although the biochemical defect has not been elucidated, a recent study reported an abnormal oligosaccharide in the urine of two unrelated patients with this condition.[137]

Histopathology[138]

There is increased pigmentation of the basal layer and some thickening of the dermis. Fibroblasts are markedly increased in number, although in late lesions there are only a few fibroblasts in the thickened masses of amorphous collagen.[135] A perivascular lymphocytic infiltrate is also present. There is no increase in mucopolysaccharides in the dermis.

Electron microscopy. This shows dilated and vacuolated mitochondria in dermal fibroblasts.[135] Cytoplasmic myofilaments, a prominent fibrous nuclear lamina and some dilatation of the rough endoplasmic reticulum have also been noted.[136]

PACHYDERMOPERIOSTOSIS

The clinical manifestations of this rare syndrome include digital clubbing, thickening of the legs and forearms resulting primarily from periosteal new bone formation at the distal ends of the long bones, and progressive coarsening of facial features with deeply furrowed, thickened skin on the cheeks, forehead and scalp (cutis verticis gyrata).[139,140] Pachydermoperiostosis has an insidious onset, usually in adolescence, and a self-limited course. There is a predilection for males.[141] A familial incidence is sometimes present and in these cases the inheritance is thought to be autosomal dominant with incomplete penetrance and variable expressivity of the gene.[142]

This condition has also been referred to as primary hypertrophic osteoarthropathy to distinguish it from a secondary form which is usually associated with an intrathoracic neoplasm.[143] Facial and scalp changes, usually less severe than in pachydermoperiostosis, have been reported in some individuals with the secondary form.[139,144,145] Finger clubbing may be the sole manifestation in some relatives of patients with pachydermoperiostosis, indicating the overlap between these conditions.[139,143,146]

The pathogenesis is unknown, although many mechanisms have been postulated for the secondary form. Increased peripheral blood flow is found in secondary hypertrophic osteoarthropathy, but not in the primary variant.[147]

Histopathology[141,148]

The epidermis may be normal or mildly acanthotic. There is a diffuse thickening of the dermis with closely packed, broad collagen bundles. Some hyalinization of the collagen is usually present. Fibroblasts are increased in number in some areas. The subcutis may also participate in the fibrosing reaction. Elastic fibres are usually normal, although variations have been recorded. Acid mucopolysaccharides are sometimes increased in the dermis. In late stages there is some thickening of capillary walls with an increase in pericapillary collagen.[147]

Other changes include a variable, usually mild, perivascular and periappendageal chronic inflammatory cell infiltrate and prominence of sebaceous and eccrine glands.[149]

ACRO-OSTEOLYSIS

Acro-osteolysis refers to lytic changes in the distal phalanges. There is a familial form, an idiopathic form with onset in early adult life and an occupational variant related to exposure to polyvinyl chloride.[150] Cutaneous lesions are described in only some idiopathic cases;[150] in contrast, they are a characteristic feature of occupational acro-osteolysis.[151] There are sclerodermoid plaques on the hands accompanied by Raynaud's phenomenon.[132] With altered work practices occupational acro-osteolysis should become a historical disease.[152]

Histopathology[150]

The dermis is thickened, with swollen collagen bundles and decreased cellularity. There is usually no significant inflammation and there is no calcinosis. Elastic fibres are often fragmented.

CHEMICAL- AND DRUG-RELATED DISORDERS

Sclerodermoid lesions may develop in the skin following occupational exposure to polyvinyl chloride (acro-osteolysis, see above), trichlorethylene,[153] perchlorethylene, aromatic hydrocarbon solvents, certain epoxy resins and silica.[152,153a] Silica has also been implicated in the aetiology of scleroderma itself.[153a]

The injection of phytomenadione (phytonadione)[154,155] or pentazocine[15] will result in a localized sclerodermatous reaction. Similarly, if silicone is extravasated into the tissues from a leaking prosthetic breast implant, a dense collagenous reaction is produced (see p. 425).

The ingestion of an olive oil substitute — rapeseed oil, denatured with aniline — produced a multisystem disease of epidemic proportions in Spain some years ago.[156] Sclerodermoid lesions developed in the skin.[157] A similar multisystem illness follows the ingestion of products containing L-tryptophan.[125a]

The chemotherapeutic agent bleomycin will produce cutaneous sclerosis, particularly involving the fingers, in addition to its other complications of alopecia, cutaneous pigmentation and pulmonary toxicity.[158,159] The cutaneous lesions produced by bleomycin in particular, and to a lesser extent by some of the other agents listed above, are self-limiting, with

some resolution of the lesions after withdrawal of the offending agent.

Histopathology

The changes resemble quite closely those found in systemic scleroderma. In bleomycin-induced lesions, the homogenized collagen is often most prominent around blood vessels and adnexal structures.

LICHEN SCLEROSUS ET ATROPHICUS

This chronic disorder has a predilection for the anogenital region of middle-aged and elderly women.[160–161] About 20% of the patients have extragenital lesions, these sometimes occurring without coexisting genital involvement.[162] Extragenital sites which are affected include the upper part of the trunk, the neck, the upper part of the arms, the flexor surfaces of the wrists and the forehead. Very rarely, palmar[163] and plantar[164,165] skin, the face,[166] scalp,[167] mouth,[168] and even a vaccination site[169] have been involved.

Lichen sclerosus et atrophicus may involve the glans, prepuce or external urethral meatus of uncircumcised prepubertal or adolescent males, resulting in phimosis.[170–172] These lesions, also known in the past as balanitis xerotica obliterans, are not associated with extragenital involvement,[170] although isolated extragenital lesions may be seen in other males.[173,174]

Lichen sclerosus et atrophicus commences as flat, ivory to white papules that coalesce to form plaques of varying size and shape. These develop follicular plugging and progressive atrophy leading to a parchment-like, wrinkled, flat, or slightly depressed scar ('cigarette paper atrophy'). Vulval lesions may have secondary lichenification from the pruritus-related scratching, or they may coexist with hypertrophic areas, the so-called mixed vulval dystrophy.[160a] Infrequently, haemorrhagic bullae form,[175,176] and these may be complicated by the subsequent development of milia.[177]

Usually, the disorder is slowly progressive with periods of quiescence. Spontaneous involution may occur, particularly in girls[178] at or about the menarche.[179-181]

There is controversy concerning the relationship of lichen sclerosus et atrophicus to morphoea.[182,183] Although many authors have reported small numbers of cases of lichen sclerosus et atrophicus coexisting with or superimposed upon morphoea,[33] it is suggested that these patients have morphoea with secondary lymphoedema and sclerosis of the superficial dermis mimicking lichen sclerosus et atrophicus both clinically and pathologically.[183] In most instances, there have been no genital lesions. Some patients with lichen sclerosus et atrophicus have had coexisting autoimmune diseases.[184,185]

Extragenital lesions never undergo malignant degeneration, although in the genital region there may, uncommonly, be coexisting, or subsequent, squamous cell carcinoma.[186-188] In these circumstances, the tumour usually arises in the hyperplastic areas of what is a mixed vulval dystrophy.[181]

Recently, *Borrelia burgdorferi* has been detected in biopsies of lichen sclerosus et atrophicus by a modified silver stain[36a] or by immunoperoxidase techniques using an antibody to this organism.[37,38] Most of these studies have been from Austria; studies from other countries have detected the organism or antibodies to it in only a limited number of cases. This spirochaete can also be detected in some cases of morphoea (see p. 327), and in Lyme disease (see p. 635).[37,38]

Glucose intolerance or diabetes mellitus is sometimes present in cases of lichen sclerosus et atrophicus. The pathogenetic significance of this finding is uncertain.[189]

Histopathology[190]

Established lesions show hyperkeratosis, follicular plugging, thinning of the epidermis and vacuolar alteration of the basal layer (Fig. 11.3). There is a broad zone of subepidermal oedema with homogenization of collagen and poor staining in haematoxylin and eosin preparations (Fig. 11.4). In later lesions, this zone becomes more sclerotic in appearance and shows more eosinophilia. There is dilatation of thin-walled

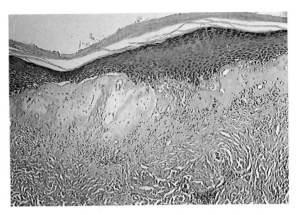

Fig. 11.3 Lichen sclerosus et atrophicus. There is orthokeratotic hyperkeratosis, some basal vacuolar change and subepidermal oedema and homogenization of collagen. Haematoxylin — eosin

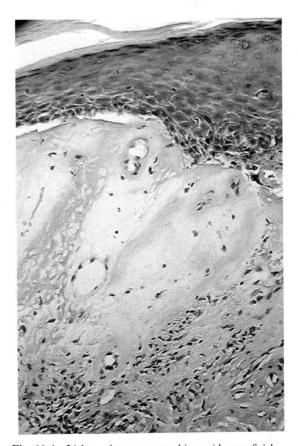

Fig. 11.4 Lichen sclerosus et atrophicus with superficial dermal oedema, telangiectasia of vessels and homogenization of collagen. Haematoxylin — eosin

vessels in the zone and sometimes haemorrhage. Beneath the oedema there is a diffuse, perivascular infiltrate of lymphocytes in the mid dermis. This infiltrate is sometimes quite sparse in established vulval lesions, and it may contain a few plasma cells and histiocytes. In vulval lesions there is also more diversity of epidermal changes, with hyperplastic areas in mixed dystrophies.[191] The appendages are usually preserved.

In the early stages, elastic fibres are pushed downwards by the oedematous zone and subsequently destroyed.[192] In contrast, elastic fibres are normal or increased in morphoea.[192a] Small amounts of acid mucopolysaccharide may be found in this zone. The basement membrane may focally fragment and PAS-positive material may be found in the subjacent dermis, partially as homogeneous clumps.[192]

In early lesions, the inflammatory infiltrate is quite heavy and is superficial and band-like, mimicking lichen planus. There may also be acanthosis and only minimal hyperkeratosis. As the oedematous zone broadens, the infiltrate is pushed downwards and becomes more dispersed and usually less intense (Fig. 11.5).

In presumptive cases with coexisting morphoea, the absence of vacuolar alteration, the lack of a well-defined inflammatory infiltrate beneath the thickened dermis, and the presence of deep dermal changes of morphoea are features supporting a diagnosis of morphoea without coexisting lichen sclerosus et atrophicus.[183]

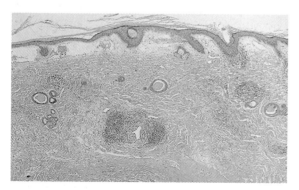

Fig. 11.5 Lichen sclerosus et atrophicus. The oedematous zone has widened. The dermal infiltrate is now more dispersed.
Haematoxylin — eosin

Electron microscopy. This has shown degeneration and regeneration of superficial dermal collagen, the presence of collagen in intercellular spaces in the epidermis, abnormalities of the basement membrane zone, and condensation of tonofilaments in the basal epidermal cells.[193,194]

OTHER HYPERTROPHIC COLLAGENOSES

Collagen is increased in several conditions, but not necessarily in the manner seen in scleroderma and the sclerodermoid disorders. Connective tissue naevi and hypertrophic scars and keloids have been arbitrarily included in this section; they could also be regarded as tumour-like proliferations of fibrous tissue, other examples of which are discussed in Chapter 34.

CONNECTIVE TISSUE NAEVUS

Connective tissue naevi are cutaneous hamartomas in which one of the components of the extracellular connective tissue — collagen, elastic fibres or glycosaminoglycans — is present in abnormal amounts.[195] They can be subclassified on the basis of the component predominantly involved:

Collagen type
  Collagenoma
  Shagreen patch
Elastin type
  Elastoma
Proteoglycan type
  Nodules in Hunter's syndrome.

Sometimes there are alterations in more than one component of connective tissue, and these lesions may simply be categorized as connective tissue naevi.[196] Only the connective tissue naevi of collagen type will be discussed in this section.

Collagenoma

Collagenomas (connective tissue naevi of collagen type) are rare hamartomas of the skin in which there is an increase in dermal collagen. They usually present as asymptomatic, firm, flesh-coloured plaques and nodules, 0.5–5.0 cm in diameter, on the trunk and upper part of the arms.[195] There may be several lesions,[197] or up to a hundred or more, with an onset in adolescence.[198] A family history is sometimes present (familial cutaneous collagenoma), and in these cases there is autosomal dominant inheritance.[198,199]

Associated clinical features have included a cardiomyopathy,[195] and Down's syndrome[200] in one patient. Uncommonly, the connective tissue naevi associated with the Buschke–Ollendorff syndrome (see p. 363) are of collagenous composition rather than of the usual elastic tissue type.[201,202]

Solitary collagenomas are sometimes quite large, as seen with the cerebriform or 'paving stone' variants on the sole of the foot.[203]

Histopathology

The epidermis is usually normal, although an overlying epidermal naevus has been reported.[204] There is thickening of the dermis, sometimes with partial replacement of the subcutis. The collagen bundles are broad and have a haphazard arrangement.[205] Elastic fibres are more widely spaced, but this may represent a dilution phenomenon.[205] Sometimes the elastic fibres are thin and fragmented. There is no increase in mucopolysaccharides. Calcification was present in one reported case.[206]

Shagreen patch

The shagreen patch is a distinct clinical variant of collagenoma, found exclusively in those with tuberous sclerosis. It consists of a slightly elevated, flesh-coloured plaque of variable size, usually on the lower part of the trunk.[207] It has the appearance of untanned leather. Smaller 'goose flesh' papules may form as satellite lesions.

Histopathology[207]

There are dense sclerotic bundles of collagen, with an interwoven pattern, in the reticular dermis.[208] Fibroblasts appear hypertrophied.[208] There is no inflammatory infiltrate or increase in vascularity. The overlying epidermis is usually flat, although sometimes it has the pattern of acanthosis nigricans.[207]

HYPERTROPHIC SCARS AND KELOIDS

Hypertrophic scars and keloids are a variation of the optimal wound healing process.[209] Keloids have been defined as cutaneous scars that extend beyond the confines of the original wound and hypertrophic scars as raised scars that remain within the boundaries of the wound.[210] Because the clinical distinction may be blurred, the usefulness of these definitions has been questioned.[211] Equally, the histopathological definitions proposed below have been criticized on the grounds that they do not always correlate with the above clinical definitions.[209] As the differences between keloids, hyperplastic scars and the optimal (normal) wound healing process are of degree only, it is not surprising that cases with overlap features exist. Because they may be quite disfiguring, keloids have attracted much more attention than hypertrophic scars.

Keloids are firm, variably pruritic masses, usually at the site of injury. They may be unevenly contoured. Early lesions are erythematous, while older lesions are usually pale, although occasionally they may be pigmented.[211] Sites of predilection are the upper part of the back, the deltoid and presternal areas and the ear lobes. Rare sites include the genitalia, eyelids and even palms and soles.[211] They usually develop over a period of weeks or months. Attempted surgical excision of a keloid results in regrowth of a larger lesion unless some concurrent effective therapeutic measures are adopted.[211,212] Recurrence is significantly less frequent in hypertrophic scars.[212,213]

Factors which lead to the formation of keloids and hypertrophic scars include race, increased skin tension in a wound, age of the patient, wound infection, site, as already mentioned, and a predisposition to scar hypertrophy.[209,210] Keloids are more common in black races. They have a predilection for individuals under 30 years of age.

There have been numerous experimental studies designed to identify the aetiology and pathogenesis of keloids. Fibroblasts isolated from keloids often synthesize normal amounts of collagen,[214] although proline hydroxylase activity, a marker of collagen synthesis, is higher in keloids than in hypertrophic scars or normal wounds.[215] The relative amounts of type III collagen are increased. Collagenase activity may be normal or increased in keloids.[216] It appears that collagen accumulates in keloids and hypertrophic scars because there are more fibroblasts present making more collagen than in normal wound healing, and this collagen may be protected from degradation by proteoglycan and specific protease inhibitors.[211,217]

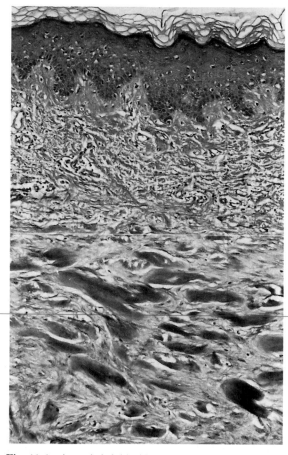

Fig. 11.6   An early keloid with thick hyaline collagen replacing the scar tissue. Haematoxylin — eosin

Histopathology[213,218]

Early *keloids* show abundant fibrillary collagen (Fig. 11.6). Mature keloids have a characteristic appearance with broad, homogeneous, brightly eosinophilic collagen bundles in haphazard array. Fibroblasts are increased and are found along the collagen bundles with an orientation similar to the accompanying collagen. There is also abundant mucopolysaccharide, particularly chondroitin-4-sulphate, between the bundles.

Keloids are usually elevated above the surrounding skin surface. The overlying epidermis may be thin, and beneath it there are often some telangiectatic vessels. A sparse, chronic inflammatory cell infiltrate may surround these peripheral vessels.

In contrast, *hypertrophic scars* are only slightly elevated, if at all, above the surrounding skin. The collagen bundles are characteristically oriented parallel to the skin surface, as are the accompanying fibroblasts. These are markedly increased in number, although there is some reduction in number with time. Capillaries are generally oriented perpendicular to the skin surface, and these may be surrounded by a sparse inflammatory cell infiltrate within the scar itself. There is little mucin except in early lesions. Elastic tissue is sparse or absent.

Subepidermal clefting sometimes develops overlying a scar.[219]

Mast cells are increased in both hypertrophic scars and keloids. Dystrophic calcification and bone may occasionally develop, particularly in abdominal scars.[220]

Electron microscopy. Keloids exhibit numerous fibroblasts with prominent Golgi complexes and abundant rough endoplasmic reticulum.[221] Myofibroblasts have usually not been demonstrated,[221] although it has been speculated that they may be present in early lesions.[222] Very fine elastic fibres can be seen in hypertrophic scars on electron microscopy, although they cannot be demonstrated by light microscopy.[223]

STRIAE DISTENSAE

Striae distensae are a common finding in adolescents of both sexes,[224,224a] particularly females, and in pregnancy (striae gravidarum).[225] They are also found following prolonged heavy lifting.[226,227] Striae form in association with the excess corticosteroid of Cushing's disease, with systemic steroid therapy, and with prolonged topical use of steroid preparations.[228,229] They develop on the abdomen, lower part of the back, buttocks, thighs, and female breasts.

Striae show a progression of clinical appearances, commencing as flat, pink lesions which broaden and lengthen and assume a violaceous colour.[228] This gradually fades to leave a white, depressed scar. The direction of the striae is conditioned by the mechanical forces responsible, but they are usually linear. They have been attributed to the stretching of corticosteroid-conditioned skin.[226] It is possible that only minimal stress is required in some circumstances, such as adolescence.[230] The proportion of cross-linked to unlinked collagen may also be of critical pathogenetic importance.[230]

Histopathology[231–233]

Striae distensae are basically scars. The epidermis is flat with loss of the normal rete ridge pattern. Dermal collagen bundles are arranged in parallel array.[231] The Verhoeff elastic stain will usually show a reduction in elastic tissue in early lesions although many additional thin fibres will be seen with the orcein or Luna stains.[232] Even these latter stains appear to underestimate the amount of elastic tissue, to judge by the scanning electron microscope which reveals a well-developed, dense network of fine fibres:[231,233] these presumably have a low elastin content precluding their demonstration with the Verhoeff stain. In older lesions, thicker elastic fibres can be seen in the affected skin.[233] Early lesions (striae rubrae) are rarely biopsied. They have been reported to show vascular dilatation and a mild perivascular inflammatory cell infiltrate.

FIBROBLASTIC RHEUMATISM

Only a few cases of this entity have been described since the initial report in 1980.[234–236] There is a sudden onset of symmetrical polyarthritis and Raynaud's phenomenon, and the development of cutaneous nodules, which are found mainly on the hands. The nature of the disease is unknown.

Histopathology

The cutaneous nodules show a fibroblastic proliferation with thickened collagen bundles having a whorling pattern.[236]

COLLAGENOSIS NUCHAE

Collagenosis nuchae is a recently delineated entity which presents clinically with diffuse induration and swelling of the back of the neck, accompanied by features suggesting low grade inflammation.[237] Two personally studied cases have had similar features.[238]

Histopathology

Thick, disorganized collagen bundles partly replace the subcutaneous fat. The collagen merges almost imperceptibly with the lower dermis and the ligamentum nuchae. There are no inflammatory cells present, despite the clinical impression of inflammation. Furthermore, there are very few fibroblasts, distinguishing the lesion from a fibromatosis. There is no increase in mucin, as seen in scleredema (see p. 389).

ATROPHIC COLLAGENOSES

The microscopical assessment of dermal atrophy can be difficult in the early stages. It requires a knowledge of the regional variability in skin thickness. The age of the patient is also relevant, since there is some atrophy of the skin in the elderly. Technical artefacts in the preparation of histological sections can also influence dermal thickness.

The following conditions, discussed below, can be associated with a decrease in dermal thickness:

Aplasia cutis congenita
Focal dermal hypoplasia
Focal facial dermal dysplasia
Pseudo-ainhum constricting bands
Keratosis pilaris atrophicans
Corticosteroid atrophy
Atrophoderma of Pasini and Pierini
Acrodermatitis chronica atrophicans.

In addition, dermal thinning can be seen in type IV Ehlers–Danlos syndrome (see p. 347) and also in some forms of the Marfan syndrome (see p. 348).

APLASIA CUTIS CONGENITA

Aplasia cutis congenita is the term applied to a heterogeneous group of disorders in which localized or widespread areas of skin are absent at birth. The defect is most often limited to the vertex of the scalp,[239,240] but other parts of the body such as the trunk or limbs may be affected, often symmetrically, with or without accompanying scalp lesions.[241,242] Other recorded associations include limb defects,[243–245] mental retardation,[246] epidermal and organoid naevi,[247,248] epidermolysis bullosa,[249–252] chromosomal abnormalities,[242] fetus papyraceus[247] and focal dermal hypoplasia.[242,246,253]

Two recent publications have attempted to define distinct clinical subtypes, based on the location of the skin defects and the presence of associated malformations.[242,247] Some cases have an autosomal dominant inheritance with reduced penetrance of the gene;[254] others appear to be the result of gene mutation.[242] The condition has been reported in one of monozygotic twins.[255] Other factors which may be aetiologically significant in individual cases include amniotic adhesions, intrauterine trauma, drugs (particularly the antithyroid drug, methimazole),[256] biomechanical forces from the hemispheric growth of the brain,[257] and

ischaemia resulting from placental infarcts[258] or associated with the condition fetus papyraceus.[247]

The defect in the skin presents as an ulcer, a membranous lesion, or an area of atrophic scarring. Lesions on the scalp usually heal with cicatricial alopecia.[259] An abnormal tendency to cutaneous scarring has been reported in two siblings with this condition.[260]

Histopathology[247]

The epidermis may be absent or thin, with only two or three layers of flattened cells. The underlying dermis is usually thin and composed of loosely arranged connective tissue in which there is some disarray of collagen fibres (Fig. 11.7).[261] The dermis may resemble a scar.[262] Elastic fibres may be reduced, increased or fragmented.[263] Appendages are absent or rudimentary.[264] The subcutis is usually thin.

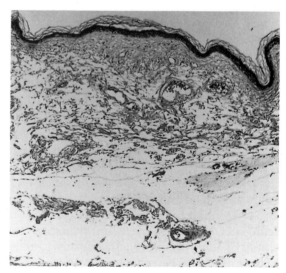

Fig. 11.7 Aplasia cutis congenita of the scalp. Appendages are lost and the dermis is composed of thin, widely-spaced bundles of collagen.
Haematoxylin — eosin

FOCAL DERMAL HYPOPLASIA

Focal dermal hypoplasia (Goltz or Goltz–Gorlin syndrome) is a rare syndrome with multiple congenital malformations of mesoderm and ectoderm, affecting particularly the skin, bones, eyes and teeth.[265–267] It is thought to be inherited as an X-linked dominant trait, which usually is lethal in the male:[268] however, this is not absolute as some male cases have been reported.[269]

Cutaneous manifestations include widespread areas of dermal thinning in a reticular, cribriform and linear pattern, soft yellowish nodules representing either herniations of subcutaneous fat through an underdeveloped dermis or heterotopic fat (a fat naevus),[269] and linear or reticular areas of hyper- or hypo-pigmentation.[265,270] Focal loss of hair, nail changes, total absence of skin from various sites, lichenoid hyperkeratotic papules and periorificial tag-like lesions may also occur.[265,270] Skeletal abnormalities include syndactyly, polydactyly and longitudinal striations of the metaphyseal region of long bones (osteopathia striata).[271–273] Rarely, only cutaneous abnormalities are present.

Experimental studies using fibroblasts from affected skin have shown that synthesis of collagen by individual fibroblasts is normal, but that there is an abnormality in cell kinetics with reduced proliferative activity of fibroblasts.[274]

Histopathology[265,269a,274]

The epidermis is usually normal. There is a marked reduction in the thickness of the dermis, with some thin, loosely arranged collagen fibres in the papillary dermis. Adipose tissue continuous with the subcutaneous fat extends almost to the undersurface of the epidermis in some areas. The extreme degree of attenuation of the collagen seen in focal dermal hypoplasia is not present in naevus lipomatosus in which mature fat also replaces part of the dermis; furthermore, the clinical presentations of the two conditions are quite distinct.

Inflammatory cells, sometimes quite numerous, have been present in biopsies of focal dermal hypoplasia taken in the neonatal period.[268,275] Other findings have included the presence of increased numbers of blood vessels and of some elastic tissue within the fat, a feature not present in normal subcutaneous fat.[276]

Electron microscopy. One study has shown fine filamentous tropocollagen within and between collagen bundles.[277] Rough endoplasmic reticulum and Golgi complexes are not prominent in dermal fibroblasts.[277] Multilocular fat cells, which are regarded as young fat cells, are often seen.[277]

FOCAL FACIAL DERMAL DYSPLASIA

This rare genodermatosis is characterized by congenital, usually symmetrical, scar-like lesions of the temple.[278] There is often a spectrum of associated facial anomalies.[278] Inheritance is usually as an autosomal dominant trait with incomplete penetrance.[279] This entity has been regarded in the past as a variant of aplasia cutis congenita[263] or as an ectodermal dysplasia.[280]

Histopathology

The epidermis is thin and usually depressed. There is more prominent thinning of the dermis, and this is usually associated with some decrease in elastic tissue and absence of adnexal structures.[278,280] Small bundles of striated muscle are sometimes present within the dermis.[263,279]

PSEUDO-AINHUM CONSTRICTING BANDS

This term refers to congenital constriction bands which may take the form of shallow depressions in the skin or deep constrictions associated with gross deformity or even amputation of a limb or digit.[281] The term ainhum is a West African name for similar constrictive lesions, usually of the fifth toe, that lead eventually to spontaneous amputation and that probably result from effects of repeated trauma in the genetically predisposed African patients.

Histopathology[281]

There is marked thinning of the dermis with finger-like projections of fibrous tissue extending into the underlying subcutis. Elastic tissue may be increased in this region.

KERATOSIS PILARIS ATROPHICANS

This term refers to a group of three related disorders in which keratosis pilaris is associated with mild perifollicular inflammation and subsequent atrophy, particularly involving the face. Differences in the location and the degree of atrophy have been used to categorize these three conditions.

Keratosis pilaris atrophicans faciei (ulerythema ophryogenes) is manifest soon after birth by follicular papules with an erythematous halo involving the lateral part of the eyebrows.[282] It may later involve the forehead and cheeks. Pitted scars and alopecia usually result.[282] Keratosis pilaris of the arms, buttocks and thighs is often present. Less common clinical associations include atopy,[283] mental retardation,[282] Noonan's syndrome[284-286] and a low serum vitamin A level.[282,287] Some reports suggest an autosomal dominant inheritance.[282]

Keratosis follicularis spinulosa decalvans is another exceedingly rare condition which begins in infancy with diffuse keratosis pilaris associated with scarring alopecia of the scalp and eyebrows.[288-290] 'Moth-eaten' scarring of the cheeks usually results. Associations include atopy, photophobia, corneal abnormalities, palmar-plantar keratoderma, and other ectodermal defects.[291] A sex-linked inheritance has been proposed.[288]

Atrophoderma vermiculata (folliculitis ulerythematosa reticulata)[292] involves the preauricular region and cheeks.[293] It develops in late childhood with the formation of horny follicular plugs which are later shed. This is followed by a reticulate atrophy with some comedones and scattered milia. Inheritance is autosomal dominant in type. Rare clinical associations include leucokeratosis oris[294] and tricho-epitheliomas with basal cell carcinomas

(ROMBO syndrome — see p. 820).[295] Keratosis pilaris of the limbs is quite commonly present. A condition described in the literature as *atrophia maculosa varioliformis cutis* affected a similar location on the cheeks[296,296a] but there was no mention in these cases of a preceding stage with follicular plugging.[296]

All three conditions are regarded as congenital follicular dystrophies with abnormal keratinization of the superficial part of the follicles. A fourth condition, *erythromelanosis follicularis faciei et colli*, has minute follicular papules resulting from small keratin plugs associated with red-brown pigmentation and fine telangiectasias.[297-299] This rare disease appears to be another follicular dystrophy but is usually not considered with the other three conditions because it lacks any atrophy.

Histopathology

In all three variants of keratosis pilaris atrophicans there is follicular hyperkeratosis with atrophy of the underlying follicle and sebaceous gland.[287] Comedones and milia may also be present.[293] There is variable perifollicular fibrosis which may extend into the surrounding reticular dermis as horizontal lamellar fibrosis.[288] The dermis may be reduced in thickness. A mild perivascular infiltrate of lymphocytes and histiocytes is usually present.

CORTICOSTEROID ATROPHY

Cutaneous atrophy is an important complication of the long-term topical application of corticosteroids, especially if occlusive dressings are used or the steroids are fluorinated preparations.[300-302] The injection of corticosteroids into the skin will also produce local atrophy;[303,304] rarely atrophic linear streaks develop along the lines of the overlying lymphatic vessels draining the injection site.[305-308] Telangiectasia and striae are other complications which may develop.[309,310]

The pathogenesis of the atrophy is not completely understood. It appears to involve diminished synthesis and enhanced degradation of collagen.[311]

Histopathology[309,312]

Epidermal thinning with loss of the rete ridges is an early change. The superficial dermis often has a loose texture and there may be telangiectasia of superficial vessels. The reticular dermis is reduced in thickness only after prolonged topical therapy. If atrophy is present the collagen bundles may appear thin and lightly stained.[313] At other times the collagen appears homogenized.[314] In some areas fibroblasts are decreased in number. Elastic fibres are focally crowded. There may also be a reduction in the size of the dermal appendages.[315]

Electron microscopy. There is disorganization of the collagen bundles and a variable thickness of the fibres.[313] Globular masses of microfibrils are also seen.

ATROPHODERMA

Atrophoderma (of Pasini and Pierini) is an uncommon yet distinctive form of dermal atrophy consisting of one or more sharply demarcated, depressed and pigmented patches.[316] The colour varies from bluish to slate grey or brown.[317] There is no induration or wrinkling.[317] Individual lesions are round or ovoid and these may coalesce to give large patches of involvement. There is a predilection for the trunk, particularly the back. The onset, which is insidious, usually occurs in adolescence.[316] Lesions may slowly progress over many years, or they may persist unchanged.

Atrophoderma is regarded by some as a variant of morphoea,[318,319] an opinion favoured by some overlapping clinical and histopathological features and by isolated reports of progression to either morphoea or systemic sclerosis.[320] Others regard it as a distinct disease entity on the basis of the dermal atrophy, and the usual absence of sclerosis.[316] Unfortunately, this controversy is based on a small spectrum of clinical experience.[321]

The aetiology and pathogenesis are unknown, but it has been suggested that macrophages and T lymphocytes that are present around the vessels in the dermis may play some role.[318]

Histopathology

There is dermal atrophy but this may not be apparent unless adjacent normal skin is included in the biopsy for comparison.[317] The collagen bundles in the mid and deep dermis are sometimes oedematous or slightly homogenized in appearance.[316,319] Elastic fibres are usually normal, although there may be some clumping and loss of fibres in the deep dermis.[316] Adnexal structures are usually preserved. There is a perivascular infiltrate of lymphocytes and a few macrophages. The infiltrate is usually mild in the upper dermis, and somewhat heavier around vessels in the deep dermis. Some superficial vessels may be mildly dilated.

The epidermis is usually normal, apart from hyperpigmentation of the basal layer. There may be a few melanophages in the superficial dermis.

Electron microscopy. In the one study that I know of, the collagen and elastic fibres were normal.[318]

ACRODERMATITIS CHRONICA ATROPHICANS

This spirochaete-induced disease (see p. 636) is characterized by atrophy of the dermis to about one half of its normal thickness or less. The pilosebaceous follicles and subcutis also undergo atrophy.

Of interest is the recent report of coexisting acrodermatitis chronica atrophicans and morphoea in a British native.[321a] The antibody titres to *Borrelia burgdorferi* were high.

PERFORATING COLLAGENOSES

The perforating collagenoses are a group of dermatoses in which altered collagen is eliminated from the dermis through the epidermis.[322] Included in this group are reactive perforating collagenosis, the closely related entity of perforating verruciform 'collagenoma' (*collagénome perforant verruciforme*), and also chondrodermatitis nodularis helicis.

Collagen elimination is also found as a secondary event in some cases of granuloma annulare (perforating granuloma annulare) and of necrobiosis lipoidica. It has also been seen in healing wounds, in resolving keratoacanthomas and following the intradermal injection of corticosteroid.[323,324]

REACTIVE PERFORATING COLLAGENOSIS

Reactive perforating collagenosis, first described in 1967, is a rare condition in which collagen is eliminated from the dermis.[325] There are two distinct clinical variants.[326] In the usual form, in which the onset is in childhood, there are recurrent, umbilicated papules up to 6 mm or so in diameter which spontaneously disappear after 6–8 weeks, leaving a hypopigmented, sometimes scarred area.[327] New lesions develop as older lesions are involuting, and this may continue into adult life.[328] The papules are found on the extremities, particularly the dorsum of the hands and forearms. There is often a history of superficial trauma, such as a scratch or insect bite.[329] Lesions have been induced experimentally by trauma.[326,330] An autosomal recessive inheritance has been proposed for some cases.[322,331]

The other clinical variant is acquired in adult life and occurs especially in diabetics with chronic renal failure.[332,333] In patients with chronic renal failure there is sometimes clinical and histological overlap with other perforating disorders such as perforating folliculitis (see p. 447) and Kyrle's disease (see p. 286).[334–336] The recent finding that both collagen and elastic fibres undergo transepithelial elimination in these circumstances suggests that a single disease process is present.[336a] The term 'acquired perforating dermatosis' has been suggested for the different expressions of transepithelial elimination associated with renal disease and/or diabetes mellitus.[336a,336b] Reactive perforating collagenosis has also been reported in association with Hodgkin's disease,[337] lichen amyloidosus, Wegener's granulomatosis, rheumatoid arthritis, Henoch–Schönlein purpura,[322] and the acquired immunodeficiency syndrome associated with end-stage renal disease.[337a]

Histopathology[322,325,329]

The appearances vary with the stage of evolution of the lesion. In early lesions, there is acanthosis of the epidermis, and an accumulation of basophilic collagen in the dermal papillae. In established lesions, there is a cup-shaped depression of the epidermis which is filled with a plug consisting of parakeratotic keratin, some collagen, and inflammatory debris. The underlying epidermis is thin with fine slits through which basophilic collagen fibres in vertical orientation are extruded. Sometimes there is a complete break in the epidermis. A few studies have shown elastic fibres in the extruded material and granulation tissue in the superficial dermis.[338] Immunohistochemical and ultrastructural studies have shown that the extruded collagen is normal.[338] There is also absence of the basal lamina at the site of the perforation.[335]

PERFORATING VERRUCIFORM 'COLLAGENOMA' (COLLAGÉNOME PERFORANT VERRUCIFORME)

This entity is closely related to reactive perforating collagenosis. Traumatically altered collagen is eliminated in a single, self-limited episode.[324,339,340] The episode of trauma is usually more substantial than in reactive perforating collagenosis and the lesion that results is more verrucous. I have seen a large plaque develop on the chest, following trauma from a motor-car seat belt, with the histological features outlined below.[341]

Histopathology[340]

There is prominent epithelial hyperplasia with some acanthotic downgrowths encompassing

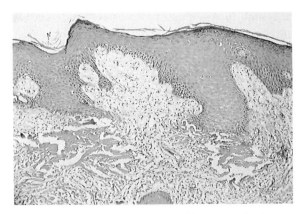

Fig. 11.8 A variant of perforating collagenosis following trauma from a seat belt in a motor car. Damaged collagen is being eliminated through the epidermal downgrowths. Haematoxylin — eosin

necrobiotic collagen and debris (Fig. 11.8). Elastic fibres are partly preserved in the central plug.[336]

CHONDRODERMATITIS NODULARIS HELICIS

Chondrodermatitis nodularis helicis is a chronic, intermittently crusted, painful or tender nodule found primarily on the upper part of the helix of the ear of males over 50 years of age. The lesions are usually solitary, and average 4–6 mm in diameter. There is a predilection for the right ear in some series.[342] The condition is infrequent in females, in whom it is more common on the antihelix.[343] The recurrence rate after treatment, which is usually curettage and cautery, can be as high as 20%.[344]

The aetiology and pathogenesis are speculative, but it has been suggested that the primary event is localized degeneration of dermal collagen with its subsequent partial extrusion through a central ulcer, or by actual transepidermal elimination. The collagen degeneration possibly results from a combination of factors which include minor trauma or pressure (during sleep),[345] poor vascularity, and sometimes solar damage.[344] Goette has called it an 'actinically induced perforating necrobiotic granuloma', but this statement appears to be an overgeneralization.[346] Recently it has been suggested that the infundibular portion of the hair follicle is primarily involved, with perforation of follicular contents into the dermis.[347,348]

Histopathology[349,350]

The characteristic changes are a central area of ulceration or erosion, or a more or less tight funnel-shaped defect, in the epidermis overlying an area of dermal collagen which shows variable oedema and fibrinoid degeneration (Fig. 11.9). Some inflammatory, keratinous and collagenous debris caps the area of degenerate collagen, forming the crust noted clinically.

At the margins of the central defect there is variable epidermal acanthosis, which rarely assumes the proportions of pseudo-epitheliomatous hyperplasia.[348] It extends peripherally over 3 to 5 rete pegs, and there is

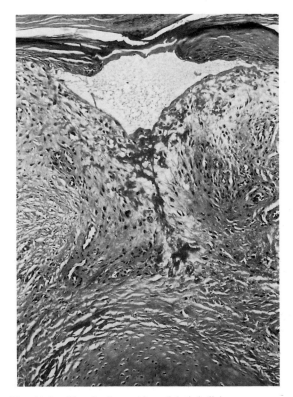

Fig. 11.9 Chondrodermatitis nodularis helicis. Haematoxylin — eosin

usually a prominent granular layer with some overlying hyperkeratotic and parakeratotic scale.[350] Richly vascularized granulation tissue borders the necrobiotic material peripherally, and sometimes the vessels have some glomus-like features. This area usually contains a mild, but sometimes moderately heavy, inflammatory cell infiltrate. The infiltrate is predominantly lymphocytic with an admixture of plasma cells, histiocytes and sometimes a few neutrophils. Rarely, the histiocytes may assume a palisaded arrangement at the margins of the necrobiotic zone.[350] Irregular slit-like spaces may extend into the degenerate collagen and other spaces containing fibrin may be found at the dermo–epidermal junction above the peripheral granulation tissue. Uncommonly, degenerate collagen will be seen in slits within the epidermis, representing true transepidermal elimination.

Beyond the lesion itself there may be some telangiectatic vessels in the upper dermis and variable solar elastosis.[346] Elastic fibres are diminished and focally absent in the area of degenerate collagen.

In nearly all cases there are changes in the perichondrium which are most marked directly beneath the degenerate collagen. These changes include fibrous thickening and very mild chronic inflammation. Degenerative changes may also be found in the cartilage, with alterations in its staining qualities, patchy hyalinization and, uncommonly, partial destruction with necrosis.[350] Calcification and even ossification have been noted in the distal part of the chondral lamina.[351]

VARIABLE COLLAGEN CHANGES

Variable changes in dermal collagen are found in Ehlers–Danlos syndrome, osteogenesis imperfecta and Marfan's syndrome. Marked thinning of the dermis can occur in some forms of all three disorders, although in other clinical variants it may appear quite normal. Defects in the biosynthesis of collagen have been detected in a number of patients with osteogenesis imperfecta and Ehlers–Danlos syndrome,

although in the majority of cases the defect has not been defined.[1]

EHLERS–DANLOS SYNDROME

Ehlers–Danlos syndrome is a heterogeneous disorder of connective tissue which combines hyperextensible fragile skin and loose-jointedness with a tendency to bruising and bleeding.[352-354] At least 11 types are now recognized, each with a characteristic clinical expression, inheritance pattern and, in some cases, a defined biochemical defect.[8] Paradoxically, specific defects in collagen biosynthesis have not been elucidated in the common forms of this disease. Syndrome delineation is still proceeding, and some cases do not fit neatly into any category.[355]

Histopathology

Contradictory results have been published on the histopathology of this condition.[356,357] More recent reports have generally stated that the dermis is normal on light microscopy.[356] Marked thinning of the dermis has been reported in some variants of type IV[14] and also in type VI, while solar elastotic changes have been documented in type IV disease.[356] Elastosis perforans serpiginosa has been reported in several cases of the syndrome, again particularly type IV.[322] Similarly, ultrastructural studies have been contradictory, with some authors reporting normal fibre diameter and others observing some variability in size.[14,358,359] A distorted arrangement of fibrils has been noted in several reports.[358] Scanning electron microscopy may offer further information in the future, as preliminary studies have shown disordered fibril aggregation and orientation.[354] Other ultrastructural findings will be mentioned below in the discussion of the specific types of the syndrome.

Subtypes of Ehlers–Danlos syndrome

Type I (gravis). Clinical features are usually

severe in this common, autosomal dominant form of the disease.[4] Herniation of fat into the dermis, with subsequent calcification, may occur at pressure points.[360] Increased fibre diameter and loosely assembled fibrils have been reported.[361] The biochemical defect is not known, although reduced type III collagen production has been reported in one case.[361] It has been normal in others.

Type II (mitis).

The molecular defect of this mild, autosomal dominant form is unknown.[4] Partial deletion of the C-terminal end of the procollagen molecule has been demonstrated in one case.[6] Minor variations in fibril diameter have been noted ultrastructurally, and in one case there was lateral fusion of fibrils.[359] It has been suggested recently that mild variants of the mitis form are not uncommon in the general population.[362]

Type III (benign hypermobile).

There is marked joint hypermobility but only minor skin changes.[4] Inheritance is autosomal dominant. The molecular defect is unknown.

Type IV (arterial, ecchymotic).

This is a heterogeneous group with at least four subtypes.[363,364] Both autosomal dominant and recessive variants occur.[363,365] There is a reduced life expectancy because of a propensity for rupture of large arteries and internal hollow viscera, particularly the colon.[8,366] Thin, translucent skin on the face and distal parts of the limbs in several subtypes gives the appearance of premature ageing (acrogeria— page 349).[364,367] In most cases, a decreased amount of type III procollagen is recovered from cultured skin fibroblasts.[8] Defective type III collagen is sometimes found.[8] However, a case with type III collagen deficiency, but with a normal phenotype, has been documented.[368]

Ultrastructural changes have included the finding of collagen fibrils with reduced diameter, the presence of dilated rough endoplasmic reticulum in fibroblasts and fragmentation of elastic fibres.[367]

Immunofluorescence of cultured skin fibroblasts has recently shown abnormal amounts of type III collagen retained in their cytoplasm.[369] This is not a feature in normal subjects or in other connective tissue diseases.

Type V (X-linked).

This rare form shows marked cutaneous extensibility.[4,353,370] A defect in lysyl oxidase was found in one kindred, but this has not been confirmed in others.[370]

Type VI (ocular).

This autosomal recessive variant is characterized by ocular fragility, kyphoscoliosis and prominent cutaneous and joint signs.[4] There is a deficiency in lysyl hydroxylase and an absence of hydroxylysine in dermal collagen.[352,371] This results in abnormal cross-links in both type I and type III collagen.[372] This variant of the syndrome is probably a biochemically heterogeneous entity, as normal levels of enzyme have been found in some individuals.[4]

Type VII (arthrochalasis congenita).

There is gross joint instability leading to multiple dislocations at birth. As a result of reduced procollagen aminoproteinase there is defective removal of the amino terminal peptides of procollagen.[373] Another subgroup has a deletion of amino acids from the alpha 1 chain of type I procollagen: this leads to resistance to cleavage by procollagen aminoproteinase.[373] Abnormal collagen fibrils with bilobed and hieroglyphic forms have been found on electron microscopy.[373]

Type VIII (periodontal).

This autosomal dominant form is marked by easy bruising, pretibial hyperpigmented scars and the early onset of periodontal disease.[352] There may be loose-jointedness of the fingers. The biochemical defect is unknown.

Type IX.

This recently recognized variant is X-linked and characterized by the presence of occipital horns and other skeletal abnormalities, and a propensity to bladder diverticula and to hernias.[370,374] Cutaneous changes are mild. There is defective activity of lysyl oxidase. It has been suggested that all disorders with deficient lysyl oxidase, including Menkes' syndrome (see

p. 375), should be classified as type IX disease,[375,376] but this ignores the absence of the usual clinical features of Ehlers–Danlos syndrome in patients with Menkes' syndrome.

Type X (fibronectin).   Some cases of the type X variant were originally classified as type IX disease.[377] There are moderately severe skin and joint changes and a defect in platelet aggregation.[377] The platelet defect can be corrected by fibronectin, which is an important adhesive glycoprotein which cross-links to collagen.[377]

Type XI (familial joint instability syndrome).   Joint changes are prominent in this autosomal dominant variant.[355,359]

Other types.   Many cases of Ehlers–Danlos syndrome defy classification. Such are the case reported with abnormalities localized to the shoulder region[378] and another with intracellular degradation of alpha 2 chains of type I procollagen.[379] This same defect is found in some cases of osteogenesis imperfecta and of Marfan's syndrome.[379]

OSTEOGENESIS IMPERFECTA

Bone fragility is the cardinal manifestation of osteogenesis imperfecta, a genetically heterogeneous entity in which various defects in type I collagen have been detected.[7,380] Other clinical manifestations include short stature, joint laxity, blue sclerae and otosclerosis. The skin may be thin in the severe variants.

Histopathology

The dermis is markedly reduced in thickness in those with clinically thin skin.[14] The fine collagen bundles which constitute the dermis are often argyrophilic.

MARFAN'S SYNDROME

The clinical features of Marfan's syndrome include tall stature, skeletal malformations, arachnodactyly and dislocation of the lens.[380a] The most severe complications relate to the cardiovascular system and include aortic dissection and mitral valve prolapse. Cutaneous manifestations are relatively insignificant. Several experimental observations indicate disordered collagen metabolism, although the specific molecular defects have not yet been elucidated.[2] Abnormalities in elastic cross-linking have also been reported in the aorta.[381]

Histopathology[14]

In some cases, thinning of the dermis, resulting from a diminished quantity of collagen and thinner collagen bundles, has been reported. This has been confirmed ultrastructurally. An increase in matrix material and fragmentation of elastic fibres have also been reported.

SYNDROMES OF PREMATURE AGEING

This disease group can be very small, or quite large, depending on the criteria used.[382] There are five conditions with prominent cutaneous findings that are usually included in any discussion on this subject — Werner's syndrome (adult progeria), progeria (Hutchinson–Gilford syndrome), acrogeria, Rothmund–Thomson syndrome (poikiloderma congenitale) and Cockayne's syndrome.[382,383] The Rothmund–Thomson syndrome includes poikiloderma as a major feature, and is accordingly discussed with the lichenoid reaction pattern (see p. 55), while in Cockayne's syndrome photosensitivity and sensitivity of cultured fibroblasts to ultraviolet light are a major feature. The other three syndromes show changes in dermal collagen, and accordingly they will be considered further in this chapter. In the two types of progeria this takes the form of sclerodermoid lesions, while in acrogeria the dermis is almost always atrophic.

WERNER'S SYNDROME (ADULT PROGERIA)

Werner's syndrome is an autosomal recessive disorder in which evidence of premature ageing becomes manifest between the ages of 15 and 30 years.[382] The clinical features include short stature, bird-like facies, juvenile cataracts, a tendency to diabetes mellitus, trophic ulcers of the legs, premature greying of the hair and balding, an increased incidence of neoplasms and acral sclerodermoid changes.[382,384] Death usually occurs in the fifth decade from the complications of arteriosclerosis.

Skin fibroblasts from patients with Werner's syndrome are difficult to culture, although in one study they produced more collagen but less glycosaminoglycans than normal.[385] A recent study has confirmed that cultured fibroblasts produce increased amounts of collagen; the levels of collagen m-RNA were also increased, suggesting an alteration in the control of collagen synthesis at the transcriptional level.[385a] Fibroblasts appear to become hyporesponsive in vitro to a stimulator of collagen synthesis that has been found in the serum of patients with Werner's syndrome.[386] The pathogenetic significance of these disparate findings remains to be elucidated.

Histopathology

There is usually some epidermal atrophy, although there may be hyperkeratosis over bony prominences.[384] In the scleroderma-like areas there is variable hyalinization of the thickened dermal collagen. There may be replacement of subcutaneous fat by connective tissue. The pilosebaceous structures and sweat glands become atrophic. Calcinosis cutis may also develop.[386]

In other areas, the dermis is thinned with a decrease in the size of the collagen bundles[386] and degenerative changes in the elastic fibres.

PROGERIA

Progeria (Hutchinson–Gilford syndrome) is a rare disease with markedly accelerated ageing, clinical features becoming apparent in the first year of life. These features include growth retardation, alopecia, craniofacial disproportion, loss of subcutaneous fat and atrophy of muscle.[382,387,388] The skin is generally thin as a result of the loss of subcutaneous fat, except for areas with scleroderma-like plaques. Acral hyperplastic scars and keloid-like nodules composed of type IV collagen have also been described.[389] Although an autosomal recessive mode of inheritance has been postulated, the majority of cases are sporadic.

The biochemical basis of this disease is unknown, but it has been shown that skin fibroblasts are difficult to culture and tropoelastin production by fibroblasts is markedly increased.[387]

Histopathology[388,390]

The scleroderma-like plaques show a diffusely thickened dermis with hyalinization of collagen.[390] This may assume a homogenized appearance in the lower dermis. Fibrous tissue often extends into the subcutis. Hair follicles are atrophic and eventually lost.[391] There are variable changes in the elastic tissue. In other areas of the body there is loss of subcutaneous fat and some atrophy of the dermis.[390]

ACROGERIA

Acrogeria (Gottron's syndrome) is an exceedingly rare disease with onset in early childhood.[392] There is atrophy, dryness and wrinkling of the skin which is most severe on the face and extremities.[382,383,392] Interesting associations include bony abnormalities and disorders of dermal elastic tissue in the form of elastosis perforans serpiginosa and perforating elastomas.[392,393] Inheritance is probably autosomal recessive. A syndrome described as metageria has features that overlap with those of acrogeria.[382,383] Acrogeria is regarded by some as a distinct subgroup of type IV Ehlers–Danlos syndrome.[394]

Histopathology[382,392,393]

There is atrophy of the dermis with degenerative changes in the collagen. Fibres may be swollen and present a 'boiled appearance'. The subcuta-neous fat is often replaced by connective tissue which is indistinguishable from the dermal collagen. Elastic fibres are disrupted and irregular, with some clumping. Changes of elastosis perforans serpiginosa may be present.

REFERENCES

Introduction

1. Spranger J. The developmental pathology of collagens in humans. Birth Defects 1987; 23: 1–16.
2. Uitto J, Lichtenstein JR. Defects in the biochemistry of collagen in diseases of connective tissue. J Invest Dermatol 1976; 66: 59–79.
3. Burgeson RE. Genetic heterogeneity of collagen. J Invest Dermatol 1982; 79: 25s–30s.
4. Krieg T, Ihme A, Weber L et al. Molecular defects of collagen metabolism in the Ehlers Danlos syndrome. Int J Dermatol 1981; 20: 415–425.
5. Prockop DJ, Kivirikko KI. Heritable diseases of collagen. N Engl J Med 1984; 311: 376–386.
6. Pope FM, Dorling J, Nicholls AC, Webb J. Molecular abnormalities of collagen: a review. J R Soc Med 1983; 76: 1050–1062.
7. Tsipouras P, Ramirez F. Genetic disorders of collagen. J Med Genet 1987; 24: 2–8.
8. Stolle CA, Pyeritz RE, Myers JC, Prockop DJ. Synthesis of an altered type III procollagen in a patient with type IV Ehlers-Danlos syndrome. J Biol Chem 1985; 260: 1937–1944.
9. Uitto J, Santa-Cruz DJ. The Ehlers-Danlos syndrome (EDS) type IV: Decreased synthesis of triple-helical type III procollagen by cultured skin fibroblasts. J Invest Dermatol 1979; 72: 274 (abstract).
10. Stanley JR, Woodley DT, Katz SI, Martin GR. Structure and function of basement membrane. J Invest Dermatol 1982; 79: 69s–72s.
11. Sage H. Collagens of basement membrane. J Invest Dermatol 1982; 79: 51s–59s.
12. Uitto J, Tan EML, Ryhanen L. Inhibition of collagen accumulation in fibrotic processes: Review of pharmacologic agents and new approaches with amino acids and their analogues. J Invest Dermatol 1982; 79: 113s–120s.
13. Prockop DJ, Kivirikko KI, Tuderman L, Guzman NA. The biosynthesis of collagen and its disorders. N Engl J Med 1979; 301: 13–23.
14. Holbrook KA, Byers PH. Structural abnormalities in the dermal collagen and elastic matrix from the skin of patients with inherited connective tissue disorders. J Invest Dermatol 1982; 79: 7s–16s.

Scleroderma

15. Young EM Jr, Barr RJ. Sclerosing dermatoses. J Cutan Pathol 1985; 12: 426–441.
16. Rodnan GP, Jablonska S, Medsger TA Jr. Classification and nomenclature of progressive systemic sclerosis. Clin Rheum Dis 1979; 5: 5–12.
17. Callen JP, Provost TT, Tuffanelli DL. Periodic synopsis on collagen vascular disease. J Am Acad Dermatol 1985; 13: 809–815.
18. LeRoy EC, Black C, Fleischmajer R et al. Scleroderma (systemic sclerosis): classification, subsets and pathogenesis. J Rheumatol 1988; 15: 202–205.
19. Jablonska S, Rodnan GP. Localized forms of scleroderma. Clin Rheum Dis 1979; 5: 215–241.
20. Ruffatti A, Peserico A, Glorioso S et al. Anticentromere antibody in localized scleroderma. J Am Acad Dermatol 1986; 15: 637–642.
21. Falanga V, Medsger TA Jr, Reichlin M. Antinuclear and anti-single-stranded DNA antibodies in morphea and generalized morphea. Arch Dermatol 1987; 123: 350–353.
22. Serup J. Clinical appearance of skin lesions and disturbances of pigmentation in localized scleroderma. Acta Derm Venereol 1984; 64: 485–492.
23. Synkowski DR, Lobitz WC Jr, Provost TT. Bullous scleroderma. Arch Dermatol 1981; 117: 135–137.
24. Winkelmann RK. Localized cutaneous scleroderma. Semin Dermatol 1985; 4: 90–103.
25. Leibovici V, Zlotogorski A, Kanner A, Shinar E. Generalized morphea and idiopathic thrombocytopenia. J Am Acad Dermatol 1988; 18: 1194–1196.
26. Cantwell AR Jr, Jones JE, Kelso DW. Pleomorphic, variably acid-fast bacteria in an adult patient with disabling pansclerotic morphea. Arch Dermatol 1983; 120: 656–661.
27. Diaz-Perez JL, Connolly SM, Winkelmann RK. Disabling pansclerotic morphea of children. Arch Dermatol 1980; 116: 169–173.
28. Doyle JA, Connolly SM, Winkelmann RK. Cutaneous and subcutaneous inflammatory sclerosis syndromes. Arch Dermatol 1982; 118: 886–890.
28a. Whittaker SJ, Smith NP, Russell Jones R. Solitary morphoea profunda. Br J Dermatol 1989; 120: 431–440.
29. Su WPD, Person JR. Morphea profunda. A new concept and a histopathologic study of 23 cases. Am J Dermatopathol 1981; 3: 251–260.
29a. Akintewe TA, Alabi GO. Scleroderma presenting with multiple keloids. Br Med J 1985; 291: 448–449.
30. Kennedy C, Leigh IM. Systemic sclerosis with subcutaneous nodules. Br J Dermatol 1979; 101: 93–96.
31. James WD, Berger TG, Butler DF, Tuffanelli DL. Nodular (keloidal) scleroderma. J Am Acad Dermatol 1984; 11: 1111–1114.
32. Synkowski DR, Lobitz WC Jr, Provost TT. Bullous

scleroderma. Arch Dermatol 1981; 117: 135–137.

33. Uitto J, Santz Cruz DJ, Bauer EA, Eisen AZ. Morphea and lichen sclerosus et atrophicus. J Am Acad Dermatol 1980; 3: 271–279.

34. Barr RJ, Siegel JM, Graham JH. Elastosis perforans serpiginosa associated with morphea. An example of "perforating morphea". J Am Acad Dermatol 1980; 3: 19–22.

35. Umbert P, Winkelmann RK. Concurrent localized scleroderma and discoid lupus erythematosus. Cutaneous 'mixed' or 'overlap' syndrome. Arch Dermatol 1978; 114: 1473–1478.

36. Freeman WE, Lesher JL Jr, Smith JG Jr. Connective tissue disease associated with sclerodermoid features, early abortion, and circulating anticoagulant. J Am Acad Dermatol 1988; 19: 932–936.

36a. Ross SA, Sanchez JL, Taboas JO. Spirochetal forms in the dermal lesions of morphea and lichen sclerosus et atrophicus. Am J Dermatopathol 1990; 12: 357–362.

37. Aberer E, Kollegger H, Kristoferitsch W, Stanek G. Neuroborreliosis in morphea and lichen sclerosus et atrophicus. J Am Acad Dermatol 1988; 19: 820–825.

38. Aberer E, Stanek G. Histological evidence of spirochetal origin of morphea and lichen sclerosus et atrophicans. Am J Dermatopathol 1987; 9: 374–379.

39. Tuffanelli D. Do some patients with morphea and lichen sclerosus et atrophicans have a Borrelia infection? Am J Dermatopathol 1987; 9: 371–373.

40. Lecerf V, Bagot M, Revuz J et al. Borrelia burgdorferi and localized scleroderma. Arch Dermatol 1989; 125: 297.

41. Hoesly JM, Mertz LE, Winkelmann RK. Localized scleroderma (morphea) and antibody to Borrelia burgdorferi. J Am Acad Dermatol 1987; 17: 455–458.

41a. Halkier-Sorensen L, Kragballe K, Hansen K. Antibodies to the Borrelia burgdorferi flagellum in patients with scleroderma, granuloma annulare and porphyria cutanea tarda. Acta Derm Venereol 1989; 69: 116–119.

41b. Garioch JJ, Rashid A, Thomson J, Seywright M. The revelance of elevated Borrelia burgdorferi titres in localized scleroderma. Clin Exp Dermatol 1989; 14: 439–441.

41c. Colver GB, Rodger A, Mortimer PS et al. Post-irradiation morphoea. Br J Dermatol 1989; 120: 831–835.

41d. Leshin B, Piette WW, Caplan RM. Morphea after bromocriptine therapy. Int J Dermatol 1989; 28: 177–179.

42. Falanga V, Medsger TA Jr, Reichlin M, Rodnan GP. Linear scleroderma. Clinical spectrum, prognosis, and laboratory abnormalities. Ann Intern Med 1986; 104: 849–857.

43. Piette WW, Dorsey JK, Foucar E. Clinical and serologic expression of localized scleroderma. Case report and review of the literature. J Am Acad Dermatol 1985; 13: 342–350.

44. Long PR, Miller OF III. Linear scleroderma. Report of a case presenting as persistent unilateral eyelid edema. J Am Acad Dermatol 1982; 7: 541–544.

45. Hulsmans RFHJ, Asghar SS, Siddiqui AH, Cormane RH. Hereditary deficiency of C2 in association with linear scleroderma 'en coup de sabre'. Arch Dermatol 1986; 122: 76–79.

46. Serup J, Serup L, Sjo O. Localized scleroderma 'en coup de sabre' with external eye muscle involvement at the same line. Clin Exp Dermatol 1984; 9: 196–200.

47. Dilley JJ, Perry HO. Bilateral linear scleroderma en coup de sabre. Arch Dermatol 1968; 97: 688–689.

48. Lakhani PJ, David TJ. Progressive hemifacial atrophy with scleroderma and ipsilateral limb wasting (Parry-Romberg syndrome). J R Soc Med 1984; 77: 138–139.

48a. Dintiman BJ, Shapiro RS, Hood AF, Guba AM. Parry-Romberg syndrome in association with contralateral Poland syndrome. J Am Acad Dermatol 1990; 22: 371–373.

49. Miyachi Y, Horio T, Yamada A, Ueo T. Linear melorheostotic scleroderma with hypertrichosis. Arch Dermatol 1979; 115: 1233–1234.

50. Wagers LT, Young AW Jr, Ryan SF. Linear melorheostotic scleroderma. Br J Dermatol 1972; 86: 297–301.

51. Serup J. Localized scleroderma (morphoea). Acta Derm Venereol (Suppl) 1986; 122: 1–61.

52. Morley SM, Gaylarde PM, Sarkany I. Epidermal thickness in systemic sclerosis and morphoea. Clin Exp Dermatol 1985; 10: 51–57.

53. Reed RJ, Clark WH, Mihm MC. The cutaneous collagenoses. Hum Pathol 1973; 4: 165–186.

54. Kobayasi T, Serup J. Nerve changes in morphea. Acta Derm Venereol 1983; 63: 321–327.

55. Handfield-Jones SE, Peachey RDG, Moss ALH, Dawson A. Ossification in linear morphoea with hemifacial atrophy — treatment by surgical excision. Clin Exp Dermatol 1988; 13: 385–388.

56. Fleischmajer R, Nedwich A. Generalized morphea. I. Histology of the dermis and subcutaneous tissue. Arch Dermatol 1972; 106: 509–514.

57. Su WPD, Greene SL. Bullous morphea profunda. Am J Dermatopathol 1986; 8: 144–147.

58. Person JR, Su WPD. Subcutaneous morphoea: a clinical study of sixteen cases. Br J Dermatol 1979; 100: 371–380.

58a. Jablonska S, Schubert H, Kikuchi I. Congenital facial dystrophy: Stiff skin syndrome — a human counterpart of the tight-skin mouse. J Am Acad Dermatol 1989; 21: 943–950.

59. Kobayasi T, Asboe-Hansen G. Ultrastructural changes in the inflammatory zone of localized scleroderma. Acta Derm Venereol 1974; 54: 105–112.

60. Fleischmajer R, Prunieras M. Generalized morphea. II. Electron microscopy of collagen, cells, and the subcutaneous tissue. Arch Dermatol 1972; 106: 515–524.

61. Krieg T, Meurer M. Systemic scleroderma. Clinical and pathophysiologic aspects. J Am Acad Dermatol 1988; 18: 457–481.

62. Chanda JJ. Scleroderma and other diseases associated with cutaneous sclerosis. Med Clin North Am 1980; 64: 969–983.

63. Furey NL, Schmid FR, Kwaan HC, Friederici HHR. Arterial thrombosis in scleroderma. Br J Dermatol 1975; 93: 683–693.

64. Thomas JR III, Winkelmann RK. Vascular ulcers in scleroderma. Arch Dermatol 1983; 119: 803–807.

65. Livingston JZ, Scott TE, Wigley FM et al. Systemic sclerosis (scleroderma): clinical, genetic, and serologic subsets. J Rheumatol 1987; 14: 512–518.

66. Reimer G, Steen VD, Penning CA et al. Correlates between autoantibodies to nucleolar antigens and

clinical features in patients with systemic sclerosis (scleroderma). Arthritis Rheum 1988; 31: 525–532.

67. Chen Z, Virella G, Tung HE et al. Immune complexes and antinuclear, antinucleolar, and anticentromere antibodies in scleroderma. J Am Acad Dermatol 1984; 11: 461–467.

68. Chen Z, Fedrick JA, Pandey JP et al. Anticentromere antibody and immunoglobulin allotypes in scleroderma. Arch Dermatol 1985; 121: 339–344.

69. Tuffanelli DL, McKeon F, Kleinsmith DM et al. Anticentromere and anticentriole antibodies in the scleroderma spectrum. Arch Dermatol 1983; 119: 560–566.

70. Chorzelski TP, Jablonska S, Beutner EH et al. Anticentromere antibody: an immunological marker of a subset of systemic sclerosis. Br J Dermatol 1985; 113: 381–389.

71. Fritzler MJ, Arlette JP, Behm AR, Kinsella TD. Hereditary hemorrhagic telangiectasia versus CREST syndrome: Can serology aid diagnosis? J Am Acad Dermatol 1984; 10: 192–196.

72. Carr RD, Heisel EB, Stevenson TD. CREST syndrome. A benign variant of scleroderma. Arch Dermatol 1965; 92: 519–525.

73. Velayos EE, Masi AT, Stevens MB, Shulman LE. The 'CREST' syndrome. Comparison with systemic sclerosis (scleroderma). Arch Intern Med 1979; 139: 1240–1244.

74. Asboe-Hansen G. Scleroderma. J Am Acad Dermatol 1987; 17: 102–108.

75. Sanchez JL, Vazquez M, Sanchez NP, Vitiligolike macules in systemic scleroderma. Arch Dermatol 1983; 119: 129–133.

76. Jawitz JC, Albert MK, Nigra TP, Bunning RD. A new skin manifestation of progressive systemic sclerosis. J Am Acad Dermatol 1984; 11: 265–268.

77. Luderschmidt C, Scholz S, Mehlhaff E et al. Association of progressive systemic scleroderma to several HLA-B and HLA-DR alleles. Arch Dermatol 1987; 123: 1188–1191.

78. Rendall JR, McKenzie AW. Familial scleroderma. Br J Dermatol 1974; 91: 517–522.

79. Greger RE. Familial progressive systemic scleroderma. Arch Dermatol 1975; 111: 81–85.

80. Kleinsmith DM, Heinzerling RH, Burnham TK. Antinuclear antibodies as immunologic markers for a benign subset and different clinical characteristics of scleroderma. Arch Dermatol 1982; 118: 882–885.

80a. Bell S, Krieg T, Meurer M. Antibodies to Ro/SSA detected by ELISA: correlation with clinical features in systemic scleroderma. Br J Dermatol 1989; 121: 35–41.

81. Fleischmajer R, Perlish JS, Duncan M. Scleroderma. A model for fibrosis. Arch Dermatol 1983; 119: 957–962.

82. Haustein UF, Herrmann K, Bohme HJ. Pathogenesis of progressive systemic sclerosis. Int J Dermatol 1986; 25: 286–293.

83. Lee EB, Anhalt GJ, Voorhees JJ, Diaz LA. Pathogenesis of scleroderma. Current concepts. Int J Dermatol 1984; 23: 85–89.

84. LeRoy EC. Pathogenesis of scleroderma (systemic sclerosis). J Invest Dermatol 1982; 79: 87s–89s.

85. Silverstein JL, Steen VD, Medsger TA Jr, Falanga V. Cutaneous hypoxia in patients with systemic sclerosis

(scleroderma). Arch Dermatol 1988; 128: 1379–1382.

86. Dowd PM, Kirby JD, Holborow EJ et al. Detection of immune complexes in systemic sclerosis and Raynaud's phenomenon. Br J Dermatol 1981; 105: 179–188.

86a. Falanga V, Soter NA, Altman RD, Kerdel FA. Elevated plasma histamine levels in systemic sclerosis (scleroderma). Arch Dermatol 1990; 126: 336–338.

87. Kahari V-M, Sandberg M, Kalimo H et al. Identification of fibroblasts responsible for increased collagen production in localized scleroderma by in situ hybridization. J Invest Dermatol 1988; 90: 664–670.

88. Perlish JS, Lemlich G, Fleischmajer R. Identification of collagen fibrils in scleroderma skin. J Invest Dermatol 1988; 90: 48–54.

89. Zachariae H, Halkier-Sorensen L, Heickendorff L. Serum aminoterminal propeptide of type III procollagen in progressive systemic sclerosis and localized scleroderma. Acta Derm Venereol 1989; 69: 66–70.

90. Lovell CR, Nicholls AC, Duance VC, Bailey AJ. Characterization of dermal collagen in systemic sclerosis. Br J Dermatol 1979; 100: 359–369.

91. Falanga V, Alstadt SP. Effect of a platelet release fraction on glycosaminoglycan synthesis by cultured dermal fibroblasts from patients with progressive systemic sclerosis. Br J Dermatol 1988; 118: 339–345.

92. Ishikawa H, Kitabatake M, Akiyama F. Biochemical characterization of scleroderma-inducing glycosaminoglycan. Acta Derm Venereol 1988; 68: 378–384.

93. Cantwell AR Jr, Rowe L, Kelso DW. Nodular scleroderma and pleomorphic acid-fast bacteria. Arch Dermatol 1980; 116: 1283–1290.

94. Cantwell AR Jr. Histologic forms resembling "large bodies" in scleroderma and "pseudoscleroderma". Am J Dermatopathol 1980; 2: 273–276.

95. Fleischmajer R, Damiano V, Nedwich A. Alteration of subcutaneous tissue in systemic scleroderma. Arch Dermatol 1972; 105: 59–66.

96. Fleischmajer R. The pathophysiology of scleroderma. Int J Dermatol 1977; 16: 310–318.

97. Fleischmajer R, Perlish JS, Shaw KV, Pirozzi DJ. Skin capillary changes in early systemic scleroderma. Arch Dermatol 1976; 112: 1553–1557.

98. Rodnan GP, Myerowitz RL, Justh GO. Morphologic changes in the digital arteries of patients with progressive systemic sclerosis (scleroderma) and Raynaud phenomenon. Medicine (Baltimore) 1980; 59: 393–408.

99. Nishioka K, Kobayashi Y, Katayama I, Takijiri C. Mast cell numbers in diffuse scleroderma. Arch Dermatol 1987; 123: 205–208.

99a. Claman HN. Mast cell changes in a case of rapidly progressive scleroderma — ultrastructural analysis. J Invest Dermatol 1989; 92: 290–295.

100. Connolly SM, Winkelmann RK. Direct immunofluorescent findings in scleroderma syndromes. Acta Derm Venereol 1981; 61: 29–36.

101. Reimer G, Huschka U, Keller J et al. Immunofluorescence studies in progressive systemic sclerosis (scleroderma) and mixed connective tissue disease. Br J Dermatol 1983; 109: 27–36.

102. Fleischmajer R, Perlish JS, West WP. Ultrastructure of cutaneous cellular infiltrates in scleroderma. Arch Dermatol 1977; 113: 1661–1666.

103. Sharp GC, Irvin WS, Tan EM et al. Mixed connective tissue disease: an apparently distinct rheumatic disease syndrome associated with a specific antibody to an extractable nuclear antigen (ENA). Am J Med 1972; 52: 148–159.
104. Sharp GC, Anderson PC. Current concepts in the classification of connective tissue diseases. Overlap syndromes and mixed connective tissue disease. J Am Acad Dermatol 1980; 2: 269–279.
105. Rasmussen EK, Ullman S, Hoier-Madsen M et al. Clinical implications of ribonucleoprotein antibody. Arch Dermatol 1987; 123: 601–605.
106. Chubick A, Gilliam JN. A review of mixed connective tissue disease. Int J Dermatol 1978; 17: 123–133.
107. Gilliam JN, Prystowsky SD. Mixed connective tissue disease syndrome. Arch Dermatol 1977; 113: 583–587.
108. Bentley-Phillips CB, Geake TMS. Mixed connective tissue disease characterized by speckled epidermal nuclear IgG deposition in normal skin. Br J Dermatol 1980; 102: 529–533.
109. Chanda JJ, Callen JP, Taylor WB. Diffuse fasciitis with eosinophilia. Arch Dermatol 1978; 114: 1522–1524.
110. Golitz LE. Fasciitis with eosinophilia: The Shulman syndrome. Int J Dermatol 1980; 19: 552–555.
111. Lupton GP, Goette DK. Localized eosinophilic fasciitis. Arch Dermatol 1979; 115: 85–87.
112. Michet CJ Jr, Doyle JA, Ginsburg WW. Eosinophilic fasciitis. Report of 15 cases. Mayo Clin Proc 1981; 56: 27–34.
113. Falanga V, Medsger TA Jr. Frequency, levels, and significance of blood eosinophilia in systemic sclerosis, localized scleroderma, and eosinophilic fasciitis. J Am Acad Dermatol 1987; 17: 648–656.
114. Fleischmajer R, Jacotot AB, Binnick SA. Scleroderma, eosinophilia, and diffuse fasciitis. Arch Dermatol 1978; 114: 1320–1325.
115. Ormerod AD, Grieve JHK, Rennie JAN, Edward N. Eosinophilic fasciitis — a case with hypogammaglobulinaemia. Clin Exp Dermatol 1984; 9: 416–418.
116. Bennett RM, Herron A, Keogh L. Eosinophilic fasciitis. Case report and review of the literature. Ann Rheum Dis 1977; 36: 354–359.
117. Lee P. Eosinophilic fasciitis — new associations and current perspectives (Editorial). J Rheumatol 1981; 8: 6–8.
118. Torres VM, George WM. Diffuse eosinophilic fasciitis. A new syndrome or a variant of scleroderma. Arch Dermatol 1977; 113: 1591–1593.
119. Jarratt M, Bybee JD, Ramsdell W. Eosinophilic fasciitis: An early variant of scleroderma. J Am Acad Dermatol 1979; 1: 221–226.
120. Cramer SF, Kent L, Abramowsky C, Moskowitz RW. Eosinophilic fasciitis. Arch Pathol Lab Med 1982; 106: 85–91.
120a. Kahari V-M, Heino J, Niskanen L et al. Eosinophilic fasciitis. Increased collagen production and type I procollagen messenger RNA levels in fibroblasts cultured from involved skin. Arch Dermatol 1990; 126: 613–617.
121. Frayha RA, Atiyah F, Karam P et al. Eosinophilic fasciitis terminating as progressive systemic sclerosis in a child. Dermatologica 1985; 171: 291–294.
122. Coyle E, Chapman RS. Eosinophilic fasciitis (Shulman syndrome) in association with morphoea and systemic sclerosis. Acta Derm Venereol 1980; 60: 181–182.
123. Stanek G, Konrad K, Jung M, Ehringer H. Shulman syndrome, a scleroderma subtype caused by Borrelia burgdorferi? Lancet 1987; 1: 1490.
124. Sepp N, Schmutzhard E, Fritsch P. Shulman syndrome associated with Borrelia burgdorferi and complicated by carpal tunnel syndrome. J Am Acad Dermatol 1988; 18: 1361–1362.
125. Janin-Mercier A, Mosser C, Souteyrand P, Bourges M. Subcutaneous sclerosis with fasciitis and eosinophilia after phytonadione injections. Arch Dermatol 1985; 121: 1421–1423.
125a. Gordon ML, Lebwohl MG, Phelps RG et al. Eosinophilic fasciitis associated with tryptophan ingestion. Arch Dermatol 1991; 127: 217–220.
126. Barnes L, Rodnan GP, Medsger TA Jr, Short D. Eosinophilic fasciitis. A pathologic study of twenty cases. Am J Pathol 1979; 96: 493–518.
127. Weinstein D, Schwartz RA. Eosinophilic fasciitis. Arch Dermatol 1978; 114: 1047–1049.
128. Keczkes K, Goode JD. The Shulman syndrome: report of a further case. Br J Dermatol 1979; 100: 381–384.
129. Kent LT, Cramer SF, Moskowitz RW. Eosinophilic fasciitis. Clinical, laboratory, and microscopic considerations. Arthritis Rheum 1981; 24: 677–683.
130. Tamura T, Saito Y, Ishikawa H. Diffuse fasciitis with eosinophilia: Histological and electron microscopic study. Acta Derm Venereol 1979; 59: 325–331.
131. Botet MV, Sanchez JL. The fascia in systemic scleroderma. J Am Acad Dermatol 1980; 3: 36–42.

Sclerodermoid disorders

132. Fleischmajer R, Pollock JL. Progressive systemic sclerosis: Pseudoscleroderma. Clin Rheum Dis 1979; 5: 243–261.
132a. Uitto J, Jimenez S. Fibrotic skin diseases. Clinical presentations, etiologic considerations, and treatment options. Arch Dermatol 1990; 126: 661–664.
133. Jablonska S, Stachow A, Suffczynska M. Skin and muscle indurations in phenylketonuria. Arch Dermatol 1967; 95: 443–450.
134. Winchester P, Grossman H, Lim WN, Danes BS. A new acid mucopolysaccharidosis with skeletal deformities simulating rheumatoid arthritis. Am J Roentgenol 1969; 106: 121–128.
135. Hollister DW, Rimoin DL, Lachman RS et al. The Winchester syndrome: A nonlysosomal connective tissue disease. J Pediatr 1974; 84: 701–709.
136. Cohen AH, Hollister DW, Reed WB. The skin in the Winchester syndrome. Histologic and ultrastructural studies. Arch Dermatol 1975; 111: 230–236.
137. Dunger DB, Dicks-Mireaux C, O'Driscoll P et al. Two cases of Winchester syndrome: with increased urinary oligosaccharide excretion. Eur J Pediatr 1987; 146: 615–619.
138. Nabai H, Mehregan AH, Mortezai A et al. Winchester syndrome: Report of a case from Iran. J Cutan Pathol 1977; 4: 281–285.
139. Mackenzie CR. Pachydermoperiostosis: a

paraneoplastic syndrome. N Y State J Med 1986; 86: 153–154.

140. Venencie PY, Boffa GA, Delmas PD et al. Pachydermoperiostosis with gastric hypertrophy, anemia, and increased serum bone Gla-protein levels. Arch Dermatol 1988; 124: 1831–1834.

141. Vogl A, Goldfischer S. Pachydermoperiostosis. Primary or idiopathic hypertrophic osteoarthropathy. Am J Med 1962; 33: 166–187.

142. Rimoin DL. Pachydermoperiostosis (idiopathic clubbing and periostosis). N Engl J Med 1965; 272: 923–931.

143. Stone OJ. Clubbing and koilonychia. Dermatol Clin 1985; 3: 485–490.

144. Gray RG, Gottlieb NL. Pseudoscleroderma in hypertrophic osteoarthropathy. JAMA 1981; 246: 2062–2063.

145. Marmelzat WL. Secondary hypertrophic ·osteoarthropathy and acanthosis nigricans. Arch Dermatol 1964; 89: 328–333.

146. Curth HO, Firschein IL, Alpert M. Familial clubbed fingers. Arch Dermatol 1961; 83: 828–836.

147. Matucci-Cerinic M, Lotti T, Jajic I et al. Cutaneous fibrinolytic activity in primary hypertrophic osteoarthropathy. Scand J Rheumatol 1987; 16: 205–212.

148. Hambrick GW Jr, Carter DM. Pachydermoperiostosis. Arch Dermatol 1966; 94: 594–608.

149. Shawarby K, Ibrahim MS. Pachydermoperiostosis. A review of literature and report on four cases. Br Med J 1962; 1: 763–766.

150. Meyerson LB, Meier GC. Cutaneous lesions in acroosteolysis. Arch Dermatol 1972; 106: 224–227.

151. Markowitz SS, McDonald CJ, Fethiere W, Kerzner MS. Occupational acroosteolysis. Arch Dermatol 1972; 106: 219–223.

152. Haustein UF, Ziegler V. Environmentally induced systemic sclerosis-like disorders. Int J Dermatol 1985; 24: 147–151.

153. Saihan EM, Burton JL, Heaton KW. A new syndrome with pigmentation, scleroderma, gynaecomastia, Raynaud's phenomenon and peripheral neuropathy. Br J Dermatol 1978; 99: 437–440.

153a. Haustein U-F, Ziegler V, Herrmann K et al. Silica-induced scleroderma. J Am Acad Dermatol 1990; 22: 444–448.

154. Brunskill NJ, Berth-Jones J, Graham-Brown RAC. Pseudosclerodermatous reaction to phytomenadione injection (Texier's syndrome). Clin Exp Dermatol 1988; 13: 276–278.

155. Robison JW, Odom RB. Delayed cutaneous reaction to phytonadione. Arch Dermatol 1978; 114: 1790–1792.

156. Iglesias JL, De Moragas JM. The cutaneous lesions of the Spanish toxic oil syndrome. J Am Acad Dermatol 1983; 9: 159–160.

157. Martinez-Tello FJ, Navas-Palacios JJ, Ricoy JR et al. Pathology of a new toxic syndrome caused by ingestion of adulterated oil in Spain. Virchows Arch (A) 1982; 397: 261–285.

158. Cohen IS, Mosher MB, O'Keefe EJ et al. Cutaneous toxicity of bleomycin therapy. Arch Dermatol 1973; 107: 553–555.

159. Mountz JD, Downs Minor MB, Turner R et al. Bleomycin-induced cutaneous toxicity in the rat: analysis of histopathology and ultrastructure compared with progressive systemic sclerosis (scleroderma). Br J Dermatol 1983; 108: 679–686.

160. Wallace HJ. Lichen sclerosus et atrophicus. Trans St John's Hosp Dermatol Soc 1971; 57: 9–30.

160a. Ridley CM. Lichen sclerosus et atrophicus. Semin Dermatol 1989; 8: 54–63.

161. Tremaine RDL, Miller RAW. Lichen sclerosus et atrophicus. Int J Dermatol 1989; 28: 10–16.

162. Sanchez NP, Mihm MC Jr. Reactive and neoplastic alterations of the vulva. J Am Acad Dermatol 1982; 6: 378–388.

163. Purres J, Krull EA. Lichen sclerosus et atrophicus involving the palms. Arch Dermatol 1971; 104: 68–69.

164. Petrozzi JW, Wood MG, Tisa V. Palmar-plantar lichen sclerosus et atrophicus. Arch Dermatol 1979; 115: 884.

165. Hammar H. Plantar lesions of lichen sclerosus et atrophicus accompanied by erythermalgia. Acta Derm Venereol 1978; 58: 91–92.

166. Dalziel K, Reynolds AJ, Holt PJA. Lichen sclerosus et atrophicus with ocular and maxillary complications. Br J Dermatol 1987; 116: 735–737.

167. Foulds IS. Lichen sclerosus et atrophicus of the scalp. Br J Dermatol 1980; 103: 197–200.

168. Miller RF. Lichen sclerosus et atrophicus with oral involvement. Arch Dermatol 1957; 76: 43–55.

169. Anderton RL, Abele DC. Lichen sclerosus et atrophicus in a vaccination site. Arch Dermatol 1976; 112: 1787.

170. Chalmers RJG, Burton PA, Bennett RF et al. Lichen sclerosus et atrophicus. A common and distinctive cause of phimosis in boys. Arch Dermatol 1984; 120: 1025–1027.

171. Rickwood AMK, Hemalatha V, Batcup G, Spitz L. Phimosis in boys. Br J Urol 1980; 52: 147–150.

172. Clemmensen OJ, Krogh J, Petri M. The histologic spectrum of prepuces from patients with phimosis. Am J Dermatopathol 1988; 10: 104–108.

173. Apisarnthanarax P, Osment LS, Montes LF. Extensive lichen sclerosus et atrophicus in a 7-year-old boy. Arch Dermatol 1972; 106: 94–96.

174. Meyrick Thomas RH, Ridley CM, Black MM. Clinical features and therapy of lichen sclerosus et atrophicus affecting males. Clin Exp Dermatol 1987; 12: 126–128.

175. Klein LE, Cohen SR, Weinstein M. Bullous lichen sclerosus et atrophicus: Treatment by tangential excision. J Am Acad Dermatol 1984; 10: 346–350.

176. Di Silverio A, Serri F. Generalized bullous and haemorrhagic lichen sclerosus et atrophicus. Br J Dermatol 1975; 93: 215–217.

177. Leppard B, Sneddon IB. Milia occurring in lichen sclerosus et atrophicus. Br J Dermatol 1975; 92: 711–714.

178. Clark JA, Muller SA. Lichen sclerosus et atrophicus in children. A report of 24 cases. Arch Dermatol 1967; 95: 476–482.

179. Shirer JA, Ray MC. Familial occurrence of lichen sclerosus et atrophicus. Arch Dermatol 1987; 123: 485–488.

180. Ridley CM. Lichen sclerosus et atrophicus. Arch Dermatol 1987; 123: 457–460.

181. Murphy FR, Lipa M, Haberman HF. Familial vulvar dystrophy of lichen sclerosus type. Arch Dermatol 1982; 118: 329–331.
182. Goltz R. Questions to the Editorial Board and other authorities. Am J Dermatopathol 1980; 2: 283.
183. Patterson JAK, Ackerman AB. Lichen sclerosus et atrophicus is not related to morphea. Am J Dermatopathol 1984; 6: 323–335.
184. Meyrick Thomas RH, Ridley CM, Black MM. The association of lichen sclerosus et atrophicus and autoimmune-related disease in males. Br J Dermatol 1983; 109: 661–664.
185. Meyrick Thomas RH, Ridley CM, McGibbon DH, Black MM. Lichen sclerosus et atrophicus and autoimmunity — a study of 350 women. Br J Dermatol 1988; 118: 41–46.
186. Leighton PC, Langley FA. A clinico-pathological study of vulval dermatoses. J Clin Pathol 1975; 28: 394–402.
187. Sloan PJM, Goepel J. Lichen sclerosus et atrophicus and perianal carcinoma: a case report. Clin Exp Dermatol 1981; 6: 399–402.
188. Hart WR, Norris HJ, Helwig EB. The malignant potential of lichen sclerosus et atrophicus of the vulva. Am J Clin Pathol 1975; 63: 758 (abstract).
189. Garcia–Bravo B, Sanchez-Pedreno P, Rodriguez-Pichardo A, Camacho F. Lichen sclerosus et atrophicus. A study of 76 cases and their relation to diabetes. J Am Acad Dermatol 1988; 19: 482–485.
190. Barker LP, Gross P. Lichen sclerosus et atrophicus of the female genitalia. Arch Dermatol 1962; 85: 362–373.
191. Suurmond D. Lichen sclerosus et atrophicus of the vulva. Arch Dermatol 1964; 90: 143–152.
192. Steigleder GK, Raab WP. Lichen sclerosus et atrophicus. Arch Dermatol 1961; 84: 219–226.
192a. Rahbari H. Histochemical differentiation of localized morphea-scleroderma and lichen sclerosus et atrophicus. J Cutan Pathol 1989; 16: 342–347.
193. Mann PR, Cowan MA. Ultrastructural changes in four cases of lichen sclerosus et atrophicus. Br J Dermatol 1973; 89: 223–231.
194. Kint A, Geerts ML. Lichen sclerosus et atrophicus. An electron microscopic study. J Cutan Pathol 1975; 2: 30–34.

Other hypertrophic collagenoses

195. Uitto J, Santa Cruz DJ, Eisen AZ. Connective tissue nevi of the skin. J Am Acad Dermatol 1980; 3: 441–461.
196. Rocha G, Winkelmann RK. Connective tissue nevus. Arch Dermatol 1962; 85: 722–729.
197. Cohen EL. Connective tissue naevus of the palm. Clin Exp Dermatol 1979; 4: 543–544.
198. Uitto J, Santa-Cruz DJ, Eisen AZ. Familial cutaneous collagenoma: genetic studies on a family. Br J Dermatol 1979; 101: 185–195.
199. Henderson RR, Wheeler CE Jr, Abele DC. Familial cutaneous collagenoma. Report of cases. Arch Dermatol 1968; 98: 23–27.
200. Kopec AV, Levine N. Generalized connective tissue nevi and ichthyosis in Down's syndrome. Arch Dermatol 1979; 115: 623–624.
201. Morrison JGL, Wilson Jones E, MacDonald DM. Juvenile elastoma and osteopoikilosis (the Buschke-Ollendorff syndrome). Br J Dermatol 1977; 97: 417–422.
202. Ledoux-Corbusier M, Achten G, De Dobbeleer G. Juvenile elastoma (Weidman). An ultrastructural study. J Cutan Pathol 1981; 8: 219–227.
203. Uitto J, Bauer EA, Santa Cruz DJ et al. Decreased collagenase production by regional fibroblasts cultured from skin of a patient with connective tissue nevi of the collagen type. J Invest Dermatol 1982; 78: 136–140.
204. Herbst VP, Kauh YC, Luscombe HA. Connective tissue nevus masquerading as a localized linear epidermal nevus. J Am Acad Dermatol 1987; 16: 264–266.
205. Pierard GE, Lapiere CM. Nevi of connective tissue. A reappraisal of their classification. Am J Dermatopathol 1985; 7: 325–333.
206. Smith LR, Bernstein BD. Eruptive collagenoma. Arch Dermatol 1978; 114: 1710–1711.
207. Nickel WR, Reed WB. Tuberous sclerosis. Special reference to the microscopic alterations in the cutaneous hamartomas. Arch Dermatol 1962; 85: 209–224.
208. Reed RJ. Cutaneous manifestations of neural crest disorders (neurocristopathies). Int J Dermatol 1977; 16: 807–826.
209. Ketchum LD. Hypertrophic scars and keloids. Clin Plast Surg 1977; 4: 301–310.
210. Ketchum LD, Cohen IK, Masters FW. Hypertrophic scars and keloids. A collective review. Plast Reconstr Surg 1974; 53: 140–154.
211. Murray JC, Pollack SV, Pinnell SR. Keloids: A review. J Am Acad Dermatol 1981; 4: 461–470.
212. Cosman B, Crikelair GF, Gaulin JC, Lattes R. The surgical treatment of keloids. Plast Reconstr Surg 1961; 27: 335–358.
213. Blackburn WR, Cosman B. Histologic basis of keloid and hypertrophic scar differentiation. Arch Pathol 1966; 82: 65–71.
214. Ala-Kokko L, Rintala A, Savolainen E-R. Collagen gene expression in keloids: Analysis of collagen metabolism and type I, III, IV and V procollagen mRNAs in keloid tissue and keloid fibroblast cultures. J Invest Dermatol 1987; 89: 238–244.
215. Cohen IK, Keiser HR, Sjoerdsma A. Collagen synthesis in human keloid and hypertrophic scar. Surg Forum 1971; 22: 488–489.
216. Milsom JP, Craig RDP. Collagen degradation in cultured keloid and hypertrophic scar tissue. Br J Dermatol 1973; 89: 635–644.
217. Abergel RP, Pizzurro D, Meeker CA et al. Biochemical composition of the connective tissue in keloids and analysis of collagen metabolism in keloid fibroblast cultures. J Invest Dermatol 1985; 84: 384–390.
218. Ackerman AB, Ragaz A. The lives of lesions. Chronology in dermatopathology. New York: Masson, 1984; 58–61.
219. Pedragosa R, Serrano S, Carol-Murillo J et al. Blisters over burn scars in a child. Br J Dermatol 1986; 115: 501–506.
220. Redmond WJ, Baker SR. Keloidal calcification. Arch Dermatol 1983; 119: 270–272.
221. Matsuoka LY, Uitto J, Wortsman J et al. Ultrastructural characteristics of keloid fibroblasts.

Am J Dermatopathol 1988; 10: 505–508.

222. James WD, Besanceney CD, Odom RB. The ultrastructure of a keloid. J Am Acad Dermatol 1980; 3: 50–57.

223. Tsuji T, Sawabe M. Elastic fibers in scar tissue: scanning and transmission electron microscopic studies. J Cutan Pathol 1987; 14: 106–113.

224. Elton RF, Pinkus H. Striae in normal men. Arch Dermatol 1966; 94: 33–34.

224a. Nigam PK. Striae cutis distensae. Int J Dermatol 1989; 28: 426–428.

225. Wong RC, Ellis CN. Physiologic skin changes in pregnancy. J Am Acad Dermatol 1984; 10: 929–940.

226. Shelley WB, Cohen W. Stria migrans. Arch Dermatol 1964; 90: 193–194.

227. Carr RD, Hamilton JF. Transverse striae of the back. Arch Dermatol 1969; 99: 26–30.

228. Arem AJ, Kischer CW. Analysis of striae. Plast Reconstr Surg 1980; 65: 22–29.

229. Chernosky ME, Knox JM. Atrophic striae after occlusive corticosteroid therapy. Arch Dermatol 1964; 90: 15–19.

230. Shuster S. The cause of striae distensae. Acta Derm Venereol (Suppl) 1979; 85: 161–169.

231. Zheng P, Lavker RM, Kligman AM. Anatomy of striae. Br J Dermatol 1985; 112: 185–193.

232. Pinkus H, Keech MK, Mehregan AH. Histopathology of striae distensae with special reference to striae and wound healing in the Marfan syndrome. J Invest Dermatol 1966; 46: 283–292.

233. Tsuji T, Sawabe M. Elastic fibers in striae distensae. J Cutan Pathol 1988; 15: 215–222.

234. Chaouat Y, Aron-Brunetiere R, Faures B et al. Une nouvelle entité: Le rhumatisme fibroblastique. A propos d'une observation. Rev Rhum Mal Osteoartic 1980; 47: 345–351.

235. Crouzet J, Amouroux J, Duterque M et al. Reumatisme fibroblastique. Un cas avec étude de l'histologie synoviale. Rev Rhum Mal Osteoartic 1982; 49: 469–472.

236. Vignon-Pennamen M-D, Naveau B, Foldes C et al. Fibroblastic rheumatism. J Am Acad Dermatol 1986; 14: 1086–1088.

237. Lister DM, Graham-Brown RAC, Burns DA et al. Collagenosis nuchae — a new entity? Clin Exp Dermatol 1988; 13: 263–264.

238. Weedon D (1989). Unpublished observations.

Atrophic collagenoses

239. Guillen PS, Pichardo AR, Martinez FC. Aplasia cutis congenita. J Am Acad Dermatol 1985; 13: 429–433.

240. Pap GS. Congenital defect of scalp and skull in three generations of one family. Plast Reconstr Surg 1970; 46: 194–196.

241. Rauschkolb RR, Enriquez SI. Aplasia cutis congenita. Arch Dermatol 1962; 86: 54–57.

242. Sybert VP. Aplasia cutis congenita: A report of 12 new families and review of the literature. Pediatr Dermatol 1985; 3: 1–14.

243. Irons GB, Olson RM. Aplasia cutis congenita. Plast Reconstr Surg 1980; 66: 199–203.

244. Scribanu N, Temtamy SA. The syndrome of aplasia cutis congenita with terminal, transverse defects of limbs. J Pediatr 1975; 87: 79–82.

245. Fryns JP, Corbeel L, Van den Berghe H. Congenital scalp defect with distal limb reduction anomalies. Eur J Pediatr 1977; 126: 289–295.

246. Ruiz-Maldonado R, Tamayo L. Aplasia cutis congenita, spastic paralysis, and mental retardation. Am J Dis Child 1974; 128: 699–701.

247. Frieden IJ. Aplasia cutis congenita: A clinical review and proposal for classification. J Am Acad Dermatol 1986; 14: 646–660.

248. Mimouni F, Han BK, Barnes L et al. Multiple hamartomas associated with intracranial malformation. Pediatr Dermatol 1986; 3: 219–225.

249. Bart BJ, Gorlin RJ, Anderson VE, Lynch FW. Congenital localized absence of skin and associated abnormalities resembling epidermolysis bullosa. Arch Dermatol 1966; 93: 296–304.

250. Wojnarowska FT, Eady RAJ, Wells RS. Dystrophic epidermolysis bullosa presenting with congenital localized absence of skin: report of four cases. Br J Dermatol 1983; 108: 477–483.

251. Skoven I, Drzewiecki KT. Congenital localized skin defect and epidermolysis bullosa hereditaria letalis. Acta Derm Venereol 1979; 59: 533–537.

252. Smith SZ, Cram DL. A mechanobullous disorder of the newborn: Bart's syndrome. Arch Dermatol 1978; 114: 81–84.

253. Deeken JH, Caplan RM. Aplasia cutis congenita. Arch Dermatol 1970; 102: 386–389.

254. Fisher M, Schneider R. Aplasia cutis congenita in three successive generations. Arch Dermatol 1973; 108: 252–253.

255. Yagupsky P, Reuveni H, Karplus M, Moses S. Aplasia cutis congenita in one of monozygotic twins. Pediatr Dermatol 1986; 3: 403–405.

256. Kalb RE, Grossman ME. The association of aplasia cutis congenita with therapy of maternal thyroid disease. Pediatr Dermatol 1986; 3: 327–330.

257. Stephan MJ, Smith DW, Ponzi JW, Alden ER. Origin of scalp vertex aplasia cutis. J Pediatr 1982; 101: 850–853.

258. Levin DL, Nolan KS, Esterly NB. Congenital absence of skin. J Am Acad Dermatol 1980; 2: 203–206.

259. Munkvad JM, Nielsen AO, Asmussen T. Aplasia cutis congenita. A follow-up evaluation after 25 years. Arch Dermatol 1981; 117: 232–233.

260. Leung RSC, Beer WE, Mehta HK. Aplasia cutis congenita presenting as a familial triad of atrophic alopecia, ocular defects and a peculiar scarring tendency of the skin. Br J Dermatol 1988; 118: 715–720.

261. Croce EJ, Purohit RC, Janovski NA. Congenital absence of skin (aplasia cutis congenita). Arch Surg 1973; 106: 732–734.

262. Harari Z, Pasmanik A, Dvoretzky I et al. Aplasia cutis congenita with dystrophic nail changes. Dermatologica 1976; 153: 363–368.

263. Rudolph RI, Schwartz W, Leyden JJ. Bitemporal aplasia cutis congenita. Occurrence with other cutaneous abnormalities. Arch Dermatol 1974; 110: 615–618.

264. Fukamizu H, Matsumoto K, Inoue K, Moriguchi T. Familial occurrence of aplasia cutis congenita. J Dermatol Surg Oncol 1982; 8: 1068–1070.

265. Goltz RW, Henderson RR, Hitch JM, Ott JE. Focal

dermal hypoplasia syndrome. A review of the literature and report of two cases. Arch Dermatol 1970; 101: 1–11.

266. Ishibashi A, Kurihara Y. Goltz's syndrome: focal dermal dysplasia syndrome (focal dermal hypoplasia). Dermatologica 1972; 144: 156–167.

267. Lever WF. Hypoplasia cutis congenita. Arch Dermatol 1964; 90: 340.

268. Prentice FM, Mackie RM. A case of focal dermal hypoplasia. Clin Exp Dermatol 1982; 7: 149–153.

269. Staughton RCD. Focal dermal hypoplasia (Goltz's syndrome) in a male. Proc R Soc Med 1976; 69: 232–233.

269a. Howell JB, Freeman RG. Cutaneous defects of focal dermal hypoplasia: an ectomesodermal dysplasia syndrome. J Cutan Pathol 1989; 16: 237–258.

270. Gottlieb SK, Fisher BK, Violin GA. Focal dermal hypoplasia. A nine-year follow-up study. Arch Dermatol 1973; 108: 551–553.

271. Larrègue M, Duterque M. Striated osteopathy in focal dermal hypoplasia. Arch Dermatol 1975; 111: 1365.

272. Happle R, Lenz W. Striation of bones in focal dermal hypoplasia: manifestation of functional mosaicism? Br J Dermatol 1977; 96: 133–138.

273. Champion RH. Focal dermal hypoplasia. Br J Dermatol (Suppl) 1975; 11: 70–71.

274. Uitto J, Bauer EA, Santa-Cruz DJ et al. Focal dermal hypoplasia: Abnormal growth characteristics of skin fibroblasts in culture. J Invest Dermatol 1980; 75: 170–175.

275. Atherton DJ, Hall M. Focal dermal hypoplasia syndrome. Clin Exp Dermatol 1979; 5: 249–252.

276. Howell JB. Nevus angiolipomatosus Vs focal dermal hypoplasia. Arch Dermatol 1965; 92: 238–248.

277. Tsuji T. Focal dermal hypoplasia syndrome. An electron microscopical study of the skin lesions. J Cutan Pathol 1982; 9: 271–281.

278. Magid ML, Prendiville JS, Esterly NB. Focal facial dermal dysplasia: Bitemporal lesions resembling aplasia cutis congenita. J Am Acad Dermatol 1988; 18: 1203–1207.

279. McGeoch AH, Reed WB. Familial focal facial dermal dysplasia. Arch Dermatol 1973; 107: 591–595.

280. Jensen NE. Congenital ectodermal dysplasia of the face. Br J Dermatol 1971; 84: 410–416.

281. Raque CJ, Stein KM, Lane JM, Reese EC Jr. Pseudoainhum constricting bands of the extremities. Arch Dermatol 1972; 105: 434–438.

282. Burnett JW, Schwartz MF, Berberian BJ. Ulerythema ophryogenes with multiple congenital anomalies. J Am Acad Dermatol 1988; 18: 437–440.

283. Mertens RLJ. Ulerythema ophryogenes and atopy. Arch Dermatol 1968; 97: 662–663.

284. Pierini DO, Pierini AM. Keratosis pilaris atrophicans faciei (ulerythema ophryogenes): a cutaneous marker in the Noonan syndrome. Br J Dermatol 1979; 100: 409–416.

284a. Snell JA, Mallory SB. Ulerythema ophryogenes in Noonan syndrome. Pediatr Dermatol 1990; 7: 77–78.

285. Neild VS, Pegum JS, Wells RS. The association of keratosis pilaris atrophicans and woolly hair, with and without Noonan's syndrome. Br J Dermatol 1984; 110: 357–362.

286. Markey AC, Tidman MJ, Sharvill DE, Wells RS.

287. Davenport DD. Ulerythema ophryogenes. Arch Dermatol 1964; 89: 74–80.

Ulerythema ophryogenes in Noonan's syndrome. Br J Dermatol (Suppl) 1988; 33: 114.

288. Rand R, Baden HP. Keratosis follicularis spinulosa decalvans. Report of two cases and literature review. Arch Dermatol 1983; 119: 22–26.

289. Britton H, Lustig J, Thompson BJ et al. Keratosis follicularis spinulosa decalvans. Arch Dermatol 1978; 114: 761–764.

290. Kuokkanen K. Keratosis follicularis spinulosa decalvans in a family from Northern Finland. Acta Derm Venereol 1971; 51: 146–150.

291. Appell ML, Sherertz EF. A kindred with alopecia, keratosis pilaris, cataracts, and psoriasis. J Am Acad Dermatol 1987; 16: 89–95.

292. Rozum LT, Mehregan AH, Johnson SAM. Folliculitis ulerythematosa reticulata. A case with unilateral lesions. Arch Dermatol 1972; 106: 388–389.

293. Frosch PJ, Brumage MR, Schuster-Pavlovic C, Bersch A. Atrophoderma vermiculatum. Case reports and review. J Am Acad Dermatol 1988; 18: 538–542.

294. Seville RH, Mumford PF. Congenital ectodermal defect. Atrophodermia vermicularis with leukokeratosis oris. Br J Dermatol 1956; 68: 310.

295. Michaelsson G, Olsson E, Westermark P. The ROMBO syndrome: a familial disorder with vermiculate atrophoderma, milia, hypotrichosis, trichoepitheliomas, basal cell carcinomas and peripheral vasodilation with cyanosis. Acta Derm Venereol 1981; 61: 497–503.

296. Marks VJ, Miller OF. Atrophia maculosa varioliformis cutis. Br J Dermatol 1986; 115: 105–109.

296a. Venencie PY, Foldes C, Cuny M et al. Atrophia maculosa varioliformis cutis with extrahepatic biliary atresia. J Am Acad Dermatol 1989; 21: 309.

297. Andersen BL. Erythromelanosis follicularis faciei et colli. Br J Dermatol 1980; 102: 323–325.

298. Whittaker SJ, Griffiths WAD. Erythromelanosis follicularis faciei et colli. Clin Exp Dermatol 1987; 12: 33–35.

299. Watt TL, Kaiser JS. Erythromelanosis follicularis faciei et colli. J Am Acad Dermatol 1981; 5: 533–534.

300. Snyder DS, Greenberg RA. Evaluation of atrophy production and vasoconstrictor potency in humans following intradermally injected corticosteroids. J Invest Dermatol 1974; 63: 461–463.

301. Stevanovic DV. Corticosteroid-induced atrophy of the skin with telangiectasia. Br J Dermatol 1972; 87: 548–556.

302. Sneddon IB. Atrophy of the skin. The clinical problems. Br J Dermatol (Suppl) 1976; 12: 121–123.

303. Fritsch WC. Deep atrophy of the skin of the deltoid area. Arch Dermatol 1970; 101: 585–587.

304. Goldman L. Reactions following intralesional and sublesional injections of corticosteroids. JAMA 1962; 182: 613–616.

305. Kikuchi I, Horikawa S. Perilymphatic atrophy of the skin. A side effect of topical corticosteroid injection therapy. Arch Dermatol 1974; 109: 558–559.

306. Gottlieb NL, Penneys NS, Brown HE Jr. Periarticular perilymphatic skin atrophy. JAMA 1978; 240: 559–560.

307. Gupta AK, Rasmussen JE. Perilesional linear atrophic streaks associated with intralesional corticosteroid

injections in a psoriatic plaque. Pediatr Dermatol 1987; 4: 259–260.

308. Friedman SJ, Butler DF, Pittelkow MR. Perilesional linear atrophy and hypopigmentation after intralesional corticosteroid therapy. J Am Acad Dermatol 1988; 19: 537–541.

309. James MP, Black MM, Sparkes CG. Measurement of dermal atrophy induced by topical steroids using a radiographic technique. Br J Dermatol 1977; 96: 303–305.

310. Dykes PJ, Marks R. An appraisal of the methods used in the assessment of atrophy from topical corticosteroids. Br J Dermatol 1979; 101: 599–609.

311. Cohen IK, Diegelmann RF, Johnson ML. Effect of corticosteroids on collagen synthesis. Surgery 1977; 82: 15–20.

312. Wilson Jones E. Steroid atrophy — a histological appraisal. Dermatologica (Suppl) 1976; 152: 107–115.

313. Jablonska S, Groniowska M, Dabroswki J. Comparative evaluation of skin atrophy in man induced by topical corticoids. Br J Dermatol 1979; 100: 193–206.

314. Fulop E. Mechanism of local skin atrophy caused by intradermally injected corticosteroids. Dermatologica (Suppl) 1976; 152: 139–146.

315. Schetman D, Hambrick GW Jr, Wilson CE. Cutaneous changes following local injection of triamcinolone. Arch Dermatol 1963; 88: 820–828.

316. Canizares O, Sachs PM, Jaimovich L, Torres VM. Idiopathic atrophoderma of Pasini and Pierini. Arch Dermatol 1958; 77: 42–59.

317. Pullara TJ, Lober CW, Fenske NA. Idiopathic atrophoderma of Pasini and Pierini. Int J Dermatol 1984; 23: 643–645.

318. Berman A, Berman GD, Winkelmann RK. Atrophoderma (Pasini–Pierini). Findings on direct immunofluorescent, monoclonal antibody, and ultrastructural studies. Int J Dermatol 1988; 27: 487–490.

319. Miller RF. Idiopathic atrophoderma. Report of a case and nosologic study. Arch Dermatol 1965; 92: 653–660.

320. Bisaccia EP, Scarborough DA, Lowney ED. Atrophoderma of Pasini and Pierini and systemic scleroderma. Arch Dermatol 1982; 118: 1–2.

321. Perry HO. Diseases that present as cutaneous sclerosis. Australas J Dermatol 1982; 23: 45–52.

321a. Coulson IH, Smith NP, Holden CA. Acrodermatitis chronica atrophicans with coexisting morphoea. Br J Dermatol 1989; 121: 263–269.

Perforating collagenoses

322. Woo TY, Rasmussen JE. Disorders of transepidermal elimination. Part 1. Int J Dermatol 1985; 24: 267–279.

323. Goette DK. Transepithelial elimination of altered collagen after intralesional adrenal steroid injections. Arch Dermatol 1984; 120: 539–540.

324. Delacretaz J, Gattlen JM. Transepidermal elimination of traumatically altered collagen. Dermatologica 1976; 152: 65–71.

325. Mehregan AH, Schwartz OD, Livingood CS. Reactive perforating collagenosis. Arch Dermatol 1967; 96: 277–282.

326. Yusuk S, Trau H, Stempler D et al. Reactive perforating collagenosis. Int J Dermatol 1985; 24: 584–586.

327. Fretzin DF, Beal DW, Jao W. Light and ultrastructural study of reactive perforating collagenosis. Arch Dermatol 1980; 116: 1054–1058.

328. Weiner AL. Reactive perforating collagenosis. Arch Dermatol 1970; 102: 540–544.

329. Cerio R, Jones EW. Reactive perforating collagenosis: a clinicopathological review of 10 cases. J Cutan Pathol 1988; 15: 301 (abstract).

330. Bovenmyer DA. Reactive perforating collagenosis. Experimental production of the lesion. Arch Dermatol 1970; 102: 313–317.

331. Nair BKH, Sarojini PA, Basheer AM, Nair CHK. Reactive perforating collagenosis. Br J Dermatol 1974; 91: 399–403.

332. Poliak SC, Lebwohl MG, Parris A, Prioleau PG. Reactive perforating collagenosis associated with diabetes mellitus. N Engl J Med 1982; 306: 81–84.

333. Cochran RJ, Tucker SB, Wilkin JK. Reactive perforating collagenosis of diabetes mellitus and renal failure. Cutis 1983; 31: 55–58.

334. Gupta AK, Gupta MA, Cardella CJ, Haberman HF. Cutaneous associations of chronic renal failure and dialysis. Int J Dermatol 1986; 25: 498–504.

335. Beck H-I, Brandrup F, Hagdrup HK et al. Adult, acquired reactive perforating collagenosis. Report of a case including ultrastructural findings. J Cutan Pathol 1988; 15: 124–128.

336. Patterson JW. The perforating disorders. J Am Acad Dermatol 1984; 10: 561–581.

336a. Rapini RP, Hebert AA, Drucker CR. Acquired perforating dermatosis. Evidence for combined transepidermal elimination of both collagen and elastic fibres. Arch Dermatol 1989; 125: 1074–1078.

336b. Patterson JW. Progress in the perforating dermatoses. Arch Dermatol 1989; 125: 1121–1123.

337. Pedragosa R, Knobel HJ, Huguet P et al. Reactive perforating collagenosis in Hodgkin's disease. Am J Dermatopathol 1987; 9: 41–44.

337a. Bank DE, Cohen PR, Kohn SR. Reactive perforating collagenosis in a setting of double disaster: Acquired immunodeficiency syndrome and end-stage renal disease. J Am Acad Dermatol 1989; 21: 371–374.

338. Millard PR, Young E, Harrison DE, Wojnarowska F. Reactive perforating collagenosis: light, ultrastructural and immunohistological studies. Histopathology 1986; 10: 1047–1056.

339. Laugier P, Woringer F. Reflexions au sujet d'un collagènome perforant verruciforme. Ann Dermatol Syph 1963; 90: 29–36.

340. Detlefs RL, Goette DK. Collagènome perforant verruciforme. Arch Dermatol 1986; 122: 1044–1046.

341. Weedon D. Unpublished observation.

342. Burns DA, Calnan CD. Chondrodermatitis nodularis antihelicis. Clin Exp Dermatol 1978; 3: 207–208.

343. Barker LP, Young AW, Sachs W. Chondrodermatitis of the ears. Arch Dermatol 1960; 81: 15–25.

344. Bard JW. Chondrodermatitis nodularis chronica helicis. Dermatologica 1981; 163: 376–384.

345. Dean E, Bernhard JD. Bilateral chondrodermatitis nodularis antihelicis. An unusual complication of cardiac pacemaker insertion. Int J Dermatol 1988; 27: 122.

346. Goette DK. Chondrodermatitis nodularis helicis: A perforating necrobiotic granuloma. J Am Acad Dermatol 1980; 2: 148–154.
347. Hurwitz RM. Painful papule of the ear: A follicular disorder. J Dermatol Surg Oncol 1987; 13: 270–274.
348. Hurwitz RM. Pseudocarcinomatous or infundibular hyperplasia. Am J Dermatopathol 1989; 11: 189–191.
349. Shuman R, Helwig EB. Chondrodermatitis helicis. Am J Clin Pathol 1954; 24: 126–144.
350. Santa Cruz DJ. Chondrodermatitis nodularis helicis: a transepidermal perforating disorder. J Cutan Pathol 1980; 7: 70–76.
351. Garcia E, Silva L, Martins O, Da Silva Picoto A et al. Bone formation in chondrodermatitis nodularis helicis. J Dermatol Surg Oncol 1980; 6: 582–585.

Variable collagen changes

352. Nelson DL, King RA. Ehlers–Danlos syndrome type VIII. J Am Acad Dermatol 1981; 5: 297–303.
353. Pinnell SR. Molecular defects in the Ehlers–Danlos syndrome. J Invest Dermatol 1982; 79: 90s–92s.
354. Black CM, Gathercole LJ, Bailey AJ, Beighton P. The Ehlers-Danlos syndrome: an analysis of the structure of the collagen fibres of the skin. Br J Dermatol 1980; 102: 85–96.
355. Maroteaux P, Frezal J, Cohen-Solal L. The differential symptomatology of errors of collagen metabolism. A tentative classification. Am J Med Genet 1986; 24: 219–230.
356. Sulica VI, Cooper PH, Pope FM et al. Cutaneous histologic features in Ehlers-Danlos syndrome. Arch Dermatol 1979; 115: 40–42.
357. Wechsler HL, Fisher ER. Ehlers–Danlos syndrome. Pathologic, histochemical, and electron microscopic observations. Arch Pathol 1964; 77: 613–619.
358. Kobayasi T, Oguchi M, Asboe-Hansen G. Dermal changes in Ehlers–Danlos syndrome. Clin Genet 1984; 25: 477–484.
359. Rizzo R, Contri MB, Micali G et al. Familial Ehlers–Danlos syndrome type II: abnormal fibrillogenesis of dermal collagen. Pediatr Dermatol 1987; 4: 197–204.
360. Pinnell SR. The skin in Ehlers–Danlos syndrome. J Am Acad Dermatol 1987; 16: 399–400.
361. De Paepe A, Nicholls A, Narcisi P et al. Ehlers–Danlos syndrome type I: a clinical and ultrastructural study of a family with reduced amounts of collagen type III. Br J Dermatol 1987; 117: 89–97.
362. Holzberg M, Hewan-Lowe KO, Olansky AJ. The Ehlers–Danlos syndrome: Recognition, characterization and importance of a milder variant of the classic form. A preliminary study. J Am Acad Dermatol 1988; 19: 656–666.
363. Sulh HMB, Steinmann B, Rao VH et al. Ehlers–Danlos syndrome type IV D: an autosomal recessive disorder. Clin Genet 1984; 25: 278–287.
364. Pope FM, Jones PM, Wells RS et al. EDS IV (acrogeria): new autosomal dominant and recessive types. J R Soc Med 1980; 73: 180–186.
365. Pope FM, Martin GR, McKusick VA. Inheritance of Ehlers–Danlos type IV syndrome. J Med Genet 1977; 14: 200–204.
366. McFarland W, Fuller DE. Mortality in Ehlers–Danlos syndrome due to spontaneous rupture of large arteries. N Engl J Med 1964; 271: 1309–1310.
367. Hernandez A, Aguirre-Negrette MG, Gonzalez-Flores S et al. Ehlers–Danlos features with progeroid facies and mild mental retardation. Clin Genet 1986; 30: 456–461.
368. Pope FM, Nicholls AC, Dorrance DE et al. Type III collagen deficiency with normal phenotype. J R Soc Med 1983; 76: 518–520.
369. Temple AS, Hinton P, Narcisi P, Pope FM. Detection of type III collagen in skin fibroblasts from patients with Ehlers–Danlos syndrome type IV by immunofluorescence. Br J Dermatol 1988; 118: 17–26.
370. Beighton P, Curtis D. X-linked Ehlers Danlos syndrome type V; the next generation. Clin Genet 1985; 27: 472–478.
371. Pinnell SR, Krane SM, Kenzora JE, Glimcher MJ. A heritable disorder of connective tissue. Hydroxylysine-deficient collagen disease. N Engl J Med 1972; 286: 1013–1020.
372. Ihme A, Krieg T, Nerlich A et al. Ehlers–Danlos syndrome type VI: collagen type specificity of defective lysyl hydroxylation in various tissues. J Invest Dermatol 1984; 83: 161–165.
373. Cole WG, Evans R, Sillence DO. The clinical features of Ehlers–Danlos type VII due to a deletion of 24 amino acids from the pro α 1 (1) chain of type I procollagen. J Med Genet 1987; 24: 698–701.
374. Zalis EG, Roberts DC. Ehlers-Danlos syndrome. Arch Dermatol 1967; 96: 540–544.
375. Prockop DJ, Kivirikko KI, Tuderman L, Guzman NA. The biosynthesis of collagen and its disorders. N Engl J Med 1979; 301: 77–85.
376. Peltonen L, Kuivaniemi H, Palotie A et al. Alterations in copper and collagen metabolism in the Menkes syndrome and a new subtype of the Ehlers–Danlos syndrome. Biochemistry 1983; 22: 6156–6163.
377. Arneson MA, Hammerschmidt DE, Furcht LT, King RA. A new form of Ehlers–Danlos syndrome. Fibronectin corrects defective platelet function. JAMA 1980; 244: 144–147.
378. Cullen SI. Localized Ehlers–Danlos syndrome. Arch Dermatol 1979; 115: 332–333.
379. Sasaki T, Arai K, Ono M et al. Ehlers-Danlos syndrome. Arch Dermatol 1987; 123: 76–79.
380. Pope FM, Nicholls AC, McPheat J et al. Collagen genes and proteins in osteogenesis imperfecta. J Med Genet 1985; 22: 466–478.
380a. Cohen PR, Schneiderman P. Clinical manifestations of the Marfan syndrome. Int J Dermatol 1989; 28: 291–299.
381. Abraham PA, Perejda AJ, Carnes WH, Uitto J. Marfan syndrome. Demonstration of abnormal elastin in aorta. J Clin Invest 1982; 70: 1245–1252.

Syndromes of premature ageing

382. Beauregard S, Gilchrest BA. Syndromes of premature aging. Dermatol Clin 1987; 5: 109–121.
383. Gilkes JJH, Sharvill DE, Wells RS. The premature ageing syndromes. Report of eight cases and description of a new entity named metageria. Br J Dermatol 1974; 91: 243–262.
384. Hrabko RP, Milgrom H, Schwartz RA. Werner's syndrome with associated malignant neoplasms. Arch Dermatol 1982; 118: 106–108.
385. Gawkrodger DJ, Priestley GC, Vijayalaxmi et al.

Werner's syndrome. Biochemical and cytogenetic studies. Arch Dermatol 1985; 121: 636–641.

385a. Arakawa M, Hatamochi A, Takeda K, Ueki H. Increased collagen synthesis accompanying elevated m-RNA levels in cultured Werner's syndrome fibroblasts. J Invest Dermatol 1990; 94: 187–190.

386. Bauer EA, Uitto J, Tan EML, Holbrook KA. Werner's syndrome. Evidence for preferential regional expression of a generalized mesenchymal cell defect. Arch Dermatol 1988; 124: 90–101.

387. Sephal GC, Sturrock A, Giro MG, Davidson JM. Increased elastin production by progeria skin fibroblasts is controlled by the steady-state levels of elastin mRNA. J Invest Dermatol 1988; 90: 643–647.

388. Badame AJ. Progeria. Arch Dermatol 1989; 125: 540–544.

389. Jimbow K, Kobayashi H, Ishii M et al. Scar and keloidlike lesions in progeria. Arch Dermatol 1988; 124: 1261–1266.

390. Fleischmajer R, Nedwich A. Progeria (Hutchinson-Gilford). Arch Dermatol 1973; 107: 253–258.

391. Ramesh V, Jain RK. Progeria in two brothers. Australas J Dermatol 1987; 28: 33–35.

392. De Groot WP, Tafelkruyer J, Woerdeman MJ. Familial acrogeria (Gottron). Br J Dermatol 1980; 103: 213–223.

393. Venencie PY, Powell FC, Winkelmann RK. Acrogeria with perforating elastoma and bony abnormalities. Acta Derm Venereol 1984; 64: 348–351.

394. Pope FM, Nicholls AC, Narcici P et al. Type III collagen mutations in Ehlers Danlos syndrome type IV and other related disorders. Clin Exp Dermatol 1988; 13: 285–302.

Disorders of elastic tissue

INTRODUCTION

Normal elastic tissue

Elastic fibres are the important resilient component of mammalian connective tissue, and their presence is necessary for the proper structure and function of the cardiovascular, pulmonary and intestinal systems.[1,2] They constitute less than 4% of the dry weight of the skin, forming a complex and extensive network in the dermis which imparts elasticity to the skin.[3]

Structure and composition

Mature elastic fibres are composed of structural glycoproteins, which contribute to the formation of microfibrils, and elastin, a fibrous protein with a molecular weight of 72 000.[3] Elastin forms an amorphous core to the elastic fibres, and this is surrounded by the microfibrils. Approximately 90% of the mature elastic fibre is elastin. It has a high concentration of alanine and valine, but less hydroxyproline than is present in collagen. Elastin is antigenic.

The papillary dermis contains fine fibres which run perpendicular to the dermo–epidermal junction and connect the basal lamina to the underlying dermal elastic tissue.[4] These oxytalan fibres, as they are called, consist of microfibrils without a core of elastin.[5] They branch to form a horizontal plexus in the upper reticular dermis, where they are known as elaunin fibres, which contain a small amount of elastin. The mature elastic fibres with their full composition of elastin are found below this in the reticular dermis. These three types of fibres probably correspond to consecutive stages of normal elastogenesis.[5]

Formation of elastic fibres

The formation of elastic fibres by fibroblasts, and in some circumstances by smooth muscle cells and chondroblasts, entails several different steps which are still poorly understood. Theoretically, these stages would include the expression of genes coding for elastin polypeptides, various intracellular processes, secretion of the precursor components, and extracellular modifications leading to the assembly of the fibres.[3] Recent work suggests that genes in chromosome 2 control the formation of elastin.[6]

Elastin is secreted in the form of a precursor tropoelastin. This is ultimately cross-linked with desmosine to form stable elastin.[7] The formation of desmosine requires the copper-dependent enzyme lysyl oxidase.[7]

Degrading of elastic tissue

There are very few enzymes which can degrade cross-linked elastin.[8] One of these is elastase, which is found in the pancreas and in neutrophils, macrophages, platelets, certain bacteria and cultured human fibroblasts.[7,8] The exact role of elastase in normal skin is uncertain, but it may play a part in the elastolysis seen in acquired cutis laxa associated with inflammatory skin lesions. Elastase inhibitors also exist; these include α_1-antitrypsin and α_2-macroglobulin. There are two factors, vitronectin and delay-accelerating factor, which appear to prevent damage to elastic fibres by complement.[8a] Further work is needed to clarify the role of these substances.

Age-related changes

There is evidence of continuing synthesis of elastic fibres throughout life, but after the age of 50 the new fibres are loosely rather than compactly assembled.[9] With age, there is some loss of the superficial dermal fibres, and a slow, progressive degradation of mature fibres.[7] Ultrastructural changes include the formation of cystic spaces and lacunae, imparting a porous look to the fibres;[10,10a] they may fragment, or develop a fuzzy indistinct border.[10] The changes are quite distinct from those seen in solar elastosis (see p. 369).

Another age-related change is the deposition on elastic fibres of terminal complement complexes and vitronectin. This latter substance is a multifunctional glycoprotein which is hypothetically involved in the prevention of tissue damage in proximity to local complement activation.[11a]

Staining of elastic tissue

The commonly used stains for elastic tissue are the orcein, aldehyde–fuchsin, Verhoeff and Weigert methods. However, the superficial fine elastic fibres do not stain with most of these methods, although they will with a modified orcein stain[7] and with Luna's stain, which incorporates aldehyde–fuchsin and Weigert's iron haematoxylin.[12] The Luna stain also demonstrates a fibrillary component in solar elastosis. Elastic fibres stain a brilliant purple against a pale lavender background with this stain.[12]

A monoclonal antibody, HB8, has recently been described as a stain for elastic fibres.[13] It has no advantages over the modified orcein or Luna stains.

Categorization of elastic tissue disorders

A simple classification of disorders of cutaneous elastic tissue divides them into those in which the elastic tissue is increased, and those in which it is reduced.[14] The solar elastotic syndromes are best considered as a discrete group. Minor alterations in elastic tissue may occur in the various collagen disorders, in line with the observation that alterations in one component of the connective tissue matrix may influence the structure and function of others.[15] This group will not be considered in great detail here.

Although not categorized separately in this chapter, it should be remembered that elastic fibres are the most important structure to undergo transepidermal elimination. This can occur in elastosis perforans serpiginosa, perforating folliculitis, perforating pseudoxanthoma elasticum, solar elastosis, keratoacanthoma, healing wounds, and hypertrophic discoid lupus erythematosus.

The clinical and pathological features of the major disorders of elastic tissue are summarized in Table 12.1 (pages 377 and 378).

INCREASED ELASTIC TISSUE

Very little is known about the mechanisms which lead to an increase in dermal elastic tissue. Besides the conditions to be considered below, a mild increase in elastic tissue has been reported in osteogenesis imperfecta,[16] chronic acidosis,[17] amyotrophic lateral sclerosis,[18] and some stages of radiation dermatitis.[19,20] The solar elastotic syndromes are also characterized by increased elastic tissue, and they will be considered after this section.

ELASTOMA

Elastoma (juvenile elastoma,[21] naevus elasticus, connective tissue naevus of Lewandowsky type)[22] is a variant of connective tissue naevus (see p. 336) in which the predominant abnormality is an increase in dermal elastic tissue.[23] The lesions may be solitary or multiple,[21] and in the latter circumstance they are often associated with multiple small foci of sclerosis of bone (osteopoikilosis). This association is known as the Buschke–Ollendorf syndrome[24,25] and the cutaneous lesions as dermatofibrosis lenticularis disseminata. In several instances, the cutaneous lesions have shown abnormalities in collagen (collagenomas) rather than elastic tissue,[26–28] and for this reason dermatofibrosis lenticularis disseminata is not entirely synonymous with the term elastoma.[29]

The Buschke–Ollendorf syndrome is inherited as an autosomal dominant trait with variable expressivity.[24] Some family members have only cutaneous lesions or only bony lesions, but not both.[26,30]

Elastomas are small, flesh-coloured or yellowish papules or discs, usually in asymmetric distribution on the lower trunk or extremities. They develop at an early age. Studies of the desmosine content of elastomas indicate a three to seven-fold increase in elastin.[31] There appears to be an abnormality of elastogenesis with faulty aggregation of elastin units associated with the overall increase in elastin.

The term 'linear focal elastosis (elastotic striae)' has been suggested for a distinctive acquired lesion composed of palpable, striae-like, yellow lines and dermal elastosis on microscopic examination.[31a] The lesions were not solar related.

Histopathology

Examination of haematoxylin and eosin stained sections usually shows a normal dermis,[24] although sometimes there is an increase in its thickness. The epidermis may have a slight wavy pattern. Elastic tissue stains show an accumulation of broad, branching and interlacing elastic fibres in the mid and lower dermis (Fig. 12.1).[27] The papillary dermis is unaffected. Sometimes the elastic fibres encase the collagen in a marble-vein configuration.[21,32] Clumped elastic fibres have been reported.[33]

Uncommon changes include an increase in acid mucopolysaccharides,[27] slight thickening of collagen bundles, or a well-developed vascular component.[34] Two cases have been reported with facial plaques and increased dermal elastic tissue;[35,36] in one, there was also perifollicular mucin.[36]

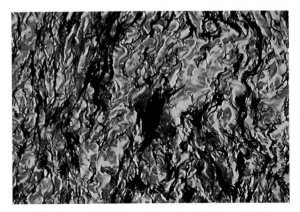

Fig. 12.1 Elastoma. There are irregular clumps of elastic tissue within the reticular dermis.
Verhoeff — Van Gieson

Electron microscopy. Ultrastructural findings have been variable.[31,37] Usually there are branched elastic fibres of variable diameter, without fragmentation. Elastic microfibrils may be replaced by granular or lucent material.[21,38] Collagen fibres are sometimes increased in diameter[37] and some fibroblasts may have dilated rough endoplasmic reticulum.[31]

ELASTOFIBROMA

Elastofibroma is a slowly growing proliferation of collagen and abnormal elastic fibres with a predilection for the subscapular fascia of older individuals.[39–40a] It is rarely found at other sites. Most elastofibromas are unilateral and asymptomatic. They are grey-white or tan in colour and measure 5–10 cm in diameter. The pathogenesis is unknown, but they may represent a reaction to prolonged mechanical stress. Subclinical elastofibromas have been found at autopsy.[41]

Histopathology

Elastofibromas are non-encapsulated lesions which blend with the surrounding fat and connective tissue.[40] They are composed of swollen collagen bundles admixed with numerous, irregular, lightly eosinophilic fibres and some mature

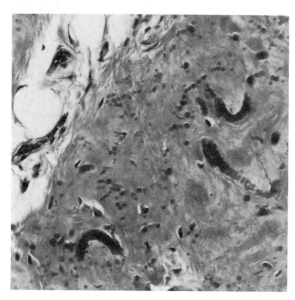

Fig. 12.2 Elastofibroma dorsi. Coarse elastic fibres are admixed with collagen and adipose tissue.
Haematoxylin — eosin

fat (Fig. 12.2). The fibres, which account for almost 50% of the tissue, stain black with the Verhoeff elastic stain. Some fibres are branched while others show a serrated edge.

Electron microscopy. This confirms the presence of abnormal elastic fibres, which result from a proliferation of elastic fibrils around the original elastic fibres.[41] Large ('active') fibroblasts[39] and cells with the features of myofibroblasts[42] have both been described.

ELASTOSIS PERFORANS SERPIGINOSA

This condition (also known as perforating elastosis) presents as small papules, either grouped or in a circinate or serpiginous arrangement, on the neck, upper extremities, upper trunk or face.[43–47] Rarely, the lesions are generalized.[48,49] There is a predilection for males, with the onset usually in the second decade. Familial cases have been reported.[50,51] In up to a third of cases there is an associated systemic condition or connective tissue disorder: these include Down's syndrome,[49,52] osteogenesis imperfecta,[53] Ehlers–Danlos syndrome, Marfan's syndrome, acrogeria, scleroderma[54,55] and chronic renal failure.[56]

Similar cutaneous lesions have been reported in patients with Wilson's disease and cystinuria receiving long-term penicillamine therapy.[57–59a] In these patients, a local copper depletion or a direct effect of penicillamine on elastin synthesis may be responsible for the formation of the abnormal elastic fibres, which are then eliminated transepidermally.[57,60] Elastic tissue damage appears to occur in other organs as well, a feature generally lacking in the usual idiopathic form of the disease.[60,61] The nature of the defect in the idiopathic form is unknown, but it is possible that perforating elastosis is the final common pathway for more than one abnormality of elastic fibres.[44,61a]

Histopathology[43–46]

In fully developed lesions, there is a localized area of hyperplastic epidermis, associated with a channel through which the basophilic nuclear debris and brightly eosinophilic fragmented elastic fibres are being eliminated (Fig. 12.3). A keratinous plug usually overlies this channel, which may take the form of a dilated infundibular structure or a more oblique canal coursing through hyperplastic epidermis, follicular epithelium or the acrosyringium (Fig. 12.4). When the canal is oblique, sections may only show a surface plug of keratinous debris and a localized area of hyperplastic epidermis which in its lower portion forms a bulbous protrusion into the dermis. This appears to envelop an area of the papillary dermis containing basophilic debris and some refractile eosinophilic elastic fibres.

Elastic tissue stains show increased numbers of coarse elastic fibres in the papillary dermis (Fig. 12.5). Some of these appear to overlap the basal

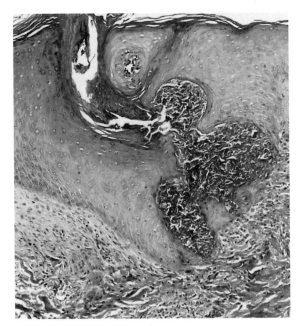

Fig. 12.3 Elastosis perforans serpiginosa. Debris is present within a channel in the epidermis.
Haematoxylin — eosin

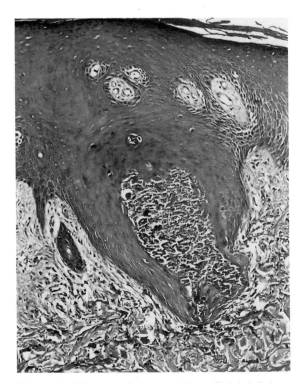

Fig. 12.4 Elastosis perforans serpiginosa. Debris is being enveloped by a bulbous protrusion of the epidermis.
Haematoxylin — eosin

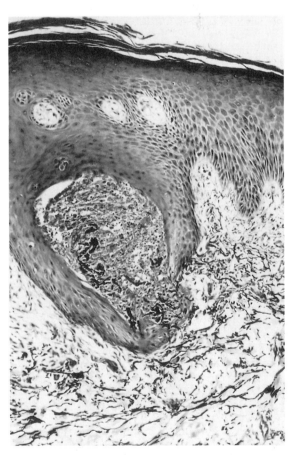

Fig. 12.5 Elastosis perforans serpiginosa. Coarse elastic fibres are being enveloped by a bulbous protrusion of the epidermis.
Verhoeff — Van Gieson

epidermal cells. In the region of their transepidermal elimination, the elastic fibres lose their staining properties as they enter the canal and become brightly eosinophilic. They will stain with the Giemsa method. A few foreign body giant cells and inflammatory cells are often present in the dermis adjacent to the channel. In older lesions, there is focal dermal scarring, and usually an absence of elastic fibres.

IgM, C3 and C4 were demonstrated on the abnormal elastic fibres in the papillary dermis in one of two cases studied by immunofluorescence.[62]

In *penicillamine-related cases*, there is an increased number of thickened elastic fibres in the reticular dermis, and less hyperplasia of elastic fibres in the papillary dermis, except in the areas of active transepidermal elimination.[63] The elastic fibres are irregular in outline with buds and serrations. This may be discerned in haematoxylin and eosin stained preparations, but it is well shown by elastic tissue stains[64] or in Epon-embedded thin sections stained with toluidine blue.[60]

Electron microscopy. Ultrastructural examination of the dermis in *penicillamine-related cases* shows that the elastic fibres have a normal core and an irregular coat with thorn-like protrusions at regular intervals, the so-called 'lumpy bumpy' or 'bramble-bush' fibres.[63–66] Collagen fibres are also abnormal with extreme variations in thickness.[66,67] Electron microscopy of *idiopathic cases* has shown increased numbers of large elastic fibres which are convoluted and branching.[68] Fine filaments, similar to those in embryonic elastic fibres, are present on the surface of the fibres.[68,69]

PSEUDOXANTHOMA ELASTICUM

Pseudoxanthoma elasticum is an inherited disorder of connective tissue in which calcification of elastic fibres occurs in certain areas of the skin, eyes, and cardiovascular system.[70–73] Skin changes are usually evident by the second decade and consist of closely set yellowish papules, with a predilection for flexural creases, particularly in the neck and axillae, and less commonly in the groins, periumbilical area and the cubital and popliteal fossae.[70–72] Oral lesions may occur.[73] The skin becomes wrinkled and thickened and eventually may become lax and redundant.[73a] The calcium content of affected skin may be up to several hundred times normal.[74] Eye changes include angioid streaks and a degenerative choroidoretinitis which may lead to blindness. Calcification of elastic fibres in arteries, and intimal and endocardial fibroelastosis develop. The vascular changes may lead to hypertension, cerebrovascular accidents and gastrointestinal haemorrhage.[75–77]

Genetic studies have shown a heterogeneous pattern.[78] There are two variants with autosomal dominant inheritance, and two with autosomal recessive inheritance. In dominant type 1, there are cutaneous changes, and often vascular complications and severe choroidoretinitis. In dominant type 2, there is an atypical yellowish macular rash, only mild retinal changes, and no vascular complications. Recessive type 1 is of intermediate severity with classic skin changes. Recessive type 2 is exceedingly rare and has generalized cutaneous laxity but no systemic complications.[79,80]

There has been one report of spontaneous resolution and repair of elastic tissue calcification.[81] Hyperphosphatasia has been present in several cases.[82] Patients purporting to have co-existing elastosis perforans serpiginosa and pseudoxanthoma elasticum have been reported; they are now regarded as having perforating pseudoxanthoma elasticum.[83–85] Many of these patients have so-called acquired pseudoxanthoma elasticum (see below).

The factors that lead to the calcification of initially normal elastic fibres in pseudoxanthoma elasticum are not known.[85a] Polyanionic material is deposited in association with the calcified material. Cultured fibroblasts from patients with this condition release a proteolytic substance, and it has been postulated that this may cause selective damage to elastin, leading to calcification.[86]

Acquired pseudoxanthoma elasticum refers to an aetiologically and clinically diverse group of patients with late onset of the disease, no family history, absence of vascular and retinal stigmata, and identical dermal histology.[87,88] The term perforating calcific elastosis has been suggested for some of these cases.[89] Included in this group are individuals exposed to calcium salts, including farmers exposed to Norwegian saltpetre (calcium and ammonium nitrate),[90,91] and obese, usually multiparous black women who develop reticulated and atrophic plaques and some discrete papules around the umbilicus [85,89,91a] or lower chest.[92] Perforation is common in this latter group. A patient with chronic renal failure on dialysis has also been reported with this acquired variant.[87]

Histopathology[72]

There are short, curled, frayed, basophilic elastic fibres in the reticular dermis, particularly in the upper and mid parts (Fig. 12.6). The papillary dermis is spared except at sites of transepidermal elimination (perforation). The elastic fibres in affected skin are stained black with the von Kossa method. They stain with the Verhoeff method, and there is intense blue staining with phosphotungstic acid haematoxylin (PTAH).

If perforation is present, there is a focal central erosion or tunnel with surrounding pseudoepitheliomatous hyperplasia or prominent acanthosis (Figs 12.7 and 12.8). Basophilic elastic fibres are extruded through this defect. Sometimes foreign body giant cells, histiocytes and a few chronic inflammatory cells are present when there is perforation or traumatic ulceration.[93] The giant cells may then engulf some elastic fibres.

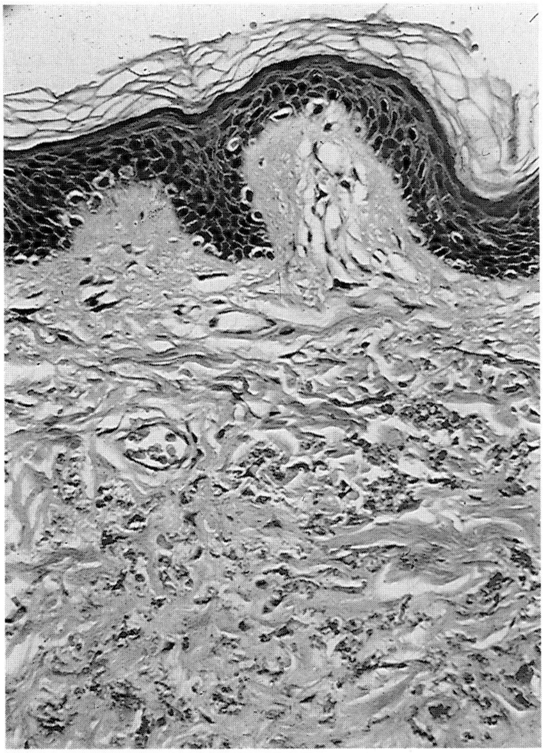

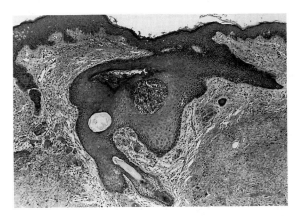

Fig. 12.7 Perforating pseudoxanthoma elasticum. There is pseudoepitheliomatous hyperplasia (enlarged follicular infundibula) overlying disordered elastic fibres. Haematoxylin — eosin

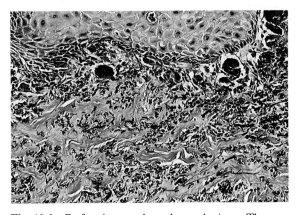

Fig. 12.8 Perforating pseudoxanthoma elasticum. The elastic fibres which are about to undergo transepithelial elimination are short, curled and frayed. Clumped elastic fibres are also present. Verhoeff — van Gieson.

Fig. 12.6 Pseudoxanthoma elasticum. Note the short, curled elastic fibres in the reticular dermis. Haematoxylin — eosin

Electron microscopy. Calcification occurs initially in the central zones of the elastic fibres.[94] There is also some calcification of intercellular spaces, and occasionally also of collagen fibres; the latter change may be reversible.[82,92] There is continuing elastogenesis with some normal elastic fibres.[82] Twisted collagen fibrils and thready material[95] which has been found to contain fibrinogen, collagenous protein and glycoprotein, are also present.[96] This indicates that the abnormality is not limited to the elastic fibres.

ELASTIC GLOBES

Elastic globes are small basophilic bodies, found in the upper dermis of clinically normal skin, which stain positively for elastic fibres (Fig. 12.9). They are considered with the other dermal cytoid bodies on page 416. Numerous elastic globes have been reported in a patient with epidermolysis bullosa whose skin was wrinkled,[96a] and in a patient with the cartilage-hair hypoplasia syndrome whose skin was hyperextensible.[96b]

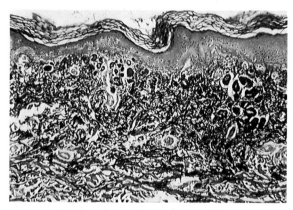

Fig. 12.9   Elastic globes. There are multiple, round and ovoid deposits in the papillary dermis. Solar elastosis is also present.
Verhoeff — van Gieson

SOLAR ELASTOTIC SYNDROMES

The term solar elastosis refers to the accumulation of abnormal elastic tissue in the dermis in response to long-term sun exposure. There are many different clinical patterns of solar elastosis, some of which form distinct clinicopathological entities.[96c] Other clinical patterns are histologically indistinguishable from one another, and they are usually grouped together under the umbrella term solar elastosis.

The following entities are regarded as solar elastotic syndromes:

Solar elastosis
Nodular elastosis with cysts and comedones
Elastotic nodules of the ears
Collagenous and elastotic plaques of the hands.

Colloid milium can also be regarded as a solar elastotic syndrome, as it appears that the colloid substance derives, at least in major part, from elastic fibres through actinic degeneration.[97] Colloid degeneration (paracolloid, colloid-milium-like solar elastosis) has overlapping features histologically with both colloid milium and solar elastosis. These topics are considered with the cutaneous deposits in Chapter 14 (pp. 413 and 414).

Solar elastotic skin is more susceptible than normal skin to chronic infections with *Staphylococcus aureus* and several other bacteria. Uncommonly, this results in a chronic suppurative process, variants of which have been reported as 'coral reef granuloma' and blastomycosis-like pyoderma (see p. 601). Actinic comedonal plaque, in which fibrous tissue and comedones are present with some residual elastosis at the periphery, can be the end stage picture of this inflammatory process.

Another secondary change that may occur in sun-damaged skin is the formation of actinic granulomas in which there is a granulomatous response to solar elastotic material and its resorption by macrophages and giant cells (elastophagocytosis, elastoclasis). Actinic granulomas present clinically as one or more annular lesions with an atrophic centre and an elevated border. They are considered with the granulomatous tissue reaction (see p. 201). Elastophagocytosis has also been reported in association with various inflammatory processes in sun-protected skin.[97a]

Ultraviolet light is usually incriminated in the aetiology of the degenerative changes.[98] However it has been suggested that infrared radiation may also contribute as changes characteristic of solar elastosis are seen in erythema ab igne.[99] Although not usually regarded as one of the elastotic syndromes, this condition will be considered in this section because of its similar histological appearances.

SOLAR ELASTOSIS (ACTINIC ELASTOSIS)

The usual clinical appearance of solar elastosis is thickened, dry, coarsely wrinkled skin. Sometimes there is a yellowish hue. There may be some telangiectasia and pigmentary changes (poikilodermatous changes) in severe cases.[100,100a] The best recognized clinical variant is cutis rhomboidalis in which there is thickened, deeply fissured skin on the back of the neck. Other clinical patterns include citrine skin, Dubreuilh's and other elastomas,[101] and solar elastotic bands of the forearm.[102]

The origin of the elastotic material has been the subject of much debate. It has been attributed to the degradation of collagen or elastic fibres or both.[103,104] Alternatively, it has been suggested by others that the material results from the actinic stimulation of fibroblasts.[104a] Recent work suggests that the elastotic material is primarily derived from elastic fibres.[105] Small amounts of type I and VI collagen and procollagen type III are present, but the significance of this finding remains uncertain.[105] The changes are qualitatively different from those seen in ageing, contrary to the assertion of some.[106]

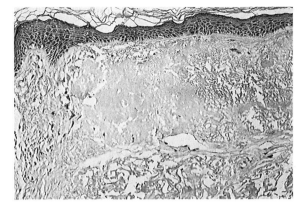

Fig. 12.10 Solar elastosis with amorphous and fibrillary material in the upper dermis. Haematoxylin — eosin

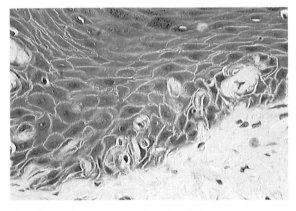

Fig. 12.11 Solar elastosis. Curled elastotic fibres are insinuating between basal keratinocytes. This represents the early stages of the transepidermal elimination of these damaged fibres. Haematoxylin — eosin

Histopathology

In mild actinic damage there is a proliferation of elastic fibres in the papillary dermis. They are normal or slightly increased in thickness. In established cases the papillary and upper reticular dermis is replaced by accumulations of thickened, curled and serpiginous fibres forming tangled masses which are basophilic in haematoxylin and eosin stained sections (Fig. 12.10).[9] Sometimes there are amorphous masses of elastotic material in which the outline of fibres is lost except at the periphery. These masses are thought to form from the tangled fibres, as transitions can be seen on electron microscopy. A thin grenz zone of normal-appearing collagen is present in the subepidermal zone.[107] This may have lost its network of fine vertical fibres. Collagen is reduced in amount in the reticular dermis. Transepidermal elimination of elastotic material can occur.[108] This process is not uncommon following cryotherapy to severely damaged skin, which seems to trigger elimination in some individuals (Fig. 12.11). The elastotic material stains

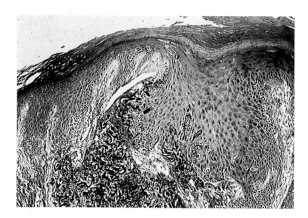

Fig. 12.12   Perforating solar elastosis. The elastic fibres being eliminated are thick, curled and serpiginous in morphology.
Verhoeff — van Gieson

black with the Verhoeff stain (Fig. 12.12). Sometimes the homogeneous deposits are less well stained.

Biopsies from individuals with chronic sunlight exposure, some of whom had persistent erythema, have been described as showing a 'perivenular histiocytic-lymphocytic infiltrate in which numerous mast cells, often in close apposition to fibroblasts, were observed': this condition has been termed chronic heliodermatitis.[109]

Epidermal changes also occur in severely damaged skin. The stratum corneum may be compact and laminated or gelatinous, and it sometimes contains vesicles full of proteinaceous material.[109a] In the malpighian layer, cell heterogeneity, vacuolization and dysplasia may be found.[109a]

Electron microscopy. A spectrum of ultrastructural changes is found which parallels the clinical degree of damage.[9,110,111] In mild cases, the elastic fibres in the papillary dermis are increased in number. The microfibrillar dense zones become irregular in outline, more electron-dense and many times larger. In severe cases the elastin matrix becomes granular and develops lucent areas around the microfibrillar dense zones.[9] Some fibres become disrupted and show a moth-eaten appearance or become transformed into finely granular bodies.[9] Similar ultrastructural findings have been reported in chronic radiodermatitis.[112] Following PUVA therapy, the elastic fibre changes include a breakdown of the microfibrils and subsequent fragmentation of the elastic fibres.[113]

Scanning electron microscopy of solar elastosis shows some normal fibres, some thick damaged cylindrical fibres and large masses of markedly changed fibres, which probably correspond to the amorphous deposits seen in severe cases.[114]

NODULAR ELASTOSIS WITH CYSTS AND COMEDONES

This solar degenerative condition, also known as the Favre–Racouchot syndrome, occurs as thickened yellowish plaques studded with cysts and open comedones.[115,116] It involves the head and neck, but particularly the skin around the eyes. Lesions may extend to the temporal and zygomatic areas. There is a predilection for males who have a history of prolonged solar exposure.

Histopathology[115,116]

In addition to the marked solar elastosis, there are dilated follicles and comedones which contain keratinous debris in the lumen. The sebaceous glands are often atrophic. A recent study of patients without much solar exposure showed multiple comedones without significant solar elastosis, suggesting that the two processes might be independent.[117]

ELASTOTIC NODULES OF THE EARS

Elastotic nodules are small, usually asymptomatic, pale papules and nodules found predominantly on the anterior crus of the antihelix in response to actinic damage.[118–120] They are often bilateral. There is a marked predilection for elderly white males. Rare cases develop on the helix where they may be painful, simulating chondrodermatitis nodularis helicis. They may be diagnosed clinically as basal cell carcinoma, amyloid or even small gouty tophi.

Histopathology[119]

There is marked elastotic degeneration of the dermis with the formation of irregular, coarse elastotic fibres, and larger clumped masses of

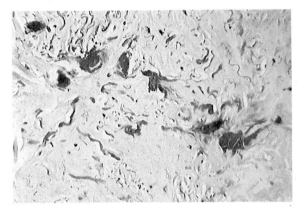

Fig. 12.13 Elastotic nodule of the ear. Clumped masses of elastotic material are present in the mid dermis. Haematoxylin — eosin

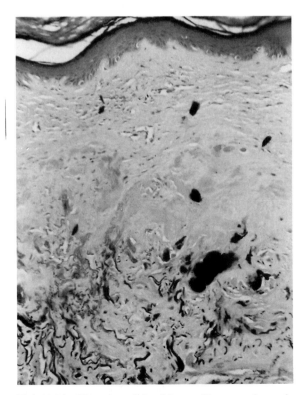

Fig. 12.14 Elastotic nodule of the ear. There are clumped masses of elastotic material. Verhoeff — van Gieson

elastotic material (Figs 12.13 and 12.14). These changes are best seen with the Verhoeff elastic stain. The overlying epidermis shows mild to moderate orthokeratosis and some irregular acanthosis. There is mild telangiectasia of vessels in the papillary dermis with some new collagen often present in this area.

COLLAGENOUS AND ELASTOTIC PLAQUES OF THE HANDS

This entity, also known as 'degenerative collagenous plaques of the hands' and 'keratoelastoidosis marginalis', is a slowly progressive, degenerative condition found predominantly in older males.[121–123] There are waxy, linear plaques at the juncture of palmar and dorsal skin of the hands. The condition particularly involves the medial aspect of the thumbs and the lateral aspect of the adjacent index finger. In this respect the lesions resemble in part those seen in the genodermatosis acrokeratoelastoidosis (see p. 275).[121] Physical trauma of a repetitive nature, and prolonged actinic exposure may play a role in the aetiology of collagenous and elastotic plaques of the hand.[123]

Histopathology

The most noticeable changes are in the dermis where there are numerous thick collagen bundles having a haphazard arrangement, but with a proportion running perpendicular to the surface (Fig. 12.15).[124] There is often a slight basophilic tint to the dermis; elastotic fibres can be seen in the lower papillary dermis and intimately admixed with the collagen bundles in the reticular dermis.

In elastic tissue stains, the elastotic material in the lower papillary dermis is confirmed. In the reticular dermis, granular and elastotic material can be seen in an intimate relationship within some of the larger collagen bundles.[121] In some cases, there are focal deposits of calcification in the dermis. The changes are distinct from those of solar elastosis.

The overlying epidermis may show mild hyperkeratosis and thickening of the granular

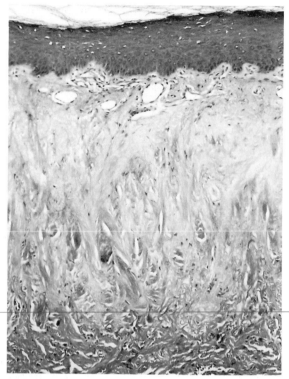

Fig. 12.15 Collagenous and elastotic plaque. The collagen bundles in the upper dermis have a characteristic haphazard arrangement with some bundles arranged vertically. Elastotic material is admixed.
Haematoxylin — eosin

layer. In some there is slight acanthosis, while in other cases there may be loss of the rete pattern.

ERYTHEMA AB IGNE

This term refers to the development of persistent areas of reticular erythema, with or without pigmentation, at the sites of repeated exposure to heat, usually from open hearths.[125,125a] The lower legs are usually involved. Erythema ab igne is now seen only rarely. Keratoses and, rarely, squamous cell carcinomas may develop in lesions of long standing.[126]

Histopathology[125,127]

There is thinning of the epidermis with efface-

ment of the rete ridges and some basal vacuolar changes. Areas of epithelial atypia, resembling that seen in actinic keratoses, are sometimes present. There is usually prominent elastotic material in the mid dermis.[128] A small amount of haemosiderin and melanin may be present in the upper dermis.[125]

DECREASED ELASTIC TISSUE

There are several distinct levels in the biosynthesis of elastic fibres at which errors can be introduced. These can lead to reduced production of elastic fibres or to the appearance of abnormal ones. Breakdown of fibres (elastolysis) is another mechanism which can lead to a reduction in the elastic tissue content of the dermis.

The reduction in dermal elastic tissue can be generalized, as in cutis laxa, or localized, as in anetoderma and blepharochalasis. Cases with features intermediate between these two types also occur. Sometimes the reduction in elastic fibres is subclinical or overshadowed by other features. This is the case in various granulomatous inflammatory disorders.

NAEVUS ANELASTICUS

This is the term suggested by Staricco and Mehregan[34] for several cases reported in the earlier literature characterized by an absence or definite reduction and/or fragmentation of elastic fibres in cutaneous lesions of early onset.[129] Further cases have been reported in which multiple papular lesions have developed, particularly on the trunk.[129–130a] The lesions are not perifollicular in distribution. Separation from the non-inflammatory type of anetoderma may be difficult (see below).

Histopathology

Sections show a localized reduction in elastic fibres, with normal collagen.[130] The elastic fibres may show intense fragmentation in some cases.[129] Fibres in the papillary dermis may be normal. There is no inflammation.

PERIFOLLICULAR ELASTOLYSIS

Perifollicular elastolysis is a not uncommon condition of the face and upper back in which 1–3 mm grey or white, finely wrinkled lesions develop in association with a central hair follicle.[131,132] Balloon-like bulging of larger lesions may develop.[131] The disorder is significantly associated with acne vulgaris.[132,132a] An elastase-producing strain of *Staphylococcus epidermidis* was found in the hair follicles located within lesions in one report.[131]

Histopathology[131]

There is an almost complete loss of elastic fibres confined to the immediate vicinity of hair follicles. There is no inflammation.

ANETODERMA

Anetoderma (macular atrophy) is a rare cutaneous disorder in which multiple, oval lesions with a wrinkled surface develop progressively over many years.[133,134] Individual lesions may bulge outwards or be slightly depressed. They usually herniate inwards with finger tip pressure. There is a predilection for the upper trunk and upper arms, but the neck and thighs may also be involved. Facial involvement may lead to chalazodermia.[133] Onset of the lesions is in late adolescence and early adult life. Familial cases are quite rare.[135]

The onset of lesions may be preceded by an inflammatory stage with erythematous macules and papules (Jadassohn–Pellizzari type), or there may be no precursor inflammatory lesions (Schweninger–Buzzi type).[134] These two types have been classified as primary anetodermas to distinguish them from the secondary anetodermas[133,134] which may develop in the course of syphilis, leprosy, sarcoidosis, tuberculosis, acrodermatitis chronica atrophicans,[133] lupus erythematosus,[133] amyloidosis, lymphocytoma cutis, or following penicillamine therapy.[136] The association with urticaria pigmentosa may be coincidental.[137] The lesions of secondary anetoderma do not always correspond with those of the primary disease process.

A variety of ocular and skeletal defects have been reported in individuals with anetoderma. They have been chronicled in a review of the extensive European literature on this condition.[133]

Theoretically anetoderma could result from increased degradation, or reduced synthesis, of elastic tissue.[138] It has been suggested that all cases have an inflammatory pathogenesis, which would tend to indicate that an elastolytic process is operative.[8a,139] The concentration of elastin, as measured by the desmosine content of the skin, is markedly reduced.[138]

Histopathology[139]

If a biopsy is taken from a clinically inflammatory lesion, the dermis will show a moderately heavy perivascular and even interstitial infiltrate, predominantly of lymphocytes. Plasma cells and eosinophils are occasionally present. Neutrophils have been noted sometimes in very early lesions.[139]

In established lesions, most reports have noted an essentially normal appearance in haematoxylin and eosin stained sections. However, in one large series, a perivascular infiltrate of lymphocytes was found in all cases.[139] There was a predominance of helper T cells.[140] The authors of that account did not attempt to reconcile their findings with earlier reports in which inflammatory cells were noted to be absent.[134,138,139]

Scattered macrophages and giant cells may also be present. Non-caseating granulomas were present in one case, in association with Takayasu's arteritis.[141]

Elastic tissue stains show a normal complement of fibres in the early inflammatory lesions. In established lesions, elastic fibres are sparse in the superficial dermis and almost completely absent in the mid dermis (Fig. 12.16).

Direct immunofluorescence in some cases of primary anetoderma shows a pattern of immune deposits similar to that of lupus erythematosus.[141a] There are no other manifestations of the latter disease in these cases.

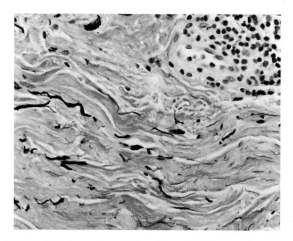

Fig. 12.16 Anetoderma. There is a mild infiltrate of lymphocytes in the mid dermis. Beneath this the elastic fibres have partly disappeared.
Verhoeff — Van Gieson

Electron microscopy. The elastic fibres which remain are fragmented and irregular in appearance but the collagen is normal.[138,142] Occasionally, macrophages can be seen enveloping the fragmented fibres.[143]

CUTIS LAXA

The term cutis laxa encompasses a group of rare disorders of elastic tissue in which the skin hangs in loose folds, giving the appearance of premature ageing.[144] In many cases, there is a more generalized loss of elastic fibres involving the lungs, gastrointestinal tract and aorta, leading to emphysema, hernias, diverticula and aneurysms.[145–147]

Congenital and acquired forms exist. *Congenital cutis laxa* is genetically heterogeneous with several different autosomal recessive forms of the disease, one of which is associated with growth retardation.[148,149] There is an autosomal dominant form which is less severe. The X-linked recessive variant,[150] in which there is a deficiency of lysyl oxidase, is now regarded as a variant of Ehlers–Danlos syndrome.[151] The congenital forms are associated with a characteristic facies, with a hooked nose and a long upper lip.

Approximately 30 cases of *acquired cutis laxa*

have been described. The changes may be generalized or localized.[152,153] Acquired cutis laxa may be of insidious onset[154] or develop after a prior inflammatory lesion of the skin[155] which may take the form of erythema, erythema multiforme, urticaria, a vesicular eruption or Sweet's syndrome.[156] Several cases have followed an allergic reaction to penicillin,[157,158] while others have been associated with isoniazid therapy,[159] myelomatosis,[160–162] systemic lupus erythematosus,[163] or the nephrotic syndrome.[144] Cutis laxa may occur as a manifestation of an autosomal dominant form of pseudoxanthoma elasticum.

The congenital cases presumably result from a defect in the synthesis or assembly of the components of the elastic fibre. Possibly a different step is involved in the various genetic types. In those acquired cases associated with severe dermal inflammation, it has been suggested that granulocytic elastase may be involved.

Localized areas of loose skin may develop in cutaneous lesions of sarcoidosis, syphilis, and neurofibromatosis.[154]

Histopathology[164]

The fine elastic fibres in the papillary dermis are lost, and there is a decrease in fibres elsewhere in the dermis. Remaining fibres are often shortened, and they vary greatly in diameter. The borders are sometimes indistinct and hazy. Fragmentation of fibres may be noted. Giant cells are rarely present, phagocytosing elastic fibres. A variable inflammatory reaction is present in the acquired cases with an associated clinical inflammatory component. In several cases, the inflammatory infiltrate has been quite heavy, with neutrophils, eosinophils and lymphocytes in the superficial and deep dermis.[158]

Electron microscopy.[144] The elastic tissue varies in content, appearance, and the proportion and manner by which elastin and the microfibrillar component associate.[165,166] There is some fragmentation of elastic fibres with accumulation of granular material.[160] Fragmented fibres are sometimes surrounded by fibroblasts or macrophages. Abnormalities of collagen structure have been noted in a few reports,[165,167] but specifically excluded in others.[160]

Atypical wrinkles and elastolysis

There have been reports from Africa and South America of a disease in young children with features intermediate between anetoderma and mild cutis laxa in which generalized wrinkling, without the redundant folds of cutis laxa, develops.[168,169] This condition has recently been reported in a North American child.[170] A preceding inflammatory stage is present. There is some dermal atrophy with fragmentation and partial loss of elastic tissue in the dermis.

Idiopathic wrinkling has also been reported associated with the loss of mid-dermal elastic tissue.[171–175]

Elastolysis of the earlobes

This condition may represent a variant of cutis laxa confined to the earlobes.[176] This is supported by a case in which spread to the face occurred.[176] *Blepharochalasis* is a similar lesion with eyelid and periorbital involvement.[163]

MENKES' SYNDROME

Menkes' kinky hair syndrome is a rare multisystem disorder of elastic tissue transmitted as an X-linked recessive trait.[177–179] Characteristically the hair is white, sparse, brittle and kinky. It resembles and feels like steel wool. Neurodegenerative changes, vascular insufficiency, hypothermia and susceptibility to infections are other manifestations of this syndrome.[19,179] Mild forms occur.[180]

The finding of reduced serum copper levels led to the view that Menkes' syndrome was a simple copper deficiency state akin to that seen in copper-deficient sheep.[181,182] It is now thought to be a storage disease in which copper is trapped in several tissues by metallothionin, a cysteine-rich metalloprotein involved in cellular copper transport, with a resultant deficiency of copper in other tissues.[179,183] There is reduced

activity of the copper-dependent enzyme lysyl oxidase in fibroblasts derived from the skin of patients with this syndrome.[184] This enzyme is necessary for the cross-linking of elastin.[3] It has been suggested that this syndrome should be reclassified with Ehlers–Danlos syndrome type IX, in which a disorder of lysyl oxidase also occurs (see p. 347).

Histopathology

There are various hair shaft abnormalities which include pili torti, monilethrix and trichorrhexis nodosa (see p. 448).[179] The internal elastic lamina of vessels is fragmented and there is intimal proliferation. Dermal elastic tissue appears to be unaffected.

FRAGILE X SYNDROME

This rare X-linked form of mental retardation is associated with a characteristic facies and connective tissue abnormalities which are clinically reminiscent of cutis laxa and the Ehlers–Danlos syndromes.[185] No specific biochemical defect has yet been identified.

Histopathology[185]

There is a reduction in dermal elastic tissue. The fibres are fragmented and curled and lack arborization. There is a reduction in stromal acid mucopolysaccharides.

GRANULOMATOUS DISEASES

Rarely, anetoderma develops as a complication of sarcoidosis, leprosy or tuberculosis. Reduced numbers of elastic fibres, not necessarily leading to clinical manifestations, may occur in the course of several other granulomatous disorders. These include the closely related conditions of elastolytic giant cell granuloma, actinic granuloma, atypical necrobiosis lipoidica of the face and scalp, and Miescher's granuloma.[186,187] Elastic tissue is reduced in active lesions of granuloma annulare. Multinucleate giant cells and macrophages appear to be responsible for the digestion of the elastic fibres.[186] These conditions are discussed further in Chapter 7 (pp. 201–203).

'GRANULOMATOUS SLACK SKIN'

This rare form of cutaneous T-cell lymphoma is characterized by progressively pendulous skin folds in flexural areas, and an abnormal cutaneous infiltrate.[188–192] The distinctive clinical appearance results from elastolysis, apparently mediated by giant cells in the infiltrate (see p. 1042).

Histopathology[188]

There is permeation of the entire dermis and subcutis by a heavy infiltrate of lymphocytes admixed with tuberculoid granulomas and giant cells with up to 30 nuclei. Foam cells may also be present.[190] There is almost complete absence of elastic tissue in the dermis, and elastic fibres may be seen within the giant cells. Loss of elastic fibres and subcutaneous granulomas are not present in the granulomatous form of mycosis fungoides which otherwise resembles this condition on histopathology (see p. 1036).[188]

MYXOEDEMA

Elastic fibres are significantly reduced in the dermis in hypothyroid myxoedema and in pretibial myxoedema.[193] Ultrastructural examination shows wide variability of elastic fibre diameter and a decrease in microfibrils.[193]

ACROKERATOELASTOIDOSIS

In this genodermatosis (see p. 275), the dermal elastic fibres are usually fragmented and decreased in number. The epidermal changes are clinically more significant than the elastic tissue changes.

VARIABLE OR MINOR ELASTIC TISSUE CHANGES

LEPRECHAUNISM

Leprechaunism is a rare disorder with characteristic facies, phallic enlargement and a deficiency· of subcutaneous fat stores.[194] Cutaneous changes include hypertrichosis, acanthosis nigricans, wrinkled loose skin and prominent rugal folds around the body orifices.[194]

Histopathology

Loss and fragmentation of elastic fibres and decreased collagen were noted in one report of this condition.[195] In contrast, in a recent study it was noted that the elastic fibres were thick and extended into the widened septa of the subcutaneous fat.[194]

SYNDROMES OF PREMATURE AGEING

The elastic tissue changes in these conditions are variable. They may be increased in Werner's syndrome (see p. 349) with granular and filamentous ultrastructural changes.[196] Elastosis perforans has been reported in acrogeria (see p. 349).[197] At other times there may be loss of elastic fibres in association with dermal atrophy or sclerosis.[198]

WRINKLES

Although of great cosmetic importance, wrinkles are of little dermatopathological interest. In general, wrinkles are bilateral and increased with ageing and sun damage. One case of unilateral wrinkles has been reported.[199]

Histopathology[200–204]

It has been stated that wrinkles are a 'configurational change' with no distinguishing histological features.[200] In contrast, it has been reported that the dermis in a deep wrinkle shows substantially less elastotic changes than the surrounding areas, and that the superficial elastic fibres appear slightly thickened and the overlying epidermis depressed.[203,204]

Electron microscopy. Electron-dense inclusions have been noted in elastic fibres in the upper dermis of the wrinkled areas, and these are thought to represent the earliest changes of solar elastosis.[203,204] More severe changes are present in the surrounding dermis.

MARFAN'S SYNDROME

Marfan's syndrome is a rare, autosomal dominant defect of connective tissue, with ocular, skeletal and cardiovascular manifestations.[205] Cutaneous manifestations are of little clinical importance; they include striae distensae and elastosis perforans serpiginosa.[206] Defects in the cross-linking and composition of collagen have been described, but abnormalities in elastic tissue also occur. One study showed that elastin isolated from the aorta was deficient in desmosine cross-links.[207]

Histopathology

The striae distensae show the usual features of this lesion (see p. 339) with regeneration of elastic fibres.[208] The lesions of elastosis perforans serpiginosa resemble those already described for this entity (see p. 364).

Clinically normal skin shows no detectable abnormality, although one study suggested that the elastic fibres looked a little tortuous and fragmented.[206]

Electron microscopy. This shows an increase in fine elastic fibres, possibly resulting from incomplete fusion of elastic fibres.[206] Degenerative changes in elastic fibres have been observed in the lung.[209]

Table 12.1 Summary of the major disorders of elastic tissue

Diagnosis	Clinical features	Pathology
Elastoma	Solitary or multiple; papules and discs; sometimes osteopoikilosis	Increased, thick, branching elastic fibres
Elastofibroma	Deep scapular region; older age	Proliferation of collagen and elastic tissue
Elastosis perforans serpiginosa	Hyperkeratotic papules on face and neck	Pappilary accumulation and transepidermal elimination of elastic tissue
Pseudoxanthoma elasticum	Yellowish papules and plaques; angioid streaks	Fragmented and calcified elastic fibres in mid dermis; may perforate
Elastic globes	Asymptomatic	Basophilic cytoid bodies in the upper dermis
Solar elastosis	Thickened, furrowed skin	Accumulation of curled basophilic elastic fibres and elastic masses in upper dermis
Nodular elastosis	Usually periorbital with cysts and comedones	Comedones and usually solar elastosis
Elastotic nodules of the ears	Asymptomatic papules on the ear	Clumped masses of elastotic material
Collagenous and elastotic plaques	Waxy, linear plaques at juncture of palmar and dorsal skin	Thick collagen, some perpendicular; admixed granular, elastotic material
Erythema ab igne	Follows repeated heat exposure	Elastotic material in dermis

Table continued on next page

Table 12.1 Summary of the major disorders of elastic tissue (*continued from page 377*)

Diagnosis	Clinical features	Pathology
Naevus anelasticus	Papular lesions on lower trunk; early onset; no inflammation	A 'minus naevus' with reduced, fragmented elastic tissue in reticular dermis
Perifollicular elastolysis	Common; face and back; often associated acne vulgaris	Loss of elastic tissue around follicles
Anetoderma	Well-circumscribed areas of soft, wrinkled skin; may have preceding inflammation or be secondary to some other disease	Loss of elastic fibres, particularly in mid dermis
Cutis laxa	Widespread, large folds of pendulous skin; often involves internal organs; congenital or acquired	Fragmentation and loss of elastic fibres
Menkes' syndrome	Copper storage disease; brittle, 'steel wool' hair; vascular and neurological changes	Pili torti, often with monilethrix and trichorrhexis nodosa
'Granulomatous slack skin'	Pendulous skin in flexural areas; T-cell lymphoma	Lymphoid cells; granulomas with multinucleate giant cells; absence of elastic fibres

There is also an increase in elastic tissue in osteogenesis imperfecta, chronic acidosis, amyotrophic lateral sclerosis, stages of radiation damage, corticosteroid therapy and Werner's syndrome.
Elastic fibres may be decreased in myxoedema, acrokeratoelastoidosis, fragile X syndrome and various granulomatous disorders.

REFERENCES

Introduction

1. Sandberg LB, Soskel NT, Wolt TB. Structure of the elastic fibre: an overview. J Invest Dermatol 1982; 79 (suppl 1): 128s–132s.
2. Davidson JM, Crystal RG. The molecular aspects of elastin gene expression. J Invest Dermatol 1982; 79 (suppl 1): 133s–137s.
3. Uitto J, Rhyanen L, Abraham PA, Perejda AJ. Elastin in diseases. J Invest Dermatol 1982; 79 (suppl 1): 160s–168s.
4. Tsuji T. Elastic fibres in the dermal papilla. Scanning and transmission electron microscopic studies. Br J Dermatol 1980; 102: 413–417.
5. Cotta-Pereira G, Rodrigo FG, Bittencourt-Sampaio S. Oxytalan, elaunin, and elastic fibers in the human skin. J Invest Dermatol 1976; 66: 143–148.
6. Patton MA, Tolmie J, Ruthnum P et al. Congenital cutis laxa with retardation of growth and development. J Med Genet 1987; 24: 556–561.
7. Frances C, Robert L. Elastin and elastic fibers in normal and pathologic skin. Int J Dermatol 1984; 23: 166–179.

8. Werb Z, Banda MJ, McKerrow JH, Sandhaus RA. Elastases and elastin degradation. J Invest Dermatol 1982; 79 (suppl 1): 154s–159s.
8a. Werth VP, Ivanov IE, Nussenzweig V. Decay-accelerating factor in human skin is associated with elastic fibers. J Invest Dermatol 1988; 91: 511–516.
9. Braverman IM, Fonferko E. Studies in cutaneous aging: 1 The elastic fiber network. J Invest Dermatol 1982; 78: 434–443.
10. Tsuji T, Hamada T. Age-related changes in human dermal elastic fibres. Br J Dermatol 1981; 105: 57–63.
10a. Herzberg AJ, Dinehart SM. Chronologic aging in black skin. Am J Dermatopathol 1989; 11: 319–328.
11. Fenske NA, Lober CW. Structural and functional changes of normal aging skin. J Am Acad Dermatol 1986; 15: 571–585.
11a. Dahlback K, Lofberg H, Alumets J, Dahlback B. Immunohistochemical demonstration of age-related deposition of vitronectin (S-protein of complement) and terminal complement complex on dermal elastic fibres. J Invest Dermatol 1989; 92: 727–733.

12. Kligman LH. Luna's technique. A beautiful stain for elastin. Am J Dermatopathol 1981; 3: 199–201.
13. Dawson JF, Brochier J, Schmitt D et al. Elastic fibres: histological correlation with orcein and a new monoclonal antibody, HB8. Br J Dermatol 1984; 110: 539–546.
14. Reed RJ, Clark WH, Mihm MC. The cutaneous elastoses. Hum Pathol 1973; 4: 187–199.
15. Holbrook KA, Byers PH. Structural abnormalities in the dermal collagen and elastic matrix from the skin of patients with inherited connective tissue disorders. J Invest Dermatol 1982; 79 (suppl 1): 7s–16s.

Increased elastic tissue

16. Stadil P. Histopathology of the corium in osteogenesis imperfecta. Danish Med Bull 1961; 8: 131–134.
17. Olmstead EG, Lunseth JH. Skin manifestations of chronic acidosis. Arch Dermatol 1958; 77: 304–313.
18. Fullmer HM, Siedler HD, Krooth RS, Kurland LT. A cutaneous disorder of connective tissue in amyotrophic lateral sclerosis. A histochemical study. Neurology 1960; 10: 717–724.
19. Bader L. Disorders of elastic tissue: a review. Pathology 1973; 5: 269–289.
20. Fisher ER, Wechsler HL. The so-called collagen diseases and elastoses of skin. In: Helwig EB, Mostofi FK, eds. The skin. Huntington, New York: Robert E Krieger, 1980; 366.
21. Ledoux-Corbusier M, Achten G, De Dobbeleer G. Juvenile elastoma (Weidman). An ultrastructural study. J Cutan Pathol 1981; 8: 219–227.
22. Raque CJ, Wood MG. Connective-tissue nevus. Arch Dermatol 1970; 102: 390–396.
23. Uitto J, Santa Cruz DJ, Eisen AZ. Connective tissue nevi of the skin. J Am Acad Dermatol 1980; 3: 441–461.
24. Atherton DJ, Wells RS. Juvenile elastoma and osteopoikilosis (the Buschke–Ollendorf syndrome). Clin Exp Dermatol 1982; 7: 109–113.
25. Reinhardt LA, Rountree CB, Wilkin JK. Buschke–Ollendorff syndrome. Cutis 1983; 31: 94–96.
26. Schorr WF, Optiz JM, Reyes CN. The connective tissue nevus–osteopoikilosis syndrome. Arch Dermatol 1972; 106: 208–214.
27. Morrison JGL, Wilson Jones E, MacDonald DM. Juvenile elastoma and osteopoikilosis (the Buschke–Ollendorff syndrome). Br J Dermatol 1977; 97: 417–422.
28. Piette-Brion B, Lowy-Motulsky M, Ledoux-Corbusier M, Achten G. Dermatofibromas, elastomas and deafness: a new case of Buschke–Ollendorff syndrome? Dermatologica 1984; 168: 255–258.
29. Verbov J. Buschke–Ollendorff syndrome (disseminated dermatofibrosis with osteopoikilosis). Br J Dermatol 1977; 96: 87–90.
30. Verbov J, Graham R. Buschke–Ollendorff syndrome — disseminated dermatofibrosis with osteopoikilosis. Clin Exp Dermatol 1986; 11: 17–26.
31. Uitto J, Santa Cruz DJ, Starcher BC et al. Biochemical and ultrastructural demonstration of elastin accumulation in the skin lesions of the Buschke–Ollendorff syndrome. J Invest Dermatol 1981; 76: 284–287.
31a. Burket JM, Zelickson AS, Padila RS. Linear focal elastosis (elastotic striae). J Am Acad Dermatol 1989; 20: 633–636.
32. Cole GW, Barr RJ. An elastic tissue defect in dermatofibrosis lenticularis disseminata. Arch Dermatol 1982; 118: 44–46.
33. Danielsen L, Midtgaard K, Christensen HE. Osteopoikilosis associated with dermatofibrosis lenticularis disseminata. Arch Dermatol 1969; 100: 465–470.
34. Staricco RG, Mehregan AH. Nevus elasticus and nevus elasticus vascularis. Arch Dermatol 1961; 84: 943–947.
35. Sosis AC, Johnson WC. Connective tissue nevus. Dermatologica 1972; 144: 57–62.
36. Becke RFA, Musso LA. An unusual epithelial-connective tissue naevus with perifollicular mucinosis. Australas J Dermatol 1978; 19: 118–120.
37. Danielsen L, Kobayasi T, Jacobsen GK. Ultrastructural changes in disseminated connective tissue nevi. Acta Derm Venereol 1977; 57: 93–101.
38. Reymond JL, Stoebner P, Beani JC, Amblard P. Buschke–Ollendorf syndrome. An electron microscopic study. Dermatologica 1983; 166: 64–68.
39. Madri JA, Dise CA, LiVolsi VA et al. Elastofibroma dorsi: an immunochemical study of collagen content. Hum Pathol 1981; 12: 186–190.
40. Enzinger FM, Weiss SW. Soft tissue tumours. St. Louis: C.V. Mosby, 1983; 33–37.
40a. Schwarz T, Oppolzer G, Duschet P et al. Ulcerating elastofibroma dorsi. J Am Acad Dermatol 1989; 21: 1142–1144.
41. Jarvi OH, Lansimies PH. Subclinical elastofibromas in the scapular region in an autopsy series. Acta Path Microbiol Scand (A). 1975; 83: 87–108.
42. Ramos CV, Gillespie W, Narconis RJ. Elastofibroma. A pseudotumor of myofibroblasts. Arch Pathol Lab Med 1978; 102: 538–540.
43. Mehregan AH. Elastosis perforans serpiginosa. A review of the literature and report of 11 cases. Arch Dermatol 1968; 97: 381–393.
44. Patterson JW. The perforating disorders. J Am Acad Dermatol 1984; 10: 561–581.
45. Woo TY, Rasmussen JE. Disorders of transepidermal elimination. Part 1. Int J Dermatol 1985; 24: 267–279.
46. White CR. The dermatopathology of perforating disorders. Semin Dermatol 1986; 5: 359–366.
47. Weidman AI, Allyn B. Elastosis perforans serpiginosa. Two cases involving the ear. Arch Dermatol 1971; 103: 324–327.
48. Pedro SD, Garcia RL. Disseminate elastosis perforans serpiginosa. Arch Dermatol 1974; 109: 84–85.
49. Rasmussen JE. Disseminated elastosis perforans serpiginosa in four mongoloids. Br J Dermatol 1972; 86: 9–13.
50. Woerdeman MJ, Bour DJH, Bijlsma JB. Elastosis perforans serpiginosa. Report of a family with a chromosomal investigation. Arch Dermatol 1965; 92: 559–560.
51. Ayala F, Donofrio P. Elastosis perforans serpiginosa. Report of a family. Dermatologica 1983; 166: 32–37.
52. Crotty G, Bell M, Estes SA, Kitzmiller KW. Cytologic features of elastosis perforans serpiginosa (EPS) associated with Down's syndrome. J Am Acad Dermatol 1983; 8: 255–256.

53. Carey TD. Elastosis perforans serpiginosa. Arch Dermatol 1977; 113: 1444–1445.

54. Barr RJ, Siegel JM, Graham JH. Elastosis perforans serpiginosa associated with morphea. An example of "perforating morphea". J Am Acad Dermatol 1980; 3: 19–22.

55. May NC, Lester RS. Elastosis perforans serpiginosa associated with systemic sclerosis. J Am Acad Dermatol 1982; 6: 945.

56. Schamroth JM, Kellen P, Grieve TP. Elastosis perforans serpiginosa in a patient with renal disease. Arch Dermatol 1986; 122: 82–84.

57. Pass F, Goldfischer S, Sternlieb I, Scheinberg IH. Elastosis perforans serpiginosa during penicillamine therapy for Wilson disease. Arch Dermatol 1973; 108: 713–715.

58. Rosenblum GA. Liquid nitrogen cryotherapy in a case of elastosis perforans serpiginosa. J Am Acad Dermatol 1983; 8: 718–721.

58a. Goldstein JB, McNutt NS, Hambrick GW Jr, Hsu A. Penicillamine dermatopathy with lymphangiectases. A clinical, immunohistologic, and ultrastructural study. Arch Dermatol 1989; 125: 92–97.

59. Levy RS, Fisher M, Alter JN. Penicillamine: Review and cutaneous manifestations. J Am Acad Dermatol 1983; 8: 548–558.

59a. van Joost T, Vuzevski VD, ten Kate FJW et al. Elastosis perforans serpiginosa: clinical, histomorphological and immunological studies. J Cutan Pathol 1988; 15: 92–97.

60. Price RG, Prentice RSA. Penicillamine-induced elastosis perforans serpiginosa. Tip of the iceberg? Am J Dermatopathol 1986; 8: 314–320.

61. Eide J. Elastosis perforans serpiginosa with widespread arterial lesions: a case report. Acta Derm Venereol 1977; 57: 533–537.

61a. Rapini RP, Hebert AA, Drucker CR. Acquired perforating dermatosis. Evidence for combined transepidermal elimination of both collagen and elastic fibers. Arch Dermatol 1989; 125: 1074–1078.

62. Bergman R, Friedman-Birnbaum R, Hazaz B. A direct immunofluorescence study in elastosis perforans serpiginosa. Br J Dermatol 1985; 113: 573–579.

63. Bardach H, Gebhart W, Niebauer G. "Lumpy-bumpy" elastic fibers in the skin and lungs of a patient with penicillamine-induced elastosis perforans serpiginosa. J Cutan Pathol 1979; 6: 243–252.

64. Gebhart W, Bardach H. The "lumpy-bumpy" elastic fiber. A marker for long-term administration of penicillamine. Am J Dermatopathol 1981; 3: 33–39.

65. Kirsch N, Hukill PB. Elastosis perforans serpiginosa induced by penicillamine. Electron microscopic observations. Arch Dermatol 1977; 113: 630–635.

66. Hashimoto K, McEvoy B, Belcher R. Ultrastructure of penicillamine-induced skin lesions. J Am Acad Dermatol 1981; 4: 300–315.

67. Reymond JL, Stoebner P, Zambelli P et al. Penicillamine induced elastosis perforans serpiginosa: an ultrastructural study of two cases. J Cutan Pathol 1982; 9: 352–357.

68. Meves C, Vogel A. Electron microscopical studies in elastosis perforans serpiginosa. Dermatologica 1973; 145: 210–221.

69. Volpin D, Pasquali-Ronchetti I, Castellani I et al. Ultrastructural and biochemical studies on a case of elastosis perforans serpiginosa. Dermatologica 1978; 156: 209–223.

70. Neldner KH. Pseudoxanthoma elasticum. Int J Dermatol 1988; 27: 98–100.

71. Woo TY, Rasmussen JE. Disorders of transepidermal elimination. Part 2. Int J Dermatol 1985; 24: 337–348.

72. Goodman RM, Smith EW, Paton D et al. Pseudoxanthoma elasticum: a clinical and histopathological study. Medicine (Baltimore) 1963; 42: 297–334.

73. Danielsen L, Kobayasi T. Pseudoxanthoma elasticum. An ultrastructural study of oral lesions. Acta Derm Venereol 1974; 54: 173–176.

73a. Rongioletti F, Bertamino R, Rebora A. Generalized pseudoxanthoma elasticum with deficiency of vitamin K-dependent clotting factors. J Am Acad Dermatol 1989; 21: 1150–1152.

74. Reeve EB, Neldner KH, Subryan V, Gordon SG. Development and calcification of skin lesions in thirty-nine patients with pseudoxanthoma elasticum. Clin Exp Dermatol 1979; 4: 291–301.

75. Mendelsohn G, Bulkley BH, Hutchins GM. Cardiovascular manifestations of pseudoxanthoma elasticum. Arch Pathol Lab Med 1978; 102: 298–302.

76. Dymock RB. Pseudoxanthoma elasticum: report of a case with reno-vascular hypertension. Australas J Dermatol 1979; 20: 82–84.

77. Akhtar M, Brody H. Elastic tissue in pseudoxanthoma elasticum. Ultrastructural study of endocardial lesions. Arch Pathol 1975; 99: 667–671.

78. Pope FM. Historical evidence for the genetic heterogeneity of pseudoxanthoma elasticum. Br J Dermatol 1975; 92: 493–509.

79. Pope FM. Two types of autosomal recessive pseudoxanthoma elasticum. Arch Dermatol 1974; 110: 209–212.

80. Macmillan DC. Pseudoxanthoma elasticum and a coagulation defect. Br J Dermatol 1971; 84: 182.

81. Martinez-Hernandez A, Huffer WE, Neldner K et al. Resolution and repair of elastic tissue calcification in pseudoxanthoma elasticum. Arch Pathol Lab Med 1978; 102: 303–305.

82. Eng AM, Bryant J. Clinical pathologic observations in pseudoxanthoma elasticum. Int J Dermatol 1975; 14: 586–605.

83. Schutt DA. Pseudoxanthoma elasticum and elastosis perforans serpiginosa. Arch Dermatol 1965; 91: 151–152.

84. Lund HZ, Gilbert CF. Perforating pseudoxanthoma elasticum. Its distinction from elastosis perforans serpiginosa. Arch Pathol Lab Med 1976; 100: 544–546.

85. Schwartz RA, Richfield DF. Pseudoxanthoma elasticum with transepidermal elimination. Arch Dermatol 1978; 114: 279–280.

85a. Walker ER, Frederickson RG, Mayes MD. The mineralization of elastic fibers and alterations of extracellular matrix in pseudoxanthoma elasticum. Ultrastructure, immunocytochemistry, and x-ray analysis. Arch Dermatol 1989; 125: 70–76.

86. Gordon SG, Overland M, Foley J. Evidence for increased protease activity secreted from cultured fibroblasts from patients with pseudoxanthoma elasticum. Connect Tissue Res 1978; 6: 61–68.

87. Nickoloff BJ, Noodleman FR, Abel EA. Perforating

pseudoxanthoma elasticum associated with chronic renal failure and hemodialysis. Arch Dermatol 1985; 121: 1321–1322.

88. Dupre A, Bonafe JL, Christol B. Chequered localized pseudoxanthoma elasticum: a variety of Christensen's exogenous pseudoxanthoma elasticum? Acta Derm Venereol 1979; 59: 539–541.

89. Hicks J, Carpenter CL, Reed RJ. Periumbilical perforating pseudoxanthoma elasticum. Arch Dermatol 1979; 115: 300–303.

90. Christensen OB. An exogenous variety of pseudoxanthoma elasticum in old farmers. Acta Derm Venereol 1978; 58: 319–321.

91. Nielsen AO, Christensen OB, Hentzer B et al. Salpeter-induced dermal changes electron-microscopically indistinguishable from pseudoxanthoma elasticum. Acta Derm Venereol 1978; 58: 323–327.

91a. Kazakis AM, Parish WR. Periumbilical perforating pseudoxanthoma elasticum. J Am Acad Dermatol 1988; 19: 384–388.

92. Neldner KH, Martinez-Hernandez A. Localized acquired cutaneous pseudoxanthoma elasticum. J Am Acad Dermatol 1979; 1: 523–530.

93. Heyl T. Pseudoxanthoma elasticum with granulomatous skin lesions. Arch Dermatol 1967; 96: 528–531.

94. McKee PH, Cameron CHS, Archer DB, Logan WC. A study of four cases of pseudoxanthoma elasticum. J Cutan Pathol 1977; 4: 146–153.

95. Danielsen L, Kobayasi T. Pseudoxanthoma elasticum. An ultrastructural study of scar tissue. Acta Derm Venereol 1974; 54: 121–128.

96. Yamamura T, Sano S. Ultrastructural and histochemical analysis of thready material in *pseudoxanthoma elasticum*. J Cutan Pathol 1984; 11: 282–291.

96a. Nakayama H, Hashimoto K, Kambe N, Eng A. Elastic globes: electron microscopic and immunohistochemical observations. J Cutan Pathol 1988; 15: 98–103.

96b. Brennan TE, Pearson RW. Abnormal elastic tissue in cartilage-hair hypoplasia. Arch Dermatol 1988; 124: 1411–1414.

Solar elastotic syndromes

96c. Salasche SJ, Clemons DE. Cutaneous manifestations of chronic solar exposure. J Assoc Milit Dermatol 1985; 11: 3–10.

97. Hashimoto K, Black M. Colloid milium: a final degeneration product of actinic elastoid. J Cutan Pathol 1985; 12: 147–156.

97a. Barnhill RL, Goldenhersh MA. Elastophagocytosis: a non-specific reaction pattern associated with inflammatory processes in sun-protected skin. J Cutan Pathol 1989; 16: 199–202.

98. Cockerell EG, Freeman RG, Knox JM. Changes after prolonged exposure to sunlight. Arch Dermatol 1961; 84: 467–472.

99. O'Brien JP. Solar and radiant damage to elastic tissue as a cause of internal vascular damage. Australas J Dermatol 1980; 21: 1–8.

100. Kocsard E. Senile elastosis: central phenomenon of aging of exposed skin. Geriatrics Digest 1970; 7: 10–18.

100a. Taylor CR, Stern RS, Leyden JJ, Gilchrest BA. Photoaging/photodamage and photoprotection. J Am Acad Dermatol 1990; 22: 1–15.

101. Degos R, Touraine R, Civatte J, Belaich S. Elastome en nappe du nez. Bull Soc Franc Derm Syph 1966; 73: 123–124.

102. Raimer SS, Sanchez RL, Hubler WR Jr, Dodson RF. Solar elastotic bands of the forearm: An unusual clinical presentation of actinic elastosis. J Am Acad Dermatol 1986; 15: 650–656.

103. Mitchell RE. Chronic solar dermatosis: a light and electron microscopic study of the dermis. J Invest Dermatol 1967; 48: 203–220.

104. Stevanovic DV. Elastotic degeneration. A light and electron microscopic study. Br J Dermatol 1976; 94: 23–29.

104a. Bouissou H, Pieraggi M-T, Julian M, Savit T. The elastic tissue of the skin. A comparison of spontaneous and actinic (solar) aging. Int J Dermatol 1988; 27: 327–335.

105. Chen VL, Fleischmajer R, Schwartz E et al. Immunochemistry of elastotic material in sun-damaged skin. J Invest Dermatol 1986; 87: 334–337.

106. Montagna W, Carlisle K. Structural changes in aging human skin. J Invest Dermatol 1979; 73: 47–53.

107. Lavker RM. Structural alterations in exposed and unexposed aged skin. J Invest Dermatol 1979; 73: 59–66.

108. Goette DK. Transepidermal elimination of actinically damaged connective tissue. Int J Dermatol 1984; 23: 669–672.

109. Lavker RM, Kligman AM. Chronic heliodermatitis: a morphologic evaluation of chronic actinic dermal damage with emphasis on the role of mast cells. J Invest Dermatol 1988; 90: 325–330.

109a. Montagna W, Kirchner S, Carlisle K. Histology of sun-damaged human skin. J Am Acad Dermatol 1989; 21: 907–918.

110. Ledoux-Corbusier M, Danis P. Pinguecula and actinic elastosis. An ultrastructural study. J Cutan Pathol 1979; 6: 404–413.

111. Danielsen L, Kobayasi T. Degeneration of dermal elastic fibres in relation to age and light-exposure. Preliminary report on electron microscopic studies. Acta Derm Venereol 1972; 52: 1–10.

112. Ledoux-Corbusier M, Achten G. Elastosis in chronic radiodermatitis. An ultrastructural study. Br J Dermatol 1974; 91: 287–295.

113. Zelickson AS, Mottaz JH, Zelickson BD, Muller SA. Elastic tissue changes in skin following PUVA therapy. J Am Acad Dermatol 1980; 3: 186–192.

114. Tsuji T. The surface structural alterations of elastic fibers and elastotic material in solar elastosis: a scanning electron microscopic study. J Cutan Pathol 1984; 11: 300–308.

115. Cuce LC, Paschoal LHC, Curban GV. Cutaneous nodular elastoidosis with cysts and comedones. Arch Dermatol 1964; 89: 798–802.

116. Helm F. Nodular cutaneous elastosis with cysts and comedones (Favre–Racouchot syndrome). Arch Dermatol 1961; 84: 666–668.

117. Hassounah A, Pierard GE. Kerosis and comedones without prominent elastosis in Favre–Racouchot disease. Am J Dermatopathol 1987; 9: 15–17.

118. Carter VH, Constantine VS, Poole WL. Elastotic

nodules of the antihelix. Arch Dermatol 1969; 100: 282–285.

119. Weedon D. Elastotic nodules of the ear. J Cutan Pathol 1981; 8: 429–433.

120. Kocsard E, Ofner F, Turner B. Elastotic nodules of the antihelix. Arch Dermatol 1970; 101: 370.

121. Rahbari H. Acrokeratoelastoidosis and keratoelastoidosis marginalis — any relation? J Am Acad Dermatol 1981; 5: 348–350.

122. Burks JW, Wise LJ, Clark WH. Degenerative collagenous plaques of the hands. Arch Dermatol 1960; 82: 362–366.

123. Kocsard E. Keratoelastoidosis marginalis of the hands. Dermatologica 1964; 131: 169–175.

124. Ritchie EB, Williams HM. Degenerative collagenous plaques of the hands. Arch Dermatol 1966; 93: 202–203.

125. Shahrad P, Marks R. The wages of warmth: changes in erythema ab igne. Br J Dermatol 1977; 97: 179–186.

125a. Milligan A, Graham-Brown RAC. Erythema ab igne affecting the palms. Clin Exp Dermatol 1989; 14: 168–169.

126. Arrington JH III, Lockman DS. Thermal keratoses and squamous cell carcinoma in situ associated with erythema ab igne. Arch Dermatol 1979; 115: 1226–1228.

127. Finlayson GR, Sams WM Jr, Smith JG Jr. Erythema ab igne: a histopathological study. J Invest Dermatol 1966; 46: 104–108.

128. Johnson WC, Butterworth T. Erythema ab igne elastosis. Arch Dermatol 1971; 104: 128–131.

Decreased elastic tissue

129. Bordas X, Ferrandiz C, Ribera M, Galofre E. Papular elastorrhexis: a variety of nevus anelasticus? Arch Dermatol 1987; 123: 433–434.

130. Crivellato E. Disseminated nevus anelasticus. Int J Dermatol 1986; 25: 171–173.

130a. Sears JK, Stone MS, Argenyi Z. Papular elastorrhexis: A variant of connective tissue nevus. Case reports and review of the literature. J Am Acad Dermatol 1988; 19: 409–414.

131. Varadi DP, Saqueton AC. Perifollicular elastolysis. Br J Dermatol 1970; 83: 143–150.

132. Taaffe A, Cunliffe WJ, Clayden AD. Perifollicular elastolysis — a common condition. Br J Dermatol (Suppl) 1983; 24: 20.

132a. Wilson BB, Dent CH, Cooper PH. Papular acne scars. A common cutaneous finding. Arch Dermatol 1990; 126: 797–800.

133. Venencie PY, Winkelmann RK, Moore BA. Anetoderma. Clinical findings, associations, and long-term follow-up evaluations. Arch Dermatol 1984; 120: 1032–1039.

134. Miller WN, Ruggles CW, Rist TE. Anetoderma. Int J Dermatol 1979; 18: 43–45.

135. Friedman SJ, Venencie PY, Bradley RR, Winkelmann RK. Familial anetoderma. J Am Acad Dermatol 1987; 16: 341–345.

136. Davis W. Wilson's disease and penicillamine-induced anetoderma. Arch Dermatol 1977; 113: 976.

137. Carr RD. Urticaria pigmentosa associated with anetoderma. Acta Derm Venereol 1971; 51: 120–122.

138. Oikarinen AI, Palatsi R, Adomian GE et al. Anetoderma: Biochemical and ultrastructural demonstration of an elastin defect in the skin of three patients. J Am Acad Dermatol 1984; 11: 64–72.

139. Venencie PY, Winkelmann RK. Histopathologic findings in anetoderma. Arch Dermatol 1984; 120: 1040–1044.

140. Venencie PY, Winkelmann RK. Monoclonal antibody studies in the skin lesions of patients with anetoderma. Arch Dermatol 1985; 121: 747–749.

141. Taieb A, Dufillot D, Pellegrin-Carloz B et al. Postgranulomatous anetoderma associated with Takayasu's arteritis in a child. Arch Dermatol 1987; 123: 796–800.

141a. Bergman R, Friedman-Birnbaum R, Hazaz B et al. An immunofluorescence study of primary anetoderma. Clin Exp Dermatol 1990; 15: 124–130.

142. Venencie PY, Winkelmann RK, Moore BA. Ultrastructural findings in the skin lesions of patients with anetoderma. Acta Derm Venereol 1984; 64: 112–120.

143. Kossard S, Kronman KR, Dicken CH, Schroeter AL. Inflammatory macular atrophy: Immunofluorescent and ultrastructural findings. J Am Acad Dermatol 1979; 1: 325–334.

144. Tsuji T, Imajo Y, Sawabe M et al. Acquired cutis laxa concomitant with nephrotic syndrome. Arch Dermatol 1987; 123: 1211–1216.

145. Schreiber MM, Tilley JC. Cutis laxa. Arch Dermatol 1961; 84: 266–272.

146. Ledoux-Corbusier M. *Cutis laxa*, congenital form with pulmonary emphysema: an ultrastructural study. J Cutan Pathol 1983; 10: 340–349.

147. Mehregan AH, Lee SC, Nabai H. Cutis laxa (generalized elastolysis). A report of four cases with autopsy findings. J Cutan Pathol 1978; 5: 116–126.

148. Sakati NO, Nyhan WL. Congenital cutis laxa and osteoporosis. Am J Dis Child 1983; 137: 452–454.

149. Agha A, Sakati NO, Higginbottom MC et al. Two forms of cutis laxa presenting in the newborn period. Acta Paediatr Scand 1978; 67: 775–780.

150. Byers PH, Siegel RC, Holbrook KA et al. X-linked cutis laxa. N Engl J Med 1980; 303: 61–65.

151. Brown FR III, Holbrook KA, Byers PH et al. Cutis laxa. Johns Hopkins Med J 1982; 150: 148–153.

152. Fisher BK, Page E, Hanna W. Acral localized acquired cutis laxa. J Am Acad Dermatol 1989; 21: 33–40.

153. Greenbaum SS, Krull EA, Rubin MG, Lee R. Localized acquired cutis laxa in one of identical twins. Int J Dermatol 1989; 28: 402–406.

154. Reed WB, Horowitz RE, Beighton P. Acquired cutis laxa. Primary generalized elastolysis. Arch Dermatol 1971; 103: 661–669.

155. Nanko H, Jepsen LV, Zachariae H, Sogaard H. Acquired cutis laxa (generalized elastolysis): light and electron microscopic studies. Acta Derm Venereol 1979; 59: 315–324.

156. Muster AJ, Bharati S, Herman JJ et al. Fatal cardiovascular disease and cutis laxa following acute febrile neutrophilic dermatosis. J Pediatr 1983; 102: 243–248.

157. Harris RB, Heaphy MR, Perry HO. Generalized elastolysis (cutis laxa). Am J Med 1978; 65: 815–822.

158. Kerl H, Burg G, Hashimoto K. Fatal, penicillin-

induced, generalized postinflammatory elastolysis (cutis laxa). Am J Dermatopathol 1983; 5: 267–276.

159. Koch SE, Williams ML. Acquired cutis laxa: case report and review of disorders of elastolysis. Pediatr Dermatol 1985; 2: 282–288.

160. Hashimoto K, Kanzaki T. Cutis laxa. Ultrastructural and biochemical studies. Arch Dermatol 1975; 111: 861–873.

161. Scott MA, Kauh YC, Luscombe HA. Acquired cutis laxa associated with multiple myeloma. Arch Dermatol 1976; 112: 853–855.

162. Ting HC, Foo MH, Wang F. Acquired cutis laxa and multiple myeloma. Br J Dermatol 1984; 110: 363–367.

163. Randle HW, Muller S. Generalized elastolysis associated with systemic lupus erythematosus. J Am Acad Dermatol 1983; 8: 869–873.

164. Goltz RW, Hult A-M, Goldfarb M, Gorlin RJ. Cutis laxa. A manifestation of generalized elastolysis. Arch Dermatol 1965; 92: 373–387.

165. Sephel GC, Byers PH, Holbrook KA, Davidson JM. Heterogeneity of elastin expression in cutis laxa fibroblast strains. J Invest Dermatol 1989; 93: 147–153.

166. Kitano Y, Nishida K, Okada N et al. Cutis laxa with ultrastructural abnormalities of elastic fiber. J Am Acad Dermatol 1989; 21: 378–380.

167. Marchase P, Holbrook K, Pinnell SR. A familial cutis laxa syndrome with ultrastructural abnormalities of collagen and elastin. J Invest Dermatol 1980; 75: 399–403.

168. Marshall J, Heyl T, Weber HW. Post-inflammatory elastolysis and cutis laxa. Sth Afr Med J 1966; 40: 1016–1022.

169. Verhagen AR, Woerdeman MJ. Post-inflammatory elastolysis and cutis laxa. Br J Dermatol 1975; 92: 183–190.

170. Lewis PG, Hood AF, Barnett NK, Holbrook KA. Postinflammatory elastolysis and cutis laxa. J Am Acad Dermatol 1990; 22: 40–48.

171. Brenner W, Gschnait F, Konrad K et al. Non-inflammatory dermal elastolysis. Br J Dermatol 1978; 99: 335–338.

172. Shelley WB, Wood MG. Wrinkles due to idiopathic loss of mid-dermal elastic tissue. Br J Dermatol 1977; 97: 441–445.

173. Rao BK, Blakely FA, Menter A, Freeman RG. Mid dermal elastolysis. J Cutan Pathol 1988; 15: 340 (abstract).

174. Rudolph RI. Mid dermal elastolysis. J Am Acad Dermatol 1990; 22: 203–206.

175. Rae V, Falanga V. Wrinkling due to middermal elastolysis. Report of a case and review of the literature. Arch Dermatol 1989; 125: 950–951.

176. Barker SM, Dicken CH. Elastolysis of the earlobes. J Am Acad Dermatol 1986; 14: 145–147.

177. Menkes JH, Alter M, Steigleder GK et al. A sex-linked recessive disorder with retardation of growth, peculiar hair, and focal cerebral and cerebellar degeneration. Pediatrics 1962; 29: 764–779.

178. Hockey A, Masters CL. Menkes' kinky (steely) hair disease. Australas J Dermatol 1977; 18: 77–80.

179. Hart DB. Menkes' syndrome: An updated review. J Am Acad Dermatol 1983; 9: 145–152.

180. Procopis P, Camakaris J, Danks DM. A mild form of Menkes' steely hair syndrome. J Pediatr 1981; 98: 97–99.

181. Danks DM, Stevens BJ, Campbell PE et al. Menkes' kinky hair syndrome. Lancet 1972; 1: 1100–1102.

182. Oakes BW, Danks DM, Campbell PE. Human copper deficiency: ultrastructural studies of the aorta and skin in a child with Menkes' syndrome. Exp Mol Pathol 1976; 25: 82–98.

183. Williams DM, Atkin CL. Tissue copper concentrations of patients with Menkes' kinky hair disease. Am J Dis Child 1981; 135: 375–376.

184. Royce PM, Camakaris J, Danks DM. Reduced lysyl oxidase activity in skin fibroblasts from patients with Menkes' syndrome. Biochem J 1980; 192: 579–586.

185. Waldstein G, Mierau G, Ahmad R et al. Fragile X syndrome: skin elastin abnormalities. Birth Defects 1987; 23: 103–114.

186. Yanagihara M, Kato F, Mori S. Extra- and intra-cellular digestion of elastic fibers by macrophages in annular elastolytic giant cell granuloma. An ultrastructural study. J Cutan Pathol 1987; 14: 303–308.

187. Boneschi V, Brambilla L, Fossati S et al. Annular elastolytic giant cell granuloma. Am J Dermatopathol 1988; 10: 224–228.

188. LeBoit PE, Zackheim HS, White CR Jr. Granulomatous variants of cutaneous T-cell lymphoma. The histopathology of granulomatous mycosis fungoides and granulomatous slack skin. Am J Dermatopathol 1988; 12: 83–95.

189. Alessi E, Crosti C, Sala F. Unusual case of granulomatous dermohypodermitis with giant cells and elastophagocytosis. Dermatologica 1986; 172: 218–221.

190. Balus L, Bassetti F, Gentili G. Granulomatous slack skin. Arch Dermatol 1985; 121: 250–252.

191. Convit J, Kerdel F, Goihman M et al. Progressive, atrophying, chronic granulomatous dermohypodermitis. Arch Dermatol 1973; 107: 271–274.

192. LeBoit PE, Beckstead JH, Bond B et al. Granulomatous slack skin: clonal rearrangement of the T-cell receptor B gene is evidence for the lymphoproliferative nature of a cutaneous elastolytic disorder. J Invest Dermatol 1987; 89: 183–186.

193. Matsuoka LY, Wortsman J, Uitto J et al. Altered skin elastic fibers in hypothyroid myxedema and pretibial myxedema. Arch Intern Med 1985; 145: 117–121.

Variable or minor elastic tissue changes

194. Roth SI, Schedewie HK, Herzberg VK et al. Cutaneous manifestations of leprechaunism. Arch Dermatol 1981; 117: 531–535.

195. Patterson JH, Watkins WL. Leprechaunism in a male infant. J Pediatr 1962; 60: 730–739.

196. Bauer EA, Uitto J, Tan EML, Holbrook KA. Werner's syndrome. Evidence for preferential regional expression of a generalized mesenchymal cell defect. Arch Dermatol 1988; 124: 90–101.

197. Venencie PY, Powell FC, Winkelmann RK. Acrogeria with perforating elastoma and bony abnormalities. Acta Derm Venereol 1984; 64: 348–351.

198. Beauregard S, Gilchrest BA. Syndromes of premature aging. Dermatol Clin 1987; 5: 109–121.

199. Shelley WB, Wood MG. Unilateral wrinkles.

blue technique at pH 2.5, and the colloidal iron stain, with which acid mucopolysaccharides are blue-green. Metachromasia of mucin is usually demonstrated with the toluidine blue or Giemsa methods. It has been suggested recently that fixation in a 1% solution of cetylpyridinium chloride in formalin, followed by colloidal iron staining of the paraffin sections, gives the best definition of glycosaminoglycans in the skin.[5]

DERMAL MUCINOSES

The distribution of the glycosaminoglycans is said to differ in the various dermal mucinoses. However, in a comparative study several years ago, Matsuoka and colleagues found that the distribution of these substances is generally not diagnostically specific.[5] Accordingly, clinico-pathological correlation is important in this group. Scleredema and scleromyxoedema differ from the other dermal mucinoses by the presence of collagen deposition and fibroblast hypertrophy and/or hyperplasia, in addition to the deposition of mucin.

GENERALIZED MYXOEDEMA

Myxoedema is one of several cutaneous changes in hypothyroidism.[3,6,7] These changes are most pronounced around the eyes, nose and cheeks, often giving a characteristic facies, and also on the distal extremities.

Palmoplantar keratoderma is a poorly recognized presentation of myxoedema.[7a] Glycosaminoglycans are deposited in other organs of the body as well as the skin and it has been suggested that there is impaired degradation, rather than increased synthesis of these substances.[4,8]

Histopathology

In most cases, the changes are subtle with only small amounts of mucin in the dermis.[4] This is predominantly hyaluronic acid. Sometimes this material is deposited only focally around vessels and hair follicles.[4] There may be mild hyper-

keratosis and keratotic follicular plugging. Elastic fibres are sometimes fragmented and reduced in amount.

PRETIBIAL MYXOEDEMA

Pretibial myxoedema is found in 1–4% of patients with Graves' disease, particularly those with exophthalmos, but it may not develop until after the correction of the hyperthyroidism.[9] It may also occur in patients with non-thyrotoxic Graves' disease,[10] and occasionally in association with autoimmune thyroiditis. It presents as sharply circumscribed nodular lesions, diffuse non-pitting oedema, or elephantiasis-like thickening of the skin. There may be overlap of these lesions, or progression from nodular to more diffuse plaques.[9] The anterior aspect of the lower legs, sometimes with spread to the dorsum of the feet, is the most usual site of involvement, although, rarely, the upper trunk, upper extremities and even the face, neck or ears have been involved.[11,12] Localization to scar tissue has been reported.[12a] Slow resolution of the lesions often occurs after many years.

The theory that pretibial myxoedema results from the stimulation of fibroblasts by LATS (long-acting thyroid stimulator) is no longer tenable, although one or multiple other substances or autoantibodies are presumably involved.[11,13] A circulating factor which stimulates increased synthesis of glycosaminoglycans by normal skin fibroblasts is present in increased amounts in patients with pretibial myxoedema.[14] Furthermore, fibroblasts from pretibial skin cultured in the presence of serum from patients with pretibial myxoedema produce increased amounts of hyaluronic acid.[15] There is no primary lymphatic abnormality.[9]

Histopathology

There are large amounts of mucin deposited in the dermis, particularly in the mid and lower thirds (Fig. 13.1). This manifests as basophilic threads and granular material with wide separation of collagen bundles.[3] There is no increase in fibroblasts although a few stellate

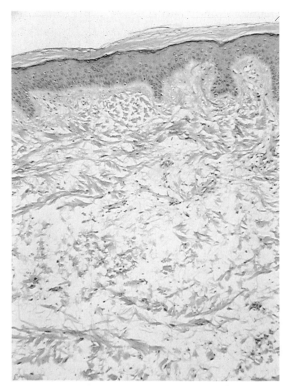

Fig. 13.1 Pretibial myxoedema. The collagen bundles in the dermis are widely spaced, a consequence of the increased amount of interstitial mucin. Haematoxylin — eosin

forms may be present. There may be mild overlying hyperkeratosis and a mild superficial perivascular chronic inflammatory cell infiltrate.[8]

Elastic tissue stains show fragmentation and a reduction in elastic tissue, a finding confirmed on electron microscopy[16] which also shows microfibrils with knobs (glycosaminoglycans)[17] or amorphous material (glycoproteins)[18] on the surface of fibroblasts that have dilated endoplasmic reticulum.[17,18]

PAPULAR MUCINOSIS AND SCLEROMYXOEDEMA

Papular mucinosis (lichen myxoedematosus) is a rare cutaneous mucinosis in which multiple, asymptomatic, pale or waxy papules, 2 to 3 mm in diameter, develop on the hands, forearms, face, neck and upper trunk.[19–21] A variant in which the lesions are restricted to the hands and wrists has been reported as acral persistent papular mucinosis.[22,22a] *Scleromyxoedema* is a variant in which lichenoid papules and plaques are accompanied by skin thickening involving almost the entire body.[20,23,24] Involvement of the glabella region may give rise to bovine facies.[20] A paraproteinaemia, particularly of IgG lambda type, is almost invariably present in scleromyxoedema and sometimes in papular mucinosis.[3] Other classes of immunoglobulins are sometimes present;[25] a few patients have a normal immunoglobulin profile.[26] Multiple myeloma and Waldenström's macroglobulinaemia are rare associations.[27–29] Bizarre neurological symptoms,[30,31] underlying carcinoma,[21] pachydermoperiostosis,[21] dermatomyositis, scleroderma,[28] atherosclerosis,[32] oesophageal aperistalsis,[33] and multiple keratoacanthomas[25] have all been reported in association with scleromyxoedema.[28]

Scleromyxoedema is usually progressive, but spontaneous resolution has been reported.[34] Mucin has been noted in other organs, in a few autopsy cases, but it has been specifically excluded in others.[21,30] Rarely, hypothyroidism has been present.[35,36]

It has been postulated that a serum factor stimulates fibroblast proliferation and increased production of glycosaminoglycans.[37] Whether this factor is identical to the monoclonal immunoglobulin is controversial.[28,38] In one study, cultured skin fibroblasts from a patient with scleromyxoedema produced an IgG immunoglobulin.[39]

Histopathology

The histopathological features of *scleromyxoedema* are the most precise of any of the mucinoses.[8,20,40] In addition to the dermal deposits of mucin, there are a marked proliferation of fibroblasts and increased collagen deposition in the upper and mid dermis (Figs 13.2 and 13.3).[8] The fibroblasts are irregularly arranged and the collagen, which is most pronounced in older lesions, has a whorled pattern. Flattening of the epidermis and atrophy of pilosebaceous follicles are secondary changes.

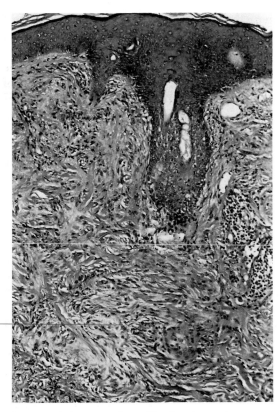

Fig. 13.2 Scleromyxoedema. The dermis contains an increase in fibroblasts, collagen and interstitial mucin. Haematoxylin — eosin

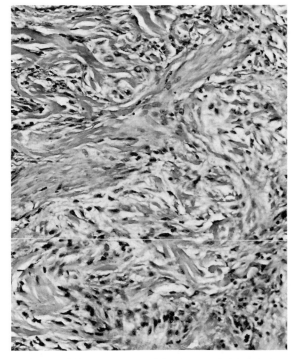

Fig. 13.3 Scleromyxoedema. The characteristic triad of an increase in fibroblasts, collagen and mucin is present. Haematoxylin — eosin

Elastic fibres are often fragmented.[39] A sparse perivascular infiltrate of lymphocytes is often present. Occasionally, eosinophils[30,33] or mast cells[41] are prominent. A similar appearance may follow the ingestion of L-tryptophan.

Ultrastructurally, the fibroblasts have prominent rough endoplasmic reticulum. Proteoglycans are present between the collagen bundles.[42]

The changes in *papular mucinosis* are not as characteristic. In the discrete form, the changes may be indistinguishable from focal mucinosis,[43] although in the more generalized cases a slight proliferation of fibroblasts is often present in addition to the mucin deposition in the upper dermis.[35]

RETICULAR ERYTHEMATOUS MUCINOSIS (REM)

This dermal mucinosis presents with erythematous maculopapules and infiltrated plaques, often with a reticulated or net-like pattern, in the midline of the back or chest, sometimes spreading to the upper abdomen.[44-48] Rarely, the face and arms[49] are involved, and one case is said to have involved the gums.[50] There is a predilection for young to middle-aged females. Sunlight may cause exacerbations and induce mild pruritus.[3] The lesions may subside after many years.

Histopathology

There is a mild superficial and mid-dermal perivascular infiltrate with variable deep perivascular extension, the latter sometimes being

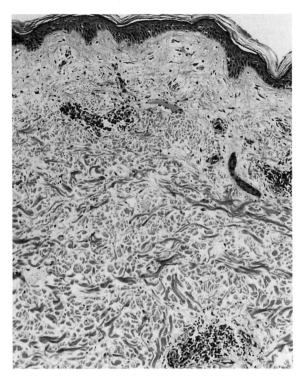

Fig. 13.4 Reticular erythematous mucinosis. There is a superficial and deep infiltrate and an increase in interstitial mucin.
Haematoxylin — eosin

restricted to the region of the eccrine glands.[46] There may be some perifollicular infiltrate as well. This infiltrate is predominantly lymphocytic with a few admixed mast cells and histiocytes. There is slight vascular dilatation and, sometimes, focal mild haemorrhage in the upper dermis.[49]

There is separation of dermal collagen bundles, and sometimes small amounts of stringy basophilic mucin can be seen in the upper and mid dermis (Fig. 13.4). A few stellate fibroblasts may be present, but this is not an obvious feature. The epidermis is usually normal, although mild exocytosis with spongiosis has been reported in one case.

The mucin gives variable staining reactions. Colloidal iron staining is superior to alcian blue which on occasions has failed to demonstrate mucin.[51,52] The material is not usually metachromatic with toluidine blue.[52] Staining with colloidal iron and alcian blue will be negative following digestion with hyaluronidase. There may be focal fragmentation of elastic fibres.[51]

Electron microscopy. There are widening of the intercollagenous spaces, focal fragmentation of elastic fibres, and some active fibroblasts.[53] Numerous tubular aggregates have also been seen in endothelial cells, pericytes and some dermal macrophages.[51,54] In one report, lesional skin showed granular basement membrane deposits of IgM, IgA and C3.[55]

SCLEREDEMA

Scleredema (scleredema adultorum of Buschke) is characterized by the development of non-pitting induration of the skin with a predilection for symmetrical involvement of the posterior neck, the shoulders, the upper trunk and the face.[56,57] In cases of more widespread involvement, the upper part of the body is always involved much more than the lower part, and the feet are spared. The condition occurs at all ages, although nearly 50% of cases develop in children and adolescents.[58,59] There is a predilection for females.

There are several different clinical settings.[60,61] In one group the onset is sudden and follows days to weeks after an acute febrile illness caused by streptococci or viruses. Spontaneous resolution occurs in approximately one-third of these patients after 6 to 18 months. This group is now seen less frequently than previously. Another clinical group has an insidious onset, without any predisposing illness, and a protracted course.[62] The third group is associated with insulin-dependent, mature onset diabetes, which is difficult to control.[63–65] Vascular complications of diabetes are common.[66,67] The scleredema is insidious in onset and prolonged in its course.

Systemic manifestations such as ECG changes, serosal effusions and involvement of skeletal, ocular and tongue musculature may develop. Paraproteinaemia[68–73] and rheumatoid arthritis[74] have been present in a few patients. There may be cutaneous abscesses or cellulitis preceding or following the onset of the condition.[75,76] Rarely, there is erythema at sites of skin thickening.[77]

Scleredema is characterized by the accumulation of glycosaminoglycans, particularly hyaluronic acid, in the dermis, with concurrent dermal sclerosis.[78] The aetiology is unknown, although a recent study using cultured fibroblasts from the fibrotic skin of a patient with scleredema showed enhanced collagen production and elevated type 1 procollagen messenger RNA levels in the cultured fibroblasts.[70]

Histopathology[56,68]

The epidermis is usually unaffected except for some effacement of the rete ridge pattern, and occasionally mild basal hyperpigmentation.[79] There is thickening of the reticular dermis, with collagen extending also into the subcutis. The collagen fibres are swollen and separated from one another. The extent of this separation, which mirrors the amount of interstitial mucopolysac-

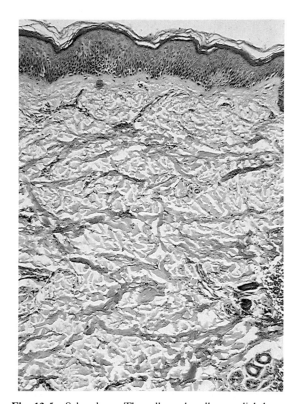

Fig. 13.5 Scleredema. The collagen bundles are slightly swollen and separated from one another. Cellularity of the dermis is normal with no increase in fibroblasts.
Haematoxylin — eosin

charide present, depends on the stage of the disease (Fig. 13.5). This material may only be present in noticeable amounts at the onset of the disease.[61] Sometimes it is most prominent in the lower dermis.[80] Cetylpyridinium has been proposed as a superior fixative to formalin for the preservation of the interstitial mucopolysaccharides.[58] These may subsequently be stained with alcian blue or toluidine blue (pH 5.0 or 7.0), or with colloidal iron. Cryostat sections of unfixed material usually result in the optimal preservation of the interstitial hyaluronic acid.

Other features of scleredema include preservation of the appendages and an increase in mast cells.[81] Other inflammatory cells are sparse. Elastic fibres are reduced and may be fragmented.[79]

The acellular fibrosis of the dermis in scleredema contrasts with the marked fibroblastic proliferation seen in scleromyxoedema, and the patchy deep inflammatory cell infiltrate seen at the advancing edge of plaques of morphoea.

Electron microscopy. This shows thickened collagen fibres with widening of the interfibrillar spaces.[68] The fibroblasts have prominent rough endoplasmic reticulum.[68]

FOCAL MUCINOSIS

Focal mucinosis usually presents as a solitary, asymptomatic, flesh-coloured papule or nodule on the face, trunk or proximal and mid extremities of adults.[82-85] The nodules average 1 cm in diameter. There has been a report of multiple nodules localized to a 'palm-wide area' of the right leg,[86] and also a report of multiple lesions in a patient with hypothyroidism, which responded to thyroxine.[35]

It is thought that increased amounts of hyaluronic acid are produced by fibroblasts at the expense of the connective tissue elements.[82]

Histopathology[82]

There is a slightly elevated or dome-shaped dermal nodule with separation and variable replacement of collagen bundles by mucinous

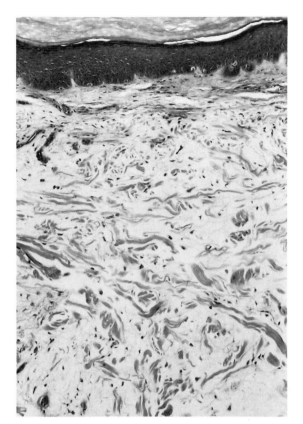

Fig. 13.6 Focal mucinosis. There is a 'pool' of mucin dispersed through the upper dermis. Admixed collagen bundles are thinner than usual.
Haematoxylin — eosin

deposits (Fig. 13.6). These may be localized to the upper dermis or extend through the full thickness of the dermis. Slit-like spaces occasionally develop. The margins of the mucinous deposition are not sharply demarcated. Spindle-shaped fibroblasts are present within the mucinous areas, and there may be an increase in small blood vessels. The appearances resemble the early stages of a digital mucous cyst (see below) and an individual lesion of papular mucinosis. The material stains with colloidal iron and alcian blue at pH 2.5 and is metachromatic with toluidine blue at pH 3.0.

Electron microscopy. The fibroblasts have a well-developed rough endoplasmic reticulum. In addition, there are large macrophages, and granular and amorphous material representing the mucinous deposits.[86]

DIGITAL MUCOUS (MYXOID) CYST

These occur as solitary, dome-shaped, shiny, tense cystic nodules on the dorsum of the fingers, usually overlying the distal interphalangeal joint but sometimes involving the base of the nail.[87] The toes are uncommonly involved. The cysts are found in the middle-aged or elderly and there is a slight female preponderance. Their origin has been controversial, but injection studies have demonstrated a connection with the underlying joint cavity.[88]

Histopathology[89]

There may be a dermal cavity devoid of an epithelial lining, with a loose connective tissue wall showing areas of myxoid change (pseudo-cyst) (Fig. 13.7). Sometimes the wall is composed of more dense connective tissue. A more frequent variant is a large myxoid area containing stellate fibroblasts, sometimes with microcystic spaces. This form resembles that seen in cutaneous myxoma (focal mucinosis). The overlying epidermis may be thinned by the expanding subepidermal collection of mucus. There may be large, thick-walled blood vessels at the base of the lesion. The mucin stains with the colloidal iron stain, as well as with alcian blue at pH 2.5, and it is digested by hyaluronidase.[89]

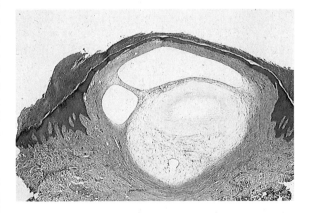

Fig. 13.7 Digital mucous cyst. The accumulation of mucin has resulted in a subepidermal pseudocyst.
Haematoxylin — eosin

MUCOCELE OF THE LIP

Mucoceles (mucous cysts) result from the rupture of a duct of a minor salivary gland with extravasation of mucus into the submucosal tissues, most commonly of the lower lip.[90] They may also develop in the buccal mucosa or tongue. They are found mostly in young adults.

Mucoceles are translucent, whitish or bluish nodules with a firm cystic consistency and varying in size up to 1 cm in diameter. They occasionally rupture spontaneously or after minor trauma.

A superficial variant of mucocele, which results in vesicular lesions that may be mistaken for mucous membrane pemphigoid, has been reported.[91] They may be single or multiple, and they arise on non-inflamed mucosa.

Histopathology

Two patterns may be seen, but there may be some overlap between the two.[90] In one, there is a cystic space with a surrounding poorly defined lining of macrophages, fibroblasts and capillaries with variable amounts of connective tissue. In the other pattern, there is granulation and fibrous tissue containing mucin-filled spaces with variable numbers of muciphages (Fig. 13.8). Small cystic spaces may be present. Numerous neutrophils and some eosinophils are present in the cystic spaces or stroma of both types. There

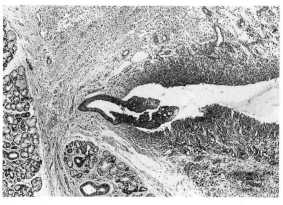

Fig. 13.8   Mucocele. A duct leads into a pseudocyst lined by granulation tissue and muciphages.
Haematoxylin — eosin

is no epithelial lining to the cyst, although occasionally a ruptured salivary duct may be seen at one edge of the cyst. Minor salivary gland tissue is present in the adjacent connective tissue.

The mucin is strongly PAS positive and diastase resistant, and is positive with alcian blue at pH 2.5 and with colloidal iron.

Superficial mucoceles are subepithelial although there may be partial or complete epithelial regeneration across the vesicle floor. They contain sialomucin. Salivary gland ducts are present in the immediate vicinity of the lesions and are a clue to the diagnosis.[91]

CUTANEOUS MYXOMA

Cutaneous myxomas have been reported in approximately 50% of the patients with the complex of cardiac myxomas, spotty pigmentation (lentigines and blue naevi), and endocrine overactivity.[92,93] The cutaneous myxomas may be the earliest manifestation of the syndrome. Similar cases have been reported as the NAME or LAMB syndrome (see Ch. 32, p. 778).

Solitary myxomas, unassociated with any systemic abnormalities, may also occur.[94,95] They are benign neoplasms, but they are included here because of their prominent stromal mucin.

Histopathology

The tumours are sharply circumscribed, non-encapsulated lesions which may be in the dermis or subcutis. They are composed of a prominent mucinous matrix containing variably shaped fibroblasts, prominent capillaries, mast cells and a few collagen and reticulin fibres (Fig. 13.9). Sometimes an epithelial component is present and this may take the form of a keratinous cyst or of epithelial strands with trichoblastic features. The lesions differ from focal mucinosis by their vascularity. Nerve sheath myxomas are more cellular, often with a distinct patterned arrangement.

The designation fibromyxoma has been applied to the lesions in a patient with multiple cutaneous tumours, resembling dermatofibromas clinically,

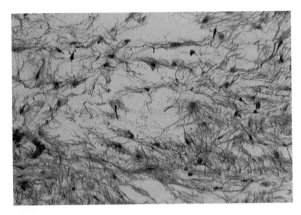

Fig. 13.9   Myxoma. There are thin collagen bundles and fibroblasts scattered through a mucinous matrix. Haematoxylin — eosin

but containing more fibroblasts than the usual cutaneous myxomas and some histiocytes, in addition to the interstitial mucin.[96] Familial myxovascular fibroma is a morphologically-related entity (see p. 876).

CUTANEOUS MUCINOSIS OF INFANCY

There have been two reports of infants presenting with multiple, small, papular lesions on the upper extremities.[97,98] There was abundant mucin in the papillary dermis, no significant increase in fibroblasts, and a few chronic inflammatory cells in a perivascular distribution.

SELF-HEALING JUVENILE CUTANEOUS MUCINOSIS

There have been several reports of a cutaneous mucinosis characterized by the rapid onset in childhood of infiltrated plaques on the head and torso, and deep nodules on the face and periarticular region with spontaneous resolution in weeks or months.[99,100] A viral aetiology, possibly involving fibroblasts, has been postulated. There was abundant mucin with a mild increase in fibroblasts and mast cells. Hyaluronic acid was the predominant mucin in one report,[100] and sialomucins in another.[99]

SECONDARY DERMAL MUCINOSES

Mucin deposited may be in a wide variety of connective tissue diseases and in some tumours. These include dermatomyositis, lupus erythematosus (see below), scleroderma, hypertrophic scars, connective tissue naevi, granuloma annulare, malignant atrophic papulosis (Degos' disease), erythema annulare centrifugum, and Jessner's lymphocytic infiltrate.[3,4] It is sometimes present in large amounts around the secretory coils of the eccrine glands of the lower leg when sweat excretion is blocked.[4] Tumours containing mucin include neurofibromas, neurilemmomas, nerve sheath myxomas, chondroid syringomas and some basal cell carcinomas.

A diffuse dermal mucinosis can be found occasionally in biopsies of lesional skin from patients with discoid and systemic lupus erythematosus (SLE).[101,102] Rarely, patients with SLE can present with papulonodules due to a diffuse mucinous deposition in the skin.[102,103] In these individuals, the deposition occurs in areas free from specific lesions of lupus erythematosus, and it produces clinically distinct manifestations.

FOLLICULAR MUCINOSES

Follicular mucinosis is a tissue reaction pattern in which hair follicles and the attached sebaceous glands accumulate mucin with some dissolution of cellular attachments (Fig. 13.10).[2] There is an accompanying perifollicular and perivascular inflammatory cell infiltrate of lymphocytes, histiocytes, and a few eosinophils. Sometimes follicles are converted into cystic cavities with disruption of much of the external root sheath. These cysts contain mucin, inflammatory cells and keratinous debris. There is often marked disparity between the amount of follicular mucin and the degree of follicular and perifollicular inflammation.[104] The material is stained by the alcian blue and colloidal iron methods.

The concept that follicular mucinosis is a

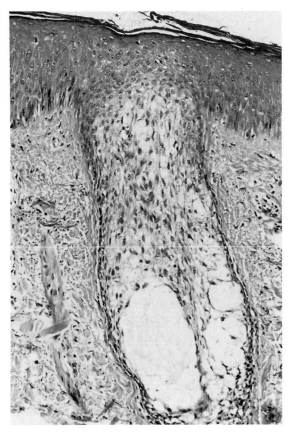

Fig. 13.10 Follicular mucinosis. The accumulation of mucin within the hair follicle has resulted in the dissolution of many cellular attachments. Haematoxylin — eosin

tissue reaction pattern and not a disease sui generis is a relatively recent one[2] and, as a consequence, most reports in the literature use the term follicular mucinosis for what Pinkus described as alopecia mucinosa in 1957.[105] In the discussion which follows, the term follicular mucinosis will be used for the histopathological pattern, and alopecia mucinosa for the idiopathic dermatosis which is the prototype for this reaction pattern.

ALOPECIA MUCINOSA

Alopecia mucinosa (follicular mucinosis) is an uncommon inflammatory dermatosis with a predilection for adults in the third and fourth decades of life.[106] Three clinical types have traditionally been recognized:[107,108] a benign transient form with one or several plaques or grouped follicular papules, usually limited to the face or scalp and with accompanying alopecia;[109,110] a more widely distributed form with follicular papules, plaques and nodules on the extremities, face and trunk and a course often exceeding two years; and a third group, accounting for 15–30% of cases, with widespread lesions and associated with malignant lymphoma of the skin or mycosis fungoides.[111-113] Rarely, patients with leukaemia cutis,[114] Hodgkin's disease,[115] familial reticuloendotheliosis,[116] Sézary syndrome,[117,118] and angiolymphoid hyperplasia[119,120] have also had this presentation. This third group was regarded by Hempstead and Ackerman[2] as belonging to the group of secondary follicular mucinoses, because of the lack, at that time, of convincing examples of alopecia mucinosa progressing to mycosis fungoides or cutaneous lymphoma.[121,122] However, cases of alopecia mucinosa progressing to mycosis fungoides have since been well documented.[123,124]

The protean clinical presentations attributed to alopecia mucinosa, such as eczematous,[125] annular, pityriasis-rosea-like,[126] and folliculitis, are in many cases examples of specific dermatoses in which secondary follicular mucinosis is present.

Although it has been postulated that follicular keratinocytes are the source of the mucopolysaccharides,[2,127] this has not been confirmed in a recent study, which proposed a role for cell-mediated immune mechanisms in the aetiology.[122]

Histopathology[108,128,129]

The major changes are those described above for follicular mucinosis (Fig. 13.11). However, the inflammatory cell infiltrate is predominantly follicular, perifollicular and perivascular in location, in contrast to the follicular mucinosis secondary to lymphomas where the infiltrate is more dispersed, often heavier and nodular, and sometimes has more plasma cells and fewer eosinophils than in alopecia mucinosa.[104,130] Furthermore, there is usually a milder mucinous

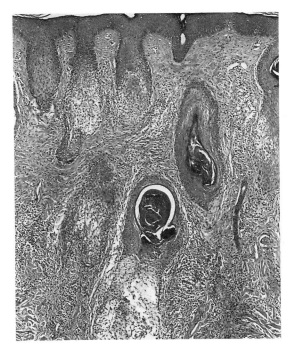

Fig. 13.11   Alopecia mucinosa. Multiple follicles show the reaction pattern of follicular mucinosis.
Haematoxylin — eosin

change in follicular mucinosis secondary to lymphomas than in alopecia mucinosa.[130] Atypical cells and Pautrier microabscesses are not seen in alopecia mucinosa,[104] but may be present in secondary follicular mucinosis with accompanying lymphoma or mycosis fungoides. Rarely, dermal mucinosis[115,131] or a proliferation of eccrine sweat duct epithelium is present.[132]

Electron microscopy. This shows disattached keratinocytes closely opposed to significant numbers of macrophages and Langerhans cells.[122] Some degeneration of keratinocytes has also been noted.[127,133] Fine granular and flocculent material is present between the keratinocytes.

SECONDARY FOLLICULAR MUCINOSES

Follicular mucinosis may be found as an incidental phenomenon in rare cases of lichen simplex chronicus, hypertrophic lichen planus,

discoid lupus erythematosus, acne vulgaris, pseudolymphoma, naevocellular naevi[134] and arthropod bite reactions.[2] The superficial follicular spongiosis seen in some cases of atopic dermatitis, Grover's disease and actinic prurigo,[135] as well as in infundibulofolliculitis, may contain small amounts of mucin.[136]

More controversial is the classification of those cases of follicular mucinosis associated with leukaemia cutis and malignant lymphoma, including mucosis fungoides. Although Hempstead and Ackerman have stated categorically that they do not think 'that alopecia mucinosa is related to any malignant lymphoma or ever eventuates in a malignant lymphoma',[2] most articles on the subject still include the lymphoma-related cases as a subgroup of alopecia mucinosa.[107,110] The very presence of prominent follicular mucin deposits is going to produce clinical lesions with some resemblance to alopecia mucinosa, so this factor should not be used in any argument for their retention as a clinical subgroup of alopecia mucinosa.

PERIFOLLICULAR MUCINOSIS

There is one report of an adolescent male who developed two plaques on the face, characterized by prominent perifollicular mucin. The lesions were regarded as being of naevoid origin.[137]

EPITHELIAL MUCINOSES

Small foci of intercellular mucin are an inconstant and incidental finding in some spongiotic dermatoses, as well as in verrucae, seborrhoeic keratoses, basal cell and squamous cell carcinomas and keratoacanthomas.[2] Epidermal mucin is sometimes a conspicuous feature in mycosis fungoides (see p. 1035).

MUCOPOLYSACCHARIDOSES

The mucopolysaccharidoses are a group of ten lysosomal storage diseases which result from the deficiency of specific lysosomal enzymes involved in the degradation of dermatan sulphate, heparan sulphate or keratan sulphate, singly or in combination.[138–140] As a consequence, mucopolysaccharides accumulate in various tissues and are excreted in the urine.[141] Because of genetic variability, heterogeneity and pleiotropism, more than ten clinical syndromes are associated with the ten enzyme deficiencies.[138]

The specific enzyme defect can be identified using cultured fibroblasts, although in many instances a tentative diagnosis is possible on the clinical features alone. Analysis of the urine for certain mucopolysaccharides will also assist in the diagnosis. The urine contains heparan sulphate in the Sanfilippo syndrome (MPS III), keratan sulphate in the Morquio syndrome (MPS IV), dermatan sulphate in the Maroteaux–Lamy syndrome (MPS VI), and an excess of dermatan and heparan sulphates in varying ratios in the others.

The mucopolysaccharidoses share many clinical features.[138] These include skeletal abnormalities characterized as dysostosis multiplex (except in Morquio's syndrome), short stature (excluding Scheie's syndrome — MPS IS), corneal clouding (except in the Hunter — MPS II and Sanfilippo — MPS III syndromes), deafness, grotesque facies (gargoylism), hirsutism, premature arteriosclerosis, hepatosplenomegaly and severe mental retardation (excluding MPS VI and MPS IS).[138] The best known of the mucopolysaccharidoses are Hurler's syndrome (MPS I), which has the worst prognosis and is due to a deficiency of α-L-iduronidase, and Hunter's syndrome (MPS II), which results from a deficiency of iduronate-2-sulphate sulphatase.

Cutaneous manifestations of the mucopolysaccharidoses include hirsutism and dryness of the skin. There may be mild thickening also, and this is most marked in Hurler's syndrome where sclerodermoid thickening of the fingers and furrowing of the skin can occur.[142,143] Firm, flesh-coloured to waxy papules and nodules can be found on the upper trunk, particularly in the scapular region, in Hunter's syndrome.[144,145]

Histopathology

Metachromatic granules are present in the cytoplasm of fibroblasts in all cases, and sometimes in eccrine sweat glands and epidermal keratinocytes.[142] Extracellular mucin of any significant amount is only found in the mid and lower dermis in the papulonodules of Hunter's syndrome.[144] The mucin is best seen in toluidine blue stained sections of alcohol-fixed material, but it can also be demonstrated with the Giemsa and colloidal iron stains.[144] The fibroblasts are slightly more prominent than usual with an oval nucleus and a definable cytoplasmic outline, but these changes are quite subtle.

Electron microscopy. The ultrastructural features are characteristic, with multiple membrane-bound vacuoles, containing some amorphous and granular material, within the cytoplasm of fibroblasts.[146,147] These are also present, to a variable extent, in endothelial cells, Schwann cells,[146] mononuclear cells[148] and eccrine glands.[149] Lamellar inclusions are sometimes observed, particularly in Schwann cells.[150,151] A single large vacuole, indenting the nucleus of keratinocytes, has been seen in some cases.[152] Vacuoles may develop in some cells as an artefact of fixation and these should not be misinterpreted as features of a mucopolysaccharidosis.[153]

REFERENCES

Introduction

1. Reed RJ, Clark WH, Mihm MC. The cutaneous mucinoses. Hum Pathol 1973; 4: 201–205.
2. Hempstead RW, Ackerman AB. Follicular mucinosis. A reaction pattern in follicular epithelium. Am J Dermatopathol 1985; 7: 245–257.
3. Truhan AP, Roenigk HH. The cutaneous mucinoses. J Am Acad Dermatol 1986; 14: 1–18.
4. Steigleder GK, Kuchmeister B. Cutaneous mucinous deposits. J Cutan Pathol 1985; 12: 334–347.
5. Matsuoka LY, Wortsman J, Dietrich JG, Kupchella CE. Glycosaminoglycans in histologic sections. Arch Dermatol 1987; 123: 862.

Dermal mucinoses

6. Christianson HB. Cutaneous manifestations of hypothyroidism including purpura and ecchymoses. Cutis 1976; 17: 45–52.

7. Warin AP. Eczéma craquelé as the presenting feature of myxoedema. Br J Dermatol 1973; 89: 289–291.

7a. Good JM, Neill SM, Rowland Payne CME, Staughton RCD. Keratoderma of myxoedema. Clin Exp Dermatol 1988; 13: 339–341.

8. Matsuoka LY, Wortsman J, Carlisle KS et al. The acquired cutaneous mucinoses. Arch Intern Med 1984; 144: 1974–1980.

9. Stewart G, Kinmonth JB, Browse NL. Pretibial myxoedema. Ann R Coll Surg Engl 1984; 66: 391–395.

10. Lynch PJ, Maize JC, Sisson JC. Pretibial myxedema and nonthyrotoxic thyroid disease. Arch Dermatol 1973; 107: 107–111.

11. Noppakun N, Bancheun K, Chandraprasert S. Unusual locations of localized myxedema in Graves' disease. Arch Dermatol 1986; 122: 85–88.

12. Slater DN. Cervical nodular localized myxoedema in a thyroidectomy scar: light and electron microscopy and histochemical findings. Clin Exp Dermatol 1987; 12: 216–219.

12a. Wright AL, Buxton PK, Menzies D. Pretibial myxedema localized to scar tissue. Int J Dermatol 1990; 29: 54–55.

13. Yeo PPB, Cheah JS, Sinniah R. Pretibial myxoedema: a clinical and pathological study. Aust NZ J Med 1978; 8: 60–62.

14. Jolliffe DS, Gaylarde PM, Brock AP, Sarkany I. Pretibial myxoedema: stimulation of mucopolysaccharide production of fibroblasts by serum. Br J Dermatol 1979; 100: 557–560.

15. Cheung HS, Nicoloff JT, Kamiel MB et al. Stimulation of fibroblast biosynthetic activity by serum of patients with pretibial myxedema. J Invest Dermatol 1978; 71: 12–17.

16. Matsuoka LY, Wortsman J, Uitto J et al. Altered skin elastic fibres in hypothyroid myxedema and pretibial myxedema. Arch Intern Med 1985; 145: 117–121.

17. Kobayasi T, Danielsen L, Asboe-Hansen G. Ultrastructure of localized myxedema. Acta Derm Venereol 1976; 56: 173–185.

18. Konrad K, Brenner W, Pehamberger H. Ultrastructural and immunological findings in Graves' disease with pretibial myxedema. J Cutan Pathol 1980; 7: 99–108.

19. Hill TG, Crawford JN, Rogers CC. Successful management of lichen myxedematosus. Arch Dermatol 1976; 112: 67–69.

20. Chanda JJ. Scleromyxedema. Cutis 1979; 24: 549–552.

21. Farmer ER, Hambrick GW, Shulman LE. Papular mucinosis. A clinicopathologic study of four patients. Arch Dermatol 1982; 118: 9–13.

22. Flowers SL, Cooper PH, Landes HB. Acral persistent papular mucinosis. J Am Acad Dermatol 1989; 21: 293–297.

22a. Crovato F, Nazzari G, Desirello G. Acral persistent papular mucinosis. J Am Acad Dermatol 1990; 23: 121–122.

23. Milam CP, Cohen LE, Fenske NA, Ling NS. Scleromyxedema: Therapeutic response to isotretinoin in three patients. J Am Acad Dermatol 1988; 19: 469–477.

24. Harris AO, Altman AR, Tschen JA, Wolf JE Jr. Scleromyxedema. Int J Dermatol 1989; 28: 661–667.

25. Penmetcha M, Highet AS, Hopkinson JM. Failure of PUVA in lichen myxoedematosus: acceleration of associated multiple keratoacanthomas with development of squamous carcinoma. Clin Exp Dermatol 1987; 12: 220–223.

26. Howsden SM, Herndon JH, Freeman RG. Lichen myxedematosus. Dermal infiltrative disorder responsive to cyclophosphamide therapy. Arch Dermatol 1975; 111: 1325–1330.

27. Lang E, Zabel M, Schmidt H. Skleromyxödem Arndt-Gottron und assoziierte Phänomene. Dermatologica 1984; 169: 29–35.

28. Kantor GR, Bergfeld WF, Katzin WE et al. Scleromyxedema associated with scleroderma renal disease and acute psychosis. J Am Acad Dermatol 1986; 14: 879–888.

29. Wright RC, Franco RS, Denton MD, Blaney DJ. Scleromyxedema. Arch Dermatol 1976; 112: 63–66.

30. Rudner EJ, Mehregan A, Pinkus H. Scleromyxedema. A variant of lichen myxedematosus. Arch Dermatol 1966; 93: 3–12.

31. Jepsen LV. Two cases of scleromyxedema. Acta Derm Venereol 1980; 60: 77–79.

32. Lowe NJ, Dufton PA, Hunter RD, Vickers CFH. Electron-beam treatment of scleromyxoedema. Br J Dermatol 1982; 106: 449–454.

33. Alligood TR, Burnett JW, Raines BL. Scleromyxedema associated with esophageal aperistalsis and dermal eosinophilia. Cutis 1981; 28: 60–66.

34. Hardie RA, Hunter JAA, Urbaniak S, Habeshaw JA. Spontaneous resolution of lichen myxoedematosus. Br J Dermatol 1979; 100: 727–730.

35. Jakubovic HR, Salama SSS, Rosenthal D. Multiple cutaneous focal mucinoses with hypothyroidism. Ann Intern Med 1982; 96: 56–58.

36. Archibald GC, Calvert HT. Hypothyroidism and lichen myxedematosus. Arch Dermatol 1977; 113: 684.

37. Bergfeld WF, Lobur D, Cathcart M. Fibroblast studies in scleromyxedema: Cellular proliferation and glycosaminoglycan metabolism. Arch Dermatol 1984; 120: 1609 (abstract).

38. Westheim AI, Lookingbill DP. Plasmapheresis in a patient with scleromyxedema. Arch Dermatol 1987; 123: 786–789.

39. Lai A Fat RFM, Suurmond D, Radl J, van Furth R. Scleromyxoedema (lichen myxoedematosus) associated with a paraprotein IgG$_1$ of type kappa. Br J Dermatol 1973; 88: 107–116.

40. Perry HO, Montgomery H, Stickney JM. Further observations on lichen myxedematosus. Ann Intern Med 1960; 53: 955–969.

41. Abd El-Ad H, Salem SS, Salem A. Lichen myxedematosus: histochemical study. Dermatologica 1981; 162: 273–276.

42. Ishii M, Furukawa M, Okada M, Hamada T. The use of improved ruthenium red staining for the ultrastructural detection of proteoglycan aggregates in normal skin and Lichen myxoedematosus. J Cutan Pathol 1984; 11: 292–295.

43. Coskey RJ, Mehregan A. Papular mucinosis. Int J Dermatol 1977; 16: 741–744.

44. Perry HO, Kierland RR, Montgomery H. Plaque-like form of cutaneous mucinosis. Arch Dermatol 1960; 82: 980–985.
45. Steigleder GK, Gartmann H, Linker U. REM syndrome: reticular erythematous mucinosis (round-cell erythematosis), a new entity? Br J Dermatol 1974; 91: 191–199.
46. Quimby SR, Perry HO. Plaquelike cutaneous mucinosis: Its relationship to reticular erythematous mucinosis. J Am Acad Dermatol 1982; 6: 856–861.
47. Kocsard E, Munro VF. Reticular erythematous mucinosis (REM syndrome) of Steigleder: its relationship to other mucinoses and to chronic erythemata. Aust J Dermatol 1978; 19: 121–124.
47a. Cohen PR, Rabinowitz AD, Ruszkowski AM, DeLeo VA. Reticular erythematous mucinosis syndrome: review of the world literature and report of the syndrome in a prepubertal child. Pediatr Dermatol 1990; 7: 1–10.
48. Braddock SW, Davis CS, Davis RB. Reticular erythematous mucinosis and thrombocytopenic purpura. Report of a case and review of the world literature, including plaquelike cutaneous mucinosis. J Am Acad Dermatol 1988; 19: 859–868.
49. Morison WL, Shea CR, Parrish JA. Reticular erythematous mucinosis syndrome. Arch Dermatol 1979; 115: 1340–1342.
50. Keczkes K, Jadhav P. REM syndrome (reticular erythematous mucinosis). Report of a further case or variant of it. Arch Dermatol 1977; 113: 335–338.
51. Bleehen SS, Slater DN, Mahood J, Church RE. Reticular erythematous mucinosis: light and electron microscopy, immunofluorescence and histochemical findings. Br J Dermatol 1982; 106: 9–18.
52. Smith NP, Sanderson KV, Crow KD. Reticular erythematous mucinosis syndrome. Clin Exp Dermatol 1976; 1: 99–103.
53. Vanuytrecht-Henderickx D, Dewolf-Peeters C, Degreef H. Morphological study of the reticular erythematous mucinosis syndrome. Dermatologica 1984; 168: 163–169.
54. Chavaz P, Polla L, Saurat JH. Paramyxovirus-like inclusions and lymphocyte type in the REM syndrome. Br J Dermatol 1982; 106: 741.
55. Dodd HJ, Sarkany I, Sadrudin A. Reticular erythematous mucinosis syndrome. Clin Exp Dermatol 1987; 12: 36–39.
56. Carrington PR, Sanusi ID, Winder PR et al. Scleredema adultorum. Int J Dermatol 1984; 23: 514–522.
57. Burke MJ, Seguin J, Bove KE. Scleredema: An unusual presentation with edema limited to scalp, upper face, and orbits. J Pediatr 1982; 101: 960–963.
58. Heilbron B, Saxe N. Scleredema in an infant. Arch Dermatol 1986; 122: 1417–1419.
59. Greenberg LM, Geppert C, Worthen HG, Good RA. Scleredema "adultorum" in children. Pediatrics 1963; 32: 1044–1054.
60. Graff R. Scleredema adultorum (discussion). Arch Dermatol 1968; 98: 320.
61. Venencie PY, Powell FC, Su WPD, Perry HO. Scleredema: a review of thirty-three cases. J Am Acad Dermatol 1984; 11: 128–134.
62. Curtis AC, Shulak BM. Scleredema adultorum. Arch Dermatol 1965; 92: 526–541.
63. Krakowski A, Covo J, Berlin C. Diabetic scleredema. Dermatologica 1973; 146: 193–198.
64. Cohn BA, Wheeler CE, Briggaman RA. Scleredema adultorum of Buschke and diabetes mellitus. Arch Dermatol 1970; 101: 27–35.
65. Parker SC, Fenton DA, Black MM. Scleredema. Clin Exp Dermatol 1989; 14: 385–386.
66. Fleischmajer R, Faludi G, Krol S. Scleredema and diabetes mellitus. Arch Dermatol 1970; 101: 21–26.
67. McNaughton F, Keczkes K. Scleredema adultorum and diabetes mellitus (scleredema diutinum). Clin Exp Dermatol 1983; 8: 41–45.
68. Ohta A, Uitto J, Oikarinen AI et al. Paraproteinemia in patients with scleredema. Clinical findings and serum effects on skin fibroblasts in vitro. J Am Acad Dermatol 1987; 16: 96–107.
69. Pajarre S. Scleroedema adultorum Buschke. Acta Derm Venereol 1975; 55: 158–159.
70. Oikarinen A, Ala-Kokko L, Palatsi R et al. Scleredema and paraproteinemia. Arch Dermatol 1987; 123: 226–229.
71. McFadden N, Ree K, Soyland E, Larsen TE. Scleredema adultorum associated with a monoclonal gammopathy and generalized hyperpigmentation. Arch Dermatol 1987; 123: 629–632.
72. Hodak E, Tamir R, David M et al. Scleredema adultorum associated with IgG-kappa multiple myeloma — a case report and review of the literature. Clin Exp Dermatol 1988; 13: 271–274.
73. Salisbury JA, Shallcross H, Leigh IM. Scleredema of Buschke associated with multiple myeloma. Clin Exp Dermatol 1988; 13: 269–270.
74. Miyagawa S, Dohi K, Tsuruta S, Shirai T. Scleredema of Buschke associated with rheumatoid arthritis and Sjögren's syndrome. Br J Dermatol 1989; 121: 517–520.
75. Rees R, Moore A, Nanney L, King L. Scleredema adultorum: The surgical implications of a rare dermatologic disorder. Plast Reconstr Surg 1983; 72: 90–93.
76. Verghese A, Noble J, Diamond RD. Scleredema adultorum. A case of the recurrent cellulitis syndrome. Arch Dermatol 1984; 120: 1518–1519.
77. Millns JL, Fenske NA. Scleredema and persistent erythema. Arch Dermatol 1982; 118: 290–291.
78. Fleischmajer R, Perlish JS. Glycosaminoglycans in scleroderma and scleredema. J Invest Dermatol 1972; 58: 129–132.
79. Holubar K, Mach KW. Scleredema (Buschke). Histological and histochemical investigations. Acta Derm Venereol 1967; 47: 102–110.
80. Roupe G, Laurent TC, Malmstrom A et al. Biochemical characterization and tissue distribution of the scleredema in a case of Buschke's disease. Acta Derm Venereol 1987; 67: 193–198.
81. Fleischmajer R, Lara JV. Scleredema. A histochemical and biochemical study. Arch Dermatol 1965; 92: 643–652.
82. Johnson WC, Helwig EB. Cutaneous focal mucinosis. Arch Dermatol 1966; 93: 13–20.
83. Hazelrigg DE. Cutaneous focal mucinosis. Cutis 1974; 14: 241–242.
84. Decroix J, Guilmot-Bruneau MM, Defresne C. Myxome cutané ou mucinose focale cutanée. Dermatologica 1981; 162: 368–371.
85. Nishiura S, Mihara M, Shimao S et al. Cutaneous focal mucinosis. Br J Dermatol 1989; 121: 511–515.
86. Suhonen R, Niemi K-M. Cutaneous focal mucinosis

with spontaneous healing. J Cutan Pathol 1983; 10: 334–339.

87. Armijo M. Mucoid cysts of the fingers. J Dermatol Surg Oncol 1981; 7: 317–322.
88. Epstein E. A simple technique for managing digital mucous cysts. Arch Dermatol 1979; 115: 1315–1316.
89. Johnson WC, Graham JH, Helwig EB. Cutaneous myxoid cyst. JAMA 1965; 191: 109–114.
90. Lattanand A, Johnson WC, Graham JH. Mucous cyst (mucocele). Arch Dermatol 1970; 101: 673–678.
91. Jensen JL. Superficial mucoceles of the oral mucosa. Am J Dermatopathol 1990; 12: 88–92.
92. Carney JA, Gordon H, Carpenter PC et al. The complex of myxomas, spotty pigmentation, and endocrine overactivity. Medicine (Baltimore) 1985; 64: 270–283.
93. Carney JA, Headington JT, Su WPD. Cutaneous myxomas. Arch Dermatol 1986; 122: 790–798.
94. Sanusi ID. Subungual myxoma. Arch Dermatol 1982; 118: 612–614.
95. Allen PW, Dymock RB, MacCormac LB. Superficial angiomyxomas with and without epithelial components. Report of 30 tumors in 28 patients. Am J Surg Pathol 1988; 12: 519–530.
96. Zina AM, Bundino S. Multiple cutaneous fibromyxomas: a light and electron microscopic study. J Cutan Pathol 1980; 7: 335–341.
97. Lum D. Cutaneous mucinosis of infancy. Arch Dermatol 1980; 116: 198–200.
98. McGrae JD. Cutaneous mucinosis of infancy. A congenital and linear variant. Arch Dermatol 1983; 119: 272–273.
99. Bonerandi JJ, Andrac L, Follana J et al. Mucinose cutanée juvénile spontanément résolutive. Ann Dermatol Venereol 1980; 107: 51–57.
100. Pucevich MV, Latour DL, Bale GF, King LE. Self-healing juvenile cutaneous mucinosis. J Am Acad Dermatol 1984; 11: 327–332.
101. Weigand DA, Burgdorf WHC, Gregg LJ. Dermal mucinosis in discoid lupus erythematosus. Report of two cases. Arch Dermatol 1981; 117: 735–738.
102. Rongioletti F, Rebora A. Papular and nodular mucinosis associated with systemic lupus erythematosus. Br J Dermatol 1986; 115: 631–636.
103. Gammon WR, Caro I, Long JC, Wheeler CE. Secondary cutaneous mucinosis with systemic lupus erythematosus. Arch Dermatol 1978; 114: 432–435.

Follicular mucinoses

104. Nickoloff BJ, Wood C. Benign idiopathic versus mycosis-fungoides-associated follicular mucinosis. Pediatr Dermatol 1985; 2: 201–206.
105. Pinkus H. Alopecia mucinosa. Arch Dermatol 1957; 76: 419–426.
106. Gibson LE, Muller SA, Peters MS. Follicular mucinosis of childhood and adolescence. Pediatr Dermatol 1988; 5: 231–235.
107. Coskey RJ, Mehregan AH. Alopecia mucinosa. A follow-up study. Arch Dermatol 1970; 102: 193–194.
108. Emmerson RW. Follicular mucinosis. A study of 47 patients. Br J Dermatol 1969; 81: 395–413.
109. Locker E, Duncan WC. Hypopigmentation in alopecia mucinosa. Arch Dermatol 1979; 115: 731–733.
110. Snyder RA, Crain WR, McNutt NS. Alopecia mucinosa. Report of a case with diffuse alopecia and normal-appearing scalp skin. Arch Dermatol 1984; 120: 496–498.
111. Binnick AN, Wax FD, Clendenning WE. Alopecia mucinosa of the face associated with mycosis fungoides. Arch Dermatol 1978; 114: 791–792.
112. Plotnick H, Abbrecht M. Alopecia mucinosa and lymphoma. Report of two cases and review of literature. Arch Dermatol 1965; 92: 137–141.
113. Wilkinson JD, Black MM, Chu A. Follicular mucinosis associated with mycosis fungoides presenting with gross cystic changes on the face. Clin Exp Dermatol 1982; 7: 333–340.
114. Thomson J, Cochran REI. Chronic lymphatic leukemia presenting as atypical rosacea with follicular mucinosis. J Cutan Pathol 1978; 5: 81–87.
115. Stankler L, Ewen SWB. Hodgkin's disease in a patient with follicular and dermal mucinosis and spontaneous ooze of mucin (mucinorrhoea). Br J Dermatol 1975; 93: 581–586.
116. Freeman RG. Familial reticuloendotheliosis with eosinophilia and follicular mucinosis. Arch Dermatol 1972; 105: 737–738.
117. Fairris GM, Kirkham N, Goodwin PG et al. Erythrodermic follicular mucinosis. Clin Exp Dermatol 1987; 12: 50–52.
118. Rivers JK, Norris PG, Greaves MW, Smith NP. Follicular mucinosis in association with Sézary syndrome. Clin Exp Dermatol 1987; 12: 207–210.
119. Wolff HH, Kinney J, Ackerman AB. Angiolymphoid hyperplasia with follicular mucinosis. Arch Dermatol 1978; 114: 229–232.
120. Bovet R, Delacrétaz J. Hyperplasie angio-lymphoïde avec mucinose folliculaire. Dermatologica 1979; 158: 343–347.
121. Kim R, Winkelmann RK. Follicular mucinosis (alopecia mucinosa). Arch Dermatol 1962; 85: 490–498.
122. Lancer HA, Bronstein BR, Nakagawa H et al. Follicular mucinosis: A detailed morphologic and immunopathologic study. J Am Acad Dermatol 1984; 10: 760–768.
123. Sentis HJ, Willemze R, Scheffer E. Alopecia mucinosa progressing into mycosis fungoides. A long-term follow-up of two patients. Am J Dermatopathol 1988; 10: 478–486.
124. Gibson LE, Muller SA, Leiferman KM, Peters MS. Follicular mucinosis: Clinical and histopathologic study. J Am Acad Dermatol 1989; 20: 441–446.
125. Rustin MHA, Bunker CB, Levene GM. Follicular mucinosis presenting as acute dermatitis and response to dapsone. Clin Exp Dermatol 1989; 14: 382–384.
126. Kubba RK, Stewart TW. Follicular mucinosis responding to dapsone. Br J Dermatol 1974; 91: 217–220.
127. Ishibashi A. Histogenesis of mucin in follicular mucinosis. An electron microscopic study. Acta Derm Venereol 1976; 56: 163–171.
128. Pinkus H. Commentary: Alopecia mucinosa. Arch Dermatol 1983; 119: 698–699.
129. Haber H. Follicular mucinosis (alopecia mucinosa. Pinkus). Br J Dermatol 1961; 73: 313–322.
130. Logan RA, Headington JT. Follicular mucinosis — a histologic review of 80 cases. J Cutan Pathol 1988; 15: 324 (abstract).

131. Okun MR, Kay F. Follicular mucinosis (alopecia mucinosa). Arch Dermatol 1964; 89: 809–814.
132. Berger TG, Goette DK. Eccrine proliferation with follicular mucinosis. J Cutan Pathol 1987; 14: 188–190.
133. Ishibashi A, Chujo T. Ultrastructure of follicular mucinosis. J Cutan Pathol 1974; 1: 126–131.
134. Jordaan HF. Follicular mucinosis in association with a melanocytic nevus. A report of two cases. J Cutan Pathol 1987; 14: 122–126.
135. Weedon D. Unpublished observation.
136. Nickoloff BJ, Wood C, Farber EM. Follicular spongiosis with intercellular deposition of mucin: observations and speculations. Am J Dermatopathol 1985; 7: 302–303.
137. Becke RFA, Musso LA. An unusual epithelial-connective tissue naevus with perifollicular mucinosis. Australas J Dermatol 1978; 19: 118–120.

Mucopolysaccharidoses

138. McKusick VA, Neufeld EF. In: The metabolic basis of inherited disease, 5th ed. New York: McGraw-Hill, 1983; 751.
139. Gebhart W. Heritable metabolic storage diseases. J Cutan Pathol 1985; 12: 348–357.
140. Fluharty AL. The mucopolysaccharidoses: a synergism between clinical and basic investigation. J Invest Dermatol 1982; 79: 38s–44s.
141. McKusick VA. The nosology of the mucopolysaccharidoses. Am J Med 1969; 47: 730–747.
142. Hambrick GW, Scheie HG. Studies of the skin in Hurler's syndrome. Arch Dermatol 1962; 85: 455–470.
143. Cole HN, Irving RC, Lund HZ et al. Gargoylism with cutaneous manifestations. Arch Dermatol 1952; 66: 371–383.
144. Freeman RG. A pathological basis for the cutaneous papules of mucopolysaccharidosis II (the Hunter syndrome). J Cutan Pathol 1977; 4: 318–328.
145. Prystowsky MD, Maumenee IH, Freeman RG et al. Cutaneous marker in the Hunter syndrome. Arch Dermatol 1977; 113: 602–605.
146. Lasser A, Carter DM, Mahoney MJ. Ultrastructure of the skin in mucopolysaccharidoses. Arch Pathol 1975; 99: 173–176.
147. Bioulac P, Mercier M, Beylot C, Fontan D. The diagnosis of mucopolysaccharidoses by electron microscopy of skin biopsies. J Cutan Pathol 1975; 2: 179–190.
148. Belcher RW. Ultrastructure and cytochemistry of lymphocytes in the genetic mucopolysaccharidoses. Arch Pathol 1972; 93: 1–7.
149. Belcher RW. Ultrastructure and function of eccrine glands in the mucopolysaccharidoses. Arch Pathol 1973; 96: 339–341.
150. O'Brien JS, Bernett J, Veath ML, Paa D. Lysosomal storage disorders: Diagnosis by ultrastructural examination of skin biopsy specimens. Arch Neurol 1975; 32: 592–599.
151. Belcher RW. Ultrastructure of the skin in the genetic mucopolysaccharidoses. Arch Pathol 1972; 94: 511–518.
152. DeCloux RJ, Friederici HHR. Ultrastructural studies of the skin in Hurler's syndrome. Arch Pathol 1969; 88: 350–358.
153. Sipe JC, O'Brien JS. Ultrastructure of skin biopsy specimens: Common sources of error in diagnosis. Clin Genet 1979; 15: 118–125.

14

David Weedon

Cutaneous deposits

INTRODUCTION

Cutaneous deposits are a heterogeneous group of substances which are not normal constituents of the skin. They are laid down, usually in the dermis, in a variety of different circumstances. There are four broad categories of deposits. The first group includes calcium salts, bone and cartilage.[1] The second category includes the hyaline deposits. These have an eosinophilic, somewhat glassy appearance in haematoxylin and eosin preparations. The third category includes various pigments, heavy metals (many of which are deposited in the form of a pigmented salt), and complex drug pigments. The fourth category, cutaneous implants, includes substances such as collagen and silicone which are inserted into the skin for cosmetic purposes.

Deposits which do not fit neatly into any of these four categories include oxalate crystals and fibreglass. Oxalate crystals, which are light yellow to brown in haematoxylin and eosin preparations, are birefringent; they may contain calcium. The crystals are sometimes found in the skin in primary oxalosis and in chronic renal failure with secondary oxalosis.[1a] Fibreglass can be identified in the stratum corneum and sometimes in the epidermis, after contact with this agent.[1b] Fibreglass dermatitis is rarely seen these days.

Some deposits evoke an inflammatory or foreign body reaction, although many of the hyaline and pigment deposits produce no significant response, except for some macrophages in the case of pigments. Hyaline deposits may blend imperceptibly with the surrounding collagen and require special histochemical staining for their positive identification.

CALCIUM, BONE AND CARTILAGE

CALCINOSIS CUTIS

The cutaneous deposition of calcium salts — calcinosis cutis — has historically been divided into a *dystrophic* variety, when the calcium is deposited in damaged or degenerate tissue, and a less common *metastatic* form associated with elevated serum levels of calcium or phosphate or both. In many cases, the pathogenetic mechanism is unknown and these have been assigned to a third *idiopathic* group. The following classification, which is a modification of the historic one, includes several recently described variants.[1]

Subepidermal calcified nodule.[2–3] This entity usually occurs as a solitary nodule on the head or the extremities of infants and young children, but it may develop in an older group of patients in whom it has a predilection for the upper extremities. Subepidermal calcified nodule is one of the idiopathic calcinoses, although it has been suggested that the calcification occurs in a pre-existing naevus or hamartoma. There is no evidence to support this view.

Idiopathic scrotal calcinosis.[4–6] Single or multiple lesions, up to 3 cm or more in diameter, develop in the scrotal skin in children or young adults. They may break down and discharge chalky material. It has been suggested recently that the lesions represent dystrophic calcification of eccrine duct milia[7] or of epidermal cysts.[5a]

Tumoral calcinosis.[8–10] This idiopathic condition consists of massive subcutaneous deposits of calcium salts, often overlying the large joints in otherwise healthy patients. There is a predilection for black races.

Auricular calcinosis .[11] This is a rare lesion of one or both ears which may be secondary to local factors such as inflammation, frost bite or trauma, or be associated with systemic diseases such as Addison's disease, ochronosis or hypopituitarism.

Infantile calcinosis of the heel.[12] This condition has been reported in infants who received multiple heel pricks for blood tests. The deposits have been recognized at 10–12 months of age and they disappear about a year later. This group should probably be regarded as a clinical variant of dystrophic calcification; the nature of the underlying damage to the dermis which leads to the deposition of the calcium salts has not been elucidated.

Milia-like calcinosis. There have been several reports of children with pinhead-sized nodules, usually in the genital area, thighs or knees, which disappeared spontaneously, to recur a few weeks later.[13,14]

Dystrophic calcification. In dystrophic calcification there may be widespread large deposits (calcinosis universalis), such as occur in dermatomyositis[15,16] and rarely in lupus erythematosus,[17–17c] or a few small deposits (calcinosis circumscripta), as seen in scleroderma (see p. 329). Also included in the dystrophic group[1] are the calcium deposits that are found, rarely, in burn scars, keloids, acne scars, and following calcium chloride burns or infusions and the use of calcium-chloride-containing electrode pastes for electro-encephalograms.[18,18a] Cutaneous calcification, of dystrophic type, may follow the percutaneous penetration of calcium salts in those exposed to industrial drilling fluids containing calcium salts.[18] It has also been reported following neonatal herpes simplex infection,[19] and in patients with the Ehlers–Danlos syndrome (see p. 346).

Metastatic calcification. Cutaneous involvement is a rare manifestation of the metastatic calcification that may accompany the hypercalcaemia associated with primary or secondary hyperparathyroidism, destructive lesions of bone, hypervitaminosis D, and other rare causes.[19a] The deposits are found in the deep dermis or subcutaneous tissue, particularly of the axillae, abdomen, medial aspect of the thighs and the flexural areas.[20,20a]

Calcification of blood vessels. Calcification may involve blood vessels in the skin in metastatic and in dystrophic calcification.[21]

Calcification of cysts and neoplasms.[1] This group includes trichilemmal cysts, pilomatrixomas, trichoepitheliomas, basal cell carcinomas and haemangiomas.

Histopathology

Calcium salts are easily recognized in haematoxylin and eosin sections by their intense, uniform basophilia; if necessary, their nature may be confirmed by von Kossa's silver stain which blackens the deposits. The subcutaneous deposits found in tumoral calcinosis (Fig. 14.1) and foci of metastatic and dystrophic calcification tend to be large and dense while those found in the dermis, as in subepidermal calcified nodule, are multiple, small and globular in type (Fig. 14.2). Scrotal deposits are more or less amorphous masses (Fig. 14.3). In subepidermal calcified nodule and in milia-like calcinosis there is often overlying pseudoepitheliomatous hyperplasia, associated with transepidermal elimination of some granules.

Foreign body giant cells and peripheral condensation of connective tissue are other features often associated with the deposition of

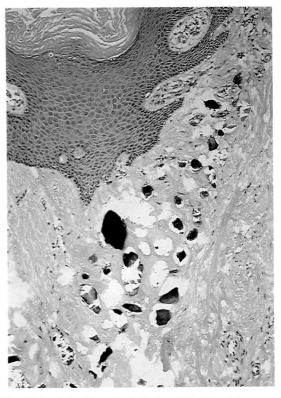

Fig. 14.2 Subepidermal calcified nodule. The calcium deposits are small and globular.
Haematoxylin — eosin

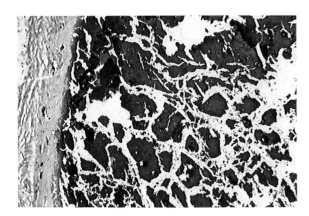

Fig. 14.1 Tumoral calcinosis. The calcium deposits are large and irregular in shape.
Haematoxylin — eosin

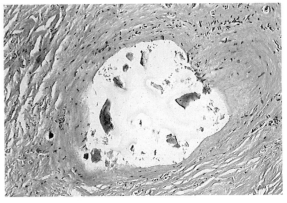

Fig. 14.3 Idiopathic scrotal calcinosis. The deposits are surrounded by hyaline fibrous tissue.
Haematoxylin — eosin

calcium salts. Chronic inflammation is mild or absent.

Epidermal and follicular calcification has been reported in the necrotic epithelium associated with toxic epidermal necrolysis in a patient who also had secondary hyperparathyroidism.[21a] There were no dermal deposits of calcium present.

CUTANEOUS OSSIFICATION

Cutaneous ossification has traditionally been classified into a primary form (osteoma cutis), where there is an absence of a pre-existing or associated lesion, and a secondary type (metaplastic ossification), where ossification develops in association with, or secondary to, a wide range of inflammatory, traumatic and neoplastic processes. There are several distinct clinical variants within the traditional primary group, and several syndromes associated with cutaneous ossification. For this reason, the following classification is suggested to cover all circumstances where bone is found in the skin:

Congenital plaque-like osteomatosis. This form consists of the slow development of a large mass of bone in the lower dermis or subcutaneous tissues.[22,23] It is present at birth or soon afterwards. It has been reported to involve the thigh,[24] scalp,[25,25a] back[26] and calf.[27] Two cases reported as 'limited dermal ossification', although much more extensive in distribution than the typical plaque-like lesion just described, are best included in this category.[28,29]

Multiple osteomas. In this variant, multiple foci of cutaneous ossification are present at birth or develop in childhood.[30–32] A family history is sometimes present.[30,32] Albright's hereditary osteodystrophy should be excluded. An acquired, late onset variant is mentioned in the literature.[23]

Multiple miliary osteomas of the face. Although there is usually a history of previous acne and/or dermabrasion of the face,[33] it

appears this may be found as a true primary condition.[34] Multiple, hard, flesh-coloured papules, a few millimetres in diameter, develop on the face.

Osteomas of the distal extremities.[23] Included in this group are the subungual exostoses[35,35a] (see p. 406), which are basically cartilage derived, and a rare group of bony tumours of the digits in which no cartilage or bony connection can be demonstrated.

Albright's hereditary osteodystrophy.[36–39] Cutaneous ossification at an early age may be a presenting feature of this condition, which includes the older clinical designations of pseudohypoparathyroidism and pseudo-pseudohypoparathyroidism. The basic abnormality is a defect in tissue responsiveness to parathormone. Hypocalcaemia may be present in some cases. The inheritance appears to be X-linked dominant in type. In addition to the ossification of dermal, subcutaneous or fascial tissues, there may also be a characteristic round facies, defective dentition, mental retardation, calcification of basal ganglia, cataracts and characteristic short, thick-set fingers with stubby hands and feet attributable to early closure of the metacarpal and metatarsal epiphyses.[38,39]

Fibrodysplasia ossificans progressiva.[40] This extremely rare condition is manifested by hallux valgus, shortening of the great toes and thumbs, and ossification in muscles and connective tissue. Dermal ossification may precede or accompany these changes. Chondral elements may also be present. The muscles of the shoulder and axial skeleton are commonly involved.

Secondary ossification.[22,23] This group accounts for the great majority of cases of cutaneous ossification. Bone may be found in naevi, particularly on the face (osteonaevus of Nanta), in basal cell carcinomas, in up to 20% of pilomatrixomas, and less commonly in trichoepitheliomas, haemangiomas, pyogenic granulomas,[41] schwannomas, lipomas, chondroid syringomas, organoid naevi,[42] epidermal and dermoid cysts, dermatofibromas, desmoplastic melanomas[43] and some cutaneous metastases. It may develop in sites of infection, trauma and scarring, such as acne scars,[44] injection sites, haematomas, and surgical scars. Myositis ossificans and the related fibro-osseous pseudotumour of the digits[45] can also be included. Abdominal wounds are particularly involved and it seems that injury to the xiphoid process or pubis may liberate bone-forming cells into the wound with subsequent ossification which appears within the first six months after surgery.[46] Other circumstances include chronic venous insufficiency of the legs,[47] scrotal calcinosis,[23] scleroderma, morphoea,[48] dermatomyositis and, rarely, gouty tophi. Secondary ossification has also been reported in neurological diseases associated with paralysis,[49] and in a plaque of alopecia in a patient with polyostotic fibrous dysplasia.[50]

Histopathology

Cutaneous bone usually develops by membranous (mesenchymal) ossification without the presence of a cartilage precursor. There are small spicules or large masses of bone in the deep dermis, and/or subcutaneous tissue (Fig. 14.4). Haversian systems and cement lines are usually present. Occasionally there is active osteoblastic activity, particularly in Albright's

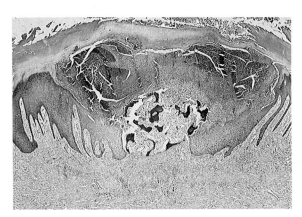

Fig. 14.4 Osteoma cutis. The spicules of bone are undergoing transepidermal elimination. There is surface crusting present.
Haematoxylin — eosin

hereditary osteodystrophy, but this is unusual in the primary solitary lesion and secondary forms associated with acne scars. Osteoclasts are also uncommon. There is often a stromal component of fat, but occasionally haemopoietic cells are also present. In the congenital plaque-like osteomatosis, bone may extend around the dermal appendages.[22] Pigmentation of the bone has been reported in acne patients receiving tetracycline: clinically these nodules may have a bluish colour.[51] The crystalline component of the bone is hydroxyapatite, as in skeletal bone.[52]

CARTILAGINOUS LESIONS OF THE SKIN

This term encompasses several different entities, which have in common the presence of cartilage of variable maturity. Some of these entities have been discussed in other sections. The following classification has been suggested by Hsueh and Santa Cruz:[53]

Chondromas. True cutaneous chondromas are an exceedingly rare dermal tumour, without bony connection.[54,55] They occur most commonly on the fingers; they have been recorded at other sites such as the ear.[55a]

Hamartomas containing cartilage. This group includes accessory tragi, the closely related Meckel's cartilage (cartilaginous rests in the neck, 'wattles'[56,57]), bronchogenic cysts and dermoid cysts. The lesions reported as elastic cartilage choristomas of the neck[58] were midline and suprasternal and therefore different from the usual laterally-placed, branchially-derived remnants.

Soft tissue tumours with cartilaginous differentiation. These extraskeletal tumours arise most frequently in the soft tissues of the extremities, especially the fingers.[59] They may have varying degrees of cytological atypia in the chondrocytes, but despite this they invariably pursue a benign course.

Skeletal tumours with cartilaginous differentiation. This group includes osteochondromas, synovial chondromatosis and subungual exostoses.[35a,60,61] Only the latter group is of dermatopathological interest. They may be very painful lesions and the great toe is the usual site. The lesion consists of mature bone with a proliferating fibrocartilaginous cap.

Miscellaneous lesions. The eccrine tumour, chondroid syringoma, may have prominent cartilaginous differentiation which may at first glance obscure its sweat gland origin.

Also included in this group are the two reports of infants with chordoma-like nodules in the subcutaneous tissues.[62,63]

HYALINE DEPOSITS

Hyaline deposits may be seen in the dermis in several 'metabolic' disorders, including amyloidosis, erythropoietic protoporphyria, lipoid proteinosis and Waldenström's macroglobulinaemia. In gouty tophi the deposits are of a crystalline nature, but when these are dissolved in an aqueous fixative the residual stromal tissue appears hyaline. Other causes of hyaline deposits are colloid milium and massive cutaneous hyalinosis; they may also occur following certain corticosteroid injections. Cytoid bodies are a heterogeneous group of hyaline deposits which are commonly overlooked in routine sections.

GOUT

Although the prevalence of gout in the community is relatively constant, the proportion of gouty patients with cutaneous manifestations — tophi — shows a continuing decline.[64] This undoubtedly results from improved clinical management of these patients, particularly the use of allopurinol, a xanthine oxidase inhibitor that blocks uric acid production. Tophi, which are endstage manifestations of primary gout, are deposits of monosodium urate crystals within and around joints, overlying the olecranon and prepatellar bursae, and in the helix of the ears.[65] Sometimes chalky white material is extruded from tophi. Smaller nodular deposits have been described on the fingers and toes, and there are two reports of a panniculitis with urate deposition as the presenting manifestation of gout.[66,67]

Histopathology

Tophi are dermal and subcutaneous deposits of urate crystals. If material is fixed in alcohol, they appear as well-demarcated deposits of closely arranged, brown, needle-shaped crystals (Fig. 14.5). The crystals are doubly refractile under polarized light. In formalin-fixed material, the crystals will usually have dissolved, and there are characteristic, amorphous pink areas corresponding to the sites of crystal deposition (Fig.

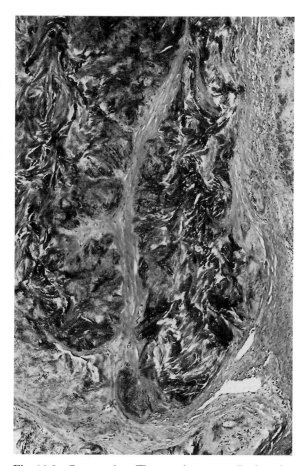

Fig. 14.5   Gouty tophus. There are brown, needle-shaped crystals forming large deposits in the dermis and subcutis. The biopsy was fixed in alcohol.
Haematoxylin — eosin

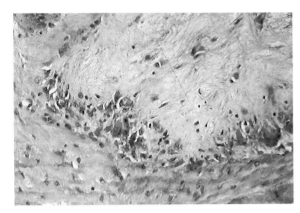

Fig. 14.6 Gouty tophus. The urate crystals have been dissolved in this formalin-fixed biopsy, leaving a hyaline area surrounded by macrophages and foreign body giant cells. Haematoxylin — eosin

14.6). Surrounding the deposits is a granulomatous reaction with macrophages and many foreign body giant cells.[67a] There is usually only a sparse chronic inflammatory cell infiltrate. Often there is some fibrosis as well, and in old lesions calcification and even ossification may occasionally develop. Transepidermal elimination of crystals is rarely seen.

It has been suggested that the primary event in the formation of a tophus is the accumulation of macrophages in an acinar arrangement followed by the centripetal transport of urate by the macrophages from the interstitial fluid to the central zone.[67a] This expands progressively as more urate crystals are deposited. The corona of macrophages commonly disappears and adjacent deposits may fuse.[67a]

AMYLOIDOSIS

Amyloidosis refers to the extracellular deposition of eosinophilic hyaline material which has characteristic staining properties and a fibrillar ultrastructure.[68–69a] The skin may be involved in the course of systemic (generalized) amyloidosis, but more commonly it is the only organ in the body to be involved — localized cutaneous (skin-limited) amyloidosis. Within each of these two major categories, several distinct clinical variants are found, as outlined in the classification which follows.

Systemic amyloidosis
  Primary and myeloma-associated
  Secondary
  Heredofamilial
  Amyloid elastosis

Localized cutaneous amyloidosis
  Lichen, macular and biphasic
  Nodular
  Poikilodermatous
  Familial cutaneous
  Secondary localized.

Because the histochemical, immunofluorescence and ultrastructural properties of the various cutaneous amyloidoses are similar, these will be discussed before the description of the individual clinical variants.

Histochemical properties

Amyloid stains pink with haematoxylin and eosin, and metachromatically with crystal violet and methyl violet.[70] It stains selectively with Congo red; in addition, amyloid stained by Congo red gives an apple-green birefringence when viewed in polarized light. Amyloid gives a bright yellow-green fluorescence with thioflavine T.[71] We have found crystal violet to be more reliable than Congo red in solar damaged skin which sometimes gives false positive staining with Congo red. The cotton dye, pagoda red No.9 (Dylon), used as a variant of the Congo red method, is said to be more specific for amyloid than Congo red because it does not stain the material in paraffin sections of lipoid proteinosis, colloid milium or solar elastosis.[72–74] Congo red staining of the deposits in secondary systemic amyloidosis can be prevented by prior treatment of the sections with potassium permanganate.[75,76] In some cases of primary systemic amyloidosis the amyloid has relatively little affinity for Congo red.

Immunoperoxidase methods using monoclonal antisera can also be used to demonstrate amyloid P component (a non-fibrillar protein derived from a glycoprotein found in the blood of all normal persons) in all cutaneous deposits.[77–78] The amyloid in lichen amyloidosis and macular amyloidosis, as well as in secondary localized cutaneous amyloidosis, stains with the monoclonal antibody EKH4 which recognizes 50kd neutral and acidic keratin.[72] The anti-keratin antibody EAB-903 which recognizes 57kd and 66kd keratin peptides reacts with the amyloid deposits in both lichen amyloidosus and macular amyloidosis, but not with the amyloid in systemic amyloidosis.[78a] Other keratin monoclonals have given mixed results.[79–82] Disulphide (S–S) bonds in the amyloid deposits can be stained with a fluorescent thiol reagent DACM, but there are no sulphydryl groups as found in living keratinocytes in the epidermis.[83,84]

Immunofluorescence

Immunoglobulins, particularly IgM, and C3 complement are found in cutaneous amyloid deposits.[85,86] Most of the studies have been confined to the localized cutaneous forms. Amyloid is thought to act like a filamentous sponge with non-specific trapping of the immunoglobulins and complement.[86a]

Ultrastructure[73]

Amyloid is composed of straight, non-branching filaments, 6–10 nm in diameter, of indefinite length, and in random array (Fig. 14.7). A close association with elastic fibres is sometimes

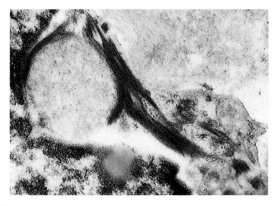

Fig. 14.7 Lichen amyloidosus. There are intracellular deposits and some dense tonofilament bundles in basal keratinocytes. The deposits appear to represent the earliest stages of amyloid formation.
Electron micrograph × 18 000

observed.[87–89] Intracellular amyloid has been noted in dermal fibroblasts,[90,91] and in keratinocytes in lichen amyloidosus.[90]

The ultrastructural studies of Hashimoto and colleagues[92,93] and other groups[94] have confirmed earlier views[95,96] that the basal epidermal cells are involved in the histogenesis of the amyloid in lichen amyloidosus and macular amyloidosis. Basal keratinocytes overlying dermal amyloid show degenerative changes with the accumulation of modified tonofilaments (thicker, but less electron-dense than normal) in the cytoplasm.[97] This process has been termed filamentous degeneration.[97] It is sometimes regarded incorrectly as being synonymous with apoptosis. The cells showing this filamentous degeneration eventually liberate the filamentous material into the upper dermis. Melanosomes may be seen within this material. How these modified tonofilaments 'transform' into mature amyloid, and in the process adopt a beta-pleated sheet pattern (as opposed to the usual alpha pattern of keratin) is still speculative.

Primary systemic amyloidosis

Cutaneous involvement is common in primary systemic amyloidosis and in the closely related myeloma-associated amyloidosis, with lesions in approximately one-third of patients.[68,98] There are non-pruritic, waxy papules on the scalp, face and neck and sometimes the genitalia.[76,99,100] There is a predilection for the periorbital areas. Plaque-like lesions may develop on the hands and flexural areas. Haemorrhage into the lesions is quite common.[100,101] Rare presentations include alopecia, occlusion of the external auditory canals,[102] bullous lesions,[98,103–104] indurated cord-like lesions resulting from thick vascular deposits[105] and elastolytic lesions.[105a]

Histopathology

Papular lesions result from deposits of amyloid in the papillary dermis; in plaques there is a more diffuse dermal infiltration, sometimes with extension into the subcutis (Fig. 14.8).[106] In this latter site, amyloid deposits around individual fat cells form 'amyloid rings' (Fig. 14.9). Dermal

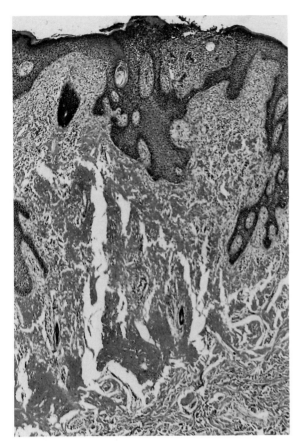

Fig. 14.8 Primary amyloidosis. The hyaline deposits in the dermis show some artifactual separation.
Haematoxylin — eosin

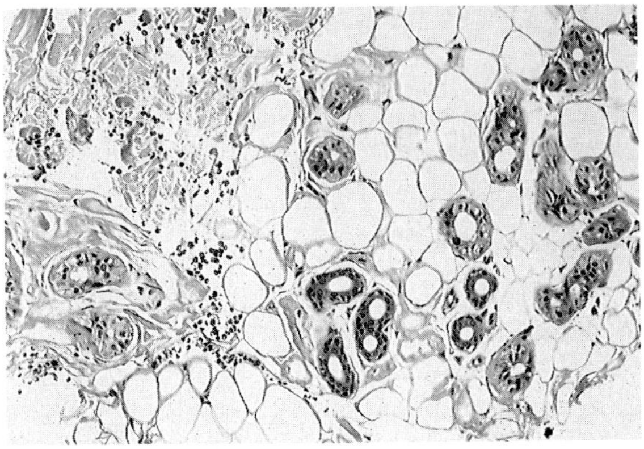

Fig. 14.9 Amyloid rings. There are fine deposits of amyloid surrounding individual fat cells.
Haematoxylin — eosin
Photomicrograph supplied by Dr G Strutton.

blood vessels are usually involved in haemorrhagic lesions, and pilosebaceous units are involved in areas of alopecia.[100,106] The rare bullous lesions are caused by intradermal cleavage within the amyloid deposits.[98,107] There is often clefting about and within the amyloid in the larger papular lesions. If the deposits are large, there is often attenuation of the overlying epidermis.[106] There are no pigmented cells, and inflammatory cells are scarce.[107]

Clinically normal skin will show deposits of amyloid in the dermis, usually in the walls of blood vessels, in about 50% of biopsies in cases of primary systemic amyloidosis.[108]

Secondary systemic amyloidosis

Clinical involvement of the skin is rare in cases of secondary systemic amyloidosis.[68,106] Uncommonly, this form of amyloidosis is the result of an underlying chronic skin disease such as lepromatous leprosy, hidradenitis suppurativa, arthropathic psoriasis,[75] or dystrophic epidermolysis bullosa.[109]

Histopathology

Amyloid has been found in several sites in the clinically normal skin of some patients with secondary amyloidosis, including the papillary dermis, the subcutis, the walls of blood vessels and around eccrine sweat glands.[106–108]

Heredofamilial amyloidosis

There are skin manifestations in certain of the heredofamilial amyloidoses.[110] These include trophic changes and amyloid deposits in the arrector pili muscles in heredofamilial amyloid polyneuropathy[69,73] and urticaria in other forms such as the Muckle–Wells syndrome (urticaria, amyloidosis and deafness).[111]

Amyloid elastosis

This is a recently described entity with cutaneous lesions and progressive systemic disease.[112] The elastic fibres in the skin and serosae are coated with the amyloid material;[112]

the amyloid is localized to the microfibrils of the elastic fibres.[112a] Why amyloid is preferentially deposited on elastic fibres, resulting in clinically-evident lesions, is unknown.

Lichen, macular and biphasic amyloidoses

Lichen amyloidosus and macular amyloidosis are clinical variants of the same process.[73] Patients with features of both variants, or transformation from one to the other (biphasic form), are well documented.[113,114] There is no visceral involvement in lichen amyloidosus or macular amyloidosis.[115]

Lichen amyloidosus presents as small, discrete, often pruritic, waxy papules with a predilection for the extensor surfaces of the lower extremities.[115] Rare clinical presentations have included similar distribution in identical twins,[116] and involvement of the glans penis.[117] Lichen amyloidosus is not uncommon in South East Asia and some South American countries.[115,118]

Macular amyloidosis is a less common variant. It occurs as poorly defined hyperpigmented and rippled patches on the trunk.[96,119] There is a predilection for the interscapular region of adult females.[120] Lesions are often pruritic. Macular amyloidosis has been reported in Japanese patients following prolonged rubbing of the skin with nylon brushes and towels.[72,120a] An unusual presentation is involvement of the knees[121] or elbows.[122]

Histopathology

Both lichen amyloidosus and macular amyloidosis are characterized by small globular deposits of amyloid in the papillary dermis (Fig. 14.10).[86] Sometimes a thin band of compressed collagen separates these from the overlying epidermis,[115] while in others the deposits are in contact with the basal cells and sometimes interspersed between them. Transepidermal elimination of the amyloid sometimes occurs.[123] Pigmented cells are often seen within the dermal deposits.

In lichen amyloidosus (Fig. 14.11) the overlying epidermis shows hyperkeratosis and

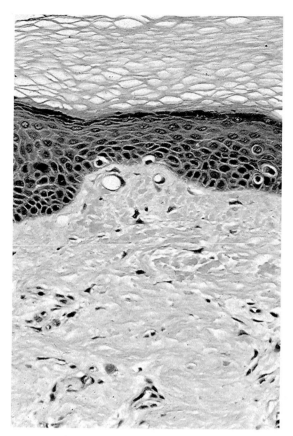

Fig. 14.10   Macular amyloidosis. Hyaline material, barely distinguishable from collagen, is present in the papillary dermis. The diagnosis can be easily missed. Haematoxylin — eosin

acanthosis, with the changes sometimes resembling those of lichen simplex chronicus (see p. 84).[124]

In both types of amyloidosis occasional apoptotic bodies are present within the epidermis.[124a] Basal vacuolar change also occurs.

Nodular amyloidosis

This uncommon form of cutaneous amyloidosis is manifested by solitary[125] or multiple waxy nodules, measuring 0.5 to 7 cm in diameter, on the lower extremities, face, scalp or genital region.[126–128] In at least 15% of cases, the patients will subsequently develop systemic amyloidosis.[124,127] A light-chain origin of the amyloid has been proved in many

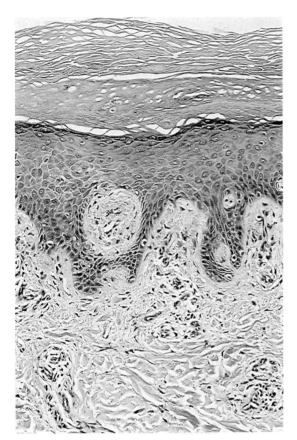

Fig. 14.11 Lichen amyloidosus. Small, hyaline deposits of amyloid are situated in the papillary dermis. There is overlying epidermal hyperplasia.
Haematoxylin — eosin

Poikilodermatous amyloidosis[131]

Poikilodermatous lesions are rare. A distinct subset of patients have short stature, early onset, light sensitivity and sometimes palmoplantar keratoderma — the *poikilodermatous cutaneous amyloidosis syndrome*.[131]

Histopathology

There is amyloid in the dermal papillae and around dermal blood vessels, resembling the pattern of primary systemic amyloidosis.

Familial primary cutaneous amyloidosis

This is an extremely rare, autosomal dominant genodermatosis with keratotic papules and/or swirled hyper- and hypopigmentation[132] on the extremities and sometimes the trunk.[100,133,134] Transepidermal elimination of the papillary dermal deposits of amyloid has been a characteristic feature.[134]

Secondary localized cutaneous amyloidosis

This refers to the finding of amyloid in the stroma of various cutaneous tumours such as basal cell carcinoma (Fig. 14.12)[135,136] and, less commonly, squamous cell carcinomas,[137] naevocellular naevi,[138] trichoblastic fibromas, cylindromas, pilomatrixomas and syringo-

cases.[126,128,128a] Lambda light chains are probably an inherent component of the amyloid filaments.[129]

Histopathology

There are large masses of amyloid in the dermis and subcutis, with accentuated deposition around deep vascular channels and adnexal structures.[100] Plasma cells, some with large Russell bodies, are usually quite prominent at the margins and within the amyloid islands.[107,127] Foreign body giant cells and focal calcification are sometimes present.[127] The amyloid may be deposited in relation to the elastica.[87,130]

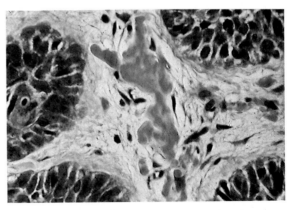

Fig. 14.12 Secondary amyloidosis. Hyaline deposits are present in the stroma of a basal cell carcinoma.
Haematoxylin — eosin

cystadenoma papilliferum.[139] Amyloid may underlie the epithelium in seborrhoeic and actinic keratoses,[140] Bowen's disease, porokeratosis, skin treated with ultraviolet-A radiation after the ingestion of psoralens (PUVA),[141] and mycosis fungoides.[73,142] Amyloid has also been reported localized to areas of severe solar elastosis:[143] amyloid A protein was identified in this latter case.[143] In all other circumstances, the amyloid appears to be of keratinocyte origin.[73]

PORPHYRIA

Porphyria is a metabolic disorder with varied cutaneous manifestations. It is considered in detail in Chapter 18, p. 532.

The characteristic histological feature of the cutaneous porphyrias is the deposition of lightly eosinophilic, hyaline material in and around small blood vessels in the upper dermis. In erythropoietic protoporphyria the hyaline material also forms an irregular cuff around these vessels but it does not encroach upon the adjacent dermis as much as the hyaline material does in lipoid proteinosis (see below). Furthermore, there is no involvement of the sweat glands in cutaneous porphyria. The hyaline material has similar staining characteristics in both diseases, although the hyaline material in porphyria tends to stain less intensely with Hale's colloidal iron method than it does in lipoid proteinosis.

LIPOID PROTEINOSIS

Lipoid proteinosis is a rare, autosomal recessive, multisystem genodermatosis which primarily affects the skin, oral cavity and larynx, with the deposition of an amorphous hyaline material.[144-145] Early clinical features are hoarseness and the development of recurrent skin infections, sometimes with vesiculobullous lesions which heal leaving atrophic pock-like scars.[146,147] Waxy papules and plaques develop progressively over several years on the face, scalp, neck and extremities. Other features include beaded papules on the eyelid margins (blepharosis)[148] and verrucous lesions on the elbows, knees and hands. Although deposits have been found in many organs of the body, resulting dysfunction is rare.[149] Epilepsy may be associated with calcification of the hippocampus.

Although one study has suggested this is a lysosomal storage disease,[150] recent work has shown the deposited material to be matrix glycoproteins with increased laminin and collagen of types IV and V, and a relative decrease in collagen type I.[151-154] The selective increase in pro-α1(IV)mRNA in lipoid proteinosis may have relevance to the accumulation of this basement membrane component in the skin in this condition.[152a]

Histopathology [155]

There is a progressive deposition of pale, eosinophilic, hyaline material in the superficial dermis, but this is initially localized around small blood vessels and at the periphery of eccrine sweat glands.[144a] Small capillaries are sometimes increased in number. In advanced lesions, the deposits around blood vessels may have an 'onion-skin' appearance (Fig. 14.13). There is also progressive atrophy of secretory sweat glands associated with increasing hyaline deposition. This material is also deposited in arrector pili muscles, and around pilosebaceous units. The epidermis may show hyperkeratosis and

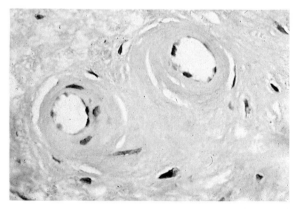

Fig. 14.13 Lipoid proteinosis. Hyaline material is arranged around blood vessels in the papillary dermis in an onion-skin pattern.
Haematoxylin — eosin

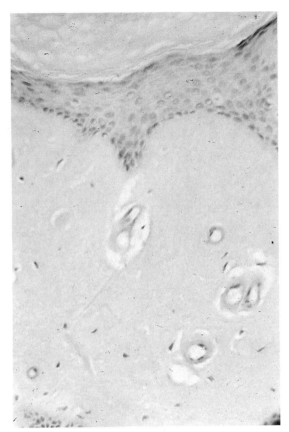

Fig. 14.14 Lipoid proteinosis. The hyaline material involving the papillary dermis and wall of blood vessels is PAS-positive.
Periodic acid — Schiff

some acanthosis in the verrucous lesions.

The hyaline deposits are PAS positive and diastase resistant (Fig. 14.14). They stain positively with colloidal iron and alcian blue at pH 2.5, and also with Sudan black and oil red O on frozen sections.[156] The accumulation of lipid is usually a late, and presumably secondary, phenomenon.[156,157]

Although histologically and histochemically similar material is found in erythropoietic protoporphyria, the deposits in the latter condition are more limited in distribution, being perivascular only.[158] Sweat glands are not involved in porphyria.

Electron microscopy. In lipoid proteinosis there are fine collagen fibrils embedded in an amorphous, granular matrix.[159–160] There is prominent reduplication of the basal lamina at the dermo–epidermal junction, and concentrically around vessels.[151,153,160] Calcium deposits may be seen. Cytoplasmic inclusions have been noted in the fibroblasts; their exact significance is unknown.[150,153]

WALDENSTRÖM'S MACROGLOBULINAEMIA

Translucent papules, formed by deposits of monoclonal IgM, are an uncommon manifestation of this disease (see page 1003). The hyaline deposits which fill the papillary and upper reticular dermis, are strongly PAS positive.

COLLOID MILIUM AND COLLOID DEGENERATION

There are at least four distinct clinicopathological conditions which can be included under the umbrella term of 'colloid milium and colloid degeneration'.[161] Regrettably, our knowledge of these conditions is limited by the paucity of reports in the literature. The four variants are:

Colloid milium — classic adult type[162–165]
Juvenile colloid milium[166]
Pigmented colloid milium (hydroquinone-related)[167]
Colloid degeneration (paracolloid).[168]

The *adult type* develops in early to mid-adult life with numerous yellow-brown, semitranslucent, dome-shaped papules, 1–4 mm or more in diameter. They may be discrete, or clustered to form plaques. The cheeks, ears, neck, and dorsum of the hands are sites of predilection. Often there is a history of exposure to petroleum products and/or excessive sunlight,[165] but obviously there is some underlying predisposition as well.[169] The material in the dermis is now thought to represent a degeneration product of elastic fibres induced by solar radiation (actinic elastoid).[170,171]

Juvenile colloid milium is exceedingly

rare.[166,172,172a] Papules or plaques develop, usually on the face and neck, prior to puberty. Some purported cases probably represent examples of erythropoietic protoporphyria.

Pigmented colloid milium[167] is found as grey to black clustered or confluent papules on the face, following the excessive use of hydroquinone bleaching creams (see ochronosis, p. 417).

Colloid degeneration (paracolloid) presents as nodular, plaque-like areas, usually on the face.[168,173] This is probably a heterogeneous group.

Histopathology

In the *adult form*, there are nodular masses of homogeneous, eosinophilic material expanding the papillary dermis and extending into the mid dermis (Fig. 14.15).[163] Fissures and clefts divide this material into smaller islands, and fibroblasts are commonly aligned along the lines of fissuring (Fig. 14.16). A thin grenz zone of uninvolved collagen usually separates the colloid material from the overlying epidermis, which is thinned.[174] Some clumped elastotic fibres are often present in this grenz zone and also between and below the colloid masses, but the colloid material itself stains only lightly or not at all with elastic stains.[171] This material has been reported to stain positively with crystal violet and Congo red and to give fluorescence with thioflavine T; such reactions are more likely to be positive on frozen than paraffin sections.[163,174] Our own material (including a few cases using frozen

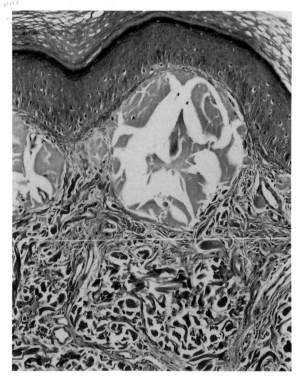

Fig. 14.16   Colloid milium. The clefted, hyaline material is hypocellular.
Haematoxylin — eosin

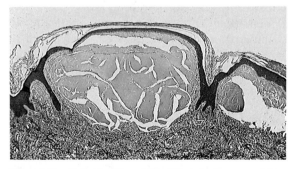

Fig. 14.15   Colloid milium. The clefted, hyaline material in the papillary dermis forms a papular lesion.
Haematoxylin — eosin

sections) has not shown these reactions. In contrast to lipoid proteinosis and primary cutaneous amyloidosis, colloid milium does not contain laminin or type IV collagen.[172a]

In the *juvenile form*, hypocellular material is present in the broadened dermal papillae; this shows some clefting with intervening spindle or stellate fibroblasts.[166] In most areas there is no grenz zone and the basal layer may show hyaline transformation with a transition towards the dermal material. The colloid is PAS positive and sometimes methyl violet positive, but it is Congo red negative.

In the *pigmented form*,[167] there are lightly pigmented colloid islands in the upper dermis (see p. 417).

In the *plaque type of colloid degeneration*,[168] there is amorphous, homogenized, dermal collagen with small fissures and clefts extending deeply into the dermis (Fig. 14.17). The material is relatively acellular. It is weakly PAS

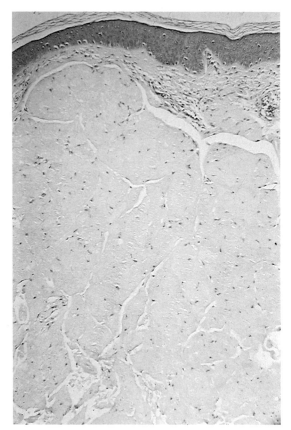

Fig. 14.17 Colloid degeneration (paracolloid). The deposits extend more deeply than in colloid milium and clefting is often less conspicious. Haematoxylin — eosin

positive, but negative with Congo red and crystal violet. There is patchy staining with elastic tissue stains, but other areas are negative.

Electron   microscopy. The ultrastructural features are different in the various types. In the *adult form*, there are large amounts of amorphous and granular material with some wavy, ill-defined, short and branching filaments.[174,175] Some components of actinic elastoid are present at the margins of the islands.[73] There are active fibroblasts. In the *juvenile form* there are fibrillary masses with some whorling, rare nuclear remnants and some melanosomes and desmosomes.[166] Fibrillary transformation of keratinocytes has been observed, leading to the concept that the dermal tonofilament-like

material is of epidermal origin.[166] This has been confirmed by positive staining using a polyclonal antikeratin antibody.[172a] *Colloid degeneration* has shown microfilaments admixed with collagen, but more studies are needed before definite conclusions are reached.

MASSIVE CUTANEOUS HYALINOSIS

This term has been used to describe the condition of a patient with massive amorphous deposits of hyaline material in the deep dermis and subcutis of the face and upper trunk.[176] The material was PAS positive, Congo red negative and ultrastructurally non-fibrillary.[176] Subsequent investigations have shown that there are three major components of this hyaline material: kappa light chains, a mannose-rich glycoprotein and type 1 collagen.[177]

CORTICOSTEROID INJECTION SITES

The local injection of corticosteroids into keloids or various soft tissue lesions results in a characteristic histological appearance should this site be biopsied subsequently.[178–181]

Histopathology

There are usually well-defined, irregularly contoured lakes of lightly staining material in the dermis or deeper tissues.[179] The material is finely granular or amorphous and is surrounded by a variable histiocytic response, sometimes with a few admixed foreign body giant cells and lymphocytes (Fig. 14.18).[181] On low power, the material resembles to some extent that seen in gouty tophi after the crystals have been dissolved by formalin fixation. Crystal-shaped empty spaces may be seen within the material, and occasionally birefringent crystals · have been present.[181] Sometimes there is no discernible reaction, while at other times a few neutrophils may be present. There is some controversy whether these differing appearances are time-related.[181].

The material may be weakly PAS positive, but

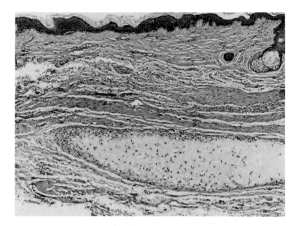

Fig. 14.18   Triamcinolone injection site. There is pale, foamy material surrounded by a palisade of macrophages. Haematoxylin — eosin

although superficially resembling mucin it does not stain for it.[180]

A rheumatoid nodule-like appearance has been reported following corticosteroid injection.[179,181] Transepidermal elimination of altered collagen has followed the intralesional injection of triamcinolone in areas of psoriasis.[182]

CYTOID BODIES

Cytoid bodies are ovoid, round or polygonal, discrete deposits which vary in size from 5–20 μm, or more, in diameter. The term has been applied to a heterogeneous group of deposits which includes amyloid, colloid bodies, Russell bodies and elastic globes.[183] With the exception of Russell bodies, which are derived from plasma cells, cytoid bodies are usually found in the papillary dermis. *Colloid bodies* are derived from degenerate keratinocytes, usually associated with the lichenoid reaction pattern. They represent tonofilament-rich bodies extruded into the dermis, but they are sometimes trapped in the epidermis and are carried upwards with normal epidermal maturation. They are considered with the lichenoid tissue reaction in Chapter 3, page 32.

Elastic globes were first described in the nineteenth century and were for a time regarded as a diagnostic sign in cutaneous lupus erythematosus or scleroderma.[183] In 1965, Pinkus and colleagues described them in normal skin and suggested that they are a structural variant of elastic fibres.[184] They can be found regularly in clinically normal skin from the face and extremities, particularly the calf. It has been suggested that elastic globes in some circumstances may represent the end stage of degenerated colloid bodies; this has not been confirmed by immunohistochemistry which shows that elastic globes have a close immunological profile to elastic fibre microfibrils.[184a]

Histopathology[183,185]

Elastic globes are usually amphophilic, PAS-positive structures found in the papillary dermis (see p. 368). They may have a slight basophilic tint in sun-damaged skin. They are usually larger than cell size (Fig. 14.19). They stain strongly with elastic tissue stains. They are weakly autofluorescent.

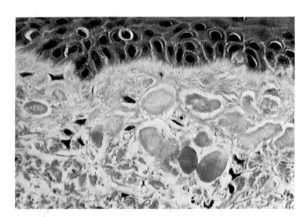

Fig. 14.19   Elastic globes in the papillary dermis. Haematoxylin — eosin

Electron microscopy. This shows electron-dense, granular, amorphous and filamentous material.[184a]

PIGMENT AND RELATED DEPOSITS

A   heterogeneous   group   of   exogenous   and

endogenous pigments may be found in the skin. For convenience, the various heavy metals and drugs which produce deposits and/or pigmentary changes are discussed here as well.

OCHRONOSIS

Ochronosis refers to the yellow-brown or ochre pigment (homogentisic acid) deposited in collagen-containing tissues in alkaptonuria. This is an autosomal recessive disorder in which the hepatic and renal enzyme homogentisic acid oxidase is absent.[186–188] The term is also used for the deposition of similar hydroquinone derivatives in certain exogenously induced conditions which sometimes followed the topical use of phenol in the treatment of leg ulcers and of picric acid in the treatment of burns (both procedures have now been abandoned), and which are still seen as a complication of the oral administration[189–191] or intramuscular injection[192] of antimalarial drugs and the topical use of hydroquinone bleaching creams in black races.[193–197] I have also seen it in a patient who consumed large quantities of quinine-containing tonic water.

There is some clinical variability in the presentation of the various types. In alkaptonuria, there is bluish and bluish-black pigmentation of the face, neck and dorsum of the hands, and bluish discoloration of the sclerae and of the cartilage of the ears and sometimes of the nose.[198] In the pigmentation associated with antimalarial therapy, the pretibial, palatal, facial and subungual areas have been involved.[189] In hydroquinone-induced lesions, the face (particularly the malar areas), neck, and sometimes the ears, corresponding to sites of application of the cream, are involved. There is hyperpigmentation, with variable development of finely papular and even colloid milium-like areas.[193–196] Of interest is the complete absence of hydroquinone-induced ochronosis in areas of vitiligo.[198a] This suggests that melanocytes are necessary for the deposition of the pigment, which is presumably derived from a melanin-hydroquinone precursor.[198a]

Histopathology[194,198]

There is a marked similarity between the ochronotic deposits in alkaptonuria and hydroquinone-induced ochronosis.[195] In the earliest stages, there is some basophilia of the collagen fibres in the upper dermis, followed by the appearance of stout, sharply defined, ochre-coloured fibres which may be crescentic, vermiform or banana-shaped (Fig. 14.20).[194] Fragmented fibres and small pigmented deposits may also be present, the latter lying free in the dermis or in macrophages. Pigment granules are also found in the endothelial cells of blood vessels and the basement membrane of sweat glands.[187] Colloid-milium-like foci often develop in the hydroquinone-induced lesions and these foci may show no visible ochronotic material, or only partial staining of the fibres.[194,196]

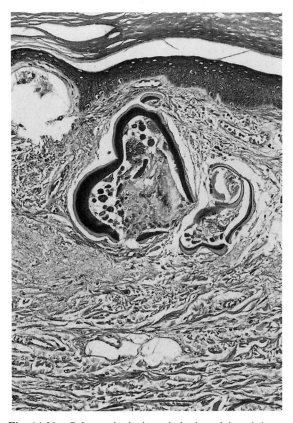

Fig. 14.20 Ochronosis. An irregularly-shaped deposit is present in the upper dermis.
Haematoxylin — eosin

Transepidermal elimination of ochronotic fibres has been observed.[196] There is a variable number of macrophages present, but they are usually infrequent in alkaptonuria. Rarely, foreign body giant cells surround the fibres, but this occurs more often in extracutaneous sites.[188]

In hydroquinone-induced pigmentation there is usually diminution in basal melanin, but prominent melanin in macrophages in the papillary dermis. In lesions induced by antimalarial drugs, the changes are usually different, with small pigment granules which are predominantly in macrophages in a perivascular position and around appendages.[189,190] Small ochre-coloured fibres can be present throughout the dermis, but large fibres in the upper dermis are not a feature. The pigment in the antimalarial-induced cases usually stains positively for melanin and haemosiderin,[190] while in the other forms the fibres and smaller deposits are usually negative with these stains, and also with elastic tissue stains.[194] They do, however, stain darkly with methylene blue.[195]

Electron microscopy. The ochronotic deposits are electron dense. They are usually homogeneous[195] but may be fibrillar.[186] There is granular, less electron-dense material at the periphery with fibroblasts investing and ramifying through it.[194] Active phagocytosis of electron-dense material is present.[195]

TATTOOS

Tattoos are produced by the mechanical introduction of insoluble pigments into the dermis. Most are decorative in type, but occasionally carbon or some other pigment is traumatically implanted in an industrial or firearm accident.[199] The incidence of complications is becoming quite rare with the declining use of mercury salts (such as cinnabar), and a greater emphasis on hygiene in tattoo parlours.

The complications have been well reviewed.[200–202] They may be grouped into several broad categories: infections introduced at the time of tattooing; cutaneous diseases that localize in tattoos, often in a Koebner-type phenomenon; allergic reactions to the tattoo pigments; photosensitivity reactions;[202,203] tumours; and miscellaneous reactions. The infections reported have included pyogenic infections, syphilis, leprosy, tuberculosis,[204] tetanus, chancroid, verruca vulgaris,[201,205] vaccinia, herpes simplex and zoster, molluscum contagiosum,[206] viral hepatitis and a dermatophyte infection.[207] Cutaneous diseases which may localize in tattoos include psoriasis, lichen planus,[208] Darier's disease and discoid lupus erythematosus, the latter in the red areas.[202] Allergic reactions can occur to mercury,[209] chromium,[210,211] manganese,[212] aluminium,[212a] cobalt and cadmium salts.[202,213,214] Photosensitivity reactions may be photoallergic or phototoxic, the latter reaction being quite common with cadmium sulphide, a yellow pigment.[213] The development of tumours such as basal cell[215] and squamous cell carcinomas, melanoma, keratoacanthoma and reticulohistiocytoma may well be coincidental.[200] Miscellaneous lesions include keloids,[201] regional lymphadenopathy and a sarcoidal reaction which may be localized or systemic.[216–218]

Recent experimental work with guinea pigs suggests that the lightening of tattoos after laser therapy results more from widespread necrosis and subsequent tissue sloughing and dermal fibrosis than from any specific changes in the pigment or its handling by macrophages.[219]

Histopathology[220]

Tattoo pigments are easily visualized in tissue sections. After several weeks they localize around vessels in the upper and mid dermis in macrophages and fibroblasts. Extracellular deposits of pigment are also found between collagen bundles. The pigment is generally refractile, but not doubly refractile. A foreign body granulomatous reaction has not been recorded except in the presence of other severe reactions.

Hypersensitivity reactions in tattoos vary from a diffuse lymphohistiocytic infiltrate in the dermis (Fig. 14.21), with an admixture of some plasma cells and eosinophils, to a lichenoid reaction,[221–223] sometimes with associated epi-

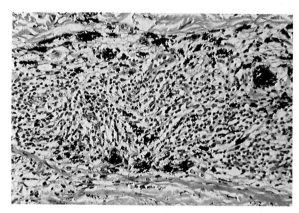

Fig. 14.21 Tattoo pigment with an associated inflammatory reaction, the result of an allergic reaction to one of the pigments.
Haematoxylin — eosin

thelial hyperplasia.[214,224,225] Other reactions include the development of sarcoidal granulomas or of a pseudolymphomatous pattern.[224,226] Epidermal spongiosis has been reported.[220]

Recently, attempts have been made to correlate the ultrastructural features with the pigment used, as determined by X-ray microanalysis techniques.[227] The pigment present in macrophages may be granular or crystalline.[227] It is sometimes membrane bound. Tattoo pigment has also been found in dermal fibroblasts.[228]

HAEMOCHROMATOSIS

Haemochromatosis is a multisystem disorder of iron metabolism in which cutaneous pigmentation is a manifestation in up to 90% of patients ('bronzed diabetes').[229,230] Although generalized, the pigmentation is most obvious on the face, especially the forehead and malar areas.[230] Some patients have been reported to have a slate-grey colour, rather than the typical bronze pigmentation.[230] Cutaneous pigmentation fades slowly with venesection of the patient.

The bronze colour results from increased melanin in the basal layers of the epidermis and, to a lesser extent, some coexisting thinning of the epidermis.[229] Patients with a slate-grey colour have been reported to show haemosiderin

deposits in the epidermis as well as the dermis, and it is assumed that the epidermal haemosiderin contributes to the skin colour in these patients.[230] The absence of pigmentation in the vitiliginous areas of patients with both vitiligo and haemochromatosis indicates that haemosiderin in the usual dermal sites does not contribute significantly to the bronze colour in patients with haemochromatosis.[231] Pigment changes are not as apparent in dark-skinned races, although the darkening of pre-existing epidermal cysts, due to increased melanin in their walls, or of keloids, may be a useful marker.[232]

The increased melanin production is thought to result from the deposition of haemosiderin in the skin, as other heavy metals will produce a similar response. The mechanism by which the heavy metals stimulate melanin production is uncertain.

Histopathology[229,233]

There may be some thinning of the epidermis and increased melanin pigment in the basal layer. Golden brown granules of haemosiderin are present in the basement membrane region of the sweat glands, and in macrophages in the loose connective tissue stroma of these glands. A small amount can often be seen associated with sebaceous glands and their stroma. In some cases, small specks of haemosiderin can be seen in the epidermis with Perls' stain.[230,234]

HAEMOSIDERIN FROM OTHER SOURCES

Haemosiderin has also been noted in the skin following the application of Monsel's solution (20% aqueous ferric subsulphate) for haemostasis in minor surgical procedures,[235-237] and the use of iron sesquioxide on a skin ulcer.[238] In both circumstances there has been ferrugination of collagen fibres with numerous siderophages[236,237] and sometimes multinucleate giant cells[238] in the interstitial tissues of the dermis. Perls' stain has been strongly positive in these areas.

Haemosiderin is conspicuous in venous stasis

of the lower legs.[238a] It is also present in the pigmented purpuric dermatoses (see p. 238), Zoon's balanitis and Zoon's vulvitis (see p. 1003), granuloma faciale (see p. 225), and the pigmented pretibial patches of diabetes mellitus (see p. 531). Haemosiderin is also present in dermatofibromas and various tumours of blood vessels.

'BRONZE BABY' SYNDROME

This refers to the transient bronze discoloration of the skin, serum and urine which is a relatively uncommon complication of photo-therapy for neonatal hyperbilirubinaemia.[239,240] The pigment is thought to be either a photo-oxidation product of bilirubin or a copper-bound porphyrin; it may even be biliverdin.[240] No histological studies have been undertaken.

SILVER DEPOSITION (ARGYRIA)

Argyria, which refers to the systemic deposition of silver salts, is an iatrogenic disease resulting from the indiscriminate ingestion of silver-containing compounds, or their application to mucous membranes or burnt skin.[241,242] Now that the availability of these preparations is restricted, argyria is very rare, and is seen only in relation to industrial exposure or bizarre dietary fads.[243–245]

Cutaneous changes of argyria are permanent blue-grey pigmentation, resembling cyanosis, which is most marked in sun-exposed areas.[246] The nail lunulae may be azure blue.[246,247] The pigmentation is thought to result from the photoactivated reduction of the absorbed silver salts to metallic silver.[243,248] There is probably some contribution from increased melanin production as well.

Localized argyria due to prolonged topical exposure has been reported.[249]

Histopathology[241]

There are multiple, minute, brown-black gran-ules deposited in a band-like fashion in relation

to the basement membranes of sweat glands. They are also found in elastic fibres in the papillary dermis, and to a lesser extent in the connective tissue sheaths around the pilosebaceous follicles, in the arrector pili muscles, and in arteriolar walls. On dark-field examination, the deposits are more easily detected, giving a 'stars in heaven' pattern.[250] In one case of localized argyria the deposits were in the papillary dermis adjacent to the intraepidermal sweat duct.[249] There is usually an increase in melanin pigment in the basal layer of the epidermis and melanophages are present in the papillary dermis.

Scanning electron microscopy has shown that the granules are larger and more abundant in exposed than non-exposed skin.[243] Transmission electron microscopy shows electron-dense bodies 13–1000 μm in diameter in relation to sweat glands and the microfibrils of elastic fibres.[244,250–252] The granules are found in macrophages in membrane-bound aggre-gates.[243,244] Histochemical studies suggested that the deposits were in the form of silver sulphide;[253] the recent use of X-ray probe microanalysis has confirmed the presence of silver and sulphur, with the addition of selenium and other metals in trace amounts.[241,244]

GOLD DEPOSITION (CHRYSIASIS)

Chrysiasis refers to the permanent blue-grey pigmentation of the skin, most pronounced in sun-exposed areas, which results from the depo-sition of gold salts in the dermis, following gold injections for the treatment of rheumatoid arthritis and pemphigus.[241,254–255a] Its develop-ment is, in part, dose-related, but light exposure appears to favour its deposition.[256]

Besides chrysiasis, gold injections may produce a non-specific eczematous or urticarial reaction, eruptions resembling lichen planus and pityriasis rosea, and, rarely, erythema nodosum or erythroderma.[257,258]

Histopathology[241,256]

Small round or oval black granules, irregular in

size, are present in dermal macrophages which tend to localize around blood vessels in the upper and mid dermis. Similar pigment may be in elongated, fibroblast-like cells in the upper dermis.[255] The gold is well visualized on darkfield examination. The granules are larger than silver granules and, unlike argyria, there is no deposition of gold on membranes.

Electron microscopy. This shows electron-dense particles in phagolysosomes of macrophages.[255,259]

MERCURY

Now that mercury-containing ointments are no longer commonly used, the slate grey pigmentation of the skin related to topical application of mercury salts is rarely seen.[254,260,261] Another manifestation of mercury intoxication which is rarely seen is acrodynia (pink disease), a condition of early childhood attributed to chronic mercury ingestion in teething powders.[262] Acral parts assume a dusky pink colour. Serious systemic symptoms and even death sometimes ensue.

A widespread allergic reaction (mercury exanthem) may follow exposure to high concentrations of mercury vapour.[263] Local sclerosing granulomatous lesions may follow the implantation of mercury associated with skin trauma from a broken thermometer,[264] or self-injection.[265]

Histopathology[261,265,266]

The pigmentation from topical applications of mercurial preparations results from the deposition of brown-black mercury granules in aggregates of up to 300 μm in macrophages around blood vessels in the upper dermis, and in linear bands following the course of elastic fibres.[241] The particles are refractile. There may be a contribution from increased melanin in the basal layer.[267]

The mercury exanthem shows subcorneal neutrophilic microabscesses with a variable perivascular neutrophilic and lymphocytic infiltrate

around vessels in the upper dermis.

The accidental or deliberate implantation of mercury into the skin results in a granulomatous foreign body giant cell reaction.[265] A zone of degenerate collagen often surrounds the black spherules of mercury in the tissues.[264,265] In older lesions there may be fibrosis around the deposits.[264] Ulceration or pseudoepitheliomatous hyperplasia may overlie dermal deposits of mercury.

Electron microscopy. Particles averaging 14 nm in diameter, but forming larger aggregates, are present in the dermis.[267]

ARSENIC

Prolonged ingestion of arsenic may result in a diffuse, macular, bronze pigmentation, most pronounced on the trunk with 'raindrop' areas of normal or depigmented skin.[241] The colour is said to arise partly from increased melanin in the basal layer and partly from the metal itself. Other manifestations of chronic arsenical poisoning include keratoses, hyperkeratosis of the palms and soles, and carcinomas of the skin.

LEAD

Lead poisoning may result in a blue line at the gingival margin due to the subepithelial deposit of lead sulphide granules.[241,268]

ALUMINIUM

Persistent subcutaneous nodules are a rare complication of the use of aluminium-adsorbed vaccines in immunization procedures.[269–271] The nodules may be painful or pruritic.[269,270] Aluminium salts used in tattooing rarely cause a granulomatous reaction in the skin.[212a]

Histopathology[271]

There is a heavy lymphoid infiltrate in the lower dermis and subcutis with well-formed lymphoid

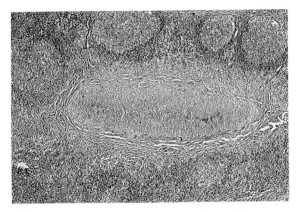

Fig. 14.22   An aluminium-adsorbed vaccine was injected at this site. There is a heavy lymphoid infiltrate, with lymphoid follicles, surrounding a central area of necrosis.
Haematoxylin — eosin
Photograph supplied by Dr G Strutton.

follicles, complete with germinal centres (Fig. 14.22). The infiltrate around the follicles includes lymphocytes, plasma cells and sometimes eosinophils. Macrophages with slightly granular cytoplasm which stains purple-grey with haematoxylin and eosin are usually present.[270] Giant cells and small areas of necrosis are sometimes seen. The aluminium can be confirmed by X-ray microanalysis,[270] or by the solochrome-azurine stain in which crystals of aluminium salts stain a deep grey-blue colour.

BISMUTH

Generalized pigmentation resembling argyria may follow systemic use of bismuth. Metallic granules are present in the dermis.[241] It has been suggested that prurigo pigmentosa, a condition seen mostly in Japan, is a persistent lichenoid reaction to bismuth with post-inflammatory melanin incontinence and pigmentation of the skin.[272]

TITANIUM

There is one report of a patient developing small papules on the penis following the application of an ointment containing titanium dioxide for the treatment of herpetic lesions.[272a] Numerous brown granules, confirmed as titanium by electron probe microanalysis, were present in the upper dermis, both free and in macrophages.[272a]

DRUG DEPOSITS AND PIGMENTATION

There are a number of mechanisms involved in the cutaneous pigmentation induced by certain drugs. These include an increased formation of melanin, the deposition of the drug or complexes derived therefrom in the dermis, and post-inflammatory pigmentation, with melanin incontinence, usually following a lichenoid reaction.[254] The exact mechanism is still unknown in many cases. Drugs, therefore, share many features with the heavy metals already considered. This subject has been well reviewed.[241]

Antimalarial drugs

The long-term use of antimalarial drugs, either for malarial prophylaxis or in the treatment of various collagen diseases and dermatoses, can result in cutaneous pigmentation. Several patterns are seen.[241] Yellow pigmentation is sometimes seen with mepacrine (quinacrine), although the histopathology has not been described. Small ochronosis-like deposits are a rare finding. Pretibial pigmentation is more common and this is slate grey to blue-black in colour. Pigment granules — some staining for haemosiderin, some for melanin and some for both — can be seen in macrophages and extracellularly.[273]

Phenothiazines

Prolonged use of phenothiazines produces a progressive grey-blue pigmentation in sun-exposed areas. Slow fading occurs with cessation of the drug.[274] Similar cutaneous pigmentation has been reported in a patient taking imipramine.[274a] Pigment with the staining properties of melanin is found in dermal macrophages, especially around vessels in the superficial vascular plexus.[241] The Perls method for iron is negative. Electron microscopy shows melanin granules in macrophages but also other bodies of varying electron densities which may represent metabolites or complexes of the drug.[275,275a]

Tetracycline

Bluish pigmentation of cutaneous osteomas has resulted from the use of tetracycline (see p. 405).[52]

Methacycline

The prolonged use of the antibiotic methacycline produces grey-black pigmentation of light-exposed areas and some conjunctival pigmentation in a small percentage of patients.[241] In addition to increased melanin in the basal layer of the epidermis there is extracellular pigment in the elastotic sun-damaged areas which stains positively with the Masson–Fontana method for melanin.[276] Some of this pigment is in macrophages. Electron microscopy shows dermal melanin granules in various states of degradation as well as electron-dense granules in the elastic fibres.[241]

Minocycline

Three different patterns[277,278] of cutaneous pigmentation may follow long-term therapy with the antibiotic minocycline:

1. a generalized muddy brown pigmentation due to increased melanin in the basal layer,[279]
2. bluish-black pigmentation of scars[280] and old inflammatory foci related to haemosiderin or an iron chelate of minocycline, and
3. blue-grey pigmentation of the lower legs and arms due to a pigment which is probably a drug metabolite–protein complex chelated with iron and calcium.

The pigmentation in all cases gradually fades after cessation of the drug.[281]

Histopathology[241,278]

The pigment in the localized types is present in

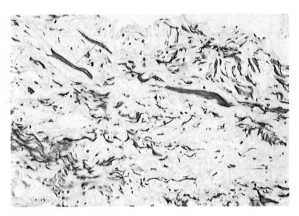

Fig. 14.23 Minocycline pigment deposited on dermal elastic fibres.
Masson Fontana

macrophages, often aggregated in perivascular areas, and in eccrine myoepithelial cells.[282] In other cases the pigment may deposit on elastic fibres (Fig. 14.23). This complex pigment is positive with both the Perls method for iron and the Masson–Fontana method for melanin, but is negative with the PAS stain. It is non-birefringent and non-fluorescent.

Electron microscopy. There are intra-cytoplasmic granules of dark homogeneous material and small fine particles containing iron.[278,283–284]

Amiodarone

Dermal lipofuscin is responsible for the blue-grey pigmentation of light-exposed skin, which is an uncommon complication of the long-term use of amiodarone, an iodinated drug used in the treatment of cardiac arrhythmias.[285–286] The cutaneous pigmentation slowly disappears after cessation of the drug.[285a]

Polyene antibiotics such as nystatin may also produce local lipofuscinosis.[285–286] The mechanism responsible for the production and deposition of the lipofuscin is unknown for both these drugs.

Histopathology[285,286]

Yellow-brown granules of lipofuscin are found in

to refract polarized light and stains a pale grey-violet colour with Masson's trichrome stain and is only lightly eosinophilic in haematoxylin and eosin preparations.[297] Bovine collagen is apparently absorbed as it can no longer be detected by light microscopy or immunofluorescence techniques once several months have passed.[298]

Following injection of the material, a mild lymphocytic and histiocytic infiltrate is found around blood vessels in the vicinity. This is followed by a slight increase in the numbers of fibroblasts and the subsequent deposition of native collagen. Calcification, which is not uncommon at the site of injection of bovine collagen into animals, has not been recorded in humans. Rare reactions include the formation of foreign body granulomas[297,299] or of necrobiotic granulomas resembling granuloma annulare (see p. 196).[295]

REFERENCES

Introduction

1. Mehregan AH. Calcinosis cutis: a review of the clinical forms and report of 75 cases. Semin Dermatol 1984; 3: 53–61.
1a. Spiers EM, Sanders DY, Omura EF. Clinical and histologic features of primary oxalosis. J Am Acad Dermatol 1990; 22: 952–956.
1b. Fisher BK, Warkentin JD. Fiber glass dermatitis. Arch Dermatol 1969; 99: 717–719.

Calcium, bone and cartilage

2. Shmunes E, Wood MG. Subepidermal calcified nodules. Arch Dermatol 1972; 105: 593–597.
2a. Azon-Masoliver A, Ferrando J, Navarra E, Mascaro JM. Solitary congenital nodular calcification of Winer located on the ear: report of two cases. Pediatr Dermatol 1989; 6: 191–193.
3. Weigand DA. Subepidermal calcified nodule. Report of a case with apparent hair follicle origin. J Cutan Pathol 1976; 3: 109–115.
4. Shapiro L, Platt N, Torres-Rodriguez VM. Idiopathic calcinosis of the scrotum. Arch Dermatol 1970; 102: 199–204.
4a. Dekio S, Tsukazaki N, Jidoi J. Idiopathic calcinosis of the scrotum presenting as a solitary pedunculated tumour. Clin Exp Dermatol 1989; 14: 60–61.
5. Moss RL, Shewmake SW. Idiopathic calcinosis of the scrotum. Int J Dermatol 1981; 20: 134–136.
5a. Song DH, Lee KH, Kang WH. Idiopathic calcinosis of the scrotum: Histopathologic observations of fifty-one nodules. J Am Acad Dermatol 1988; 19: 1095–1101.
6. Swinehart JM, Golitz LE. Scrotal calcinosis. Dystrophic calcification of epidermoid cysts. Arch Dermatol 1982; 118: 985–988.
7. Dare AJ, Axelsen RA. Scrotal calcinosis: origin from dystrophic calcification of eccrine duct milia. J Cutan Pathol 1988; 15: 142–149.
8. Whiting DA, Simson IW, Kallmeyer JC, Dannheimer IPL. Unusual cutaneous lesions in tumoral calcinosis. Arch Dermatol 1970; 102: 465–473.
9. Pursley TV, Prince MJ, Chausmer AB, Raimer SS. Cutaneous manifestations of tumoral calcinosis. Arch Dermatol 1979; 115: 1100–1102.
10. McKee PH, Liomba NG, Hutt MSR. Tumoral calcinosis: a pathological study of fifty-six cases. Br J Dermatol 1982; 107: 669–674.

11. Chadwick JM, Downham TF. Auricular calcification. Int J Dermatol 1978; 17: 799–801.
12. Sell EJ, Hansen RC, Struck-Pierce S. Calcified nodules on the heel: A complication of neonatal intensive care. J Pediatr 1980; 96: 473–475.
13. Eng AM, Mandrea E. Perforating calcinosis cutis presenting as milia. J Cutan Pathol 1981; 8: 247–250.
14. Neild VS, Marsden RA. Pseudomilia — widespread cutaneous calculi. Clin Exp Dermatol 1985; 10: 398–401.
15. Nielsen AO, Johnson E, Hentzer B, Kobayasi T. Dermatomyositis with universal calcinosis. J Cutan Pathol 1979; 6: 486–491.
16. Kawakami T, Nakamura C, Hasegawa H et al. Ultrastructural study of calcinosis universalis with dermatomyositis. J Cutan Pathol 1986; 13: 135–143.
17. Kabir DI, Malkinson FD. Lupus erythematosus and calcinosis cutis. Arch Dermatol 1969; 100: 17–22.
17a. Johansson E, Kanerva L, Niemi K-M, Valimaki MM. Diffuse soft tissue calcifications (calcinosis cutis) in a patient with discoid lupus erythematosus. Clin Exp Dermatol 1988; 13: 193–196.
17b. Rothe MJ, Grant-Kels JM, Rothfield NF. Extensive calcinosis cutis with systemic lupus erythematosus. Arch Dermatol 1990; 126: 1060–1063.
17c. Nomura M, Okada N, Okada M, Yoshikawa K. Large subcutaneous calcification in systemic lupus erythematosus. Arch Dermatol 1990; 126: 1057–1059.
18. Wheeland RG, Roundtree JM. Calcinosis cutis resulting from percutaneous penetration and deposition of calcium. J Am Acad Dermatol 1985; 12: 172–175.
18a. Goldminz D, Barnhill R, McGuire J, Stenn KS. Calcinosis cutis following extravasation of calcium chloride. Arch Dermatol 1988; 124: 922–925.
19. Beers BB, Flowers FP, Sherertz EF, Selden S. Dystrophic calcinosis cutis secondary to intrauterine herpes simplex. Pediatr Dermatol 1986; 3: 208–211.
19a. Grattan CEH, Buist L, Hubscher SG. Metastatic calcification and cytomegalovirus infection. Br J Dermatol 1988; 119: 785–788.
20. Cochran RJ, Wilkin JK. An unusual case of calcinosis cutis. J Am Acad Dermatol 1983; 8: 103–106.
20a. Grob JJ, Legre R, Bertocchio P et al. Calcifying panniculitis and kidney failure. Considerations on pathogenesis and treatment of calciphylaxis. Int J Dermatol 1989; 28: 129–131.

21. Kossard S, Winkelmann RK. Vascular calcification in dermatopathology. Am J Dermatopathol 1979; 1: 27–34.

21a. Solomon AR, Comite SL, Headington JT. Epidermal and follicular calciphylaxis. J Cutan Pathol 1988; 15: 282–285.

22. Roth SI, Stowell RE, Helwig EB. Cutaneous ossification. Arch Pathol 1963; 76: 44–54.

23. Burgdorf W, Nasemann T. Cutaneous osteomas: a clinical and histopathologic review. Arch Derm Res 1977; 260: 121–135.

24. Worret WI, Burgdorf W. Congenital plaque-like cutaneous osteoma. Hautarzt 1978; 29: 590–596.

25. Combes FC, Vanina R. Osteosis cutis. Arch Dermatol 1954; 69: 613–615.

25a. Alegre VA, Pujol C, Martinez A, Aliaga A. Cutaneous ossification: report of three cases. J Cutan Pathol 1989; 16: 293 (abstract).

26. Takato T, Yanai A, Tanaka H, Nagata S. Primary osteoma cutis of the back. Plast Reconstr Surg 1986; 77: 309–311.

27. Voncina D. Osteoma cutis. Dermatologica 1974; 148: 257–261.

28. Foster CM, Levin S, Levine M et al. Limited dermal ossification: Clinical features and natural history. J Pediatr 1986; 109: 71–76.

29. Lim MO, Mukherjee AB, Hansen JW. Dysplastic cutaneous osteomatosis. Arch Dermatol 1981; 117: 797–799.

30. Maclean GD, Main RA, Anderson TE, Best PV. Connective tissue ossification presenting in the skin. Arch Dermatol 1966; 94: 168–174.

30a. Gardner RJM, Yun K, Craw SM. Familial ectopic ossification. J Med Genet 1988; 25: 113–117.

31. O'Donnell TF, Geller SA. Primary osteoma cutis. Arch Dermatol 1971; 104: 325–326.

32. Peterson WC, Mandel SL. Primary osteomas of skin. Arch Dermatol 1963; 87: 626–632.

33. Rossman RE, Freeman RG. Osteoma cutis, a stage of preosseous calcification. Arch Dermatol 1964; 89: 68–73.

34. Helm F, De La Pava S, Klein E. Multiple miliary osteomas of the skin. Arch Dermatol 1967; 96: 681–682.

35. Matthewson MH. Subungual exostoses of the fingers. Are they really uncommon? Br J Dermatol 1978; 98: 187–189.

35a. Miller-Breslow A, Dorfman HD. Dupuytren's (subungual) exostosis. Am J Surg Pathol 1988; 12: 368–378.

36. Piesowicz AT. Pseudo-pseudo-hypoparathyroidism with osteoma cutis. Proc R Soc Med 1965; 58: 126–128.

37. Brook CGD, Valman HB. Osteoma cutis and Albright's hereditary osteodystrophy. Br J Dermatol 1971; 85: 471–475.

38. Barranco VP. Cutaneous ossification in pseudohypoparathyroidism. Arch Dermatol 1971; 104: 643–647.

39. Eyre WG, Reed WB. Albright's hereditary osteodystrophy with cutaneous bone formation. Arch Dermatol 1971; 104: 634–642.

40. Rogers JG, Geho WB. Fibrodysplasia ossificans progressiva. A survey of forty-two cases. J Bone Joint Surg 1979; 61A: 909–914.

41. Fulton RA, Smith GD, Thomson J. Bone formation in a cutaneous pyogenic granuloma. Br J Dermatol 1980; 102: 351–352.

42. Wilson Jones E, Heyl T. Naevus sebaceus. A report of 140 cases with special regard to the development of secondary malignant tumours. Br J Dermatol 1970; 82: 99–117.

43. Moreno A, Lamarca J, Martinez R, Guix M. Osteoid and bone formation in desmoplastic malignant melanoma. J Cutan Pathol 1986; 13: 128–134.

44. Basler RSW, Watters JH, Taylor WB. Calcifying acne lesions. Int J Dermatol 1977; 16: 755–758.

45. Dupree WB, Enzinger FM. Fibro-osseous pseudotumor of the digits. Cancer 1986; 58: 2103–2109.

46. Marteinsson BTH, Musgrove JE. Heterotopic bone formation in abdominal incisions. Am J Surg 1975; 130: 23–25.

47. Lippmann HI, Goldin RR. Subcutaneous ossification of the legs in chronic venous insufficiency. Radiology 1960; 74: 279–288.

48. Monroe AB, Burgdorf WHC, Sheward S. Platelike cutaneous osteoma. J Am Acad Dermatol 1987; 16: 481–484.

49. Kewalramani LD, Orth MS. Ectopic ossification. Am J Phys Med 1977; 56: 99–121.

50. Shelley WB, Wood MG. Alopecia with fibrous dysplasia and osteomas of skin. A sign of polyostotic fibrous dysplasia. Arch Dermatol 1976; 112: 715–719.

51. Walter JF, Macknet KD. Pigmentation of osteoma cutis caused by tetracycline. Arch Dermatol 1979; 115: 1087–1088.

52. Basler RSW, Taylor WB, Peacor DR. Postacne osteoma cutis. X-ray diffraction analysis. Arch Dermatol 1974; 110: 113–114.

53. Hsueh S, Santa Cruz DJ. Cartilaginous lesions of the skin and superficial soft tissue. J Cutan Pathol 1982; 9: 405–416.

54. Holmes HS, Bovenmeyer DA. Cutaneous cartilaginous tumor. Arch Dermatol 1976; 112: 839–840.

55. Ayala F, Lembo G, Montesano M. A rare tumor: subungual chondroma. Dermatologica 1983; 167: 339–340.

55a. Quercetani R, Gelli R, Pimpinelli N, Reali UM. Bilateral chondroma of the auricle. J Dermatol Surg Oncol 1988; 14: 436–438.

56. Hogan D, Wilkinson RD, Williams A. Congenital anomalies of the head and neck. Int J Dermatol 1980; 19: 479–486.

57. Clarke JA. Are wattles of auricular or branchial origin? Br J Plast Surg 1976; 29: 238–244.

58. Rachman R, Heffernan AH. Elastic cartilage choristoma of the neck. Plast Reconstr Surg 1979; 63: 424–425.

59. Dahlin DC, Salvador AH. Cartilaginous tumors of the soft tissues of the hands and feet. Mayo Clin Proc 1974; 49: 721–726.

60. Landon GC, Johnson KA, Dahlin DC. Subungual exostoses. J Bone Joint Surg 1979; 61A: 256–259.

61. Cohen HJ, Frank SB, Minkin W, Gibbs RC. Subungual exostoses. Arch Dermatol 1973; 107: 431–432.

62. Ackerman AB, Koch K, Pardo V. Chordoma-like subcutaneous nodules in an infant. Arch Dermatol 1974; 109: 247–250.

131. Ogino A, Tanaka S. Poikiloderma-like cutaneous amyloidosis. Dermatologica 1977; 155: 301–309.

132. Eng AM, Cogan L, Gunnar RM, Blekys I. Familial generalized dyschromic amyloidosis cutis. J Cutan Pathol 1976; 3: 102–108.

133. Vasily DB, Bhatia SG, Uhlin SR. Familial primary cutaneous amyloidosis. Arch Dermatol 1978; 114: 1173–1176.

134. Newton JA, Jagjivan A, Bhogal B et al. Familial primary cutaneous amyloidosis. Br J Dermatol 1985; 112: 201–208.

135. Hashimoto K, Brownstein MH. Localized amyloidosis in basal cell epitheliomas. Acta Derm Venereol 1973; 53: 331–339.

136. Weedon D, Shand E. Amyloid in basal cell carcinomas. Br J Dermatol 1979; 101: 141–146.

137. Malak JA, Smith EW. Secondary localized cutaneous amyloidosis. Arch Dermatol 1962; 86: 465–477.

138. MacDonald DM, Black MM. Secondary localized cutaneous amyloidosis in melanocytic naevi. Br J Dermatol 1980; 103: 553–556.

139. Jennings RC, Ahmed E. An amyloid forming nodular syringocystadenoma. Arch Dermatol 1970; 101: 224–226.

140. Hashimoto K, King LE. Secondary localized cutaneous amyloidosis associated with actinic keratosis. J Invest Dermatol 1973; 61: 293–299.

141. Hashimoto K, Kumakiri M. Colloid-amyloid bodies in PUVA-treated human psoriatic patients. J Invest Dermatol 1979; 72: 70–80.

142. Brownstein MH, Helwig EB. The cutaneous amyloidoses. I. Localized forms. Arch Dermatol 1970; 102: 8–19.

143. Tsuji T, Asai Y, Hamada T. Secondary localized cutaneous amyloidosis in solar elastosis. Br J Dermatol 1982; 106: 469–476.

144. Caro I. Lipoid proteinosis. Int J Dermatol 1978; 17: 388–393.

144a. Pierard GE, Van Cauwenberge D, Budo J, Lapiere CM. A clinicopathologic study of six cases of lipoid proteinosis. Am J Dermatopathol 1988; 10: 300–305.

145. Heyl T. Lipoid proteinosis. I. The clinical picture. Br J Dermatol 1963; 75: 465–477.

146. Pursley TV, Apisarnthanarax P. Lipoid proteinosis. Int J Dermatol 1981; 20: 137–139.

147. Buchan NG, Harvey Kemble JV. Successful surgical treatment of lipoid proteinosis. Br J Dermatol 1974; 91: 561–566.

148. Barthelemy H, Mauduit G, Kanitakis J et al. Lipoid proteinosis with pseudomembranous conjunctivitis. J Am Acad Dermatol 1986; 14: 367–371.

149. Caplan RM. Visceral involvement in lipoid proteinosis. Arch Dermatol 1967; 95: 149–155.

150. Bauer EA, Santa Cruz DJ, Eisen AZ. Lipoid proteinosis: In vivo and in vitro evidence for a lysosomal storage disease. J Invest Dermatol 1981; 76: 119–125.

151. Fleischmajer R, Krieg T, Dziadek M et al. Ultrastructure and composition of connective tissue in hyalinosis cutis et mucosae skin. J Invest Dermatol 1984; 82: 252–258.

152. Harper JI, Duance VC, Sims TJ, Light ND. Lipoid proteinosis: an inherited disorder of collagen metabolism? Br J Dermatol 1985; 113: 145–151.

152a. Olsen DR, Chu M-L, Uitto J. Expression of basement membrane zone genes coding for type IV procollagen and laminin by human skin fibroblasts in vitro: elevated α1(IV) collagen mRNA levels in lipoid proteinosis. J Invest Dermatol 1988; 90: 734–738.

153. Moy LS, Moy RL, Matsuoka LY et al. Lipoid proteinosis: Ultrastructural and biochemical studies. J Am Acad Dermatol 1987; 16: 1193–1201.

154. Ishibashi A. Hyalinosis cutis et mucosae. Dermatologica 1982; 165: 7–15.

155. Hofer P-A. Urbach-Wiethe disease. Acta Derm Venereol (Suppl) 1973; 71: 5–37.

156. Harper JI, Filipe MI, Staughton RCD. Lipoid proteinosis: variations in the histochemical characteristics. Clin Exp Dermatol 1983; 8: 135–141.

157. Shore RN, Howard BV, Howard WJ, Shelley WB. Lipoid proteinosis. Demonstration of normal lipid metabolism in cultured cells. Arch Dermatol 1974; 110: 591–594.

158. van der Walt JJ, Heyl T. Lipoid proteinosis and erythropoietic protoporphyria: a histologic and histochemical study. Arch Dermatol 1971; 104: 501–507.

159. Hashimoto K, Klingmuller G, Rodermund O-E. Hyalinosis cutis et mucosae. An electron microscopic study. Acta Derm Venereol 1972; 52: 179–195.

159a. Aubin F, Blanc D, Badet J-M, Chobaut J-C. Lipoid proteinosis: case report. Pediatr Dermatol 1989; 6: 109–113.

160. Fabrizi G, Porfiri B, Borgioli M, Serri F. Urbach-Wiethe disease. Light and electron microscopic study. J Cutan Pathol 1980; 7: 8–20.

161. Agius JRG. Colloid pseudomilium. Br J Dermatol 1963; 74: 55–59.

162. Zoon JJ, Jansen LH, Hovenkamp A. The nature of colloid milium. Br J Dermatol 1955; 67: 212–217.

163. Graham JH, Marques AS. Colloid milium: a histochemical study. J Invest Dermatol 967; 49: 497–507.

164. Guin JD, Seale ER. Colloid degeneration of the skin (colloid milium). Arch Dermatol 1959; 80: 533–537.

165. Gilbert TM, Cox CB. Colloid degeneration of the skin: report of eight cases. Med J Aust 1946: 2: 21–22.

166. Ebner H, Gebhart W. Colloid milium: light and electron microscopic investigations. Clin Exp Dermatol 1977; 2: 217–226.

167. Findlay GH, Morrison JGL, Simson IW. Exogenous ochronosis and pigmented colloid milium from hydroquinone bleaching creams. Br J Dermatol 1975; 93: 613–622.

168. Dupre A, Bonafe JF, Pieraggi MT, Perrot H. Paracolloid of the skin. J Cutan Pathol 1979; 6: 304–309.

169. Holzberger PC. Concerning adult colloid milium. Arch Dermatol 1960; 82: 711–716.

170. Hashimoto K, Black M. Colloid milium: a final degeneration product of actinic elastoid. J Cutan Pathol 1985; 12: 147–156.

171. Kobayashi H, Hashimoto K. Colloid and elastic fibre: ultrastructural study on the histogenesis of colloid milium. J Cutan Pathol 1983; 10: 111–122.

172. Wooldridge WE, Frerichs JB. Amyloidosis: a new clinical type. Arch Dermatol 1960; 82: 230–234.

172a. Hashimoto K, Nakayama H, Chimenti S et al. Juvenile colloid milium. Immunohistochemical and ultrastructural studies. J Cutan Pathol 1989; 16: 164–174.

173. Sullivan M, Ellis FA. Facial colloid degeneration in plaques. Arch Dermatol 1961; 84: 816–823.

174. Hashimoto K, Miller F, Bereston ES. Colloid milium. Histochemical and electron microscopic studies. Arch. Dermatol 1972; 105: 684–694.

175. Hashimoto K, Katzman RL, Kang AH, Kanzaki T. Electron microscopical and biochemical analysis of colloid milium. Arch Dermatol 1975; 111: 49–59.

176. Niemi K-M, Stenman S, Borgstrom GH et al. Massive cutaneous hyalinosis. A newly recognized disease. Arch Dermatol 1980; 116: 580–583.

177. Maury CPJ, Teppo A-M. Massive cutaneous hyalinosis. Am J Clin Pathol 1984; 82: 543–551.

178. Santa Cruz DJ, Ulbright TM. Mucin-like changes in keloids. Am J Clin Pathol 1981; 75: 18–22.

179. Weedon D, Gutteridge BH, Hockly RG, Emmett AJJ. Unusual cutaneous reactions to injections of corticosteroids. Am J Dermatopathol 1982; 4: 199-203.

180. Bhawan J. Steroid-induced 'granulomas' in hypertrophic scar. Acta Derm Venereol 1983; 63: 560–563.

181. Balogh K. The histologic appearance of corticosteroid injection sites. Arch Pathol Lab Med 1986; 110: 1168–1172.

182. Goette DK. Transepithelial elimination of altered collagen after intralesional adrenal steroid injections. Arch Dermatol 1984; 120: 539–540.

183. Ebner H, Gebhart W. Light and electron microscopic studies on colloid and other cytoid bodies. Clin Exp Dermatol 1977; 2: 311–322.

184. Pinkus H, Mehregan AH, Staricco RG. Elastic globes in human skin. J Invest Dermatol 1965; 45: 81–85.

184a. Nakayama H, Hashimoto K, Kambe N, Eng A. Elastic globes: electron microscopic and immunohistochemical observations. J Cutan Pathol 1988; 15: 98–103.

185. Gebhart W. Zytoide Korperchen in der menschlichen Haut. Wien Klin Wschr (Suppl) 1976; 60: 3–24.

Pigment and related deposits

186. Cullison D, Abele DC, O'Quinn JL. Localized exogenous ochronosis. J Am Acad Dermatol 1983; 8: 882–889.

187. Lichtenstein L, Kaplan L. Hereditary ochronosis. Pathologic changes observed in two necropsied cases. Am J Pathol 1954; 30: 99–125.

188. Kutty MK, Iqbal QM, Teh E-C. Ochronotic arthropathy. Arch Pathol 1973; 96: 100–103.

189. Tuffanelli D, Abraham RK, Dubois EI. Pigmentation from antimalarial therapy. Arch Dermatol 1963; 88: 419–426.

190. Mahler R, Sissons W, Watters K. Pigmentation induced by quinidine therapy. Arch Dermatol 1986; 122: 1062–1064.

191. Egorin MJ Trump DL, Wainwright CW. Quinacrine ochronosis and rheumatoid arthritis. JAMA 1976; 236: 385–386.

192. Bruce S, Tschen JA, Chow D. Exogenous ochronosis resulting from quinine injections. J Am Acad Dermatol 1986; 15: 357–361.

193. Hoshaw RA, Zimmerman KG, Menter A.

194. Phillips JI, Isaacson C, Carman H. Ochronosis in black South Africans who used skin lighteners. Am J Dermatopathol 1986; 8: 14–21.

195. Tidman MJ, Horton JJ, MacDonald DM. Hydroquinone-induced ochronosis — light and electron microscopic features. Clin Exp Dermatol 1986; 11: 224–228.

196. Findlay GH, Morrison JGL, Simson IW. Exogenous ochronosis and pigmented colloid milium from hydroquinone bleaching creams. Br J Dermatol 1975; 93: 613–622.

196a. Hardwick N, van Gelder LW, van der Merwe CA, van der Merwe MP. Exogenous ochronosis: an epidemiological study. Br J Dermatol 1989; 120: 229–238.

196b. Lawrence N, Bligard CA, Reed R, Perret WJ. Exogenous ochronosis in the United States. J Am Acad Dermatol 1988; 18: 1207–1211.

197. Findlay GH. Ochronosis following skin bleaching with hydroquinone. J Am Acad Dermatol 1982; 6: 1092–1093.

198. Attwood HD, Clifton S, Mitchell RE. A histological, histochemical and ultrastructural study of dermal ochronosis. Pathology 1971; 3: 115–121.

198a. Hull PR, Procter PR. The melanocyte: An essential link in hydroquinone–induced ochronosis. J Am Acad Dermatol 1990; 22: 529–531.

199. Hanke CW, Conner AC, Probst EL, Fondak AA. Blast tattoos resulting from black powder firearms. J Am Acad Dermatol 1987; 17: 819–825.

200. Beerman H, Lane RAG. 'Tattoo'. A survey of some of the literature concerning the medical complications of tattooing. Am J Med Sci 1954; 227: 444–465.

201. Scutt RWB. The medical hazards of tattooing. Br J Hosp Med 1972; 8: 195–202.

202. Goldstein N. IV. Complications from tattoos. J Dermatol Surg Oncol 1979; 5: 869–878.

203. Lamb JH, Jones PE, Morgan RJ et al. Further studies in light-sensitive eruptions. Arch Dermatol 1961; 83: 568–581.

204. Horney DA, Gaither JM, Lauer R et al. Cutaneous inoculation tuberculosis secondary to 'jailhouse tattooing'. Arch Dermatol 1985; 121: 648–650.

205. Watkins DB. Viral disease in tattoos: verruca vulgaris. Arch Dermatol 1961; 84: 306–309.

206. Hallam R, Foulds IS. Molluscum contagiosum: an unusual complication of tattooing. Br Med J 1982; 285: 607.

207. Brancaccio RR, Berstein M, Fisher AA, Shalita AR. Tinea in tattoos. Cutis 1981; 28: 541–542.

208. Taaffe A, Wyatt EH. The red tattoo and lichen planus. Int J Dermatol 1980; 19: 394–396.

209. McGrouther DA, Downie PA, Thompson WD. Reactions to red tattoos. Br J Plast Surg 1977; 30: 84–85.

210. Rostenberg A, Brown RA, Caro MR. Discussion of tattoo reactions with report of a case showing a reaction to a green color. Arch Dermatol 1950; 62: 540–547.

211. Cairns RJ, Calnan CD. Green tattoo reactions associated with cement dermatitis. Br J Dermatol 1962; 74: 288–294.

212. Nguyen LQ, Allen HB. Reactions to manganese and cadmium in tattoos. Cutis 1979; 23: 71–72.

212a. McFadden N, Lyberg T, Hensten-Pettersen A. Aluminum-induced granulomas in a tattoo. J Am Acad Dermatol 1989; 20: 903–908.

213. Bjornberg A. Reactions to light in yellow tattoos from cadmium sulfide. Arch Dermatol 1963; 88: 267–271.

214. Goldstein N. Mercury-cadmium sensitivity in tattoos. A photoallergic reaction in red pigment. Ann Intern Med 1967; 67: 984–989.

215. Earley MJ. Basal cell carcinoma arising in tattoos: a clinical report of two cases. Br J Plast Surg 1983; 36: 258–259.

216. Hanada K, Chiyoya S, Katabira Y. Systemic sarcoidal reaction in tattoo. Clin Exp Dermatol 1985; 10: 479–484.

217. Blobstein SH, Weiss HD, Myskowski PL. Sarcoidal granulomas in tattoos. Cutis 1985; 32: 423–424.

218. Dickinson JA. Sarcoidal reactions in tattoos. Arch Dermatol 1969; 100: 315–319.

219. Diette KM, Bronstein BR, Parrish JA. Histologic comparison of argon and tunable dye lasers in the treatment of tattoos. J Invest Dermatol 1985; 85: 368–373.

220. Goldstein AP. VII. Histologic reactions in tattoos. J Dermatol Surg Oncol 1979; 5: 896–900.

221. Taaffe A, Knight AG, Marks R. Lichenoid tattoo hypersensitivity. Br Med J 1978; 1: 616–618.

222. Clarke J, Black MM. Lichenoid tattoo reactions. Br J Dermatol 1979; 100: 451–454.

223. Winkelmann RK, Harris RB. Lichenoid delayed hypersensitivity reactions in tattoos. J Cutan Pathol 1979; 6: 59–65.

224. Blumental G, Okun MR, Ponitch JA. Pseudolymphomatous reaction to tattoos. J Am Acad Dermatol 1982; 6: 485–488.

225. Biro L, Klein WP. Unusual complication of mercurial (cinnabar) tattoo. Arch Dermatol 1967; 96: 165–167.

226. Zinberg M, Heilman E, Glickman F. Cutaneous pseudolymphoma resulting from a tattoo. J Dermatol Surg Oncol 1982; 8: 955–958.

227. Slater DN, Durrant TE. Tattoos: light and transmission electron microscopy studies with X-ray microanalysis. Clin Exp Dermatol 1984; 9: 167–173.

228. Lea PJ, Pawlowski A. Human tattoo. Int J Dermatol 1987; 26: 453–458.

229. Cawley EP, Hsu YT, Wood BT, Weary PE. Hemochromatosis and the skin. Arch Dermatol 1969; 100: 1–6.

230. Milder MS, Cook JD, Stray S, Finch CA. Idiopathic hemochromatosis, an interim report. Medicine (Baltimore) 1980; 59: 34–49.

231. Perdrup A, Poulsen H. Hemochromatosis and vitiligo. Arch Dermatol 1964; 90: 34–37.

232. Leyden JJ, Lockshin NA, Kriebel S. The black keratinous cyst. A sign of hemochromatosis. Arch Dermatol 1972; 106: 379–381.

233. Chevrant-Breton J, Simon M, Bourel M, Ferrand B. Cutaneous manifestations of idiopathic hemochromatosis. Study of 100 cases. Arch Dermatol 1977; 113: 161–165.

234. Weintraub LR, Demis DJ, Conrad ME, Crosby WH. Iron excretion by the skin. Selective localization of iron[59] in epithelial cells. Am J Pathol 1965; 46: 121–126.

235. Olmstead PM, Lund HZ, Leonard DD. Monsel's solution: a histologic nuisance. J Am Acad Dermatol 1980; 3: 492–498.

236. Amazon K, Robinson MJ, Rywlin AM. Ferrugination caused by Monsel's solution. Am J Dermatopathol 1980; 2: 197–205.

237. Wood C, Severin GL. Unusual histiocytic reaction to Monsel's solution. Am J Dermatopathol 1980; 2: 261–264.

238. Hanau D, Grosshans E. Monsel's solution and histological lesions. Am J Dermatopathol 1981; 3: 418–419.

238a. Ackerman Z, Seidenbaum M, Loewenthal E, Rubinow A. Overload of iron in the skin of patients with varicose ulcers. Arch Dermatol 1988; 124: 1376–1378.

239. Ashley JR, Littler CM, Burgdorf WHC, Brann BS. Bronze baby syndrome. Report of a case. J Am Acad Dermatol 1985; 12: 325–328.

240. Purcell SM, Wians FH, Ackerman NB, Davis BM. Hyperbiliverdinemia in the bronze baby syndrome. J Am Acad Dermatol 1987; 16: 172–177.

241. Granstein RD, Sober AJ. Drug– and heavy metal-induced hyperpigmentation. J Am Acad Dermatol 1981; 5: 1–18.

242. Gaul LE, Staud AH. Clinical spectroscopy. Seventy cases of generalized argyrosis following organic and colloidal silver medication. JAMA 1935; 104: 1387–1388.

243. Shelley WB, Shelley ED, Burmeister V. Argyria: The intradermal 'photograph', a manifestation of passive photosensitivity. J Am Acad Dermatol 1987; 16: 211–217.

244. Bleehen SS, Gould DJ, Harrington CI et al. Occupational argyria; light and electron microscopic studies and X-ray microanalysis. Br J Dermatol 1981; 104: 19–26.

245. East BW, Boddy K, Williams ED et al. Silver retention, total body silver and tissue silver concentrations in argyria associated with exposure to an anti-smoking remedy containing silver acetate. Clin Exp Dermatol 1980; 5: 305–311.

246. Pariser RJ. Generalized argyria. Clinicopathologic features and histochemical studies. Arch Dermatol 1978; 114: 373–377.

247. Koplon BS. Azure lunulae due to argyria. Arch Dermatol 1966; 94: 333–334.

248. Marshall JP, Schneider RP. Systemic argyria secondary to topical silver nitrate. Arch Dermatol 1977; 113: 1077–1079.

249. Buckley WR. Localized argyria. Arch Dermatol 1963; 88: 531–539.

250. Johansson EA, Kanerva L, Niemi K-M, Lakomaa E-L. Localized argyria with low ceruloplasmin and copper levels in the serum. A case report with clinical and microscopical findings and a trial of penicillamine treatment. Clin Exp Dermatol 1982; 7: 169–176.

251. Mehta AC, Dawson-Butterworth K, Woodhouse MA. Argyria. Electron microscopic study of a case. Br J Dermatol 1966; 78: 175–179.

252. Prose PH. An electron microscopic study of human generalized argyria. Am J Pathol 1963; 42: 293–297.

253. Buckley WR, Oster CF, Fassett DW. Localized argyria. II. Chemical nature of the silver containing particles. Arch Dermatol 1965; 92: 697–705.

254. Levantine A, Almeyda J. Drug induced changes in pigmentation. Br J Dermatol 1973; 89: 105–112.

255. Cox AJ, Marich KW. Gold in the dermis following gold therapy for rheumatoid arthritis. Arch Dermatol 1973; 108: 655–657.

255a. Millard PR, Chaplin AJ, Venning VA et al. Chrysiasis: transmission electron microscopy, laser microprobe mass spectrometry and epipolarized light as adjuncts to diagnosis. Histopathology 1988; 13: 281–288.

256. Beckett VL, Doyle JA, Hadley GA, Spear KL. Chrysiasis resulting from gold therapy in rheumatoid arthritis. Mayo Clin Proc 1982; 57: 773–777.

257. Penneys NS, Ackerman AB, Gottlieb NL. Gold dermatitis. A clinical and histopathological study. Arch Dermatol 1974; 109: 372–376.

258. Penneys NS. Gold therapy: Dermatologic uses and toxicities. J Am Acad Dermatol 1979; 1: 315–320.

259. Schultz Larsen F, Boye H, Hage E. Chrysiasis: electron microscopic studies and X-ray microanalysis. Clin Exp Dermatol 1984; 9: 174–180.

260. Kern AB. Mercurial pigmentation. Arch Dermatol 1969; 99: 129–130.

261. Lamar LM, Bliss BO. Localized pigmentation of the skin due to topical mercury. Arch Dermatol 1966; 93: 450–453.

262. Dinehart SM, Dillard R, Raimer SS et al. Cutaneous manifestations of acrodynia (Pink disease). Arch Dermatol 1988; 124: 107–109.

263. Rogers M, Goodhew P, Szafraniec T, McColl I. Mercury exanthem. Australas J Dermatol 1986; 27: 70–75.

264. Rachman R. Soft-tissue injury by mercury from a broken thermometer. Am J Clin Pathol 1974; 61: 296–300.

265. Lupton GP, Kao GF, Johnson FB et al. Cutaneous mercury granuloma. A clinicopathologic study and review of the literature. J Am Acad Dermatol 1985; 12: 296–303.

266. Kennedy C, Molland EA, Henderson WJ, Whiteley AM. Mercury pigmentation from industrial exposure. Br J Dermatol 1977; 96: 367–374.

267. Burge KM, Winkelmann RK. Mercury pigmentation. An electron microscopic study. Arch Dermatol 1970; 102: 51–61.

268. Allan BR, Moore MR, Hunter JAA. Lead and the skin. Br J Dermatol 1975; 92: 715–719.

269. Pembroke AC, Marten RH. Unusual cutaneous reactions following diphtheria and tetanus immunization. Clin Exp Dermatol 1979; 4: 345–348.

270. Slater DN, Underwood JCE, Durrant TE et al. Aluminium hydroxide granulomas: light and electron microscopic studies and X-ray microanalysis. Br J Dermatol 1982; 107: 103–108.

271. Fawcett HA, Smith NP. Injection-site granuloma due to aluminum. Arch Dermatol 1984; 120: 1318–1322.

272. Dijkstra JWE, Bergfeld WF, Taylor JS, Ranchoff RE. Prurigo pigmentosa. A persistent lichenoid reaction to bismuth? Int J Dermatol 1987; 26: 379–381.

272a. Dupre A, Touron P, Daste J et al. Titanium pigmentation. An electron probe microanalysis study. Arch Dermatol 1985; 121: 656–658.

273. Tuffanelli D, Abraham RK, Dubois EI. Pigmentation from antimalarial therapy. Arch Dermatol 1963; 88: 419–426.

274. Almeyda J. Cutaneous side effects of phenothiazines. Br J Dermatol 1971; 84: 605–607.

274a. Hashimoto K, Joselow SA, Tye MJ. Slate-gray hyperpigmentation caused by long term administration of imipramine. J Cutan Pathol 1989; 16: 306 (abstract).

275. Hashimoto K, Weiner W, Albert J, Nelson RG. An electron microscopic study of chlorpromazine pigmentation. J Invest Dermatol 1966; 47: 296–306.

275a. Benning TL, McCormack KM, Ingram P et al. Microprobe analysis of chlorpromazine pigmentation. Arch Dermatol 1988; 124: 1541–1544.

276. Dyster-Aas K, Hansson H, Miorner G et al. Pigment deposits in eyes and light-exposed skin during long-term methacycline therapy. Acta Derm Venereol 1974; 54: 209–222.

277. Basler RSW. Minocycline-related hyperpigmentation. Arch Dermatol 1985; 121: 606–608.

278. Argenyi ZB, Finelli L, Bergfeld WF et al. Minocycline-related cutaneous hyperpigmentation as demonstrated by light microscopy, electron microscopy and X-ray energy spectroscopy. J Cutan Pathol 1987; 14: 176–180.

279. Simons JJ, Morales A. Minocycline and generalized cutaneous pigmentation. J Am Acad Dermatol 1980; 3: 244–247.

280. Butler JM, Marks R, Sutherland R. Cutaneous and cardiac valvular pigmentation with minocycline. Clin Exp Dermatol 1985; 10: 432–437.

281. Fenske NA, Millns JL. Cutaneous pigmentation due to minocycline hydrochloride. J Am Acad Dermatol 1980; 3: 308–310.

282. Gordon G, Sparano BM, Iatropoulos MJ. Hyperpigmentation of the skin associated with minocycline therapy. Arch Dermatol 1985; 121: 618–623.

283. Sato S, Murphy GF, Bernhard JD et al. Ultrastructural and X-ray microanalytical observations of minocycline-related hyperpigmentation of the skin. J Invest Dermatol 1981; 77: 264–271.

283a. Okada N, Moriya K, Nishida K et al. Skin pigmentation associated with minocycline therapy. Br J Dermatol 1989; 121: 247–254.

284. McGrae JD Jr, Zelickson AS. Skin pigmentation secondary to minocycline therapy. Arch Dermatol 1980; 116: 1262–1265.

285. Miller RAW, McDonald ATJ. Dermal lipofuscinosis associated with amiodarone therapy. Arch Dermatol 1984; 120: 646–649.

285a. Rappersberger K, Honigsmann H, Ortel B et al. Photosensitivity and hyperpigmentation in amiodarone-treated patients: incidence, time course, and recovery. J Invest Dermatol 1989; 93: 201–209.

286. Alinovi A, Reverberi C, Melissari M, Gabrielli M. Cutaneous hyperpigmentation induced by amiodarone hydrochloride. J Am Acad Dermatol 1985; 12: 563–566.

287. Kossard S, Doherty E, McColl I, Ryman W. Autofluorescence of clofazimine in discoid lupus erythematosus. J Am Acad Dermatol 1987; 17: 867–871.

288. Rademaker M, Meyrick Thomas RH, Lowe DG, Munro DD. Linear streaking due to bleomycin. Clin Exp Dermatol 1987; 12: 457–459.

289. Fernandez–Obregon AC, Hogan KP, Bibro MK.

Flagellate pigmentation from intrapleural bleomycin. J Am Acad Dermatol 1985; 13: 464–468.

Cutaneous implants

290. Clark DP, Hanke CW, Swanson NA. Dermal implants: Safety of products injected for soft tissue augmentation. J Am Acad Dermatol 1989; 21: 992–998.

290a. Postlethwait RW, Willigan DA, Ulin AW. Human tissue reaction to sutures. Ann Surg 1975; 181: 144–150.

291. Travis WD, Balogh K, Abraham JL. Silicone granulomas: report of three cases and review of the literature. Hum Pathol 1985; 16: 19–27.

292. Rae V, Pardo RJ, Blackwelder PL, Falanga V. Leg ulcers following subcutaneous injection of a liquid silicone preparation. Arch Dermatol 1989; 125: 670–673.

293. Symmers W St C. Silicone mastitis in topless waitresses and some other varieties of foreign body mastitis. Br Med J 1968; 3: 19–22.

294. Charriere G, Bejot M, Schnitzler L et al. Reactions to a bovine collagen implant. Clinical and immunologic study in 705 patients. J Am Acad Dermatol 1989; 21: 1203–1208.

295. Barr RJ, King DF, McDonald RM, Bartlow GA. Necrobiotic granulomas associated with bovine collagen test site injections. J Am Acad Dermatol 1982; 6: 867–869.

296. Brooks N. A foreign body granuloma produced by an injectable collagen implant at a test site. J Dermatol Surg Oncol 1982; 8: 111–114.

297. Robinson JK, Hanke CW. Injectable collagen implant: histopathologic identification and longevity of correction. J Dermatol Surg Oncol 1985; 11: 124–130.

298. Stegman SJ, Chu S, Bensch K, Armstrong R. A light and electron microscopic evaluation of Zyderm collagen and Zyplast implants in aging human facial skin. Arch Dermatol 1987; 123: 1644–1649.

299. Burke KE, Naughton G, Waldo E, Cassai N. Bovine collagen implant: histologic chronology in pig dermis. J Dermatol Surg Oncol 1983; 9: 889–895.

15

David Weedon

Diseases of cutaneous appendages

INTRODUCTION

This chapter covers the non-tumorous disorders of the cutaneous appendages, the great majority of which are inflammatory diseases of the pilosebaceous apparatus. Inflammation of the apocrine and eccrine glands is quite uncommon by comparison. Hamartomas and some related congenital malformations are included with the appendageal tumours in Chapter 33 (pages 817–872) .

The following categories of appendageal diseases will be considered in this chapter:

1. Inflammatory diseases of the pilosebaceous apparatus
2. Hair shaft abnormalities
3. Alopecias
4. Miscellaneous disorders.

1. INFLAMMATORY DISEASES OF THE PILOSEBACEOUS APPARATUS

Inflammatory diseases of the pilosebaceous apparatus are a common problem in dermatological practice, although it is unusual for biopsies to be taken in many of the entities included in this category. It often assists in arriving at a specific diagnosis if the various inflammatory diseases are subdivided into six categories, although it should be recognized at the outset that this subdivision is somewhat arbitrary. These categories are as follows:

Acneiform lesions
Superficial folliculitides
Deep infectious folliculitides
Deep scarring folliculitides
Follicular occlusion triad
Miscellaneous folliculitides.

Acneiform lesions combine inflammation of the pilosebaceous apparatus with the presence of comedones, and often scarring as well. Comedones are dilated and plugged hair follicles which may have a small infundibular orifice (closed comedo) or a wide patulous opening (open comedo). Comedones are not confined to acne, being found in senile skin and certain other circumstances (see below).

The other categories in this section are all folliculitides. The term *folliculitis* refers to the presence of inflammatory cells within the wall and lumen of a hair follicle, while *perifolliculitis* denotes their presence in the perifollicular connective tissue, sometimes extending into the adjacent reticular dermis. Folliculitis and perifolliculitis are often found together because an inflammatory process in the follicle spills over into the adjacent connective tissue. If the inflammatory process is severe enough, destruction of the hair follicle will ensue. Scarring may also result if the inflammatory process is severe and/or persistent. Five major categories of folliculitis can be defined although, as already mentioned, this subdivision is somewhat arbitrary. They will be considered after the acneiform lesions have been discussed.

ACNEIFORM LESIONS

Acneiform lesions are characterized by the presence of comedones, as well as inflammation of the hair follicle. Frequently, the inflammatory process extends into the adjacent dermis with the formation of pustules, draining sinuses and subsequent scarring. The most important entity in this group is acne vulgaris.

ACNE VULGARIS

Acne vulgaris, an inflammatory disease of sebaceous follicles, is a common disorder which affects a large proportion of the teenage population.[1,2] It is usually a mild affliction which improves spontaneously after adolescence.[3] In a small proportion, it produces considerable disfigurement.

Acne is a polymorphic disorder with such diverse lesions as comedones, papules, pustules, cysts, sinuses and scars.[1] The comedones may take the form of tiny white papules known as 'whiteheads' (closed comedones), or small papules with a central core, the surface of which is black. These lesions are known as 'blackheads' (open comedones). Comedones are not confined to acne, being found in senile skin,[4] in naevus comedonicus, and following exposure to certain chemicals such as coal tar. Only a few inflammatory lesions are present at any one time in mild acne, although comedones may be present and dormant for years.[5]

Acne affects the face and, less frequently, the upper part of the trunk. These are sites of maximum density of sebaceous follicles.[2] In one report, acne presented in a zosteriform distribution ('acne naevus').[6]

Acne vulgaris is of multifactorial origin with both intrinsic and extrinsic factors contributing to the final outcome. There are four principal pathogenetic events: abnormal follicular keratinization with retention of keratinous material in the follicle, increased sebum production, the presence of the Gram-positive anaerobic diphtheroid, *Propionibacterium acnes*, and inflammation.[2,7] These various factors are, in part, interrelated.

The initial event is abnormal keratinization of the infra-infundibular portion of sebaceous follicles leading to the impaction of adherent horny lamellae within the follicle.[8] The cause of this retention hyperkeratosis is unknown although both the formation of free fatty acids and the follicular deficiency of the fatty acid linoleic acid[9] have been implicated at different times. Impacted follicles, which are the precursors of comedones and inflammatory lesions, are not detectable clinically.[8] They are termed microcomedones.

The role of sebum is poorly understood.[10] Acne patients have increased sebum secretion by the sebaceous follicles.[9] Sebum production is known to be under the influence of androgens,[11] which are increased in some patients, particularly females, with acne.[12–16] Of interest is the recent finding that most women with acne have polycystic ovaries.[16a] Furthermore, the injection of sebum into the skin produces inflammatory lesions that mimic those of acne.[17]

P. acnes is the bacterial species most consistently isolated from lesions of acne,[18] although it is present in only 70% of early inflammatory lesions.[19] Bacteria are not essential for the formation of comedones.[20] *P. acnes* produces several factors which may have pathogenetic importance.[21–23] These include lipases and proteases, and chemotactic factors. *P. acnes* can, in some way, activate the complement system, and it may stimulate the release of hydrolases from neutrophils.[22] These substances may in turn damage the follicular wall leading to the liberation of the contents of the follicle into the dermis and the consequent inflammatory reaction. Antibiotic-resistant strains of *P. acnes* are present in some cases of recalcitrant acne vulgaris.[24]

Many external factors may influence the course of acne vulgaris.[25] These include drugs (halides, various hormones,[26] barbiturates, lithium and diphenylhydantoin), cosmetics, soaps and shampoos,[27] industrial chemicals, ultraviolet light, and friction or trauma.[28]

Acneiform lesions are seen in Apert's syndrome (acrocephalosyndactyly)[29] and pyoderma faciale, although in the latter there are cysts and draining sinuses but no comedones.[30] An acneiform eruption may complicate the use of topical and systemic corticosteroid therapy ('steroid acne').[30a]

Histopathology[1,31]

The three major components of acne vulgaris are comedones, inflammatory lesions and scars. A *comedo* is an impaction of horny cells in the lumen of a sebaceous follicle.[1,32] Preceding this is the microcomedo, a clinically invisible lesion in which there is only minimal distension of the infra-infundibular canal of a sebaceous follicle, accompanied by increased retention of horny cells and a prominent underlying granular layer.[8,33] There are two types of comedo: a closed comedo ('whitehead') with only a small orifice, and an open comedo ('blackhead') which in contrast has a wide patulous orifice.[31] Both consist of a cyst-like cavity filled with a compact mass of keratinous material and numerous bacteria.[31] In the closed comedo there are one or two hairs trapped in the lumen and atrophic sebaceous acini, while in the open comedo there are up to 10–15 hairs in the lumen and the sebaceous acini are atrophic or absent.[1,31] The epithelial lining of comedones is usually thin.

The source of the pigmentation in open comedones ('blackheads') is disputed. It has been attributed to the presence of active melanocytes in the uppermost follicle,[34] but a more recent study failed to confirm this.[35] It is now suggested that densely packed, often concentric, horny material, interspersed with sebaceous material and bacterial breakdown products may be responsible for the observed pigmentation.[35]

If comedones rupture, re-epithelialization may eventually occur, producing secondary comedones which may be distorted in shape as a consequence of the residual inflammation and dermal scarring.[1,31] Epidermal cysts may also form, particularly on the neck. They differ from comedones by their often larger size, and the complete absence of sebaceous acini and a pilary unit.[31] Comedones of all types may be dormant for a long period. At any time they may become inflamed.

Inflammatory lesions have traditionally been attributed to the accumulation of neutrophils within microcomedones or comedones with subsequent rupture of the follicle and the formation of a pustule in the dermis.[36] It now appears that there is an even earlier stage which involves the transmigration of lymphocytes into the wall of the follicle associated with increasing spongiosis of the follicular epithelium (Fig. 15.1).[33] This change has been likened to an allergic contact sensitivity reaction.[33] This is followed after 24–72 hours by the accumulation

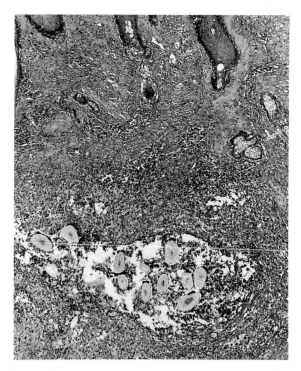

Fig. 15.2   Acne vulgaris. A perifollicular pustule is present in the dermis. It contains liberated hair shafts. Haematoxylin — eosin

of neutrophils within the follicle, leading to its distension and subsequent rupture.[33] There may be a localized loss of the granular layer in the region of the eventual rupture, suggesting a defect in keratinization in this region.[37] A perifollicular pustule develops following the rupture of the comedo (Fig. 15.2). Lymphocytes, plasma cells and foreign body giant cells subsequently appear. The follicular epithelium tends to encapsulate the inflammatory mass; sometimes this is followed by the formation of draining sinuses lined by remnants of the follicular epithelium. When the inflammatory process subsides, distorted secondary comedones may result.

Scars in acne vulgaris may take the form of localized dermal fibrosis or of hypertrophic scars, even with keloidal changes. Small atrophic pits are quite common.[31,36] A thin fibrotic dermis, devoid of appendages, is found directly beneath the epidermis-lined pit. Perifollicular fibrosis and elastolysis,[37a] dystrophic calcification, osteoma

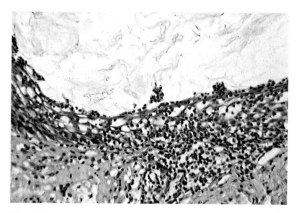

Fig. 15.1   Acne vulgaris (early lesion). There is transmigration of lymphocytes through the spongiotic epithelium lining a microcomedone. A few neutrophils are present along the inner edge. Haematoxylin — eosin

cutis[38,39] and localized haemosiderosis[40] are other complications of inflammatory acne lesions.

Electron microscopy. Comedones contain keratinized cells, sebum, organisms and hairs.[41] Treatment with isotretinoin leads to a reduction in the quantity of this material and a loss of cohesion between the keratinized cells.[42]

ACNE FULMINANS

Acne fulminans is a rare, acute form of acne, found usually in young adult males.[43] There is a sudden onset of painful, ulcerated and crusted lesions accompanied by fever, musculoskeletal pain and leucocytosis.[43] Lytic lesions of bone develop in 25% of cases.[43–45] Acne fulminans has been reported in association with Crohn's disease,[46] erythema nodosum[47] and the use of testosterone.[48]

The aetiology of this condition is unknown, although there is speculation that immune mechanisms are involved.[44]

Histopathology[49]

Comedones are uncommon in acne fulminans. There are extensive inflammatory lesions in the dermis associated with necrosis of follicles and the overlying epidermis. Follicles distended with neutrophils are also present. Severe dermal scarring usually follows the subsidence of the inflammation.

CHLORACNE

Chloracne is an acneiform eruption due to systemic poisoning by halogenated aromatic compounds.[50] Industrial exposure is the usual source of the chloracnegens, although exposure to defoliants containing dioxin was encountered in the Vietnam War.[51,52] Cutaneous lesions may persist for long periods after the last exposure to the offending chemical.

Chloracne is distinct from other forms of acne.[50] It most often involves the malar crescent, the retroauricular region and the scrotum and

penis. Erythema and pigmentation of the face may also occur.[50] The primary lesion is the comedo, which is intermingled with small cysts.[50] Inflammatory lesions are sparse. Dioxins have also produced areas resembling granuloma annulare and atrophoderma vermiculatum.[50]

Histopathology[50,51]

There is follicular hyperkeratosis with infundibular dilatation forming bottle-shaped and columnar funnels containing keratinous debris. Comedones and keratinous cysts with an attachment to the epidermis also form.[51] Small inflammatory foci may be present.

SUPERFICIAL FOLLICULITIDES

In this group of folliculitides, the inflammatory infiltrate is found beneath the stratum corneum overlying a hair follicle, and/or in the follicular infundibulum. Disruption of the follicle wall may lead to inflammation of the upper dermis adjacent to the affected hair follicle.

ACUTE SUPERFICIAL FOLLICULITIS

This condition, also known as impetigo of Bockhart, is characterized by small pustules developing around follicular ostia, and frequently pierced by a hair.[53] *Staphylococcus aureus* has been implicated in the aetiology.

Histopathology

There is a subcorneal pustule overlying the follicular infundibulum. In addition to neutrophils, there are also lymphocytes and macrophages in the infiltrate, which usually extends into the upper follicle and the surrounding dermis. A morphologically similar entity, confined to the scalp, and possibly related to infection with *Propionibacterium acnes*,[54] has been reported as chronic non-scarring folliculitis of the scalp.[55]

ACTINIC FOLLICULITIS

There have been several reports of a pustular folliculitis of the face and upper part of the trunk following exposure to sunlight.[56-58] The mechanism by which exposure to ultraviolet light results in folliculitic lesions remains to be elucidated, although the condition may be related to acne vulgaris and acne aestivalis.[58]

Histopathology

In one report, the microscopic changes resembled those of an acute superficial folliculitis.[56] No organisms are seen, and bacterial cultures have been negative.

ACNE NECROTICA

Acne necrotica (acne varioliformis) is a rare dermatosis of adults, consisting of crops of erythematous, follicle-based papules that become superficially necrotic, umbilicated and crusted, with subsequent healing which produces a depressed varioliform scar.[59-61] Only a small number of active lesions may be present at any time. They develop on the frontal hairline, forehead and face, and sometimes on the upper part of the trunk.

Acne necrotica miliaris has been regarded as a pruritic, non-scarring variant of acne necrotica in which follicular vesiculopustules develop on the scalp.[59] This condition has been regarded as nothing more than neurotic excoriations superimposed on a bacterial folliculitis, an aetiology that has also been proposed for acne necrotica itself.[62]

Histopathology[59]

Early lesions show an intense perivascular and perifollicular lymphocytic infiltrate extending to the mid dermis and associated with prominent subepidermal oedema. The infiltrate also extends into the wall of the upper part of the follicle and into the epidermis, where there is associated spongiosis and death of individual keratinocytes. Later, there is confluent necrosis of the upper follicle, the epidermis and dermis. At this stage neutrophils are seen in the upper follicle and the adjacent dermis. A florid superficial folliculitis and perifolliculitis are sometimes present.

Biopsies of acne necrotica miliaris may show superficially inflamed excoriations, centred on hair follicles.[62] It is unusual to have an intact lesion biopsied; presumably a superficial folliculitis would be seen.

NECROTIZING FOLLICULITIS OF AIDS

A necrotizing folliculitis is a rare cutaneous manifestation of the acquired immunodeficiency syndrome (AIDS) or its prodromes.[63]

Histopathology

Although the folliculitis and perifolliculitis may not be confined to the superficial follicle, this condition is classified with the superficial folliculitides because the accompanying necrosis is confined to the upper part of the follicle and the adjacent epidermis and superficial dermis, characteristically in a wedge-shaped area.[63] There is fibrinoid necrosis of vessels at the apex of the wedge.

EOSINOPHILIC PUSTULAR FOLLICULITIS

Eosinophilic pustular folliculitis (Ofuji's disease) is a rare, chronic dermatosis, first described in the Japanese,[64,65] but now reported occasionally in Caucasians.[66-68] There are recurrent, sterile, often pruritic follicular papules and pustules with a tendency to form circinate plaques.[69-71] These may show central clearing with residual hyperpigmentation. 'Seborrhoeic areas', such as the face, trunk, and extensor surface of the proximal part of the limbs[72] are usually involved, but in 20% of cases the non-hair-bearing palms and soles may also be involved.[70] For this reason, the designations 'eosinophilic pustular dermatosis'[73] and 'sterile eosinophilic pustulosis'[74] have been suggested as more appropriate titles. A peripheral leucocytosis and eosinophilia are often present.

Scarring alopecia was present in one case.[74] The condition reported in two brothers as circinate eosinophilic dermatosis has some similarities.[75]

The aetiology of eosinophilic pustular folliculitis is unknown. Interestingly, a similar lesion has been reported in dogs.[76] Various immunological abnormalities have been reported in some patients, but this is not a constant feature.[77] The condition has developed in several patients with the acquired immunodeficiency syndrome.[78,78a] Circulating antibodies to basal cell cytoplasm[79] and intercellular antigens have been noted.[80] Chemotactic factors have also been isolated from the skin.[81]

Histopathology[67,68,70]

There is eosinophilic spongiosis and pustulosis involving particularly the infundibular region of the hair follicle. The infiltrate often extends into the attached sebaceous gland. Most follicles are preserved, but some show disruption or destruction of the wall by the inflammatory infiltrate.[67] In addition to the eosinophils, there are variable numbers of neutrophils and some mononuclear cells. There is also a moderately dense, perivascular and perifollicular inflammatory cell infiltrate composed of lymphocytes, eosinophils and macrophages. A PAS or silver methenamine preparation should always be examined, as dermatophyte infections occasionally give a similar appearance.[79,82]

Lesions on the palms and soles show subcorneal and intraepidermal pustules. There is a variable inflammatory infiltrate in the underlying dermis.

INFUNDIBULOFOLLICULITIS

This entity is mentioned here for completeness, although it is discussed in further detail with the spongiotic tissue reaction (see p. 100). The histopathological changes are those of follicular spongiosis. A few neutrophils may be found in the spongiotic infundibulum, or in the keratin plug which is sometimes present in the involved follicle.

DEEP INFECTIOUS FOLLICULITIDES

In this group of folliculitides the inflammatory process involves the deep portion of the hair follicle, although both superficial and deep inflammation may be present (Fig. 15.3). The aetiological agents include bacteria, fungi and the herpes virus, and are not always easily identified in routine tissue sections. Although not considered further in this section, a folliculitis is an uncommon presentation of secondary syphilis (see p. 633).

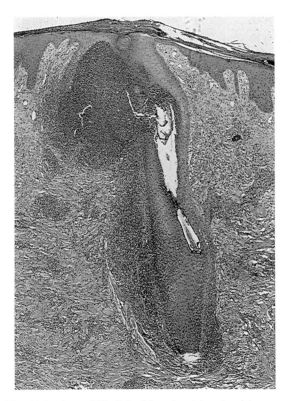

Fig. 15.3 Acute folliculitis of fungal aetiology involving both the superficial and deep portion of the follicle. Haematoxylin — eosin

FURUNCLE

A furuncle (boil) is a deep-seated infection centred on the pilosebaceous unit.[83] Boils commonly occur at sites of friction by clothing such as the back of the neck, the buttocks and inner aspect of the thighs. The lesion begins as a painful, follicular papule with surrounding erythema and induration.[83] The centre usually becomes yellow, softens and discharges pus. Healing takes place with minimal scarring. A carbuncle is a coalescence of multiple furuncles which may lead to multiple points of drainage on the skin surface. There are often constitutional symptoms.

Staphylococcus aureus is the organism most often involved.

Histopathology[84]

A furuncle consists of a deep dermal abscess centred on a hair follicle. This is usually destroyed, although a residual hair shaft is sometimes present in the centre of the abscess. There is often extension of the inflammatory process into the subcutis. The overlying epidermis is eventually destroyed and the surface is covered by an inflammatory crust.

PSEUDOMONAS FOLLICULITIS

Pseudomonas folliculitis is usually caused by *Pseudomonas aeruginosa*. It presents as an erythematous follicular eruption which may be maculopapular, vesicular, pustular or polymorphous.[85,86] It usually involves the trunk, axillae and proximal parts of the extremities. There may be constitutional symptoms.[87] Lesions develop 8–48 hours after recreational exposure to the organism, which is found in contaminated whirlpools and hot tubs.[88] Spontaneous clearing usually occurs within a week.

Histopathology[85]

There is an acute suppurative folliculitis which may be both superficial and deep. If disruption of the follicular wall occurs, dermal suppuration may result. Attempts to demonstrate organisms in conventional histological preparations are usually unsuccessful.

OTHER BACTERIAL FOLLICULITIDES

A folliculitis caused by Gram-negative bacteria may occur as a complication of prolonged antibiotic therapy in patients with acne vulgaris.[89] Most of these infections are caused by a subgroup of lactose-fermenting bacteria, resulting in superficial pustules grouped around the nose.[90] *Pseudomonas aeruginosa* has also been implicated in this clinical setting.[91] In others, deep nodular and cystic lesions occur as a result of infection by species of *Proteus*.[89]

Bacteria, possibly complicating the application of various oils to the skin, have been implicated in a pustular eruption of the legs, seen in parts of Africa and India, and known as dermatitis cruris pustulosa et atrophicans.[92]

Salmonella dublin was isolated from one case of widespread folliculitis.[93]

Histopathology

Both a superficial and deep folliculitis may be present in these bacterial folliculitides. There is variable involvement of the perifollicular dermis.

HERPES FOLLICULITIS

The pilosebaceous follicle may be infected with herpes simplex virus type I (see p. 683). Vesicular lesions may not be obvious clinically.

Histopathology

There is partial or complete necrosis of the follicle with exocytosis of lymphocytes into the follicular wall and the attached sebaceous gland. Sometimes there is adjacent dermal necrosis. The epidermis sometimes shows the typical features of herpetic infection. At other times, a 'bottom heavy', perivascular and interstitial dermal inflammatory cell infiltrate is the only clue. This finding necessitates the cutting of multiple deeper sections in search of an involved hair follicle. Inclusion bodies and multinucleate cells are not always found in the follicular epithelium.

DERMATOPHYTE FOLLICULITIS

Fungal elements may be seen on or within the hair shafts in certain dermatophyte infections, particularly tinea capitis (see p. 644). Various organisms may be involved, particularly *Trichophyton tonsurans*, *Microsporum canis* and *M. audouinii*. Sometimes an inflamed boggy mass, known as a kerion, develops.

Histopathology

There is variable inflammation of the follicle and perifollicular dermis. If disruption of the hair follicle occurs, a few foreign body giant cells may be present. Hyphae and arthrospores may be found within the hair shaft, or on the surface, depending on the nature of the infection. PAS or methenamine silver preparations are usually required in order to demonstrate the fungal elements.

Abscess formation with partial or complete destruction of hair follicles occurs in a kerion.

PITYROSPORUM FOLLICULITIS

This entity, resulting from infection of the follicle by *Malassezia furfur* (*Pityrosporum*), has been described on page 650. The small oval yeast responsible can be seen within the inflamed follicle and may be found in the adjacent dermis following rupture of the follicle.

DEEP SCARRING FOLLICULITIDES

In this group there is severe folliculitis involving the deep part of the follicle and often the upper part as well. Rupture of the follicle and its contents into the dermis leads to eventual scarring of variable severity. It is usually mild in folliculitis decalvans, but quite marked in folliculitis keloidalis nuchae. A similar picture can be seen following severe petrol burns of the skin.[94]

FOLLICULITIS DECALVANS

This chronic form of deep folliculitis usually occurs on the scalp as oval patches of scarring alopecia at the expanding margins of which are follicular pustules.[53,95] Any or all of the hairy areas of the body may be involved. Folliculitis barbae (lupoid sycosis) is a related condition confined to the beard area,[96] while epilating folliculitis of the glabrous skin is the name used in the earlier literature for a related condition involving the legs.[97]

Folliculitis decalvans usually runs a prolonged course of variable severity. The aetiology is unknown, although *Staphylococcus aureus* is sometimes cultured from the lesions.

Histopathology[53,95]

Initially there is a folliculitis, which is followed by disruption of the follicular wall and liberation of the contents of the follicle into the dermis (Fig. 15.4). The dermis adjacent to the destroyed follicle contains a mixed inflammatory cell infiltrate. Plasma cells are sometimes present in the infiltrate, particularly in resolving lesions. Foreign body giant cells may form around the hair shafts lying free in the dermis. Variable scarring results, but this is never as severe as in folliculitis keloidalis nuchae.

FOLLICULITIS KELOIDALIS NUCHAE

This condition, also known as acne keloidalis, is a rare, idiopathic, inflammatory condition of the nape of the neck, restricted to adult males.[98–99] It is more common in blacks. There are follicular papules and pustules which enlarge, forming confluent, thickened plaques, sometimes with discharging sinuses.[98,100] Scarring results from this chronic inflammatory process.

Histopathology[98,98a]

There is an initial folliculitis with subsequent rupture and destruction of the follicle and liberation of hair shafts into the dermis (Fig. 15.5).[98a] Usually, by the time a biopsy is taken,

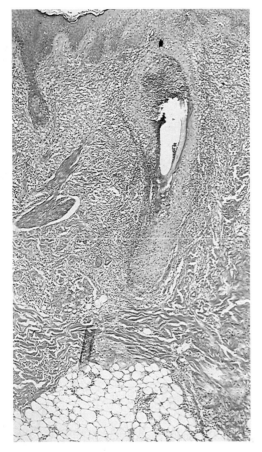

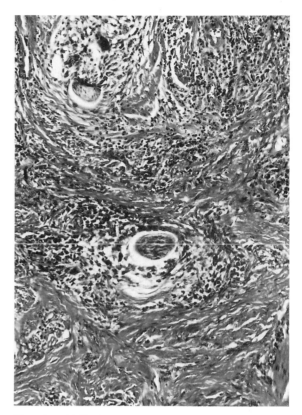

Fig. 15.5   Folliculitis keloidalis. A hair shaft lies free in the scarred and inflamed dermis.
Haematoxylin — eosin

Fig. 15.4   Folliculitis decalvans. The patient had a scarring alopecia. There is early disruption of the wall of an inflamed follicle.
Haematoxylin — eosin

there is already dense dermal fibrosis with a chronic inflammatory cell infiltrate which includes numerous plasma cells. Hair shafts are present in the dermis and these are surrounded by microabscesses and/or foreign body giant cells. Sinus tracts may lead to the surface. Sometimes there are claw-like epidermal downgrowths associated with the transepidermal elimination of hair shafts and inflammatory debris.[101] Intact follicles at the margins may show polytrichia.[98] Keloid fibres develop within the dense fibrous tissue in some cases.[98]

FOLLICULAR OCCLUSION TRIAD

The follicular occlusion triad refers to hidradenitis suppurativa, dissecting cellulitis of the scalp and acne conglobata. These three conditions constitute a form of deep scarring folliculitis: they are grouped together on the basis of their presumed common pathogenesis of poral occlusion[102] followed by bacterial infection.[103] The presence of draining sinuses is a further characteristic feature of this group. It has been suggested that pilonidal sinus is a related entity. These follicular occlusion disorders may coexist.[104]

HIDRADENITIS SUPPURATIVA

Hidradenitis suppurativa is a chronic, relapsing, inflammatory disorder involving one or more apocrine-gland-bearing areas, which include the axillae, groins, pubic region and perineum.[105–107] There are recurrent, deep-seated inflammatory nodules, complicated by draining sinuses and subsequent scarring. The development of squamous cell carcinoma is a late and rare complication.[108,109] Other clinical features include the presence of comedones in retroauricular and apocrine sites,[110] a female predominance,[111] and a genetic predisposition.[112,113] Host defence mechanisms are usually normal,[114] except in some severe cases, where a reduction in T lymphocytes has been documented.[115] There is now good evidence that hidradenitis suppurativa is an androgen-dependent disorder,[116–118] although how this relates to the presumed pathogenesis of poral occlusion with subsequent infection is uncertain.

Histopathology

In established lesions, there is a heavy, mixed inflammatory cell infiltrate in the lower half of the dermis, usually with extension into the subcutis.[119] Chronic abscesses are present in active cases and these may connect with sinus tracts leading to the skin surface (Fig. 15.6). The sinuses are usually lined by stratified squamous epithelium in their outer part. They contain inflammatory and other debris.[120] Some of these tracts are probably residual follicular structures.[120a]

Granulation tissue containing inflammatory cells and occasional foreign body giant cells may be present in some cases. Extensive fibrosis with destruction of pilosebaceous follicles and of apocrine and eccrine glands usually ensues. Uncommonly, inflammation of the apocrine glands is present (Fig. 15.7).

In early lesions, there is folliculitis and perifolliculitis involving the lower part of the follicle. The infundibulum is usually dilated and contains keratinous material and inflammatory debris.

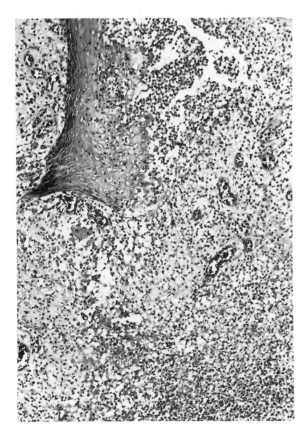

Fig. 15.6 Hidradenitis suppurativa. There is acute and chronic inflammation in the deep dermis and an epithelium-lined tract (probably of follicular origin) draining the area. Haematoxylin — eosin

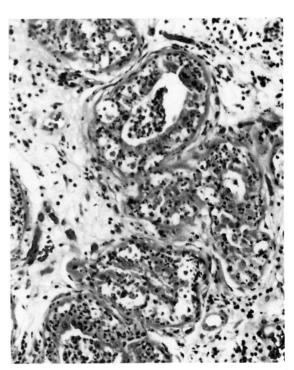

Fig. 15.7 Hidradenitis suppurativa. Inflammation of the apocrine glands is present in this unusual case. Haematoxylin — eosin

DISSECTING CELLULITIS OF THE SCALP

This extremely rare disease, also known as perifolliculitis capitis abscedens et suffodiens (Hoffmann's disease), is characterized by the appearance of tender, suppurative nodules with interconnecting draining sinuses and subsequent scarring.[121-123] Patchy alopecia usually overlies the lesions, which have a predilection for the vertex and occipital scalp.[124] There is a predilection for young adult black males. Dissecting cellulitis may occur alone, or in association with the other follicular occlusion diseases — hidradenitis suppurativa and acne conglobata.[104]

The development of squamous cell carcinoma is a rare complication.[125]

Histopathology[126,127]

The earliest lesion is a folliculitis and perifolliculitis with a heavy infiltrate of neutrophils leading to abscess formation in the dermis. Draining sinuses may develop and in later lesions the infiltrate becomes mixed. Variable destruction of follicles ensues.

ACNE CONGLOBATA

Acne conglobata is an uncommon dermatosis, occurring almost exclusively in males, and commencing after puberty. There are small and large, tender, inflamed nodules, cysts and discharging sinuses that eventually heal leaving disfiguring scars.[128] Lesions may develop in any hair-bearing area, particularly the trunk, buttocks and proximal parts of the extremities. The distribution is much wider than in hidradenitis suppurativa.

Malignant degeneration has been reported in lesions of acne conglobata of long standing.[128]

Histopathology

The appearances are similar to hidradenitis suppurativa, with deep abscesses and mixed inflammation, foreign body granulomas and discharging sinuses.[120] Comedones are often present.

MISCELLANEOUS FOLLICULITIDES

There are several folliculitides that do not fit appropriately into the categories already discussed. They include pseudofolliculitis, pruritic folliculitis of pregnancy and perforating folliculitis. Follicular pustules have also been reported in association with toxic erythema,[129] and in young individuals with acne treated with systemic steroids (see p. 437).[53]

PSEUDOFOLLICULITIS

Pseudofolliculitis is a common disorder of adult black males, usually confined to the beard area of the face and neck.[130,131] Rarely the scalp,[132] pubic area[133] and legs[134] may be involved. It consists of papules and pustules in close proximity to hair follicles. Scarring and keloid formation sometimes result.[135]

Pseudofolliculitis is an inflammatory response to an ingrown hair. Hair shafts in black people have a tendency to form tight coils, and following shaving the sharp ends may pierce the skin adjacent to the orifice of the follicles.[132]

Histopathology[130]

Surprisingly little has been written about the histopathology of this common disorder. There are parafollicular inflammatory foci which are initially suppurative. Small foreign body granulomas and a mixed inflammatory cell infiltrate are present in older lesions. Variable scarring may ensue. In some instances, epithelium grows down from the surface to encase both the hair and the inflammatory response, assisting in their eventual transepithelial elimination.

PRURITIC FOLLICULITIS OF PREGNANCY

This is a rare dermatosis of pregnancy in which

pruritic, erythematous papules develop in a widespread distribution in the latter half of pregnancy.[136] The lesions clear spontaneously at delivery or in the postpartum period. The aetiology is unknown.

Histopathology[136]

The appearances are those of an acute folliculitis, sometimes resulting in destruction of follicular walls and abscess formation in the adjacent dermis. No organisms have been noted in the cases reported so far.

PERFORATING FOLLICULITIS

Perforating folliculitis is manifested by discrete, keratotic, follicular papules with a predilection for the extensor surfaces of the extremities and the buttocks.[137,138] It may persist for months or years, although periods of remission often occur. Disease associations have included psoriasis,[139] juvenile acanthosis nigricans, primary sclerosing cholangitis[140] and renal failure, often in association with haemodialysis.[138,141]

The features of perforating folliculitis associated with renal failure (see page 286) may overlap those of reactive perforating collagenosis and Kyrle's disease[138] (the latter disease has been regarded by some as a variant of perforating folliculitis).[142] Lesions associated with renal failure are often pruritic, in contrast to the asymptomatic lesions of the majority of cases.[143]

The aetiology of perforating folliculitis is unknown, although minor mechanical trauma may play a role. It has been suggested that perforation of the epithelium is the primary event and that it is not a disorder of transepithelial elimination (see p. 26).[143]

Histopathology[53,137,138]

There is a dilated follicular infundibulum filled with keratinous and cellular debris. A curled hair shaft is sometimes present. The follicular epithelium is disrupted in one or more areas in the infundibulum. The adjacent dermis shows degenerative changes involving the connective

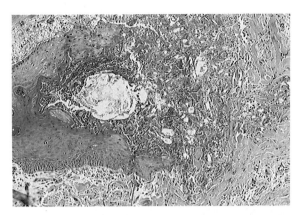

Fig. 15.8 Perforating folliculitis. Degenerate collagen and elastic tissue are entering the perforated follicle. The patient had chronic renal failure.
Haematoxylin — eosin

tissue, and sometimes collagen and elastic fibres are seen entering the perforation (Fig. 15.8). The elastic fibres are not increased as in elastosis perforans serpiginosa. A variable inflammatory reaction is present in the dermis in this region and sometimes a granulomatous perifolliculitis develops. Although a few neutrophils may be present in the infiltrate, they are never as plentiful as in pityrosporum folliculitis, which often ruptures into the dermis (see p. 650). Sometimes the follicular localization of perforating folliculitis is not appreciated unless serial sections are examined.

In chronic renal failure the lesion begins as a follicular pustule which perforates, resulting in a suppurative and granulomatous perifolliculitis.[144] Late lesions may develop epidermal features of prurigo nodularis (see p. 732).[144,145]

2. HAIR SHAFT ABNORMALITIES

Hair shafts may be abnormal as a result of an intrinsic defect, either congenital or acquired, in the hair shaft itself, or because of the deposition or attachment of extraneous matter such as fungi, bacteria or lacquer.[146] In either case, structural weakness of the hair shaft may occur; the resulting hair breakage and loss may be severe enough to produce alopecia.

Several clinical classifications of hair shaft abnormalities have been proposed.[146–148] One such classification distinguishes the structural defects with increased fragility from those without this characteristic, as only the cases in the former group (monilethrix, pili torti, trichorrhexis nodosa, trichothiodystrophy, Netherton's syndrome and Menkes' syndrome) present clinically with patchy or diffuse alopecia.[147] Another clinical approach has been to separate off those conditions associated with 'unruly hair', namely woolly hair, acquired progressive kinking of hair, pili torti, and rare cases associated with brain-growth deficiency.[149]

The classification to be followed here is morphologically based, and it is similar to the one proposed by Whiting.[146] Four major groups exist:

Fractures of hair shafts
Irregularities of hair shafts
Coiling and twisting abnormalities
Extraneous matter on hair shafts.

FRACTURES OF HAIR SHAFTS

This is the most important group of hair shaft abnormalities because it may lead to alopecia. However, sometimes these abnormalities occur sporadically or intermittently,[150] involving only isolated hairs as an incidental phenomenon. This is particularly likely to occur in those who subject their hair to physical or chemical trauma. More than one type of fracture may be present in these cases.[151] The following types of fractures will be considered:

Trichorrhexis nodosa
Trichoschisis
Trichoclasis
Trichorrhexis invaginata
Tapered fracture
Trichoptilosis.

TRICHORRHEXIS NODOSA

This condition is characterized by one or more small, beaded swellings along the hair shaft,

corresponding to sites that fracture easily. Scalp hair is most often involved although the genital region may also be affected.[152] Because the hairs fracture easily, alopecia may result.

The basic cause of trichorrhexis nodosa is prolonged mechanical trauma or chemical insults,[153] although a contributing factor in some instances is an inherent weakness of the hair shaft.[154] This weakness may result from a specific pilar dystrophy such as pili torti, monilethrix and trichorrhexis invaginata, or from an inborn error of metabolism affecting the hair such as arginosuccinic aminoaciduria, Menkes' syndrome[155] or trichothiodystrophy.[148,156–157a] This latter group of abnormalities is quite rare but they usually form the basis of hereditary cases of trichorrhexis nodosa.[157]

Histopathology

The expanded areas of the hair shaft are composed of frayed cortical fibres which usually remain attached.[151,158] This appearance has been likened to the splayed bristles of two paint brushes (or brooms) thrust into one another (Fig. 15.9).[159] The cuticular cells become disrupted prior to this splaying of the cortical fibres.

In black people, trauma-related cases of trichorrhexis nodosa usually affect the proximal part of the hair shaft, whereas in white and oriental races the distal part is more often affected.[146]

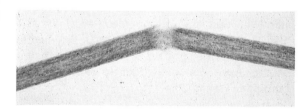

Fig. 15.9   Trichorrhexis nodosa with its characteristic fracturing of the hair shaft.

TRICHOSCHISIS

Trichoschisis is a clean transverse fracture of the hair shaft through the cuticle and cortex.[146] It is usually seen in the brittle hair associated with trichothiodystrophy, a condition in which the sulphur content of the hair is less than 50% of normal.[146,159] This results from a deficiency of the sulphur-containing amino acid cystine in the cuticle and cortex.[160,161] Trichothiodystrophy is often associated with *b*rittle hair, *i*mpaired *i*ntelligence, *d*ecreased fertility and *s*hort stature (BIDS syndrome), sometimes combined with *i*chthyosis (IBIDS syndrome).[160,162]

Histopathology

Trichoschisis involves a clean transverse break in the shaft.[146] In those with underlying trichothiodystrophy there are striking bright and dark bands seen with polarized light.[162] Lesions resembling trichorrhexis nodosa may also be present.

On scanning electron microscopy, the cuticle scales are often damaged or absent and there may be abnormal ridging of the surface.

TRICHOCLASIS

There is a transverse or oblique fracture of the shaft with irregular borders and a cuticle which is partly intact.[146] As such it resembles a greenstick fracture.[146] It does not indicate any specific underlying systemic disease, but rather it may follow trauma to the hair or be associated with pili torti, monilethrix or other hair shaft abnormalities (see below).

TRICHORRHEXIS INVAGINATA

Trichorrhexis invaginata (bamboo hair) is a rare, but unique abnormality of the hair shaft in which there are nodose swellings that give the hair an appearance reminiscent of a bamboo stem.[163] The scalp hair is usually short, dull and friable and the eyebrows and eyelashes may be sparse.[159] It is one of the hair anomalies associated with Netherton's syndrome, an autosomal recessive disorder in which there is also ichthyosis linearis circumflexa or some other ichthyosiform dermatosis (see page 270).[148,163]

This hair shaft anomaly is seen less characteristically as a sporadic change following trauma, or in association with other hair shaft abnormalities.[146,163]

Trichorrhexis invaginata may result from a transient defect of keratinization of the hair shaft due to incomplete cystine linkages, leading to softness of the cortex at the point of disruption.[163]

Histopathology

There is a cup-like expansion of the proximal part of the hair shaft which surrounds the club-shaped distal segment in the manner of a ball and socket joint.[146]

Transmission electron microscopy shows cleavages and electron-dense depositions in the cortex.[163]

TAPERED FRACTURE

This refers to a progressive narrowing of the emerging hair shaft as a result of inhibition of protein synthesis in the hair root.[146] Fracture of the shaft may occur near the skin surface. Tapered fractures ('pencil-pointing') are seen in anagen effluvium (see p. 464) caused by cytotoxic drugs.[146]

TRICHOPTILOSIS

Trichoptilosis refers to longitudinal splitting or fraying of the distal part of the hair shaft as a result of persistent trauma.[164] It results from separation of the longitudinal cortical fibres following loss of the cuticle from wear and tear.[146] A rare variant with the split in the centre of the hair and reconstitution of the shaft distal to this has been reported.[165]

IRREGULARITIES OF HAIR SHAFTS

This group of hair shaft abnormalities is characterized by various morphological irregularities in the hair. A common change, which is sometimes classified as a discrete abnormality, is longitudinal grooving of the hair. It is usually an isolated phenomenon of no clinical importance, although rarely it is widespread and associated with a form of congenital hypotrichosis or with trichothiodystrophy.[146] It will not be considered further.

Included in this group are the following entities:

Pili canaliculati et trianguli
Pili bifurcati
Pili multigemini
Trichostasis spinulosa
Pili annulati
Monilethrix
Tapered hairs
Bubble hair.

Each of these entities will be considered in turn.

PILI CANALICULATI ET TRIANGULI

This rare disorder of the hair shaft is also known as the uncombable hair syndrome and the spunglass hair syndrome.[166–168] The hair is drier, glossier and lighter, and it is unmanageable in that it does not lie flat when combed.[169,170] The condition derives its name from the longitudinal canalicular depression in one side of the shaft and its triangular or kidney shape in cross section.[169] It may result from a disorder of keratinization of the hair.[148]

Straight hair naevus, a localized disorder in which the involved hairs are short and straight, in contrast to the usual woolly hair of black people, in whom this condition has been described, has been regarded as a localized form of uncombable hair.[171] However, it should be noted that in straight hair naevus there may be an associated epidermal naevus; furthermore, the hairs are normal in cross section, in contrast to pili canaliculati et trianguli.[172,173]

Histopathology

The hairs appear normal on light microscopy.[167] However, under polarized light they have a diagnostic homogeneous band on one edge.[167]

Paraffin-blocked hairs have a triangular or kidney-shaped appearance on transverse section.[167] The shape is confirmed by scanning electron microscopy which also shows the longitudinal depression of the shaft resembling a canal.[159,167]

PILI BIFURCATI

In the condition known as pili bifurcati, hairs show intermittent bifurcations of the shaft which subsequently rejoin further along the shaft to form a normal structure.[174] Unlike trichoptilosis, which it superficially resembles, each ramus of the bifurcated segments is invested by its own cuticle.[174] This abnormality has been regarded as a restricted form of pili multigemini.[146]

PILI MULTIGEMINI

This rare malformation of the pilary apparatus is associated with the emergence of multiple hairs from a follicular canal which in turn is composed of as many papillae as there are hairs.[175] These multigeminate follicles may arise on the face or the scalp. It differs from *tufted folliculitis*[175a,175b] in which distinctive tufts of multiple hairs emerge from a single follicular orifice into which several complete follicles open. Tufted folliculitis has been regarded as the consequence of bacterial folliculitis with scarring, and as a naevoid abnormality of hair follicles which are prone to inflammation.[175b]

TRICHOSTASIS SPINULOSA

This condition presents either as asymptomatic, comedone-like lesions on the nose,[176] or as mildly pruritic hyperkeratotic papules on the upper trunk or arms.[146,177,178] With a hand lens, multiple vellus hairs can sometimes be seen protruding from the patulous follicles. There is retention of telogen hairs within the follicles, although the reason for this is unknown.[177]

Histopathology[178]

Multiple hairs are enveloped in a keratinous sheath within a dilated hair follicle. The keratin plug may protrude above the skin surface. There is only one hair matrix and papilla at the base of the follicle,[146] in contrast to pili multigemini. Sometimes there is mild perifollicular inflammation.

PILI ANNULATI

The condition of pili annulati (ringed hairs) is a rare, familial or sporadic anomaly in which there are alternating light and dark bands along the shaft, when viewed by reflected light.[179,180] Axillary hair is occasionally affected.

The light bands are due to clusters of abnormal, air-filled cavities which appear to result from insufficient production of the interfibrillar matrix.[179,181]

The term *pseudopili annulati* refers to the presence of light and dark bands when slightly flattened or twisted hair is examined under reflected light.[182] It is thought to be a variant of normal hair and to have no clinical significance.[146]

Histopathology

The alternating light and dark bands occur approximately every 0.5 mm along the shaft when viewed by reflected light.[158,181,183] Scanning electron microscopy reveals the presence of many small holes within the cortex as well as an irregular arrangement of the cuticular scales.[181]

MONILETHRIX

In monilethrix the hairs have a beaded or moniliform appearance as a result of a periodic decrease in the diameter of the hair.[184] Inheritance is usually as an autosomal dominant trait with high gene penetrance but variable expressivity.[146]

The hair is susceptible to fracture at the narrower internodal regions, leading to short hair

and hair loss.[153] The occipital region is usually involved soon after birth and the affected area slowly extends.[148] Other hairy areas may also be involved. Some improvement occurs with age, and occasionally there is spontaneous remission at puberty.[159]

The defect leading to monilethrix may result from a periodic dysfunction of the hair matrix.[184,185] Abnormalities also exist in the inner root sheath adjacent to the zones of abnormal shaft thinning.

Pseudomonilethrix is now considered to be an artefact in which irregularly placed nodes develop at irregular intervals along the hair shaft as a result of the compression of normal or fragile hairs between glass slides, prior to their microscopic examination.[186–188]

Histopathology

The elliptical nodes of monilethrix, which are 0.7–1 mm apart, are separated by tapered internodes lacking a medulla (Fig. 15.10).[148] Scanning electron microscopy shows weathering changes with loss of cuticular cells and the presence of longitudinal grooves on the internodal shaft.[146,184]

Fractures and trichorrhexis nodosa may also be present.

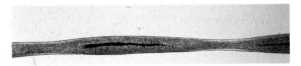

Fig. 15.10   Monilethrix. The tapered internodal regions lack a medulla.

TAPERED HAIRS

Tapered hairs can arise in the same way as tapered fractures (see p. 449), and they may also occur in association with other abnormalities of the hair shaft.[146] Several distinct variants have been described. The *Pohl–Pinkus mark* is an isolated narrowing of the hair shaft which coincides with a surgical operation, or some other traumatic episode.[146] This narrowing is not as abrupt in the *bayonet hair*, which may possibly be a form of the Pohl–Pinkus mark.[146] Newly growing anagen hairs often have a tapered, hypopigmented top.

BUBBLE HAIR

This rare abnormality is characterized by a large cavity in the shaft on scanning electron microscopy and an unusual 'bubble' appearance on light microscopy. It presents with a localized area of brittle, easily broken hairs on the scalp.[189]

COILING AND TWISTING ABNORMALITIES

As the heading suggests, the hair shafts in this group of disorders adopt various configurations.[146] The following are involved:

Pili torti
Woolly hair
Acquired progressive kinking
Trichonodosis
Circle hair.

The condition of pili torti is the most important member of this group, while trichonodosis and circle hairs are of little consequence.

PILI TORTI

Pili torti result from a structural defect in which the hair shaft is twisted on its axis at irregular intervals, with flattening of the hair at the sites of twisting.[190] This leads to increased fragility, particularly in areas subjected to trauma.[149] There are several clinical settings in which pili torti can occur.[146]

The rare congenital (Ronchese) type presents at birth or soon after, with a localized area of alopecia or short hair which gradually spreads.[146] Sites other than the scalp may be affected. Pili torti may occur alone or in association with other syndromes, particularly of ectodermal type. These include Bazex's,

Crandall's and Bjornstad's syndromes[191] as well as hypohidrotic ectodermal dysplasia.[149] They also occur in citrullinaemia[190] and in Menkes' kinky hair syndrome.[148,159]

Postpubertal onset has also been recorded (Beare type).[149] Involvement of multiple hair-bearing sites and mental retardation are usually a feature of this variant. An acquired form of pili torti has been described as a result of trauma, associated with cicatricial alopecia, following the use of synthetic retinoids (isotretinoin),[192] and on the abdomen and thighs of hirsute males and females.[193] Pili torti of early onset may improve with age.

Histopathology

The twisting of the shaft is easily appreciated on light microscopy (Fig. 15.11). Fractures and trichorrhexis nodosa are sometimes present as well.[153,194] Corkscrew hairs, with the shaft coiled into a double spiral, have been seen in pili torti.[146]

Curvatures and twisting have been recorded in the hair follicles that produce pili torti.[146,148]

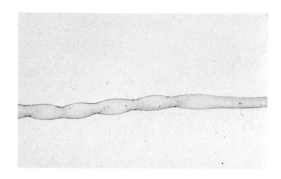

Fig. 15.11   Pilus tortus. Twisting of the hair shaft is present.

WOOLLY HAIR

Woolly hair is very curly hair that is difficult to style.[195] It is normal in most black races but in white races it occurs in several different clinical settings.[146,196] These include an autosomal dominant form which affects the entire scalp (the hereditary type), an autosomal recessive form (the familial type), a diffuse partial form where shorter, finer, curly hair is interspersed with normal hair,[196] and a well-demarcated localized form (woolly hair naevus) which may be associated with an ipsilateral epidermal naevus.[197–198a] Acquired progressive kinking of the hair (see below) is sometimes included as a variant of woolly hair.[148]

Histopathology

The hairs are usually normal on light microscopy, although on cross section the shaft diameter is sometimes reduced.[146] In woolly hair naevus the hairs are more oval on cross section than normal hairs;[196] a case with triangular hairs has been reported.[197] The follicles may be somewhat curved in woolly hair naevus.

ACQUIRED PROGRESSIVE KINKING

This rare disorder of the hair shaft is sometimes considered to be a variant of woolly hair, but it is best regarded as a distinct entity on the basis of its onset at or after puberty, the involvement of certain regions of the scalp rather than the entire scalp and the tendency for affected hair to resemble pubic hair both in texture and colour.[199–201] Acquired progressive kinking of the hair tends to occur in males who subsequently develop a male pattern alopecia of fairly rapid onset.[199,202] 'Whisker hair', which occurs not uncommonly about the ears, is probably a variant.[146,199,203]

Histopathology

There is usually some flattening of the hair shafts with partial twisting at irregular intervals.[202] Longitudinal canalicular grooves can be demonstrated on scanning electron microscopy.[202,204]

TRICHONODOSIS

Trichonodosis (knotted hair) is usually an incidental finding in individuals with various lengths and types of scalp hair, particularly those with curly or kinky hair.[205,206] There may be a single or a double knot. Various hair shaft abnormalities of a secondary nature may be present in and adjacent to the knots.[146]

CIRCLE HAIR

Circle hair (rolled hair) presents as a black circle related to hair follicles as the result of a hair shaft becoming coiled into a circle under a thin transparent roof of stratum corneum.[207,208] The cause of this abnormality is unknown but it may be seen in middle-aged men on the back, abdomen and thighs.[208]

Histopathology

Keratotic plugs containing a coiled or broken hair are a characteristic feature of keratosis pilaris (see p. 467).[208] Similar changes are seen in some cases of circle hair, although keratotic follicular plugging is not always present.[208]

EXTRANEOUS MATTER ON HAIR SHAFTS

Hair shafts may be colonized by fungi (tinea capitis and piedra), bacteria (trichomycosis axillaris) and the eggs (nits) of the lice causing pediculosis capitis.[146] Casts resembling nits (hair casts, pseudo-nits) may occur in association with various scaly dermatoses of the scalp or as a rare, idiopathic phenomenon. Deposits such as lacquer, paint and glue form another category of extraneous matter.

TINEA CAPITIS

In tinea capitis (see p. 642), fungal elements may be found on the surface of the hair shaft (ectothrix) or within the substance of the hair (endothrix).[146] In both cases the affected hairs are fragile and break near the skin surface.

PIEDRA

The condition known as piedra occurs in two forms, white piedra and black piedra.[146] They are characterized by the formation of minute concretions on the affected hair (the Spanish word *piedra* means stone).

White piedra (trichosporonosis, trichosporosis)[209–211] is a rare superficial infection of the terminal part of the hair caused by the yeast-like fungus *Trichosporon beigelii* (see p. 650). It occurs particularly in South America, parts of Europe, Japan and the USA.[212] There are numerous discrete or coalescing cream-coloured nodules, just visible to the naked eye, forming sleeve-like concretions attached to the hair shaft.[213,214] White piedra may affect hairs on the face, scalp or scrotum.[213] Fracture of the hair shaft may result.

Black piedra, which is caused by the ascomycete *Piedraia hortai*, consists of gritty black nodules which are darker, firmer and more adherent than those found in white piedra.[214] Black piedra is prevalent in tropical climates.

Histopathology

In *white piedra*, a potassium hydroxide preparation of a hair shows that the concretions are composed of numerous fungal arthrospores in compact masses encasing the hair shaft.[214] In *black piedra*, the nodules are composed of brown hyphae with ovoid asci containing 2–8 ascospores.[214]

TRICHOMYCOSIS AXILLARIS

In this condition, there are tiny, cream to yellow nodules attached to axillary or pubic hair (Fig. 15.12).[146] It is not a mycosis but the result of infection by species of *Corynebacterium* (see p. 602).

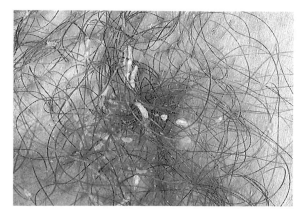

Fig. 15.12   Trichomycosis. Small pale nodules are attached to some of the hair shafts.

PEDICULOSIS CAPITIS

Nits are small, white to brown ovoid structures attached to the hair shaft.[146] They are the eggs of the lice responsible for pediculosis capitis (see p. 723).

Histopathology

The egg lies to one side of the hair shaft, to which it is attached by a sheath that envelops both the shaft and the base of the egg.[146]

HAIR CASTS

Hair casts (peripilar casts, pseudo-nits) are firmish, yellow-white concretions, 3–7 mm long, ensheathing hairs and movable along them.[215] Two types of hair casts exist.[216,217] The more common type (*parakeratotic hair cast*) is associated with various inflammatory scalp disorders such as psoriasis, seborrhoeic dermatitis and pityriasis capitis.[216] The second type (*peripilar keratin cast*), which is quite uncommon, occurs predominantly in female children without any underlying disease as a diffuse disorder of scalp hair.[217] Hair casts appear to be nothing more than portions of root sheath pulled out of the follicle by a hair shaft itself.[218]

Histopathology[218,219]

In both types of hair casts the follicular openings contain parakeratotic keratinous material which breaks off at intervals to form the hair casts. In casts associated with parakeratotic disorders it seems that only external sheath is present in the casts. In the uncommon peripilar casts both inner and outer root sheaths are demonstrable on transverse section of the cast. Scanning electron microscopy has confirmed the presence of an inner, incomplete layer and an outer, thicker, but less compact layer.[218]

DEPOSITS

Various substances may become adherent to hair shafts causing an unusual appearance on microscopy.[146] These include paint, hair spray, lacquer and glue. Microscopy reveals that the deposits are not inherent parts of the hair shaft.[146]

3. ALOPECIAS

There are several hundred disease states or events which may precipitate abnormal hair loss.[220] As a consequence, any aetiological classification of the alopecias is invariably comprised of long lists of causative factors.[221] From a clinical viewpoint, alopecias are usually divided into those that are patterned and those that diffusely involve the scalp. Further subclassification into scarring and non-scarring types is usually made.[220] Because scarring alopecias are almost invariably irreversible, they are of great clinical importance. Biopsies are not often taken from alopecias which are diffuse and non-scarring as the aetiology is often apparent to the clinician, or the alopecia is subclinical or not of cosmetic significance.

A more useful approach for the dermatopathologist is a classification based on the mechanisms involved in the hair loss.[222] This has some shortcomings in that our knowledge of these mechanisms is not complete, particularly in some of the congenital/hereditary alopecias. Furthermore, some of the early reports of this group lack histological descriptions of the skin and hair shafts. For this reason, the congenital/hereditary alopecias will be considered together until further knowledge allows a more accurate subdivision based on the mechanism involved.

The following classification of alopecias will be used in the account which follows:

Congenital/hereditary alopecias
Premature catagen/telogen
Premature telogen with anagen arrest
Vellus follicle formation
Anagen defluvium
Scarring alopecias
Hair shaft abnormalities (see p. 447).

Before discussing the various mechanisms of hair loss, brief mention will be made of the normal hair cycle.

The normal hair cycle

The formation of hairs is a cyclical phenomenon which results from successive periods of growth, involution and rest by hair follicles.[223,224] The phase of active hair production is known as *anagen*. It lasts for a period of 2–6 years on the scalp, although the average duration is usually quoted as 1000 days.[146] At any one time, 85–90% of the 100 000 hair follicles on the scalp are in the anagen phase. There is regional variation in the duration of anagen. For example, anagen lasts for approximately 1 year in the beard region, while its duration in the axilla and pubic region is only a few months.[225]

The involutionary stage, *catagen*, is quite short, lasting for less than 2 weeks in each hair follicle on the scalp. There is very little regional variation in the duration of catagen, although in some animals this period may be as short as 24 hours. Approximately 1% of scalp follicles are in the catagen phase at any time. In humans, the entry of follicles into catagen is a random process, in contrast to its synchronous onset in animals (moulting). Seasonal factors, including temperature and light intensity, play some role in precipitating moulting in certain animals. In other animals, and in humans, the factors which normally precipitate catagen are not known.[226] It follows a set period of anagen which is presumably genetically determined in some way for each particular region. The mechanism by which hair follicles shorten during catagen was an enigma for a long time. It was in part attributed to the cessation of mitoses in the hair matrix and also to 'collapse', 'regression', 'disintegration' and 'involution' of the lower follicle.[227] It is now known that massive cell loss by apoptosis is the mechanism responsible for catagen involution.[226-228] The apoptotic fragments are quickly phagocytosed by adjacent cells in the lower follicle and by macrophages.[226] With progressive retraction of the follicle resulting from this cell loss, there is wrinkling and thickening of the fibrous root sheath.

The resting phase, *telogen*, lasts for approximately 3–4 months. During this period, there is no active hair production.[225] At any one time, approximately 10–15% of scalp follicles are in this phase. Telogen is followed by regrowth of the hair follicle and a new anagen phase. The telogen hair (club hair) is extruded and shed at this time.

Each stage of the hair cycle has a characteristic morphological appearance.[223]

Catagen follicles are characterized by loss of mitotic activity in the matrix and the cessation of pigment production by melanocytes in the hair bulb. Scattered apoptotic cells develop in the outer root sheath, an easily recognizable sign of catagen (Fig. 15.13).[227] The inner root sheath disappears and there is progressive thickening and corrugation of the fibrous root sheath. The lower end of the follicle gradually retracts upwards with a trailing connective tissue streamer beneath it.

Telogen follicles consist of a short protrusion of basaloid, undifferentiated cells below the epithelial sac which surrounds the club hair. This is situated not far below the entrance of the sebaceous duct. The telogen hair, if plucked, has a short, club-shaped root which lacks root sheaths and a keratogenous zone. There is also depigmentation of the proximal part of the shaft.[146,225]

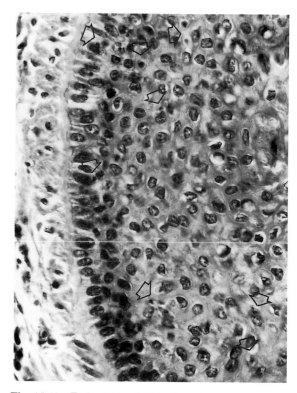

Fig. 15.13 Early catagen follicle. Note the numerous apoptotic cells.
Haematoxylin — eosin

Anagen growth recapitulates to some extent the changes present in the original development of the follicle.[229] There is increased mitotic activity in the germinal cells at the base of the telogen follicle. This ball of cells extends downwards, partly enclosing the dermal papilla.[230] Both descend into the dermis along the path of the connective tissue streamer which formed during the previous catagen phase. The matrix cells of the new anagen bulb form a new inner root sheath and hair.[230] Melanocytes lining the papillae form melanin again. The new hair eventually dislodges the club hair of the previous cycle. Plucked anagen hairs have long indented roots with intact inner and outer root sheaths and are fully pigmented.[225]

CONGENITAL/HEREDITARY ALOPECIAS

The rare alopecias of this clinical grouping are considered together because the mechanism involved in the pathogenesis of the hair loss is not known for some of the conditions.[230,231] Furthermore, biopsies have not been carried out on some of the entities listed, while in other instances the biopsy findings have not been consistent from one report to another. Several different clinical groups of congenital/hereditary alopecias are usually recognized:[159]

1. Alopecias without associated defects
2. Alopecias in association with ectodermal dysplasia
3. Alopecias as a characteristic or inconstant feature of a named syndrome.

Alopecia or hypotrichosis occurs without any associated defect in alopecia congenitalis, hereditary hypotrichosis (Marie–Unna type) and atrichia with papular lesions, and in keratosis pilaris atrophicans. They are considered further below. Localized alopecia, possibly occurring as a naevoid state, has been reported.[232] Another localized form of alopecia, congenital triangular alopecia, involves the presence of vellus follicles and is discussed on page 463.

Alopecia is a characteristic feature of one subgroup of the ectodermal dysplasias, a heterogeneous group of congenital diseases involving the epidermis and at least one appendage. Absence or hypoplasia of hair follicles has been recorded in some of these rare syndromes,[233] while in others no detailed studies have been made. The ectodermal dysplasias have been discussed on page 289. They will not be considered further here.

There is a long list of rare syndromes in which alopecia is a characteristic or inconstant feature. Skeletal abnormalities are present in one subgroup.[159,234] These have been reviewed elsewhere.[159] Little is known about the mechanism of the alopecia in this group. One entity, the Hallermann–Streiff syndrome, will be discussed briefly below because something is known of its pathology.

ALOPECIA CONGENITALIS

This diagnosis has been applied to cases of congenital alopecia without associated defects.[159,235] Hair loss occurs at birth or shortly after in one subgroup with autosomal recessive inheritance, while in those with autosomal dominant inheritance the hair is normal until mid childhood.[236,237]

Histopathology

Hair follicles are hypoplastic and reduced in number.[159] In the dominant form, follicles are said to be normal in number initially, but they fail progressively to re-enter anagen.[230]

HEREDITARY HYPOTRICHOSIS

Hereditary hypotrichosis (Marie–Unna type) presents with short, sparse hair at birth and progressive loss of hair resembling androgenic alopecia, commencing during adolescence.[159,238]

Histopathology

There are no specific features although progressive destruction of hair follicles is the probable mechanism.[159] Follicles are reduced in number.[238] Milia and perifollicular granulomas have been recorded.[159]

ATRICHIA WITH PAPULAR LESIONS

This is a rare disorder in which progressive shedding of scalp and body hair occurs in the first few months of life.[239,240] Eyelashes are typically spared. Numerous, small, milia-like cysts develop on the face, neck, scalp and extremities in childhood and early adult life.[240] Both autosomal dominant and recessive inheritance have been reported.

Histopathology[240]

The small follicular cysts resemble milia. They contain keratinous material, which is sometimes calcified, but there are no vellus hairs in the lumen. Scattered foreign body giant cells may be present around some of the cysts. In the scalp the infundibulum of the follicle is normally developed, although it often contains a keratin plug. There is a lack of development of the germinal end of the follicle, with no shaft formation.[239]

KERATOSIS PILARIS ATROPHICANS

Keratosis pilaris atrophicans refers to a group of clinically related syndromes in which inflammatory keratosis pilaris leads to atrophic scarring (see p. 342). This condition is mentioned here because it is a cause of scarring alopecia.

HALLERMANN–STREIFF SYNDROME

The Hallermann–Streiff syndrome (mandibulo-oculofacial dyscephaly) is a branchial arch syndrome which combines a characteristic facies with ocular abnormalities and alopecia, which may have an unusual sutural distribution on the scalp.[241] Atrophic patches of skin, which may be limited to the areas of alopecia, also occur.[241] Most cases appear to occur as new mutations.[230]

Histopathology

Very little is known about the histological characteristics of the alopecia, although the atrophic areas are composed of loosely woven collagen.[230] The hair shafts show some cuticular weathering on scanning electron microscopy.[241] Circumferential grooving of the shaft has also been noted in some cases.[242]

PREMATURE CATAGEN/TELOGEN

At any one time, approximately 10–15% of the hair follicles of the scalp are in the resting (telogen) phase, and, because of its shorter duration, only a small number of follicles are in the preceding involutionary stage of catagen. Under certain circumstances an abnormal

number of hair follicles is in the telogen phase. This results from the premature termination of anagen.[243] After a latent period of approximately 3 months from the onset of catagen/telogen, club hairs are lost, leading to thinning of the hair.[243] It is surprising how much hair can be lost before this thinning becomes noticeable.[243]

Numerous telogen follicles are found in telogen effluvium (see below), a condition which results from various stressful circumstances and from some drugs, such as heparin.[243] Because such conditions are not biopsied until the hair loss becomes noticeable, some 3 months after the onset, catagen hairs are not usually found.

In trichotillomania (see below) and certain traumatic alopecias, the insult is usually continuous and, accordingly, catagen follicles are seen in addition to telogen ones.[244] Catagen follicles are sometimes prominent at the rapidly advancing edge of a patch of alopecia areata.

In summary, catagen follicles are prominent in trichotillomania and related traumatic alopecias resulting from traction associated with hairstyles and the like. They are often seen at the edge of a patch of alopecia areata. Telogen follicles are prominent in telogen effluvium, in alopecia areata and in a rare disorder with onset in childhood, familial focal alopecia.[245] In this latter condition there is telogen arrest with prolonged persistence of telogen follicles in contrast to the transient nature of the process in telogen effluvium.[245]

TRICHOTILLOMANIA AND TRAUMATIC ALOPECIA

Trichotillomania is a rare form of alopecia resulting from the deliberate, although at times unconscious, avulsion of hairs by patients who may be under psychosocial stress.[246] In adults it is more common in women, although in children there has been no sex predilection in some series.

Although the crown and occipital scalp are primarily affected, other areas of the scalp, as well as the eyebrows, trunk and pubic areas, may also be involved. Similar features can result from traction of hair associated with hairstyles, and from prolonged pressure.[247] The term 'traumatic alopecia' can be applied to such cases, including trichotillomania.[248]

Clinical differentiation from alopecia areata can be difficult.

Histopathology[220,249–251a]

The histological features are characteristic, but not all of the recognized features are present in every biopsy. There is a greater chance of observing them if multiple sections are examined. The two most specific features are the presence of increased numbers of catagen hairs, associated usually with the presence of early and late anagen hairs, and the presence of empty hair ducts. Other changes include dilated follicular infundibula which may contain melanin casts

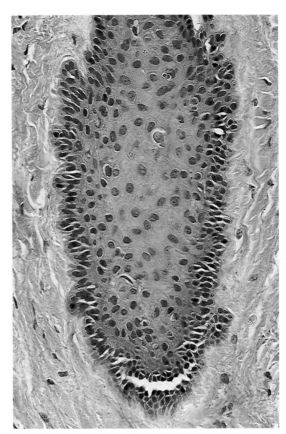

Fig. 15.15 Trichotillomania. Clefting has occurred at the dermal interface of the hair follicle which is showing early changes of catagen. Haematoxylin — eosin

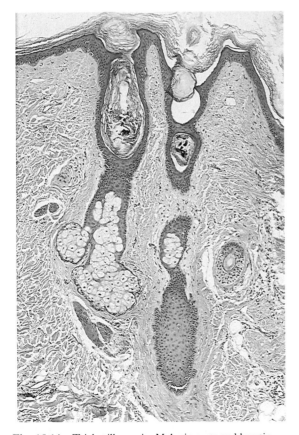

Fig. 15.14 Trichotillomania. Melanin casts and keratin plugs are present in the dilated follicular infundibula. Haematoxylin — eosin

and keratin plugs, clefts around the lower end of hair follicles, distortion of the hair bulb with dissociation of cells in the hair matrix, the release of melanin pigment within the papilla and surrounding connective tissue sheaths, traumatized connective tissue sheaths, small areas of dermal haemorrhage, and empty spaces in the sebaceous glands (Figs 15.14 and 15.15).[249] Sometimes there is even extrusion of sebaceous lobules. Only a very sparse inflammatory infiltrate is present.

TELOGEN EFFLUVIUM

Telogen effluvium has been regarded as a syndrome and as a non-specific reaction pattern, rather than as a disease sui generis.[243,252] It is nevertheless a useful term to apply to those cases of diffuse hair loss in which various stressful circumstances precipitate the premature termination of anagen. Telogen effluvium can follow febrile illness, parturition, systemic illnesses, chronic infections, air travellers' 'jet lag', psychogenic illnesses, 'crash diets', and sudden severe stress. It may also be associated with an internal cancer.[222,253] Loss of hair in the newborn is a physiological example of this process.[243] Exceptionally, drugs such as heparin, oral contraceptives, excess vitamin A and the antihypertensive agent minoxidil[254] have been implicated in the aetiology of telogen effluvium.[244]

Telogen effluvium presents as a diffuse thinning of the scalp hair, although the hair loss is not always obvious clinically. Sometimes this hair loss unmasks small areas of alopecia, of other causes, which had previously gone unnoticed.

Histopathology

A biopsy of the affected scalp will show a proportionately greater number of normal telogen follicles than usual. There is no inflammation in the dermis. An examination of plucked hairs will reveal telogen counts greater than 25%.

PREMATURE TELOGEN WITH ANAGEN ARREST

Alopecia areata is the only type of hair loss in which this mechanism applies. At the expanding edge, follicles in late catagen and telogen are characteristic findings, although in older lesions follicles in an arrested anagen phase are also present.

ALOPECIA AREATA

Alopecia areata is a relatively common condition affecting individuals of any age, but particularly those between the ages of 15 and 40.[255] Although mild cases may escape clinical detection, alopecia areata usually has a sudden onset with the development of one or more discrete, asymptomatic patches of non-scarring hair loss.[256] Exclamation mark hairs are found near the advancing margins.[256] The clinical course is variable. There may be spontaneous remission, sometimes followed by exacerbations, or there may be relentless progression to involve the entire scalp (alopecia totalis) and, uncommonly, all body hair (alopecia universalis).[257] Progression to alopecia totalis is more likely in children.[258] Regeneration is heralded by the development of fine white or tan hair.[256] A family history of alopecia areata is present in 10–25% of affected individuals.[255,258–260]

There are conflicting data on the clinical associations of alopecia areata. Many reports have documented an increased incidence of autoimmune diseases such as Hashimoto's thyroiditis, Addison's disease, vitiligo and lupus erythematosus, but not others.[256,257,261] Autoantibodies to various thyroid antigens,[262–264] gastric parietal cells[259] and smooth muscle[265] have been reported,[266,267] although not all of these findings have been confirmed by others.[268] No consistent HLA type has been found.[269] There are also conflicting results on the various cell-mediated functions in alopecia areata, but this may in part reflect the different techniques that have been used and the heterogeneous nature of this condition.[264,270] Other clinical associations have included atopic states,[271] Down's syndrome[272] and following vasectomy.[273] Various nail changes have been reported in 10% of patients.[274]

Although the pathogenesis of alopecia areata is not understood, the evidence for an immunological basis comes from five sources:[257,274a] the clinical association of other autoimmune diseases, the presence in some patients of circulating organ-specific autoantibodies (although none has been detected to any hair follicle component),[275] altered cellular immune functions,[276,277] the favourable effects of treatment with synthetic immunomodulators,[278,279] and the histopathological finding of activated T cells and HLA-DR expression[280] in the vicinity of the hair bulb.[281–284]

The basic disturbance is the premature entry

of anagen follicles into telogen, although some follicles survive for a time in a dystrophic anagen state.[285,286]

The term 'nanogen' has been proposed for the morphologically-distorted telogen follicle that is produced in alopecia areata.[287] Follicles may re-enter anagen, but growth appears to be halted in anagen stage III[288] and not IV as originally proposed.[289] Interestingly, follicles producing non-pigmented hair are less susceptible to premature telogen.[255] Cell deletion by apoptosis, probably cell-mediated, is the mechanism by which premature catagen and telogen come about. Apoptosis may also play a role in the anagen arrest which occurs.[288] Graft experiments suggest that hair growth ability in situ is normal and the causation is mediated humorally.[290]

Histopathology[285]

The appearances vary according to the duration of the process at the biopsy site (Figs 15.16 and 15.17). At the expanding edge the majority of the follicles are in late catagen and telogen. A few anagen follicles are in the subcutis while small mid-dermal ones may also be seen. The larger anagen follicles show a peribulbar infiltrate of lymphocytes (likened to a swarm of bees) and macrophages, and sometimes a few eosinophils and plasma cells.[285] The majority of the

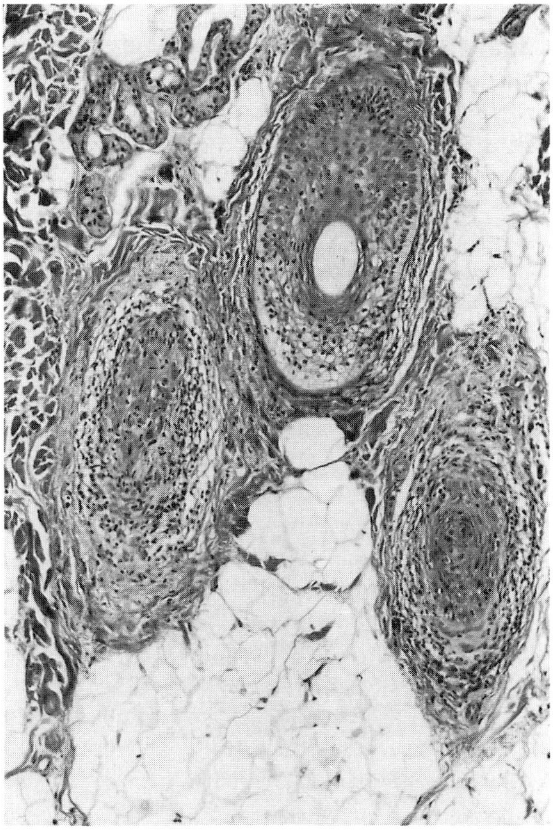

Fig. 15.17 Alopecia areata. There is a mild peribulbar infiltrate of lymphocytes — the so-called 'swarm of bees' appearance.
Haematoxylin — eosin

lymphocytes are small and mature.[281] The small anagen follicles show a disproportionate reduction in the size of the epithelial matrix relative to that of the dermal papilla.

In established cases and in alopecia totalis there are many telogen follicles and some small anagen follicles with mid-dermal bulbs.[285] The anagen/telogen ratio is variable. Although routine sections give the impression of marked follicle loss because of the absence of follicles in the subcutis, the use of transverse sections allows a better assessment of follicle density.[291,292] A transverse section at the level of the sebaceous gland will usually show a normal number of pilar units. This has prognostic significance because it indicates that normal regrowth of hair is theoretically possible in these circumstances.[291] There is only a mild peribulbar inflammatory cell

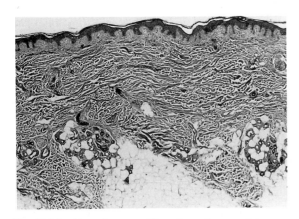

Fig. 15.16 Alopecia areata. There is an absence of the deeply-extending terminal hair follicles. A small anagen follicle (barely discernible) remains.
Haematoxylin — eosin

infiltrate around these small anagen follicles. Occasional apoptotic cells and mitoses can be seen. Atrophy of sebaceous glands is seen sometimes in longstanding cases.

In regenerating areas, the number of melanocytes and the degree of pigmentation of the cells in the hair bulb are much less than in the normal pigmented follicle.[285,288]

In all stages, a non-sclerotic fibrous tract extends along the site of the previous follicle into the subcutis. This fibrous tract contains a few small vessels, and small deposits of melanin. In cases of long standing there is widespread damage and fibrosis of the follicular sheath structures. There may be only a few lymphocytes and macrophages at the site of the previous hair bulb. There are no Arão–Perkins elastic bodies along this connective tissue tract, such as are seen in male pattern alopecia (see opposite).[293]

Immunofluorescence shows deposits of C3 and occasionally of IgG and IgM along the basement zone of the inferior segment of hair follicles.[294–296] Careful ultrastructural studies are needed to assess the role of lymphocyte-mediated apoptosis in the pathogenesis of this disease.

VELLUS FOLLICLE FORMATION

This group of alopecias is characterized by the presence of small vellus follicles in the dermis. In common baldness, which is the most important member of this group, an early biopsy may only show a progressive diminution in the size of follicles which are not truly vellus. In established lesions typical vellus follicles will be seen. Vellus follicles are also a feature of congenital triangular (temporal) alopecia but this presumably represents the development of vellus follicles in the affected site ab initio rather than the progressive reversion of terminal hair follicles to vellus follicles.

COMMON BALDNESS

Common baldness (androgenic alopecia) is a physiological event which may commence in males soon after puberty.[297] It occurs less often in females and its onset is a decade or so later than in males. Clinically there is progressive replacement of terminal hairs by fine, virtually unpigmented vellus hairs, with hair loss in distinct geographical areas of the scalp.[298] Increased shedding of hairs is usually noted.[297] In females, there may be features of hyperandrogenism such as hirsutism and acne.[299]

In males, the hair loss is patterned and involves the frontal, central and temporal regions. Various categories of male baldness have been defined, based on which of the above areas are involved.[297]

In females, three distinct patterns of baldness have been recognized.[300,301] The most common type is a diffuse fronto-vertical thinning without temporal recession.[299] The second type is similar to that seen in the male (male pattern alopecia). It is often associated with virilism, although in one study it was found in a significant number of normal postmenopausal women.[302] The third pattern is diffuse thinning confined to the vertex, and developing after the menopause.[300] In endocrinologically normal females, the rate of progression of baldness is very slow. However, it should always be kept in mind that common baldness, in both sexes, may be accompanied or unmasked by other forms of hair loss such as alopecia areata, telogen effluvium or the hair loss associated with hypothyroidism and even with iron deficiency.[303]

Common baldness results from a progressive diminution in the size of terminal follicles with each successive cycle and their eventual conversion to vellus follicles.[297,303a] This vellus conversion occurs under the influence of androgenic stimulation or in individuals with genetic predisposition.[299] The method of inheritance has not been clearly defined. Racial influences also play a part.[299]

Elevated urinary[304] and sometimes serum dehydroepiandrosterone levels have been noted in male pattern alopecia.[305] Hair follicles from sites involved with baldness have shown altered levels in the activity of the enzyme responsible for the conversion of certain androgens to their more active metabolites.[306,307] Hyperandrogenism has been detected in approximately 40% of females with the diffuse type of alopecia.[300,308] Polycystic ovaries are frequently the cause of this hyperandrogenic state.[308]

Histopathology[309,310]

The earliest change in common baldness is focal basophilic degeneration of the connective tissue sheath of the lower one-third of otherwise normal anagen follicles.[297] The terminal follicles become progressively smaller and a proportion regress to the vellus state (Fig. 15.18). Only in very advanced stages do the vellus follicles disappear leaving thin hyaline strands in the dermis.[222] Some quiescent terminal follicles are present until a late stage, and it is these follicles which produce hairs under the influence of minoxidil.[311]

There is also an increase in the number of telogen and catagen hairs relative to the number of anagen hairs.[297] This results from a shortening of the anagen cycle. This altered telogen/anagen ratio cannot be appreciated in conventional sections because only a small number of follicles is present in the plane of section. However, if transverse sections are taken of the biopsy then a greater number of follicles is available for study.[291] The decreased hair diameter can also be quantified in these sections.

In the connective tissue streamers that lie beneath the vellus follicles, small elastin bodies can be seen. They are known as Arão–Perkins bodies and they indicate the sites of the papillae of each preceding generation of follicles.[221] They can be stained with the acid orcein method, but not the Verhoeff elastic stain.[221]

It is usually suggested that the sebaceous glands are increased in size, number and lobulation.[310] However, planimetric studies have shown that the total number of sebaceous glands is significantly decreased.[297] The arrectores eventually diminish in size, but this lags behind the follicles. Accordingly, relatively large arrectores can usually be seen attached to the connective tissue streamers below the small vellus follicles.

Other changes that may be present include mild vascular dilatation and a mild perivascular round cell infiltrate which often includes mast cells.[310] Multinucleate giant cells are present in up to one-third of biopsies.[312] Small nerve networks, resembling encapsulated end organs, may be seen. Solar elastosis and some thinning of the dermis may also be present in cases of long standing.

Female pattern alopecia is usually regarded as having similar morphological features to those seen in males.[309] A recent study showed frequent catagen follicles in the female type with a paucity of telogen follicles.[313] Numerous vellus follicles were also present.

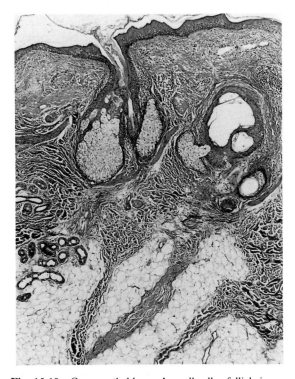

Fig. 15.18 Common baldness. A small vellus follicle is dwarfed by the adjacent sebaceous gland. Haematoxylin — eosin

CONGENITAL TRIANGULAR ALOPECIA

Congenital triangular (temporal) alopecia consists of a triangular patch of alopecia with its base extending to the fronto-temporal hairline.[314,315] It is usually unilateral. Fine vellus hairs are often present in the area.[315]

Histopathology

There is replacement of the normal abundant terminal follicles of the scalp by sparse vellus follicles.[316] Sebaceous glands and the dermis appear normal.

ANAGEN DEFLUVIUM

Anagen defluvium (anagen effluvium) is the loss of anagen hairs, either because they are defective and break or, rarely, because they are easily detached from the hair follicles.[222] The hair loss may be patterned or diffuse and it appears one month or less after the causative event, much faster than the hair loss in telogen effluvium (see p. 459).[220]

Defective hairs which break easily occur in several hair shaft abnormalities such as pili torti, trichorrhexis nodosa and monilethrix.[222] They also develop following antimitotic agents, various drugs, thallium, arsenic, vitamin A intoxication and X-ray therapy.[222] Other causes include trauma, thyroid disease, hypopituitarism, deficiency states, infections of the follicle or hair shaft and alopecia areata.[220,222]

Easy detachment of anagen hairs is a rare cause of anagen defluvium, occurring in follicular mucinosis, lymphomatous infiltration of the hair follicles and the rare loose anagen syndrome (see below).

In most instances, the diagnosis is made on clinical grounds and scalp biopsies are rarely performed. Two disorders, the loose anagen syndrome and drug alopecia, will be considered in further detail. It should be noted that various mechanisms may be involved in drug alopecias.

LOOSE ANAGEN SYNDROME

This is a recently delineated entity of childhood in which anagen hairs are easily pulled from the scalp of affected individuals, who present with diffuse hair loss.[317,318] Some improvement in the alopecia occurs with increasing age.

Histopathology

Abnormal keratinization of Huxley's and Henle's layers of the inner root sheath has been found in some samples.[318] Marked cleft formation between hair shafts and regressively altered inner root sheaths were noted in another study.[317] The easily extracted hairs are misshapen anagen hairs without external root sheaths.[318]

DRUG-INDUCED ALOPECIA

Alopecia induced by drugs usually presents as diffuse, non-scarring hair loss that is reversible upon withdrawal of the drug.[319,320] It is a common complication of the various antimitotic agents used in the chemotherapy of cancer, but it may also occur as a rare complication of other therapeutic drugs.

Drugs may interfere with hair growth in a number of different ways. For example, thallium, excess vitamin A, retinoids and certain cholesterol-lowering drugs interfere with the keratinization of the hair follicle.[319] The antimitotic drugs interfere with hair growth in the anagen phase by interrupting the normal replication of the hair matrix cells.[320] Other drugs induce telogen effluvium and the follicles remain in the resting phase.

Besides those already listed, the drugs which may induce alopecia include anticoagulants, antithyroid drugs, anticonvulsants, hormone-related substances such as clomiphene, heavy metals such as lead, bismuth, arsenic, gold, mercury and lithium, antibacterial agents such as gentamicin, nitrofurantoin and ethambutol, and non-steroidal anti-inflammatory or anti-hyper-uricaemic agents such as naproxen, ibuprofen, allopurinol, probenecid and indometh-acin.[319–321] Drugs which have been incriminated rarely include amphetamines, beta-blocking agents, cimetidine, levodopa, methysergide, penicillamine, bromocriptine, borates, quinacrine, selenium and tricyclic antidepressants.[320]

Histopathology

Those drugs producing telogen effluvium will induce catagen changes in many of the follicles. By the time a biopsy is taken, the follicles have usually entered the telogen phase. The antimitotic agents also induce premature catagen transformation. At a later stage the follicles enter anagen but their growth is then arrested at various stages of development.

SCARRING ALOPECIAS

The scarring (cicatricial) alopecias are an aetiologically diverse group which share in common the destruction of hair follicles associated with atrophy and/or scarring of the affected area, usually leading to permanent hair loss. They may result from intrinsic inflammation of the hair follicle (folliculitis) or destruction of follicles by an inflammatory or neoplastic process external to them.[322] The scarring alopecias may be classified on an aetiological basis, as follows:[322]

Developmental and related disorders
   Epidermal naevus
   Aplasia cutis
   Incontinentia pigmenti
   Keratosis pilaris atrophicans
   Porokeratosis of Mibelli
   Ichthyosis vulgaris
   Darier's disease
   Epidermolysis bullosa (recessive dystrophic)
   Polyostotic fibrous dysplasia

Physical injuries
   Mechanical trauma
   Thermal, electric and petrol burns
   Radiodermatitis

Specific infections
   Certain fungal infections (including kerion and favus)
   Herpes zoster and varicella
   Pyogenic folliculitides
   Lupus vulgaris
   Syphilis (late stages)
   Leishmaniasis

Specific dermatoses
   Lichen planus
   Lupus erythematosus
   Scleroderma
   Necrobiosis lipoidica
   Lichen sclerosus et atrophicus
   Sarcoidosis
   Cicatricial pemphigoid
   Follicular mucinosis
   Folliculitis decalvans
   Dissecting cellulitis of the scalp

Neoplasms (alopecia neoplastica)
   Basal and squamous cell carcinomas
   Secondary tumours

Idiopathic
   Idiopathic scarring alopecia (pseudopelade).

With the exception of idiopathic scarring alopecia (pseudopelade), these conditions have all been discussed in other sections of this volume.

IDIOPATHIC SCARRING ALOPECIA (PSEUDOPELADE)

Idiopathic scarring alopecia (fibrosing alopecia,[221,293] alopecia cicatrisata, pseudopelade) is a rare, asymptomatic form of scarring alopecia in which there is patchy hair loss not accompanied by any clinical evidence of folliculitis, lichen planus, lupus erythematosus or any of the specific diseases listed above.[323] The term idiopathic scarring alopecia is preferred to the more commonly employed name *pseudopelade*, which has been used in the past in a variety of contexts:[324] it has been applied to end stage scarring alopecias following known dermatoses such as lichen planus and lupus erythematosus.[324] It is conceded that the term pseudopelade has some use in a clinical setting to refer to a scarring alopecia, the cause of which is not yet known, but it should not be used to refer to a clinicopathological entity.

Idiopathic scarring alopecia tends to affect females over the age of 40 years. It has an insidious onset and a chronic, usually slowly progressive course. It results in slightly depressed patches of irreversible hair loss which may occur singly, or in groups that have been described as resembling 'footprints in the snow'.[222] The small patches may coalesce to form larger patches of scarring alopecia. As the designation idiopathic implies, the aetiology is unknown.

Histopathology[221,293]

In established lesions there is loss of hair follicles and sebaceous glands and these are replaced by bands of fibrous tissue containing elastic fibres (Fig. 15.19). These bands extend above the level of the attachment of the arrectores pilorum, in contrast to normal telogen where the fibrous tissue replaces only the deeper part of the hair follicle.

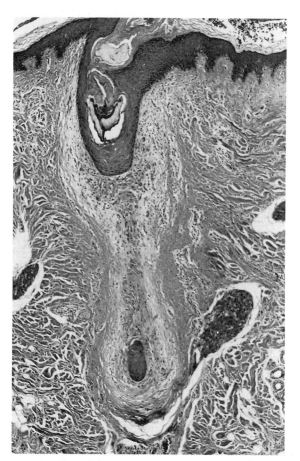

Fig. 15.19   Idiopathic scarring alopecia. A band of fibrous tissue is present at the site of a destroyed hair follicle. Haematoxylin — eosin

In early lesions, a moderately heavy infiltrate of lymphocytes surrounds the upper two-thirds of the follicle. It has been suggested that these may extend into the follicle, producing its massive apoptotic involution.[325] The epidermis is not involved by the inflammatory infiltrate. In late lesions the epidermis may show some atrophic changes with loss of the rete ridge pattern.

The orcein elastic stain may provide useful information in the scarring alopecias.[293] Whereas the fibrous tracts associated with the scarring alopecia of lichen planus and lupus erythematosus are usually devoid of elastic fibres, there are elastic fibres in the fibrous tracts of idiopathic scarring alopecia. In a proportion of cases elastic fibres develop around the lower cyclic portion of the hair follicle.[293] Following atrophy of the follicle a streak of elastic fibres and collagen is found in the subcutaneous tissue as well as at higher levels in the dermis.[293]

Direct immunofluorescence may also assist in the diagnosis of the scarring alopecias.[326] In idiopathic scarring alopecia this is negative, in contrast to lupus erythematosus in which a band of immunoglobulins and complement may be found along the basement membrane zone and surrounding hair follicles.[326] In lichen planus, colloid bodies containing IgM, and often C3, are present beneath the epidermis and around hair follicles.[326] In 'burnt-out' lesions, direct immunofluorescence may be negative.

FOLLICULITIS DECALVANS

This entity is sometimes considered to be a primary scarring alopecia. However, because inflammation of the follicle is a major feature, it has been considered with the folliculitides on page 443.

4. MISCELLANEOUS DISORDERS

PILOSEBACEOUS DISORDERS

There are several diseases of the pilosebaceous glands which do not fit readily into any of the categories discussed above. They include hypertrichosis, keratosis pilaris, lichen spinulosus and rosacea. Rosacea is traditionally included with the pilosebaceous disorders although there is increasing evidence that it is not a primary disease of the appendages.

HYPERTRICHOSIS

Hypertrichosis refers to the growth of hair on any part of the body in excess of the amount usually present in persons of the same age, race and sex.[327] Androgen-induced hair growth (hirsutism) is not included in this definition. Several distinct clinical forms exist.

Congenital hypertrichosis lanuginosa. This is an exceedingly rare familial disorder, often inherited as an autosomal dominant trait, in which there is excessive growth of lanugo hair.[328] Dental abnormalities may also be present.

Acquired hypertrichosis lanuginosa. This form of hypertrichosis is usually generalized, except for the palms and soles. An important cause is an underlying cancer, usually of epithelial type,[329-331] although rarely a lymphoma is present.[332] Hair growth may antedate the appearance of the tumour by months to several years.[333,334] The pathogenesis is unknown. Vellus hairs, intermediate forms and terminal hairs may be increased in cases of porphyria, malnutrition and brain injury and, usually reversibly, in patients taking streptomycin, diphenylhydantoin, cortico-steroids, penicillamine, psoralens, benoxa-profen, the vasodilators diazoxide and minoxidil,[335] and cyclosporin A.[327,336]

Congenital circumscribed hypertricho-sis.[327] Localized areas of hypertrichosis can be seen in congenital pigmented naevi, Becker's naevus, naevoid hypertrichosis[337] and spinal dysraphism ('faun-tail').[338]

Acquired circumscribed hypertrichosis.[327] Hypertrichosis may develop at sites of persistent friction and irritation in association with plaster casts, and at sites of inflammation, including insect bites.[339]

Histopathology

Little has been written on the histopathology of hypertrichosis.[336,340] In the acquired form, the follicles have been reported to be small and deviated from their normal vertical position. They extend obliquely or even parallel to the epidermis and contain thin unmedullated hairs. The follicles are surrounded by small lipidized mantles representing sebaceous ducts showing early glandular differentiation.[340]

KERATOSIS PILARIS

Keratosis pilaris is a disorder of keratinization involving the infundibulum of the hair follicle. It is a common condition which is found in up to 5% of adult males, and in 30% of females, particularly those showing hyperandrogenism and obesity.[341,342] The lesions, which vary from subtle follicular excrescences to more prominent follicular spikes, are found most often on the posterior aspect of the upper part of the arms and on the lateral aspect of the thighs and buttocks.[341] Follicular keratotic plugs resem-bling keratosis pilaris may be found in keratosis pilaris atrophicans (see p. 342), lichen spinulosus (see below), pityriasis rubra pilaris, ichthyosis, psoriasis, some eczemas and urae-mia.[342,343] Unusual follicular plugs containing cryoglobulin have been reported in a patient with multiple myeloma who developed horny spicules on his face.[341a]

It is thought that androgenic stimulation of the pilosebaceous follicle may result in the hyperkeratinization of the infundibulum.[342]

Histopathology

A keratin plug fills the infundibulum of the hair follicle and protrudes above the surface for a variable distance (Fig. 15.20). Serial sections are sometimes necessary to show the plug to best advantage. A very sparse lymphocytic infiltrate may be present in the dermis adjacent to the follicular infundibulum.

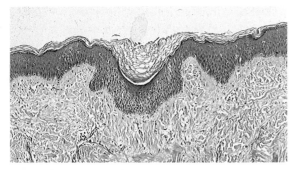

Fig. 15.20   Keratosis pilaris. A small keratin plug fills the infundibulum of the follicle and protrudes a short distance above the surface. A hair shaft emerges from the keratin plug.
Haematoxylin — eosin

LICHEN SPINULOSUS

Lichen spinulosus is a rare dermatosis of unknown aetiology characterized by follicular keratotic papules that are grouped into plaques, 2–6 cm in diameter.[343a] The horny spines protrude 1–2 mm above the surface. Lesions are distributed symmetrically on the extensor surfaces of the arms and legs and on the back, chest, face and neck. Onset of the disease is in adolescence.

Histopathology[343a]

In lichen spinulosus, there is a keratotic plug in the follicular infundibulum as in keratosis pilaris. However, there is a heavier perifollicular infiltrate of lymphocytes in lichen spinulosus, particularly adjacent to the infundibulum of the follicle, which is often dilated. Less constant changes include perifollicular fibrosis and atrophy of the sebaceous glands.

Lichen spinulosus is best regarded as a variant of keratosis pilaris in which the lesions are more papular, a consequence of the more pronounced dermal inflammation.

ROSACEA

Rosacea (acne rosacea) is a fairly common disorder of adults, involving primarily the face.[344-346] It exists in four clinical forms,[347] although cases with overlapping features are common:

1. an erythematous, telangiectatic type,
2. a papulopustular type,
3. a granulomatous type (see p. 187), and
4. a hyperplastic glandular type which results in irregular, bulbous enlargement of the nose, the condition known as rhinophyma.[348]

Rosacea is a difficult entity to classify, not only because its pathogenesis is poorly understood, but also because of the broad spectrum of histopathological changes found. Rosacea has been variously regarded as a folliculitis, a sebaceous gland disorder, a response to overabundant demodex mites, and a functional disorder of superficial dermal blood vessels associated with prominent flushing.[349] The last of these possibilities is currently the most favoured, although some of the evidence supporting it is somewhat circumstantial.[350] Vasodilator drugs may also exacerbate rosacea.[351] Rosacea-like eruptions can be seen in response to heavy local infestations by *Demodex folliculorum* (rosacea-like demodicidosis — see p. 719) and following the topical application of potent fluorinated steroids.[352] Perioral dermatitis (see p. 188) is a related entity.[353-356]

Histopathology[357]

Rosacea is characterized by a combination of several histopathological features. In the erythematous-telangiectatic group there is telangiectasia, sometimes prominent, of superficial dermal vessels (Figs 15.21 and 15.22). There is a perivascular infiltrate of lymphocytes, usually mild to moderate in intensity. A small number of plasma cells is usually present, and is an important clue to the diagnosis. Inconstant features include mild dermal oedema, solar elastosis and mild perifolliculitis. The papulopustular lesions have a more pronounced inflammatory cell infiltrate which is both perivascular and peripilar, involving the superficial and mid dermis. The infiltrate may include a few neutrophils as well as lymphocytes and plasma cells. Active pustular lesions show a

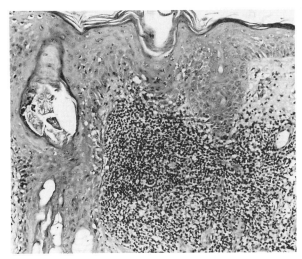

Fig. 15.21 Rosacea. A perivascular and perifollicular infiltrate of lymphocytes and plasma cells is present. Several demodex mites are present in the hair follicle.
Haematoxylin — eosin

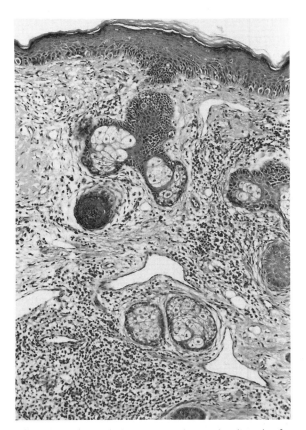

Fig. 15.22 Rosacea. There is prominent telangiectasia of vessels. The infiltrate includes plasma cells.
Haematoxylin — eosin

superficial folliculitis while in older lesions a granulomatous perifolliculitis is often present. Keratotic follicular plugging, but not comedones, may be present. Demodex mites are present in 20–50% of cases. The granulomatous form[358] is usually characterized by a tuberculoid reaction, often in the vicinity of damaged hair follicles (see p. 187).

Sebaceous gland hypertrophy and scattered follicular plugging are present in most cases of rhinophyma.[359] Telangiectasia of superficial dermal vessels is also quite common, a feature which is not present in senile sebaceous gland hyperplasia. Demodex may be present in the pilosebaceous follicles. Inconstant features include solar elastosis, dilatation of follicles, focal folliculitis and perifolliculitis. Sometimes, finger-like acanthotic downgrowths extend from the epidermis and follicular walls.[359] The infiltrate of lymphocytes and plasma cells around superficial vessels varies from sparse to moderately heavy in intensity.

Direct immunofluorescence has demonstrated the presence of immunoglobulins and complement in the region of the dermo–epidermal junction in some cases.[360,361]

APOCRINE DISORDERS

Diseases of the apocrine glands are exceedingly uncommon. Only apocrine miliaria and apocrine chromhidrosis have dermatopathological interest.

APOCRINE MILIARIA (FOX–FORDYCE DISEASE)

Apocrine miliaria (Fox–Fordyce disease) presents as a chronic papular eruption limited to areas bearing apocrine glands such as the axillae, the pubic and perineal regions and the areolae of the breasts.[362,363] There is intense pruritus which is sometimes intermittent.[364] The condition affects, almost exclusively, young adult females, although males are not exempt.[365] Axillary lesions have occasionally resulted from the prolonged use of topical antiperspirants.[366]

Apocrine miliaria results from rupture of the intraepidermal portion of the apocrine duct. This appears to result from keratotic plugging of the duct, producing an outflow obstruction.

Histopathology[362,363,367]

Serial sections are often required to demonstrate the spongiosis and spongiotic vesiculation of the follicular infundibulum adjacent to the point of entry of the apocrine duct. A keratotic plug is sometimes seen above this area.[364,367] There is an associated mild to moderate inflammatory cell infiltrate which may contain some neutrophils as well as chronic inflammatory cells.

APOCRINE CHROMHIDROSIS

Chromhidrosis refers to the production of coloured sweat by apocrine or eccrine sweat glands.[368] Slight colouration of apocrine sweat is not uncommon.

Histopathology

Orange-brown cytoplasmic granules, predominantly in an apical location, are present in apocrine sweat glands in apocrine chromhidrosis (Fig. 15.23). The pigment may not always be lipofuscin, as originally believed.[368]

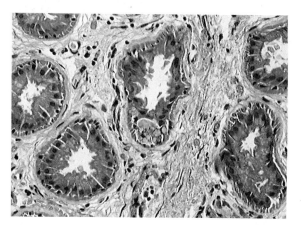

Fig. 15.23 Apocrine chromhidrosis. Granular material is present in the cytoplasm of some apocrine cells. Haematoxylin — eosin

ECCRINE DISORDERS

Excessive sweating (hyperhidrosis) is an important clinical problem but it is not related to any morphological changes in the sweat glands. Accordingly it will not be considered further. Obstruction of the eccrine duct produces small vesicular lesions known as miliaria. The various types of miliaria are discussed on p. 98. Eccrine glands may be absent in some types of ectodermal dysplasia and following radiation to the skin.

Four histopathological entities will be considered — eccrine duct hyperplasia, eccrine metaplasias, neutrophilic eccrine hidradenitis and sweat gland necrosis.

ECCRINE DUCT HYPERPLASIA

The proliferation of eccrine ducts is not a distinct clinical entity but a histological reaction pattern that can be seen in a variety of circumstances.[369,370] The best documented of these is in keratoacanthomas,[371] in which the epithelium of the lower duct and of the secretory coil may show atypical hyperplasia or squamous metaplasia (see below). Rarely, eccrine ducts are prominent, and presumably hyperplastic, overlying an intradermal naevus or adjacent to epithelial tumours on the dorsum of the hand and on the lower leg.[372] Branching ducts can also be seen in these circumstances.

Hyperplastic sweat ducts sleeved by a dense lymphocytic infiltrate (*syringolymphoid hyperplasia*) have been reported in patients with multiple reddish-brown papules, forming a plaque of alopecia.[373,374] Proliferation of ducts, without any inflammation, has been seen in a biopsy from the scalp of a patient with alopecia areata.[375]

Eruptive lesions resulting from eccrine duct hyperplasia have been reported following the use of benoxaprofen (Opren), a drug which has been withdrawn from the market.[376]

ECCRINE METAPLASIAS

Clear cell metaplasia, not due to glycogen or lipid, is occasionally an incidental finding in eccrine glands and, to a lesser extent, eccrine ducts.[377] This and other minor histological variations in the morphology of the eccrine apparatus have been reviewed on two occasions in the last 40 years.[378,379]

Squamous metaplasia of glandular and ductal epithelium (*squamous syringometaplasia*) is a not uncommon histological finding in areas of ischaemia, and adjacent to ulcers or healing surgical wounds; it may follow radiation,[379a] cryotherapy or curettage.[370,380] This change has also been reported in pyoderma gangrenosum and lobular panniculitis.[381] The occurrence of squamous metaplasia in patients receiving chemotherapy for various malignant tumours[382,383] has led to the suggestion that squamous syringometaplasia is at the non-inflammatory end of the spectrum of eccrine gland reactions induced by chemotherapy, and neutrophilic eccrine hidradenitis (see below) is at the inflammatory end.[383] Squamous syringometaplasia may simulate squamous cell carcinoma because of the islands of atypical squamous epithelium in the dermis, but careful inspection will show a normal architectural pattern of sweat glands and the presence of a lumen with a hyaline inner cuticle. This condition is analogous to necrotizing sialometaplasia, an entity found in minor salivary glands.[384]

Mucinous syringometaplasia is a rare entity which presents as a verruca-like lesion on the sole of the foot or on a finger, or as an ulcerated nodule in other sites.[385–389] Histologically, there is usually a shallow depression in the epidermis with one or several duct-like structures leading into the invagination. The ducts and portions of the surface epithelium are lined by low columnar, mucin-containing cells admixed with squamous epithelium (Fig. 15.24). The goblet cells in one reported case also extended into the sweat glands in the deep dermis.[385] The staining characteristics suggest that a sialomucin is present. The adjacent dermis contains a variable chronic inflammatory cell infiltrate with lymphocytes and plasma cells.

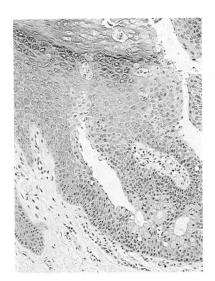

Fig. 15.24 Mucinous syringometaplasia. Mucin-containing cells are admixed with squamous epithelium in the duct-like structure which enters the epidermis from below. Haematoxylin — eosin

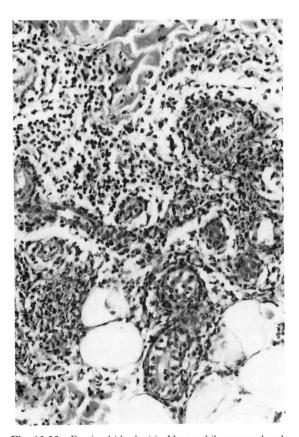

Fig. 15.25 Eccrine hidradenitis. Neutrophils surround and engulf the eccrine secretory glands. Haematoxylin — eosin

NEUTROPHILIC ECCRINE HIDRADENITIS

This is a rare complication of induction chemotherapy used in the treatment of an underlying cancer.[390] The first reports concerned patients with acute myelogenous leukaemia receiving cytarabine therapy,[390,391] but other cancers[392–394] and other chemotherapeutic agents[393,395] have now been implicated. Clinically there are plaques and nodules, often on the trunk. The lesions may resolve after 2–3 weeks.

Histopathology[390–393]

There is an infiltrate of neutrophils around and within the eccrine secretory coils, associated with vacuolar degeneration and even necrosis of the secretory epithelium (Fig. 15.25). Squamous metaplasia is sometimes present. There may be oedema and mucinous change in the loose connective tissue and fat surrounding the coils. An epidermal lichenoid tissue reaction with prominent basal vacuolar change is sometimes present as well.

SWEAT GLAND NECROSIS

Sweat gland necrosis occurs in association with vesiculobullous skin lesions in patients with drug-induced and carbon-monoxide-induced coma. This entity is discussed in further detail on p. 162.

REFERENCES

INFLAMMATORY DISEASES OF THE PILOSEBACEOUS APPARATUS

Acneiform lesions

1. Kligman AM. An overview of acne. J Invest Dermatol 1974; 62: 268–287.
2. Cunliffe WJ, Clayden AD, Gould D, Simpson NB. Acne vulgaris — its aetiology and treatment. Clin Exp Dermatol 1981; 6: 461–469.
3. Puhvel SM, Amirian D, Weintraub J, Reisner RM. Lymphocyte transformation in subjects with nodulo-cystic acne. Br J Dermatol 1977; 97: 205–211.
4. Kumar P, Marks R. Sebaceous gland hyperplasia and senile comedones: a prevalence study in elderly hospitalized patients. Br J Dermatol 1987; 117: 231–236.
5. Shalita AR, Lee W-L. Inflammatory acne. Dermatol Clin 1983; 1: 361–364.
6. Hughes BR, Cunliffe WJ. An acne naevus. Clin Exp Dermatol 1987; 12: 357–359.
7. Shalita AR, Leyden JE Jr, Pochi PE, Strauss JS. Acne vulgaris. J Am Acad Dermatol 1987; 16: 410–412.
8. Heilman ER, Lavker RM. Abnormal follicular keratinization. Dermatol Clin 1983; 1: 353–359.
9. Downing DT, Stewart ME, Wertz PW, Strauss JS. Essential fatty acids and acne. J Am Acad Dermatol 1986; 14: 221–225.
10. Marsden JR, Middleton B, Mills C. Is remission of acne due to changes in sebum composition? Clin Exp Dermatol 1987; 12: 18–20.
11. Pochi PE. Hormones and acne. Semin Dermatol 1982; 1: 265–273.
12. van der Meeren HLM, Thijssen JHH. Circulating androgens in male acne. Br J Dermatol 1984; 110: 609–611.
13. Steinberger E, Rodriguez-Rigau LJ, Smith KD, Held B. The menstrual cycle and plasma testosterone levels in women with acne. J Am Acad Dermatol 1981; 4: 54–58.
14. Lawrence D, Shaw M, Katz M. Elevated free testosterone concentration in men and women with acne vulgaris. Clin Exp Dermatol 1986; 11: 263–273.
15. Lookingbill DP, Horton R, Demers LM et al. Tissue production of androgens in women with acne. J Am Acad Dermatol 1985; 12: 481–487.
16. Marynick SP, Chakmakjian ZH, McCaffree DL, Herndon JH Jr. Androgen excess in cystic acne. N Engl J Med 1983; 308: 981–986.
16a. Bunker CB, Newton JA, Kilborn J et al. Most women with acne have polycystic ovaries. Br J Dermatol 1989; 121: 675–680.
17. Strauss JS, Pochi PE. Intracutaneous injection of sebum and comedones. Histological observations. Arch Dermatol 1965; 92: 443–456.
18. Kersey P, Sussman M, Dahl M. Delayed skin test reactivity to *Propionibacterium acnes* correlates with severity of inflammation in acne vulgaris. Br J Dermatol 1980; 103: 651–655.
19. Leeming JP, Holland KT, Cunliffe WJ. The microbial colonization of inflamed acne vulgaris lesions. Br J Dermatol 1988; 118: 203–208.
20. Lavker RM, Leyden JJ, McGinley KJ. The relationship between bacteria and the abnormal follicular keratinization in acne vulgaris. J Invest Dermatol 1981; 77: 325–330.
21. Webster GF, Leyden JJ. Mechanisms of *Propionibacterium acnes* - mediated inflammation in

acne vulgaris. Semin Dermatol 1982; 1: 299–304.

22. Puhvel SM. *Propionibacterium acnes* and acne vulgaris. Semin Dermatol 1982; 1: 293–298.

23. Ingham E, Gowland G, Ward RM et al. Antibodies to *P. acnes* and *P. acnes* exocellular enzymes in the normal population at various ages and on patients with acne vulgaris. Br J Dermatol 1987; 116: 805–812.

24. Eady EA, Cove JH, Blake J et al. Recalcitrant acne vulgaris. Clinical, biochemical and microbiological investigation of patients not responding to antibiotic treatment. Br J Dermatol 1988; 118: 415–423.

25. Mills OH Jr, Kligman AM. External factors aggravating acne. Dermatol Clin 1983; 1: 365–370.

26. Bierman SM. Autoimmune progesterone dermatitis of pregnancy. Arch Dermatol 1973; 107: 896–901.

27. Mills OH Jr, Kligman AM. Acne detergicans. Arch Dermatol 1975; 111: 65–68.

28. Mills OH Jr, Kligman A. Acne mechanica. Arch Dermatol 1975; 111: 481–483.

29. Steffen C. The acneform eruption of Apert's syndrome is not acne vulgaris. Am J Dermatopathol 1984; 6: 213–220.

30. Massa MC, Su WPD. Pyoderma faciale: A clinical study of twenty-nine patients. J Am Acad Dermatol 1982; 6: 84–91.

30a. Hurwitz RM. Steroid acne. J Am Acad Dermatol 1989; 21: 1179–1181.

31. Plewig G. Morphologic dynamics of acne vulgaris. Acta Derm Venereol (Suppl) 1980; 89: 9–16.

32. Invitational Symposium on Comedogenicity. J Am Acad Dermatol 1989; 20: 272–277.

33. Norris JFB, Cunliffe WJ. A histological and immunocytochemical study of early acne lesions. Br J Dermatol 1988; 118: 651–659.

34. Kaidbey KH, Kligman AM. Pigmentation in comedones. Arch Dermatol 1974; 109: 60–62.

35. Zelickson AS, Mottaz JH. Pigmentation of open comedones. An ultrastructural study. Arch Dermatol 1983; 119: 567–569.

36. Strauss JS, Kligman AM. The pathologic dynamics of acne vulgaris. Arch Dermatol 1960; 82: 779–790.

37. Vasarinsh P. Keratinization of pilar structures in acne vulgaris and normal skin. Br J Dermatol 1969; 81: 517–524.

37a. Wilson BB, Dent CH, Cooper PH. Papular acne scars. A common cutaneous finding. Arch Dermatol 1990; 126: 797–800.

38. Basler RSW, Watters JH, Taylor WB. Calcifying acne lesions. Int J Dermatol 1977; 16: 755–758.

39. Brodkin RH, Abbey AA. Osteoma cutis: a case of probable exacerbation following treatment of severe acne with isotretinoin. Dermatologica 1985; 170: 210–212.

40. Basler RSW, Kohnen PW. Localized haemosiderosis as a sequela of acne. Arch Dermatol 1978; 114: 1695–1697.

41. Wilborn WH, Montes LF, Lyons RE, Battista GW. Ultrastructural basis for the assay of topical acne treatments. Transmission and scanning electron microscopy of untreated comedones. J Cutan Pathol 1978; 5: 165–183.

42. Zelickson AS, Strauss JS, Mottaz J. Ultrastructural changes in open comedones following treatment of cystic acne with isotretinoin. Am J Dermatopathol 1985; 7: 241–244.

43. Nault P, Lassonde M, St-Antoine P. Acne fulminans with osteolytic lesions. Arch Dermatol 1985; 121: 662–664.

44. Pauli S-L, Kokko M-L, Suhonen R, Reunala T. Acne fulminans with bone lesions. Acta Derm Venereol 1988; 68: 351–355.

45. Jemec GBE, Rasmussen I. Bone lesions of acne fulminans. Case report and review of the literature. J Am Acad Dermatol 1989; 20: 353–357.

46. McAuley D, Miller RA. Acne fulminans associated with inflammatory bowel disease. Arch Dermatol 1985; 121: 91–93.

47. Kellett JK, Beck MH, Chalmers RJG. Erythema nodosum and circulating immune complexes in acne fulminans after treatment with isotretinoin. Br Med J 1985; 290: 820.

48. Traupe H, von Muhlendahl KE, Bramswig J, Happle R. Acne of the fulminans type following testosterone therapy in three excessively tall boys. Arch Dermatol 1988; 124: 414–417.

49. Goldschmidt H, Leyden JJ, Stein KH. Acne fulminans. Investigation of acute febrile ulcerative acne. Arch Dermatol 1977; 113: 444–449.

50. Tindall JP. Chloracne and chloracnegens. J Am Acad Dermatol 1985; 13: 539–558.

51. Crow KD. Chloracne. Semin Dermatol 1982; 1: 305–314.

52. Moses M, Prioleau PG. Cutaneous histologic findings in chemical workers with and without chloracne with past exposure to 2,3,7,8–tetrachlorodibenzo-p-dioxin. J Am Acad Dermatol 1985; 12: 497–506.

Superficial folliculitides

53. Golitz L. Follicular and perforating disorders. J Cutan Pathol 1985; 12: 282–288.

54. Maibach HI. Scalp pustules due to *Corynebacterium acnes*. Arch Dermatol 1967; 96: 453–455.

55. Hersle K, Mobacken H, Moller A. Chronic non-scarring folliculitis of the scalp. Acta Derm Venereol 1979; 59: 249–253.

56. Nieboer C. Actinic superficial folliculitis; a new entity? Br J Dermatol 1985; 112: 603–606.

57. Verbov J. Actinic folliculitis. Br J Dermatol 1985; 112: 630–631.

58. Norris PG, Hawk JLM. Actinic folliculitis — response to isotretinoin. Clin Exp Dermatol 1989; 14: 69–71.

59. Kossard S, Collins A, McCrossin I. Necrotizing lymphocytic folliculitis: The early lesion of acne necrotica (varioliformis). J Am Acad Dermatol 1987; 16: 1007–1014.

60. Rook A, Dawber R. Diseases of the hair and scalp. Oxford: Blackwell Scientific Publications, 1982; 475–477.

61. Maibach HI. Acne necroticans (varioliformis) versus *Propionibacterium acnes* folliculitis. J Am Acad Dermatol 1989; 21: 323.

62. Fisher DA. Acne necroticans (varioliformis) and *Staphylococcus aureus*. J Am Acad Dermatol 1988; 18: 1136–1137.

63. Barlow RJ, Schulz EJ. Necrotizing folliculitis in AIDS-related complex. Br J Dermatol 1987; 116: 581–584.

64. Ise S, Ofuji S. Subcorneal pustular dermatosis. A follicular variant? Arch Dermatol 1965; 92: 169–171.

65. Ofuji S, Ogino A, Horio T et al. Eosinophilic pustular

folliculitis. Acta Derm Venereol 1970; 50: 195–203.

66. Holst R. Eosinophilic pustular folliculitis. Report of a European case. Br J Dermatol 1976; 95: 661–664.

67. Jaliman HD, Phelps RG, Fleischmajer R. Eosinophilic pustular folliculitis. J Am Acad Dermatol 1986; 14: 479–482.

68. Dinehart SM, Noppakun N, Solomon AR, Smith EB. Eosinophilic pustular folliculitis. J Am Acad Dermatol 1986; 14: 475–479.

69. Ishibashi A, Nishiyama Y, Miyata C, Chujo T. Eosinophilic pustular folliculitis (Ofuji). Dermatologica 1974; 149: 240–247.

70. Takematsu H, Nakamura K, Igarashi M, Tagami H. Eosinophilic pustular folliculitis. Report of two cases with a review of the Japanese literature. Arch Dermatol 1985; 121: 917–920.

71. Colton AS, Schachner L, Kowalczyk AP. Eosinophilic pustular folliculitis. J Am Acad Dermatol 1986; 14: 469–474.

72. Cutler TP. Eosinophilic pustular folliculitis. Clin Exp Dermatol 1981; 6: 327–332.

73. Saruta T, Nakamizo Y. Eosinophilic pustular folliculitis. Rinsho Dermatol 1979; 21: 689–697.

74. Orfanos CE, Sterry W. Sterine eosinophile pustulose. Dermatologica 1978; 157: 193–205.

75. Beer WE, Emslie ES, Lanigan S. Circinate eosinophilic dermatosis. Int J Dermatol 1987; 26: 192–193.

76. Scott DW. Sterile eosinophilic pustulosis in dog and man. Comparative aspects. J Am Acad Dermatol 1987; 16: 1022–1026.

77. Lucky AW, Esterly NB, Heskel N et al. Eosinophilic pustular folliculitis in infancy. Pediatr Dermatol 1984; 1: 202–206.

78. Soeprono FF, Schinella RA. Eosinophilic pustular folliculitis in patients with acquired immunodeficiency syndrome. Report of three cases. J Am Acad Dermatol 1986; 14: 1020–1022.

78a. Frentz G, Niordson A-M, Thomsen K. Eosinophilic pustular dermatosis: an early skin marker of infection with human immunodeficiency virus? Br J Dermatol 1989; 121: 271–274.

79. Nunzi E, Parodi A, Rebora A. Ofuji's disease: High circulating titers of IgG and IgM directed to basal cell cytoplasm. J Am Acad Dermatol 1985; 12: 268–273.

80. Vakilzadeh F, Suter L, Knop J, Macher E. Eosinophilic pustulosis with pemphigus-like antibody. Dermatologica 1981; 162: 265–272.

81. Takematsu H, Tagami H. Eosinophilic pustular folliculitis. Studies on possible chemotactic factors involved in the formation of pustules. Br J Dermatol 1986; 114: 209–215.

82. Kuo T-T, Chen S-Y, Chan H-L. Tinea infection histologically simulating eosinophilic pustular folliculitis. J Cutan Pathol 1986; 13: 118–122.

Deep infectious folliculitides

83. Tunnessen WW Jr. Practical aspects of bacterial skin infections in children. Pediatr Dermatol 1985; 2: 255–265.

84. Pinkus H. Furuncle. J Cutan Pathol 1979; 6: 517–518.

85. Fox AB, Hambrick GW Jr. Recreationally associated *Pseudomonas aeruginosa* folliculitis. Report of an epidemic. Arch Dermatol 1984; 120: 1304–1307.

86. Chandrasekar PH, Rolston KVI, Kannangara DW et al. Hot tub-associated dermatitis due to *Pseudomonas aeruginosa*. Case report and review of the literature. Arch Dermatol 1984; 120: 1337–1340.

87. Feder HM Jr, Grant-Kels JM, Tilton RC. Pseudomonas whirlpool dermatitis. Report of an outbreak in two families. Clin Pediatr (Phila) 1983; 22: 638–642.

88. Silverman AR, Nieland ML. Hot tub dermatitis: A familial outbreak of *Pseudomonas* folliculitis. J Am Acad Dermatol 1983; 8: 153–156.

89. Blankenship ML. Gram-negative folliculitis. Follow-up observations in 20 patients. Arch Dermatol 1984; 120: 1301–1303.

90. Leyden JJ, Marples RR, Mills OH Jr, Kligman AM. Gram-negative folliculitis — a complication of antibiotic therapy in acne vulgaris. Br J Dermatol 1973; 88: 533–538.

91. Leyden JJ, McGinley KJ, Mills OH. *Pseudomonas aeruginosa* gram-negative folliculitis. Arch Dermatol 1979; 115: 1203–1204.

92. Jacyk WK. Clinical and pathologic observations in dermatitis cruris pustulosa et atrophicans. Int J Dermatol 1978; 17: 802–807.

93. Gillians JA, Palmer HW, Dyte PH. Follicular dermatitis caused by *Salmonella dublin*. Med J Aust 1982; 1: 390–391.

Deep scarring folliculitides

94. Weedon D. Unpublished observations.

95. Rook A, Dawber R. Diseases of the hair and scalp. Oxford: Blackwell Scientific Publications, 1982; 314–315.

96. Loewenthal LJA. A case of lupoid sycosis or ulerythema sycosiforme beginning in infancy. Br J Dermatol 1957; 69: 443–449.

97. Miller RF. Epilating folliculitis of the glabrous skin. Arch Dermatol 1961; 83: 777–784.

98. Cosman B, Wolff M. Acne keloidalis. Plast Reconstr Surg 1972; 50: 25–30.

98a. Herzberg AJ, Dinehart SM, Kerns BJ, Pollack SV. Acne keloidalis. Transverse microscopy, immunohistochemistry, and electron microscopy. Am J Dermatopathol 1990; 12: 109–121.

99. Dinehart SM, Herzberg AJ, Kerns BJ, Pollack SV. Acne keloidalis: a review. J Dermatol Surg Oncol 1989; 15: 642–647.

100. Rook A, Dawber R. Diseases of the hair and scalp. Oxford: Blackwell Scientific Publications, 1982; 477–478.

101. Goette DK, Berger TG. Acne keloidalis nuchae. A transepithelial elimination disorder. Int J Dermatol 1987; 26: 442–444.

Follicular occlusion triad

102. Shelley WB, Cahn MM. The pathogenesis of hidradenitis suppurativa in man. Arch Dermatol 1955; 72: 562–565.

103. Highet AS, Warren RE, Weekes AJ. Bacteriology and antibiotic treatment of perineal suppurative hidradenitis. Arch Dermatol 1988; 124: 1047–1051.

104. Chicarilli ZN. Follicular occlusion triad: hidradenitis suppurativa, acne conglobata, and dissecting cellulitis of the scalp. Ann Plast Surg 1987; 18: 230–237.

105. Bell BA, Ellis H. Hidradenitis suppurativa. J R Soc Med 1978; 71: 511–515.
106. Watson JD. Hidradenitis suppurativa — a clinical review. Br J Plast Surg 1985; 38: 567–569.
107. Broadwater JR, Bryant RL, Petrino RA et al. Advanced hidradenitis suppurativa. Review of surgical treatment in 23 patients. Am J Surg 1982; 144: 668–670.
108. Humphrey LJ, Playforth H, Leavell UW Jr. Squamous cell carcinoma arising in hidradenitis suppurativum. Arch Dermatol 1969; 100: 59–62.
109. Alexander SJ. Squamous cell carcinoma in chronic hidradenitis suppurativa. A case report. Cancer 1979; 43: 745–748.
110. Jemec GBE. The symptomatology of hidradenitis suppurativa in women. Br J Dermatol 1988; 119: 345–350.
111. Jemec GBE. Effect of localized surgical excisions in hidradenitis suppurativa. J Am Acad Dermatol 1988; 18: 1103–1107.
112. Fitzsimmons JS, Guilbert PR, Fitzsimmons EM. Evidence of genetic factors in hidradenitis suppurativa. Br J Dermatol 1985; 113: 1–8.
113. Fitzsimmons JS, Guilbert PR. A family study of hidradenitis suppurativa. J Med Genet 1985; 22: 367–373.
114. Dvorak VC, Root RK, MacGregor RR. Host-defense mechanisms in hidradenitis suppurativa. Arch Dermatol 1977; 113: 450–453.
115. O'Loughlin S, Woods R, Kirke PN et al. Hidradenitis suppurativa. Glucose tolerance, clinical, microbiologic, and immunologic features and HLA frequencies in 27 patients. Arch Dermatol 1988; 124: 1043–1046.
116. Ebling FJG. Hidradenitis suppurativa: an androgen dependent disorder. Br J Dermatol 1986; 115: 259–262.
117. Mortimer PS, Dawber RPR, Gales MA, Moore RA. Mediation of hidradenitis suppurativa by androgens. Br Med J 1986; 292: 245–248.
118. Mortimer PS, Dawber RPR, Gales MA, Moore RA. A double-blind controlled cross-over trial of cyproterone acetate in females with hidradenitis suppurativa. Br J Dermatol 1986; 115: 263–268.
119. Thomas R, Barnhill D, Bibro M, Hoskins W. Hidradenitis suppurativa: a case presentation and review of the literature. Obstet Gynecol 1985; 66: 592–595.
120. Hyland CH, Kheir SM. Follicular occlusion disease with elimination of abnormal elastic tissue. Arch Dermatol 1980; 116: 925–928.
120a. Yu CC-W, Cook MG. Hidradenitis suppurativa: a disease of follicular epithelium, rather than apocrine glands. Br J Dermatol 1990; 122: 763–769.
121. Berne B, Venge P, Ohman S. Perifolliculitis capitis abscedens et suffodiens (Hoffman). Complete healing associated with oral zinc therapy. Arch Dermatol 1985; 121: 1028–1030.
122. Adrian RM, Arndt KA. Perifolliculitis capitis: successful control with alternate-day corticosteroids. Ann Plast Surg 1980; 4: 166–169.
123. Glass LF, Berman B, Laub D. Treatment of perifolliculitis capitis abscedens et suffodiens with the carbon dioxide laser. J Dermatol Surg Oncol 1989; 15: 673–676.
124. Moschella SL, Klein MH, Miller RJ. Perifolliculitis capitis abscedens et suffodiens. Report of a successful therapeutic scalping. Arch Dermatol 1967; 96: 195–197.
125. Curry SS, Gaither DH, King LE Jr. Squamous cell carcinoma arising in dissecting perifolliculitis of the scalp. A case report and review of secondary squamous cell carcinomas. J Am Acad Dermatol 1981; 4: 673–678.
126. Jolliffe DS, Sarkany I. Perifolliculitis capitis abscedens et suffodiens (dissecting cellulitis of the scalp). Clin Exp Dermatol 1977; 2: 291–293.
127. Moyer DG, Williams RM. Perifolliculitis capitis abscedens et suffodiens. A report of six cases. Arch Dermatol 1962; 85: 378–384.
128. Weinrauch L, Peled I, Hacham-Zadeh S, Wexler MR. Surgical treatment of severe acne conglobata. J Dermatol Surg Oncol 1981; 7: 492–494.

Miscellaneous folliculitides

129. Kushimoto H, Aoki T. Toxic erythema with generalized follicular pustules caused by streptomycin. Arch Dermatol 1981; 117: 444–445.
130. Strauss JS, Kligman AM. Pseudofolliculitis of the beard. Arch Dermatol 1956; 74: 533–542.
131. Kligman AM, Mills OH Jr. Pseudofolliculitis of the beard and topically applied tretinoin. Arch Dermatol 1973; 107: 551–552.
132. Smith JD, Odom RB. Pseudofolliculitis capitis. Arch Dermatol 1977; 113: 328–329.
133. Alexander AM. Pseudofolliculitis diathesis. Arch Dermatol 1974; 109: 729–730.
134. Dilaimy M. Pseudofolliculitis of the legs. Arch Dermatol 1976; 112: 507–508.
135. Brauner GJ, Flandermeyer KL. Pseudofolliculitis barbae. 2. Treatment. Int J Dermatol 1977; 16: 520–525.
136. Zoberman E, Farmer ER. Pruritic folliculitis of pregnancy. Arch Dermatol 1981; 117: 20–22.
137. Mehregan AH, Coskey RJ. Perforating folliculitis. Arch Dermatol 1968; 97: 394–399.
138. Patterson JW. The perforating disorders. J Am Acad Dermatol 1984; 10: 561–581.
139. Patterson JW, Graff GE, Eubanks SW. Perforating folliculitis and psoriasis. J Am Acad Dermatol 1982; 7: 369–376.
140. Kahana M, Trau H, Delev E. Perforating folliculitis in association with primary sclerosing cholangitis. Am J Dermatopathol 1985; 7: 271–276.
141. Hurwitz RM, Melton ME, Creech FT III et al. Perforating folliculitis in association with hemodialysis. Am J Dermatopathol 1982; 4: 101–108.
142. Ackerman AB. Histologic diagnosis of inflammatory skin diseases. Philadelphia: Lea & Febiger, 1978; 685–687.
143. Burkhart CG. Perforating folliculitis. A reappraisal of its pathogenesis. Int J Dermatol 1981; 20: 597–599.
144. Hurwitz RM. The evolution of perforating folliculitis in patients with chronic renal failure. Am J Dermatopathol 1985; 7: 231–239.
145. White CR Jr, Heskel NS, Pokorny DJ. Perforating folliculitis of hemodialysis. Am J Dermatopathol 1982; 4: 109–116.

HAIR SHAFT ABNORMALITIES

146. Whiting DA. Structural abnormalities of the hair shaft. J Am Acad Dermatol 1987; 16: 1–25.
147. Rook A, Dawber R. Diseases of the hair and scalp. Oxford: Blackwell Scientific Publications, 1982; 179–232.
148. Camacho-Martinez F, Ferrando J. Hair shaft dysplasias. Int J Dermatol 1988; 27: 71–80.
149. Mortimer PS. Unruly hair. Br J Dermatol 1985; 113: 467–473.

Fractures of hair shafts

150. Birnbaum PS, Baden HP, Bronstein BR et al. Intermittent hair follicle dystrophy. J Am Acad Dermatol 1986; 15: 54–60.
151. Chetty GN, Kamalam A, Thambiah AS. Acquired structural defects of the hair. Int J Dermatol 1981; 20: 119–121.
152. Chernosky ME, Owens DW. Trichorrhexis nodosa. Clinical and investigative studies. Arch Dermatol 1966; 94: 577–585.
153. Dawber RPR. Weathering of hair in monilethrix and pili torti. Clin Exp Dermatol 1977; 2: 271–277.
154. Owens DW, Chernosky ME. Trichorrhexis nodosa. *In vitro reproduction.* Arch Dermatol 1966; 94: 586–588.
155. Ricci MA, Tunnessen WW Jr, Pergolizzi JJ, Hellems MA. Menkes' kinky hair syndrome. Cutis 1982; 30: 55–58.
156. Papa CM, Mills OH Jr, Hanshaw W. Seasonal trichorrhexis nodosa. Arch Dermatol 1972; 106: 888–892.
156a. Itin PH, Pittelkow MR. Trichothiodystrophy: Review of sulfur-deficient brittle hair syndromes and association with the ectodermal dysplasias. J Am Acad Dermatol 1990; 22: 705–717.
157. Leonard JN, Gummer CL, Dawber RPR. Generalized trichorrhexis nodosa. Br J Dermatol 1980; 103: 85–90.
157a. Rushton DH, Norris MJ, James KC. Amino-acid composition in trichorrhexis nodosa. Clin Exp Dermatol 1990; 15: 24–28.
158. Dawber R, Comaish S. Scanning electron microscopy of normal and abnormal hair shafts. Arch Dermatol 1970; 101: 316–322.
159. Birnbaum PS, Baden HP. Heritable disorders of hair. Dermatol Clin 1987; 5: 137–153.
160. Price VH, Odom RB, Ward WH, Jones FT. Trichothiodystrophy. Sulfur-deficient brittle hair as a marker for a neuroectodermal symptom complex. Arch Dermatol 1980; 116: 1375–1384.
161. Gummer CL, Dawber RPR. Trichothiodystrophy: an ultrastructural study of the hair follicle. Br J Dermatol 1985; 113: 273–280.
162. Jorizzo JL, Atherton DJ, Crounse RG, Wells RS. Ichthyosis, brittle hair, impaired intelligence, decreased fertility and short stature (IBIDS syndrome). Br J Dermatol 1982; 106: 705–710.
163. Ito M, Ito K, Hashimoto K. Pathogenesis in trichorrhexis invaginata (bamboo hair). J Invest Dermatol 1984; 83: 1–6.
164. Yesudian P, Srinivas K. Ichthyosis with unusual hair shaft abnormalities in siblings. Br J Dermatol 1977; 96: 199–203.
165. Burkhart CG, Huttner JJ, Bruner J. Central trichoptilosis. J Am Acad Dermatol 1981; 5: 703–705.

Irregularities of hair shafts

166. Matis WL, Baden H, Green R et al. Uncombable-hair syndrome. Pediatr Dermatol 1986; 4: 215–219.
167. Shelley WB, Shelley ED. Uncombable hair syndrome: Observations on response to biotin and occurrence in siblings with ectodermal dysplasia. J Am Acad Dermatol 1985; 13: 97–102.
168. Ravella A, Pujoi RM, Noguera X, de Moragas JM. Localized pili canaliculi and trianguli. J Am Acad Dermatol 1987; 17: 377–380.
169. Zegpi M, Roa I. The uncombable hair syndrome. Arch Pathol Lab Med 1987; 111: 754–755.
170. Baden HP, Schoenfeld RJ, Stroud JO, Happle R. Physicochemical properties of "spun glass" hair. Acta Derm Venereol 1981; 61: 441–444.
171. Downham TF II, Chapel TA, Lupulescu AP. Straight-hair nevus syndrome: a case report with scanning electron microscopic findings of hair morphology. Int J Dermatol 1976; 15: 438–443.
172. Gibbs RC, Berger RA. The straight-hair nevus. Int J Dermatol 1970; 9: 47–49.
173. Day TL. Straight-hair nevus, ichthyosis hystrix, leukokeratosis of the tongue. Arch Dermatol 1967; 96: 606.
174. Weary PE, Hendricks AA, Wawner F, Ajgaonkar G. Pili bifurcati. Arch Dermatol 1973; 108: 403–407.
175. Mehregan AH, Thompson WS. Pili multigemini. Br J Dermatol 1979; 100: 315–322.
175a. Dalziel KL, Telfer NR, Wilson CL, Dawber RPR. Tufted folliculitis. A specific bacterial disease? Am J Dermatopathol 1990; 12: 37–41.
175b. Tong AKF, Baden HP. Tufted folliculitis. J Am Acad Dermatol 1989; 21: 1096–1099.
176. Kailasam V, Kamalam A, Thambiah AS. Trichostasis spinulosa. Int J Dermatol 1979; 18: 297–300.
177. Sarkany I, Gaylarde PM. Trichostasis spinulosa and its management. Br J Dermatol 1971; 84: 311–315.
178. Young MC, Jorizzo JL, Sanchez RL et al. Trichostasis spinulosa. Int J Dermatol 1985; 24: 575–580.
179. Gummer CL, Dawber RPR. Pili annulati: electron histochemical studies on affected hairs. Br J Dermatol 1981; 105: 303–309.
180. Musso LA. Pili annulati. Aust J Dermatol 1970; 11: 67–75.
181. Dini G, Casigliani R, Rindi L et al. Pili annulati. Optical and scanning electron microscopic studies. Int J Dermatol 1988; 27: 256–257.
182. Price VH, Thomas RS, Jones FT. Pseudopili annulati. An unusual variant of normal hair. Arch Dermatol 1970; 102: 354–358.
183. Price VH, Thomas RS, Jones FT. Pili annulati. Optical and electron microscopic studies. Arch Dermatol 1968; 98: 640–647.
184. Gummer CL, Dawber RPR, Swift JA. Monilethrix: an electron microscopic and electron histochemical study. Br J Dermatol 1981; 105: 529–541.
185. Ito M, Hashimoto K, Yorder FW. Monilethrix: an ultrastructural study. J Cutan Pathol 1984; 11: 513–521.

186. Bentley-Phillips B, Bayles MAH. A previously undescribed hereditary hair anomaly (pseudo-monilethrix). Br J Dermatol 1973; 89: 159–167.

187. Zitelli JA. Pseudomonilethrix. An artifact. Arch Dermatol 1986; 122: 688–690.

188. Zitelli JA. Pseudomonilethrix. Arch Dermatol 1987; 123: 564.

189. Brown VM, Crounse RG, Abele DC. An unusual new hair shaft abnormality: "Bubble hair". J Am Acad Dermatol 1986; 15: 1113–1117.

Coiling and twisting abnormalities

190. Patel HP, Unis ME. Pili torti in association with citrullinemia. J Am Acad Dermatol 1985; 12: 203–206.

191. Scott MJ Jr, Bronson DM, Esterly NB. Bjornstad syndrome and pili torti. Pediatr Dermatol 1983; 1: 45–50.

192. Hays SB, Camisa C. Acquired pili torti in two patients treated with synthetic retinoids. Cutis 1985; 35: 466–468.

193. Barth JH, Dawber RPR. Pili torti and hirsuties: are twisted hairs a normal variant? Acta Derm Venereol 1987; 67: 455–457.

194. Lyon JB, Dawber RPR. A sporadic case of dystrophic pili torti. Br J Dermatol 1977; 96: 197–198.

195. Hutchinson PE, Wells RS. Woolly hair. Br J Dermatol (Suppl) 1973; 9: 17.

196. Ormerod AD, Main RA, Ryder ML, Gregory DW. A family with diffuse partial woolly hair. Br J Dermatol 1987; 116: 401–405.

197. Hasper MF, Klokke AH. Woolly hair naevus with triangular hairs. Br J Dermatol 1983; 108: 111–113.

197a. Peteiro C, Perez Oliva N, Zulaica A, Toribio J. Woolly-hair nevus: report of a case associated with a verrucous epidermal nevus in the same area. Pediatr Dermatol 1989; 6: 188–190.

198. Lantis SDH, Pepper MC. Woolly hair nevus. Arch Dermatol 1978; 114: 233–238.

198a. Reda AM, Rogers RS III, Peters MS. Woolly hair nevus. J Am Acad Dermatol 1990; 22: 377–380.

199. Mortimer PS, Gummer C, English J, Dawber RPR. Acquired progressive kinking of hair. Arch Dermatol 1985; 121: 1031–1033.

200. English JSC, Mortimer PS. Acquired progressive kinking of the hair. Clin Exp Dermatol 1984; 9: 102–104.

201. Cullen SI, Fulghum DD. Acquired progressive kinking of the hair. Arch Dermatol 1989; 125: 252–255.

202. Esterly NB, Lavin MP, Garancis JC. Acquired progressive kinking of the hair. Arch Dermatol 1989; 125: 813–815.

203. Norwood OT. Whisker hair. Arch Dermatol 1979; 115: 930–931.

204. Rebora A, Guarrera M. Acquired progressive kinking of the hair. J Am Acad Dermatol 1985; 12: 933–936.

205. English DT, Jones HE. Trichonodosis. Arch Dermatol 1973; 107: 77–79.

206. Dawber RPR. Knotting of scalp hair. Br J Dermatol 1974; 91: 169–173.

207. Fergusson AG, Derblay PR. Rolled hairs. A possible complication of corticosteroid therapy. Arch Dermatol 1963; 87: 311–314.

208. Levit F, Scott MJ Jr. Circle hairs. J Am Acad Dermatol 1983; 8: 423–425.

Extraneous matter on hair shafts

209. Gold I, Sommer B, Urson S, Schewach-Millet M. White piedra. A frequently misdiagnosed infection of hair. Int J Dermatol 1984; 23: 621–623.

210. Benson PM, Lapins NA, Odom RB. White piedra. Arch Dermatol 1983; 119: 602–604.

211. Smith JD, Murtishaw WA, McBride ME. White piedra (trichosporosis). Arch Dermatol 1973; 107: 439–442.

212. Lassus A, Kanerva L, Stubb S, Salonen A. White piedra. Report of a case evaluated by scanning electron microscopy. Arch Dermatol 1982; 118: 208–211.

213. Kalter DC, Tschen JA, Cernoch PL et al. Genital white piedra: Epidemiology, microbiology, and therapy. J Am Acad Dermatol 1986; 14: 982–993.

214. Steinman HK, Pappenfort RB. White piedra — a case report and review of the literature. Clin Exp Dermatol 1984; 9: 591–598.

215. Dawber RPR. Hair casts. Arch Dermatol 1979; 100: 417–421.

216. Taieb A, Surleve-Bazeille JE, Maleville J. Hair casts. A clinical and morphologic study. Arch Dermatol 1985; 121: 1009–1013.

217. Keipert JA. Hair casts. Review and suggestion regarding nomenclature. Arch Dermatol 1986; 122: 927–930.

218. Fabbri P, Difonzo EM, Palleschi GM, Pacini P. Hair casts. Int J Dermatol 1988; 27: 319–321.

219. Scott MJ Jr, Roenigk HH Jr. Hair casts: Classification, staining characteristics, and differential diagnosis. J Am Acad Dermatol 1983; 8: 27–32.

ALOPECIAS

220. Steck WD. The clinical evaluation of pathologic hair loss with a diagnostic sign in trichotillomania. Cutis 1979; 24: 293–301.

221. Pinkus H. Alopecia. Clinicopathologic correlations. Int J Dermatol 1980; 19: 245–253.

222. Ioannides G. Alopecia: a pathologist's view. Int J Dermatol 1982; 21: 316–328.

223. Montagna E, Parakkal PF. The structure and function of skin. New York: Academic Press, 1974.

224. Rook A, Dawber R. Diseases of the hair and scalp. Oxford: Blackwell Scientific Publications, 1982; 1–17.

225. Braun-Falco O, Heilgemeir GP. The trichogram. Structural and functional basis, performance, and interpretation. Semin Dermatol 1985; 4: 40–52.

226. Weedon D, Strutton G. Apoptosis as the mechanism of the involution of hair follicles in catagen transformation. Acta Derm Venereol 1981; 61: 335–339.

227. Weedon D, Strutton G. The recognition of early stages of catagen. Am J Dermatopathol 1984; 6: 553–555.

228. Hollis DE, Chapman RE. Apoptosis in wool follicles during mouse epidermal growth factor (mEGF)-induced catagen regression. J Invest Dermatol 1987; 88: 455–458.

229. Barth JH. Normal hair growth in children. Pediatr Dermatol 1987; 4: 173–184.
230. Rook A, Dawber R. Diseases of the hair and scalp. Oxford: Blackwell Scientific Publications, 1982; 146–178.

Congenital/hereditary alopecias

231. Muller SA. Alopecia: syndromes of genetic significance. J Invest Dermatol 1973; 60: 475–491.
232. Barth JH, Dawber RPR. Focal naevoid hypotrichosis. Acta Derm Venereol 1987; 67: 178–179.
233. Vogt BR, Traupe H, Hamm H. Congenital atrichia with nail dystrophy, abnormal facies, and retarded psychomotor development in two siblings: a new autosomal recessive syndrome? Pediatr Dermatol 1988; 5: 236–242.
234. Kulin P, Sybert VP. Hereditary hypotrichosis and localized morphea: a new clinical entity. Pediatr Dermatol 1986; 3: 333–338.
235. Baden HP, Kubilus J. Analysis of hair from alopecia congenita. J Am Acad Dermatol 1980; 3: 623–626.
236. Bentley-Phillips B, Grace HJ. Hereditary hypotrichosis. A previously undescribed syndrome. Br J Dermatol 1979; 101: 331–339.
237. Toribio J, Quinones PA. Hereditary hypotrichosis simplex of the scalp. Evidence for autosomal dominant inheritance. Br J Dermatol 1974; 91: 687–696.
238. Stevanovic DV. Hereditary hypotrichosis congenita: Marie Unna type. Br J Dermatol 1970; 83: 331–337.
239. del Castillo V, Ruiz-Maldonado R, Carnevale A. Atrichia with papular lesions and mental retardation in two sisters. Int J Dermatol 1974; 13: 261–265.
240. Kanzler MH, Rasmussen JE. Atrichia with papular lesions. Arch Dermatol 1986; 122: 565–567.
241. Grattan CEH, Liddle BJ, Willshaw HE. Atrophic alopecia in the Hallermann–Streiff syndrome. Clin Exp Dermatol 1989; 14: 250–252.
242. Golomb RS, Porter PS. A distinct hair shaft abnormality in the Hallermann–Streiff syndrome. Cutis 1975; 16: 122–128.

Premature catagen/telogen

243. Kligman AM. Pathologic dynamics of human hair loss. I. Telogen effluvium. Arch Dermatol 1961; 83: 175–198.
244. Steck WD. Telogen effluvium. A clinically useful concept, with traction alopecia as an example. Cutis 1978; 21: 543–548.
245. Headington JT, Astle N. Familial focal alopecia. A new disorder of hair growth clinically resembling pseudopelade. Arch Dermatol 1987; 123: 234–237.
246. Oranje AP, Peereboom-Wynia JDR, De Raeymaecker DMJ. Trichotillomania in childhood. J Am Acad Dermatol 1986; 15: 614–619.
247. Wiles JC, Hansen RC. Postoperative (pressure) alopecia. J Am Acad Dermatol 1985; 12: 195–198.
248. Dawber R. Self-induced hair loss. Semin Dermatol 1985; 4: 53–57.
249. Lachapelle JM, Pierard GE. Traumatic alopecia in trichotillomania: a pathogenic interpretation of histologic lesions in the pilosebaceous unit. J Cutan Pathol 1977; 4: 51–67.
250. Mehregan AH. Trichotillomania. A clinicopathologic study. Arch Dermatol 1970; 102: 129–133.

251. Muller SA, Winkelmann RK. Trichotillomania. A clinicopathologic study of 24 cases. Arch Dermatol 1972; 105: 535–540.
251a. Muller SA. Trichotillomania: A histopathologic study in sixty-six patients. J Am Acad Dermatol 1990; 23: 56–62.
252. Rook A, Dawber R. Diseases of the hair and scalp. Oxford: Blackwell Scientific Publications, 1982; 115–125.
253. Klein AW, Rudolph RI, Leyden JJ. Telogen effluvium as a sign of Hodgkin's disease. Arch Dermatol 1973; 108: 702–703.
254. Bardelli A, Rebora A. Telogen effluvium and minoxidil. J Am Acad Dermatol 1989; 21: 572–573.

Premature telogen with anagen arrest

255. Friedmann PS. Clinical and immunologic associations of alopecia areata. Semin Dermatol 1985; 4: 9–15.
256. Nelson DA, Spielvogel RL. Alopecia areata. Int J Dermatol 1985; 24: 26–34.
257. Mitchell AJ, Krull EA. Alopecia areata: Pathogenesis and treatment. J Am Acad Dermatol 1984; 11: 763–775.
258. Muller SA, Winkelmann RK. Alopecia areata. An evaluation of 736 patients. Arch Dermatol 1963; 88: 290–297.
259. Friedman PS. Alopecia areata and auto-immunity. Br J Dermatol 1981; 105: 153–157.
260. Hordinsky MK, Hallgren H, Nelson D, Filipovich AH. Familial alopecia areata. HLA antigens and autoantibody formation in an American family. Arch Dermatol 1984; 120: 464–468.
261. Muller HK, Rook AJ, Kubba R. Immunohistology and autoantibody studies in alopecia areata. Br J Dermatol 1980; 102: 609–610.
262. Korkij W, Soltani K, Simjee S et al. Tissue-specific autoantibodies and autoimmune disorders in vitiligo and alopecia areata: a retrospective study. J Cutan Pathol 1984; 11: 522–530.
263. Galbraith GMP, Thiers BH, Vasily DB, Fudenberg HH. Immunological profiles in alopecia areata. Br J Dermatol 1984; 110: 163–170.
264. Hordinsky MK, Hallgren H, Nelson D, Filipovich AH. Suppressor cell number and function in alopecia areata. Arch Dermatol 1984; 120: 188–194.
265. Main RA, Robbie RB, Gray ES et al. Smooth muscle antibodies and alopecia areata. Br J Dermatol 1975; 92: 389–393.
266. Milgraum SS, Mitchell AJ, Bacon GE, Rasmussen JE. Alopecia areata, endocrine function, and autoantibodies in patients 16 years of age or younger. J Am Acad Dermatol 1987; 17: 57–61.
267. Kern F, Hoffman WH, Hambrick GW Jr, Blizzard RM. Alopecia areata. Immunologic studies and treatment with prednisone. Arch Dermatol 1973; 107: 407–412.
268. Cochran REI, Thomson J, MacSween RNM. An auto-antibody profile in alopecia totalis and diffuse alopecia. Br J Dermatol 1976; 95: 61–65.
269. Kianto U, Reunala T, Karvonen J et al. HLA-B12 in alopecia areata. Arch Dermatol 1977; 113: 1716.
270. Baadsgaard O, Lindskov R. Circulating lymphocyte subsets in patients with alopecia areata. Acta Derm Venereol 1986; 66: 266–268.

271. De Weert J, Temmerman L, Kint A. Alopecia: a clinical study. Dermatologica 1984; 168: 224–229.

272. Carter DM, Jegasothy BV. Alopecia areata and Down syndrome. Arch Dermatol 1976; 112: 1397–1399.

273. Brown AC. Alopecia areata: a neuroendocrine disorder. Semin Dermatol 1985; 4: 16–28.

274. Shelley WB. The spotted lunula. A neglected nail sign associated with alopecia areata. J Am Acad Dermatol 1980; 2: 385–387.

274a. Perret CM, Steijlen PM, Happle R. Alopecia areata. Pathogenesis and topical immunotherapy. Int J Dermatol 1990; 29: 83–88.

275. Friedman PS. Decreased lymphocyte reactivity and auto-immunity in alopecia areata. Br J Dermatol 1981; 105: 145–151.

276. Majewski BBJ, Koh MS, Taylor DR et al. Increased ratio of helper to suppressor T cells in alopecia areata. Br J Dermatol 1984; 110: 171–175.

277. Lutz G, Niedecken H, Bauer R, Kreysel HW. Natural killer cell and cytotoxic/suppressor T cell deficiency in peripheral blood in subjects with alopecia areata. Australas J Dermatol 1988; 29: 29–32.

278. Galbraith GMP, Thiers BH, Jensen J, Hoehler F. A randomized double-blind study of inosiplex (Isoprinosine) therapy in patients with alopecia totalis. J Am Acad Dermatol 1987; 16: 977–983.

279. Swanson NA, Mitchell AJ, Leahy MS et al. Topical treatment of alopecia areata. Arch Dermatol 1981; 117: 384–387.

280. Baadsgaard O, Lindskov R, Clemmensen OJ. *In situ* lymphocyte subsets in alopecia areata before and during treatment with a contact allergen. Clin Exp Dermatol 1987; 12: 260–264.

281. Ranki A, Kianto U, Kanerva L et al. Immunohistochemical and electron microscopic characterization of the cellular infiltrate in alopecia (areata, totalis, and universalis). J Invest Dermatol 1984; 83: 7–11.

282. Todes-Taylor N, Turner R, Wood GS et al. T cell subpopulations in alopecia areata. J Am Acad Dermatol 1984; 11: 216–223.

283. Peereboom-Wynia JDR, van Joost T, Stolz E, Prins MEF. Markers of immunologic injury in progressive alopecia areata. J Cutan Pathol 1986; 13: 363–369.

284. Khoury EL, Price VH, Greenspan JS. HLA-DR expression by hair follicle keratinocytes in alopecia areata: evidence that it is secondary to the lymphoid infiltration. J Invest Dermatol 1988; 90: 193–200.

285. Messenger AG, Slater DN, Bleehen SS. Alopecia areata: alterations in the hair growth cycle and correlation with the follicular pathology. Br J Dermatol 1986; 114: 337–347.

286. Eckert J, Church RE, Ebling FJ. The pathogenesis of alopecia areata. Br J Dermatol 1968; 80: 203–210.

287. Headington JT, Mitchell A, Swanson N. New histopathologic findings in alopecia areata studied in transverse sections. J Invest Dermatol 1981; 76: 325 (abstract).

288. Messenger AG, Bleehen SS. Alopecia areata: light and electron microscopic pathology of the regrowing white hair. Br J Dermatol 1984; 110: 155–162.

289. Van Scott EJ. Morphologic changes in pilosebaceous units and anagen hairs in alopecia areata. J Invest Dermatol 1958; 31: 35–43.

290. Gilhar A, Krueger GG. Hair growth in scalp grafts from patients with alopecia areata and alopecia universalis grafted onto nude mice. Arch Dermatol 1987; 123: 44–50.

291. Headington JT. Transverse microscopic anatomy of the human scalp. A basis for a morphometric approach to disorders of the hair follicle. Arch Dermatol 1984; 120: 449–456.

292. Whiting DA. Diagnostic and predictive value of transverse sections of scalp biopsies in alopecia areata. J Cutan Pathol 1988; 15: 350 (abstract).

293. Pinkus H. Differential patterns of elastic fibers in scarring and non-scarring alopecias. J Cutan Pathol 1978; 5: 93–104.

294. Klaber MR, Munro DD. Alopecia areata: immunofluorescence and other studies. Br J Dermatol 1978; 99: 383–386.

295. Igarashi R, Morohashi M, Takeuchi S, Sato Y. Immunofluorescence studies on complement components in the hair follicles of normal scalp and of scalp affected by alopecia areata. Acta Derm Venereol 1981; 61: 131–135.

296. Bystryn J-C, Orentreich N, Stengel F. Direct immunofluorescence studies in alopecia areata and male pattern alopecia. J Invest Dermatol 1979; 73: 317–320.

Vellus follicle formation

297. Rook A, Dawber R. Diseases of the hair and scalp. Oxford: Blackwell Scientific Publications, 1982; 90–114.

298. Rushton H, James KC, Mortimer CH. The unit area trichogram in the assessment of androgen-dependent alopecia. Br J Dermatol 1983; 109: 429–437.

299. Alexander S. Common baldness in women. Semin Dermatol 1985; 4: 1–3.

300. De Villez RL, Dunn J. Female androgenic alopecia. Arch Dermatol 1986; 122: 1011–1015.

301. Ludwig E. Classification of the types of androgenetic alopecia (common baldness) occurring in the female sex. Br J Dermatol 1977; 97: 247–254.

302. Venning VA, Dawber RPR. Patterned alopecia in women. J Am Acad Dermatol 1988; 18: 1073–1077.

303. Dawber RPR. Alopecia and hirsutism. Clin Exp Dermatol 1982; 7: 177–182.

303a. Olsen EA, Buller TA, Weiner S, Delong ER. Natural history of androgenetic alopecia. Clin Exp Dermatol 1990; 15: 34–36.

304. Phillipou G, Kirk J. Significance of steroid measurements in male pattern alopecia. Clin Exp Dermatol 1981; 6: 53–56.

305. Pitts RL. Serum elevation of dehydroepiandrosterone sulfate associated with male pattern baldness in young men. J Am Acad Dermatol 1987; 16: 571–573.

306. Hay JB. A study of the *in vitro* metabolism of androgens by human scalp and pubic skin. Br J Dermatol 1977; 97: 237–246.

307. Lucky AW. The paradox of androgens and balding: where are we now? J Invest Dermatol 1988; 91: 99–100.

308. Futterweit W, Dunaif A, Yeh H-C, Kingsley P. The prevalence of hyperandrogenism in 109 consecutive female patients with diffuse alopecia. J Am Acad Dermatol 1988; 19: 831–836.

309. Dawber RPR. Common baldness in women. Int J

Dermatol 1981; 20: 647–650.

310. Lattanand A, Johnson WC. Male pattern alopecia. A histopathologic and histochemical study. J Cutan Pathol 1975; 2: 58–70.

311. Pestana A, Olsen EA, Delong ER, Murray JC. Effect of ultraviolet light on topical minoxidil-induced hair growth in advanced male pattern baldness. J Am Acad Dermatol 1987; 16: 971–976.

312. Domnitz JM, Silvers DN. Giant cells in male pattern alopecia: a histologic marker and pathogenetic clue. J Cutan Pathol 1979; 6: 108–112.

313. Scott GS, Stenn KS, Savin R. Diffuse female pattern alopecia — a histological study of 40 cases. J Cutan Pathol 1988; 15: 341 (abstract).

314. Kubba R, Rook A. Congenital triangular alopecia. Br J Dermatol 1976; 95: 657–659.

315. Tosti A. Congenital triangular alopecia. Report of fourteen cases. J Am Acad Dermatol 1987; 16: 991–993.

316. Minars N. Congenital temporal alopecia. Arch Dermatol 1974; 109: 395–396.

Anagen defluvium

317. Hamm H, Traupe H. Loose anagen hair of childhood: The phenomenon of easily pluckable hair. J Am Acad Dermatol 1989; 20: 242–248.

318. Price VH, Gummer CL. Loose anagen syndrome. J Am Acad Dermatol 1989; 20: 249–256.

319. Rook A, Dawber R. Diseases of the hair and scalp. Oxford: Blackwell Scientific Publications, 1982; 133–145.

320. Stroud JD. Drug-induced alopecia. Semin Dermatol 1985; 4: 29–34.

321. Levantine A, Almeyda J. Drug induced alopecia. Br J Dermatol 1973; 89: 549–553.

Scarring alopecias

322. Rook A, Dawber R. Diseases of the hair and scalp. Oxford: Blackwell Scientific Publications, 1982; 307–341.

323. Roenigk RK, Wheeland RG. Tissue expansion in cicatricial alopecia. Arch Dermatol 1987; 123: 641–646.

324. Ronchese F. Pseudopelade. Arch Dermatol 1960; 82: 336–343.

325. Pierard-Franchimont C, Pierard GE. Massive lymphocyte-mediated apoptosis during the early stage of pseudopelade. Dermatologica 1986; 172: 254–257.

326. Jordon RE. Subtle clues to diagnosis by immunopathology. Scarring alopecia. Am J Dermatopathol 1980; 2: 157–159.

MISCELLANEOUS DISORDERS

Pilosebaceous disorders

327. Fenton DA. Hypertrichosis. Semin Dermatol 1985; 4: 58–67.

328. Beighton P. Congenital hypertrichosis lanuginosa. Arch Dermatol 1970; 101: 669–672.

329. Fretzin DF. Malignant down. Arch Dermatol 1967; 95: 294–297.

330. Sindhuphak W, Vibhagool A. Acquired hypertrichosis lanuginosa. Int J Dermatol 1982; 21: 599–601.

331. McLean DI, Macaulay JC. Hypertrichosis lanuginosa acquisita associated with pancreatic carcinoma. Br J Dermatol 1977; 96: 313–316.

332. Jemec GBE. Hypertrichosis lanuginosa acquisita. Report of a case and review of the literature. Arch Dermatol 1986; 122: 805–808.

333. Wadskov S, Bro-Jorgensen A, Sondergaard J. Acquired hypertrichosis lanuginosa. A skin marker of internal malignancy. Arch Dermatol 1976; 112: 1442–1444.

334. Goodfellow A, Calvert H, Bohn G. Hypertrichosis lanuginosa acquisita. Br J Dermatol 1980; 103: 431–433.

335. Burton JL, Marshall A. Hypertrichosis due to minoxidil. Br J Dermatol 1979; 101: 593–595.

336. Kassis V, Sondergaard J. Hypertrichosis lanuginosa. Semin Dermatol 1984; 3: 282–286.

337. Cox NH, McClure JP, Hardie RA. Naevoid hypertrichosis — report of a patient with multiple lesions. Clin Exp Dermatol 1989; 14: 62–64.

338. Harris HW, Miller OF. Midline cutaneous and spinal defects. Midline cutaneous abnormalities associated with occult spinal disorders. Arch Dermatol 1976; 112: 1724–1728.

339. Tisocco LA, Del Campo DV, Bennin B, Barsky S. Acquired localized hypertrichosis. Arch Dermatol 1981; 117: 127–128.

340. Hegedus SI, Schorr WF. Acquired hypertrichosis lanuginosa and malignancy. Arch Dermatol 1972; 106: 84–88.

341. Forman L. Keratosis pilaris. Br J Dermatol 1954; 66: 279–282.

341a. Bork K, Bockers M, Pfeifle J. Pathogenesis of paraneoplastic follicular hyperkeratotic spicules in multiple myeloma. Arch Dermatol 1990; 126: 509–513.

342. Barth JH, Wojnarowska F, Dawber RPR. Is keratosis pilaris another androgen-dependent dermatosis? Clin Exp Dermatol 1988; 13: 240–241.

343. Garcia-Bravo B, Rodriguez-Pichardo A, Camacho F. Uraemic follicular hyperkeratosis. Clin Exp Dermatol 1985; 10: 448–454.

343a. Friedman SJ. Lichen spinulosus. Clinicopathologic review of thirty-five cases. J Am Acad Dermatol 1990; 22: 261–264.

344. Ayres S Jr. Extrafacial rosacea is rare but does exist. J Am Acad Dermatol 1987; 16: 391–392.

344a. Rebora A. Rosacea. J Invest Dermatol (Suppl) 1987; 88: 56s–60s.

345. Marks R, Wilson Jones E. Disseminated rosacea. Br J Dermatol 1969; 81: 16–28.

346. Wilkin JK. Rosacea. Int J Dermatol 1983; 22: 393–400.

347. Rosen T, Stone MS. Acne rosacea in blacks. J Am Acad Dermatol 1987; 17: 70–73.

348. Dotz W, Berliner N. Rhinophyma. A master's depiction, a patron's affliction. Am J Dermatopathol 1984; 6: 231–235.

349. Marks R. Concepts in the pathogenesis of rosacea. Br J Dermatol 1968; 80: 170–177.

350. Findlay GH, Simson IW. Leonine hypertrophic

rosacea associated with a benign bronchial carcinoid tumour. Clin Exp Dermatol 1977; 2: 175–176.

351. Wilkin JK. Vasodilator rosacea. Arch Dermatol 1980; 116: 598.

352. Leyden JJ, Thew M, Kligman AM. Steroid rosacea. Arch Dermatol 1974; 110: 619–622.

353. Marks R, Black MM. Perioral dermatitis. A histopathological study of 26 cases. Br J Dermatol 1971; 84: 242–247.

354. Cotterill JA. Perioral dermatitis. Br J Dermatol 1979; 101: 259–262.

355. Wilkinson DS, Kirton V, Wilkinson JD. Perioral dermatitis: a 12–year review. Br J Dermatol 1979; 101: 245–257.

356. Wilkinson D. What is perioral dermatitis? Int J Dermatol 1981; 20: 485–486.

357. Marks R, Harcourt-Webster JN. Histopathology of rosacea. Arch Dermatol 1969; 100: 683–691.

358. Mullanax MG, Kierland RR. Granulomatous rosacea. Arch Dermatol 1970; 101: 206–211.

359. Acker DW, Helwig EB. Rhinophyma with carcinoma. Arch Dermatol 1967; 95: 250–254.

360. Nunzi E, Rebora A, Hamerlinck F, Cormane RH. Immunopathological studies on rosacea. Br J Dermatol 1980; 103: 543–551.

361. Manna V, Marks R, Holt P. Involvement of immune mechanisms in the pathogenesis of rosacea. Br J Dermatol 1982; 107: 203–208.

Apocrine disorders

362. Shelley WB, Levy EJ. Apocrine sweat retention in man: II. Fox–Fordyce disease (apocrine miliaria). Arch Dermatol 1956; 73: 38–49.

363. MacMillan DC, Vickers HR. Fox–Fordyce disease. Br J Dermatol 1971; 84: 181.

364. Giacobetti R, Caro WA, Roenigk HH Jr. Fox–Fordyce disease. Control with tretinoin cream. Arch Dermatol 1979; 115: 1365–1366.

365. Graham JH, Shafer JC, Helwig EB. Fox–Fordyce disease in male identical twins. Arch Dermatol 1960; 82: 212–221.

366. Carleton AB, Hall GS, Wigley JEM, Symmers W St C. Cited in Systemic Pathology, 2nd ed. Edinburgh: Churchill Livingstone, 1980; 6: 2636.

367. Montes LF, Cortes A, Baker BL, Curtis AC. Fox–Fordyce disease. A report with endocrinological and histopathological studies, of a case which developed after surgical menopause. Arch Dermatol 1959; 80: 549–553.

368. Mali-Gerrits MMG, van de Kerkhof PCM, Mier PD, Happle R. Axillary apocrine chromhidrosis. Arch Dermatol 1988; 124: 494–496.

Eccrine disorders

369. Mehregan AH. Proliferation of sweat ducts in certain diseases of the skin. Am J Dermatopathol 1981; 3: 27–31.

370. Freeman RG. On the pathogenesis of pseudoepitheliomatous hyperplasia. J Cutan Pathol 1974; 1: 231–237.

371. Santa Cruz DJ, Clausen K. Atypical sweat duct hyperplasia accompanying keratoacanthoma. Dermatologica 1977; 154: 156–160.

372. Weedon D. Eccrine tumors: a selective review. J Cutan Pathol 1984; 11: 421–436.

373. Vakilzadeh F, Brocker EB. Syringolymphoid hyperplasia with alopecia. Br J Dermatol 1984; 110: 95–101.

374. Kossard S, Munro V, King R. Syringolymphoid hyperplasia with alopecia. J Cutan Pathol 1988; 15: 322 (abstract).

375. Barnhill RL, Goldberg B, Stenn KS. Proliferation of eccrine sweat ducts associated with alopecia areata. J Cutan Pathol 1988; 15: 36–39.

376. Lerner TH, Barr RJ, Dolezal JF, Stagnone JJ. Syringomatous hyperplasia and eccrine squamous syringometaplasia associated with benoxaprofen therapy. Arch Dermatol 1987; 123: 1202–1204.

377. Burket JM, Brooks R, Burket DA. Eccrine gland reticulated cytoplasm. J Am Acad Dermatol 1985; 13: 497–500.

378. Holyoke JB, Lobitz WC Jr. Histologic variations in the structure of human eccrine sweat glands. J Invest Dermatol 1952; 18: 147–167.

379. Luther H, Altmeyer P. Eccrine sweat gland reaction. A histological and immunocytochemical study. Am J Dermatopathol 1988; 10: 390–398.

379a. Leshin B, White WL, Koufman JA. Radiation-induced squamous sialometaplasia. Arch Dermatol 1990; 126: 931–934.

380. King DT, Barr RJ. Syringometaplasia: mucinous and squamous variants. J Cutan Pathol 1979; 6: 284–291.

381. Metcalf JS, Maize JC. Squamous syringometaplasia in lobular panniculitis and pyoderma gangrenosum. Am J Dermatopathol 1990; 12: 141–149.

382. Bhawan J, Malhotra R. Syringosquamous metaplasia. A distinctive eruption in patients receiving chemotherapy. Am J Dermatopathol 1990; 12: 1–6.

383. Hurt MA, Halvorsen RD, Petr FC Jr et al. Eccrine squamous syringometaplasia. Arch Dermatol 1990; 126: 73–77.

384. Kinney RB, Burton CS, Vollmer RT. Necrotizing sialometaplasia: a sheep in wolf's clothing. Arch Dermatol 1986; 122: 208–210.

385. Scully K, Assaad D. Mucinous syringometaplasia. J Am Acad Dermatol 1984; 11: 503–508.

386. Walker AN, Morton BD. Acral mucinous syringometaplasia. A benign cutaneous lesion associated with verrucous hyperplasia. Arch Pathol Lab Med 1986; 110: 248–249.

387. Kwittken J. Muciparous epidermal tumor. Arch Dermatol 1974; 109: 554–555.

388. Mehregan AH. Mucinous syringometaplasia. Arch Dermatol 1980; 116: 988–989.

389. Poomeechaiwong S, Hahn DC, Golitz LE. Mucinous and squamous syringometaplasia. J Cutan Pathol 1988; 15: 339 (abstract).

390. Harrist TJ, Fine JD, Berman RS et al. Neutrophilic eccrine hidradenitis. Arch Dermatol 1982; 118: 263–266.

391. Flynn TC, Harrist TJ, Murphy GF et al. Neutrophilic eccrine hidradenitis: a distinctive rash associated with cytarabine therapy and acute leukemia. J Am Acad Dermatol 1984; 11: 584–590.

392. Beutner KR, Packman CH, Markowitch W. Neutrophilic eccrine hidradenitis associated with Hodgkin's disease and chemotherapy. Arch Dermatol 1986; 122: 809–811.

393. Fitzpatrick JE, Bennion SD, Reed OM et al. Neutrophilic eccrine hidradenitis associated with induction chemotherapy. J Cutan Pathol 1987; 14: 272–278.

394. Bailey DL, Barron D, Lucky AW. Neutrophilic eccrine hidradenitis: a case report and review of the literature. Pediatr Dermatol 1989; 6: 33–38.

395. Scallan PJ, Kettler AH, Levy ML, Tschen JA. Neutrophilic eccrine hidradenitis. Evidence implicating bleomycin as a causative agent. Cancer 1988; 62: 2532–2536.

Cysts and sinuses

INTRODUCTION

A cyst is an enclosed space within a tissue, usually containing fluid and lined by epithelium. Cysts are usually classified on the basis of their pathogenesis. In the skin, the most important cysts are derived from the dermal appendages as retention cysts. The developmental cysts, which result from the persistence of vestigial remnants, are much less common. The term 'pseudocyst' is sometimes applied to cyst-like structures without an epithelial lining.

The important histological features of the various cutaneous cysts are shown in Table 16.1 (page 496).

APPENDAGEAL CYSTS

EPIDERMAL (INFUNDIBULAR) CYST

Epidermal cysts are solitary, slowly growing cysts with a predilection for the trunk, neck and face. They measure 1–4 cm or more in diameter. Epidermal cysts are usually located in the mid and lower dermis but they do not shell out like the tricholemmal cyst. There is often a surface punctum.

They are thought to be derived from the pilosebaceous follicle, but they may arise from implantation of the epidermis,[1] particularly on the palms and soles,[2] and in the subungual region.[3] Epidermal cysts have also developed following chronic dermabrasion.[4] Multiple cysts may be found in Gardner's syndrome.[5] Epidermal cysts may become infected, and this may be followed by rupture of the cyst, usually into

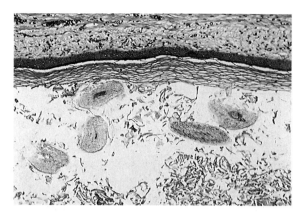

Fig. 16.3   Pigmented follicular cyst. The lumen of the cyst contains a number of pigmented hair shafts.
Haematoxylin — eosin

pigmented hair shafts (Fig. 16.3). The cyst is lined by stratified squamous epithelium showing epidermal keratinization, but in addition the lining may show rete ridges and dermal papillae, a feature not seen in epidermal cysts.

CUTANEOUS KERATOCYST

Cutaneous cysts are a feature of the basal cell naevus syndrome (see p. 750). Usually these cysts are of epidermal type, but there is a recent report of a patient with this syndrome in whom two of the cutaneous cysts resembled keratocysts of the jaw.[36] They contained a thick brown fluid.

Histopathology[36]

The cysts had a corrugated or festooned configuration with a lining of several layers of squamous epithelium, but with no granular layer. Lanugo hairs were present in one cyst. There was a superficial resemblance to steatocystoma multiplex (see below), but there were no sebaceous lobules in the wall.

VELLUS HAIR CYST

Eruptive vellus hair cysts, first reported in 1977,[37] occur as multiple, small, asymptomatic papules with a predilection for the chest and axilla of children or young adults.[38] They are also found on the face,[39] neck and extremities. They may have an autosomal dominant inheritance or occur sporadically.[40,41] Spontaneous regression of the cysts has been reported, probably following the transepidermal elimination of the cyst contents.[42]

An eruptive vellus hair cyst has been reported in a patient with a steatocystoma, suggesting that these two entities are in some way related;[43] both may be derived from the sebaceous duct.[44]

Histopathology[37]

These small dermal cysts are lined by stratified squamous epithelium which may show focal tricholemmal as well as epidermoid keratinization. The lumen contains keratin and numerous transversely and obliquely sectioned vellus hair shafts (Fig. 16.4). These are doubly refractile

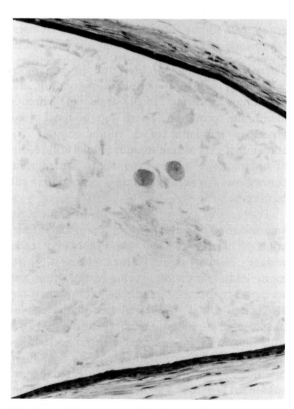

Fig. 16.4   Vellus hair cyst. The lumen of the cyst contains small vellus hairs.
Haematoxylin — eosin

with polarized light. A rudimentary hair follicle may be attached to the wall. There may be focal rupture of the cyst wall with a foreign body granulomatous reaction and associated dermal fibrosis and mild chronic inflammation.

Some cysts may show a connecting pore at the skin surface, the likely mechanism of the spontaneous regression mentioned above.

STEATOCYSTOMA MULTIPLEX

This condition is characterized by multiple yellowish to skin-coloured papules[45] or cysts measuring from less than 3 mm in diameter to 3 cm or more. They may be found on the face,[45-47] scalp,[48] trunk, axillae and proximal parts of the extremities, but they have a predilection for the chest. They are mostly sporadic, but familial cases with autosomal dominant inheritance are well documented.[49] Other abnormalities may be present in the inherited cases.[46] Patients with only a solitary lesion (steatocystoma simplex) are seen rarely.[50] The cysts usually present in adolescents as asymptomatic lesions, but infected cysts may be painful.[51] Steatocystoma is thought to represent a naevoid malformation of the pilosebaceous duct.

Histopathology[49]

The lining of the dermal cysts is usually undulating due to collapse of the cyst. It is composed of stratified squamous epithelium, only a few cells thick, and without a granular layer. The characteristic feature is the presence of sebaceous glands of varying size in or adjacent to the wall (Fig. 16.5). A ribbon-like cord of epithelial cells connects the cyst with the epidermis, but this may not be seen in the plane of section. One pilar unit is associated with each cyst and the cyst may contain one or more lanugo hairs.

Electron microscopy. The keratinization takes place without the formation of keratohyaline granules, a feature which is characteristic of the sebaceous duct.[45]

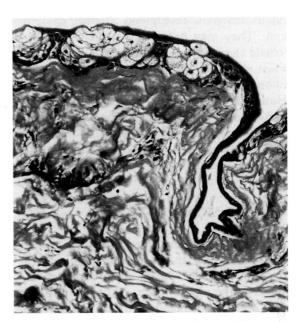

Fig. 16.5 Steatocystoma multiplex. The cyst wall has an undulating appearance. An occasional sebaceous gland is present within the epithelial lining.
Haematoxylin — eosin

MILIUM

A milium is a small (1 or 2 mm in diameter) dermal cyst which may arise from the pilosebaceous apparatus or eccrine sweat ducts.[52] Milia may be seen in the newborn as congenital lesions or they may develop later in life secondary to dermabrasion, to the topical application of corticosteroids,[52] and to radiotherapy, and as a consequence of subepidermal bullous disorders such as porphyria cutanea tarda, epidermolysis bullosa dystrophica and second-degree burns. They have also been reported in association with some inherited disorders.[53]

Milia most commonly occur as multiple lesions on the cheeks and forehead, but they may involve the genitalia or other sites depending on the predisposing lesion. A rare erythematous plaque variant has been reported.[53,54]

Histopathology

The small cysts are lined by several layers of stratified squamous epithelium with central kera-

squamous epithelium present in the outer part of the cyst in those presenting as a sinus on the skin surface.[74] Smooth muscle and even mucous glands are found commonly in the wall, but cartilage is present only occasionally. There may be some inflammation and fibrosis adjacent to the cyst.

BRANCHIAL CLEFT CYST

Branchial cleft remnants present clinically as cysts, sinus tracts, skin tags or combinations of these lesions.[73a,75] Those derived from the second branchial pouch are usually found along the anterior border of the sternomastoid muscle of children or young adults, while those of first pouch origin arise near the angle of the mandible. They may be found at any depth between the skin and pharynx. Secondary infection may cause sudden swelling of the lesions.

The cysts contain turbid fluid, rich in cholesterol crystals. Squamous cell carcinoma is a rare complication in lesions of long standing.[76,77]

Histopathology

The cysts are mostly lined by stratified squamous epithelium, but deeper parts may have a lining of ciliated columnar epithelium. A heavy lymphoid infiltrate invests the cyst or sinus wall, and this includes lymphoid follicles. Mucinous glands and cartilage are occasionally present in the wall.[73]

THYROGLOSSAL CYST

Most examples of thyroglossal cyst are deep lesions in the midline of the neck and therefore beyond the scope of this volume. There is one report of a depressed lesion in the midline of the neck, present since birth, which consisted of tubular glands lined by respiratory epithelium, opening on to the skin surface.[73] Deeper branching tubules penetrated into the underlying striated muscle. The lesion was presumed to be of thyroglossal duct origin.

THYMIC CYST

These rare cysts are found in the mediastinum or neck. The cervical lesions usually present as painless swellings in children or adolescents.[78-80] Thymic cysts are thought to arise from remnants of the thymopharyngeal duct, a derivative of the third pouch. They are most often found posterior to a lateral lobe of the thyroid, more often on the left-hand side.

The cysts are unilocular or multilocular and measure from 1 to 15 cm in diameter. The contents are variable, ranging from yellow-brown fluid to cloudy or gelatinous material. Cholesterol crystals may be present.

Histopathology

Thymic cysts are lined by one or more of the following epithelia: squamous, columnar, cuboidal or pseudostratified columnar. Occasionally, the cyst is devoid of an epithelial lining and has a fibrous tissue lining only. The wall characteristically contains Hassall's corpuscles and in addition there may be lymphoid tissue, cholesterol granulomas and sometimes parathyroid tissue.[78]

Thymic remnants, without cyst formation, have been reported in the skin of the neck.[80a]

CUTANEOUS CILIATED CYST OF THE LOWER LIMBS

The term 'cutaneous ciliated cyst' is sometimes applied to several varieties of developmental cysts that are lined by ciliated epithelium but that are of quite different origin (see above). It is best restricted to a rare cyst which usually arises on the lower extremities of women in the second and third decade.[81,81a] The cysts are less than 3 cm in diameter. They have been thought to be of Müllerian origin, but the occurrence of a case in a male has raised the possibility of an origin from an eccrine sweat gland.[82]

Histopathology

The cyst is lined by ciliated cuboidal to

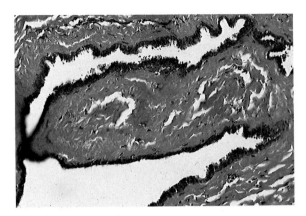

Fig. 16.9 Cutaneous ciliated cyst. The cyst is collapsed with some infolding of the wall. The lining epithelium is ciliated.
Haematoxylin — eosin

columnar epithelium with pseudostratified areas (Fig. 16.9). Focal squamous metaplasia is sometimes present. The cysts may be multilocular and there are often papillary projections into the lumen. Glandular and smooth muscle elements are absent.[83]

VULVAL MUCINOUS AND CILIATED CYST

These cysts are found in the vestibule of the vulva.[84] They vary in size from 0.5 to 3.0 cm or more. Included among the cases reported have been several instances of Bartholin's cyst. Vulval mucinous and ciliated cysts are presumed to be of urogenital sinus origin.

Histopathology

The cysts are lined by pseudostratified ciliated columnar epithelium and/or mucinous epithelium. There may be areas of squamous metaplasia.

MEDIAN RAPHE CYST

This is the preferred term for midline developmental cysts found at any point from the external urethral meatus to the anus, including the ventral aspect of the penis, the scrotal raphe and the perineal raphe, but most commonly near the glans penis.[85] They are thought to arise as a result of defective embryological closure of the median raphe, but some may result from the anomalous outgrowth of the entodermal urethral lining (urethroid cyst).[86] They are most commonly diagnosed in the first three decades of life. Canals coursing longitudinally in the line of the median raphe are sometimes found.[87]

Most raphe cysts are less than 1 cm in diameter. The contents are usually clear, but they may be turbid if there are abundant mucous glands in the wall.

Histopathology[85]

Median raphe cysts are situated in the dermis, but they do not connect with the overlying surface epithelium. They are lined by pseudostratified columnar epithelium, which may be

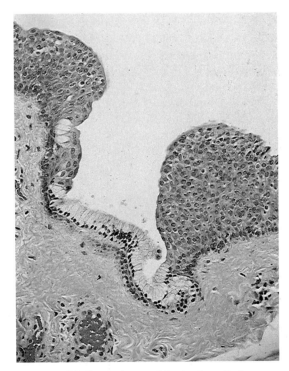

Fig. 16.10 Median raphe cyst. Islands of stratified squamous epithelium are interspersed between mucin-secreting epithelium in the lining of this cyst removed from near the urethral meatus.
Haematoxylin — eosin

quite attenuated in some areas. Occasionally, mucous glands are present in the wall. In cysts situated near the meatus, the lining is usually of stratified squamous epithelium (Fig. 16.10).

DERMOID CYST

Dermoid cysts are rare subcutaneous cysts of ectodermal origin found along lines of embryonic fusion, particularly at the lateral angle of the eye or the midline of the forehead or neck.[88] Those arising in the midline of the dorsum of the nose frequently have an overlying fistula communicating with the skin surface and the underlying cyst, which is sometimes quite deep.[89–92] A tuft of hair usually protrudes from the central pit.

Dermoid cysts are usually asymptomatic masses present at birth, but inflammation, secondary often to trauma, may draw attention to a pre-existing lesion in an older person.

The cysts are unilocular structures between 1 and 4 cm in diameter, containing fine hair shafts admixed with variable amounts of thick yellowish sebum.

The subcutaneous cyst on the back, reported recently as a *cystic teratoma*, had features of both a dermoid and bronchogenic cyst (see below).[93]

Histopathology[88]

Dermoid cysts are lined by keratinizing squamous epithelium with attached pilosebaceous structures (Fig. 16.11). Sebaceous glands may empty directly into the cyst, the lumen of which contains hair shafts and keratinous debris. Eccrine and apocrine glands, as well as smooth muscle, may be present in the wall of up to one-quarter of the cases. Partial rupture of the cyst, resulting in a local foreign body granulomatous reaction, may be found. Focal calcification is a rare finding.

The fistulous tract sometimes found in association with midline dermoids of the nose is lined by the same elements as those found in the cyst wall.[90]

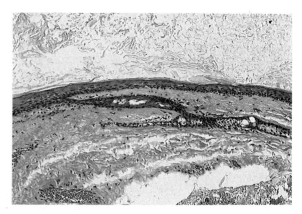

Fig. 16.11 Dermoid cyst. A pilosebaceous structure is attached to the cyst lining, which otherwise resembles an epidermal cyst. Haematoxylin — eosin

CYSTIC TERATOMA

Two cases of cystic teratoma of the skin have been reported in the English language literature.[93,94] Both lesions were present at birth, one in the glabellar region[94] and the other on the back.[93] One was composed of respiratory epithelium, thyroid and nervous tissue, and striated and smooth muscle.[94] The other resembled a dermoid cyst with the addition of areas lined by pseudostratified, ciliated epithelium with goblet cells and occasional seromucinous glands and some surrounding smooth muscle.[93]

MISCELLANEOUS CYSTS

PARASITIC CYSTS

Parasitic cysts are considered in Chapter 29. The most important is cysticercosis, the larval form of *Taenia solium*, which may present as one or more subcutaneous cysts[95] (see p. 712). Sparganosis may also present as a subcutaneous 'cyst' (see p. 713).

PHAEOMYCOTIC CYSTS

A phaeomycotic cyst (phaeohyphomycosis) is a subcutaneous cystic granuloma resulting from infection by hyphae with brown walls.[96] A wood splinter is sometimes present in the lumen and is the source of this opportunistic fungus (see p. 655).

DIGITAL MUCOUS CYST

This lesion is usually found as a tense cystic nodule overlying the distal phalanx of a finger or thumb. Although a single cystic space may be present, there is usually a large myxoid (mucinous) area with multiple microcystic spaces. Accordingly, digital mucous cysts are considered in detail with other mucinoses (see p. 391).

MUCOUS CYST (MUCOCELE)

Mucous cysts, found usually on the lower lip or buccal mucosa, result from the rupture of a duct of a minor salivary gland with extravasation of mucus. Large mucinous pools are formed with a variable inflammatory and fibroblastic response. These lesions are considered with the mucinoses (see p. 392).

METAPLASTIC SYNOVIAL CYST

Metaplastic synovial cysts are intradermal cysts lined by a membrane that resembles hyperplastic synovium.[97,98] The lesions usually arise in surgical scars or at sites of trauma,[98a] unrelated to joints or other synovial structures.[98]

Histopathology[97,98]

The cyst lining resembles hyperplastic synovium with partly hyalinized synovial villi. Sometimes only slit-like spaces lined by synovium are present (Fig. 16.12). The cystic cavities may communicate with the surface epidermis.

PSEUDOCYST OF THE AURICLE

This is an uncommon, non-inflammatory, intracartilaginous lesion affecting the upper half

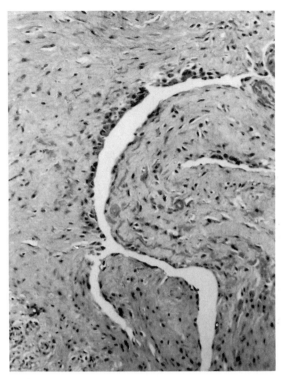

Fig. 16.12   Metaplastic synovial cyst. A slit-like cavity lined by synovium is present below an area of scar tissue in the dermis.
Haematoxylin — eosin

or third of the ear, most often in young or middle-aged males.[99–101] There is usually no clear-cut history of preceding trauma.[102] Ischaemia has been suggested as a possible cause of the cartilaginous degeneration which is followed by the accumulation of yellowish fluid to form a pseudocyst. The term 'seroma' has been used for a closely related entity in which the accumulation of fluid was thought on clinical grounds to be outside the cartilage.[103]

Histopathology

There is an intracartilaginous cavity without an epithelial lining.[99,101] The wall is composed of eosinophilic, amorphous material which may contain smaller clefts (Fig. 16.13). There is focal fibrosis within the cavity, particularly at the margins, and this probably increases with the duration of the lesion.

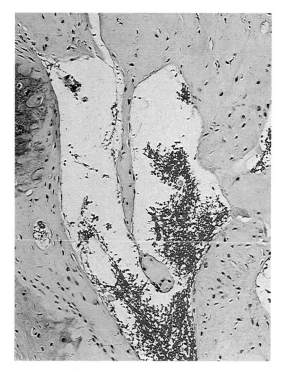

Fig. 16.13 Pseudocyst of the auricle. A cavity is present within the cartilage of the ear. Some operative haemorrhage is also present.
Haematoxylin — eosin

ENDOMETRIOSIS

Endometriosis may be found in the umbilicus, in operation scars of the lower abdomen, particularly those associated with caesarean sections, and rarely in the inguinal region, thighs, and neck.[104–109] Cutaneous endometriosis accounts for less than 1% of cases of ectopic endometrial tissue. The endometrium in most lesions responds to the normal hormonal influences of the menstrual cycle. It presents as a bluish-black tumour of the umbilicus that enlarges about the time of the menses. There may be an associated bloody discharge from the lesion. Most lesions measure from 1 to 3 cm in diameter. Endometriosis arising in scars is usually less well delineated. Such lesions are only partly cystic.

Theories of aetiology include implantation, coelomic metaplasia, lymphatic dissemination and haematogenous spread.

Histopathology[108]

There are multiple endometrial glands with surrounding endometrial stroma (Fig. 16.14). The glands may show the usual cyclical changes of the endometrium. Decidualization of the stroma is occasionally present.[110] The glands show variable cystic dilatation and may contain blood or debris. There is usually haemosiderin pigment in the functioning cases. There may be dense fibrosis between the endometriotic foci. Adenocarcinoma has been reported as a very rare complication.[111]

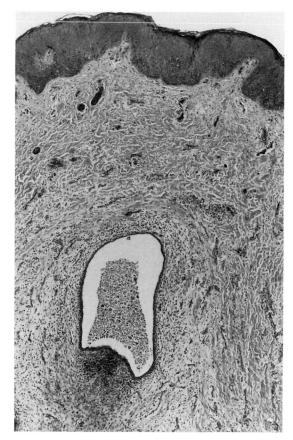

Fig. 16.14 Endometriosis of the umbilicus. An endometrial gland with stroma is set in fibrous tissue. The gland is dilated with luminal haemorrhage.
Haematoxylin — eosin

CUTANEOUS ENDOSALPINGIOSIS

A patient has been reported with multiple

papules around the umbilicus following salpingectomy.[69] The small dermal cysts were lined by tubal epithelium. This appears to be an example of endosalpingiosis, the aberrant growth of Fallopian tube epithelium outside its normal location.

Histopathology

The small cysts were unilocular and filled with granular material. There were some papillary projections into the cyst. The epithelium was composed of columnar, ciliated and secretory cells of endosalpingial type.

LYMPHATIC CYSTS

CYSTIC HYGROMA

This usually presents as a cystic swelling of the subcutaneous tissue of the lower neck of neonates and infants. It is a variant of lymphangioma, with large cavernous spaces in the subcutis lined by flattened endothelium (see p. 962). Islands of connective tissue, and sometimes smooth muscle, are found between the channels.

SINUSES

Sinus tracts may develop in relation to infected wounds, inflamed and ruptured cysts, in association with thyroglossal or branchial cleft vestiges, chronic osteomyelitis and various chronic infections such as tuberculosis, mycetomas and actinomycosis. Two sinuses of dermatopathological importance are the pilonidal sinus and the cutaneous dental sinus.

CUTANEOUS DENTAL SINUS

An intermittently suppurating, chronic sinus tract may develop on the face or neck as a result of a chronic infection of dental origin.[112,113] This is usually an apical abscess.

Histopathology

The sinus tract is lined by heavily inflamed granulation and fibrous tissue. An epithelial lining is sometimes present in part of the tract, in cases of long standing. There are no grains as seen in actinomycosis. Rarely, a squamous cell carcinoma may develop from this epithelium.[112]

PILONIDAL SINUS

This entity occurs most commonly as a sinus in the sacrococcygeal region of hirsute males. Other sites include the umbilicus,[114] axilla, scalp,[115] genital region, eyelid and the finger webs of barbers' hands. Sometimes small cysts may be found in the scalp following hair transplants.[116]

Malignancy, usually a squamous cell carcinoma, may develop as a rare complication in lesions of long standing.

Histopathology

There is usually a sinus tract lined by granulation tissue, with areas of stratified squamous epithelium in the wall in about half the cases. This leads to a bulbous expansion in the lower dermis and subcutaneous tissues where there is a chronic abscess cavity. This contains one or more hair shafts which may be in the lumen, in branches of the main cavity or in the wall itself. There are usually foreign body granulomas in the vicinity of the hairs. There is variable fibrosis in the wall of the sinus and the deeper cavity.

72. Ambiavagar PC, Rosen Y. Cutaneous ciliated cyst of the chin. Probable bronchogenic cyst. Arch Dermatol 1979; 115: 895–896.
73. Shareef DS, Salm R. Ectopic vestigial lesions of the neck and shoulders. J Clin Pathol 1981; 34: 1155–1162.
73a. Coleman WR, Homer RS, Kaplan RR. Branchial cleft heterotopia of the lower neck. J Cutan Pathol 1989; 16: 353–358.
74. Miller OF III, Tyler W. Cutaneous bronchogenic cyst with papilloma and sinus presentation. J Am Acad Dermatol 1984; 11: 367–371.
75. Foote JE, Anderson PC. Branchial cleft remnants suggesting tuberculous lymphadenitis. Arch Dermatol 1968; 97: 536–539.
76. Bernstein A, Scardino PT, Tomaszewski M-M, Cohen MH. Carcinoma arising in a branchial cleft cyst. Cancer 1976; 37: 2417–2422.
77. Compagno J, Hyams VJ, Safavian M. Does branchiogenic carcinoma really exist? Arch Pathol Lab Med 1976; 100: 311–314.
78. Sanusi ID, Carrington PR, Adams DN. Cervical thymic cyst. Arch Dermatol 1982; 118: 122–124.
79. Mikal S. Cervical thymic cyst. Case report and review of the literature. Arch Surg 1974; 109: 558–562.
80. Guba AM Jr, Adam AE, Jaques DA, Chambers RG. Cervical presentation of thymic cysts. Am J Surg 1978; 136; 430–436.
80a. Barr RJ, Santa Cruz DJ, Pearl RM. Dermal thymus. A light microscopic and immunohistochemical study. J Cutan Pathol 1989; 125: 1681–1684.
81. Farmer ER, Helwig EB. Cutaneous ciliated cysts. Arch Dermatol 1978; 114: 70–73.
81a. Al-Nafussi AI, Carder P. Cutaneous ciliated cyst: a case report and immunohistochemical comparison with fallopian tube. Histopathology 1990; 16: 595–598.
82. Leonforte JF. Cutaneous ciliated cystadenoma in a man. Arch Dermatol 1982; 118: 1010–1012.
83. True L, Golitz LE. Ciliated plantar cyst. Arch Dermatol 1980; 116: 1066–1067.
84. Robboy SJ, Ross JS, Prat J et al. Urogenital sinus origin of mucinous and ciliated cysts of the vulva. Obstet Gynecol 1978; 51: 347–351.
85. Asarch RG, Golitz LE, Sausker WF, Kreye GM. Median raphe cysts of the penis. Arch Dermatol 1979; 115: 1084–1086.
86. Paslin D. Urethroid cyst. Arch Dermatol 1983; 119: 89–90.
87. Quiles DR, Mas IB, Martinez AJ et al. Gonococcal infection of the penile median raphe. Int J Dermatol 1987; 26: 242–243.
88. Brownstein MH, Helwig EB. Subcutaneous dermoid cysts. Arch Dermatol 1973; 107: 237–239.
89. Littlewood AHM. Congenital nasal dermoid cysts and fistulas. Plast Reconstr Surg 1961; 27: 471–488.
90. Brownstein MH, Shapiro L, Slevin R. Fistula of the dorsum of the nose. Arch Dermatol 1974; 109: 227–229.
91. Graham–Brown RAC, Shuttleworth D. Median nasal dermoid fistula. Int J Dermatol 1985; 24: 181–182.
92. Szalay GC, Bledsoe RC. Congenital dermoid cyst and fistula of the nose. Am J Dis Child 1972; 124: 392–394.
93. Moreno A, Muns R. A cystic teratoma in skin. Am J Dermatopathol 1985; 7: 383–386.
94. Camacho F. Benign cutaneous cystic teratoma. J Cutan Pathol 1982; 9: 345–351.

Miscellaneous cysts

95. Raimer S, Wolf JE Jr. Subcutaneous cysticercosis. Arch Dermatol 1978; 114: 107–108.
96. Iwatsu T, Miyaji M. Phaeomycotic cyst. A case with a lesion containing a wood splinter. Arch Dermatol 1984; 120: 1209–1211.
97. Gonzalez JG, Ghiselli RW, Santa Cruz DJ. Synovial metaplasia of the skin. Am J Surg Pathol 1987; 11: 343–350.
98. Stern DR, Sexton FM. Metaplastic synovial cyst after partial excision of nevus sebaceous. Am J Dermatopathol 1988; 10: 531–535.
98a. Bhawan J, Dayal Y, Gonzales-Serva A, Eisen R. Cutaneous metaplastic synovial cyst. J Cutan Pathol 1990; 17: 22–26.
99. Glamb R, Kim R. Pseudocyst of the auricle. J Am Acad Dermatol 1984; 11: 58–63.
100. Fukamizu H, Imaizumi S. Bilateral pseudocysts of the auricles. Arch Dermatol 1984; 120: 1238–1239.
101. Heffner DK, Hyams VJ. Cystic chondromalacia (endochondral pseudocyst) of the auricle. Arch Pathol Lab Med 1986; 110: 740–743.
102. Grabski WJ, Salasche SJ, McCollough ML, Angeloni VL. Pseudocyst of the auricle associated with trauma. Arch Dermatol 1989; 125: 528–530.
103. Lapins NA, Odom RB. Seroma of the auricle. Arch Dermatol 1982; 118: 503–505.
104. Michowitz M, Baratz M, Stavorovsky M. Endometriosis of the umbilicus. Dermatologica 1983; 167: 326–330.
105. Williams HE, Barsky S, Storino W. Umbilical endometrioma (silent type). Arch Dermatol 1976; 112: 1435–1436.
106. Premalatha S, Augustine SM, Thambiah AS. Umbilical endometrioma. Clin Exp Dermatol 1978; 3: 35–37.
107. Beirne MF, Berkheiser SW. Umbilical endometriosis. A case report. Am J Obstet Gynecol 1955; 69: 895–897.
108. Tidman MJ, MacDonald DM. Cutaneous endometriosis: A histopathologic study. J Am Acad Dermatol 1988; 18: 373–377.
109. Symmers W St C. Endometriosis occurring in the neck. Personal communication, 1989.
110. Pellegrini AE. Cutaneous decidualized endometriosis. A pseudomalignancy. Am J Dermatopathol 1982; 4: 171–174.
111. Popoff L, Raitchev R, Andreev VC. Endometriosis of the skin. Arch Dermatol 1962; 85: 186–189.

Sinuses

112. Cioffi GA, Terezhalmy GT, Parlette HL. Cutaneous draining sinus tract. An odontogenic etiology. J Am Acad Dermatol 1986; 14: 94–100.
113. Lewin-Epstein J, Taicher S, Azaz B. Cutaneous sinus tracts of dental origin. Arch Dermatol 1978; 114: 1158–1161.
114. Eby CS, Jetton RL. Umbilical pilonidal sinus. Arch Dermatol 1972; 106: 893.
115. Moyer DG. Pilonidal cyst of the scalp. Arch Dermatol 1972; 105: 578–579.
116. Lepaw MI. Therapy and histopathology of complications from synthetic fiber implants for hair replacement. J Am Acad Dermatol 1980; 3: 195–204.

17

David Weedon

Panniculitis

INTRODUCTION

Inflammatory lesions of the subcutaneous fat can be classified into three distinct categories:

Septal panniculitis
Lobular panniculitis
Panniculitis associated with large vessel vasculitis.

Within each group, the histological appearances will depend on the stage of the disease at which the biopsy is taken. In early lesions there are often neutrophils in the inflammatory infiltrate, while later lesions have a chronic infiltrate composed predominantly of lymphocytes, but with a variable admixture of giant cells and lipid-containing macrophages. At an even later stage there is some fibrosis.

Inflammation of small venules will result in a *septal panniculitis* with some spillover of the inflammatory process into the lower dermis.[1] Involvement of the arterial supply, for example by vasculitis, will produce a *lobular panniculitis*. There are other mechanisms involved in some of the diseases that result in a lobular panniculitis. These will be considered in the appropriate sections. The *panniculitis associated with large vessel involvement*, such as polyarteritis nodosa and migratory thrombophlebitis, is usually localized to the immediate vicinity of the involved vessel. It often has mixed lobular and septal features.

Unless an adequate biopsy is received, it may be difficult to reach a specific diagnosis.[2,3] A diagnosis of 'lobular panniculitis, ? type' may have to suffice in these cases. Another problem with the panniculitides is the considerable confusion that exists in the literature.[4] In some reports

Histopathology

Nodular vasculitis produces a lobular panniculitis, often associated with areas of fat necrosis (Fig. 17.3). This latter change results from ischaemia produced by vasculitis which involves small, medium-sized and sometimes large arteries and even veins in the fibrous septa (Fig. 17.4). Involved vessels show endothelial swelling and a mixed inflammatory cell infiltrate in the wall and periadventitial tissue. Necrotizing vasculitis may be present. Sometimes it is difficult to distinguish nodular vasculitis from the cutaneous form of polyarteritis nodosa. Some pathologists diagnose polyarteritis nodosa when large vessels are involved, and restrict 'nodular vasculitis' to those cases with involvement of small and medium-sized vessels. As a

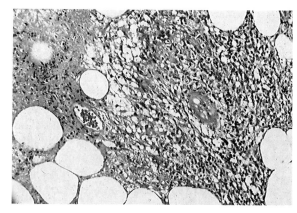

Fig. 17.4 Nodular vasculitis. There is a lobular panniculitis with focal necrosis. A small blood vessel shows fibrinoid change.
Haematoxylin — eosin

rule, nodular vasculitis involves many contiguous lobules, whereas cutaneous polyarteritis nodosa produces a more localized panniculitis restricted to the vicinity of the involved vessel.

In nodular vasculitis the inflammatory infiltrate consists of neutrophils, lymphocytes, some plasma cells and histiocytes. Neutrophils predominate in areas of recent fat necrosis; sometimes focal suppuration is present. In older lesions there are lipophage collections, multinucleate giant cells, epithelioid cells and even tuberculoid granulomas. There is variable and often progressive fibrosis.

In erythema induratum there are usually well-formed granulomas, which may extend into the lower dermis.[21]

ERYTHEMA INDURATUM

Erythema induratum of Bazin is a rare entity characterized by the presence of painful, indurated nodules, 1–2 cm in diameter, with a predilection for the lower legs, particularly the calves, of middle-aged women.[20,20a] Individual lesions may ulcerate and heal with scarring.[20b]

The existence of this entity has been questioned by some, although a recent review of 26 presumptive cases concluded that 'there is sufficient circumstantial evidence to support the

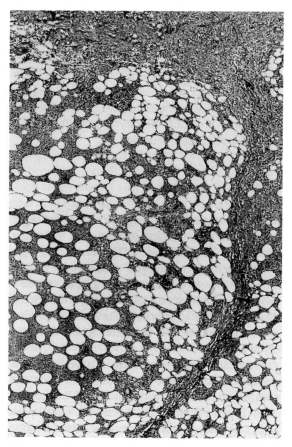

Fig. 17.3 Nodular vasculitis. There is inflammation in the septa and fat lobules.
Haematoxylin — eosin

hypothesis that erythema induratum is a true tuberculid'.[20a]

Histopathology

The diagnosis of erythema induratum is a clinicopathological one, as there are no pathognomonic features.[20a] There is usually a lobular panniculitis, although in some cases the infiltrate is predominantly paraseptal. In severe cases, the interlobular septa are also involved. Erythema induratum shares many features with nodular vasculitis, including the presence of a vasculitis. Usually venules, and sometimes arterioles, are involved.

Fat necrosis is often present, and this may be more prominent than in nodular vasculitis. Another characteristic feature is the presence of small tuberculoid granulomas in the interlobular septa and lower dermis, particularly around the eccrine glands.

SUBCUTANEOUS FAT NECROSIS OF THE NEWBORN

Subcutaneous fat necrosis of the newborn is a self-limited condition, present at birth or appearing in the first few days of life.[22,22a] It is characterized by indurated areas and distinct nodules with a predilection for the cheeks, shoulders, buttocks, thighs and calves.[23] Sometimes only solitary lesions are discernible. Hypercalcaemia has been reported in some cases.[24,25] Obstetrical trauma and cold have been incriminated in the aetiology. It has been suggested that trauma to fragile adipose tissue low in oleic acid and with a compromised circulation, and with the subsequent release of hydrolases, leads to the breakdown of unsaturated fatty acids.[22] It should be remembered that infant fat already has a greater ratio of saturated to unsaturated fatty acids than exists in adult fat.

Histopathology[22a,26,27]

There is a normal epidermis and dermis with an underlying lobular panniculitis. Focal fat

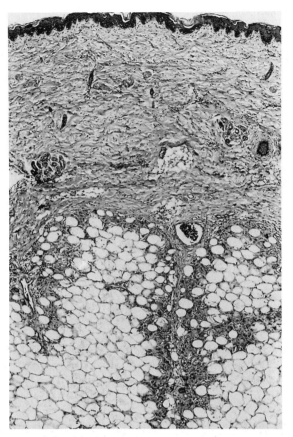

Fig. 17.5   Subcutaneous fat necrosis of the newborn. There is a paraseptal panniculitis with lymphocytes, macrophages and multinucleate giant cells wedged between the fat cells. Haematoxylin — eosin

necrosis is present and this may lead to fat cyst formation. There is an inflammatory infiltrate of lymphocytes, histiocytes, foreign body giant cells and sometimes a few eosinophils wedged between the fat cells (Fig. 17.5). Many of the fat cells retain their outline but contain fine, eosinophilic cytoplasmic strands, between which are narrow clefts radiating from a point near the periphery of the cell (Fig. 17.6). The clefts contain doubly refractile crystals, representing triglycerides, on frozen section. Similar fine, needle-like crystals can be seen in relation to some of the giant cells. Cases have been reported without the needle-like crystals.[28] In older lesions there is some fibrosis between the fat cells, and there may be foci of calcification.

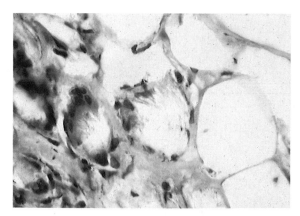

Fig. 17.6 Subcutaneous fat necrosis of the newborn. Narrow strands of tissue radiate from a point near the periphery of several of the fat cells. The intervening clefts represent the site of deposition of 'fat crystals'. Haematoxylin — eosin

Electron microscopy.[26,27] There are intact and necrotic fat cells containing needle-shaped crystals arranged radially or in parallel. Dense granular material is also present in the necrotic fat cells, which are surrounded by macrophages.

SCLEREMA NEONATORUM

Sclerema neonatorum has a pathogenetic relationship to subcutaneous fat necrosis of the newborn and was at one stage regarded as a diffuse form of the latter condition.[29] It is also characterized by intracellular microcrystallization of triglyceride in the subcutaneous and sometimes also in the visceral fat of neonates. Sclerema neonatorum produces wax-like, hard skin which is also dry and cold. It is rarely seen these days, presumably because of improved neonatal care.

Histopathology

There are fine, needle-like crystals in the fat cells, but unlike subcutaneous fat necrosis of the newborn, there is very little inflammation, few giant cells and no calcification. The subcutaneous septa are often widened by oedema which might explain the 'wide intersecting fibrous bands' formerly reported. Fat cells have been reported as increased in size, but a personally studied case showed small, immature fat cells.

COLD PANNICULITIS

Panniculitis may occur following exposure to severe cold, particularly in infants.[30-32] It has occurred in older children and on the thighs of women who have ridden horses in cold weather.[33,34] In the latter instance it has been suggested that tight pants may restrict the blood supply, contributing to the injury. The lesions are indurated, somewhat tender plaques and nodules.

Histopathology

There is a lobular panniculitis with a mixed inflammatory cell infiltrate. Changes are most marked near the dermo–subcutaneous junction where the vessels show a perivascular infiltrate of lymphocytes and histiocytes. There is some thickening of vessel walls. There is overlap with the changes described in deep perniosis (see p. 241).[35]

WEBER–CHRISTIAN DISEASE

The diagnosis of Weber–Christian disease has engendered more confusion in dermatopathology than practically any other. A major review of the literature was published in 1985.[36] It has been regarded by some as a clinical entity with non-specific pathological features, by others as an idiopathic clinicopathological entity, and even as a very useful 'concept'. It has been applied by some to all cases of panniculitis with systemic symptoms, or to all cases of fatal panniculitis with visceral involvement[37] (although some of these[38] would now be reclassifiable as cytophagic histiocytic panniculitis).[39] It has been applied also to the changes in the subcutis seen in association with malignancy, α_1-antitrypsin deficiency,[40-41a] jejuno-ileal bypass,[42] Crohn's disease,[43] autoimmune diseases,[44] immunological abnormalities,[45] factitial lesions and even various infections.[5] This confusion has arisen because there are only very limited ways in which the panniculus can respond to a wide range of stimuli. Furthermore, an underlying enzyme deficiency or systemic disease may not have been detected at the time the patient first presented with the panniculitis. The term Weber–Christian disease has been a convenient 'pigeon hole' for these undiagnosable cases.

Weber–Christian disease has been defined as a rare disorder with recurrent subcutaneous nodules and plaques with a predilection for the extremities and buttocks, commonly associated with fever.[46] It may have a short self-limited course, be recurrent, or follow an unremitting course with a fatal outcome and visceral involvement.[43,47,48] Involvement of the fatty marrow may lead to haematological aspects such as anaemia. The term 'relapsing febrile nodular non-suppurative panniculitis' has also been used.

The term 'Rothmann–Makai syndrome' was formerly applied to a range of conditions characterized by a lobular panniculitis and should no longer be used.[49]

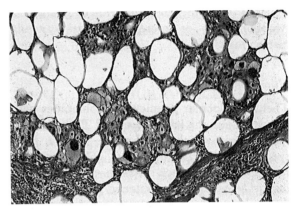

Fig. 17.7 Weber–Christian disease. Numerous foamy lipophages are distributed throughout the fat lobule. A few larger lipophages are also present. Haematoxylin — eosin

Histopathology

Weber–Christian disease produces a lobular panniculitis which varies in appearance according to the duration of the lesion. In the early stages, which are rarely seen on biopsy, there is a heavy neutrophil infiltrate between the fat cells, associated with focal degeneration of the fat.[50] There are also lymphocytes and histiocytes present. In the next stage there is an abundance of foam cells (Fig. 17.7). These are macrophages which have ingested lipid material. They are of varying size and some of the larger cells are multinucleate. There is also a sprinkling of other inflammatory cells including lymphocytes and plasma cells. Necrosis of fat cells with liquefaction may occur in this stage. In the third stage there is progressive fibrosis with replacement of foam cells by fibrous tissue. A patchy chronic inflammatory cell infiltrate is also present. Other reported features include inflammatory involvement of the septa and vasculitis.[36]

Panniculitis associated with α_1-antitrypsin deficiency is often preceded by trauma. There is usually an acute panniculitis, sometimes septal

as well as lobular, with masses of neutrophils and some necrosis of fat cells.[51] Dissolution of dermal collagen with transepidermal elimination of 'liquefied' dermis may occur. There may also be collagenolysis of the fibrous septa of the subcutis resulting in isolated adipocyte lobules.[41a] Destruction of elastic tissue may also be present.[40a] Vasculitis is sometimes present in the subcutis. Later lesions show collections of histiocytic cells and lipophages and variable fibrosis.

CYTOPHAGIC HISTIOCYTIC PANNICULITIS

Winkelmann and colleagues coined this term for a fatal syndrome which included a chronic and recurring panniculitis with an infiltrate of cytophagic histiocytes with eventual multisystem involvement, terminating usually with a haemorrhagic diathesis.[39,52–55] Other cases have been included in the past with systemic Weber–Christian disease.[38] Panniculitis can be a feature of malignant histiocytosis, but the histiocytes have the cytological features of neoplastic cells, in contrast to cytophagic histiocytic panniculitis where the cells have the morphological features of mature histiocytes, often with marked haemophagocytosis.[39]

This condition appears to begin as a reactive histiocytosis, although cases are now being

a lobular or mixed lobular and septal panniculitis.[3,108] These include cryptococcosis, mycetoma, actinomycosis, nocardiosis, chromomycosis, sporotrichosis and histoplasmosis,[109] infections with *Mycobacterium marinum*,[109a] *Mycobacterium leprae* (erythema nodosum leprosum — see p. 612), *Mycobacterium avium–intracellulare*[110] and other bacteria,[108] bites of the brown recluse spider (*Loxosceles reclusa*),[5] and metazoal infestations (myiasis, cysticercosis, sparganosis and infestations by some other helminths). Most cases of infection-induced panniculitis occur in patients who are immunosuppressed.[108]

Histopathology[108]

The presence of a lobular or mixed lobular and septal panniculitis in which there is a heavy infiltrate of neutrophils, often with extension into the dermis, should raise the suspicion of an infective aetiology (Fig. 17.12). Haemorrhage and necrosis are often present.

EOSINOPHILIC PANNICULITIS

This term has been applied to several different disease entities. It has been used for a mixed lobular and septal panniculitis with numerous eosinophils and flame figures and features resembling those seen in the dermis in Wells' syndrome (see p. 998):[111] in these cases, the panniculitis was thought to have followed inflammation or infection of the upper aerodigestive tract.[111,112] The term has been used for a panniculitis with numerous eosinophils in the infiltrate.[113] As such it is not a specific entity but a non-specific pattern seen in a diverse range of systemic diseases including erythema nodosum, vasculitis, parasitic infestation (Fig. 17.13), malignant lymphoma, atopy, and narcotic dependency with injection granulomas.[113] Finally, the term has been used for a nodular migratory panniculitis which may accompany infestations with the larva of the nematode *Gnathostoma spinigerum* (deep larva migrans):[114] in this variety eosinophils make up 95% of the infiltrate.

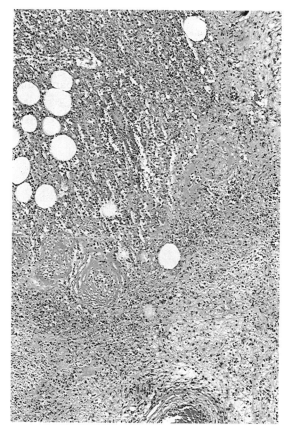

Fig. 17.12 Mycobacterium ulcerans. The presence of a widespread suppurative panniculitis, as shown here, warrants exclusion of an infective aetiology. Numerous acid-fast bacilli were present.
Haematoxylin — eosin

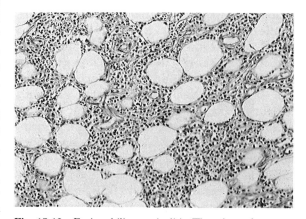

Fig. 17.13 Eosinophilic panniculitis. There is an almost pure infiltrate of eosinophils throughout the lobules of fat. A helminth was found nearby.
Haematoxylin — eosin

MISCELLANEOUS LESIONS

A focal non-specific panniculitis may be found in some cases of dermatomyositis, particularly in relation to underlying calcified deposits.[115,116] In one case a larger plaque form of lobular panniculitis was present.[117] A calcifying panniculitis resulting from calciphylaxis has been reported in chronic renal failure.[117a] Metastatic calcification in renal failure differs by its dermal localization and the absence of a panniculitis.[117a]

Panniculitis with urate crystal deposition and necrosis of fat has been reported as the only cutaneous manifestation of gout.[118,119]

A haemorrhagic panniculitis has followed atheromatous embolization of vessels of the skin.[120]

Non-caseating granulomas may be found in the subcutaneous tissue in sarcoidosis and, rarely, in Crohn's disease.[121,122]

The panniculitis which is found in about 5% of patients undergoing jejuno-ileal bypass for morbid obesity has been described as erythema nodosum-like[123] complicated by lobular fat necrosis, and as Weber–Christian-like.[42] Published photomicrographs suggest a lobular panniculitis with some resemblance to nodular vasculitis.

Fat cysts surrounded by a thin, eosinophilic membrane (so-called 'lipomembranous change') have been reported in patients with vascular insufficiency. Clinically, the lesions present as nodules or sclerotic plaques on the lower legs.[124]

Other rare causes of a panniculitis include malignancies,[125] particularly lymphomas,[3,125a] drugs such as phenytoin,[5] iodides and bromides, and low calorie diets and nutritional abnormalities.[126] Granuloma annulare may also involve the subcutis.

Cases which defy an aetiological classification are sometimes seen. Such a case was reported as 'suppressor-cytotoxic T-lymphocyte panniculitis'. The patient was febrile and had a lobular panniculitis with many OKT8 (CD8)-positive lymphocytes in the infiltrate.[127]

PANNICULITIS SECONDARY TO LARGE VESSEL VASCULITIS

A localized area of panniculitis is almost invariable in the immediate vicinity of an inflamed large artery or vein, as it courses through the subcutaneous fat. There is no lobular panniculitis of contiguous lobules as is seen in nodular vasculitis.

CUTANEOUS POLYARTERITIS NODOSA

There is a benign cutaneous form of polyarteritis nodosa which is distinct from the systemic form (Fig. 17.14). It presents with painful subcutaneous nodules in crops, mainly on the lower

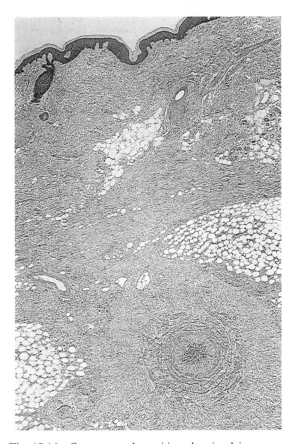

Fig. 17.14 Cutaneous polyarteritis nodosa involving a small artery in the subcutis. Sometimes an elastic tissue stain is needed to distinguish between small arteries and veins in biopsies from the lower legs.
Haematoxylin — eosin

39. Crotty CP, Winkelmann RK. Cytophagic histiocytic panniculitis with fever, cytopenia, liver failure, and terminal hemorrhagic diathesis. J Am Acad Dermatol 1981; 4: 181–194.

40. Breit SN, Clark P, Robinson JP et al. Familial occurrence of α_1-antitrypsin deficiency and Weber–Christian disease. Arch Dermatol 1983; 119: 198–202.

40a. Smith KC, Su WPD, Pittelkow MR, Winkelmann RK. Clinical and pathologic correlations in 96 patients with panniculitis, including 15 patients with deficient levels of α_1-antitrypsin. J Am Acad Dermatol 1989; 21: 1192–1196.

41. Bleumink E, Klokke HA. Protease-inhibitor deficiencies in a patient with Weber–Christian panniculitis. Arch Dermatol 1984; 120: 936–940.

41a. Hendrick SJ, Silverman AK, Solomon AR, Headington JT. α_1-antitrypsin deficiency associated with panniculitis. J Am Acad Dermatol 1988; 18: 684–692.

42. Williams HJ, Samuelson CO, Zone JJ. Nodular nonsuppurative panniculitis associated with jejunoileal bypass surgery. Arch Dermatol 1979; 115: 1091–1093.

43. Ciclitira PJ, Wight DGD, Dick AP. Systemic Weber–Christian disease: a case report with lipoprotein profile and immunological evaluation. Br J Dermatol 1980; 103: 685–692.

44. Allen-Mersh TG. Weber–Christian panniculitis and auto-immune disease: a case report. J Clin Pathol 1976; 29: 144–149.

45. Iwatsuki K, Tagami H, Yamada M. Weber–Christian panniculitis with immunological abnormalities. Dermatologica 1982; 164: 181–188.

46. Albrectsen B. The Weber–Christian syndrome, with particular reference to etiology. Acta Derm Venereol 1960; 40: 474–484.

47. Wilkinson PJ, Harman RRM, Tribe CR. Systemic nodular panniculitis with cardiac involvement. J Clin Pathol 1974; 27: 808–812.

48. Stewart CA. Systemic form of Weber–Christian disease. Pathology 1978; 10: 165–168.

49. Chan HL. Panniculitis (Rothmann–Makai) with good response to tetracycline. Br J Dermatol 1975; 92: 351–354.

50. Hendricks WM, Ahmad M, Gratz E. Weber–Christian syndrome in infancy. Br J Dermatol 1978; 98: 175–186.

51. Su WPD, Smith KC, Pittelkow MR, Winkelmann RK. α_1-antitrypsin deficiency panniculitis. A histopathologic and immunopathologic study of four cases. Am J Dermatopathol 1987; 9: 483–490.

52. Winkelmann RK, Bowie EJW. Hemorrhagic diathesis associated with benign histiocytic cytophagic panniculitis and systemic histiocytosis. Arch Intern Med 1980; 140: 1460–1463.

53. White JW Jr, Winkelmann RK. Cytophagic histiocytic panniculitis is not always fatal. J Cutan Pathol 1989; 16: 137–144.

54. Alegre VA, Winkelmann RK. Histiocytic cytophagic panniculitis. J Am Acad Dermatol 1989; 20: 177–185.

55. Alegre VA, Fortea JM, Camps C, Aliaga A. Cytophagic histiocytic panniculitis. Case report with resolution after treatment. J Am Acad Dermatol 1989; 20: 875–878.

56. Aronson IK, West DP, Variakojis D et al. Panniculitis associated with cutaneous T-cell lymphoma and cytophagocytic histiocytosis. Br J Dermatol 1985; 112: 87–96.

57. Peters MS, Winkelmann RK. Cytophagic panniculitis and B cell lymphoma. J Am Acad Dermatol 1985; 13: 882–885.

58. Willis SM, Opal SM, Fitzpatrick JE. Cytophagic histiocytic panniculitis. Arch Dermatol 1985; 121: 910–913.

59. Barron DR, Davis BR, Pomeranz JR et al. Cytophagic histiocytic panniculitis. A variant of malignant histiocytosis. Cancer 1985; 55: 2538–2542.

60. Levine N, Lazarus GS. Subcutaneous fat necrosis after paracentesis. Report of a case in a patient with acute pancreatitis. Arch Dermatol 1976; 112: 993–994.

61. Detlefs RL. Drug-induced pancreatitis presenting as subcutaneous fat necrosis. J Am Acad Dermatol 1985; 13: 305–307.

62. Hughes PSH, Apisarnthanarax P, Mullins JF. Subcutaneous fat necrosis associated with pancreatic disease. Arch Dermatol 1975; 111: 506–510.

63. Berman B, Conteas C, Smith B et al. Fatal pancreatitis presenting with subcutaneous fat necrosis. J Am Acad Dermatol 1987; 17: 359–364.

64. Bennett RG, Petrozzi JW. Nodular subcutaneous fat necrosis. A manifestation of silent pancreatitis. Arch Dermatol 1975; 111: 896–898.

65. Haber RM, Assaad DM. Panniculitis associated with a pancreas divisum. J Am Acad Dermatol 1986; 14: 331–334.

66. Millns JL, Evans HL, Winkelmann RK. Association of islet cell carcinoma of the pancreas with subcutaneous fat necrosis. Am J Dermatopathol 1979; 1: 273–280.

67. Forstrom L, Winkelmann RK. Acute, generalized panniculitis with amylase and lipase in skin. Arch Dermatol 1975; 111: 497–502.

68. Cannon JR, Pitha JV, Everett MA. Subcutaneous fat necrosis in pancreatitis. J Cutan Pathol 1979; 6: 501–506.

69. Tuffanelli DL. Lupus erythematosus panniculitis (profundus). Commentary and report on four more cases. Arch Dermatol 1971; 103: 231–242.

70. Sanchez NP, Peters MS, Winkelmann RK. The histopathology of lupus erythematosus panniculitis. J Am Acad Dermatol 1981; 5: 673–680.

71. Winkelmann RK. Panniculitis in connective tissue disease. Arch Dermatol 1983; 119: 336–344.

72. Izumi AK, Takiguchi P. Lupus erythematosus panniculitis. Arch Dermatol 1983; 119: 61–64.

73. Tuffanelli DL. Lupus panniculitis. Semin Dermatol 1985; 4: 79–81.

74. Fox JN, Klapman MH, Rowe L. Lupus profundus in children: Treatment with hydroxychloroquine. J Am Acad Dermatol 1987; 16: 839–844.

75. Harris RB, Duncan SC, Ecker RI, Winkelmann RK. Lymphoid follicles in subcutaneous inflammatory disease. Arch Dermatol 1979; 115: 442–443.

76. Winkelmann RK, Padilha-Gonclaves A. Connective tissue panniculitis. Arch Dermatol 1980; 116: 291–294.

77. Moragon M, Jorda E, Ramon MD et al. Atrophic connective tissue panniculitis. Int J Dermatol 1988; 27: 185–186.

77a. Newton J, Wojnarowska FT. Pustular panniculitis in rheumatoid arthritis. Br J Dermatol (Suppl) 1988; 30: 97–98.

78. Jaffe N, Hann HWL, Vawter GF. Post-steroid panniculitis in acute leukemia. N Engl J Med 1971; 284: 366–367.

79. Peters MS, Winkelmann RK. Localized lipoatrophy

(atrophic connective tissue disease panniculitis). Arch Dermatol 1980; 116: 1363–1368.

80. Aronson IK, Zeitz HJ, Variakojis D. Panniculitis in childhood. Pediatr Dermatol 1988; 5: 216–230.

81. Winkelmann RK, McEvoy MT, Peters MS. Lipophagic panniculitis of childhood. J Am Acad Dermatol 1989; 21: 971–978.

82. Samadaei A, Hashimoto K, Tanay A. Insulin lipodystrophy, lipohypertrophic type. J Am Acad Dermatol 1987; 17: 506–507.

83. Eadie MJ, Sutherland JM, Tyrer JH. The clinical features of hemifacial atrophy. Med J Aust 1963; 2: 177–180.

84. Chartier S, Buzzanga JB, Paquin F. Partial lipodystrophy associated with a type 3 form of membranoproliferative glomerulonephritis. J Am Acad Dermatol 1987; 16: 201–205.

84a. Font J, Herrero C, Bosch X et al. Systemic lupus erythematosus in a patient with partial lipodystrophy. J Am Acad Dermatol 1990; 22: 337–340.

85. Rongioletti F, Rebora A. Annular and semicircular lipoatrophies. Report of three cases and review of the literature. J Am Acad Dermatol 1989; 20: 433–436.

86. Jablonska S, Szczepanski A, Gorkiewicz A. Lipo-atrophy of the ankles and its relation to other lipo-atrophies. Acta Derm Venereol 1987; 55: 135–140.

87. Nelson HM. Atrophic annular panniculitis of the ankles. Clin Exp Dermatol 1988; 13: 111–113.

88. Roth DE, Schikler KN, Callen JP. Annular atrophic connective tissue panniculitis of the ankles. J Am Acad Dermatol 1989; 21: 1152–1156.

89. Karkavitsas C, Miller JA, Kirby JD. Semicircular lipoatrophy. Br J Dermatol 1981; 105: 591–593.

90. Caputo R. Lipodystrophia centrifugalis sacralis infantilis. Acta Derm Venereol 1989; 69: 442–443.

91. Imamura S, Yamada M, Yamamoto K. Lipodystrophia centrifugalis abdominalis infantilis. J Am Acad Dermatol 1984; 11: 203–209.

91a. Hiraiwa A, Takai K, Fukui Y et al. Nonregressing lipodystrophia centrifugalis abdominalis with angioblastoma (Nakagawa). Arch Dermatol 1990; 126: 206–209.

92. Zachary CB, Wells RS. Centrifugal lipodystrophy. Br J Dermatol 1984; 110: 107–110.

93. Giam YC, Rajan VS, Hock OB. Lipodystrophia centrifugalis abdominalis. Br J Dermatol 1982; 106: 461–464.

94. Furukawa F. Lipodystrophia centrifugalis abdominalis infantilis. A possible sequel to Kawasaki disease. Int J Dermatol 1989; 28: 338–339.

95. Serup J, Weismann K, Kobayasi T et al. Local panatrophy with linear distribution: a clinical, ultrastructural and biochemical study. Acta Derm Venereol 1982; 62: 101–105.

96. Peters MS, Winkelmann RK. The histopathology of localized lipoatrophy. Br J Dermatol 1986; 114: 27–36.

97. Tsuji T, Kosaka K, Terao J. Localized lipodystrophy with panniculitis: light and electron microscopic studies. J Cutan Pathol 1989; 16: 359–364.

98. Kossard S, Ecker RI, Dicken CH. Povidone panniculitis. Polyvinylpyrrolidone panniculitis. Arch Dermatol 1980; 116: 704–706.

99. Forstrom L, Winkelmann RK. Factitial panniculitis. Arch Dermatol 1974; 110: 747–750.

100. Parks DL, Perry HO, Muller SA. Cutaneous complications of pentazocine injections. Arch

Dermatol 1971; 104: 231–235.

101. Klein JA, Cole G, Barr RJ et al. Paraffinomas of the scalp. Arch Dermatol 1985; 121: 382–385.

102. Oertel YC, Johnson FB. Sclerosing lipogranuloma of male genitalia. Arch Pathol 1977; 101: 321–326.

103. Claudy A, Garcier F, Schmitt D. Sclerosing lipogranuloma of the male genitalia: ultrastructural study. Br J Dermatol 1981; 105: 451–455.

104. Hirst AE, Heustis DG, Rogers-Neufeld B, Johnson FB. Sclerosing lipogranuloma of the scalp. A report of two cases. Am J Clin Pathol 1984; 82: 228–231.

105. Delage C, Shane JJ, Johnson FB. Mammary silicone granuloma. Arch Dermatol 1973; 108: 104–107.

106. Winkelmann RK, Barker SM. Factitial traumatic panniculitis. J Am Acad Dermatol 1985; 13: 988–994.

107. Hurt MA, Santa Cruz DJ. Nodular-cystic fat necrosis. A reevaluation of the so-called mobile encapsulated lipoma. J Am Acad Dermatol 1989; 21: 493–498.

108. Patterson JW, Brown PC, Broecker AH. Infection-induced panniculitis. J Cutan Pathol 1989; 16: 183–193.

109. Abildgaard WH Jr, Hargrove RH, Kalivas J. Histoplasma panniculitis. Arch Dermatol 1985; 121: 914–916.

109a. Larson K, Glanz S, Bergfeld WF. Neutrophilic panniculitis caused by Mycobacterium marinum. J Cutan Pathol 1989; 16: 315 (abstract).

110. Sanderson TL, Moskowitz L, Hensley GT et al. Disseminated Mycobacterium avium–intracellulare infection appearing as a panniculitis. Arch Pathol Lab Med 1982; 106: 112–114.

111. Burket JM, Burket BJ. Eosinophilic panniculitis. J Am Acad Dermatol 1985; 12: 161–164.

112. Glass LA, Zaghloul AB, Solomon AR. Eosinophilic panniculitis associated with chronic recurrent parotitis. Am J Dermatopathol 1989; 11: 555–559.

113. Winkelmann RK, Frigas E. Eosinophilic panniculitis: a clinicopathologic study. J Cutan Pathol 1986; 13: 1–12.

114. Ollague W, Ollague J, Guevara de Veliz A, Penaherrera S. Human gnathostomiasis in Ecuador (nodular migratory eosinophilic panniculitis). Int J Dermatol 1984; 23: 647–651.

115. Janis JF, Winkelmann RK. Histopathology of the skin in dermatomyositis. Arch Dermatol 1968; 97: 640–650.

116. Raimer SS, Solomon AR, Daniels JC. Polymyositis presenting with panniculitis. J Am Acad Dermatol 1985; 13: 366–369.

117. Richens G, Piepkorn MW, Krueger GG. Calcifying panniculitis associated with renal failure. A case of Selye's calciphylaxis in man. J Am Acad Dermatol 1982; 6: 537–539.

117a. Lugo-Somolinos A, Sanchez JL, Mendez-Coll J, Joglar F. Calcifying panniculitis associated with polycystic kidney disease and chronic renal failure. J Am Acad Dermatol 1990; 22: 743–747.

118. Niemi K-M. Panniculitis of the legs with urate crystal deposition. Arch Dermatol 1977; 113: 655–656.

119. Le Boit PE, Schneider S. Gout presenting as lobular panniculitis. Am J Dermatopathol 1987; 9: 334–338.

120. Day LL, Aterman K. Hemorrhagic panniculitis caused by atheromatous embolization. A case report and brief review. Am J Dermatopathol 1984; 6: 471–478.

121. Vainsencher D, Winkelmann RK. Subcutaneous

ing parenteral nutrition, results in alopecia, xerosis and intertriginous erosions.[3]

Riboflavin and pyridoxine deficiency both lead to glossitis, angular stomatitis, cheilosis and a condition resembling seborrhoeic dermatitis.[3] In riboflavin deficiency there may be a scrotal dermatitis, while in pyridoxine deficiency there may be pellagra-like features.[3]

SCURVY

Scurvy results from a deficiency of vitamin C (ascorbic acid), which is a water-soluble vitamin necessary for proline hydroxylation in the formation of collagen.[2] It also plays a role in normal hair growth. Loss of the integrity of collagen leads to inadequate support for small vessels, resulting in haemorrhage from minor trauma.[4] This is characteristically perifollicular in distribution, but spontaneous petechiae and ecchymoses may also develop.[2,5] Other features include follicular hyperkeratosis, abnormal hair growth with the formation of corkscrew hairs, bleeding gums, and poor wound healing.[2,6] Woody oedema of the lower limbs with some surface scaling may be the only manifestation.[4,7] Scurvy may be seen in alcoholics, and those with dietary fads and inadequacies and, accordingly, associated deficiencies of other factors may contribute to the appearance of the cutaneous lesions.[7]

Histopathology

A characteristic feature is the presence of extravasated red cells around vessels in the upper dermis.[5] This is often in a perifollicular distribution initially. Haemosiderin, a legacy of earlier haemorrhages, is sometimes found. There may also be follicular hyperkeratosis with coiled, fragmented, corkscrew-like hairs buried in the keratotic follicular material.[6] Ulceration of the skin is sometimes seen.

Electron microscopy. Affected skin may show alterations in fibroblasts, with defective collagen formation.[8] There may also be alterations in the endothelial cells of vessels and their junctions.[8]

VITAMIN A DEFICIENCY

Vitamin A is a fat-soluble vitamin; its active form is retinol. Deficiencies are rare, and usually related to malabsorption states.[2] The skin becomes dry and scaly with follicular keratotic papules (phrynoderma).[9,10] Ocular changes include night blindness.[11]

Histopathology

Sections show hyperkeratosis and prominent keratotic follicular plugging.[11] Sweat glands may be atrophic; in severe cases they show squamous metaplasia.[10]

HYPERVITAMINOSIS A

Hypervitaminosis A is usually a result of self-administration of excess amounts of the vitamin.[12,13] Acute symptoms include vomiting, diarrhoea and desquamation of skin. In the chronic form of vitamin A toxicity there is dry skin, cheilitis and patchy alopecia. Histological changes are non-specific.

VITAMIN K DEFICIENCY

Vitamin K is a fat-soluble vitamin which is necessary for the hepatic synthesis or secretion of various coagulation factors.[2] A deficiency may result from liver disease and from malabsorption; in infants it may be associated with diarrhoea. Purpura is a common manifestation of vitamin K deficiency.

The parenteral injection of vitamin K may rarely give rise to an erythematous plaque at the site of injection, apparently due to a delayed hypersensitivity reaction.[14] A late sclerodermatous reaction is a rare complication.

VITAMIN B$_{12}$ DEFICIENCY

Vitamin B$_{12}$ deficiency may be associated with poikilodermatous pigmentation. This clinical pattern results from basal pigmentation and some melanin incontinence. The nuclei of keratinocytes were reported to be larger than normal in one patient.[15]

PELLAGRA

Pellagra is a multisystem nutritional disorder caused by inadequate amounts of nicotinic acid (niacin) in the tissues. This may result from a primary dietary deficiency,[16] malabsorption, certain chemotherapeutic agents such as isoniazid,[17,18] 6-mercaptopurine, 5-fluorouracil and chloramphenicol, or from abnormalities of tryptophan metabolism.[2,19] In this latter category is the carcinoid syndrome, in which tumour cells divert tryptophan metabolism towards serotonin and away from nicotinic acid, and Hartnup disease, in which there is a congenital defect in tryptophan absorption and transfer (see p. 528).[2]

Pellagra is traditionally remembered as the 'disease of the four Ds': dermatitis, diarrhoea, dementia and, if untreated, death.[20] The skin lesions commence as a burning erythema in sun-exposed areas, particularly the dorsum of the hands and the face and neck.[21] Blistering may occur. This is followed by intense hyperpigmentation with sharp margination, and areas of epithelial desquamation.[2] There may also be glossitis, angular cheilitis and vulvitis.[20]

Histopathology

The findings are not diagnostic. They include hyperkeratosis, parakeratosis, epidermal atrophy with pallor of the upper epidermis, and hyperpigmentation of the basal layer (Fig. 18.1).[2,22] There is usually a mild, superficial dermal infiltrate of lymphocytes. Mild keratotic follicular plugging is sometimes seen in biopsies from the face.[17,18] Bullae may be either intraepidermal or subepidermal.[21]

Similar histopathological changes are seen in Hartnup disease (see p. 528).[23]

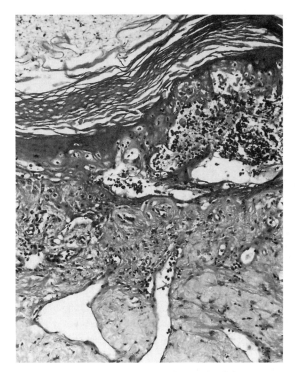

Fig. 18.1 Pellagra. There is partial necrosis of the epidermis, pallor of a few keratinocytes and haemorrhage. Haematoxylin — eosin

LYSOSOMAL STORAGE DISEASES

The lysosomal storage diseases are a specific subset of the inborn errors of metabolism: they are characterized by a deficiency in a specific lysosomal hydrolase or of a protein essential for the normal function of lysosomes.[24] As a consequence of this deficiency there is accumulation of the specific substrate in various organs of the body. The distribution of this stored material corresponds to the site where degradation of the substrate usually occurs. Lysosomes are particularly plentiful in macrophages and other cells of the mononuclear phagocyte system: organs rich in these cells, such as the liver and spleen, are frequently enlarged. In one subgroup of lysosomal storage diseases, the sphingolipidoses, there is an accumulation of certain glycolipids or phospholipids in various organs, particularly the brain.

The lysosomal storage diseases can be diagnosed by assaying for the specific enzyme, thought to be deficient, in serum, leucocytes or cultured fibroblasts.[24] In many of these diseases inclusions can be found on ultrastructural examination of the skin (Fig. 18.2). The inclusions are sometimes distinctive enough to be diagnostic of a particular disease, although in many instances they are not. Accordingly, ultrastructural examination of the skin in the diagnosis of the lysosomal storage diseases is usually no more than a useful adjunct to enzyme assay.[25]

Care must be taken, with ultrastructural studies of the skin, to avoid overdiagnosis.[25] Many cells in the skin may, at times, contain a few vacuoles, fat globules or other inclusions.[25] These must not be misinterpreted as indicative of a lysosomal storage disease.

The lysosomal storage diseases can be divided into several categories on the basis of the biochemical nature of the accumulated substrate:

Sphingolipidoses
Oligosaccharidoses
Mucolipidoses
Mucopolysaccharidoses
Others.

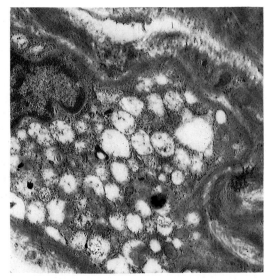

Fig. 18.2 Vacuolated fibroblasts in the skin in a lysosomal storage disease. The type of vacuole present is not diagnostic of a particular condition.
Electron micrograph × 5000

SPHINGOLIPIDOSES

The sphingolipidoses are a heterogeneous group of lysosomal storage diseases that result from a variety of enzyme deficiencies affecting different levels in the metabolism of complex lipids. There is accumulation of certain glycolipids or phospholipids in various tissues of the body, particularly the brain.[26] Cutaneous changes are present in many of the sphingolipidoses.[25]

G_{M2}-gangliosidoses

The G_{M2}-gangliosidoses are a subgroup of sphingolipidoses in which there is an accumulation of the ganglioside G_{M2}, as a result of a defect in some aspect of the hexosaminidase system.[24,27] The most common clinical variant is Tay–Sachs disease in which there is progressive psychomotor deterioration and blindness. In Sandhoff's disease, which is phenotypically similar, the gangliosides are deposited in nearly all cells of the body, in contrast to Tay–Sachs disease, in which deposits do not occur outside the nervous system.[25,28]

Histopathology

Cytoplasmic inclusions can be seen in a number of cells in osmificated, semi-thin, Epon-embedded sections in Sandhoff's disease.[29]

Electron microscopy. Membrane-bound inclusions can be found in endothelial cells, smooth muscle cells, pericytes, Schwann cells and eccrine secretory cells. There are lamellar and vacuolar structures and 'zebra bodies' (vacuoles with transverse membranes). In Tay–Sachs disease, lesions are confined to nerve axons, which may be distended by residual bodies, a change also seen in Sandhoff's disease.[25]

Inclusion bodies are also found in cultured fibroblasts in Sandhoff's disease, but they are quite sparse in Tay–Sachs disease.[30]

G_{M1}-gangliosidoses

There are two major clinical variants of G_{M1}-

gangliosidosis, of which Norman–Landing disease (pseudo-Hurler's syndrome) is the more severe.[27] This infantile form is characterized clinically by a gargoyle-like appearance, psycho-motor regression, blindness, hirsutism, hepato-splenomegaly and deformities of the hands and feet.[25,31] As in G_{M2}-gangliosidosis, a 'cherry-red spot' is often present.

The diagnosis can be made by measuring β-galactosidase activity in leucocytes or cultured skin fibroblasts.[24]

Histopathology

Vacuolation of fibroblasts, endothelial cells and eccrine secretory cells is sometimes discernible in sections stained with haematoxylin and eosin.[31]

Electron microscopy. There is vacuolation of fibroblasts, endothelial cells, smooth muscle cells and sweat gland epithelium. Schwann cells are less severely affected.[25] The vacuoles are empty or contain fine fibrillar or flocculent material.[32] Inclusions are also found in cultured fibroblasts.[30]

Gaucher's disease

In this sphingolipidosis, glucocerebroside accumulates in the cells of the mononuclear macrophage system (reticuloendothelial system).[33,34] It will not be discussed further as skin biopsies have consistently been negative, with no evidence of stored lipid in sweat ducts, fibroblasts or cutaneous nerves.[25,32]

Fabry's disease

Fabry's disease (angiokeratoma corporis diffusum) is an uncommon X-linked recessive disorder of glycosphingolipid metabolism in which there is a deficiency of the lysosomal hydrolase, α-galactosidase A (formerly called ceramide trihexosidase).[35,36] This leads to the accumulation of ceramide trihexoside in various tissues of the body, particularly the vascular and supporting elements.

The disease usually presents in late adoles-cence with recurrent fevers associated with pain in the fingers and toes, and intermittent oedema.[35,37] Characteristic whorled opacities are usually present in the cornea (cornea vert-icillata).[35,36] Cerebrovascular and cardiovascular disturbances are common, and progressive renal damage leading to renal failure in the fourth and fifth decades of life is almost invariable.[37] Heterozygous females are often asymptomatic, but they may show evidence of the disease to different degrees.[38–40]

The cutaneous lesions (angiokeratoma corporis diffusum) are multiple, deep red telangiec-tasias clustered on the lower part of the trunk, buttocks, thighs, scrotum and the shaft of the penis (see p. 945).[35] Most sites can be involved, although the face and scalp are usually spared. Cutaneous lesions are occasionally absent.[36] There may be anhidrosis.[36]

Histopathology

There are large and small thin-walled vessels in the upper dermis (see p. 946). The overlying epidermis is often thinned, with variable overlying hyperkeratosis. There are often acan-thotic or elongated portions of rete ridge at the periphery of the lesions.[41] The vessels are angi-ectatic and not a new growth.[42] Fibrin thrombi are sometimes present in the lumen.[43] There may be patchy vacuolization of the media of vessels in the deep dermis both in affected and normal skin. If frozen sections are examined, doubly refractile material may be seen in the vicinity of these vacuoles.[35] The material will also stain with Sudan black and the PAS stain.[44] Recently, the peroxidase-labelled lectins of *Ricinus communis* and *Bandeiraea simplicifolia* have been found to be strongly reactive with the material in frozen sections.[45] Fine PAS-positive granules are sometimes seen in the sweat glands.[43]

In semi-thin sections, fine intracytoplasmic granules can be seen in eccrine glands, vessel walls and fibroblasts in the dermis.

Electron microscopy.[44,46] Diagnostic intracytoplasmic inclusions having a lamellar structure can be found in endothelial cells, pericytes, fibroblasts, myoepithelial cells of sweat glands and macrophages. Involvement of eccrine secretory cells is uncommon[36] and of Schwann cells, rare.[29] The inclusions, which are sometimes membrane-bound, may also be found in heterozygotes in skin biopsies[44] and cultured fibroblasts.[30]

Metachromatic leucodystrophy

Metachromatic leucodystrophy results from a deficiency in the activity of arylsulphatase A and the accumulation of metachromatic sulphatides in the nervous system and certain other organs.[24,47] Clinically, there is progressive psychomotor retardation.

Histopathology

Vacuolated cells are sometimes seen in the endoneurium of cutaneous nerves. Brown metachromatic material can be seen in these nerves after cresyl violet staining of frozen sections.[48]

Electron microscopy.[48] The Schwann cells of myelinated nerves contain so-called 'tuff-stone' or 'herring bone' inclusions which are membrane-bound.[25,29] Macrophages containing myelin breakdown products are found within the nerves. Inclusions with a concentric lamellar structure have been reported in cultured fibroblasts.[30]

Krabbe's disease

Krabbe's disease (globoid cell leucodystrophy) results from a deficiency of galactocerebroside-β-galactosidase.[24] There are progressive neurological symptoms, beginning usually in childhood.

Histopathology

Globoid cells with PAS-positive cytoplasm are found in the central nervous system, particularly in the white matter.[49] Cutaneous nerves appear normal on light microscopy.

Electron microscopy. Tubular and crystalloid

inclusions have been reported in Schwann cells in cutaneous nerves,[29,49] but not consistently.[32] Cultured fibroblasts do not contain specific inclusions.[30]

Disseminated lipogranulomatosis (Farber's disease)

Disseminated lipogranulomatosis (Farber's disease) is a rare, autosomal recessive disorder of lipid metabolism in which there is a deficiency of acid ceramidase leading to an accumulation of ceramide and its degradation products.[50–53] The main clinical features usually appear at the age of two to four months and comprise progressive arthropathy, the development of subcutaneous, often periarticular, nodules, hoarseness, irritability and pulmonary failure.[54] The disease is progressive with death usually occurring in early childhood.[54]

The diagnosis can be made by demonstrating a deficiency in ceramidase in cultured fibroblasts or in white blood cells.[55,56]

Histopathology[57]

There is extensive fibrosis of the reticular dermis and subcutis with collagen bundles of variable thickness traversing the nodules in various directions. Within the fibrotic areas are many histiocytes with distended, somewhat foamy cytoplasm.[53,58] Some cells are multinucleate. A few lymphocytes and plasma cells are often present. Histochemical stains have given variable results, depending on whether paraffin or frozen sections have been used. The oil red 0 stain and Baker's reaction for phospholipid may be positive.[57]

Electron microscopy.[55,58] There are characteristic curvilinear bodies (Farber bodies) within the cytoplasm of fibroblasts and occasionally of endothelial cells. They are also found within phagosomes of histiocytes at various stages of degradation. Banana-like bodies can be found within Schwann cells. 'Zebra bodies' (vacuoles with transverse membranes) may be seen in some endothelial cells. They represent gangliosides and may be found in other storage diseases.[55]

Niemann–Pick disease

Niemann–Pick disease is a rare autosomal recessive disorder in which sphingomyelin accumulates in many organs due to a deficiency of sphingomyelinase.[59] Recent work suggests that it is a heterogeneous entity with more than one enzyme defect probably involved.[60] It has an unremitting course with death usually occurring in early childhood. Cutaneous lesions have been reported in a small number of cases and include diffuse tan brown hyperpigmentation, indurated brown plaques,[61] xanthomas[59] and juvenile xanthogranulomas.[62,63]

Histopathology

It is now thought that the lesions reported clinically as juvenile xanthogranulomas in Niemann–Pick disease are xanthomas associated with the basic phospholipid abnormality.[62] This view is based on the presence of cytoplasmic zebra bodies on electron microscopy of one case.[62] In the cutaneous lesions described there are large numbers of foamy histiocytes in the dermis admixed with a few lymphocytes. The vacuoles may impart a mulberry appearance. The cytoplasmic lipids stain with oil red 0 and Sudan black.[59] Scattered multinucleate cells are present.

Electron microscopy. Cultured fibroblasts from patients with Niemann–Pick disease show characteristic membrane-bound myelin-like inclusions.[30] 'Washed-out' inclusions with a lamellar structure have been reported in endothelial cells and Schwann cells in the skin.[32]

OLIGOSACCHARIDOSES

The oligosaccharidoses (glycoproteinoses) are characterized by excess urinary excretion of oligosaccharides as a consequence of a deficiency in one of the lysosomal enzymes responsible for the degradation of the oligosaccharide portion of glycoproteins.[24] The four disorders included in this subgroup of lysosomal storage diseases are sialidosis, fucosidosis, mannosidosis and aspartyl-

glycosaminuria. The cutaneous manifestations of this last condition have not been studied extensively and it will not be considered further.

Sialidosis

Sialidosis (mucolipidosis I) results from a deficiency of sialidase (neuraminidase).[64] Clinical features include coarse facies, ataxia, myoclonus and a cherry-red spot in the macula.[64]

Galactosialidosis is a slowly progressive neurodegenerative disease, with similar phenotypic features, which results from the combined deficiency of sialidase and β-galactosidase.[65,66] Angiokeratomas have been reported in patients with this combined deficiency state.[66]

Histopathology

Skin biopsies in sialidosis appear normal in sections stained with haematoxylin and eosin. In the combined deficiency, angiokeratomas may be present (see p. 946): the endothelium of these vessels is sometimes vacuolated.[66]

Electron microscopy. Cultured fibroblasts from patients with *sialidosis* contain cytoplasmic vacuoles similar to those observed in various mucopolysaccharidoses and in mannosidosis.[67]

In galactosialidosis, vacuoles are seen in the endothelium of vessels and also in fibroblasts, sweat-gland epithelium and the Schwann cells of non-myelinated nerves. The vacuoles are mostly empty, but some contain floccular material.[66] Lamellar inclusions also occur. Vacuolar and lamellar inclusions are present in cultured fibroblasts.[67]

Fucosidosis

Fucosidosis is a rare, autosomal recessive disorder in which a deficiency of the lysosomal enzyme α-L-fucosidase leads to the accumulation of fucose-containing glycolipids and other substances in various tissues.[68,69] There is early onset of psychomotor retardation and other neurological signs. Three clinical variants have been reported, but only Type 3 is associated with cutaneous lesions.[70] They are indistinguishable

bypass procedures,[110] advanced alcoholic cirrhosis[111,112] and cystic fibrosis.[113]

Although the pathogenetic mechanisms have not been fully elucidated, it appears that zinc transport and absorption in the gut are partially impaired. Acrodermatitis enteropathica is responsive to zinc therapy.[114,115] Several different factors may be implicated in transient symptomatic zinc deficiency. These include diminished tissue stores of zinc in premature infants, the decreased bioavailability of zinc in cow's milk when compared to human breast milk, and the rare, idiopathic occurrence of low zinc levels in breast milk, despite normal serum levels.[95]

Histopathology[102,116]

The histological changes, which vary with the age of the lesion, are similar to those seen in the necrolytic migratory erythema of the glucagonoma syndrome (see below). In early lesions, there is confluent parakeratosis overlying a normal basket-weave stratum corneum.[116] The granular layer is absent, and there is mild spongiosis and acanthosis. There is increasing pallor of the cells in the upper layers of the epidermis and variable psoriasiform epidermal hyperplasia.[117] Subcorneal or intraepidermal clefts may develop. Sometimes there is necrosis of the upper epidermis, but this was not encountered in one detailed study.[118]

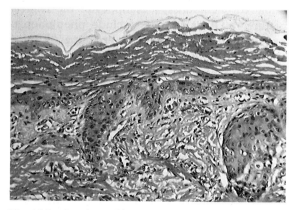

Fig. 18.3 Acrodermatitis enteropathica. This late lesion is characterized by confluent parakeratosis overlying an acanthotic epidermis.
Haematoxylin — eosin

In late lesions, there is confluent parakeratosis overlying psoriasiform epidermal hyperplasia, but there is no significant epidermal pallor (Fig. 18.3). Less common findings include dyskeratotic cells, a few acantholytic cells in vesiculobullous lesions[119] and neutrophils within the epidermis. Secondary infection may complicate the picture.

Blood vessels in the papillary dermis are often dilated, and there is a mild perivascular infiltrate of chronic inflammatory cells.

Pallor of the epidermal cells is also seen in the exceedingly rare deficiency of the M-subunit of lactate dehydrogenase, reported from Japan.[120]

Electron microscopy. Findings include lipid droplets and multiple cytoplasmic vacuoles in keratinocytes in the upper dermis.[103,116,121] Desmosomes may be diminished, associated often with widening of the intercellular space.[116]

GLUCAGONOMA SYNDROME

The clinical features of this rare syndrome include a distinctive cutaneous eruption, glossitis, stomatitis, a diabetic type of glucose intolerance, scotoma, anaemia, weight loss, venous thrombosis, elevated glucagon levels and decreased plasma amino acids.[122–125] A glucagon-secreting islet cell tumour of the pancreas is usually present, and is malignant in the majority of cases.[123,126] The syndrome has also been reported in association with a jejunal adenocarcinoma,[127] in advanced cirrhosis of the liver,[128] in association with villous atrophy of the small intestine,[129] and in a patient with elevated glucagon levels but no detectable tumour.[130]

The cutaneous lesions, called *necrolytic migratory erythema*[131] because of their similarities to both toxic epidermal necrolysis and annular erythema, are manifest by waves of extending annular or circinate erythema and superficial epidermal necrosis with shedding of the skin leading to flaccid bullae and crusted erosions. There is usually complete resolution of involved areas within 10–14 days.[132,133] The lesions primarily affect the trunk, groin, perineum, thighs and buttocks, but the legs, perioral skin[133] and sites of minor trauma may also be involved.[134] Cutaneous lesions are not invariably present in the syndrome.[124]

The pathogenesis of the skin lesions is uncertain, but their histological similarities to those seen in other deficiency states, such as pellagra and acrodermatitis enteropathica, and their disappearance with intravenous administration of supplemental amino acids suggest that profound amino acid deficiency induced by the catabolic effects of hyperglucagonaemia may be important.[133] Elevated levels of arachidonic acid, an inflammatory mediator, have been found in affected skin.[135]

Histopathology[136–140]

Several histological patterns may be seen in necrolytic migratory erythema, depending on the stage of evolution of the lesion which is biopsied (Fig. 18.4). The most distinctive pattern is the presence of pale, vacuolated keratinocytes in the upper dermis, leading to focal or confluent necrosis.[130] This process has been termed 'necrolysis'.[132] Subcorneal or intraepidermal clefts may result; acantholytic cells are rarely found in these clefts.[137] Subcorneal pustules are sometimes found adjacent to the areas of necrosis, but they may also be the only manifestation of disease in the biopsy specimen.[136]

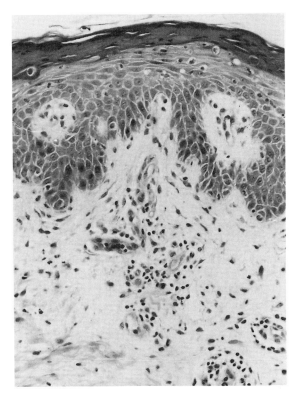

Fig. 18.5 Glucagonoma syndrome. Confluent parakeratosis overlies an epidermis in which there is mild psoriasiform hyperplasia. Haematoxylin — eosin

Diffuse neutrophilic infiltration of the epidermis may accompany this pattern.[139]

The least common histological pattern is psoriasiform hyperplasia of the epidermis with overlying confluent parakeratosis and vascular dilatation with some angioplasia in the papillary dermis (Fig. 18.5).[130,140]

In all biopsies there is usually a mild to moderate perivascular infiltrate of lymphocytes in the upper dermis. Sometimes there are occasional neutrophils as well, particularly if subcorneal pustules are present.

Uncommon histological findings include a suppurative folliculitis and the presence of concomitant candidosis.[141]

Electron microscopy. In one study, there was widening of the intercellular spaces in the upper epidermis and a reduction in the number of desmosomes.[142] The cytoplasm of affected cells

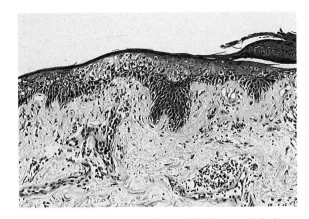

Fig. 18.4 Glucagonoma syndrome. This is an early lesion with pale, vacuolated keratinocytes in the upper dermis. Clefting has not yet developed. Haematoxylin — eosin

showed vacuolar degeneration with lysis or absence of organelles.[142] Scattered dyskeratotic cells were noted.

HARTNUP DISEASE

Hartnup disease, named after the first family to be described with this condition,[23] results from defective intestinal absorption of tryptophan and impaired renal tubular reabsorption of neutral amino acids.[143] There is a photosensitive, pellagra-like skin rash, cerebellar ataxia, mental disturbances, aminoaciduria and indicanuria.[144,145] Symptoms commence in childhood; there is often some improvement in later life. Sometimes the disease is inherited as an autosomal recessive condition.[146] Other genetic defects of tryptophan metabolism, resulting in some symptoms in common with Hartnup disease, have been described.[147]

Histopathology

The changes in the skin are similar to those seen in pellagra (see p. 519).

PROLIDASE DEFICIENCY

Prolidase deficiency is an exceedingly rare, autosomal recessive, inborn error of metabolism in which recalcitrant leg ulcers are the most characteristic feature.[148,149] Other clinical features that may be present include mental retardation, splenomegaly, recurrent infections, a characteristic facies and premature greying of the hair.[150–152] Telangiectasias, photosensitivity, lymphoedema and erosive cystitis[149] are rare manifestations.[148] Onset of symptoms occurs in childhood. Large amounts of iminodipeptides are present in the urine.[153]

Histopathology

The cutaneous ulcers may show secondary infection and variable fibrosis in chronic cases. Two reports have mentioned the presence of amyloid-like material in vessel walls and in the immediately adjacent dermis.[154,155] The significance of these findings remains to be clarified. Although the dermal collagen in non-ulcerated areas appears normal on light microscopy, the fibres are seen to be smaller and to be irregularly patterned[152] on electron microscopy. Elastic fibres are fragmented.[152]

TANGIER DISEASE

Tangier disease is a rare disorder of plasma lipid transport in which there is a deficiency of normal high density lipoproteins in the plasma and an accumulation of cholesterol esters in many organs, particularly in the reticuloendothelial system.[156] The presence of enlarged yellowish tonsils and a low plasma cholesterol level is pathognomonic. The skin usually appears clinically normal, although small papular lesions have been described.[157]

Histopathology

Biopsies from clinically normal skin show perivascular and interstitial nests of foam cells admixed with a few lymphocytes and plasma cells.[158] In frozen sections, the cytoplasm of the foam cells stains with oil red 0 and Sudan black.[158] Doubly-refractile cholesterol esters are demonstrable in both an intracellular and an extracellular location.[158] In semi-thin sections there is extensive vacuolization of the cytoplasm of Schwann cells in small, unmyelinated cutaneous nerves.[156]

Electron microscopy. The deposits are electron lucent and vary from spherical to crystalline in shape. They are not membrane bound. Lipid deposits are present in the cytoplasm of Schwann cells.[156]

LAFORA DISEASE

Lafora disease (Unverricht's disease, myoclonic epilepsy) is a familial, degenerative disorder with the clinical triad of seizures, myoclonus and dementia.[159] Cutaneous lesions are rarely present.[159] The enzyme defect is currently unknown, but the disease is usually regarded as an inborn error of carbohydrate metabolism.[160] The intracytoplasmic inclusion bodies found in various organs, particularly in ganglion cells in parts of the brain, are glucose polymers;[159] they were first described by Lafora, who considered them to consist of amyloid.

Histopathology

The inclusion bodies (Lafora bodies, polyglucosan bodies) are well seen in the excretory ducts of eccrine and apocrine sweat glands of clinically normal skin.[160,161] They are PAS positive and diastase resistant. The number of inclusions may vary with the biopsy site.[159]

Electron microscopy. The inclusions are round or oval, non-membrane-bound, and often juxtanuclear in position.[160] They are composed of fine filamentous material, dark-staining granules, and vacuoles.[159]

ULCERATIVE COLITIS AND CROHN'S DISEASE

Ulcerative colitis and Crohn's disease (regional enteritis) have many cutaneous manifestations in common.[162–164] Skin lesions occur in 10–20% of patients with either disease, but the incidence varies widely from one study to another, depending on the inclusion or otherwise of oral, perianal and non-specific lesions.[162,163,165] In the case of Crohn's disease, cutaneous manifestations are more common in patients with colonic rather than ileal disease. The onset of skin lesions occasionally precedes the symptoms and signs of the inflammatory bowel disease. There is no correlation, as a rule, with the severity or activity of the bowel disease.

Erythema nodosum and pyoderma gangrenosum[166] are the most common and specific cutaneous manifestations of *both diseases*, although pyoderma gangrenosum is more frequent in ulcerative colitis.[167] Finger clubbing, aphthous ulcers of the mouth,[168] psoriasis,[169] pyostomatitis vegetans,[170–171] erythema multiforme[172]

and vitiligo[173,174] have been reported in both conditions.[162] Cutaneous complications of therapy sometimes develop.

In *Crohn's disease*, the perianal manifestations include skin tags, fistulas and abscesses.[175] They are found in up to 80% of individuals with colonic involvement.[176] Mucosal 'cobblestoning' and fissuring may occur in the mouth.[177,178] Other lesions described in Crohn's disease include erythema elevatum diutinum,[178a] a neutrophilic dermatosis of the malar regions,[178b] epidermolysis bullosa acquisita,[179] acne fulminans,[180] cutaneous polyarteritis nodosa,[181,182] granulomatous vasculitis (Fig. 18.6),[183] and nutritional deficiency states related to zinc, nicotinic acid (niacin) and vitamin C.[162,177] The occurrence of granulomas in nodular, ulcerated or plaque-like lesions, at sites well removed from involved mucosal surfaces, has been called 'metastatic Crohn's disease'.[184–187] Some lesions are in intertriginous areas;[188] the limbs are another favoured site. There are non-caseating granulomas, similar to those seen in the bowel, scattered through the dermis and sometimes the subcutis. Sometimes there are only occasional granulomas in a perivascular distribution.[189]

Uncommon manifestations of *ulcerative colitis* include thromboembolic phenomena, cutaneous vasculitis[167,190] and a vesiculopustular eruption.[165,191] Some of the pustular lesions

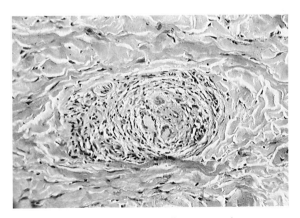

Fig. 18.6 Crohn's disease. A small, non-caseating granuloma is in intimate contact with a small blood vessel in the lower dermis. There is extravasation of fibrin into the vessel wall.
Haematoxylin — eosin

described in ulcerative colitis probably represent evolving lesions of pyoderma gangrenosum, but other non-specific pustular eruptions occur.[190, 192,193] These may show either a suppurative folliculitis or intraepidermal abscesses with an underlying mixed dermal inflammatory cell infiltrate.

WHIPPLE'S DISEASE

Whipple's disease is a rare, multisystem, bacterial infection characterized by malabsorption, abdominal pain, arthritis and neurological manifestations. The cutaneous changes include hyperpigmentation of scars and sun-exposed skin, observed in approximately 40% of patients,[194] as well as erythema nodosum and, rarely, subcutaneous nodules.[195,196]

Histopathology[195]

The subcutaneous nodules show a non-specific panniculitis with pockets of foamy macrophages containing PAS-positive, diastase-resistant material and resembling those seen in small bowel biopsies.

DIABETES MELLITUS

Cutaneous manifestations are common in diabetics, occurring at some time in approximately 30% of all people who have the disease. Most of these skin complications and associations have been discussed elsewhere in this volume, but they are listed below for completeness. Three complications which have not been considered elsewhere — microangiopathic changes, pigmented pretibial patches (diabetic dermopathy) and bullous eruption of diabetes mellitus (bullosis diabeticorum) — are discussed, in detail, below.

There are many ways of subclassifying the cutaneous manifestations and associations of diabetes mellitus.[197–199] The one used here is based on the review published some years ago by Huntley.[200]

Vascular and neuropathic complications. Both large and small vessels are affected in diabetes.[200] Atherosclerosis of large vessels contributes to the ischaemic complications, such as gangrene of the lower leg, but small vessel (microangiopathic) changes also play an important role. These latter changes are considered below. Other vascular-related phenomena include facial rubeosis[199] and the erysipelas-like areas of erythema sometimes seen on the lower parts of the legs, including the feet. Reduced sweating, loss of hair and glazed skin are, in part, related to vascular changes.

Sensory, motor and autonomic neuropathies may occur in diabetes. Autonomic dysfunction is sometimes associated with disturbances of sweating and vasomotor phenomena. Neuropathic ulcers may result from the sensory neuropathy.

Infections. These are seen less commonly than before, probably due to better control of diabetes. Bacterial infections that may occur include furuncles, non-clostridial gas gangrene, *Pseudomonas* infections of the ears, and erythrasma (see p. 602). Infections with *Candida albicans* are still common in diabetics and they may result in paronychia, stomatitis, vulvitis and balanitis (see p. 645). Dermatophyte infections may not be increased, as previously thought. Rare mycotic infections in diabetics include nocardiosis (see p. 659), cryptococcosis (see p. 648) and the zygomycoses (see p. 661).

Distinct cutaneous manifestations. Diabetes mellitus may be associated with the following conditions: necrobiosis lipoidica (see p. 192), granuloma annulare of the disseminated type (see p. 191), scleredema (also known as diabetic thick skin[201] — see p. 389), pigmented pretibial patches (see below), bullous eruption of diabetes mellitus (see below), finger 'pebbles' which resemble knuckle pads histopathologically[202] (see p. 878) and eruptive xanthomas (see p. 1018). In some diabetics, the skin is waxy and thickened, particularly over the proximal interphalangeal joints of the hands, leading to stiffness of the joints.[200] Another manifestation is yellow skin, due in part to the carotenaemia which is present in some diabetics.[199] A reduced threshold to suction-induced blisters has also been found in insulin-dependent diabetics.[203]

Less well documented associations[200] include skin tags (see p. 877), peripheral oedema, yellow nails and perforating disorders associated with diabetic renal failure and haemodialysis (see p. 447).

Diabetes mellitus or an abnormal glucose tolerance test is present in a small number of patients with Werner's syndrome (see p. 349), scleroderma (see p. 329), vitiligo (see p. 305), lichen planus (see p. 33) and Cockayne's syndrome (see p. 288), and in relatives of patients with lipoid proteinosis (see p. 412).

Secondary diabetes mellitus.[200] Diabetes mellitus may occur as a secondary process in the course of a number of diseases, such as haemochromatosis (see p. 419), lipodystrophy (see p. 507), acanthosis nigricans (see p. 552), Cushing's syndrome, acromegaly and the hepatic porphyrias, particularly porphyria cutanea tarda (see p. 536). These disorders have their own cutaneous expressions, in addition to any related to the diabetic state.

Complications of therapy.[200] The use of oral hypoglycaemic agents may be complicated by a maculopapular eruption, urticaria, photo-sensitivity, and flushing when alcohol is consumed (with chlorpropamide), and very rarely by erythema multiforme, exfoliative dermatitis or a lichenoid eruption.

Localized reactions to the injection of insulin are not uncommon and include allergic react-ions, localized induration, anaesthetic nodules composed of hypertrophied fat and some fibrous tissue, focal dermal atrophy, ulceration and necrosis, brown hyperkeratotic papules, keloid formation and localized hyperpigmentation. Insulin-induced lipoatrophy is another compli-cation which may develop 6–24 months after the onset of therapy.[198] It is more common in young females, particularly in areas of substantial fat deposition. The atrophy sometimes occurs at sites remote from injections.[197] Lipohypertrophy presents as a soft swelling resembling a lipoma. It is more common in males.[197] Generalized

allergic reactions may also occur, and these are more common with beef insulin than pork insulin.[198]

Diabetic microangiopathy

Diabetic microangiopathy refers to the abnormal small vessels found in many organs and tissues in diabetes mellitus. The kidneys, eyes, skin and muscles are particularly affected by this disease process which is the principal factor determining the prognosis of individuals with diabetes mellitus.[197]

Microangiopathy may be involved in the pathogenesis of the pigmented pretibial patches, the erysipelas-like erythema and the necrobiosis lipoidica which may occur in diabetes mellitus. It may contribute to the neuropathy that some-times occurs. Small vessel disease may be as important as atherosclerosis of large vessels in producing gangrene of the feet and lower limbs in diabetics. In many instances the micro-angiopathy is clinically silent.

Histopathology

There is thickening of the walls of small blood vessels in the dermis and subcutis and some proliferation of their endothelial cells. The thickening of the walls, and subsequent luminal narrowing, is due to the deposition of PAS-positive material in the basement membrane region. This material is partially diastase labile, although most of it is not.[204] Membranocystic lesions, in which a thin hyaline zone surrounds a small 'cystic' space, have been reported in the subcutaneous fat.[205]

Electron microscopy. The walls of the small vessels are thickened by multiple layers of veil cells (a fibroblast-like cell) and of basement membrane material.[205,206] There may also be some deposition of collagen in the walls of small vessels in the dermis.[206]

Pigmented pretibial patches

Pigmented pretibial patches (diabetic dermo-pathy, skin spots) are the most common cuta-

Table 18.1   Summary of the biosynthesis of haem and the associated clinical disorders

Metabolites	Enzymes	Porphyrias
Glycine + Succinyl COA		
- - - - - - - - - - - - - - - - - - ALA synthase		
↓		
Aminolaevulinic acid		
- - - - - - - - - - - - - - - - - - ALA-dehydratase	————	ALA-dehydratase deficiency
↓		
Porphobilinogen		
- - - - - - - - - - - - - - - - - - Porphobilinogen deaminase	————	Acute intermittent porphyria
↓		
Hydroxymethylbilane*		
- - - - - - - - - - - - - - - - - - Uroporphyrinogen III cosynthase	————	Congenital erythropoietic porphyria
↓		
Uroporphyrinogen III		
- - - - - - - - - - - - - - - - - - Uroporphyrinogen decarboxylase	———— (Homozygous)	Porphyria cutanea tarda Hepatoerythropoietic porphyri
↓		
Coproporphyrinogen III		
- - - - - - - - - - - - - - - - - - Coproporphyrinogen oxidase	————	Hereditary coproporphyria
↓		
Protoporphyrinogen IX		
- - - - - - - - - - - - - - - - - - Protoporphyrinogen oxidase	————	Variegate porphyria
↓		
Protoporphyrin IX		
- - -+Fe++- - - - - - - - - - - - Ferrochelatase	————	Erythropoietic protoporphyria
↓		
Haem		

*Hydroxymethylbilane may undergo spontaneous conversion to uroporphyrinogen I.

Hereditary coproporphyria

This is an autosomal dominant variant of acute porphyria which results from a deficiency of coproporphyrinogen oxidase.[231] Latent disease is more usual than the symptomatic form, which is characterized by episodic attacks of abdominal pain and neurological and psychiatric disturbances. These acute episodes are less severe than in acute intermittent porphyria. Cutaneous photosensitivity occurs in approximately 30% of cases, and this becomes manifest chiefly in association with the acute attacks.[231,237] The lesions resemble those seen in porphyria cutanea tarda (see below).

Laboratory findings include greatly elevated levels of urinary and faecal coproporphyrins.[238] Porphobilinogen and ALA are increased, as in variegate porphyria (see below), during acute episodes.[237]

Variegate porphyria

Variegate porphyria, like hereditary coproporphyria, may be associated with acute episodes (as seen in acute intermittent porphyria) and with photocutaneous manifestations (as seen in porphyria cutanea tarda).[239,240] It is an autosomal dominant disorder in which the activity of the enzyme protoporphyrinogen oxidase is reduced by approximately 50%. This disorder is quite common in Afrikaners and much less so in other white people and in people of other races.[239]

Only a minority of those with the enzyme defect develop clinical manifestations, and only after puberty. Acute episodes are precipitated by exogenous factors such as the ingestion of various drugs.[229,241] Cutaneous changes include skin fragility, blistering and milia formation in sun-exposed areas, as in porphyria cutanea tarda, although very occasionally an acute phototoxic reaction (as seen in erythropoietic protoporphyria) may develop.[231] Variegate porphyria is not usually associated with liver dysfunction, although it has been reported in association with a hepatocellular carcinoma.[242]

Laboratory findings are somewhat variable, depending on the activity of the disease.[231] There is usually an elevated plasma porphyrin level with plasma fluorescence that is maximal at a wavelength of 626±1 nm.[243] In practice the diagnosis is most often suggested by finding elevated levels of faecal protoporphyrin and coproporphyrin.[241] Urinary ALA and porphobilinogen are usually increased during acute episodes.

It has been reported in one homozygote that the erythrocyte protoporphyrin was raised, and that this was predominantly zinc chelated.[244]

Congenital erythropoietic porphyria (Günther's disease)

This rare, autosomal recessive disorder of haem synthesis results from a deficiency of uroporphyrinogen III cosynthase (URO-synthase) leading to an accumulation of porphyrins, particularly uroporphyrinogen I and III in the bone marrow, blood and other organs.[245] This leads to a chronic photobullous dermatosis, intermittent haemolysis and massive porphyrinuria.[245] Presentation is usually in infancy with red urine which stains diapers a pink colour.[231] Late onset of the disease has been recorded.[246]

The severe photosensitivity leads to the formation of bullae within a day or two of exposure to the sun. Recurrent eruptions may lead to mutilating deformities of the hands and face and sclerodermoid thickening of affected parts.[247,248] Other clinical features include the pathognomonic characteristic of erythrodontia (discoloration of the teeth under normal light and red fluorescence with ultraviolet light), hypertrichosis, patchy scarring alopecia, and nail changes.[245,249–251]

There are large amounts of uroporphyrins in the urine and coproporphyrins in the stool, and these are predominantly type I isomers.[247] The plasma and erythrocytes contain increased levels of uroporphyrinogen and, to a lesser extent, coproporphyrinogen.[248] Heterozygotes have blood levels of URO-synthase activity intermediate between affected individuals and controls.[247]

Erythropoietic protoporphyria

Erythropoietic protoporphyria, more recently termed simply protoporphyria,[231,252] is an autosomal dominant disorder in which the defect is in the terminal step of haem synthesis at which protoporphyrin IX and iron combine to form haem.[253–255] It is associated with a deficiency of ferrochelatase (haem synthase).

It generally becomes manifest in early childhood with episodes of acute photosensitivity accompanied by a painful, burning sensation.[254] Often there is oedema and erythema, and rarely there may be urticaria and petechiae.[231] The changes develop within a few hours of exposure to the sun. In the chronic stages there is waxy scarring of the nose, radial scars around the lips and pits or scars on the forehead, nose and cheeks.[231,256] The skin on the dorsum of the hands has a leathery texture and it may also show 'cobblestone' thickening.[231] Deaths from cirrhosis accompanying heavy accumulation of protoporphyrin in the liver have been reported.[257–259]

Rare clinical presentations have included late onset,[256] the presence of scarring bullae and milia,[260] a clinical picture resembling hydroa aestivale[261] (see p. 581), and the presence of a fibrous band involving a digit (pseudo-ainhum).[262] In one group of patients with proto-porphyria the disease appears to be exacerbated by the ingestion of iron.[253]

Protoporphyria is the only disorder of porphyrin metabolism with normal urinary porphyrins.[231] There are markedly increased levels of protoporphyrin in the faeces and blood. The erythrocytes show a red fluorescence which decays more rapidly than that in congenital erythropoietic porphyria (see above).[231]

Porphyria cutanea tarda

Porphyria cutanea tarda is the commonest form of porphyria in Europe and North America.[231] It is not a single disorder but an aetiologically diverse group which share in common reduced activity of uroporphyrinogen decarboxylase (URO-D), the enzyme which catalyses the sequential decarboxylation of uroporphyrinogen to coproporphyrinogen in a two-stage process.[231,263,264] In most forms there is a reduction in hepatic URO-D, leading to over-production of porphyrins in the liver.[265] In the uncommon familial form there is usually a deficiency of this enzyme in erythrocytes as well as in other tissues.

There are three major forms of porphyria cutanea tarda: familial, sporadic and toxic. In addition, the porphyria resulting from porphyrin-producing tumours of the liver,[263,266] and

that associated with chronic renal failure and URO-D deficiency are sometimes categorized as two further clinical variants of porphyria cutanea tarda.[265,267] Hepatoerythropoietic porphyria (see below) is regarded as the homozygous deficiency of URO-D.[265]

The *familial form* is inherited as an autosomal dominant trait.[265] It was previously thought to be associated, invariably, with a deficiency of URO-D in erythrocytes as well as in the liver, but cases with a normal level of erythrocyte URO-D have been documented.[268] Sometimes overt disease is precipitated by some exogenous factor such as childbirth, exposure to ultraviolet radiation in tanning parlours, iron overload or excessive alcohol intake.[269] Its onset is usually earlier than that of the sporadic form.

The *sporadic form* usually has its onset in mid-life. More than 70% of cases are associated with alcohol abuse and liver damage.[265,270,271] Oestrogen therapy for carcinoma of the prostate[272,273] or for menopausal symptoms is sometimes the precipitating event. Oral contraceptives have also been incriminated. Rare associations have included diabetes mellitus,[270] hepatitis, Wilson's disease,[274] hepatocellular carcinoma,[263] lymphoma,[275] AIDS,[276] agnogenic myeloid metaplasia[277] and lupus erythematosus.[278–280] The sporadic form appears to result from inactivation of URO-D in the liver[264] although this appears to be independent of, rather than the consequence of, liver injury.[265]

The *toxic form* results from exposure to polychlorinated aromatic hydrocarbons.[281] Other hepatotoxins have rarely been incriminated.

The cutaneous changes occur predominantly on light-exposed areas such as the face, arms and dorsum of the hands.[282] Their severity is highly variable. They include increased vulnerability to mechanical trauma and the formation of subepidermal vesicles or bullae measuring 0.5 – 3 cm in diameter.[270] Erosions, milia, scars and areas of hyperpigmentation are common.[270] Hypertrichosis, patchy alopecia, infections,[283] dystrophic calcification and sclerodermoid changes may occur but do so less frequently than the other cutaneous manifestations.[270] The sclerodermoid changes, which may be present in up to 20% of cases, do not always occur in light-exposed areas. They are not associated with sclerodactyly and they are not invariably permanent. It has been suggested that they are related to high levels of uroporphyrinogen.[284]

Hepatic changes are common in porphyria cutanea tarda. There is an increased risk of developing hepatocellular carcinoma.[263]

Laboratory findings include increased amounts of uroporphyrins in the urine and plasma and of coproporphyrins in the faeces. The urine contains a predominance of 8-carboxyl and 7-carboxyl porphyrins, while the faeces contain isocoproporphyrin, which is not found in significant amounts in other porphyrias.[264]

Hepatoerythropoietic porphyria

This rare, severe variant of porphyria is manifested clinically by photosensitivity commencing in early childhood.[285–288] Like porphyria cutanea tarda (PCT) there is a deficiency of uroporphyrinogen decarboxylase, but the activity of this enzyme is much less than in PCT, reflecting a homozygous state.[289,290] Hepatic involvement is common. The cutaneous features resemble those of PCT.[291]

Laboratory findings are similar to those in PCT, but an additional feature is the presence of elevated levels of protoporphyrins in erythrocytes.[285]

Pseudoporphyria

This term is used for a phototoxic bullous dermatosis which resembles porphyria cutanea tarda. However, there are normal levels of porphyrins in the serum, urine and faeces.[292] The term 'therapy-induced bullous photosensitivity' has been suggested as more appropriate[293] as this condition has been reported following the use of a number of drugs including tetracyclines,[294,295] sulphonamides, frusemide (furosemide),[296] nalidixic acid,[297] naproxen,[298–300] pyridoxine,[301] chlorthalidone[302] and etretinate.[303] A few cases have followed the prolonged use of tanning beds.[304,305] Blistering has also been reported in patients with chronic renal failure undergoing haemodialysis.[306,307] In some patients pseudoporphyria has been associated with a deficiency of uroporphyrinogen decarboxylase with increased levels of porphyrins; in others, many of whom were also receiving frusemide (furosemide), the porphyrin levels have been normal.[306,308,309]

The lesions in pseudoporphyria, which consist of spontaneous blisters and skin fragility, usually involving the dorsum of the hands, may develop as early as one week, or as late as several months, after commencement of the drug.[298] In contrast to porphyria cutanea tarda, few patients with pseudoporphyria develop hypertrichosis, hyperpigmentation or sclerodermoid features.

Histopathology[310,311]

There are remarkable similarities in the cutaneous changes in the various porphyrias: the differences are quantitative rather than qualitative.[311] The hallmarks of porphyria are the presence of lightly eosinophilic hyaline material in and around small vessels in the upper dermis, reduplication of vascular and sometimes epidermal basement membrane and the deposition of fibrillar and amorphous material around the superficial vessels and at the dermo–epidermal junction.[310,311] The hyaline material seen on light microscopy is reduplicated basement membrane associated with the fibrillar and amorphous material just mentioned. These various features will be discussed in further detail.

In *erythropoietic protoporphyria* (EPP) the hyaline material not only involves the walls of small vessels in the papillary dermis, but it also forms an irregular cuff around these vessels (Fig. 18.7). There is variable thickening of the vessel walls as a consequence of the presence of this hyaline material and this is sometimes associated with luminal narrowing. The hyaline material does not usually encroach on the adjacent dermis as much as it does in lipoid proteinosis (see p. 412) and furthermore it does not involve the sweat glands.[312] The hyaline material is strongly PAS positive and diastase resistant. It stains with Sudan black in frozen sections and it

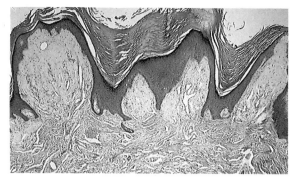

Fig. 18.7 Erythropoietic protoporphyria with hyaline material surrounding vessels in the papillary dermis. This case was initially misdiagnosed as a variant of colloid milium. Haematoxylin — eosin

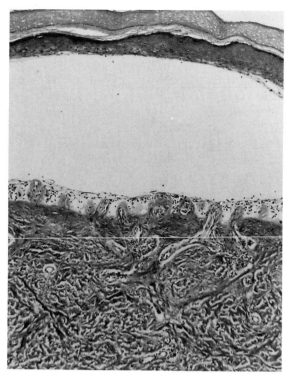

Fig. 18.8 Porphyria cutanea tarda. There is a cell-poor, subepidermal bulla with some 'festooning' in the base. Haematoxylin — eosin

is weakly positive with Hale's colloidal iron method.[313] Elastic fibres are pushed aside by the hyaline material.[313] Uninvolved areas of skin in EPP show minimal or undetectable changes. Sometimes, a few neutrophils with foci of leucocytoclasis are present in the papillary dermis.

In *porphyria cutanea tarda* (PCT), the hyaline material is restricted to the vessel walls and their immediate vicinity. It does not form a significant cuff as in EPP. Again, the material is PAS positive and diastase resistant. In some cases, there is PAS-positive thickening of the basement membrane. These changes are not usually present in early lesions of pseudoporphyria, although some PAS-positive material is found in vessel walls. Small amounts of this material may be found in vessel walls in clinically-uninvolved skin in PCT.[310] Solar elastosis is usually present in PCT, a change which is not often seen in patients with EPP, a reflection of their younger age.[311]

In *sclerodermoid lesions* there is thickening of the dermis which may be indistinguishable from that seen in scleroderma, although a looser arrangement of the collagen fibres is usually discernible in PCT.[310,311]

The *blisters* which form in the various forms of porphyria and in pseudoporphyria are subepidermal (dermolytic) with the dermal papillae projecting into the floor (festooning) (Fig. 18.8).[298,314,315] This latter change is not always prominent in pseudoporphyria.[298] There is only a very sparse inflammatory cell infiltrate which in pseudoporphyria may sometimes include a rare eosinophil. Focal haemorrhage is sometimes present in the upper dermis. The PAS-positive basement membrane is usually found in the roof of the blister.[298]

Epidermal changes are usually mild in the various porphyrias. The epidermis in PCT may be normal, acanthotic or atrophic.[311] There is sometimes hyperkeratosis and mild hypergranulosis. In sclerodermoid lesions and in EPP there is sometimes effacement of the rete ridge pattern.

Direct immunofluorescence in the porphyrias reveals deposits of IgG and, less commonly, IgM and complement in and around the upper dermal vessels.[316] Small deposits may also be found at the dermo–epidermal junction.[254] Type IV collagen and laminin are additional components of the vascular and perivascular hyaline material which may be detected using monoclonal antibodies.[304,311]

Electron microscopy.[310,311] There is prominent reduplication of the basal laminae with encasement of the vessels in a concentric fashion. External to the laminae there is finely fibrillar material which also extends into the vessel wall.[310] Irregular clumps of amorphous material are also found in the perivascular regions.

Fine collagen fibrils are present within and around the vessels in the upper dermis, while the sclerodermoid lesions have fibrils with a bimodal size throughout the dermis.[317]

Another ultrastructural finding in some of the porphyrias is reduplication of the basal lamina at the dermo–epidermal junction. This is seen in PCT and variegate porphyria, but not usually in EPP.

In blisters the cleavage is usually dermolytic, with the roof containing a thin layer of dermal fibres still attached to the anchoring fibrils.[311] Early lesions appear to develop from the enlargement of membrane-limited vacuoles in the upper dermis.[318] Some of these appear to form in the pseudopodia of basal cells which protrude into the dermis.[318]

Finally, in one study of an acute flare reaction in EPP, endothelial cell damage was noted, leading to the suggestion that leakage of vascular contents contributes to the hyaline material.[319,320] The reduplication of the basal lamina may represent a reparative reaction to repeated endothelial injury.

REFERENCES

Vitamin and dietary disturbances

1. Gupta MA, Gupta AK, Haberman HF. Dermatologic signs in anorexia nervosa and bulimia nervosa. Arch Dermatol 1987; 123: 1386–1390.
2. Barthelemy H, Chouvet B, Cambazard F. Skin and mucosal manifestations in vitamin deficiency. J Am Acad Dermatol 1986; 15: 1263–274.
3. Miller SJ. Nutritional deficiency and the skin. J Am Acad Dermatol 1989; 21: 1–30.
4. Connelly TJ, Becker A, McDonald JW. Bachelor scurvy. Int J Dermatol 1982; 21: 209–211.
5. Price NM. Vitamin C deficiency. Cutis 1980; 26: 375–377.
6. Ellis CN, Vanderveen EE, Rasmussen JE. Scurvy. A case caused by peculiar dietary habits. Arch Dermatol 1984; 120: 1212–1214.
7. Walker A. Chronic scurvy. Br J Dermatol 1968; 80: 625–630.
8. Hashimoto K, Kitabchi AE, Duckworth WC, Robinson N. Ultrastructure of scorbutic human skin. Acta Derm Venereol 1970; 50: 9–21.
9. Klein-Szanto AJP, Martin DH, Pine AH. Cutaneous manifestations in rats with advanced vitamin A deficiency. J Cutan Pathol 1980; 7: 260–270.
10. Logan WS. Vitamin A and keratinization. Arch Dermatol 1972; 105: 748–753.
11. Wechsler HL. Vitamin A deficiency following small-bowel bypass surgery for obesity. Arch Dermatol 1979; 115: 73–75.
12. Silverman AK, Ellis CN, Voorhees JJ. Hypervitaminosis A syndrome: A paradigm of retinoid side effects. J Am Acad Dermatol 1987; 16: 1027–1039.
13. Inkeles SB, Connor WE, Illingworth DR. Hepatic and dermatologic manifestations of chronic hypervitaminosis A in adults. Am J Med 1986; 80: 491–496.

14. Sanders MN, Winkelmann RK. Cutaneous reactions to vitamin K. J Am Acad Dermatol 1988; 19: 699–704.
15. Gilliam JN, Cox AJ. Epidermal changes in vitamin B_{12} deficiency. Arch Dermatol 1973; 107: 231–236.
16. Rapaport MJ. Pellagra in a patient with anorexia nervosa. Arch Dermatol 1985; 121: 255–257.
17. Comaish JS, Felix RH, McGrath H. Topically applied niacinamide in isoniazid-induced pellagra. Arch Dermatol 1976; 112: 70–72.
18. Cohen LK, George W, Smith R. Isoniazid-induced acne and pellagra. Arch Dermatol 1974; 109: 377–381.
19. Stratigos JD, Katsambas A. Pellagra: a still existing disease. Br J Dermatol 1977; 96: 99–106.
20. Castiello RJ, Lynch PJ. Pellagra and the carcinoid syndrome. Arch Dermatol 1972; 105: 574–577.
21. El Zawahry M. Pellagra: notes and comments. Int J Dermatol 1973; 12: 158–162.
22. Findlay GH, Rein L, Mitchell D. Reactions to light on the normal and pellagrous Bantu skin. Br J Dermatol 1969; 81: 345–351.
23. Baron DN, Dent CE, Harris H et al. Hereditary pellagra-like skin rash with temporary cerebellar ataxia, constant renal amino-aciduria, and other bizarre biochemical features. Lancet 1956; 2: 421–428.

Lysomal storage diseases

24. Glewe RH, Basu A, Prence EM, Remaley AT. Biology of disease. Lysosomal storage diseases. Lab Invest 1985; 53: 250–269.
25. Dolman CL. Diagnosis of neurometabolic disorders by examination of skin biopsies and lymphocytes. Semin Diagn Pathol 1984; 1: 82–97.
26. Brady RO. The sphingolipidoses. N Engl J Med 1966; 275: 312–318.

27. Volk DW, Adachi M, Schneck L. The gangliosidoses. Hum Pathol 1975; 6: 555–569.
28. Dolman CL, Chang E, Duke RJ. Pathologic findings in Sandhoff disease. Arch Pathol 1973; 96: 272–275.
29. Gebhart W. Heritable metabolic storage diseases. J Cutan Pathol 1985; 12: 348–357.
30. Takahashi K, Naito M, Suzuki Y. Lipid storage disease: Part III. Ultrastructural evaluation of cultured fibroblasts in sphingolipidoses. Acta Pathol Jpn 1987; 37: 261–272.
31. Drut R. Eccrine sweat gland involvement in G_{M1} gangliosidosis. J Cutan Pathol 1978; 5: 35–36.
32. O'Brien JS, Bernett J, Veath ML, Paa D. Lysosomal storage diseases. Diagnosis by ultrastructural examination of skin biopsy specimens. Arch Neurol 1975; 32: 592–599.
33. Peters SP, Lee RE, Glew RH. Gaucher's disease, a review. Medicine (Baltimore) 1977; 56: 425–442.
34. Lee RE, Robinson DB, Glew RH. Gaucher's disease. I. Modern enzymatic and anatomic methods of diagnosis. Arch Pathol Lab Med 1981; 105: 102–104.
35. Wallace HJ. Anderson-Fabry disease. Br J Dermatol 1973; 88: 1–23.
36. Kang WH, Chun SI, Lee S. Generalized anhidrosis associated with Fabry's disease. J Am Acad Dermatol 1987; 17: 883–887.
37. Burkholder PM, Updike SJ, Ware RA, Reese OG. Clinicopathologic, enzymatic, and genetic features in a case of Fabry's disease. Arch Pathol Lab Med 1980; 104: 17–25.
38. Burda CD, Winder PR. Angiokeratoma corporis diffusum universale (Fabry's disease) in female subjects. Am J Med 1967; 42: 293–301.
39. Hashimoto K, Lieberman P, Lamkin N Jr. Angiokeratoma corporis diffusum. Arch Dermatol 1976; 112: 1416–1423.
40. Voglino A, Paradisi M, Dompé G et al. Angiokeratoma corporis diffusum (Fabry's disease) with unusual features in a female patient. Light- and electron-microscopic investigation. Am J Dermatopathol 1988; 10: 343–348.
41. Sagebiel RW, Parker F. Cutaneous lesions of Fabry's disease: glycolipid lipidosis. J Invest Dermatol 1968; 50: 208–213.
42. von Gemmingen G, Kierland RR, Opitz JM. Angiokeratoma corporis diffusum (Fabry's disease). Arch Dermatol 1965; 91: 206–218.
43. Nakamura T, Kaneko H, Nishino I. Angiokeratoma corporis diffusum (Fabry disease): Ultrastructural studies of the skin. Acta Derm Venereol 1981; 61: 37–41.
44. Luderschmidt C, Wolff HH. Subtle clues to diagnosis of skin diseases by electron microscopy. Intracytoplasmic granules with lamellae as signs of heterozygous Fabry's disease. Am J Dermatopathol 1980; 2: 57–61.
45. Faraggiana T, Churg J, Grishman E et al. Light- and electron-microscopic histochemistry of Fabry's disease. Am J Pathol 1981; 103: 247–262.
46. Strayer DS, Santa Cruz D. Subtle clues to diagnosis of skin diseases by electron microscopy. Intracytoplasmic granules with lamellae in Fabry's disease. Am J Dermatopathol 1980; 2: 63–64.
47. Fensom AH, Marsh J, Jackson M et al. First-trimester diagnosis of metachromatic leucodystrophy. Clin Genet 1988; 34: 122–125.
48. Gebhart W, Lassmann H, Niebauer G. Demonstration of specific storage material within cutaneous nerves in metachromatic leukodystrophy. J Cutan Pathol 1978; 5: 5–14.
49. Takahashi K, Naito M. Lipid storage disease: Part II. Ultrastructural pathology of lipid storage cells in sphingolipidoses. Acta Pathol Jpn 1985; 35: 385–408.
50. Farber S. A lipid metabolic disorder—"disseminated lipogranulomatosis". A syndrome with similarity to, and important difference from Niemann–Pick and Hand–Schüller–Christian disease. Am J Dis Child 1952; 84: 499–500.
51. Sugita M, Dulaney JT, Moser HW. Ceramidase deficiency in Farber's disease (lipogranulomatosis). Science 1972; 178: 1100–1102.
52. Knobler RM, Becerano S, Gebhart W. Inborn errors of lipid metabolism — dermatological aspects. Clin Exp Dermatol 1988; 13: 365–370.
53. Chanoki M, Ishii M, Fukai K et al. Farber's lipogranulomatosis in siblings: light and electron microscopic studies. Br J Dermatol 1989; 121: 779–785.
54. Pavone L, Moser HW, Mollica F et al. Farber's lipogranulomatosis: Ceramidase deficiency and prolonged survival in three relatives. Johns Hopkins Med J 1980; 147: 193–196.
55. Rauch HJ, Aubock L. "Banana bodies" in disseminated lipogranulomatosis (Farber's disease). Am J Dermatopathol 1983; 5: 263–266.
56. Rutsaert J, Tondeur M, Vamos-Hurwitz E, Dustin P. The cellular lesions of Farber's disease and their experimental reproduction in tissue culture. Lab Invest 1977; 36: 474–480.
57. Amirhakimi GH, Haghighi P, Ghalambor MA, Honari S. Familial lipogranulomatosis (Farber's disease). Clin Genet 1976; 9: 625–630.
58. Schmoeckel C. Subtle clues to diagnosis of skin diseases by electron microscopy. "Farber bodies" in disseminated lipogranulomatosis (Farber's disease). Am J Dermatopathol 1980; 2: 153–156.
59. Crocker AC, Farber S. Niemann–Pick disease: A review of eighteen patients. Medicine (Baltimore) 1958; 37: 1–95.
60. Vanier MT, Wenger DA, Comly ME et al. Niemann–Pick disease group C: clinical variability and diagnosis based on defective cholesterol esterification. Clin Genet 1988; 33: 331–348.
61. Mardini MK, Gergen P, Akhtar M, Ghandour M. Niemann–Pick disease: Report of a case with skin involvement. Am J Dis Child 1982; 136: 650–651.
62. Wood WS, Dimmick JE, Dolman CL. Niemann–Pick disease and juvenile xanthogranuloma. Are they related? Am J Dermatopathol 1987; 9: 433–437.
63. Sibulkin D, Olichney JJ. Juvenile xanthogranuloma in a patient with Niemann–Pick disease. Arch Dermatol 1973; 108: 829–831.
64. Young ID, Young EP, Mossman J et al. Neuraminidase deficiency: case report and review of the phenotype. J Med Genet 1987; 24: 283–290.
65. Sakuraba H, Suzuki Y, Akagi M et al. β-galactosidase-neuraminidase deficiency (galactosialidosis): clinical, pathological, and enzymatic studies in a postmortem case. Ann Neurol 1983; 13: 497–503.
66. Loonen MCB, Reuser AJJ, Visser P, Arts WFM. Combined sialidase (neuraminidase) and β-galactosidase deficiency. Clinical, morphological and

enzymological observations in a patient. Clin Genet 1984; 26: 139–149.
67. Takahashi K, Naito M, Suzuki Y. Genetic mucopolysaccharidoses, mannosidosis, sialidosis, galactosialidosis, and I-cell disease. Ultrastructural analysis of cultured fibroblasts. Acta Pathol Jpn 1987; 37: 385–400.
68. Dvoretzky I, Fisher BK. Fucosidosis. Int J Dermatol 1979; 18: 213–216.
69. Willems PJ, Garcia CA, De Smedt MCH et al. Intrafamilial variability in fucosidosis. Clin Genet 1988; 34: 7–14.
70. Smith EB, Graham JL, Ledman JA, Snyder RD. Fucosidosis. Cutis 1977; 19: 195–198.
71. Kornfeld M, Snyder RD, Wenger DA. Fucosidosis with angiokeratoma. Electron microscopic changes in the skin. Arch Pathol Lab Med 1977; 101: 478–485.
72. Epinette WW, Norins AL, Drew AL et al. Angiokeratoma corporis diffusum with α-L-fucosidase deficiency. Arch Dermatol 1973; 107: 754–757.
73. Kistler JP, Lott IT, Kolodny EH et al. Mannosidosis. New clinical presentation, enzyme studies, and carbohydrate analysis. Arch Neurol 1977; 34: 45–51.
74. Dickersin GR, Lott IT, Kolodny EH, Dvorak AM. A light and electron microscopic study of mannosidosis. Hum Pathol 1980; 11: 245–256.
75. Okada S, Kato T, Oshima T et al. Heterogeneity in mucolipidosis II (I-cell disease). Clin Genet 1983; 23: 155–159.
76. Ben-Yoseph Y, Mitchell DA, Nadler HL. First trimester prenatal evaluation for I-cell disease by N-acetyl-glucosamine I-phosphotransferase assay. Clin Genet 1988; 33: 38–43.
77. Hanai J, Leroy J, O'Brien JS. Ultrastructure of cultured fibroblasts in I-cell disease. Am J Dis Child 1971; 122: 34–38.
78. Endo H, Miyazaki T, Asano S, Sagami S. Ultrastructural studies of the skin and cultured fibroblasts in I-cell disease. J Cutan Pathol 1987; 14: 309–317.
79. Kamiya M, Tada T, Kuhara H et al. I-cell disease. A case report and review of the literature. Acta Pathol Jpn 1986; 36: 1679–1692.
80. Dyken P, Krawiecki N. Neurodegenerative diseases of infancy and childhood. Ann Neurol 1983; 13: 351–364.
81. Ishii M, Takahashi K, Hamada T et al. Cutaneous ultrastructural diagnosis of ceroid-lipofuscinosis. Br J Dermatol 1981; 104: 581–585.
82. Farrell DF, Sumi SM. Skin punch biopsy in the diagnosis of juvenile neuronal ceroid-lipofuscinosis. A comparison with leukocyte peroxidase assay. Arch Neurol 1977; 34: 39–44.
82a. Manca V, Kanitakis J, Zambruno G et al. Ultrastructural study of the skin in a case of juvenile ceroid-lipofuscinosis. Am J Dermatopathol 1990; 12: 412–416.

Miscellaneous metabolic and systemic diseases

83. Danbolt N. Acrodermatitis enteropathica. Br J Dermatol 1979; 100: 37–40.
84. Neldner KH, Hambidge KM, Walravens PA. Acrodermatitis enteropathica. Int J Dermatol 1978; 17: 380–387.
85. Weston WL, Huff JC, Humbert JR et al. Zinc correction of defective chemotaxis in acrodermatitis enteropathica. Arch Dermatol 1977; 113: 422–425.
86. Traupe H, Happle R, Gröbe H, Bertram HP. Polarization microscopy of hair in acrodermatitis enteropathica. Pediatr Dermatol 1986; 3: 300–303.
87. Deffner NF, Perry HO. Acrodermatitis enteropathica and failure to thrive. Arch Dermatol 1973; 108: 658–662.
88. Neldner KH, Hagler L, Wise WR et al. Acrodermatitis enteropathica. A clinical and biochemical survey. Arch Dermatol 1974; 110: 711–721.
89. Sharma NL, Sharma RC, Gupta KR, Sharma RP. Self-limiting acrodermatitis enteropathica. A follow-up study of three interrelated families. Int J Dermatol 1988; 27: 485–486.
90. Bronson DM, Barsky R, Barsky S. Acrodermatitis enteropathica. Recognition at long last during a recurrence in a pregnancy. J Am Acad Dermatol 1983; 9: 140–144.
91. Tompkins RR, Livingood CS. Acrodermatitis enteropathica persisting into adulthood. Arch Dermatol 1969; 99: 190–195.
92. Graves K, Kestenbaum T, Kalivas J. Hereditary acrodermatitis enteropathica in an adult. Arch Dermatol 1980; 116: 562–564.
93. Owens CWI, Al-Khader AA, Jackson MJ, Prichard BNC. A severe 'stasis eczema', associated with low plasma zinc, treated successfully with oral zinc. Br J Dermatol 1981; 105: 461–464.
94. Bonifazi E, Rigillo N, De Simone B, Meneghini CL. Acquired dermatitis to zinc deficiency in a premature infant. Acta Derm Venereol 1980; 60: 449–451.
95. Bilinski DL, Ehrenkranz RA, Cooley-Jacobs J, McGuire J. Symptomatic zinc deficiency in a breast-fed, premature infant. Arch Dermatol 1987; 123: 1221–1224.
96. Connors TJ, Czarnecki DB, Haskett MI. Acquired zinc deficiency in a breast-fed premature infant. Arch Dermatol 1983; 119: 319–321.
97. Zimmerman AW, Hambidge KM, Lepow ML et al. Acrodermatitis in breast-fed premature infants: Evidence for a defect of mammary zinc secretion. Pediatrics 1982; 69: 176–183.
98. Munro CS, Lazaro C, Lawrence CM. Symptomatic zinc deficiency in breast-fed premature infants. Br J Dermatol 1989; 121: 773–778.
99. Glover MT, Atherton DJ. Transient zinc deficiency in two full-term breast-fed siblings associated with low maternal breast milk zinc concentration. Pediatr Dermatol 1988; 5: 10–13.
100. Kuramoto Y, Igarashi Y, Kato S, Tagami H. Acquired zinc deficiency in two breast-fed mature infants. Acta Derm Venereol 1986; 66: 359–361.
101. Bye AME, Goodfellow A, Atherton DJ. Transient zinc deficiency in a full-term breast-fed infant of normal birth weight. Pediatr Dermatol 1985; 2: 308–311.
102. Niemi KM, Anttila PH, Kanerva L, Johansson E. Histopathological study of transient acrodermatitis enteropathica due to decreased zinc in breast milk. J Cutan Pathol 1989; 16: 382–387.
103. Weismann K, Kvist N, Kobayasi T. Bullous acrodermatitis due to zinc deficiency during total

parenteral nutrition: an ultrastructural study of the epidermal changes. Acta Derm Venereol 1983; 63: 143–146.

104. Katoh T, Igarashi M, Ohhashi E et al. Acrodermatitis enteropathica-like eruption associated with parenteral nutrition. Dermatologica 1976; 152: 119–127.

105. van Vloten WA, Bos LP. Skin lesions in acquired zinc deficiency due to parenteral nutrition. Dermatologica 1978; 156: 175–183.

106. Arlette JP, Johnston MM. Zinc deficiency dermatosis in premature infants receiving prolonged parenteral alimentation. J Am Acad Dermatol 1981; 5: 37–42.

107. Abou-Mourad NN, Farah FS, Steel D. Dermopathic changes in hypozincemia. Arch Dermatol 1979; 115: 956–958.

108. McClain C, Soutor C, Zieve L. Zinc deficiency: a complication of Crohn's disease. Gastroenterology 1980; 78: 272–279.

109. Weismann K, Hjorth N, Fischer A. Zinc depletion syndrome with acrodermatitis during longterm intravenous feeding. Clin Exp Dermatol 1976; 1: 237–242.

110. Weismann K, Wadskov S, Mikkelsen HI et al. Acquired zinc deficiency dermatosis in man. Arch Dermatol 1978; 114: 1509–1511.

111. Weismann K, Hoyer H, Christensen E. Acquired zinc deficiency in alcoholic liver cirrhosis: report of two cases. Acta Derm Venereol 1980; 60: 447–449.

112. Ecker RI, Schroeter AL. Acrodermatitis and acquired zinc deficiency. Arch Dermatol 1978; 114: 937–939.

113. Hansen RC, Lemen R, Revsin B. Cystic fibrosis manifesting with acrodermatitis enteropathica-like eruption. Arch Dermatol 1983; 119: 51–55.

114. Moynahan EJ. Acrodermatitis enteropathica: a lethal inherited human zinc-deficiency disorder. Lancet 1974; 2: 399–400.

115. Lynch WS, Roenigk HH Jr. Acrodermatitis enteropathica. Successful zinc therapy. Arch Dermatol 1976; 112: 1304–1307.

116. Gonzalez JR, Botet MV, Sanchez JL. The histopathology of acrodermatitis enteropathica. Am J Dermatopathol 1982; 4: 303–311.

117. Sjolin K-E. Zinc deficiency syndrome. J Cutan Pathol 1979; 6: 88–89.

118. Brazin SA, Taylor Johnson W, Abramson LJ. The acrodermatitis enteropathica-like syndrome. Arch Dermatol 1979; 115: 597–599.

119. Juljulian HH, Kurban AK. Acantholysis: a feature of acrodermatitis enteropathica. Arch Dermatol 1971; 103: 105–106.

120. Yoshikuni K, Tagami H, Yamada M et al. Erythematosquamous skin lesions in hereditary lactate dehydrogenase M-subunit deficiency. Arch Dermatol 1986; 122: 1420–1424.

121. Ginsburg R, Robertson A Jr, Michel B. Acrodermatitis enteropathica. Arch Dermatol 1976; 112: 653–660.

122. Mallinson CN, Bloom SR, Warin AP et al. A glucagonoma syndrome. Lancet 1974; 2: 1–5.

123. Leichter SB. Clinical and metabolic aspects of glucagonoma. Medicine (Baltimore) 1980; 59: 100–113.

124. Parr JH, Ramsay ID, Keeling PWN et al. Glucagonoma without cutaneous manifestations. Postgrad Med J 1985; 61: 737–738.

125. Hashizume T, Kiryu H, Noda K et al. Glucagonoma syndrome. J Am Acad Dermatol 1988; 19: 377–383.

126. Vandersteen PR, Scheithauer BW. Glucagonoma syndrome. A clinicopathologic immunocytochemical, and ultrastructural study. J Am Acad Dermatol 1985; 12: 1032–1039.

127. Walker NPJ. Atypical necrolytic migratory erythema in association with a jejunal adenocarcinoma. J R Soc Med 1982; 75: 134–135.

128. Doyle JA, Schroeter AL, Rogers RS III. Hyperglucagonaemia and necrolytic migratory erythema in cirrhosis — possible pseudoglucagonoma syndrome. Br J Dermatol 1979; 100: 581–587.

129. Goodenberger DM, Lawley TJ, Strober W et al. Necrolytic migratory erythema without glucagonoma. Report of two cases. Arch Dermatol 1979; 115: 1429–1432.

130. Franchimont C, Piergard GE, Luyckx AS et al. Angioplastic necrolytic migratory erythema. Am J Dermatopathol 1982; 4: 485–495.

131. Wilkinson DS. Necrolytic migratory erythema with pancreatic carcinoma. Proc R Soc Med 1971; 64: 1197–1198.

132. Binnick AN, Spencer SK, Dennison WL Jr, Horton ES. Glucagonoma syndrome. Report of two cases and literature review. Arch Dermatol 1977; 113: 749–754.

133. van der Loos TLJM, Lambrecht ER, Lambers JCCA. Successful treatment of glucagonoma-related necrolytic migratory erythema with decarbazine. J Am Acad Dermatol 1987; 16: 468–472.

134. Sweet RD. A dermatosis specifically associated with a tumour of pancreatic alpha cells. Br J Dermatol 1974; 90: 301–308.

135. Peterson LL, Shaw JC, Acott KM et al. Glucagonoma syndrome: In vitro evidence that glucagon increases epidermal arachidonic acid. J Am Acad Dermatol 1984; 11: 468–473.

136. Kheir SM, Omura EF, Grizzle WE et al. Histologic variation in the skin lesions of the glucagonoma syndrome. Am J Surg Pathol 1986; 10: 445–453.

137. Swenson KH, Amon RB, Hanifin JM. The glucagonoma syndrome. A distinctive cutaneous marker of systemic disease. Arch Dermatol 1978; 114: 224–228.

138. Ackerman AB. Histologic diagnosis of inflammatory skin diseases. Philadelphia: Lea & Febiger, 1978; 512.

139. Parker CM, Hanke CW, Madura JA, Liss EC. Glucagonoma syndrome: case report and literature review. J Dermatol Surg Oncol 1984; 10: 884–889.

140. Kahan RS, Perez-Figaredo RA, Neimanis A. Necrolytic migratory erythema. Distinctive dermatosis of the glucagonoma syndrome. Arch Dermatol 1977; 113: 792–797.

141. Katz R, Fischmann AB, Galotto J et al. Necrolytic migratory erythema, presenting as candidiasis, due to a pancreatic glucagonoma. Cancer 1979; 44: 558–563.

142. Ohyama K, Kitoh M, Arao T. Ultrastructural studies of necrolytic migratory erythema. Arch Dermatol 1982; 118: 679–682.

143. Wong PWK, Pillai PM. Clinical and biochemical observations in two cases of Hartnup disease. Arch Dis Child 1966; 41: 383–388.

144. Ashurst PJ. Hydroa vacciniforme occurring in association with Hartnup disease. Br J Dermatol 1969; 81: 486–492.

145. Fleischmajer R, Hyman AB. Clinical significance of

derangements of tryptophan metabolism. Arch Dermatol 1961; 84: 563–573.

146. Halvorsen K, Halvorsen S. Hartnup disease. Pediatrics 1963; 31: 29–38.

147. Freundlich E, Statter M, Yatziv S. Familial pellagra-like skin rash with neurological manifestations. Arch Dis Child 1981; 56: 146–148.

148. Freij BJ, Der Kaloustian VM. Prolidase deficiency. A metabolic disorder presenting with dermatologic signs. Int J Dermatol 1986; 25: 431–433.

149. Milligan A, Graham-Brown RAC, Burns DA, Anderson I. Prolidase deficiency: a case report and literature review. Br J Dermatol 1989; 121: 405–409.

150. Der Kaloustian VM, Freij BJ, Kurban AK. Prolidase deficiency: an inborn error of metabolism with major dermatological manifestations. Dermatologica 1982; 164: 293–304.

151. Sheffield LJ, Schlesinger P, Faull K et al. Iminopeptiduria, skin ulcerations, and edema in a boy with prolidase deficiency. J Pediatr 1977; 91: 578–583.

152. Leoni A, Cetta G, Tenni R et al. Prolidase deficiency in two siblings with chronic leg ulcerations. Arch Dermatol 1987; 123: 493–499.

153. Arata J, Umemura S, Yamamoto Y et al. Prolidase deficiency. Its dermatological manifestations and some additional biochemical studies. Arch Dermatol 1979; 115: 62–67.

154. Pierard GE, Cornil F, Lapiere CM. Pathogenesis of ulcerations in deficiency of prolidase. The role of angiopathy and of deposits of amyloid. Am J Dermatopathol 1984; 6: 491–497.

155. Ogata A, Tanaka S, Tomoda T et al. Autosomal recessive prolidase deficiency. Three patients with recalcitrant leg ulcers. Arch Dermatol 1981; 117: 689–694.

156. Ferrans VJ, Fredrickson DS. The pathology of Tangier disease. A light and electron microscopic study. Am J Pathol 1975; 78: 101–158.

157. Herbert PN, Forte T, Heinen RJ, Fredrickson DS. Tangier disease. One explanation of lipid storage. N Engl J Med 1978; 299: 519–521.

158. Waldorf DS, Levy RI, Fredrickson DS. Cutaneous cholesterol ester deposition in Tangier disease. Arch Dermatol 1967; 95: 161–165.

159. White JW Jr, Gomez MR. Diagnosis of Lafora disease by skin biopsy. J Cutan Pathol 1988; 15: 171–175.

160. Busard BLSM, Renier WO, Gabreels FJM et al. Lafora's disease. Arch Neurol 1986; 43: 296–299.

161. Carpenter S, Karpati G. Sweat gland duct cells in Lafora disease: Diagnosis by skin biopsy. Neurology 1981; 31: 1564–1568.

162. Paller AS. Cutaneous changes associated with inflammatory bowel disease. Pediatr Dermatol 1986; 3: 439–445.

163. Greenstein AJ, Janowitz HD, Sachar DB. The extra-intestinal complications of Crohn's disease and ulcerative colitis: a study of 700 patients. Medicine (Baltimore) 1976; 55: 401–412.

164. Verbov JL. The skin in patients with Crohn's disease and ulcerative colitis. Trans St John's Hosp Dermatol Soc 1973; 59: 30–36.

165. Basler RSW, Dubin HV. Ulcerative colitis and the skin. Arch Dermatol 1976; 112: 531–534.

166. Stathers GM, Abbott LG, McGuinness AE. Pyoderma gangrenosum in association with regional enteritis. Arch Dermatol 1967; 95: 375–380.

167. Johnson ML, Wilson HTH. Skin lesions in ulcerative colitis. Gut 1969; 10: 255–263.

168. Croft CB, Wilkinson AR. Ulceration of the mouth, pharynx, and larynx in Crohn's disease of the intestine. Br J Surg 1972; 59: 249–252.

169. Yates VM, Watkinson G, Kelman A. Further evidence for an association between psoriasis, Crohn's disease and ulcerative colitis. Br J Dermatol 1982; 106: 323–330.

170. Nevile BW, Laden SA, Smith SE et al. Pyostomatitis vegetans. Am J Dermatopathol 1985; 7: 69–77.

170a. Ballo FS, Camisa C, Allen CM. Pyostomatitis vegetans. Report of a case and review of the literature. J Am Acad Dermatol 1989; 21: 381–387.

171. VanHale HM, Rogers RS III, Zone JJ, Greipp PR. Pyostomatitis vegetans. A reactive mucosal marker for inflammatory disease of the gut. Arch Dermatol 1985; 121: 94–98.

172. Brenner SM, Delany HM. Erythema multiforme and Crohn's disease of the large intestine. Gastroenterology 1972; 62: 479–482.

173. Monroe EW. Vitiligo associated with regional enteritis. Arch Dermatol 1976; 112: 833–834.

174. McPoland PR, Moss RL. Cutaneous Crohn's disease and progressive vitiligo. J Am Acad Dermatol 1988; 19: 421–425.

175. McCallum DI, Kinmont PDC. Dermatological manifestations of Crohn's disease. Br J Dermatol 1968; 80: 1–8.

176. Rankin GB, Watts HD, Melnyk CS, Kelley ML Jr. National Cooperative Crohn's Disease Study: extraintestinal manifestations and perianal complications. Gastroenterology 1979; 77: 914–920.

177. Burgdorf W. Cutaneous manifestations of Crohn's disease. J Am Acad Dermatol 1981; 5: 689–695.

178. Frankel DH, Mostofi RS, Lorincz AL. Oral Crohn's disease: Report of two cases in brothers with metallic dysgeusia and a review of the literature. J Am Acad Dermatol 1985; 12: 260–268.

178a. Walker KD, Badame AJ. Erythema elevatum diutinum in a patient with Crohn's disease. J Am Acad Dermatol 1990; 22: 948–952.

178b. Smoller BR, Weishar M, Gray MH. An unusual cutaneous manifestation of Crohn's disease. Arch Pathol Lab Med 1990; 114: 609–610.

179. Ray TL, Levine JB, Weiss W, Ward PA. Epidermolysis bullosa acquisita and inflammatory bowel disease. J Am Acad Dermatol 1982; 6: 242–252.

180. McAuley D, Miller RA. Acne fulminans associated with inflammatory bowel disease. Report of a case. Arch Dermatol 1985; 121: 91–93.

181. Dyer NH, Dawson AM, Verbov JL et al. Cutaneous polyarteritis nodosa associated with Crohn's disease. Lancet 1970; 1: 648–650.

182. Goslen JB, Graham W, Lazarus GS. Cutaneous polyarteritis nodosa. Report of a case associated with Crohn's disease. Arch Dermatol 1983; 119: 326–329.

183. Chalvardjian A, Nethercott JR. Cutaneous granulomatous vasculitis associated with Crohn's disease. Cutis 1982; 30: 645–655.

184. Levine N, Bangert J. Cutaneous granulomatosis in Crohn's disease. Arch Dermatol 1982; 118: 1006–1009.

185. Witkowski JA, Parish LC, Lewis JE. Crohn's disease

— non-caseating granulomas on the legs. Acta Derm Venereol 1977; 57: 181–183.

186. Lebwohl M, Fleischmajer R, Janowitz H et al. Metastatic Crohn's disease. J Am Acad Dermatol 1984; 10: 33–38.

186a. Shum DT, Guenther L. Metastatic Crohn's disease. Case report and review of the literature. Arch Dermatol 1990; 126: 645–648.

186b. Buckley C, Bayoumi A-HM, Sarkany I. Metastatic Crohn's disease. Clin Exp Dermatol 1990; 15: 131–133.

187. Mountain JC. Cutaneous ulceration in Crohn's disease. Gut 1970; 11: 18–26.

188. McCallum DI, Gray WM. Metastatic Crohn's disease. Br J Dermatol 1976; 95: 551–554.

189. Burgdorf W, Orkin M. Granulomatous perivasculitis in Crohn's disease. Arch Dermatol 1981; 117: 674–675.

190. Callen JP. Severe cutaneous vasculitis complicating ulcerative colitis. Arch Dermatol 1979; 115: 226–227.

191. Basler RSW. Ulcerative colitis and the skin. Med Clin North Am 1980; 64: 941–954.

192. Fenske NA, Gern JE, Pierce D, Vasey FB. Vesiculopustular eruption of ulcerative colitis. Arch Dermatol 1983; 119: 664–669.

193. O'Loughlin S, Perry HO. A diffuse pustular eruption associated with ulcerative colitis. Arch Dermatol 1978; 114: 1061–1064.

194. Comer GM, Brandt LJ, Abissi CJ. Whipple's disease: a review. Am J Gastroenterol 1983; 78: 107–114.

195. Good AE, Beals TF, Simmons JL, Ibrahim MAH. A subcutaneous nodule with Whipple's disease: key to early diagnosis? Arthritis Rheum 1980; 23: 856–859.

196. Kwee D, Fields JP, King LE Jr. Subcutaneous Whipple's disease. J Am Acad Dermatol 1987; 16: 188–190.

197. Haroon TS. Diabetes and skin — a review. Scott Med J 1974; 19: 257–267.

198. Sibbald RG, Schachter RK. The skin and diabetes mellitus. Int J Dermatol 1984; 23: 567–584.

199. Gouterman IH, Sibrack LA. Cutaneous manifestations of diabetes. Cutis 1980; 25: 45–56.

200. Huntley AC. The cutaneous manifestations of diabetes mellitus. J Am Acad Dermatol 1982; 7: 427–455.

201. Hanna W, Friesen D, Bombardier C et al. Pathologic features of diabetic thick skin. J Am Acad Dermatol 1987; 16: 546–553.

202. Huntley AC. Finger pebbles: A common finding in diabetes mellitus. J Am Acad Dermatol 1986; 14: 612–617.

203. Bernstein JE, Levine LE, Medenica MM et al. Reduced threshold to suction-induced blister formation in insulin-dependent diabetics. J Am Acad Dermatol 1983; 8: 790–791.

204. Cox NH, McCruden D, McQueen A et al. Histological findings in clinically normal skin of patients with insulin-dependent diabetes. Clin Exp Dermatol 1987; 12: 250–255.

205. Sueki H. Diabetic microangiopathy in subcutaneous fatty tissue. J Cutan Pathol 1987; 14: 217–222.

206. Cox NH, More IA, McCruden D et al. Electron microscopy of clinically normal skin of diabetic patients. Clin Exp Dermatol 1988; 13: 11–15.

207. Danowski TS, Sabeh G, Sarver ME et al. Skin spots and diabetes mellitus. Am J Med Sci 1966; 251: 570–575.

208. Bauer M, Levan NE. Diabetic dermopathy. Br J Dermatol 1970; 83: 528–535.

209. Binkley GW. Dermopathy in the diabetic syndrome. Arch Dermatol 1965; 92: 625–634.

210. Bauer MF, Levan NE, Frankel A, Bach J. Pigmented pretibial patches. A cutaneous manifestation of diabetes mellitus. Arch Dermatol 1966; 93: 282–286.

211. Fisher ER, Danowski TS. Histologic, histochemical, and electron microscopic features of the skin spots of diabetes mellitus. Am J Clin Pathol 1968; 50: 547–554.

212. Toonstra J. Bullosis diabeticorum. Report of a case with a review of the literature. J Am Acad Dermatol 1985; 13: 799–805.

213. Rocca FF, Pereyra E. Phlyctenar lesions in the feet of diabetic patients. Diabetes 1963; 12: 220–223.

214. Bernstein JE, Medenica M, Soltani K, Griem SF. Bullous eruption of diabetes mellitus. Arch Dermatol 1979; 115: 324–325.

215. Chuang T-Y, Korkij W, Soltani K et al. Increased frequency of diabetes mellitus in patients with bullous pemphigoid: A case-control study. J Am Acad Dermatol 1984; 11: 1099–1102.

216. Paltzik RL. Bullous eruption of diabetes mellitus. Bullosis diabeticorum. Arch Dermatol 1980; 116: 475–476.

217. Cantwell AR Jr, Martz W. Idiopathic bullae in diabetics. Bullosis diabeticorum. Arch Dermatol 1967; 96: 42–44.

218. Allen GE, Hadden DR. Bullous lesions of the skin in diabetics (bullosis diabeticorum). Br J Dermatol 1970; 82: 216–220.

219. James WD, Odom RB, Goette DK. Bullous eruption of diabetes mellitus. A case with positive immunofluorescence microscopy findings. Arch Dermatol 1980; 116: 1191–1192.

220. Kurwa A, Roberts P, Whitehead R. Concurrence of bullous and atrophic skin lesions in diabetes mellitus. Arch Dermatol 1971; 103: 670–675.

221. Goodfield MJD, Millard LG, Harvey L, Jeffcoate WJ. Bullosis diabeticorum. J Am Acad Dermatol 1986; 15: 1292–1294.

222. Bear CL, Wall LM. Idiopathic bullae in diabetics (bullosis diabeticorum). Australas J Dermatol 1969; 10: 33–37.

223. Magnus IA. The porphyrias. Semin Dermatol 1982; 1: 197–210.

224. Elder GH. Enzymatic defects in porphyria: an overview. Semin Liver Dis 1982; 2: 87–99.

224a. Elder GH. The cutaneous porphyrias. Semin Dermatol 1990; 9: 63–69.

225. Moore MR, Disler PB. Chemistry and biochemistry of the porphyrins and porphyrias. Clin Dermatol 1985; 3: 7–23.

226. Elder GH. Recent advances in the identification of enzyme deficiencies in the porphyrias. Br J Dermatol 1983; 108: 729–734.

227. Elder GH. Metabolic abnormalities in the porphyrias. Semin Dermatol 1986; 5: 88–98.

228. Thiers BH. The porphyrias. J Am Acad Dermatol 1981; 5: 621–625.

229. Targovnik SE, Targovnik JH. Cutaneous drug reactions in porphyrias. Clin Dermatol 1986; 4: 110–117.

230. Harber LC, Poh-Fitzpatrick M, Walther RR, Grossman ME. Cutaneous aspects of the porphyrias. Acta Derm Venereol (Suppl) 1982; 100: 9–15.
231. Poh-Fitzpatrick MB. Porphyrin-sensitized cutaneous photosensitivity. Pathogenesis and treatment. Clin Dermatol 1985; 3: 41–82.
232. Hunter GA. Clinical manifestations of the porphyrias: a review. Australas J Dermatol 1979; 20: 120–122.
233. Poh-Fitzpatrick MB. Pathogenesis and treatment of photocutaneous manifestations of the porphyrias. Semin Liver Dis 1982; 2: 164–176.
234. Batlle AM del C. Tetrapyrrole biosynthesis. Semin Dermatol 1986; 5: 70–87.
235. Mustajoki P. Acute intermittent porphyria. Semin Dermatol 1986; 5: 155–160.
236. Doss M. Enzymatic deficiencies in acute hepatic porphyrias: porphobilinogen synthase deficiency. Semin Dermatol 1986; 5: 161–168.
237. Roberts DT, Brodie MJ, Moore MR et al. Hereditary coproporphyria presenting with photosensitivity induced by the contraceptive pill. Br J Dermatol 1977; 96: 549–554.
238. Hunter JAA, Khan SA, Hope E et al. Hereditary coproporphyria. Photosensitivity, jaundice and neuropsychiatric manifestations associated with pregnancy. Br J Dermatol 1971; 84: 301–310.
239. Day RS. Variegate porphyria. Semin Dermatol 1986; 5: 138–154.
240. Corey TJ, DeLeo VA, Christianson H, Poh-Fitzpatrick MB. Variegate porphyria. Clinical and laboratory features. J Am Acad Dermatol 1980; 2: 36–43.
241. Quiroz-Kendall E, Wilson FA, King LE Jr. Acute variegate porphyria following a Scarsdale Gourmet Diet. J Am Acad Dermatol 1983; 8: 46–49.
242. Tidman MJ, Higgins EM, Elder GH, MacDonald DM. Variegate porphyria associated with hepatocellular carcinoma. Br J Dermatol 1989; 121: 503–505.
243. Poh-Fitzpatrick MB. A plasma porphyrin fluorescence marker for variegate porphyria. Arch Dermatol 1980; 116: 543–547.
244. Norris PG, Elder GH, Hawk JLM. Homozygous variegate porphyria: a case report. Br J Dermatol 1990; 122: 253–257.
245. Nordmann Y, Deybach JC. Congenital erythropoietic porphyria. Semin Liver Dis 1982; 2: 154–163.
246. Horiguchi Y, Horio T, Yamamoto M et al. Late onset erythropoietic porphyria. Br J Dermatol 1989; 121: 255–262.
247. Murphy GM, Hawk JLM, Nicholson DC, Magnus IA. Congenital erythropoietic porphyria (Günther's disease). Clin Exp Dermatol 1987; 12: 61–65.
248. Nordmann Y, Deybach JC. Congenital erythropoietic porphyria. Semin Dermatol 1986; 5: 106–114.
249. Kaufman BM, Vickers HR, Rayne J, Ryan TJ. Congenital erythropoietic porphyria. Br J Dermatol 1966; 79: 210–220.
250. Bhutani LK, Sood SK, Das PK et al. Congenital erythropoietic porphyria. An autopsy report. Arch Dermatol 1974; 110: 427–431.
251. Stretcher GS. Erythropoietic porphyria. Two cases and the results of metabolic alkalinization. Arch Dermatol 1977; 113: 1553–1557.
252. Bloomer JR. Protoporphyria. Semin Liver Dis 1982; 2: 143–153.
253. Milligan A, Graham-Brown RAC, Sarkany I, Baker H. Erythropoietic protoporphyria exacerbated by oral iron therapy. Br J Dermatol 1988; 119: 63–66.
254. Poh-Fitzpatrick MB. Erythropoietic protoporphyria. Int J Dermatol 1978; 17: 359–369.
255. Poh-Fitzpatrick MB. Erythropoietic protoporphyria. Semin Dermatol 1986; 5: 99–105.
256. Murphy GM, Hawk JLM, Magnus IA. Late-onset erythropoietic protoporphyria with unusual cutaneous features. Arch Dermatol 1985; 121: 1309–1312.
257. MacDonald DM, Germain D, Perrot H. The histopathology and ultrastructure of liver disease in erythropoietic protoporphyria. Br J Dermatol 1981; 104: 7–17.
258. Romslo I, Gadeholt HG, Hovding G. Erythropoietic protoporphyria terminating in liver failure. Arch Dermatol 1982; 118: 668–671.
259. Wells MM, Golitz LE, Bender BJ. Erythropoietic protoporphyria with hepatic cirrhosis. Arch Dermatol 1980; 116: 429–432.
260. Schmidt H, Snitker G, Thomsen K, Lintrup J. Erythropoietic protoporphyria. A clinical study based on 29 cases in 14 families. Arch Dermatol 1974; 110: 58–64.
261. Redeker AG, Bronow RS. Erythropoietic protoporphyria presenting as hydroa aestivale. Arch Dermatol 1964; 89: 104–109.
262. Christopher AP, Grattan CEH, Cowan MA. Pseudoainhum and erythropoietic protoporphyria. Br J Dermatol 1988; 118: 113–116.
263. O'Reilly K, Snape J, Moore MR. Porphyria cutanea tarda resulting from primary hepatocellular carcinoma. Clin Exp Dermatol 1988; 13: 44–48.
264. Mascaro JM, Herrero C, Lecha M, Muniesa AM. Uroporphyrinogen-decarboxylase deficiencies: porphyria cutanea tarda and related conditions. Semin Dermatol 1986; 5: 115–124.
265. Pimstone NR. Porphyria cutanea tarda. Semin Liver Dis 1982; 2: 132–142.
266. Keczkes K, Barker DJ. Malignant hepatoma associated with acquired hepatic cutaneous porphyria. Arch Dermatol 1976; 112: 78–82.
267. Lichtenstein JR, Babb EJ, Felsher BF. Porphyria cutanea tarda (PCT) in a patient with chronic renal failure on haemodialysis. Br J Dermatol 1981; 104: 575–578.
268. Held JL, Sassa S, Kappas A, Harber LC. Erythrocyte uroporphyrinogen decarboxylase activity in porphyria cutanea tarda: a study of 40 consecutive patients. J Invest Dermatol 1989; 93: 332–334.
269. Malina L, Lim CK. Manifestation of familial porphyria cutanea tarda after childbirth. Br J Dermatol 1988; 118: 243–245.
270. Grossman ME, Bickers DR, Poh-Fitzpatrick MB et al. Porphyria cutanea tarda. Clinical features and laboratory findings in 40 patients. Am J Med 1979; 67: 277–286.
271. Topi GC, Amantea A, Griso D. Recovery from porphyria cutanea tarda with no specific therapy other than avoidance of hepatic toxins. Br J Dermatol 1984; 111: 75–82.
272. Roenigk HH Jr, Gottlob ME. Estrogen-induced porphyria cutanea tarda. Report of three cases. Arch Dermatol 1970; 102: 260–266.
273. Malina L, Chlumsky J. Oestrogen-induced familial

porphyria cutanea tarda. Br J Dermatol 1975; 92: 707–709.

274. Chesney T McC, Wardlaw LL, Kaplan RJ, Chow JF. Porphyria cutanea tarda complicating Wilson's disease. J Am Acad Dermatol 1981; 4: 64–66.

275. Maughan WZ, Muller SA, Perry HO. Porphyria cutanea tarda associated with lymphoma. Acta Derm Venereol 1979; 59: 55–58.

276. Hogan D, Card RT, Ghadially R et al. Human immunodeficiency virus infection and porphyria cutanea tarda. J Am Acad Dermatol 1989; 20: 17–20.

277. Fivenson DP, King AJ. Porphyria cutanea tarda in a patient with agnogenic myeloid metaplasia. Arch Dermatol 1984; 120: 538–539.

278. Callen JP, Ross L. Subacute cutaneous lupus erythematosus and porphyria cutanea tarda. Report of a case. J Am Acad Dermatol 1981; 5: 269–273.

279. Clemmensen O, Thomsen K. Porphyria cutanea tarda and systemic lupus erythematosus. Arch Dermatol 1982; 118: 160–162.

280. Cram DL, Epstein JH, Tuffanelli DL. Lupus erythematosus and porphyria. Coexistence in seven patients. Arch Dermatol 1973; 108: 779–784.

281. Crips DJ, Peters HA, Gocmen A, Dogramici I. Porphyria turcica due to hexachlorobenzene: a 20 to 30 year follow-up study on 204 patients. Br J Dermatol 1984; 111: 413–422.

282. Muhlbauer JE, Pathak MA. Porphyria cutanea tarda. Int J Dermatol 1979; 18: 767–780.

283. Kranz KR, Reed OM, Grimwood RE. Necrotizing fasciitis associated with porphyria cutanea tarda. J Am Acad Dermatol 1986; 14: 361–367.

284. Friedman SJ, Doyle JA. Sclerodermoid changes of porphyria cutanea tarda: Possible relationship to urinary uroporphyrin levels. J Am Acad Dermatol 1985; 13: 70–74.

285. Lim HW, Poh-Fitzpatrick MB. Hepatoerythropoietic porphyria: A variant of childhood-onset porphyria cutanea tarda. Porphyrin profiles and enzymatic studies of two cases in a family. J Am Acad Dermatol 1984; 11: 1103–1111.

286. Smith SG. Hepatoerythropoietic porphyria. Semin Dermatol 1986; 5: 125–137.

287. Koszo F, Elder GH, Roberts A, Simon N. Uroporphyrinogen decarboxylase deficiency in hepatoerythropoietic porphyria: further evidence for genetic heterogeneity. Br J Dermatol 1990; 122: 365–370.

288. Simon N, Berko GY, Schneider I. Hepato-erythropoietic porphyria presenting as scleroderma and acrosclerosis in a sibling pair. Br J Dermatol 1977; 96: 663–668.

289. Bundino S, Topi GC, Zina AM, D'Alessandro Gandolfo L. Hepatoerythropoietic porphyria. Pediatr Dermatol 1987; 4: 229–233.

290. Day RS, Strauss PC. Severe cutaneous porphyria in a 12-year-old boy. Hepatoerythropoietic or symptomatic porphyria? Arch Dermatol 1982; 118: 663–667.

291. Czarnecki DB. Hepatoerythropoietic porphyria. Arch Dermatol 1980; 116: 307–311.

292. Harber LC, Bickers DR. Porphyria and pseudoporphyria. J Invest Dermatol 1984; 82: 207–209.

293. Poh-Fitzpatrick MB. Porphyria, pseudoporphyria, pseudopseudoporphyria ...? Arch Dermatol 1986; 122: 403–404.

294. Hawk JLM. Skin changes resembling hepatic cutanea porphyria induced by oxytetracycline photosensitization. Clin Exp Dermatol 1980; 5: 321–325.

295. Epstein JH, Tuffanelli DL, Siebert JS, Epstein WL. Porphyria-like cutaneous changes induced by tetracycline hydrochloride photosensitization. Arch Dermatol 1976; 112: 661–666.

296. Burry JN, Lawrence JR. Phototoxic blisters from high frusemide dosage. Br J Dermatol 1976; 94: 495–499.

297. Ramsay CA, Obreshkova E. Photosensitivity from nalidixic acid. Br J Dermatol 1974; 91: 523–528.

298. Judd LE, Henderson DW, Hill DC. Naproxen-induced pseudoporphyria. A clinical and ultrastructural study. Arch Dermatol 1986; 122: 451–454.

299. Burns DA. Naproxen pseudoporphyria in a patient with vitiligo. Clin Exp Dermatol 1987; 12: 296–297.

300. Rivers JK, Barnetson R St C. Naproxen-induced bullous photodermatitis. Med J Aust 1989; 151: 167–168.

301. Baer RL, Stillman MA. Cutaneous skin changes probably due to pyridoxine abuse. J Am Acad Dermatol 1984; 10: 527–528.

302. Baker EJ, Reed KD, Dixon SL. Chlorthalidone-induced pseudoporphyria: Clinical and microscopic findings of a case. J Am Acad Dermatol 1989; 21: 1026–1029.

303. McDonagh AJG, Harrington CI. Pseudoporphyria complicating etretinate therapy. Clin Exp Dermatol 1989; 14: 437–438.

304. Murphy GM, Wright J, Nicholls DSH et al. Sunbed-induced pseudoporphyria. Br J Dermatol 1989; 120: 555–562.

305. Poh-Fitzpatrick MB, Ellis DL. Porphyrialike bullous dermatosis after chronic intense tanning bed and/or sunlight exposure. Arch Dermatol 1989; 125: 1236–1238.

306. Poh-Fitzpatrick MB, Masullo AS, Grossman ME. Porphyria cutanea tarda associated with chronic renal disease and hemodialysis. Arch Dermatol 1980; 116: 191–195.

307. Shelley WB, Shelley ED. Blisters of the fingertips: A variant of bullous dermatosis of hemodialysis. J Am Acad Dermatol 1989; 21: 1049–1051.

308. Rotstein H. Photosensitive bullous eruption associated with chronic renal failure. Australas J Dermatol 1978; 19: 58–64.

309. Keczkes K, Farr M. Bullous dermatosis of chronic renal failure. Br J Dermatol 1976; 95: 541–546.

310. Epstein JH, Tuffanelli DL, Epstein WL. Cutaneous changes in the porphyrias. A microscopic study. Arch Dermatol 1973; 107: 689–698.

311. Wolff K, Honigsmann H, Rauschmeier W et al. Microscopic and fine structural aspects of porphyrias. Acta Derm Venereol (Suppl) 1982; 100: 17–28.

312. van der Walt JJ, Heyl T. Lipoid proteinosis and erythropoietic protoporphyria. A histological and histochemical study. Arch Dermatol 1971; 104: 501–507.

313. Peterka ES, Fusaro RM, Goltz RW. Erythropoietic protoporphyria. II. Histological and histochemical studies of cutaneous lesions. Arch Dermatol 1965; 92: 357–361.

314. Cormane RH, Szabo E, Hoo TT. Histopathology of the skin in acquired and hereditary porphyria cutanea tarda. Br J Dermatol 1971; 85: 531–539.

315. Grossman ME, Poh-Fitzpatrick MB. Porphyria cutanea tarda. Diagnosis and management. Med Clin North Am 1980; 64: 807–827.

316. Ahmed AR. Diagnosis of bullous disease and studies in the pathogenesis of blister formation using immunopathological techniques. J Cutan Pathol 1984; 11: 237–248.

317. Parra CA, Pizzi de Parra N. Diameter of the collagen fibrils in the sclerodermatous skin of porphyria cutanea tarda. Br J Dermatol 1979; 100: 573–578.

318. Caputo R, Berti E, Gasparini G, Monti M. The morphologic events of blister formation in porphyria cutanea tarda. Int J Dermatol 1983; 22: 467–472.

319 Schnait FG, Wolff K, Konrad K. Erythropoietic protoporphyria — submicroscopic events during the acute photosensitivity flare. Br J Dermatol 1975; 92: 545–557.

320. Baart de la Faille H. Erythropoietic protoporphyria. A photodermatosis. Utrecht: Oosthoek, Scheltema and Holkema, 1975.

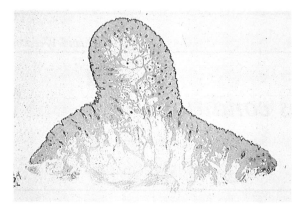

Fig. 19.1 Accessory tragus. In this case there is adipose tissue but no cartilage in the core.
Haematoxylin — eosin

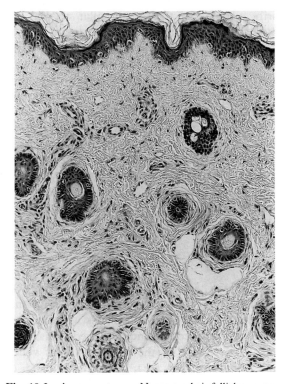

Fig. 19.2 Accessory tragus. Numerous hair follicles, some of vellus type, are present. Sebaceous glands are not developed.
Haematoxylin — eosin

least their presence is not mentioned in the reports.

The rare condition described as dermatorynchus geneae is a related first arch abnor-mality in which large amounts of striated muscle, and sometimes bone, form the central core of the elongated polypoid lesion.[8] The lesions reported as striated muscle hamartomas are closely related[9] morphologically; they were not in the preauricular region (see p. 919).

SUPERNUMERARY NIPPLE

Polythelia, as the presence of supernumerary nipples is sometimes called, is a developmental abnormality found in approximately 1% of the population.[10] There is a predilection for females. The supernumerary structure is usually a solitary, asymptomatic, slightly pigmented, nodular lesion, often with a small, central, nipple-like elevation. It may occur anywhere along the pathway of the embryonic milk line, particularly on the anterior aspect of the chest or the upper abdomen. Rarely, it is outside this line.[11,12] Clinically, it resembles a naevus or fibroma. There is an increased incidence of renal abnor-malities in patients with a supernumerary nipple.[13]

Histopathology[10]

The appearances resemble those seen in the normal nipple and include epidermal thickening with mild papillomatosis and basal hyper-pigmentation, the presence of pilosebaceous structures, variable amounts of smooth muscle, and mammary ducts, which open into pilo-sebaceous ducts or enter the epidermis. There may be underlying breast tissue, but complete supernumerary breasts are very rare.[13]

CHEILITIS GLANDULARIS

Cheilitis glandularis appears to be a hetero-geneous entity, which has been attributed in the past to hyperplasia of labial salivary glands.[14–16] However, a critical review of reported cases does not support this explanation[17] except in a few cases.[18] It has been suggested that the condition includes cases of factitious cheilitis,[19–21] pre-mature and exaggerated actinic cheilitis, and cases with a coexisting atopic diathesis in which mouth breathing may play a role.[17] It should be noted that only mild swelling of the lip is needed to produce eversion, which in itself exaggerates the appearance of swelling.[17]

The patients present with macrocheilia, usually confined to the lower lip. There is often crusting and fissuring with a mucoid discharge. Salivary duct orifices may be prominent. Clinically, the lesions need to be distinguished from plasma cell cheilitis,[22] cheilitis granulomatosa (Melkersson–Rosenthal syndrome) — (see p. 200) and Ascher's syndrome, in which there is acute swelling of the lips and eyelids (usually the upper) resulting from oedema, inflammation and a possible increase in size of labial and lacrimal glands respectively.[15]

Squamous cell carcinoma may sometimes supervene, further evidence that many cases have an actinic aetiology.[14,16]

Histopathology

There is usually hyperkeratosis, focal parakeratosis and sometimes inflammatory crusting. There is underlying oedema, variable but usually mild chronic inflammation, and variable solar elastosis.[17] Although the minor salivary glands are usually said to be hyperplastic, a recent study showed no increase in their size or appearance when compared to controls. Notwithstanding, enlargement of salivary glands with dilated ducts and some chronic inflammation has been present in some cases reported as cheilitis glandularis.[18]

UMBILICAL LESIONS

The umbilicus is an important embryological structure, into which the vitelline (omphalomesenteric) duct and urachus enter. Remnants of either structure may give rise to lesions at the umbilicus and, rarely, vestiges of both may coexist.[23]

The omphalomesenteric duct normally becomes obliterated early in embryonic life, but remnants may persist, producing an enteric fistula, an umbilical sinus, a subcutaneous cyst

or an umbilical polyp.[24] The latter presents as a bright red polyp or fleshy nodule, 0.5 – 2 cm in diameter;[25] it may discharge a mucoid secretion.

Urachal anomalies usually present at, or shortly after, birth.[23] A patent urachus will result in the passage of urine from the umbilicus. Urachal sinuses and deeper cysts result from partial obliteration of the urachus, with small persistent areas.

Other lesions presenting at the umbilicus include endometriosis (see p. 494), primary and secondary tumours (see p. 983),[26] and inflammatory granulomas.[27] The granulomas result from inflammatory changes associated with persistent epithelialized tracts, or simply from accumulation of debris in a deep umbilicus with resulting ulceration and inflammation.[23] Sometimes a pilonidal sinus is present.[28]

Histopathology

Umbilical (omphalomesenteric duct) polyps are covered by epithelium which is usually of small bowel or colonic type, but occasionally of gastric type. Ectopic pancreatic tissue has also been described.[24] There is usually an abrupt transition from epidermis to the intestinal or gastric type of epithelium. Urachal remnants are lined by transitional epithelium;[23] sometimes smooth muscle bundles are present in their wall. There may be a mild inflammatory cell infiltrate both in umbilical polyps and in urachal remnants.

Umbilical granulomas show variable inflammatory changes ranging from abscess formation to granulomatous areas.[23] Sometimes hair shafts or debris are present with associated foreign body giant cells. There is variable fibrosis.

Primary tumours of the umbilicus may take the form of adenocarcinoma, sarcoma, melanoma, squamous cell carcinoma or, rarely, basal cell carcinoma.[26] Rarely, umbilical adenocarcinomas assume a papillary pattern with psammoma bodies.[29]

RELAPSING POLYCHONDRITIS

Relapsing polychondritis is a rare disorder of unknown aetiology manifesting recurrent inflammation of the cartilaginous tissues of different organs, particularly the ear, but also the nasal septum and tracheobronchial cartilage.[30-33] A frequent presentation is with tenderness and reddening of one or both ears.[34] Onset is usually in middle age. Other manifestations include polyarthritis, ocular inflammation, audio-vestibular damage, cardiac lesions and a vasculitis.[30,35,36] A few patients have been reported with polychondritis and psoriasis.[37] The course of the disease is variable, but there is usually progressive destruction of cartilage, with consequent deformities. Death ensues in up to 25% of patients as a result of respiratory and cardiovascular complications.

There are pointers to an immunological pathogenesis. These include the detection of cell-mediated immunity to cartilage, the presence of antibodies to type II collagen[38] and the demonstration by direct immunofluorescence of immunoglobulins and C3 in the chondrofibrous junction and around chondrocytes.[39]

Colchicine,[40] dapsone[41,42] and corticosteroids have been used in the management.

Histopathology[30]

The initial changes are a decrease in the basophilia of the involved cartilage, degeneration of marginal chondrocytes which become vacuolated with pyknotic nuclei, and a florid perichondritis with obscuring of the chondrofibrous interface. The inflammatory cell infiltrate initially contains many neutrophils, but progressively there are more lymphocytes, plasma cells and histiocytes in the infiltrate, with occasional eosinophils. With time there is derangement of the cartilaginous matrix and replacement by fibrous tissue. Calcification and even metaplastic bone may develop in the late stages when only a scattering of chronic inflammatory cells remains.

Electron microscopy. There are a large number of dense granules and vesicles, compatible with matrix vesicles or lysosomes, surrounding the affected chondrocytes.[43]

ACANTHOSIS NIGRICANS

Acanthosis nigricans is a cutaneous manifestation of a diverse group of diseases which includes internal cancers, and various endocrine and congenital syndromes.[44,45] It may occur as an inherited disorder. It may also be related to the ingestion of certain drugs. In all these circumstances, acanthosis nigricans presents as symmetrical, pigmented, velvety plaques and verrucous excrescences confined usually to the flexural areas of the body, particularly the axillae.[44,45] It may also involve the back of the neck, and the periumbilical and anogenital regions. Rarely, there is generalized involvement of the skin.[46] The oral mucosa, particularly of the lips and tongue, is affected also in 25% or more of cases.[47] Hyperkeratotic lesions may develop on the palms, soles and knuckles.[48,49]

The *paraneoplastic type* of acanthosis nigricans is a rare manifestation of an internal cancer, usually an adenocarcinoma of the stomach or other part of the alimentary tract.[50-52] Lymphomas[53] and squamous cell carcinomas[54] are occasionally associated. Acanthosis nigricans may precede or follow the diagnosis of the cancer but in most instances the two are diagnosed simultaneously.[51,55] There are some reports of the reversibility of the skin lesions upon removal or treatment of the accompanying malignant disease.[51,55]

The various *endocrine disorders* and *congenital syndromes* which may be complicated by acanthosis nigricans appear to have in common a resistance of the tissues to the action of insulin.[56-62] This is so in the case of lipoatrophy,[63-66] the Prader–Willi syndrome,[67] leprechaunism,[64] pineal hyperplasia and the type A and B insulin resistance symptoms.[56,57,68] A combination of acanthosis nigricans and insulin resistance is found in approximately 5% of hyperandrogenic females, often in association with polycystic ovaries.[57,60,69]

Onset of the rare *familial cases* is in early childhood.[70] There may be accentuation of symptoms at puberty. This variant is inherited as an autosomal dominant trait, although there may be variable phenotypic expression.[70]

Drugs which have been incriminated in the

causation of acanthosis nigricans include corticosteroids,[71] nicotinic acid (niacin),[72] oral contraceptives, stilboestrol (diethylstilboestrol), the folic-acid antagonist triazemate,[73] and methyltestosterone.[74]

Although the molecular basis of acanthosis nigricans remains an enigma, the disease appears to represent an abnormal epidermal proliferation in response to various factors.[66] In the case of the paraneoplastic group, the factor may be a tumour-produced peptide, while in the group related to tissue insulin resistance, the tissue growth factors may include insulin itself, which may be increased in some of these conditions.[60,66]

Histopathology

There is hyperkeratosis, papillomatosis and mild acanthosis (Fig. 19.3).[45] The papillomatosis results from the upward projection of finger-like dermal papillae which are covered by thinned epidermis.[47] In the 'valleys' between these papillary projections the epithelium shows mild acanthosis with overlying hyperkeratosis.[47] There may be some hyperpigmentation of the basal layer, but it should be noted that the pigmentation of the lesions noted clinically results largely from the hyperkeratosis. In some instances, there is hypertrophy of all layers of the epidermis, and the pattern resembles that seen in

epidermal naevi. A resemblance to seborrhoeic keratoses has been noted in some cases. There is usually no dermal inflammation.

Oral lesions differ from the cutaneous ones by showing marked thickening of the epithelium with papillary hyperplasia and acanthosis.[47] There is a superficial resemblance to the lesions of condyloma acuminatum. There is usually mild chronic inflammation in the submucosal tissues.[47]

Finally, it is worth noting that a pattern resembling acanthosis nigricans has been reported at the site of repeated insulin injections.[75]

CONFLUENT AND RETICULATED PAPILLOMATOSIS

Confluent and reticulated papillomatosis (Gougerot and Carteaud) is a rare form of papillomatosis characterized by the development of asymptomatic, small red to brown, slightly verrucous papules with a tendency to central confluence and a reticulate pattern peripherally.[76,77] It involves particularly the upper part of the chest, and the intermammary region and back; the neck, chin, upper parts of the arms and the axillae may also be involved. It has been regarded as a variant of acanthosis nigricans, as a genodermatosis, as an unusual response to ultraviolet light[78] or to *Pityrosporum orbiculare* infection,[79–81] and a result of some unidentified endocrine imbalance.[76,82] Familial occurrence has been reported.[83]

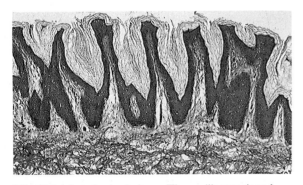

Fig. 19.3 Acanthosis nigricans. The papillomatosis and intervening 'valleys' are conspicuous in this case. Haematoxylin — eosin

Histopathology[76]

The epidermis is undulating with hyperkeratosis, low papillomatosis, and some acanthotic downgrowths from the bases of the 'valleys' between the papillomatous areas (Fig. 19.4). There may also be mild basal hyperpigmentation and focal atrophy of the malpighian layer. These changes resemble acanthosis nigricans,[84] although they are not usually as well developed as in this condition.

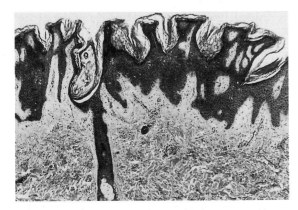

Fig. 19.4 Confluent and reticulated papillomatosis. The epidermis is undulating with papillomatosis and acanthosis. Haematoxylin — eosin

ACROKERATOSIS PARANEOPLASTICA

Acrokeratosis paraneoplastica (Bazex's syndrome) is a skin condition associated with cancers which are usually supradiaphragmatic[85,86] in origin, although tumours at other sites have also been incriminated.[87] It commences with violaceous erythema and psoriasiform scaling on the fingers and toes with later extension to the ears and nose.[88] Violaceous keratoderma of the hands and feet develops and ill-defined psoriasiform lesions eventually form at other sites on the arms and legs.[86] These changes in the skin usually precede the onset of symptoms related to the associated cancer.[89]

Histopathology[89]

The changes are somewhat variable and not diagnostically specific. There is hyperkeratosis, focal parakeratosis and acanthosis. Variable epidermal changes include spongiosis with associated exocytosis of lymphocytes, basal vacuolar change and scattered degenerate keratinocytes.[85,86] There is a mild perivascular lymphocytic infiltrate in the papillary dermis. Fibrinoid degeneration of small vessels and scattered 'pyknotic' neutrophils have been described in some reports, but specifically excluded in others.[85,89,90]

ERYTHRODERMA

Erythroderma (exfoliative dermatitis) is a cutaneous reaction pattern that can occur in a wide variety of benign and malignant diseases.[91,92] It is uncommon, with an incidence of 1–2 per 100 000 of the population.[91] Clinically, it is characterized by erythema and exfoliation which involve all or most of the skin surface.[92] Distressing pruritus is often present.[91] Other clinical features include fever, malaise, keratoderma, alopecia and a mild, generalized lymphadenopathy. Laboratory findings include blood eosinophilia, elevated levels of IgE and, in some, a polyclonal gammopathy.[91,93] The mean age of onset is approximately 60 years, although cases in infancy, often associated with ichthyosiform dermatoses (see p. 269), have been reported.[94,95] There is a male predominance, particularly in the idiopathic group (see below).

Erythroderma is most often seen as an exacerbation of a pre-existing dermatological condition but it may also be drug-related, or be associated with cutaneous T-cell lymphoma or some other malignant tumours. Approximately 15–30% of cases are idiopathic.

A *pre-existing dermatosis* is present in approximately one third of all cases. Psoriasis is the most common of these.[96] Various factors, including the use of systemic steroid therapy, have been incriminated in precipitating an erythrodermic crisis in psoriasis.[96] Other underlying dermatoses include atopic dermatitis, seborrhoeic dermatitis, contact allergic dermatitis, photosensitivity syndromes, pityriasis rubra pilaris and, rarely, stasis dermatitis, pemphigus foliaceus and even bullous pemphigoid.[97,98]

Drug-induced cases may follow topical sensitization to neomycin, ethylenediamine or vioform.[99] Usually it follows the *ingestion* of a drug such as phenytoin, penicillin, isoniazid, trimethoprim and sulphonamides, antimalarials,[100] thiazide diuretics, gold, chlorpromazine, nifedipine[101] or allopurinol.[97,102] There are a few case reports of erythroderma following the use of certain non-steroidal anti-inflammatory drugs such as sulindac, meclofenamate sodium and phenylbutazone.[103] Drug-related cases usually have a rapid onset and relatively quick resolution over 2–6 weeks, in contrast to the more prolonged course of the idiopathic and lymphoma-related cases.[97]

Approximately 20% of cases are associated with a *cutaneous T-cell lymphoma*, in the form of the Sézary syndrome or erythrodermic mycosis fungoides.[104] The erythroderma may precede or occur concurrently with the diagnosis of the cancer.[92,105] Uncommonly, erythroderma is associated with an extracutaneous lymphoma or some other tumour.[106]

The *idiopathic group*, also known as 'the red man syndrome' is associated more often with keratoderma and dermatopathic lymphadenitis than the other groups.[107] It is also more likely to persist than some of the other types. Some cases may progress to mycosis fungoides after many years.[107]

The pathogenetic mechanisms involved in erythroderma are not known. The erythema results from vascular dilatation and proliferation and it has been suggested that inter-reactions between lymphocytes and endothelium may play a role.[108]

Histopathology[109]

Skin biopsies in erythroderma have been regarded as 'largely unrewarding',[102] 'of variable usefulness',[97] 'of little value'[110] and 'misleading'.[110] However, in one series, an aetiological diagnosis was made on the skin biopsy in 43% of cases.[97] Biopsies are most often diagnostic in erythroderma associated with cutaneous T-cell lymphoma. In cases related to an underlying dermatosis, the nature of this is not always discernible in the erythrodermic phase.[109]

Usually, there is variable parakeratosis and hypogranulosis. The epidermis shows moderate acanthosis and, at times, there is psoriasiform hyperplasia, but this finding does not always correlate with the presence of underlying psoriasis.[110] Mild spongiosis is quite common. Blood vessels in the upper dermis are usually dilated and sometimes there is endothelial swelling.[109]

There is a moderately heavy chronic inflammatory cell infiltrate in the upper dermis: this is sometimes perivascular in distribution and at other times more diffuse.[111] Atypical cells with cerebriform nuclei are present in the infiltrate in cases of erythroderma related to cutaneous T-cell lymphomas. Eosinophils may be present in the infiltrate and occasionally they are plentiful.[112] Exocytosis of lymphocytes is a frequent finding.

Drug-related cases may sometimes simulate the picture of mycosis fungoides, with prominent exocytosis and scattered atypical cells with cerebriform nuclei in the infiltrate.[109,112] However, in contrast to mycosis fungoides, Pautrier microabscesses are not present in the benign erythrodermas. Eosinophils are not always present in drug-related cases, as might be expected.[112] A very occasional apoptotic keratinocyte may be a clue to the drug aetiology. Rarely, the picture is frankly lichenoid in type.[101]

Electron microscopy. One study showed a close association between lymphocytes and endothelial cells, although the significance of this finding remains to be evaluated.[108] Some lymphocytes were described as showing 'blastoid'-transformation.[108]

REFERENCES

1. Brownstein MH, Wanger N, Helwig EB. Accessory tragi. Arch Dermatol 1971; 104: 625–631.
2. Sebben JE. The accessory tragus — no ordinary skin tag. J Dermatol Surg Oncol 1989; 15: 304–307.
3. Hsueh S, Santa Cruz DJ. Cartilaginous lesions of the skin and superficial soft tissue. J Cutan Pathol 1982; 9: 405–416.
4. Sperling LC. Congenital cartilaginous rests of the neck. Int J Dermatol 1986; 25: 186–187.
5. Hogan D, Wilkinson RD, Williams A. Congenital anomalies of the head and neck. Int J Dermatol 1980; 19: 479–486.
6. Clarke JA. Are wattles of auricular or branchial origin? Br J Plast Surg 1976; 29: 238–244.

patients. J Am Acad Dermatol 1989; 21: 985–991.

97. King LE Jr, Dufresne RG Jr, Lovett GL, Rosin MA. Erythroderma: review of 82 cases. South Med J 1986; 79: 1210–1215.

98. Tappeiner G, Konrad K, Holubar K. Erythrodermic bullous pemphigoid. Report of a case. J Am Acad Dermatol 1982; 6: 489–492.

99. Petrozzi JW, Shore RN. Generalized exfoliative dermatitis from ethylenediamine. Sensitization and induction. Arch Dermatol 1976; 112: 525–526.

100. Slagel GA, James WD. Plaquenil-induced erythroderma. J Am Acad Dermatol 1985; 12: 857–862.

101. Reynolds NJ, Jones SK, Crossley J, Harman RRM. Exfoliative dermatitis due to nifedipine. Br J Dermatol 1989; 121: 401–404.

102. Sehgal VN, Srivastava G. Exfoliative dermatitis. A prospective study of 80 patients. Dermatologica 1986; 173: 278–284.

103. Bigby M, Stern R. Cutaneous reactions to nonsteroidal anti-inflammatory drugs. A review. J Am Acad Dermatol 1985; 12: 866–876.

104. Duangurai K, Piamphongsant T, Himmungnan T. Sézary cell count in exfoliative dermatitis. Int J Dermatol 1988; 27: 248–252.

105. Winkelmann RK, Buecher SA, Diaz-Perez JL. Pre-Sézary syndrome. J Am Acad Dermatol 1984; 10: 992–999.

106. Leong ASY, Cowled PA, Zalewski PD et al. Erythroderma, an unusual manifestation of B cell lymphoma. Br J Dermatol 1978; 99: 99–106.

107. Thestrup-Pedersen K, Halkier-Sorensen L, Sogaard H, Zachariae H. The red man syndrome. Exfoliative dermatitis of unknown etiology: A description and follow-up of 38 patients. J Am Acad Dermatol 1988; 18: 1307–1312.

108. Heng MCY, Heng CY, Kloss SG, Chase DG. Erythroderma associated with mixed lymphocyte-endothelial cell interaction and *Staphylococcus aureus* infection. Br J Dermatol 1986; 115: 693–705.

109. Nicolis GD, Helwig EB. Exfoliative dermatitis. A clinicopathologic study of 135 cases. Arch Dermatol 1973; 108: 788–797.

110. Abrahams I, McCarthy JT, Sanders SL. 101 cases of exfoliative dermatitis. Arch Dermatol 1963; 87: 96–101.

111. Abel EA, Lindae ML, Hoppe RT, Wood GS. Benign and malignant forms of erythroderma: Cutaneous and immunophenotypic characteristics. J Am Acad Dermatol 1988; 19: 1089–1095.

112. Sentis HJ, Willemze R, Scheffer E. Histopathologic studies in Sézary syndrome and erythrodermic mycosis fungoides: A comparison with benign forms of erythroderma. J Am Acad Dermatol 1986; 15: 1217–1226.

Cutaneous drug reactions

INTRODUCTION

A drug reaction can be defined as an undesirable response evoked by a medicinal substance. Any drug is a potential cause of an adverse reaction, although certain classes of drugs can be incriminated more often than others. Major offenders include antibiotics, non-steroidal anti-inflammatory drugs, psychotropic agents, beta blockers and gold.[1] Preservatives and colouring agents in foodstuffs, as well as chemicals used in industry, may sometimes produce cutaneous reactions that are indistinguishable from those produced by medicinal substances. These other agents should always be kept in mind in the aetiology of an apparent drug reaction.

Although some drugs cause only one clinical pattern of reaction, most drugs are capable of producing several different types of reaction.[2] While most of these adverse reactions involve the skin, other organs such as the lungs, kidneys, liver and lymph nodes may be affected singly or in various combinations.[3,4] Drug fever is another clinical manifestation of an adverse drug reaction.

Continuing advances in pharmacology have resulted in the introduction of an ever increasing number of drugs for therapeutic purposes with a consequent avalanche of case reports detailing adverse reactions.[5,6] The true prevalence of cutaneous drug reactions is difficult to determine as most studies have been based on hospital inpatients, many of whom are receiving several drugs simultaneously.[1,7] In these inpatient series, drug reactions have occurred in approximately 2% of patients;[8] this figure is probably

EXANTHEMATOUS DRUG REACTIONS

Exanthematous eruptions (also described as morbilliform, and as erythematous maculopapular eruptions) are the most common type of drug reaction, accounting for approximately 40% of all reactions.[1] The rash develops 1 day to 3 weeks after the offending drug is first given, although the timing depends on previous sensitization.[13] Uncommonly, the onset is much later in the course of the drug therapy and rarely it may develop after administration of the drug has ended.

There are erythematous macules and papules that resemble a viral exanthem. Lesions usually appear first on the trunk or in areas of pressure or trauma.[9] They spread to involve the extremities, usually in a symmetrical fashion. Pruritus and fever are sometimes present. The eruption usually lasts for 1–2 weeks and clears with cessation of the drug.[9]

Exanthematous eruptions occur in 50–80% of patients who are given ampicillin while suffering from infectious mononucleosis, cytomegalovirus infection, or chronic lymphatic leukaemia or who are also taking allopurinol.[16] Amoxycillin may sometimes produce a similar reaction in the same circumstances. An exanthematous eruption also occurs commonly in patients with AIDS who are given co-trimoxazole (trimethoprim–sulphamethoxazole).[20] Other drugs which cause an exanthematous reaction include penicillin, erythromycin, streptomycin, tetracyclines, bleomycin, amphotericin B, sulphonamides, oral hypoglycaemic agents, thiazide diuretics, barbiturates, chloral hydrate, benzodiazepines, phenothiazines, allopurinol, thiouracil, quinine, quinidine, gold, captopril and the non-steroidal anti-inflammatory drugs.[13,21] Codeine and pseudoephedrine have produced an eruption resembling scarlet fever.[22]

The mechanisms involved in exanthematous reactions are unclear, although immunological mechanisms have been suggested.[16] The eruption does not always recur on rechallenge.[9]

Histopathology

At first glance, the histological changes in the exanthematous drug reactions appear non-specific, but they are in fact quite characteristic. There are small foci of spongiosis and vacuolar change involving the basal layer with mild spongiosis extending one or two cells above this (Fig. 20.1).[23] A few lymphocytes are usually present in these foci.[23] A characteristic feature is the presence of rare apoptotic keratinocytes (Civatte bodies) in the basal layer (Fig. 20.2). Very focal parakeratosis may be present in lesions of some duration.

The papillary dermis is usually mildly oedematous and there may be vascular dilatation. The inflammatory cell infiltrate, which consists of lymphocytes (some with large nuclei suggesting activation), macrophages, mast cells, occasional eosinophils and, rarely, a few plasma cells, is usually mild and localized around the superficial vascular plexus.[23]

Epidermal changes may be minimal or even absent in scarlatiniform eruptions and in some non-specific maculopapular eruptions categorized as exanthematous for convenience.

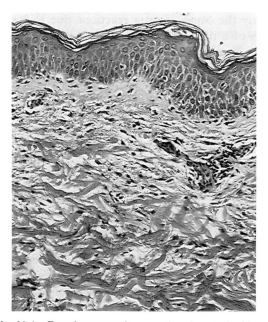

Fig. 20.1   Exanthematous drug reaction characterized by subtle basal spongiosis, mild exocytosis of lymphocytes and a mild perivascular infiltrate of lymphocytes in the upper dermis.
Haematoxylin — eosin

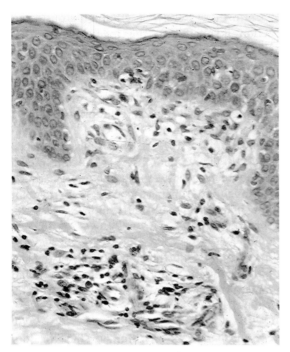

Fig. 20.2 Exanthematous drug reaction. A Civatte body (apoptotic keratinocyte) and a few lymphocytes are present in the basal layer.
Haematoxylin — eosin

HALOGENODERMAS

This term includes iododerma, bromoderma[24] and the rare fluoroderma which result from the ingestion of iodides, bromides and fluorides.[25] Iododerma is an uncommon disorder, while the other two are now exceedingly rare.

The usual source of the iodide is the potassium salt used in expectorants and some tonics.[26] Rarely, radiocontrast media[25] and amiodarone[27] have been implicated. The characteristic lesion is a papulopustule which progresses to a vegetating nodular lesion. This may be crusted and ulcerated. There are usually a number of lesions, 0.5–2 cm in diameter, on the face, neck, back or upper extremities.[25–26a] The lesions clear with cessation of the halide. The mechanism involved in their pathogenesis is uncertain.[25]

In addition to vegetating lesions, iodides may also produce erythematous papules, urticaria, vesicles, carbuncular lesions, erythema multiforme, vasculitis, polyarteritis nodosa, and ery-thema-nodosum-like lesions.[28] Iodides may also aggravate dermatitis herpetiformis, pyoderma gangrenosum, pustular psoriasis, erythema nodosum and blastomycosis-like pyoderma.[28]

Histopathology[28]

The vegetating lesions show pseudo-epitheliomatous hyperplasia with intraepidermal and some dermal abscesses.[29] The abscesses contain a few eosinophils and desquamated epithelial cells in addition to the neutrophils. There may be occasional multinucleate cells in the dermis, but this is never the prominent feature that it is in chromomycosis and sporotrichosis, which the reaction superficially resembles. In early lesions the 'intraepidermal' abscesses can be seen to be related to follicular infundibula.

OTHER CLINICOPATHOLOGICAL REACTIONS

The following account details in alphabetical order the various clinicopathological patterns that have been associated with drugs.[9] The reader should refer to the appropriate page, listed for each reaction below, for an account of the clinical and histopathological features of each particular pattern and of the drugs that may be responsible.

Acanthosis nigricans. Various hormones and corticosteroids have been implicated in the aetiology of some cases of acanthosis nigricans (see p. 552). There are no features that are specific for drug-induced lesions.

Acne. A number of drugs, cosmetics and industrial chemicals may precipitate and influence the course of acne vulgaris (see p. 436). Sometimes pustular acneiform lesions develop without the presence of comedones.

Alopecia. Numerous drugs have been implicated in the aetiology of alopecia. Several different mechanisms may be involved (see p. 464). The best understood of these is the alopecia produced by the various antimitotic

reactions and in systemic contact dermatitis[34] (see p. 113). Uncommonly, drugs may exacerbate or precipitate a named spongiotic disorder such as seborrhoeic dermatitis or nummular dermatitis. The pityriasis-rosea-like reactions (see p. 113) can also be included in this group. Certain drugs may produce a spongiotic reaction with histopathological features (Fig. 20.4) that enable it to be distinguished from other spongiotic disorders (see p. 114).

Sweat gland necrosis. Sweat gland necrosis may occur in certain drug-induced comas (see p. 472).

Toxic epidermal necrolysis. This is the most serious cutaneous reaction to drugs. Large areas of the skin are sloughed, and this is usually preceded by the development of large flaccid bullae[13] (see p. 45). Sulphonamides, allopurinol and the non-steroidal anti-inflammatory drugs are most often implicated.

Urticaria. Urticaria is second only to drug exanthems as a manifestation of drug reactions. Numerous drugs have been responsible (see p. 216). The mechanisms involved include IgE-dependent reactions, immune complexes and the non-immunological activation of effector pathways involved in mast cell degranulation.[9]

Vasculitis. The usual presentation of vasculitis is with 'palpable purpura' on the lower parts of the legs.[35] Immune mechanisms, particularly a type III reaction, are involved. Numerous drugs may produce a vasculitis (see p. 219).

OFFENDING DRUGS

The drugs which most often produce cutaneous reactions are the antibiotics, the non-steroidal anti-inflammatory drugs, psychotropic agents, the beta blockers and gold.[1,2] Other important drugs are the thiazide diuretics,[36] phenytoin and derivatives, and anti-cancer chemotherapeutic agents.[37]

Some drugs have a low incidence of reactions. Knowledge of these drugs may assist in determining the offending drug in patients receiving multiple therapeutic agents. Drugs in this category include antacids, antihistamines, atropine, digitalis glycosides,[36] insulin (regular), nystatin, potassium chloride, steroids, tetracycline, theophylline, thyroxine, vitamin preparations and warfarin.[13,16]

Brief mention will be made below of the major categories of offending drugs.

Antibiotics

Antibiotics are the major cause of drug reactions, accounting for 42% of all reactions in one series involving hospital inpatients.[2] Co-trimoxazole (trimethoprim–sulphamethoxazole) produced the highest number of reactions in one study (59 reactions/1000 recipients) while the frequency for ampicillin was 52/1000 and for the semi-synthetic penicillins 36/1000.[3] In another study, amoxycillin resulted in the highest number of reactions (51/1000 patients exposed).[7]

The most common pattern of skin reaction caused by antibiotics is an exanthematous one, but most other clinicopathological patterns have been reported at some time.[38,39] In the case of the tetracyclines, photosensitivity and fixed drug eruptions are sometimes seen.[9] The high incidence of reactions in patients taking ampicillin, who also have infectious mononucleosis, cytomegalovirus infection or chronic lymphatic leukaemia has been referred to, above. In the case of co-trimoxazole, two distinct eruptions have been recorded: an urticarial reaction with onset a few days after the onset of treatment and an exanthematous (morbilliform) reaction with its onset after one week of treatment. Toxic epidermal necrolysis has also been reported with this drug.

Non-steroidal anti-inflammatory drugs

This chemically-heterogeneous group of compounds can produce a variety of cutaneous reactions ranging from mild exanthematous eruptions to life-threatening toxic epidermal necrolysis.[40,41] They are among the most commonly prescribed class of drugs, accounting for approximately 5% of prescriptions dispensed in the United States.[21,41] Several drugs in this category have already been withdrawn from the market because of their cutaneous reactions.

The following categories of non-steroidal anti-inflammatory drugs are in use:[41]

1. *Salicylic acid derivatives*: aspirin and various compound analgesics.
2. *Heterocyclic acetic acids*: indomethacin, sulindac and tolmetin.
3. *Propionic acid derivatives*: ibuprofen, naproxen and fenoprofen.
4. *Anthranilic acids*: mefenamic acid, flufenamic acid and meclofenamate sodium.
5. *Pyrazole derivatives* (pyrazolones): phenylbutazone and oxyphenbutazone.
6. *Oxicams*: piroxicam.

Drugs belonging to any given chemical group frequently share similar mechanisms of action and toxicity. The non-steroidal anti-inflammatory drugs inhibit the enzyme cyclo-oxygenase and thus reduce production of prostaglandins and thromboxanes; this action is not solely responsible for their therapeutic actions.[21]

Exanthematous eruptions are commonly seen with phenylbutazone and indomethacin but they have been reported at some time or other with most of the other non-steroidal anti-inflammatory drugs.[9] Aspirin is an important cause of acute urticaria; it also aggravates chronic urticaria.[41] Ibuprofen may produce a vasculitis or lupus-erythematosus-like eruption; naproxen may produce a fixed drug eruption, a lichenoid reaction or a vesiculobullous reaction.[41] Piroxicam may result in a vesiculobullous eruption in areas exposed to the sun.[21] Most of the non-steroidal anti-inflammatory drugs have been reported to give toxic epidermal necrolysis and/or erythema multiforme at some time, although the substances most frequently responsible are the pyrazolones.[9,21]

Psychotropic drugs

The psychotropic drugs include the tricyclic antidepressants, antipsychotic drugs, lithium and the hypnotic and anxiolytic (tranquillizer) agents.[42] This group of drugs produces the most diverse range of reactions which include exacerbation of porphyria (chlordiazepoxide), blue-grey discoloration of the skin (chlorpromazine) and an acneiform eruption (lithium).[42,43] Further mention of the specific complications of the various drugs in this category is made in the description of the appropriate tissue reaction.

Phenytoin sodium

Phenytoin sodium is a widely prescribed anticonvulsant with a relatively low rate of side-effects. Nevertheless, a broad spectrum of cutaneous reactions has been reported.[44] These include exanthematous eruptions, acneiform lesions, exfoliative dermatitis, erythema multiforme, toxic epidermal necrolysis, vasculitis, hypertrichosis, gingival hyperplasia, coarse facies, heel-pad thickening, a lupus-erythematosus-like reaction, digital deformities[45] (the fetal hydantoin syndrome), a hypersensitivity syndrome[46] and a pseudolymphoma syndrome.[44]

Gold

Gold produces a variety of cutaneous reactions which are most commonly 'eczematous' or maculopapular in type.[47] These reactions may occur as long as two years after the initiation of therapy.[9] The lesions may take months to resolve.[9] Other reactions produced by gold include cutaneous pigmentation (see p. 420), exfoliative dermatitis, vasomotor flushing, a lichenoid drug reaction, erythema nodosum and an eruption resembling pityriasis rosea.[48]

Cytotoxic drugs

Cytotoxic drugs used in the treatment of cancer have many mucocutaneous complications. As combination chemotherapy is often used, it may be difficult to determine which drug is specifically responsible for a particular reaction. Because of their action on rapidly dividing cells, cytotoxic drugs commonly produce alopecia, stomatitis and Beau's lines on the nails.[37,49] Chemical cellulitis, ulceration and phlebitis may

Reactions to physical agents

INTRODUCTION

In this chapter, the cutaneous lesions that result from various physical agents such as trauma, heat and cold, radiation and light will be discussed.[1] This is not an exhaustive account of all the reactions that can theoretically result from physical injuries, as some are of little dermatopathological importance. Several entities produced by physical agents have been discussed in other chapters because they possess a distinctive histopathological pattern. For completeness, brief mention is made of these entities in the introductory discussion of the relevant physical agent.

REACTIONS TO TRAUMA AND IRRITATION

There are many cutaneous lesions which result from trauma and irritation in the broadest meaning of the words.[1a] However, some of these, such as abrasions, bruises, lacerations and the like are of no dermatopathological interest. In contrast, calcaneal petechiae ('black heel') and related traumatic haemorrhages in some other sites are important because they are sometimes mistaken clinically for a melanocytic lesion. Dermatitis artefacta is also an important entity because its clinical recognition is often delayed. Many quite diverse lesions can result, particularly when foreign materials are injected into the skin.

Entities discussed in other sections include scars (see p. 337), corns and calluses (see p. 756) and acanthoma fissuratum, a reaction to chronic friction from ill-fitting spectacles or other prostheses. Granuloma fissuratum presents with irregular acanthosis bordering on pseudo-epitheliomatous hyperplasia and is accordingly discussed with that tissue reaction pattern on p. 732.

DERMATITIS ARTEFACTA

Dermatitis artefacta is a self-inflicted dermatosis occurring in malingerers, the mentally retarded, and in association with various psychiatric disturbances, particularly personality disorders.[2,3] The definition is sometimes extended to include factitious lesions resulting from child abuse.[4]

The lesions may take many different forms, depending on the injurious agent used.[2,5-7] Their distribution and shape may be bizarre. Usually there are lesions in different stages of evolution. Deep abscesses, cellulitis and granulomatous lesions may result from the injection of various substances.

Histopathology

A diagnosis of dermatitis artefacta is not often made in the absence of supporting evidence from the clinician. The reasons for this include the lack of histopathological specificity in most instances, the medicolegal implications of making such a diagnosis and the traditional fear among doctors of missing an organic disease.

There is little limit to the type of lesion that may be found. This may take the form of abrasions, excoriations, ulcers and burns. There may be abscesses, cellulitis, suppurative panniculitis, irritant and allergic contact dermatitis, alopecia (trichotillomania) or haemorrhage. In the presence of granulomas or abscesses a search should always be made for foreign material, including an examination for doubly-refractile particles. Electron-probe microanalysis may assist in the identification of foreign material found in tissue sections.[8]

Telangiectasia of vessels in the dermis has been reported as a response to persistent local trauma, although in the cases reported the trauma was not intentional but resulted from recreational pursuits.[9]

DECUBITUS ULCER

A decubitus ulcer (bedsore) usually develops over pressure areas such as the sacrum, the greater trochanter and the heels, usually in individuals confined to bed for long periods.[9a] Prolonged pressure is thought to compromise the vascular supply of the affected areas. Several clinical stages have been identified. There is a preceding erythematous stage (blanching and non-blanching) and a late stage in which a black eschar forms.[10]

Histopathology[10]

The earliest changes are in the upper dermis where the vessels become dilated and the endothelial cells swollen. A perivascular round cell infiltrate forms in the papillary dermis together with vascular engorgement, formation of platelet aggregates and perivascular haemorrhage. The epidermis and appendages become necrotic. A subepidermal bulla forms prior to epidermal necrosis, if the process is acute. In some cases of low-grade, chronic pressure, epidermal atrophy will result. Full-thickness dermal necrosis with the formation of an eschar may develop where the skin is thin and bony prominences are close to the surface.[10] Re-epithelialization is always very slow when the epidermis and appendages have both been destroyed, and grafting is usually required.

FRICTION BLISTERS

Friction blisters are produced at sites where the epidermis is thick and firmly attached to the underlying dermis, such as the palms, soles, heels and backs of the fingers.[11,12] A common site is the heel, where blisters are caused by ill-fitting foot wear. Friction blisters are an uncommon manifestation of dermatitis artefacta.[11] If the trauma is prolonged and severe, or the skin is thin, erosions will occur. Recovery is rapid and complete within a few days.[13]

Histopathology[11]

There is an intraepidermal blister due to a wide cleft which is usually sited just beneath the stratum granulosum. The roof of the blister consists of stratum corneum and stratum granulosum and a thin layer of amorphous cellular debris.[14] The keratinocytes in the base of the blister show variable oedema, pallor and even degenerative changes.[15] There is only a sparse perivascular inflammatory cell infiltrate in the papillary dermis. Friction blisters differ from suction blisters which are subepidermal in position.[16]

Mitotic activity commences in the base within 30 hours and there is rapid regeneration with the return of a granular layer in 48 hours.[13]

Electron microscopy.[17] The earliest change is intracellular oedema, most noticeable at the cell periphery. The membranes of some cells rupture, allowing escape of some of their contents into the extracellular space.

CALCANEAL PETECHIAE ('BLACK HEEL')

This entity, which is usually bilateral and roughly symmetrical, consists of a painless, petechial eruption on the heels.[18–20] There is speckled, brownish-black pigmentation which may be mistaken for a plantar wart, or even a melanoma.[21]

Calcaneal petechiae appear to be traumatic in origin. Their formation probably follows a pinching force imparted by shoes at the time of sudden stopping, such as occurs in the course of basketball, tennis and other sports.[21,22]

Lesions comparable in appearance, pathogenesis and pathology occur in other situations.

Histopathology[20,23]

The pigmentation in calcaneal petechiae results from lakes of haemorrhage in the stratum

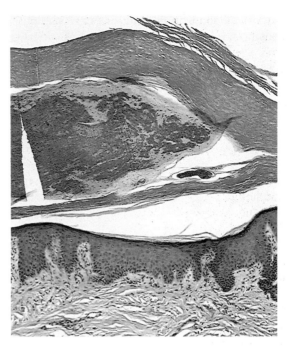

Fig. 21.1   Traumatic haemorrhage involving the stratum corneum. The lesion was removed because of a clinical suspicion that this was a melanoma.
Haematoxylin — eosin

corneum (Fig. 21.1). The red cells are extravasated into the lower epidermis from dilated vessels in the papillary dermis. They undergo transepidermal elimination during the progressive maturation of the epidermis and overlying stratum corneum.

Red cells may also be found in the stratum corneum following trauma to the palms, soles and subungual region. Haemorrhage also occurs into the parakeratotic layer overlying the digitate papillomatous projections in warts.

REACTIONS TO RADIATION

The early (acute) effects of X-irradiation differ markedly from those that develop many months or years later. In the skin, the terms acute radiodermatitis and chronic radiodermatitis have traditionally been used for these respective stages. Recently, a subacute form has been described with features resembling those of acute graft-versus-host disease.[24] All three stages are discussed below under the general heading of radiation dermatitis.

The effects of ultraviolet radiation are quite different. Ultraviolet-B radiation produces apoptosis of keratinocytes ('sunburn cells'), spongiosis and eventual parakeratosis. Endothelial cells in the superficial vascular plexus enlarge and there is some perivenular oedema.[24a] Langerhans cells in the epidermis are reduced in number for several days after the exposure. Ultraviolet-A radiation produces only mild swelling of keratinocytes and mild spongiosis but no sunburn cells.[24a]

RADIATION DERMATITIS

There is a common response to the different types of radiation that affect the skin, although the severity of the changes varies with the total dose, its fractionation and the depth of penetration of the radiation.[25–27] The use now of megavoltage therapy for deep tumours has resulted in some sparing of the skin, although fibrosis in the deep subcutaneous tissues may result.[27,28]

There is a well-defined progression of changes which follow irradiation of the skin.[27] These are usually divided into early changes (acute radiodermatitis) and chronic changes (chronic radiodermatitis) arising many months or years after the initial exposure.[29,30]

Early changes. In the weeks following irradiation there is variable erythema, accompanied by oedema in the more severe cases.[27] This is followed by epilation and hyperpigmentation. Severe changes such as vesiculation, erosion and ulceration are not seen very often in these days of more precisely controlled dosage.

Late changes.[27] The chronic effects progress slowly and are usually subclinical in the early stages. It seems that at least 1000 rads are required to produce chronic radiodermatitis.[31] The final changes resemble poikiloderma, with atrophy, telangiectasias, hypopigmentation with focal hyperpigmentation, and loss of

appendages. The affected skin is very susceptible to minor trauma, which may lead to persistent ulceration.

A small proportion of patients develop squamous[32] or basal cell carcinoma 15 years or more after irradiation.[33,34] Rarely, fibrosarcomas have been reported: their diagnosis might not stand up to scrutiny with the immunoperoxidase markers available today. Basal cell carcinomas are more common following irradiation to the head and neck region.[35] Sometimes the tumours which develop are quite aggressive, and there is a higher risk of metastasis with any squamous cell carcinoma that develops in the skin following irradiation than with cutaneous squamous cell carcinoma in general.[30] An absorbed dose of at least 2000 rads is required.[36] The risk of cutaneous cancer following superficial grenz therapy is very small indeed.[37,38]

Histopathology[27]

The early changes of radiation dermatitis are not commonly seen as there is usually little reason to perform a biopsy. There is some vacuolization of epidermal nuclei and cytoplasm with some degenerate keratinocytes. Inhibition of mitosis occurs in the germinal cells of the epidermis and pilosebaceous follicles. The follicles soon pass into the catagen phase. Later there is hyperpigmentation of the basal layer. The blood vessels in the papillary dermis are dilated and their endothelial cells are swollen. There is oedema of the papillary dermis and extravasation of red blood cells and fibrin. Thrombi composed of fibrin and platelets may form in some vessels. Only a small number of inflammatory cells is present and these are usually dispersed and not perivascular in location.

In the late stages the epidermis may be atrophic with loss of the normal rete ridge pattern and the development of focal basal vacuolar change. Sometimes there is overlying hyperkeratosis. Dyskeratotic cells are usually present. The main changes are in the dermis where there is swollen, hyalinized collagen showing irregular eosinophilic staining (Fig. 21.2). Atypical stellate fibroblasts with large nuclei containing clumped chromatin (radiation fibroblasts) are invariably present.[39] There are telangiectatic vessels in the upper dermis with marked dilatation of their lumen and swelling of the endothelial cells. Vessels are generally reduced in number. Those near the dermal–subcutaneous junction may show varying degrees of myointimal proliferation. Small arterioles and venules often show hyaline change in their walls, with narrowing of the lumen.

Pilosebaceous structures are absent and there is some atrophy of eccrine sweat glands. The arrector pili muscles remain, in contrast to the changes following thermal burns, when they are lost. The surviving muscle fibres are often embedded in a pear-shaped mass of collagen, giving the appearance of a bulbous scar.

Less common findings include ulceration, secondary infection and inflammation, and dysplastic epidermal changes resembling an actinic

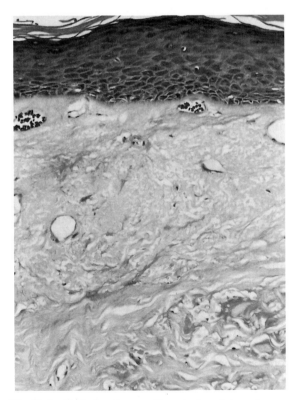

Fig. 21.2 Radiation damage. There is altered dermal collagen. Blood vessels are telangiectatic. Haematoxylin — eosin

keratosis. Basal or squamous cell carcinomas may supervene. The deep subcutaneous fibrosis which may follow megavoltage therapy overlies atrophic and degenerated skeletal muscle fibres.[28]

Recently, the concept of subacute radiation dermatitis has been discussed. The changes were present weeks to months after the exposure.[24] A biopsy showed an interface (lichenoid) dermatitis with lymphocytes in close apposition with degenerate epidermal cells (satellite cell necrosis).[24]

REACTIONS TO HEAT AND COLD

There are two broad groups of temperature-dependent skin disorders.[40] The first involves the physiological responses that occur in everyone subjected to extremes of temperature. This group includes thermal burns and cold-related disorders such as frostbite. The other group of disorders involves an abnormal response to heat and cold. Abnormal reactions to heat include erythema ab igne (see p. 372), cholinergic urticaria (see p. 216), heat urticaria (see p. 216) and erythermalgia.[40] There are numerous abnormal reactions to cold such as perniosis (see p. 241), livedo reticularis, cold urticaria (see p. 216), sclerema neonatorum (see p. 504), subcutaneous fat necrosis of the newborn (see p. 503), Raynaud's phenomenon (see p. 329) and cryoglobulinaemia (see p. 214).[40]

The following reactions to heat and cold will be considered further:

Thermal burns
Electrical burns
Frostbite
Cryotherapy effects.

THERMAL BURNS

Thermal burns are an important cause of morbidity and mortality. In children, most burns are scalds from hot liquids, while in adults accidents with flammable liquids are more

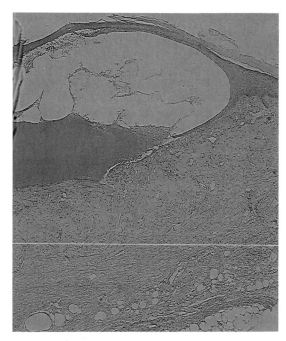

Fig. 21.4 Cryotherapy blister. The lesion is subepidermal with luminal haemorrhage.
Haematoxylin — eosin

damaged collagen and elastic fibres.[55] These changes may lead to a clinical suspicion that the initial lesion has not responded to the cryotherapy.

Another change which follows cryotherapy is localized hypopigmentation, sometimes with a halo of hyperpigmentation.[56] In either case, there may be some melanin lying free, or in macrophages, in the upper dermis.

REACTIONS TO LIGHT (PHOTODERMATOSES)

The photodermatoses are a heterogeneous group of cutaneous disorders in which light plays a significant pathogenetic role. This group is sometimes expanded by the inclusion of those conditions, both congenital and acquired, which are exacerbated in some way by light but which are not directly produced by it.[57] This expanded concept of light-sensitive dermatoses includes the following diseases:

Genodermatoses
  Xeroderma pigmentosum
  Cockayne's syndrome
  Bloom's syndrome
  Hartnup disease
  Rothmund–Thomson disease
Metabolic/nutritional dermatoses
  Porphyria
  Disorders of tryptophan metabolism
  Pellagra
Light-sensitive dermatoses
  Lupus erythematosus
  Lichen planus variants
  Rosacea
  Hailey–Hailey disease
  Darier's disease
  Seborrhoeic dermatitis
  Atopic dermatitis
  Erythema multiforme
  Pityriasis rubra pilaris
  Disseminated actinic porokeratosis
  Herpes simplex infections
Photodermatoses
  Phototoxic dermatitis
  Photoallergic dermatitis
  Hydroa vacciniforme
  Polymorphous light eruption
  Actinic prurigo
  Solar urticaria
Chronic photodermatoses
  Persistent light reaction
  Photosensitive eczema
  Actinic reticuloid.

The account which follows will be confined to the photodermatoses. Solar urticaria has been discussed with the urticarial reactions (see p. 216). The following entities will be discussed in turn:
  Phototoxic dermatitis
  Photoallergic dermatitis
  Hydroa vacciniforme
  Polymorphous light eruption
  Actinic prurigo
  Chronic photodermatoses
  Persistent light reaction
  Photosensitive eczema
  Actinic reticuloid.

PHOTOTOXIC DERMATITIS

Phototoxicity is the damage induced by ultraviolet and/or visible radiation as a result of contact with, or the ingestion of, a photosensitizing substance.[58] It does not depend on an allergic reaction and is therefore akin to an irritant contact dermatitis.[59] Phytophotodermatitis is a photosensitivity reaction, usually phototoxic in type, which results from contact with plants containing psoralens and other furocoumarins.[60,61] The families Umbelliferae and Rutaceae contain many phototoxic species. They include celery,[60] parsnips, carrots, fennel, dill, limes and lemons.[62]

Clinically, phototoxic reactions resemble an exaggerated sunburn reaction with dusky erythema; when severe, vesiculation may occur, followed by desquamation and hyperpigmentation.[63–65] Two patterns of reaction are seen: an immediate reaction, which follows the ingestion of the photosensitizing agent and involves exposed areas such as the face, ears, V-area of the neck and dorsum of the hands;[66] and a delayed reaction, which follows contact with psoralens and peaks after two or three days. The reaction is limited to the site of contact with the photosensitizing agent. Prominent pigmentation lasting for weeks or months may follow phytophotodermatitis.[60] In some instances, the preceding erythematous phase may go unnoticed.[61] Chronic changes include wrinkling, atrophy, telangiectasia and the formation of keratoses.

Another presumed phototoxic reaction is the formation of subepidermal bullae, first reported in patients with chronic renal failure receiving high doses of frusemide (furosemide).[67] Other drugs which may produce this pseudoporphyria reaction (see p. 537) include naproxen,[68] dapsone, tetracycline, pyridoxine, nalidixic acid[69] and vinblastine.[70] Prolonged sunbed exposure of chronically sun-damaged skin has also been incriminated, although whether there is any phototoxic component remains to be seen.[71]

Ingested drugs capable of causing a phototoxic reaction include, in addition to those mentioned above, phenothiazines, thiazides,[72,73] amiodarone,[74] carbamazepine and sulphonamides.[63,75] Topical agents associated with phototoxicity include coal tar and derivatives, psoralens[61] and textile dyes,[76] as well as some perfumes and sun barrier preparations.[77]

A phototoxic reaction requires the absorption of photons of specific wavelengths by the photosensitizing substance.[75] Energy is dissipated as it returns from an excited state to its ground state. Free radicals, peroxides and other substances are formed which may potentially damage cellular and subcellular membranes.[75,78] The action spectrum is usually in the ultraviolet-A range, although with some ingested substances (e.g. thiazides) it is in the shorter ultraviolet-B wavelengths.[63,72]

Phototoxicity is more common than photoallergy from which it differs by being dose-related and by its subsidence on removal of the photosensitizer or the ultraviolet radiation. Some drugs produce both toxic and allergic reactions.

Histopathology

If the photosensitizing agent is applied to the skin there is some ballooning of keratinocytes in the upper dermis, with epidermal necrosis in severe reactions[59] and scattered apoptotic keratinocytes ('sun-burn cells') in mild reactions (Fig. 21.5). There is variable spongiosis. A similar picture is seen in biopsies taken

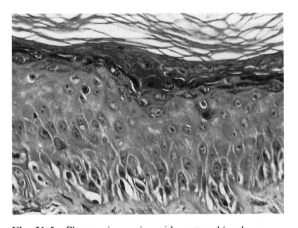

Fig. 21.5 Phototoxic reaction with scattered 'sunburn cells'. The reaction followed contact with a psoralen-containing plant (phytophotodermatitis). Haematoxylin — eosin

REFERENCES

Introduction

1. Sutton RL Jr. Dermatoses due to physical agents. Cutis 1977; 19: 513–529.

Reactions to trauma and irritation

1a. Basler RSW. Skin injuries in sports medicine. J Am Acad Dermatol 1989; 21: 1257–1262.
2. Lyell A. Cutaneous artifactual disease. A review, amplified by personal experience. J Am Acad Dermatol 1979; 1: 391–407.
3. Lyell A. Dermatitis artefacta in relation to the syndrome of contrived disease. Clin Exp Dermatol 1976; 1: 109–126.
4. Stankler L. Factitious skin lesions in a mother and two sons. Br J Dermatol 1977; 97: 217–219.
5. Van Moffaert M, Vermander F, Kint A. Dermatitis artefacta. Int J Dermatol 1985; 24: 236–238.
6. Brodland DG, Staats BA, Peters MS. Factitial leg ulcers associated with an unusual sleep disorder. Arch Dermatol 1989; 125: 1115–1118.
7. Sneddon I, Sneddon J. Self-inflicted injury: a follow-up study of 43 patients. Br Med J 1975; 3: 527–530.
8. Jackson RM, Tucker SB, Abraham JL, Millns JL. Factitial cutaneous ulcers and nodules: The use of electron-probe microanalysis in diagnosis. J Am Acad Dermatol 1984; 11: 1065–1069.
9. Tsuji T, Sawabe M. A new type of telangiectasia following trauma. J Cutan Pathol 1988; 15: 22–26.
9a. Parish LC, Witkowski JA. The infected decubitus ulcer. Int J Dermatol 1989; 28: 643–647.
10. Witkowski JA, Parish LC. Histopathology of the decubitus ulcer. J Am Acad Dermatol 1982; 6: 1014–1021.
11. Brehmer-Andersson E, Goransson K. Friction blisters as a manifestation of pathomimia. Acta Derm Venereol 1975; 55: 65–71.
12. Naylor PFD. Experimental friction blisters. Br J Dermatol 1955; 67: 327–342.
13. Epstein WL, Fukuyama K, Cortese TA. Autoradiographic study of friction blisters. Arch Dermatol 1969; 99: 94–106.
14. Sulzberger MB, Cortese TA Jr, Fishman L, Wiley HS. Studies on blisters produced by friction. I. Results of linear rubbing and twisting technics. J Invest Dermatol 1966; 47: 456–465.
15. Cortese TA Jr, Griffin TB, Layton LL, Hutsell TC. Experimental friction blisters in Macaque monkeys. J Invest Dermatol 1969; 53: 172–177.
16. Hunter JAA, McVittie E, Comaish JS. Light and electron microscopic studies of physical injury to the skin. I. Suction. Br J Dermatol 1974; 90: 481–490.
17. Hunter JAA, McVittie E, Comaish JS. Light and electron microscopic studies of physical injury to the skin. II. Friction. Br J Dermatol 1974; 90: 491–499.
18. Crissey JT, Peachey JC. Calcaneal petechiae. Arch Dermatol 1961; 83: 501.
19. Kirton V, Price MW. Black heel. Trans St John's Hosp Dermatol Soc 1965; 51: 80–84.
20. Mehregan AH. Black heel: A report of two cases. Can Med Assoc J 1966; 96: 584–585.
21. Ganpule M. Pinching trauma in "black heel". Br J Dermatol 1967; 79: 654–655.
22. Ayres S Jr, Mihan R. Calcaneal petechiae. Arch Dermatol 1972; 106: 262.
23. Apted JH. Calcaneal petechiae (black heel). Australas J Dermatol 1973; 14: 132–135.

Reactions to radiation

24. LeBoit PE. Subacute radiation dermatitis: A histologic imitator of acute cutaneous graft-versus-host disease. J Am Acad Dermatol 1989; 20: 236–241.
24a. Soter NA. Acute effects of ultraviolet radiation on the skin. Semin Dermatol 1990; 9: 11–15.
25. Fajardo LF, Berthrong M. Radiation injury in surgical pathology. Part I. Am J Surg Pathol 1978; 2: 159–199.
26. Price NM. Radiation dermatitis following electron beam therapy. Arch Dermatol 1978; 114: 63–66.
27. Fajardo LF, Berthrong M. Radiation injury in surgical pathology. Part III. Salivary glands, pancreas and skin. Am J Surg Pathol 1981; 5: 279–296.
28. James WD, Odom RB. Late subcutaneous fibrosis following megavoltage radiotherapy. J Am Acad Dermatol 1980; 3: 616–618.
29. Young EM Jr, Barr RJ. Sclerosing dermatoses. J Cutan Pathol 1985; 12: 426–441.
30. Goldschmidt H, Sherwin WK. Reactions to ionizing radiation. J Am Acad Dermatol 1980; 3: 551–579.
31. Goldschmidt H. Dermatologic radiotherapy. The risk–benefit ratio. Arch Dermatol 1986; 122: 1385–1388.
32. Volden G, Larsen TE. Squamous cell carcinoma appearing in X-ray-treated mycosis fungoides. Acta Derm Venereol 1977; 57: 341–343.
33. Lazar P, Cullen SI. Basal cell epithelioma and chronic radiodermatitis. Arch Dermatol 1963; 88: 172–175.
34. Totten RS, Antypas PG, Dupertuis SM et al. Pre-existing roentgen-ray dermatitis in patients with skin cancer. Cancer 1957; 10: 1024–1030.
35. Sarkany I, Fountain RB, Evans CD et al. Multiple basal-cell epithelioma following radiotherapy of the spine. Br J Dermatol 1968; 80: 90–96.
36. Rowell NR. A follow-up study of superficial radiotherapy for benign dermatoses: recommendations for the use of X-rays in dermatology. Br J Dermatol 1973; 88: 583–590.
37. Brodkin RH, Bleiberg J. Neoplasia resulting from Grenz radiation. Arch Dermatol 1968; 97: 307–309.
38. Lindelof B, Eklund G. Incidence of malignant skin tumors in 14140 patients after grenz-ray treatment for benign skin disorders. Arch Dermatol 1986; 122: 1391–1395.
39. Jacoby RA, Burgoon CF Jr. Atypical fibroblasts as a clue to radiation injury. Am J Dermatopathol 1985; 7: 53–56.

Reactions to heat and cold

40. Page EH, Shear NH. Temperature-dependent skin disorders. J Am Acad Dermatol 1988; 18: 1003–1019.
41. Dembling RH. Burns. N Engl J Med 1985; 313: 1389–1398.
42. Raimer BG, Raimer SS, Hebeler JR. Cutaneous signs of child abuse. J Am Acad Dermatol 1981; 5: 203–212.
43. Sutton RL Jr, Waisman M. Dermatoses due to physical

agents. Cutis 1977; 19: 513–529.

43a. Hendricks WM. The classification of burns. J Am Acad Dermatol 1990; 22: 838–839.

44. Huang TT, Larson DL, Lewis SR. Burn alopecia. Plast Reconstr Surg 1977; 60: 763–767.

45. Novick M, Gard DA, Hardy SB, Spira M. Burn scar carcinoma: a review and analysis of 46 cases. Trauma 1977; 17: 809–817.

46. Abbas JS, Beecham JE. Burn wound carcinoma: case report and review of the literature. Burns 1988; 14: 222–224.

47. Lund HZ. How often does squamous cell carcinoma of the skin metastasize? Arch Dermatol 1965; 92: 635–637.

48. Goldberg NS, Robinson JK, Peterson C. Gigantic malignant melanoma in a thermal burn scar. J Am Acad Dermatol 1985; 12: 949–952.

49. Muhlemann MF, Griffiths RW, Briggs JC. Malignant melanoma and squamous cell carcinoma in a burn scar. Br J Plast Surg 1982; 35: 474–477.

50. Foley FD. Pathology of cutaneous burns. Surg Clin North Am 1970; 50: 1201–1210.

51. Warren S. Radiation effect on the skin. In: Helwig EB, Mostofi FK, eds. The skin. Huntington, New York: Robert E Krieger, 1980; 261–278.

52. Xuewei W, Wanrhong Z. Vascular injuries in electrical burns — the pathologic basis for mechanism of injury. Burns 1983; 9: 335–339.

53. Ackerman AB, Goldfaden GL. Electrical burns of the mouth in children. Arch Dermatol 1971; 104: 308–311.

54. Kee CE. Liquid nitrogen cryotherapy. Arch Dermatol 1967; 96: 198–203.

55. Weedon D. Unpublished observations.

56. Kuflik EG, Lubritz RR, Torre D. Cryosurgery. Dermatol Clin 1984; 2: 319–332.

Reactions to light (photodermatoses)

57. White HAD. The diagnosis of the photodermatoses: a review. Australas J Dermatol 1979; 20: 123–126.

58. Emmett EA. Drug photoallergy. Int J Dermatol 1978; 17: 370–379.

59. Epstein JH. Photoallergy. A review. Arch Dermatol 1972; 106: 741–748.

60. Seligman PJ, Mathias CGT, O'Malley MA et al. Phytophotodermatitis from celery among grocery store workers. Arch Dermatol 1987; 123: 1478–1482.

61. Stoner JG, Rasmussen JE. Plant dermatitis. J Am Acad Dermatol 1983; 9: 1–15.

62. Pathak MA. Phytophotodermatitis. Clin Dermatol 1986; 4: 102–121.

63. Wintroub BU, Stern R. Cutaneous drug reactions: Pathogenesis and clinical classification. J Am Acad Dermatol 1985; 13: 167–179.

64. Wennersten G, Thune P, Jansen CT, Brodthagen H. Photocontact dermatitis: current status with emphasis on allergic contact photosensitivity (CPS) occurrence, allergens, and practical phototesting. Semin Dermatol 1986; 5: 277–289.

65. Toback AC, Anders JE. Phototoxicity from systemic agents. Dermatol Clin 1986; 4: 223–230.

66. Willis I. Photosensitivity. Int J Dermatol 1975; 14: 326–337.

67. Rotstein H. Photosensitive bullous eruption associated with chronic renal failure. Australas J Dermatol 1987; 19: 58–64.

68. Rivers JK, Barnetson R St C. Naproxen-induced bullous photodermatitis. Med J Aust 1989; 151: 167–168.

69. Ramsay CA, Obreshkova E. Photosensitivity from nalidixic acid. Br J Dermatol 1974; 91: 523–528.

70. Breza TS, Halprin KM, Taylor JR. Photosensitivity reaction to vinblastine. Arch Dermatol 1975; 111: 1168–1170.

71. Murphy GM, Wright J, Nicholls DSH et al. Sunbed-induced pseudoporphyria. Br J Dermatol 1989; 120: 555–562.

72. Addo HA, Ferguson J, Frain-Bell W. Thiazide-induced photosensitivity: a study of 33 subjects. Br J Dermatol 1987; 116: 749–760.

73. Diffey BL, Langtry J. Phototoxic potential of thiazide diuretics in normal subjects. Arch Dermatol 1989; 125: 1355–1358.

74. Ferguson J, Addo HA, Jones S et al. A study of cutaneous photosensitivity induced by amiodarone. Br J Dermatol 1985; 113: 537–549.

75. Harber LC, Bickers DR, Armstrong RB, Kochevar IE. Drug photosensitivity: phototoxic and photoallergic mechanisms. Semin Dermatol 1982; 1: 183–195.

76. Hjorth N, Moller H. Phototoxic textile dermatitis ("bikini dermatitis"). Arch Dermatol 1976; 112: 1445–1447.

77. Hawk JLM. Photosensitizing agents used in the United Kingdom. Clin Exp Dermatol 1984; 9: 300–302.

78. Kochevar IE. Phototoxicity mechanisms: chlorpromazine photosensitized damage to DNA and cell membranes. J Invest Dermatol 1981; 76: 59–64.

79. Epstein S. Chlorpromazine photosensitivity. Phototoxic and photoallergic reactions. Arch Dermatol 1968; 98: 354–363.

80. Epstein JH. Phototoxicity and photoallergy in man. J Am Acad Dermatol 1983; 8: 141–147.

81. Elmets CA. Drug-induced photoallergy. Dermatol Clin 1986; 4: 231–241.

82. Horio T. Photoallergic reactions. Classification and pathogenesis. Int J Dermatol 1984; 23: 376–382.

83. Larsen WG, Maibach HI. Fragrance contact allergy. Semin Dermatol 1982; 1: 85–90.

84. Kaidbey KH, Kligman AM. Photosensitization by coumarin derivatives. Structure-activity relationships. Arch Dermatol 1981; 117: 258–263.

85. Knobler E, Almeida L, Ruzkowski AM et al. Photoallergy to benzophenone. Arch Dermatol 1989; 125: 801–804.

86. Kaidbey KH, Allen H. Photocontact allergy to benzocaine. Arch Dermatol 1981; 117: 77–79.

87. Jarratt M. Drug photosensitization. Int J Dermatol 1976; 15: 317–325.

88. Ljunggren B, Sjovall P. Systemic quinine photosensitivity. Arch Dermatol 1986; 122: 909–911.

89. Diffey BL, Farr PM, Adams SJ. The action spectrum in quinine photosensitivity. Br J Dermatol 1988; 118: 679–685.

90. Armstrong RB, Leach EE, Whitman G et al. Quinidine photosensitivity. Arch Dermatol 1985; 121: 525–528.

91. Pariser DM, Taylor JR. Quinidine photosensitivity. Arch Dermatol 1975; 111: 1440–1443.

92. Horio T. Chlorpromazine allergy. Coexistence of immediate and delayed type. Arch Dermatol 1975; 111: 1469–1471.

Cutaneous infections and infestations — *histological patterns*

In this age of international travel it is necessary for dermatopathologists to be familiar with the appearances of all cutaneous infections, including those which are sometimes dismissed euphemistically as 'infections of other countries'. Unfortunately, there is a bewildering number of these infections, making it difficult to commit to memory the details of all of them. Further problems result from the variable morphological appearances which a particular infectious agent may produce. Factors which may influence the histopathological features of a cutaneous infection include the number and virulence of the organism, the host's immunological response, the stage of evolution of the disease, prior treatment, and the presence of secondary changes resulting from rubbing and scratching or superimposed further infection. Because certain infections may produce different histopathological changes under these various circumstances, it seems prudent to categorize the infections and infestations on an aetiological rather than a morphological basis in the succeeding chapters. This traditional approach reduces unnecessary duplication.

Table 22.1 provides an outline of the morphological approach to infections of the skin. It lists the various diseases which should be considered when a particular morphological feature is encountered in a biopsy. The list does not include some of the very rare presentations of certain infections. These various infections and infestations are the subject of the following eight chapters (Chapters 23 – 30).

Table 22.1 Histological patterns in infections and infestations

Morphological feature	Diseases to be considered
Tuberculoid granulomas	Tuberculosis (p. 604); tuberculids (p. 607); tuberculoid leprosy (p. 612); syphilis [late secondary or tertiary] (p. 634); dermatophytosis [Majocchi's granuloma] (p. 644); cryptococcosis (p. 648); alternariosis (p. 657); histoplasmosis (p. 652); keloidal blastomycosis (p. 663); prototheccosis (p. 664); leishmaniasis (p. 702); acanthamoebiasis (p. 702); echinoderm injury (p. 708).
Suppurative granulomas	Atypical mycobacterial infections (p. 608); lymphogranuloma venereum (p. 620); blastomycosis-like pyoderma* (p. 601); actinomycosis* (p. 660); nocardiosis* (p. 659); mycetoma* (p. 658); cryptococcosis (p. 648), aspergillosis (p. 662) and other deep fungal infections** (p. 651); prototheccosis (p. 664).
Histiocyte granulomas	Infections by atypical mycobacteria (p. 608); lepromatous leprosy (p. 614); leishmaniasis (p. 702); malakoplakia [Michaelis–Gutmann bodies in cytoplasm] (p. 619).
Histiocytes and plasma cells	Rhinoscleroma (p. 617); syphilis [cells prominent] (p. 632); yaws (p. 634); granuloma inguinale [often abscesses also] (p. 616).
Plasma cells prominent	Syphilis (p. 632); yaws (p. 634); lymphogranuloma venereum (p. 620); chancroid (p. 617); visceral leishmaniasis (p. 702); trypanosomiasis (p. 702); arthropod bites [an uncommon pattern]; vibrio infection (p. 600).
Eosinophils prominent	Arthropod bites (p. 725); helminth infestation (p. 711); coelenterate contact (p. 708); subcutaneous phycomycosis (p. 661).
Neutrophils prominent	Impetigo [subcorneal neutrophils] (p. 596); ecthyma (p. 598); cellulitis (p. 600); erysipelas [prominent superficial oedema also] (p. 599); granuloma inguinale [microabscesses] (p. 616); chancroid [superficial neutrophils] (p. 617); erythema nodosum leprosum (p. 614); Lucio's phenomenon (p. 614); anthrax (p. 615); yaws (p. 634) and pinta (p. 635) [both have intraepidermal abscesses]; blastomycosis-like pyoderma (p. 601); actinomycosis (p. 660); nocardiosis (p. 659); mycetoma (p. 658); fungal kerion (p. 644); phaeohyphomycosis (p. 654); aspergillosis (p. 662); mucormycosis [also infarction present] (p. 661); flea bites (p. 725).
Parasitized macrophages	Rhinoscleroma (p. 617); granuloma inguinale (p. 616); lepromatous leprosy (p. 614); histoplasmosis (p. 652); leishmaniasis (p. 702); toxoplasmosis [pseudocysts present] (p. 705).
Parasitized multinucleate giant cells or foreign body reaction	Various fungal infections; prototheccosis (p. 664); schistosomiasis (p. 711); demodex within tissues; some other mite infestations.
Superficial and deep dermal perivascular lymphocytic inflammation	Leprosy [indeterminate stage] (p. 612); secondary syphilis [often plasma cells present] (p. 633); arthropod bites (p. 725) and coral reactions (p. 708) [usually interstitial eosinophils also]; onchocercal dermatitis [microfilariae in lymphatics] (p. 713).
Psoriasiform epidermal hyperplasia	Chronic candidosis (p. 646); tinea imbricata (p. 644); chronic dermatophytoses [rare] (p. 644).

Continued opposite

Table 22.1 Histological patterns in infections and infestations (cont'd)

Pseudoepitheliomatous or irregular epidermal hyperplasia	Amoebiasis (p. 701); toxoplasmosis [rare] (p. 705); mucocutaneous leishmaniasis (p. 702); schistosomiasis (p. 711); chronic arthropod bite reactions [rare] (p. 725); yaws (p. 634); rhinoscleroma (p. 617); granuloma inguinale (p. 616); blastomycosis-like pyoderma [oblique follicles and draining sinuses] (p. 601); tuberculosis [tuberculosis verrucosa and some infections by atypical mycobacteria] (p. 604); vibrio infection (p. 600); certain deep fungal infections⋆⋆; human papilloma virus infections (p. 687); milker's nodule (p. 680) and orf (p. 681) [both these may have thin, long rete pegs].
Folliculitis and/or perifolliculitis	Syphilis [rare cases] (p. 633); dermatophytoses (p. 643); pityrosporum folliculitis (p. 650); pyogenic bacterial infections (p. 442); herpes simplex (p. 683); herpes zoster (p. 685); demodex infestations (p. 719); larva migrans [eosinophilic folliculitis] (p. 714).
Vasculitis	Erythema nodosum leprosum (p. 614); Lucio's phenomenon (p. 614); ecthyma gangrenosum (p. 598); necrotizing fasciitis (p. 600); meningococcal and gonococcal septicaemia (p. 603); cytomegalovirus infection [endothelial cell inclusion bodies] (p. 685); rickettsial infections [lymphocytic vasculitis] (p. 620); spider bites (p. 718); papulonecrotic tuberculid (p. 607).
Tissue necrosis	Ecthyma gangrenosum (p. 598); necrotizing fasciitis (p. 600); diphtheria (p. 602); anthrax (p. 615); tularaemia (p. 618); cat-scratch disease (p. 618); severe lepra reactional states (p. 614); scrofuloderma (p. 606); *Mycobacterium ulcerans* infections (p. 608); papulonecrotic tuberculid (p. 607); chancroid [superficial necrosis only] (p. 617); rickettsial infections [eschar present] (p. 620); mucormycosis (p. 661); gnat, spider and beetle bites (p. 718); acute tick bites (p. 718); stonefish and stingray contact (p. 709); orf (p. 681); amoebiasis (p. 701).
Epidermal spongiosis	Dermatophytoses (p. 643); candidosis (p. 645); cercarial dermatitis [eosinophils and neutrophils also] (p. 712); larva migrans (p. 714); chigger bites (p. 722); other arthropod bites; contact with moths of the genus *Hylesia* (p. 725); delayed reactions to coelenterates (p. 708).
Intraepidermal vesiculation	Herpes simplex, herpes zoster, varicella [all three have ballooning degeneration and intranuclear inclusions] (p. 683); orf (p. 681) and milker's nodule (p. 680) [both have pale superficial cytoplasm]; hand-foot-and-mouth disease (p. 692); erysipeloid [also superficial dermal oedema] (p. 599); beetle bites (p. 725); certain other arthropod bites [may be bullous in hypersensitive persons]; dermatophytoses (p. 643); candidosis (p. 645).
Parasite in tissue sections	Helminth and arthropod infestations; certain injuries from forms of marine life.
'Invisible dermatoses' (section stained with H&E appears normal at first glance)	Erythrasma (p. 602); pityriasis versicolor [spores and hyphae usually easily seen] (p. 649); dermatophytoses [compact orthokeratosis, neutrophils in the stratum corneum or the 'sandwich sign' often present] (p. 643); pitted keratolysis [crateriform defects, pits or pallor of the stratum corneum are usually obvious, as are bacteria] (p. 603).

⋆   These infections are more suppurative than granulomatous; the latter component is not always present.

⋆⋆   'Deep fungal infections' is used here to include North American blastomycosis, sporotrichosis, chromomycosis, coccidioidomycosis, paracoccidioidomycosis, subcutaneous phycomycosis and phaeohyphomycosis.

Bacterial and rickettsial infections (other than spirochaetal infections)

INTRODUCTION

Various bacteria form part of the normal resident flora of the skin. In certain circumstances some of these may assume pathogenic importance. Other bacteria are present only in pathological circumstances. In this chapter the following categories of bacterial infections will be considered — pyogenic, corynebacterial, neisserial, mycobacterial, miscellaneous, chlamydial and rickettsial. *Pyogenic infections*, usually caused by *Staphylococcus aureus* and strains of *Streptococcus*, are numerically the most important bacterial infections of the skin. Two distinct groups (superficial and deep) can be distinguished on the basis of the anatomical level of involvement of the skin. The pyogenic infections, with the exception of the staphylococcal 'scalded skin' syndrome which results from the effects of a bacterial exotoxin, are characterized histologically by a heavy infiltrate of neutrophils. These organisms may also infect hair follicles, resulting in folliculitis (see Ch. 15, pp. 439 & 442).

Corynebacterial infections, with the exception of diphtheria, are usually limited to the stratum corneum and, as a consequence, there is no significant inflammatory response: at first glance, the biopsy may appear normal.

Neisserial infections of the skin are rare, although they are an important cause of urethritis. Cutaneous lesions may occur in neisserial septicaemias.

Mycobacterial infections usually result in a granulomatous tissue reaction, but this depends on the immune status of the individual, including the development of delayed hypersensitivity.

Exceptions include lepromatous leprosy, in which a histiocytic response occurs, and some infections by atypical mycobacteria, in which suppurative granulomas, suppuration, and even non-specific chronic inflammation may result at various times.

A variety of inflammatory reactions can be seen in the group of *miscellaneous bacterial infections* of the skin. This chapter closes with a brief discussion of *chlamydial infections* and *rickettsial infections*. Each group will be discussed in turn.

Infections by the actinomycetes are considered in Chapter 25 (pages 658–660).

SUPERFICIAL PYOGENIC INFECTIONS

The superficial pyogenic infections of the skin (pyodermas) include impetigo and its variants and ecthyma. They also include the superficial infections of the hair follicles which are dealt with in Chapter 15 (pages 439–441). In addition, the staphylococcal 'scalded skin' syndrome can be included in this category, although the lesions result from the action of bacterial toxin rather than local infection itself.

IMPETIGO

Impetigo is an acute, superficial pyoderma which heals without scar formation. It is the most common bacterial infection of the skin in childhood.[1] Adults are sometimes affected, particularly athletes, military personnel and those in institutions.[2] Minor trauma, especially from insect bites, as well as poor hygiene and a warm, humid climate, all predispose to this infection.[3]

There are two clinical forms of impetigo, a common, vesiculopustular type and a bullous variant which is considerably less frequent.[4,5] Recent studies have shown that *Staphylococcus aureus* is now the usual organism isolated from the common type of impetigo,[6,7] which in the past was caused mostly by a Group A beta-haemolytic streptococcus, sometimes with *S. aureus* as a secondary invader.[2,8] The bullous form has always been related exclusively to *S. aureus*, usually of phage group II.[9]

Common impetigo ('school sores') commences as thin-walled vesicles or pustules on an erythematous base: the lesions rapidly rupture to form a thick, golden crust.[10] Common impetigo occurs as a solitary lesion or a cluster of several lesions which may coalesce. It is found on the face or extremities.[7] Local lymphadenopathy may be present.

Bullous impetigo is composed of shallow erosions and flaccid bullae, 0.5 – 3 cm in diameter, with an erythematous rim.[2] This has a thin roof which soon ruptures, resulting in a thin crust.[9] There may be a localized collection of a few bullae, or more generalized lesions.[11] Bullous impetigo is included with the staphylococcal epidermolytic toxin syndrome as the lesions result from the production in situ of an epidermolytic toxin by staphylococci.[2]

Histopathology

Common impetigo is rarely biopsied as the diagnosis can be made on clinical grounds. An early lesion will show a subcorneal collection of neutrophils with exocytosis of these cells through the underlying epidermis. A few acantholytic cells are sometimes seen but this is never a prominent feature. Established lesions show a thick surface crust composed of serum, neutrophils in various stages of breakdown and some parakeratotic material. Gram-positive cocci can

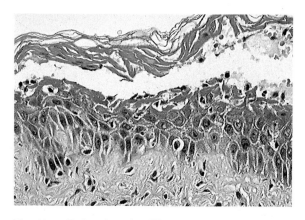

Fig. 23.1 Bullous impetigo. There is a subcorneal blister containing a few inflammatory cells and degenerate keratinocytes. Gram-positive cocci were found. Dermal inflammation is unusually mild.
Haematoxylin — eosin

usually be found without difficulty in the surface crust.

In *bullous impetigo*, the subcorneal bulla contains a few acantholytic cells, a small number of neutrophils and some Gram-positive cocci (Fig. 23.1).[9] In contrast to the lesions of the staphylococcal 'scalded skin' syndrome there is usually a mild to moderate mixed inflammatory cell infiltrate in the underlying papillary dermis.[9]

STAPHYLOCOCCAL 'SCALDED SKIN' SYNDROME (SSSS)

This condition results from the production of an epidermolytic toxin by certain strains of *Staphylococcus aureus*, most notably type 71 of phage group II.[2] These organisms are responsible for a preceding upper respiratory tract infection, conjunctivitis or carrier state. Rarely, the syndrome follows a staphylococcal infection complicating varicella or measles.[12,13]

The SSSS predominantly affects healthy infants and children younger than six years, apparently reflecting an inability to handle and excrete the toxin.[14] Rarely neonates are involved, a condition which was known in the past as Ritter's disease (Ritter von Rittershain's disease).[15-17] A few cases have been reported in adults in whom there has usually been underlying immunosuppression (including the acquired immunodeficiency syndrome)[18] and/or renal insufficiency.[19-23]

There is sudden onset of skin tenderness and a scarlatiniform eruption which is followed by the development of large, easily-ruptured, flaccid bullae and a positive Nikolsky sign.[17,24] Desquamation of large areas of the skin occurs in sheets and ribbons.[23] Occasionally, only the scarlatiniform eruption develops. The usual sites of involvement are the face, neck and trunk, including the axillae and groins. Mucous membranes are not involved.

The disease has a good prognosis in children, with spontaneous healing after several days, as a consequence of the formation of neutralizing antibodies to the epidermolytic toxin.[25] In adults, a staphylococcal septicaemia, sometimes fatal, may ensue.

Desquamation results from effects of an exotoxin of low molecular weight, produced by certain strains of *Staphylococcus aureus*. The condition can be reproduced in newborn mice by the subcutaneous or intraperitoneal injection of these organisms.[26]

Staphylococcal epidermolytic toxin syndrome

The SSSS, which was historically considered (incorrectly) to be a variant of toxic epidermal necrolysis (see p. 45), has been regarded as belonging to the staphylococcal epidermolytic toxin syndrome.[27-29] Also included in this concept are localized and generalized bullous impetigo, which result from the local production (as opposed to production at a distant site, as in SSSS) of a similar staphylococcal epidermolytic toxin.[12] Consequently, in bullous impetigo, the organisms may be demonstrated within the lesion. Impetigo is discussed in further detail above.

Histopathology[24]

In the SSSS, there is subcorneal splitting of the epidermis. A few acantholytic cells and sparse neutrophils may be present within the blister, although it is often difficult to obtain an intact lesion. A sparse, mixed inflammatory cell infiltrate is present in the underlying dermis. This is in contrast to generalized bullous impetigo and even pemphigus foliaceus, in which the dermal infiltrate is heavier.

Immunofluorescence is negative, in contrast to pemphigus foliaceus in which intercellular immunoreactants are usually demonstrable.

Electron microscopy. There is widening of the intercellular spaces followed by disruption of desmosome attachments through their central density.[2,26] There are no cytotoxic changes.

TOXIC SHOCK SYNDROME

The toxic shock syndrome was first recognized a decade ago in healthy menstruating women who used tampons.[29a] It results from a toxin produced by certain strains of *Staphylococcus aureus* which proliferate in the vagina and cervix. The toxic shock syndrome can also complicate wound infections with *S. aureus*.[29b] The clinical features of this syndrome include a fever, hypotension, inflammation of mucous membranes, vomiting and diarrhoea, and cutaneous lesions that resemble viral exanthemata or erythema multiforme.[29c] The skin lesions undergo desquamation in time.

Histopathology[29c]

The characteristic features of the toxic shock syndrome are small foci of epidermal spongiosis containing a few neutrophils, scattered degenerate keratinocytes, sometimes arranged in clusters, and a superficial perivascular and interstitial cell infiltrate.[29c] The infiltrate contains lymphocytes, neutrophils and sometimes eosinophils.[29c] Inflammatory cells often extend into the walls of the superficial dermal vessels, as seen in vasculitis, but there is no fibrin extravasation. Less constant features include irregular epidermal acanthosis, oedema of the papillary dermis, extravasation of erythrocytes, and nuclear 'dust' in the vicinity of the blood vessels.[29c] Focal parakeratosis, containing neutrophils and serum, may also be present.

ECTHYMA

Ecthyma is a deeper pyoderma than impetigo and much less frequent.[4] It has a predilection for the extremities of children, often at sites of minor trauma, which allows entry of the causative bacteria. Group A streptococci, particularly *Streptococcus pyogenes*, are usually implicated, although coagulase-positive staphylococci are sometimes isolated as well.[5,30] The lesions, which are sometimes multiple, consist of a dark crust adherent to a shallow ulcer and surrounded by a rim of erythema. Scarring usually results when the lesions heal.[5]

Ecthyma gangrenosum is a severe variant of ecthyma seen in 5% or more of immunosuppressed individuals who develop a septicaemia with *Pseudomonas aeruginosa*.[31] It com-

mences as an erythematous macule on the trunk or limbs: the lesion rapidly becomes vesicular, then pustular, and finally develops into a gangrenous ulcer with a dark eschar and an erythematous halo.[32,33] Constitutional symptoms are usually present. Patients with solitary lesions have a better prognosis than those with multiple lesions. Similar necrotic ulcers have been reported in association with aspergillus infection, candidosis, and following pseudomonas folliculitis (but usually without septicaemia).[31] *Pseudomonas aeruginosa* septicaemia may result in the development of bullae[34] or of a nodular cellulitis[35] rather than ecthyma gangrenosum.

Histopathology

In ecthyma, there is ulceration of the skin with an inflammatory crust on the surface. There is a heavy infiltrate of neutrophils in the reticular dermis which forms the base of the ulcer. Gram-positive cocci may be seen within the inflammatory crust.

Ecthyma gangrenosum shows necrosis of the epidermis and the upper dermis with some haemorrhage into the dermis.[32] The epidermis may separate from the dermis. A mixed inflammatory cell infiltrate surrounds the infarcted region. In some cases, there is a paucity of inflammation.[32,33] A necrotizing vasculitis with vascular thrombosis is present in the margins.[35] Numerous Gram-negative bacteria are usually present between the collagen bundles, and sometimes in the media and adventitia of small blood vessels.

DEEP PYOGENIC INFECTIONS (CELLULITIS)

Cellulitis is a diffuse inflammation of the connective tissue of the skin and/or the deeper soft tissues.[5,36,37] It is therefore a deeper pyoderma than impetigo and some cases of ecthyma, although ecthyma gangrenosum could be included in this category. Clinically, cellulitis presents as an expanding area of erythema which is usually oedematous and tender.[38] Necrosis sometimes supervenes.[39] In the past, these infections were usually caused by beta-haemolytic streptococci and/or coagulase-positive staphylococci.[5] A diverse range of organisms is now implicated in the causation of cellulitis.[36,39a]

Many different clinical variants of cellulitis have been reported, some with overlapping clinical features and causative bacteria.[38] This has led to a proliferation of terms for these different variants. The term 'gangrenous and crepitant cellulitis' has been used for a subset with prominent skin necrosis and/or the discernible presence of gas in the tissues.[39]

The cellulitides are characterized histopathologically by an infiltrate of neutrophils throughout the dermis and/or the subcutaneous tissue with variable subepidermal oedema and vascular ectasia. In those variants with necrosis there is usually a necrotizing vasculitis, which may be associated with fibrin thrombi in the lumen.[40,41] Bacteria are often numerous in the group with necrosis, although usually only a few can be isolated in the other variants.[42]

ERYSIPELAS

Erysipelas is a distinctive type of cellulitis which has an elevated border and spreads rapidly.[5] Vesiculation may develop, particularly at the edge of the lesion. The condition occurs particularly on the lower extremities, and less commonly on the face.[43,44] Underlying diabetes mellitus, peripheral vascular disease or lymphoedema may be present.[43] The causative group A streptococci,[37,45] or other organisms[46] gain entry through superficial abrasions. Bacteriaemia is uncommon.[5]

Histopathology

There is marked subepidermal oedema which may lead to the formation of vesiculobullous lesions. Beneath this zone there is a diffuse and usually heavy infiltrate of neutrophils, but abscesses do not form. The infiltrate is sometimes accentuated around blood vessels. There is often vascular and lymphatic dilatation. In healing lesions, the dermal infiltrate diminishes and

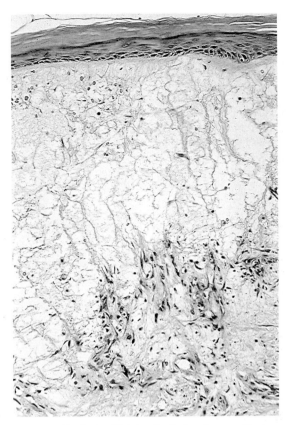

Fig. 23.2 Erysipelas. This healing lesion shows residual subepidermal oedema and underlying granulation tissue. The inflammatory cell infiltrate was deep to this zone. Haematoxylin — eosin

granulation tissue may form immediately below the zone of subepidermal oedema (Fig. 23.2). Direct immunofluorescence has been used to confirm the streptococcal aetiology of most cases of erysipelas.[45]

ERYSIPELOID

Erysipeloid is an uncommon infection, usually found on the hands, which clinically resembles erysipelas.[47] The causative organism, *Erysipelothrix rhusiopathiae*, is a contaminant of dead organic matter, and infection with this organism is an occupational hazard for fish and meat handlers. Less commonly, multiple cutaneous lesions or systemic spread of the organism may occur.

Histopathology[47]

There is usually massive oedema of the papillary dermis overlying a diffuse and polymorphous infiltrate composed of lymphocytes, plasma cells and variable numbers of neutrophils. Sometimes there is spongiosis of the epidermis leading to intraepidermal vesiculation. Organisms are not demonstrable in tissue sections, even with a Gram stain, possibly because they are present in the L form (without a cell wall).[47]

BLISTERING DISTAL DACTYLITIS

This is an uncommon, yet distinctive infection localized to the volar fat pad of the distal phalanx of the fingers.[5,48,48a] Group A streptococci are usually implicated.[48b] The blistering results from massive subepidermal oedema.

CELLULITIS

In addition to its use as a synonym for 'deep pyogenic infection' (see above), the term cellulitis is sometimes used in a more restricted sense for spreading inflammation of the cheek,[49–51] periorbital area[52] or perineum,[53] or in the margins of wounds.[5] The lesions lack the distinct border of erysipelas.[5] Various organisms have been implicated as the cause of this condition, including *Haemophilus influenzae* type b in the case of facial lesions[51] and *Vibrio vulnificus* in some infections of the extremities.[54] The latter organism can produce various lesions, including haemorrhagic bullae,[55,55a] cellulitis and necrotizing fasciitis.[56]

Histopathology

The appearances are similar to those of erysipelas; focal necrosis is sometimes present. Involvement of the subcutis may lead to a predominantly septal panniculitis.[40,54]

NECROTIZING FASCIITIS

This is a rare and distinct form of cellulitis that rapidly progresses to necrosis of the skin and underlying tissues.[57,57a] It involves tissues at a deeper level than erysipelas and may spread into the underlying muscle.[58] Necrotizing fasciitis commences as a poorly defined area of erythema, usually on the leg;[57] serosanguineous blisters develop and subsequently necrosis occurs at their centre.[59,60] Constitutional symptoms may be present, and there is a significant mortality.[58] Various organisms have been isolated, particularly Group A streptococci.[60] *Fournier's gangrene of the scrotum* is a closely related entity.[59]

Histopathology[57,57a]

Necrotizing fasciitis is a form of septic vasculitis with inflammation of the walls of vessels, sometimes associated with occlusion of the lumen by thrombi.[41] There is a mixed inflammatory cell infiltrate in the viable tissues bordering the areas of necrosis. The necrosis involves the epidermis, dermis and upper subcutis.

MISCELLANEOUS SYNDROMES

There are several rare but distinct clinicopathological entities which belong to the category of deep pyogenic infections. They include clostridial myonecrosis (gas gangrene), progressive bacterial synergistic gangrene and erosive pustular dermatosis of the scalp.[39]

Clostridial myonecrosis (gas gangrene) is associated with muscle and soft tissue necrosis. Cutaneous lesions, including bullae and necrosis, may overlie the deeper lesions. Large Gram-positive bacilli are present in the affected tissues.[39]

Progressive bacterial synergistic gangrene is characterized by indurated, ulcerated areas with a gangrenous margin, usually developing in operative wounds.[39,60a] This condition, also known as Meleney's ulcer, is often associated with a mixed growth of peptostreptococci and *Staphylococcus aureus* or enterobacteriaceae.[39]

Erosive pustular dermatosis of the scalp consists of widespread erosions and crusted pustules leading to scarring alopecia.[61–63] Its exact nosological position is uncertain, and there are some morphological similarities to blastomycosis-like pyoderma (see below). The inflammatory infiltrate is usually mixed unless acute areas of pustulation are biopsied.[62] Trauma has been implicated as a predisposing factor, and *Staphylococcus aureus* is sometimes isolated.[62]

BLASTOMYCOSIS-LIKE PYODERMA

Blastomycosis-like pyoderma is an unusual form of pyoderma which presents with large verrucous plaques studded with multiple pustules and draining sinuses.[64,65] There may be an underlying disturbance of immunological function in some cases.[65] A variant of this condition is found in subtropical areas of Australia in the actinically-damaged skin of the elderly, particularly on the forearm.[66,67] This has been known as 'coral reef granuloma' on the basis of its clinical appearance.[68] Actinic comedonal plaque, in which plaques and nodules with a cribriform appearance develop in sun-damaged skin,[69] appears to be the end stage of a similar but milder inflammatory process.[66,67] Similar lesions have been reported at the margins of tattoos.[66,70]

Bacteria, particularly *Staphylococcus aureus* and species of *Pseudomonas* and *Proteus*, have been isolated from biopsies.[65,66] Sun-damaged skin is known to diminish local immune responses and this factor is probably important in the variant found in Australia.[71]

Histopathology

There is a heavy inflammatory infiltrate throughout the dermis with multiple small abscesses set in a background of chronic inflammation (Fig. 23.3).[65] Occasionally a few granulomas are present, but these are usually related to elastotic fibres. There is prominent pseudoepitheliomatous hyperplasia which in some areas appears to result from hypertrophy of the follicular infundibulum. Intraepidermal microabscesses are present and these probably represent the attempted transepidermal elimination of the dermal inflammatory process. Solar-elastotic fibres are present

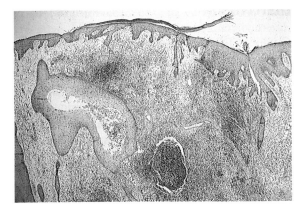

Fig. 23.3 Blastomycosis-like pyoderma. There is dermal suppuration adjacent to enlarged follicular structures which become draining sinuses. Haematoxylin — eosin

in the variants known as 'coral reef granuloma' and 'actinic comedonal plaque'.[69] There may be some dermal fibrosis in healing lesions, although actinic-damaged fibres usually persist in the upper dermis.

CORYNEBACTERIAL INFECTIONS

The corynebacteria are a diverse group of Gram-positive bacilli which include *Corynebacterium diphtheriae*, the causative organism of diphtheria, as well as a bewildering number of species that are found on the skin as part of the normal flora and that defy classification.[72] These latter organisms are usually referred to as diphtheroids or coryneforms. Certain strains have the ability to produce malodour of the axilla.[73] Three skin conditions appear to be related to an overabundance of these coryneforms — erythrasma, trichomycosis and pitted keratolysis.[72] Interestingly, the three conditions have been reported to coexist in the same person.[74] Rarely, other species of corynebacteria have been incriminated as a source of infection in diabetics[75] or immunocompromised patients, the most important being the JK group.[76] These organisms have been found in patients with heart prostheses and endocarditis, and recently as a cause of cutaneous lesions in immunocompromised patients.[76]

In pustular lesions of chronic meningo-coccaemia there are intraepidermal and subepidermal collections of neutrophils. A vasculitis is present in the dermis; the infiltrate contains some lymphocytes in addition to neutrophils.

GONOCOCCAL INFECTIONS

Urethritis ('gonorrhoea') is the usual manifestation of infection with *Neisseria gonorrhoeae*. This sexually transmitted disease may also infect the accessory glands of the vulva and the median raphe of the penis.[101a] Primary infections of extragenital skin are very rare, although pustular lesions on the digits have been reported.[101b]

Gonococcal septicaemia, both acute and chronic, may result in a cutaneous vasculitis; the lesions resemble those seen in meningococcal septicaemia (see above).

Histopathology

Primary pustular lesions on the penis or extragenital skin are usually ulcerated with a heavy inflammatory cell infiltrate in the underlying dermis. There are numerous neutrophils, often forming small abscesses. Gram-negative, intracellular diplococci can usually be found in tissue sections, but they are more easily found in smears made from the purulent exudate on the surface of the lesion.

In gonococcal septicaemia the cutaneous lesions resemble those seen in meningococcal septicaemia (see above); the appearances are those of a septic vasculitis (see p. 223).

MYCOBACTERIAL INFECTIONS

The cutaneous mycobacterioses include leprosy and tuberculosis, as well as a diverse group of infections caused by various environmental (atypical) mycobacteria. Within these three categories there are clinicopathological variants which are sometimes given the status of distinct entities; for example, infections by *Mycobacterium ulcerans* and *M. marinum* (Buruli ulcer and swimming pool granuloma, respectively) are often considered separately from infections caused by other atypical mycobacteria.

Established mycobacterial infections, in general, give rise to a granulomatous tissue reaction, although considerable variability exists in the histopathological appearances of individual lesions.[102] These aspects will be considered further below.

TUBERCULOSIS

Tuberculosis of the skin is declining in incidence all over the world, although it is still an important infective disorder in India and parts of Africa.[103–104a] With the eradication of tuberculosis in cattle, human infections with *Mycobacterium bovis* are rarely seen these days.[105–107] Accordingly, cutaneous tuberculosis can be categorized into two major aetiological groups — infections caused by *Mycobacterium tuberculosis* and those caused by atypical mycobacteria. Infections by atypical mycobacteria will be considered separately. In some of the so-called 'developed countries' such infections are more numerous than those due to *M. tuberculosis*.

Classification

Infections with *M. tuberculosis* have traditionally been classified into primary tuberculosis, when there has been no previous exposure to the organism, and secondary tuberculosis, resulting from reinfection with the tubercle bacillus.[103] Reinfection (secondary) tuberculosis of the skin is subdivided on the basis of various clinical features into lupus vulgaris, tuberculosis verrucosa, scrofuloderma, orificial tuberculosis and disseminated cutaneous tuberculosis.[108] The tuberculids are a further category and are thought to represent a cutaneous reaction to a tuberculous infection elsewhere in the body, there being no detectable bacilli in the tuberculid skin lesions.

Recently, this traditional classification has been disparaged somewhat, and a classification based on the presumed route of infection has been proposed.[109,110] Several modifications have already been suggested, but its basic format remains as follows:[111,112]

a. infections due to inoculation from an *exogenous* source;
b. infections from an *endogenous* source, both contiguous (scrofuloderma in the traditional classification) and from autoinoculation (orificial tuberculosis); and
c. infections resulting from *haematogenous* spread.

The last of these three categories can be further subdivided into lupus vulgaris, acute disseminated tuberculosis, and the formation of cutaneous nodules or abscesses.

This new system of classification has the advantage of applying to infections with atypical mycobacteria as well as those caused by *M. tuberculosis*. However, it still requires assumptions to be made when an attempt is made to classify an individual case. Furthermore, as infections with certain atypical mycobacteria (Buruli ulcer and swimming pool granuloma) are established clinical entities, it seems unlikely that this new classification will offer many advantages over the traditional one. It should also be emphasized that cases occur which defy classification by any means, and it is quite appropriate to diagnose 'cutaneous tuberculosis' in these cases, pending the completion of cultural identification (if obtained).[108,113]

Any classification of cutaneous tuberculosis should also make provision for the complications of BCG vaccination.[114] These include local abscesses and secondary bacterial infections, lupus vulgaris,[115] lymphadenitis, scrofuloderma-like lesions and local keloid formation.[115a] Fatalities have been recorded following BCG vaccination of individuals who are immunocompromised.[116]

The following classification of tuberculosis will be followed here:

Primary tuberculosis
Lupus vulgaris
Tuberculosis verrucosa
Scrofuloderma
Orificial tuberculosis

Disseminated cutaneous tuberculosis
Tuberculids.

Primary tuberculosis

Primary (inoculation) tuberculosis of the skin is the cutaneous analogue of the pulmonary Ghon focus.[117] One to three weeks after introduction of the organism by way of a penetrating injury, a red indurated papule appears.[118–120] This subsequently ulcerates, forming a so-called tuberculoid chancre. Ulcerated lesions may also be a manifestation of secondary (reinfection) tuberculosis when the source of infection may be endogenous or from inoculation, although secondary inoculation tuberculosis usually presents as tuberculosis verrucosa (see below). Regional lymphadenopathy usually develops in primary tuberculosis.

Primary tuberculosis may be associated with tattooing,[118] ritual circumcision or injury by contaminated objects to laboratory workers[121] or to prosectors.[117,122] Atypical mycobacteria are now implicated more often than *M. tuberculosis* in the aetiology of primary tuberculous infection of the skin.

Histopathology[117]

Early lesions show a mixed dermal infiltrate of neutrophils, lymphocytes and plasma cells. This is followed by superficial necrosis and ulceration. After some weeks tuberculoid granulomas form and these may be accompanied by caseation necrosis.[108] Acid-fast bacilli are usually easy to find in the early lesions but there are very few bacilli once granulomas develop.

Lupus vulgaris

Lupus vulgaris is the commonest form of reinfection tuberculosis, occurring predominantly in young adults.[123] It is caused almost exclusively by *M. tuberculosis* although rare reports implicating *M. bovis* have been published in recent years.[106] Lupus vulgaris affects primarily the head and neck region although in South-East Asia it appears to be more common on the extremities and buttocks.[124,125] Lesions involving the nose and face can be destructive.[126] The usual picture is of multiple erythematous papules forming a plaque, which on diascopy shows small 'apple jelly' nodules.[127] Crusted ulcers and dry verrucous plaques are sometimes seen.[124] The disease runs a chronic course and may result in significant scarring. Late complications include the development of contractures, lymphoedema, squamous carcinoma,[102,109,128] and, rarely, basal cell carcinoma,[129] malignant melanoma[130] and cutaneous lymphomas.[131,132]

Histopathology[124]

In lupus vulgaris there are tuberculoid granulomas with a variable mantle of lympho-

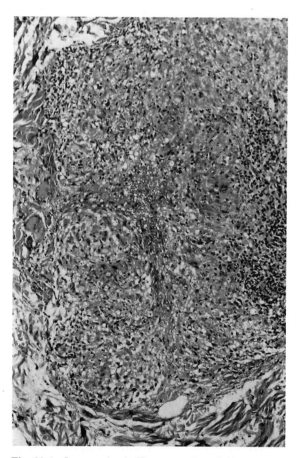

Fig. 23.6 Lupus vulgaris. There are tuberculoid granulomas, with a tendency to confluence, throughout the dermis.
Haematoxylin — eosin

cytes in the upper and mid dermis.[123] The granulomas have a tendency to confluence (Fig. 23.6). Rarely they have a perifollicular arrangement.[132a] Caseation is sometimes present. Multinucleate giant cells are not always numerous. Langerhans cells are present in moderate numbers in the granulomas.[132b] The overlying epidermis may be atrophic or hyperplastic, but only rarely is there pseudoepitheliomatous hyperplasia. Transepidermal elimination of granulomas through a hyperplastic epidermis is rarely seen.[133] Bacilli are usually sparse and difficult to demonstrate in sections stained to show acid-fast organisms.[131] In one report, Michaelis–Gutmann bodies were present in macrophages in the infiltrate.[134]

Sometimes the histological appearances resemble sarcoidosis, with only a relatively sparse lymphocytic mantle around the granulomas: consequent delay in making the correct diagnosis is common in such cases.[109]

Tuberculosis verrucosa

This uncommon form of cutaneous tuberculosis results from inoculation of organisms into the skin in individuals with good immunity.[135] It may occur as an occupational hazard in the autopsy room. A verrucous plaque forms on the back of the hand or fingers.[108,136] The lower extremities are more often involved in cases occurring in India and Hong Kong.[103,135]

Histopathology[136]

There is hyperkeratosis and hyperplasia of the epidermis, often of pseudoepitheliomatous proportions. In the mid dermis there are caseating granulomas.[104] Acid-fast bacilli can usually be found on careful examination of tissue sections.

Scrofuloderma

Scrofuloderma is tuberculous involvement of the skin resulting from direct extension from an underlying tuberculous lesion in lymph nodes or bone.[104] The neck and submandibular region are the most common sites. Scrofuloderma usually presents as an undermined ulcer or discharging sinus with surrounding induration and dusky red discoloration.[104,108]

Atypical mycobacteria are often responsible for this type of infection.

Histopathology[104]

The epidermis is usually atrophic or ulcerated, an underlying abscess and/or caseation necrosis involving the dermis and subcutis.[108] At the periphery of the necrotic tissue there are granulomas. These have fewer lymphocytes than is usual in tuberculosis. Acid-fast bacilli can usually be found in smears taken from the affected area, although they are not always demonstrable in tissue sections.[104]

Orificial tuberculosis

This rare form of cutaneous tuberculosis presents as shallow ulcers at mucocutaneous junctions in patients with advanced internal (usually pulmonary) tuberculosis.[108] It results from autoinoculation.[137]

Histopathology

There is ulceration with underlying caseating granulomas and numerous acid-fast bacilli.

Disseminated cutaneous tuberculosis

This form of cutaneous tuberculosis results from the dissemination of tubercle bacilli from pulmonary, meningeal or other tuberculous foci,[138] particularly in children.[139–142] There may be an underlying disturbance of the immune system predisposing to this widespread infection.[143] The usual presentation is with papules, pustules and vesicles that become necrotic, forming small ulcers.[108,143]

Histopathology[139]

In early lesions there is focal necrosis and abscess formation, with numerous acid-fast bacilli, surrounded by a zone of non-specific chronic inflammation.[108,143] In older lesions granulomas usually develop in this outer zone.

Tuberculids

Tuberculids are a heterogeneous group of cutaneous lesions which occur in association with tuberculous infections elsewhere in the body, or in other parts of the skin,[103] in patients with a high degree of immunity and allergic sensitivity to the organism.[144] Bacteria cannot be isolated from tuberculids.

The concept of tuberculids has been challenged from time to time, but they are usually considered to include erythema induratum, lichen scrofulosorum and papulonecrotic tuberculid;[111] granulomatous phlebitis is possibly a fourth type (phlebitic tuberculid).[144a]

Erythema induratum (Bazin's disease). This is a panniculitis (see p. 502) which presents with bluish-red plaques and nodules with a predilection for the lower part of the legs, particularly the calves.[145] The coexistence of erythema induratum and papulonecrotic tuberculid has been reported.[145a]

Lichen scrofulosorum. This tuberculid is characterized by asymptomatic, slightly scaly papules which measure 0.5 – 3 mm in diameter.[146,147] They are often follicular in distribution, mainly affecting the trunk of children and young adults.[147] Lichen scrofulosorum usually occurs in association with tuberculosis of bone or of lymph nodes, but it may be associated with tuberculous infection in other sites;[146,147] rarely, it may follow BCG vaccination.

Papulonecrotic tuberculid. This presents as dusky papules or nodules that sometimes undergo central necrosis, and that leave varioliform scars on healing.[148] There is a predilection for the extremities although the ears and genital region may also be involved.[135,149,150] In one study, a focus of tuberculosis was identified elsewhere in the body in 38% of cases.[145] The tuberculin test is usually strongly positive and the lesions respond to antituberculous drugs.

increasing number of disseminated infections due to the *M. avium–intracellulare* complex is being reported in patients with the acquired immunodeficiency syndrome (AIDS), although cutaneous lesions are uncommon in these cases.[199]

Histopathology[102]

The changes are not species specific. They include tuberculoid granulomas, poorly formed granulomas, non-specific chronic inflammation, suppuration and intermediate forms.[102] Rare patterns include a septal[205a] or mixed lobular and septal panniculitis,[102] and a diffuse histiocytic infiltrate in the dermis resembling lepromatous leprosy.[197,198] The presence of poorly formed granulomas with intervening chronic inflammation and foci of suppuration should always raise the suspicion of an infection by atypical mycobacteria. The location of the inflammation is inconstant with no specific relationship to the organism or the type of inflammation.[102] Mostly, the inflammation is centred on the dermis with some extension into the subcutis.

Organisms are difficult to find even in preparations stained to demonstrate acid-fast bacilli. They may be plentiful in cases with a histiocytoid pattern and in some infections with *M. avium* and *M. intracellulare*, although they are rarely as plentiful as in infections with *M. ulcerans*. Grains formed of bacillary clumps and somewhat resembling those seen in mycetomas have been reported in a case of *M. chelonei* infection.[204] Intracellular atypical mycobacteria have been said to be PAS positive, according to one report.[206] It should be noted that *Vibrio extorquens*, a rare cause of skin ulcers, is weakly acid-fast in tissue sections;[206a] granulomas may also be present.

LEPROSY

Leprosy (lepra) is a chronic infection caused by *Mycobacterium leprae*. It affects mainly the skin, nasal mucosa and peripheral nerves. There are estimated to be 12–15 million affected persons, worldwide.[207] Leprosy is most prevalent in tropical countries, particularly India, South-East Asia, Central Africa and Central and South America.

M. leprae is an obligate, intracellular, Gram-positive organism which is also acid fast, though less so than *M. tuberculosis*. The organism cannot be grown in vitro, although claims of successful cultivation are made from time to time.[208] *M. leprae* can be grown in the foot-pads of mice and in the nine-banded armadillo, an animal in which natural infection also occurs. *M. leprae* shares many antigens with other mycobacteria; it also possesses a unique antigen, phenolic glycolipid-1 (PG-1).[209]

The incubation period of leprosy is not known with certainty, but is thought to average five years.[209] This uncertainty and the long period make any study of the mode of transmission difficult. The organism is of low infectivity and prolonged and/or close contact with patients who have the disease is considered necessary for transmission to occur.[210] The incidence of conjugal leprosy is low, further testimony to its low infectivity.[207] There may also be a genetic predisposition to the disease. The portal of entry of the organism is not known but the skin and upper respiratory tract, particularly the nasal mucosa, are probable sites.[211] Droplet infection is the most likely mode of transmission, although rare cases of inoculation infection have been recorded.[211,212]

Clinical classification of leprosy

Leprosy exhibits a spectrum of clinical characteristics which correlate with the histopathological changes and the immunological status of the individual.[209,213,214] At one end of the spectrum is tuberculoid leprosy (TT) which is a highly resistant form with few lesions and a paucity of organisms.[215] At the other end is lepromatous leprosy (LL), in which there are numerous lesions with myriad bacilli, and an associated defective cellular immune response.[215] In between these poles there are clinical forms which are classified as borderline-tuberculoid (BT), borderline (BB), and borderline-lepromatous (BL) leprosy. The clinical state of an individual may alter along this scale, although the polar forms (TT and LL) are the most stable and the borderline form (BB) the most labile. This categorization, known as the Ridley–Jopling classification,[214,216] is sometimes modified by the addition of subpolar forms at either end of the spectrum (TTs and LLs). There is also an indeterminate form of leprosy which is classically the first lesion to develop, although it may be overlooked clinically.

Indeterminate leprosy is most often recognized in endemic regions.[217] It presents as single or multiple, slightly hypopigmented or faintly erythematous macules, usually on the limbs.[218] Sensation is normal or slightly impaired. Indeterminate lesions often heal spontaneously, but in approximately 25% of cases this form develops into one of the determinate types, usually in the borderline region of the spectrum.[207] The clinical features of the determinate forms will now be considered in further detail.

Tuberculoid leprosy (TT) is a relatively stable form of leprosy, and the most common type in India and Africa.[207] There are one or several sharply defined, reddish-brown, anaesthetic plaques which are distributed asymmetrically on the trunk or limbs.[219] An enlarged nerve may be seen entering and leaving the plaque; other superficial nerves, such as the ulnar and popliteal nerves, may also be enlarged, leading to nerve palsy.[219] The lepromin test is positive.

Borderline-tuberculoid leprosy (BT) is usually associated with more numerous lesions than tuberculoid leprosy and these are usually smaller. Daughter (satellite) patches may develop. Hypoaesthesia and impairment of hair growth within the lesions are often present.[207]

Borderline leprosy (BB) is an unstable form with erythematous or copper-coloured infiltrated patches which are often annular. Margins are often ill defined.

Borderline-lepromatous leprosy (BL) is associated with more numerous lesions which are less well defined, more shiny, and less anaesthetic than those at the tuberculoid end of the spectrum. Nodular lesions resembling those seen in lepromatous leprosy may be present. A rare subepidermal bullous form has been reported.[220]

Lepromatous leprosy (LL) usually develops from borderline or borderline-lepromatous forms by a downgrading reaction. It is a systemic disease although the primary clinical manifestations are in the skin.[221] Mucosal involvement may lead to ulceration of the nasal septum while nerve lesions may result in acral anaesthesia, claw hand and foot drop.[207] The cutaneous lesions, which are usually symmetrical, include multiple small macules, infiltrated plaques and nodules with poorly defined borders. Multiple facial nodules give a bovine appearance and this is usually accompanied by sparse eyebrows.[207] Various autoantibodies have been demonstrated in this form of leprosy.[222]

Histoid leprosy is a rare variant of the nodular variety of lepromatous leprosy and is characterized by the presence of cutaneous and/or subcutaneous nodules and plaques which are present on apparently normal skin.[223,224] It may be due to a drug-resistant strain of *M. leprae*, as it usually develops in cases of long standing.[224]

Although only a few instances of leprosy have been reported in patients with the acquired immunodeficiency syndrome (AIDS), the long incubation period of leprosy and its occurrence in areas of central Africa where AIDS is also endemic suggest that leprosy complicating AIDS may be a problem in the future.[225]

Reactional states in leprosy[207]

Reactional states are acute episodes which interrupt the usual chronic course and clinical stability of leprosy.[226,227] They are expressions of immunological instability. The reactions, which are major causes of tissue injury and morbidity, have been subdivided into three variants — the lepra reaction (type I), erythema nodosum leprosum (type II), and Lucio's phenomenon (sometimes included with type II reactions, at other times designated type III).[226,228]

Lepra (type I) reactions occur in borderline leprosy and are usually associated with a shift towards the tuberculoid pole (upgrading) as a result of an increase in delayed hypersensitivity. Uncommonly the shift is towards the lepromatous pole (a downgrading reaction).[227,229] Lepra reactions are often seen in the first six months or so of therapy, but they may occur in untreated patients or be associated with pregnancy, stress or intercurrent infections. They are characterized by oedema and increased erythema of skin lesions, sometimes accompanied by ulceration and the development of new lesions. Constitutional symptoms and neuritis may be present.

Erythema nodosum leprosum (type II reaction) occurs in 25–70% of all cases of lepromatous leprosy[226] and occasionally in association with the borderline-lepromatous form.[230,231] There are crops of painful, erythematous and violaceous nodules, particularly involving the extremities.[232] Individual lesions last 7–20 days.[233] Severe constitutional symptoms may be present.[233] The pattern varies somewhat in severity in different ethnic groups,[228] necrotizing lesions sometimes developing.[234] Type II reactions are the result of an immune-complex-mediated vasculitis.[230]

Lucio's phenomenon is seen mainly in Mexicans with the diffuse non-nodular form of lepromatous leprosy.[233,235] It is rare in other ethnic groups.[236] Haemorrhagic ulcers form as a result of the underlying necrotizing vasculitis[237] or of vascular occlusion from endothelial swelling and thrombosis.[235]

Histopathology[207,216]

Skin biopsies should include the full thickness of the dermis and should be taken from the most active edge of a lesion. The bacilli may be detected in tissue sections using the Fite–Faraco staining method or an immunofluorescent technique.[238]

Two distinct types of histological change are found in leprosy — the *lepromatous reaction*, in which there are large numbers of macrophages in the dermis parasitized with acid-fast bacilli (Fig. 23.8), and the *tuberculoid reaction*, in which there are tubercle-like aggregates of epithelioid cells, multinucleate giant cells and lymphocytes bacilli being difficult to find. These histological patterns are seen at either end of the clinical spectrum of leprosy; features overlapping with those of borderline forms may be present. Sometimes there is a disparity between the clinical and histological subclassification of

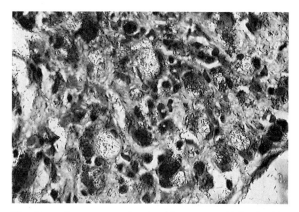

Fig. 23.8 Lepromatous leprosy. Numerous acid-fast bacilli are present within macrophages and lying free in the dermis. Wade–Fite

leprosy.[239] Early lesions of leprosy are mostly of indeterminate or tuberculoid type.[240]

Indeterminate leprosy is characterized by a superficial and deep dermal infiltrate around blood vessels, dermal appendages and nerves; the infiltrate is composed predominantly of lymphocytes with a few macrophages.[214] Mast cells are markedly increased in number and they may extend into the small nerves in the deep dermis.[241] Less than 5% of the dermis is involved by the infiltrate.[241] Mild proliferation of Schwann cells may occur, but marked neural thickening is quite uncommon.[218] There may be a few lymphocytes in the epidermis; this is one of the earliest changes to occur in leprosy.[240] Bacilli are usually quite difficult to find,[240] but if serial sections are cut and a small dermal nerve is followed, sooner or later a single bacillus or a small group of bacilli will be discovered.[217] The mechanism of the hypopigmentation in this and other forms of leprosy is still not clear. There is a reduction in melanin in the basal layer; in some reports a decreased number of melanocytes has also been recorded.[242]

Tuberculoid leprosy shows a tuberculoid reaction throughout the dermis with non-caseating granulomas composed of epithelioid cells, some Langhans giant cells and lymphocytes (Fig. 23.9).[219] The predominant lymphocyte present is the T-helper cell which is found throughout the granuloma while T-suppressor cells predominate in the lymphocyte mantle which surrounds

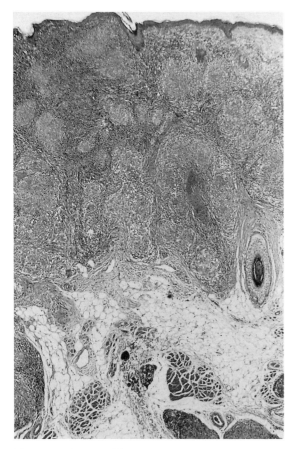

Fig. 23.9 Tuberculoid leprosy. Non-caseating granulomas extend throughout the dermis.
Haematoxylin — eosin

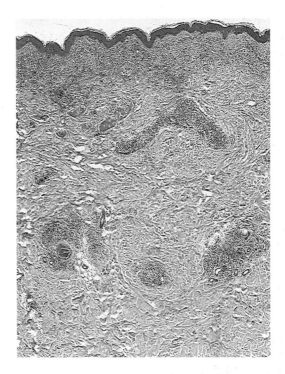

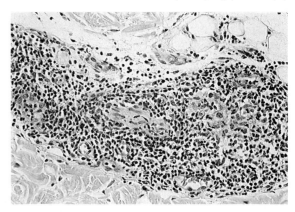

Fig. 23.10a,b Borderline leprosy. There is a superficial and deep infiltrate of lymphocytes with periappendageal and perineural extension. Epithelioid cells are present.
Haematoxylin — eosin

the granulomas.[243,244] Granulomas may erode the undersurface of the epidermis and they may also extend into peripheral nerves and into the arrectores pilorum.[219] Inflammation often engulfs the sweat glands.[240] Bacilli are found in less than 50% of cases.[219]

Borderline-tuberculoid leprosy differs from tuberculoid leprosy in several ways.[207] Tubercle formation may be less evident and nerve destruction is not as complete. A subepidermal grenz zone is invariably present. Lymphocytes and Langhans cells are usually not as plentiful in the granulomas as in tuberculoid leprosy.

In *borderline leprosy* there are collections of epithelioid cells without the formation of well-defined granulomas. Langhans giant cells are absent and lymphocytes are more dispersed.

Occasional bacilli can be found (Fig. 23.10).

In borderline-lepromatous leprosy there are small collections of macrophages rather than epithelioid cells. These large cells have abundant granular cytoplasm, although a few may have foamy cytoplasm as seen in lepromatous leprosy.[207] A variable number of lymphocytes is present and some of these are in the vicinity of small dermal nerves. A grenz zone is present in both borderline-lepromatous and true lepromatous biopsy. Bacilli are easily found.

Lepromatous leprosy is characterized by collections and sheets of heavily parasitized macrophages with a sparse sprinkling of lymphocytes, the majority of which are of suppressor type.[244] In older lesions, the macrophages have a foamy appearance (lepra cells, Virchow cells). Numerous acid-fast bacilli are present in macrophages, sweat glands, nerves, Schwann cells and vascular endothelium,[245] a finding which has been confirmed by electron microscopy.[246] The organisms in the macrophages may be arranged in parallel array, forming clusters, or in large masses known as globi (Fig. 23.11).

In *histoid leprosy* there are circumscribed nodular lesions consisting predominantly of spindle-shaped cells with some polygonal forms.

The cells are arranged in an intertwining pattern.[223,224] Small collections of foamy macrophages may also be present. The component cells contain numerous acid-fast bacilli which are longer than the usual bacilli of leprosy and are aligned along the long axis of the cell.[224]

Lepra (type I) reactions show oedema, an increase in lymphocytes and sometimes giant cells as well as the formation of small clusters of epithelioid cells.[247,248] In severe cases, fibrinoid necrosis may be present and this is followed by scarring.[229] This is the picture seen in the usual upgrading reaction. In downgrading reactions there is replacement of lymphocytes and epithelioid cells by collections of macrophages, and there is a corresponding increase in the number of bacilli.[229]

Erythema nodosum leprosum is characterized by oedema of the papillary dermis and a mixed dermal infiltrate of neutrophils and lymphocytes superimposed on collections of macrophages.[230] There are relatively more T lymphocytes of helper-inducer type than in non-reactive lepromatous leprosy.[243,249] A vasculitis may also be present.[230,233] There may be involvement of the subcutis, with the development of a mixed lobular and septal panniculitis; however, in the majority of cases involvement of the dermis is the primary and predominant finding.[234] Macrophages in the dermis contain fragmented organisms.[250] Direct immunofluorescence reveals the presence of C3 and IgG in the walls of dermal blood vessels.[230]

Lucio's phenomenon is usually the result of a necrotizing vasculitis of the small vessels in the upper and mid dermis with associated infarction of the epidermis.[233] At other times there is prominent endothelial swelling and thrombosis of superficial vessels without a vasculitis.[235] The endothelial cells and macrophages in the dermis contain numerous bacilli.[233,236] There is usually only a mild inflammatory infiltrate, with fewer neutrophils than in erythema nodosum leprosum.[236]

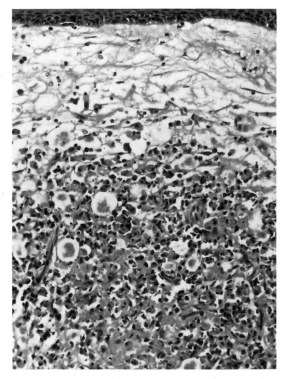

Fig. 23.11   Lepromatous leprosy with masses of organisms (globi) in the cytoplasm of macrophages. Haematoxylin — eosin

MISCELLANEOUS BACTERIAL INFECTIONS

ANTHRAX

Anthrax is mainly an occupational disease occurring in those who handle hair, wool, hide or carcasses of infected animals.[251] The causative organism, *Bacillus anthracis*, may enter the body by the skin or by inhalation or ingestion. Anthrax is now an exceedingly rare infection.[252]

The initial cutaneous lesion is usually on an exposed site. It begins as a papule which soon becomes bullous and then ulcerates, with the formation of a haemorrhagic crust (eschar). A ring of satellite vesicles may form. Haemorrhagic lymphadenopathy, constitutional symptoms, and even a fatal septicaemia may accompany the cutaneous lesion.

Histopathology[251]

There is necrosis of the epidermis and upper dermis with surrounding oedema, fibrin extravasation and haemorrhage. The blood vessels are conspicuously dilated. Inflammatory cells are often surprisingly sparse, although sometimes a florid cellulitis is present. Spongiosis and vesiculation may occur in the epidermis adjacent to the ulceration.

B. anthracis can be seen, usually in large numbers, in the exudate. It is easily recognized by its large size, square-cut ends and a tendency to be in chains. It is Gram-positive. If antibiotic therapy has been given organisms are sparse and often do not stain positively by the Gram procedure.

BRUCELLOSIS

Cutaneous involvement occurs in from 5–10% of patients with brucellosis.[253] This takes the form of a disseminated papulonodular eruption or a maculopapular rash.[253,254] Occasionally erythema-nodosum-like nodules develop. Skin lesions may not develop for many weeks after the onset of symptoms of brucellosis.[253] A dermatitis has also been reported on the forearms of veterinarians involved in the manual removal of placentas from aborting cows infected with *Brucella abortus*.[254]

Histopathology[253,254]

The maculopapular lesions usually have a non-specific appearance with a mild perivascular infiltrate of lymphocytes in the upper dermis.[254] The papulonodules have an infiltrate of lymphocytes and histiocytes which is both perivascular and periadnexal. There is also focal granulomatous change; multinucleate giant cells are uncommon. Focal exocytosis of inflammatory cells and keratinocyte necrosis may also be present.

The erythema-nodosum-like lesions show a septal panniculitis, with considerable extension of the infiltrate into the fat lobules accompanied by focal necrosis. Plasma cells are also abundant. These features are not usually associated with lesions of typical erythema nodosum.

YERSINIOSIS

Yersiniosis is a generally accepted term for diseases caused by *Yersinia pseudotuberculosis* and *Y. enterocolitica*. The incidence of cutaneous manifestations in yersiniosis is not known, although in some countries the disease is responsible for 10% or more of cases of erythema nodosum.[255,256] Erythema multiforme and figurate and non-specific erythemas may also occur.[255,257]

Histopathology

As in brucellosis, the erythema-nodosum-like lesions may show some extension of the infiltrate into the fat lobules, as well as a necrotizing vasculitis and some necrosis.[255] The appearances in some cases are more in keeping with nodular vasculitis than erythema nodosum.

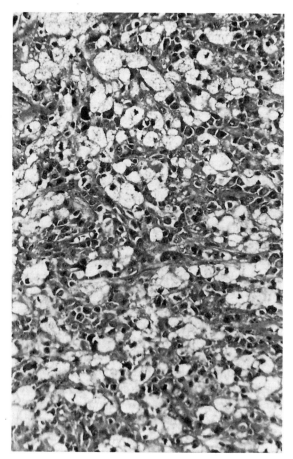

Fig. 23.14 Rhinoscleroma. The inflammatory infiltrate consists of an admixture of plasma cells and vacuolated macrophages (Mikulicz cells).
Haematoxylin — eosin

ulceration or atrophy of the overlying mucosa. Sometimes the mucosa is hyperplastic, even to the extent of pseudoepitheliomatous hyperplasia.[278]

Electron microscopy. The vacuolated Mikulicz cells are macrophages with phagosomes containing bacterial mucopolysaccharide as well as some bacteria.[277] There is often fragmentation of the limiting membrane of some of the phagosomes.[277] Plasma cells are sometimes vacuolated to a limited extent. Russell bodies are readily seen in the plasma cells and extracellularly.

TULARAEMIA

Tularaemia is named after Tulare County, California, where its occurrence was first recognized.[279] It is caused by *Francisella tularensis*, a minute Gram-negative coccobacillus which produces a fatal insect-borne septicaemic infection in ground squirrels and other rodents. The disease is transmitted to man either by the bite of an infected vector, such as mosquitoes or ticks,[280] or by contact with an infected rodent or rabbit.[279-281] It has been recognized in parts of the United States of America,[282,283] Canada[284] and the Soviet Union, and rarely in the British Isles and other parts of Europe. Skin lesions occur only in the ulceroglandular form of the disease. This is characterized by a papule at the site of the initial inoculation, followed by an ascending lymphangitis. Nodules develop along the course of the affected lymphatics, as in the lymphangitic type of sporotrichosis.[279] The occurrence of erythema nodosum and erythema multiforme has been described. Severe constitutional symptoms are usual.[285]

Histopathology

The primary lesion is an ulcer with necrosis involving the epidermis and upper dermis. The adjacent epidermis is usually acanthotic with some spongiosis. In acute lesions there is focal necrosis and suppuration, while in more chronic lesions a granulomatous picture has been described around the necrotic focus in the dermis.

The causative organism cannot be seen in conventional histological preparations. It can be demonstrated in histological sections and in films of exudate by direct immunofluorescence, following treatment with fluorescein-labelled specific antiserum.[282] *F. tularensis* is a hazard to laboratory workers.[283]

CAT-SCRATCH DISEASE

Cat-scratch disease is a self-limited illness characterized by the development at the site of a scratch by a cat of a papule or crusted nodule, which is followed approximately two weeks later by regional lymphadenitis.[286–290] In 1–2% of patients, severe systemic illness may develop: this may include an oculoglandular syndrome, pleurisy, encephalitis, osteomyelitis[291] and splenomegaly.[292] Other cutaneous manifestations have included erythema nodosum, urticaria, erythema marginatum and purpura.[290,293]

Recently, small Gram-negative bacilli have been demonstrated in the skin[287,292] and lymph nodes[292–296] of most cases, using the Warthin–Starry silver stain or the Brown–Hopps modification of the Gram stain. An organism thought to be related to the genus *Rothia* has been isolated,[297] but this remains to be confirmed.

It is now thought that the bacillus responsible for cat-scratch disease, or a related organism, has an aetiological role in the causation of bacillary angiomatosis (epithelioid angiomatosis), a rare vascular proliferation seen in patients with the acquired immunodeficiency syndrome (see p. 955).[298]

Histopathology[287,299]

The epidermal changes are variable and include acanthosis and ulceration. There is usually a zone of necrosis in the upper dermis, and this is surrounded by a mantle of macrophages and lymphocytes. Neutrophils and eosinophils are often present around zones of necrosis. Multinucleate cells and well-defined granulomas may be present. Organisms are seen within macrophages and lying free, particularly in areas of necrosis and suppuration.[292]

MALAKOPLAKIA

Malakoplakia is a rare chronic inflammatory disease which occurs predominantly in the urogenital tract, especially the bladder. More than ten cases involving the skin and subcutaneous tissue have been reported.[300–302] Several of these patients have been immunosuppressed.[303] Cutaneous involvement is usually in the vulva[304] and perianal region,[305,306] where yellow-pink indurated or polypoid masses have been described.

Although the pathogenesis of malakoplakia is uncertain, it appears to result from an acquired defect in the intracellular destruction of phagocytosed bacteria, usually *Escherichia coli*. In the skin, *Staphylococcus aureus* has also been isolated.[307]

Histopathology[300]

Malakoplakia is a chronic inflammatory process characterized by sheets of closely packed macrophages containing PAS-positive, diastase-resistant inclusions (von Hansemann cells). A variable proportion of these cells contains calcospherites with a homogeneous or target-like appearance — the Michaelis–Gutmann bodies. These stain with the von Kossa method.[307] There is a scattering of lymphocytes and plasma cells as well.

CHLAMYDIAL INFECTIONS

Chlamydiae are obligate intracellular organisms which share many features with bacteria, including a discrete cell wall. There are two morphologically distinct species, *C. trachomatis* and *C. psittaci*. The latter species is responsible for psittacosis, a pneumonia derived from infected birds, while different serotypes of *C. trachomatis* are responsible for trachoma, urethritis and lymphogranuloma venereum. The diagnosis can be confirmed by culture of the organism or by serology.

PSITTACOSIS

Psittacosis, caused by *Chlamydia psittaci*, usually presents as a pneumonic illness with various constitutional symptoms. Some patients develop a morbilliform rash or lesions resembling the rose spots of typhoid fever. Erythema nodosum,[308] erythema multiforme, erythema marginatum[309] and disseminated intravascular coagulation[310] with cutaneous manifestations have also been reported. The findings are not specific for psittacosis, either clinically or histopathologically.

LYMPHOGRANULOMA VENEREUM

Lymphogranuloma venereum (LGV, lympho-granuloma inguinale) is a sexually transmitted infection by certain immunotypes of *Chlamydia trachomatis*. Worldwide in distribution,[311] it is most frequent in parts of Asia, Africa and South America. Clinically, three stages are recognized.[312] The initial lesion, which follows a few days or weeks after exposure to the organism, consists of a small papule, ulcer or herpetiform vesicle on the penis, labia or vaginal wall. Extragenital sites of involvement have been recorded.[313] The primary lesion is transient, and often imperceptible. The secondary stage, which follows several weeks after the initial exposure, consists of regional lymphadenopathy. If the inguinal nodes are involved, enlarging buboes develop with draining sinuses. There may be constitutional symptoms at this stage. Erythema multiforme and erythema nodosum rarely develop. The tertiary stage, which is more common in women, encompasses the sequelae of the earlier inflammatory stages. There may be rectal strictures, fistula formation, and rarely genital elephantiasis related to lymphoedema.[314,315]

The organism can be isolated in a tissue culture system or in the yolk sac of eggs.[312] Serological methods are most commonly used to establish a diagnosis. A microimmunofluorescence test can detect antichlamydial antibodies to a range of serological variants of *C. trachomatis*.[312]

Histopathology

The primary lesion is not commonly biopsied. Ulceration is usually present with a dense underlying infiltrate of plasma cells and lymphocytes.[316] There is thickening of vessel walls and some endothelial swelling. Small sinus tracts may lead to the surface. A few epithelioid cell collections may be present.[316]

The characteristic lesions occur in the lymph nodes in the second stage, with the development of stellate abscesses with a poorly formed palisade of epithelioid cells and histiocytes. Sinus formation also occurs. In later lesions there is variable fibrosis.

Direct immunofluorescence, using a fluorescein-labelled antibody to *Chlamydia trachomatis*, has been used to confirm the diagnosis.[317]

RICKETTSIAL INFECTIONS

Rickettsiae are small, obligate intracellular bacteria which are transmitted in most instances by the bite of an arthropod. The various species of rickettsia are endemic in different geographical locations, and this has influenced the naming of some of the infections. Table 23.1 lists the various rickettsial infections of humans, the corresponding aetiological species, and the mode of transmission.

Rickettsiae usually produce an acute febrile illness accompanied by headache, myalgia, malaise and morbidity. Rocky Mountain spotted fever has a mortality of approximately 5%.[318–321] A specific diagnosis is usually made by serological methods, as the attempted isolation of rickettsiae in the laboratory is potentially highly hazardous for the laboratory staff.[322]

Cutaneous lesions are present in most rickettsial infections, with the exception of Q fever. Usually there is a macular or maculo-papular rash; in rickettsialpox the rash may be

Table 23.1   Rickettsial infections

Disease	Organism	Mode of Transmission
Rocky Mountain spotted fever	*R. rickettsi*	Tick
Boutonneuse fever	*R. conori*	Tick
Rickettsialpox	*R. akari*	Mite
Siberian tick typhus	*R. sibirica*	Tick
Queensland tick typhus	*R. australis*	Tick
Epidemic typhus	*R. prowazeki*	Louse faeces
Murine typhus	*R. typhi*	Flea faeces
Scrub typhus	*R. tsutsugamushi*	Mite
Q fever	*Coxiella burneti*	Aerosol

papulovesicular.[323] A more characteristic lesion is the eschar (tache noire), a crusted ulcer, 1 cm or more in diameter, which develops at the site of the arthropod bite.[324] It is thought to result not from the bite but from the inoculation of rickettsiae, which invade vascular endothelial cells.[325] Eschars are characteristic of rickettsialpox,[323] scrub typhus,[326] boutonneuse fever,[327,328] Queensland tick typhus[329] and Siberian tick typhus.[324,327] An eschar is not found in epidemic typhus or in murine typhus, and only rarely in Rocky Mountain spotted fever.[324,327]

Histopathology

The pathological basis for the cutaneous lesions of rickettsial infections is a lymphocytic vasculitis. The eschars result from coagulative necrosis of the epidermis and underlying dermis.[330,331] A crust overlies this region. Bordering the area of necrosis there is a lymphocytic vasculitis with some fibrinoid necrosis of vessels and related dermal haemorrhage.[327] Thrombosis of vessels is sometimes present.[327]

There are often a few neutrophils in the inflammatory infiltrate. Numerous organisms can be demonstrated in vascular endothelium and vessel walls using fluorescein-labelled antisera to the appropriate rickettsial species.

The maculopapular lesions of Rocky Mountain spotted fever show a focal lymphocytic vasculitis with patchy fibrinoid necrosis of small vessels and extravasation of erythrocytes.[332,333] *R. rickettsi* can be demonstrated in endothelium and vascular walls using fluorescein-labelled antisera.[334]

The papulovesicular lesions of rickettsialpox show subepidermal oedema associated with exocytosis of mononuclear cells into the epidermis.[323] These tend to obscure the dermo–epidermal interface. There is a dense perivascular infiltrate in the underlying dermis with prominence of the endothelial cells of the blood vessels and changes indicative of a mild vasculitis.[323] Fibrin thrombi are sometimes present and there may be extravasation of red cells. The causative organism, *R. akari*, has not been identified in tissue sections other than by immunofluorescent techniques.[323]

REFERENCES

Superficial pyogenic infections

1. Hayden GF. Skin diseases encountered in a pediatric clinic. Am J Dis Child 1985; 139: 36–38.
2. Melish ME. Staphylococci, streptococci and the skin. Review of impetigo and the staphylococcal scalded skin syndrome. Semin Dermatol 1982; 1: 101–109.
3. Maddox JS, Ware JC, Dillon HC Jr. The natural history of streptococcal skin infection: Prevention with topical antibiotics. J Am Acad Dermatol 1985; 13: 207–212.
4. Tunnessen WW Jr. Cutaneous infections. Pediatr Clin North Am 1983; 30: 515–532.
5. Tunnessen WW Jr. Practical aspects of bacterial skin infections in children. Pediatr Dermatol 1985; 2: 255–265.
6. Barton LL, Friedman AD. Impetigo: a reassessment of etiology and therapy. Pediatr Dermatol 1987; 4: 185–188.
7. Coskey RJ, Coskey LA. Diagnosis and treatment of impetigo. J Am Acad Dermatol 1987; 17: 62–63.
8. Dajani AS, Ferrieri P, Wannamaker L. Endemic superficial pyoderma in children. Arch Dermatol 1973; 108: 517–522.
9. Elias PM, Levy SW. Bullous impetigo. Occurrence of localized scalded skin syndrome in an adult. Arch Dermatol 1976; 112: 856–858.
10. El Zawahry M, Aziz AA, Soliman M. The aetiology of impetigo contagiosa. Br J Dermatol 1972; 87: 420–424.
11. Bronstein SW, Bickers DR, Lamkin BC. Bullous dermatosis caused by *Staphylococcus aureus* in locus minoris resistentiae. J Am Acad Dermatol 1984; 10: 259–263.
12. Lyell A. Toxic epidermal necrolysis: the scalded skin syndrome. JCE Dermatol 1978; 16 (11): 15–26.
13. Oranje AP, Vuzevski VD, Muntendam J, Rongen-Westerlaken C. Varicella complicated by staphylococcal scalded skin syndrome with unusual necrosis. Int J Dermatol 1988; 27: 38–39.
14. Fritsch P, Elias P, Varga J. The fate of Staphylococcal exfoliatin in newborn and adult mice. Br J Dermatol 1976; 95: 275–284.
15. Benson PF, Rankin GLS, Rippey JJ. An outbreak of exfoliative dermatitis of the newborn (Ritter's disease). Lancet 1962; 1: 999–1002.
16. Koblenzer PJ. Acute epidermal necrolysis (Ritter von Rittershain-Lyell). Arch Dermatol 1967: 95; 608–617.
17. Rasmussen JE. Toxic epidermal necrolysis. A review of 75 cases in children. Arch Dermatol 1975; 111: 1135–1139.
18. Richard M, Mathieu-Serra A. Staphylococcal scalded skin syndrome in a homosexual adult. J Am Acad Dermatol 1986; 15: 385–389.

19. Reid LH, Weston WL, Humbert JR. Staphylococcal scalded skin syndrome. Adult onset in a patient with deficient cell-mediated immunity. Arch Dermatol 1974; 109: 239–241.

20. Sturman SW, Malkinson FD. Staphylococcal scalded skin syndrome in an adult and a child. Arch Dermatol 1976; 112: 1275–1279.

21. Diem E, Konrad K, Graninger W. Staphylococcal scalded skin syndrome in an adult with fatal disseminated staphylococcal sepsis. Acta Derm Venereol 1982; 62: 295–299.

22. Ridgway HB, Lowe NJ. Staphylococcal scalded skin syndrome in an adult with Hodgkin's disease. Arch Dermatol 1979; 115: 589–590.

23. Borchers SL, Gomez EC, Isseroff RR. Generalized staphylococcal scalded skin syndrome in an anephric boy undergoing hemodialysis. Arch Dermatol 1984; 120: 912–918.

24. Elias PM, Fritsch P, Epstein EH Jr. Staphylococcal scalded skin syndrome. Clinical features, pathogenesis, and recent microbiological and biochemical developments. Arch Dermatol 1977; 113: 207–219.

25. Baker DH, Wuepper KD, Rasmussen JE. Staphylococcal scalded skin syndrome: detection of antibody to epidermolytic toxin by a primary binding assay. Clin Exp Dermatol 1978; 3: 17–24.

26. Dimond RL, Wolff HH, Braun-Falco O. The staphylococcal scalded skin syndrome. An experimental histochemical and electron microscopic study. Br J Dermatol 1977; 96: 483–492.

27. Lyell A. Toxic epidermal necrolysis (the scalded skin syndrome): A reappraisal. Br J Dermatol 1979; 100: 69–86.

28. Lyell A. The staphylococcal scalded skin syndrome in historical perspective: Emergence of dermopathic strains of Staphylococcus aureus and discovery of the epidermolytic toxin. J Am Acad Dermatol 1983; 9: 285–294.

29. Falk DK, King LE Jr. Criteria for the diagnosis of staphylococcal scalded skin syndrome in adults. Cutis 1983; 31: 421–424.

29a. Tofte RW, Williams DN. Toxic shock syndrome: clinical and laboratory features in 15 patients. Ann Intern Med 1981; 94: 149–156.

29b. Huntley AC, Tanabe JL. Toxic shock syndrome as a complication of dermatologic surgery. J Am Acad Dermatol 1987; 16: 227–229.

29c. Hurwitz RM, Ackerman AB. Cutaneous pathology of the toxic shock syndrome. Am J Dermatopathol 1985; 7: 563–578.

30. Kelly C, Taplin D, Allen AM. Streptococcal ecthyma. Arch Dermatol 1971; 103: 306–310.

31. El Baze P, Thyss A, Caldani C et al. Pseudomonas aeruginosa 0-11 folliculitis. Development into ecthyma gangrenosum in immunosuppressed patients. Arch Dermatol 1985; 121: 873–876.

32. Greene SL, Su WPD, Muller SA. Ecthyma gangrenosum: Report of clinical, histopathologic, and bacteriologic aspects of eight cases. J Am Acad Dermatol 1984; 11: 781–787.

33. Fast M, Woerner S, Bowman W et al. Ecthyma gangrenosum. Can Med Assoc J 1979; 120: 332–334.

34. Fleming MG, Milburn PB, Prose NS. Pseudomonas septicemia with nodules and bullae. Pediatr Dermatol 1987; 4: 18–20.

35. Schlossberg D. Multiple erythematous nodules as a manifestation of Pseudomonas aeruginosa septicemia. Arch Dermatol 1980; 116: 446–447.

Deep pyogenic infections (cellulitis)

36. Fleisher G, Ludwig S, Campos J. Cellulitis: bacterial etiology, clinical features, and laboratory findings. J Pediatr 1980; 97: 591–593.

37. Leyden JJ. Cellulitis. Arch Dermatol 1989; 125: 823–824.

38. Hook EW III. Acute cellulitis. Arch Dermatol 1987; 123: 460–461.

39. Feingold DS. Gangrenous and crepitant cellulitis. J Am Acad Dermatol 1982; 6: 289–299.

39a. Grob JJ, Bollet C, Richard MA et al. Extensive skin ulceration due to EF-4 bacterial infection in a patient with AIDS. Br J Dermatol 1989; 121: 507–510.

40. Beckman EN, Leonard GL, Castillo LE et al. Histopathology of marine vibrio wound infections. Am J Clin Pathol 1981; 76: 765–772.

41. Hurwitz RM, Leaming RD, Horine RK. Necrotic cellulitis. A localized form of septic vaculitis. Arch Dermatol 1984; 120: 87–92.

42. Musher DM. Cutaneous and soft-tissue manifestations of sepsis due to Gram-negative enteric bacilli. Rev Infect Dis 1980; 2: 854–866.

43. Ronnen M, Suster S, Schewach-Millet M, Modan M. Erysipelas. Changing faces. Int J Dermatol 1985; 24: 169–172.

44. Keefe M, Wakeel RA, Kerr REI. Erysipelas complicating chronic discoid lupus erythematosus of the face — a case report and review of erysipelas. Clin Exp Dermatol 1989; 14: 75–78.

45. Bernard P, Bedane C, Mounier M et al. Streptococcal cause of erysipelas and cellulitis in adults. A microbiologic study using a direct immunofluorescence technique. Arch Dermatol 1989; 125: 779–782.

46. Shama S, Calandra GB. Atypical erysipelas caused by Group B streptococci in a patient with cured Hodgkin's disease. Arch Dermatol 1982; 118: 934–936.

47. Barnett JH, Estes SA, Wirman JA et al. Erysipeloid. J Am Acad Dermatol 1983; 9: 116–123.

48. McCray MK, Esterly NB. Blistering distal dactylitis. J Am Acad Dermatol 1981; 5: 592–594.

48a. Telfer NR, Barth JH, Dawber RPR. Recurrent blistering distal dactylitis of the great toe associated with an ingrowing toenail. Clin Exp Dermatol 1989; 14: 380–381.

48b. Frieden IJ. Blistering dactylitis caused by Group B streptococci. Pediatr Dermatol 1989; 6: 300–302.

49. Hauger SB. Facial cellulitis: an early indicator of Group B streptococcal bacteremia. Pediatrics 1981; 67: 376–377.

50. Rasmussen JE. Haemophilus influenzae cellulitis. Case presentation and review of the literature. Br J Dermatol 1973; 88: 547–550.

51. Ginsburg CM. Haemophilus influenzae type B buccal cellulitis. J Am Acad Dermatol 1981; 4: 661–664.

52. Thirumoorthi MC, Asmar BI, Dajani AS. Violaceous discolouration in pneumococcal cellulitis. Pediatrics 1978; 62: 492–493.

53. Rehder PA, Eliezer ET, Lane AT. Perianal cellulitis. Cutaneous Group A streptococcal disease. Arch

Dermatol 1988; 124: 702–704.

54. Wickboldt LG, Sanders CV. *Vibrio vulnificus* infection. Case report and update since 1970. J Am Acad Dermatol 1983; 9: 243–251.

55. Tyring SK, Lee PC. Hemorrhagic bullae associated with *Vibrio vulnificus* septicemia. Report of two cases. Arch Dermatol 1986; 122: 818–820.

55a. Nip-Sakamoto CJ, Pien FD. *Vibrio vulnificus* infection in Hawaii. Int J Dermatol 1989; 28: 313–316.

56. Woo ML, Patrick WGD, Simon MTP, French GL. Necrotising fasciitis caused by *Vibrio vulnificus*. J Clin Pathol 1984; 37: 1301–1304.

57. Hammar H, Wanger L. Erysipelas and necrotizing fasciitis. Br J Dermatol 1977; 96: 409–419.

57a. Umbert IJ, Winkelmann RK, Oliver GF, Peters MS. Necrotizing fasciitis: A clinical, microbiologic, and histopathologic study of 14 patients. J Am Acad Dermatol 1989; 20: 774–781.

58. Goldberg GN, Hansen RC, Lynch PJ. Necrotizing fasciitis in infancy: report of three cases and review of the literature. Pediatr Dermatol 1984; 2: 55–63.

59. Tharakaram S, Keczkes K. Necrotizing fasciitis. A report of five patients. Int J Dermatol 1988; 27: 585–588.

60. Koehn GG. Necrotizing fasciitis. Arch Dermatol 1978; 114: 581–583.

60a. Horgan-Bell C, From L, Ramsay C et al. Meleney's synergistic gangrene: pathological features. J Cutan Pathol 1989; 16: 307 (abstract).

61. Pye RJ, Peachey RDG, Burton JL. Erosive pustular dermatosis of the scalp. Br J Dermatol 1979; 100: 559–566.

62. Grattan CEH, Peachey RD, Boon A. Evidence for a role of local trauma in the pathogenesis of erosive pustular dermatosis of the scalp. Clin Exp Dermatol 1988; 13: 7–10.

63. Ikeda M, Arata J, Isaka H. Erosive pustular dermatosis of the scalp successfully treated with oral zinc sulphate. Br J Dermatol 1982; 106: 742–743.

64. Williams HM Jr, Stone OJ. Blastomycosis-like pyoderma. Arch Dermatol 1966; 93: 226–228.

65. Su WPD, Duncan SC, Perry HO. Blastomycosis-like pyoderma. Arch Dermatol 1979; 115: 170–173.

66. Weedon D. Actinic comedonal plaque. J Am Acad Dermatol 1981; 5: 611.

67. Kocsard E. Actinic comedonal plaque. J Am Acad Dermatol 1981; 5: 611–612.

68. Georgouras K. Coral reef granuloma. Cutis 1967; 3: 37–39.

69. Eastern JS, Martin S. Actinic comedonal plaque. J Am Acad Dermatol 1980; 3: 633–636.

70. Yaffee HS. Localized blastomycosis-like pyoderma occurring in a tattoo. Arch Dermatol 1960; 82: 99–100.

71. O'Dell BL, Jessen T, Becker LE et al. Diminished immune response in sun-damaged skin. Arch Dermatol 1980; 116: 559–561.

Corynebacterial infections

72. Pitcher DG. Aerobic cutaneous coryneforms: recent taxonomic findings. Br J Dermatol 1978; 98: 363–370.

73. Leyden JJ, McGinley KJ, Holzle E et al. The microbiology of the human axilla and its relationship to axillary odor. J Invest Dermatol 1981; 77: 413–416.

74. Shelley WB, Shelley ED. Coexistent erythrasma, trichomycosis axillaris, and pitted keratolysis: An overlooked corynebacterial triad? J Am Acad Dermatol 1982; 7: 752–757.

75. Ceilley RI. Foot ulceration and vertebral osteomyelitis with *Corynebacterium haemolyticum*. Arch Dermatol 1977; 113: 646–647.

76. Jerdan MS, Shapiro RS, Smith NB et al. Cutaneous manifestations of *Corynebacterium* group JK sepsis. J Am Arch Dermatol 1987; 16: 444–447.

77. Bader M, Pedersen AHB, Spearman J, Harnisch JP. An unusual case of cutaneous diphtheria. JAMA 1978; 240: 1382–1383.

78. Sarkany I, Taplin D, Blank H. Erythrasma — common bacterial infection of the skin. JAMA 1961; 177: 130–132.

79. Cochran RJ, Rosen T, Landers T. Topical treatment for erythrasma. Int J Dermatol 1981; 20: 562–564.

80. Sinduphak W, MacDonald E, Smith EB. Erythrasma. Overlooked or misdiagnosed? Int J Dermatol 1985; 24: 95–96.

81. Somerville DA, Seville RH, Cunningham RC et al. Erythrasma in a hospital for the mentally subnormal. Br J Dermatol 1970; 82: 355–360.

82. Engber PB, Mandel EH. Generalized disciform erythrasma. Int J Dermatol 1979; 18: 633–635.

83. Schlappner OLA, Rosenblum GA, Rowden G, Phillips TM. Concomitant erythrasma and dermatophytosis of the groin. Br J Dermatol 1979; 100: 147–151.

84. Svejgaard E, Christophersen J, Jelsdorf H-M. Tinea pedis and erythrasma in Danish recruits. J Am Acad Dermatol 1986; 14: 993–999.

85. Montes LF, Black SH. The fine structure of diphtheroids of erythrasma. J Invest Dermatol 1967; 48: 342–349.

86. Montes LF, Black SH, McBride ME. Bacterial invasion of the stratum corneum in erythrasma. J Invest Dermatol 1967; 49: 474–485.

87. White SW, Smith J. Trichomycosis pubis. Arch Dermatol 1979; 115: 444–445.

88. Shelley WB, Miller MA. Electron microscopy, histochemistry, and microbiology of bacterial adhesion in trichomycosis axillaris. J Am Acad Dermatol 1984; 10: 1005–1014.

89. Freeman RG, McBride ME, Knox JM. Pathogenesis of trichomycosis axillaris. Arch Dermatol 1969; 100: 90–95.

90. McBride ME, Freeman RG, Knox JM. The bacteriology of trichomycosis axillaris. Br J Dermatol 1968; 80: 509–513.

91. Levit F. Trichomycosis axillaris: A different view. J Am Acad Dermatol 1988; 18: 778–779.

92. Orfanos CE, Schloesser E, Mahrle G. Hair destroying growth of *Corynebacterium tenuis* in the so-called trichomycosis axillaris. Arch Dermatol 1971; 103: 632–639.

93. Tilgen W. Pitted keratolysis (keratolysis plantare sulcatum). J Cutan Pathol 1979; 6: 18–30.

94. Zaias N. Pitted and ringed keratolysis. A review and update. J Am Acad Dermatol 1982; 7: 787–791.

95. Rubel LR. Pitted keratolysis and *Dermatophilus congolensis*. Arch Dermatol 1972; 105: 584–586.

96. Lamberg SI. Symptomatic pitted keratolysis. Arch Dermatol 1969; 100: 10–11.

97. Emmerson RW, Wilson Jones E. Ringed keratolysis of

173. Glickman FS. Sporotrichoid mycobacterial infections. Case report and review. J Am Acad Dermatol 1983; 8: 703–707.

174. Gombert ME, Goldstein EJC, Corrado ML et al. Disseminated *Mycobacterium marinum* infection after renal transplantation. Ann Intern Med 1981; 94: 486–487.

175. King AJ, Fairley JA, Rasmussen JE. Disseminated cutaneous *Mycobacterium marinum* infection. Arch Dermatol 1983; 119: 268–270.

176. Even-Paz Z, Haas H, Sacks T, Rosenmann E. *Mycobacterium marinum* skin infections mimicking cutaneous leishmaniasis. Br J Dermatol 1976; 94: 435–442.

177. Dickey RF. Sporotrichoid mycobacteriosis caused by *M. marinum (balnei)*. Arch Dermatol 1968; 98: 385–391.

178. Smith AG, Jiji RM. Cutaneous infection due to a rough variant of *Mycobacterium marinum*. Am J Clin Pathol 1975; 64: 263–270.

179. Travis WD, Travis LB, Roberts GD et al. The histopathologic spectrum in *Mycobacterium marinum* infection. Arch Pathol Lab Med 1985; 109: 1109–1113.

180. Shelley WB, Folkens AT. *Mycobacterium gordonae* infection of the hand. Arch Dermatol 1984; 120: 1064–1065.

181. Drabick JJ, Hoover DL, Roth RE et al. Ulcerative perineal lesions due to *Mycobacterium kansasii*. J Am Acad Dermatol 1988; 18: 1146–1147.

182. Fenske NA, Millns JL. Resistant cutaneous infection caused by *Mycobacterium chelonei*. Arch Dermatol 1981; 117: 151–153.

183. Bolivar R, Satterwhite TK, Floyd M. Cutaneous lesions due to *Mycobacterium kansasii*. Arch Dermatol 1980; 116: 207–208.

184. Rosen T. Cutaneous *Mycobacterium kansasii* infection presenting as cellulitis. Cutis 1983; 31: 87–89.

185. Dore N, Collins J-P, Mankiewicz E. A sporotrichoid-like *Mycobacterium kansasii* infection of the skin treated with minocycline hydrochloride. Br J Dermatol 1979; 101: 75–79.

186. Higgins EM, Lawrence CM. Sporotrichoid spread of *Mycobacterium chelonei*. Clin Exp Dermatol 1988; 13: 234–236.

186a. Murdoch ME, Leigh IM. Sporotrichoid spread of cutaneous *Mycobacterium chelonei* infection. Clin Exp Dermatol 1989; 14: 309–312.

187. Greer KE, Gross GP, Martensen SH. Sporotrichoid cutaneous infection due to *Mycobacterium chelonei*. Arch Dermatol 1979; 115: 738–739.

188. Figuerora LD, Gonzalez JR. Primary inoculation complex of skin by *Mycobacterium chelonei*. J Am Acad Dermatol 1984; 10: 333–336.

189. Kelly SE. Multiple injection abscesses in a diabetic caused by *Mycobacterium chelonei*. Clin Exp Dermatol 1987; 12: 48–49.

190. Heironimus JD, Winn RE, Collins CB. Cutaneous nonpulmonary *Mycobacterium chelonei* infection. Arch Dermatol 1984; 120: 1061–1063.

191. Owens DW, McBride ME. Sporotrichoid cutaneous infection with *Mycobacterium kansasii*. Arch Dermatol 1969; 100: 54–58.

192. Hirsh FS, Saffold OE. *Mycobacterium kansasii* infection with dermatologic manifestations. Arch Dermatol 1976; 112: 706–708.

193. Murray-Leisure KA, Egan N, Weitekamp MR. Skin lesions caused by *Mycobacterium scrofulaceum*. Arch Dermatol 1987; 123: 369–370.

194. Cross GM, Guill MA, Aton JK. Cutaneous *Mycobacterium szulgai* infection. Arch Dermatol 1985; 121: 247–249.

195. Gengoux P, Portaels F, Lachapelle JM et al. Skin granulomas due to *Mycobacterium gordonae*. Int J Dermatol 1987; 26: 181–184.

196. Noel SB, Ray MC, Greer DL. Cutaneous infection with *Mycobacterium avium – intracellulare scrofulaceum intermediate*: A new pathogenic entity. J Am Acad Dermatol 1988; 19: 492–495.

197. Cole GW, Gebhard J. *Mycobacterium avium* infection of the skin resembling lepromatous leprosy. Br J Dermatol 1979; 101: 71–74.

198. Wood C, Nickoloff BJ, Todes-Taylor NR. Pseudotumor resulting from atypical mycobacterial infection. A "histoid" variety of *Mycobacterium avium-intracellulare* complex infection. Am J Clin Pathol 1985; 83: 524–527.

199. Maurice PDL, Bunker C, Giles F et al. *Mycobacterium avium-intracellulare* infection associated with hairy-cell leukemia. Arch Dermatol 1988; 124: 1545–1549.

200. Cox SK, Strausbaugh LJ. Chronic cutaneous infection caused by *Mycobacterium intracellulare*. Arch Dermatol 1981; 117: 794–796.

201. Ward JM. *M. fortuitum* and *M. chelonei* — fast growing mycobacteria. A review with a case report. Br J Dermatol 1975; 92: 453–459.

202. Beck A. *Mycobacterium fortuitum* in abscesses of man. J Clin Pathol 1965; 18: 307–313.

203. Yip SY, Wu PC, Chan WC, Teoh-Chan CH. Tuberculoid cutaneous infection due to a niacin-positive *Mycobacterium chelonei*. Br J Dermatol 1979; 101: 63–69.

204. Onate JM, Madero S, Vanaclocha F, Gil-Martin R. An unusual form of *Mycobacterium chelonei* infection. Am J Dermatopathol 1986; 8: 73–78.

205. Nelson BR, Rapini RP, Wallace RJ Jr, Tschen JA. Disseminated *Mycobacterium chelonae* sp. *abscessus* in an immunocomponent host and with a known portal of entry. J Am Acad Dermatol 1989; 20: 909–912.

205a. Hoss DM, McNutt NS, Kreuger JG et al. Cutaneous tuberculosis mimicking erythema nodosum. J Cutan Pathol 1989; 16: 307 (abstract).

206. Pappolla MA, Mehta VT. PAS reaction stains phagocytosed atypical mycobacteria in paraffin sections. Arch Pathol Lab Med 1984; 108: 372–373.

206a. Lambert WC, Pathan AK, Imaeda T et al. Culture of *Vibrio extorquens* from severe, chronic skin ulcers in a Puerto Rican woman. J Am Acad Dermatol 1983; 9: 262–268.

207. Thangaraj RH, Yawalkar SJ. Leprosy for medical practitioners and paramedical workers. Basle: Ciba-Geigy, 1987; 15.

208. Hutchinson J. The *in vitro* cultivation of *Mycobacterium leprae*. In: Ryan TJ, McDougall AC, eds. Essays on leprosy. Oxford: St Francis Leprosy Guild, 1988; 30–51.

209. Modlin RL, Rea TH. Leprosy: New insight into an ancient disease. J Am Acad Dermatol 1987; 17: 1–13.

210. Sehgal VN, Srivastava G. Leprosy in children. Int J

Dermatol 1987; 26: 557–566.

211. Machin M. The mode of transmission of human leprosy. In: Ryan TJ, McDougall AC, eds. Essays on leprosy. Oxford: St Francis Leprosy Guild, 1988; 1–29.

212. Sehgal VN. Inoculation leprosy. Current status. Int J Dermatol 1988; 27: 6–9.

213. Rea TH, Levan NE. Current concepts in the immunology of leprosy. Arch Dermatol 1977; 113: 345–352.

214. Ridley DS, Jopling WH. Classification of leprosy according to immunity. A five-group system. Int J Lepr 1966; 34: 255–273.

215. Narayanan RB. Immunopathology of leprosy granulomas — current status: a review. Lepr Rev 1988; 59: 75–82.

216. Ridley DS. Histological classification and the immunological spectrum of leprosy. Bull WHO 1974; 51: 451–465.

217. Browne SG. Indeterminate leprosy. Int J Dermatol 1985; 24: 555–559.

218. Murray KA, McLelland BA, Job CK. Early leprosy with perineural proliferation. Arch Dermatol 1984; 120: 360–361.

219. Ramasoota T, Johnson WC, Graham JH. Cutaneous sarcoidosis and tuberculoid leprosy. A comparative histopathologic and histochemical study. Arch Dermatol 1967; 96: 259–268.

220. Singh K. An unusual bullous reaction in borderline leprosy. Lepr Rev 1987; 58: 61–67.

221. El-Shiemy S, El-Hefnawi H, Abdel-Fattah A et al. Testicular and epididymal involvement in leprosy patients, with special reference to gynecomastia. Int J Dermatol 1976; 15: 52–58.

222. Frey FLP, Gottlieb AB, Levis WR. A patient with lepromatous leprosy and anticytoskeletal antibodies. J Am Acad Dermatol 1988; 18: 1179–1184.

223. Mansfield RE. Histoid leprosy. Arch Pathol 1969; 87: 580–585.

224. Sehgal VN, Srivastava G. Histoid leprosy. Int J Dermatol 1985; 24: 286–292.

225. Turk JL, Rees RJW. Aids and leprosy. Lepr Rev 1988; 59: 193–194.

226. Sehgal VN. Reactions in leprosy. Clinical aspects. Int J Dermatol 1987; 26: 278–285.

227. Sehgal VN, Srivastava G, Sundharam JA. Immunology of reactions in leprosy. Current status. Int J Dermatol 1988; 27: 157–162.

228. Kuo T-T, Chan H-L. Severe reactional state in lepromatous leprosy simulating Sweet's syndrome. Int J Dermatol 1987; 26: 518–520.

229. Ridley DS, Radia KB. The histological course of reactions in borderline leprosy and their outcome. Int J Lepr 1981; 49: 383–392.

230. Murphy GF, Sanchez NP, Flynn TC et al. Erythema nodosum leprosum: Nature and extent of the cutaneous microvascular alterations. J Am Acad Dermatol 1986; 14: 59–69.

231. Modlin RL, Bakke AC, Vaccaro SA et al. Tissue and blood T-lymphocyte subpopulations in erythema nodosum leprosum. Arch Dermatol 1985; 121: 216–219.

232. Rea TH, Levan NE. Erythema nodosum leprosum in a general hospital. Arch Dermatol 1975; 111: 1575–1580.

233. Vazquez-Botet M, Sanchez JL. Erythema nodosum leprosum. Int J Dermatol 1987; 26: 436–437.

234. Ridley DS, Rea TH, McAdam KPWJ. The histology of erythema nodosum leprosum. Variant forms in New Guineans and other ethnic groups. Lepr Rev 1981; 52: 65–78.

235. Pursley TV, Jacobson RR, Apisarnthanarax P. Lucio's phenomenon. Arch Dermatol 1980; 116: 201–204.

236. Rea TH, Ridley DS. Lucio's phenomenon: a comparative histological study. Int J Lepr 1979; 47: 161–166.

237. Moschella SL. The lepra reaction with necrotizing skin lesions. A report of six cases. Arch Dermatol 1967; 95: 565–575.

238. Jariwala HJ, Kelkar SS. Fluorescence microscopy for detection of M. leprae in tissue sections. Int J Lepr 1979; 47: 33–36.

239. Sehgal VN, Koranne RV, Nayyar M, Saxena HMK. Application of clinical and histopathological classification of leprosy. Dermatologica 1980; 161: 93–96.

240. Nayar A, Narayanan JS, Job CK. Histopathological study of early skin lesions in leprosy. Arch Pathol 1972; 94: 199–204.

241. Tze-Chun L, Li-Zung Y, Gan-yun Y, Gu-Jing D. Histology of indeterminate leprosy. Int J Lepr 1982; 50: 172–176.

242. Parker M. Hypopigmentation in leprosy: its mechanism and significance. In: Ryan TJ, McDougall AC, eds. Essays on leprosy. Oxford: St Francis Leprosy Guild, 1988; 101–123.

243. Modlin RL, Gebhard JF, Taylor CR, Rea TH. In situ characterization of T lymphocyte subsets in the reactional states of leprosy. Clin Exp Immunol 1983; 53: 17–24.

244. Van Voorhis WC, Kaplan G, Sarno EN et al. The cutaneous infiltrates of leprosy. N Engl J Med 1982; 307: 1593–1597.

245. Coruh G, McDougall AC. Untreated lepromatous leprosy: histopathological findings in cutaneous blood vessels. Int J Lepr 1979; 47: 500–511.

246. Job CK. Mycobacterium leprae in nerve lesions in lepromatous leprosy. An electron microscopic study. Arch Pathol 1970; 89: 195–207.

247. Klenerman P. Aetiological factors in delayed-type hypersensitivity reactions in leprosy. In: Ryan TJ, McDougall AC, eds. Essays on leprosy. Oxford: St Francis Leprosy Guild, 1988; 52–63.

248. Moschella SL. Leprosy today. Australas J Dermatol 1983; 24: 47–54.

249. Modlin RL, Hofman FM, Taylor CR, Rea TH. T lymphocyte subsets in skin lesions of patients with leprosy. J Am Acad Dermatol 1983; 8: 182–189.

250. Jolliffe DS. Leprosy reactional states and their treatment. Br J Dermatol 1977; 97: 345–352.

Miscellaneous bacterial infections

251. Dutz W, Kohout-Dutz E. Anthrax. Int J Dermatol 1981; 20: 203–206.

252. Human cutaneous anthrax — North Carolina, 1987. Arch Dermatol 1988; 124: 1324.

253. Ariza J, Servitje O, Pallares R et al. Characteristic cutaneous lesions in patients with brucellosis. Arch Dermatol 1989; 125: 380–383.

254. Berger TG, Guill MA, Goette DK. Cutaneous lesions in brucellosis. Arch Dermatol 1981; 117: 40–42.

255. Niemi K-M, Hannuksela M, Salo OP. Skin lesions in human yersiniosis. A histopathological and immunohistological study. Br J Dermatol 1976; 94: 155–160.

256. Baldock NE, Catterall MD. Erythema nodosum from *Yersinia enterocolitica*. Br J Dermatol 1975; 93: 719–720.

257. Hannuksela M. Human yersiniosis: a common cause of erythematous skin eruptions. Int J Dermatol 1977; 16: 665–666.

258. Sehgal VN, Prasad ALS. Donovanosis. Current concepts. Int J Dermatol 1986; 25: 8–16.

259. Sehgal VN, Sharma NL, Bhargava NC et al. Primary extragenital disseminated cutaneous donovanosis. Br J Dermatol 1979; 101: 353–356.

260. Davis CM. Granuloma inguinale. A clinical, histological, and ultrastructural study. JAMA 1970; 211: 632–636.

261. Rosen T, Tschen JA, Ramsdell W et al. Granuloma inguinale. J Am Acad Dermatol 1984; 11: 433–437.

262. Fritz GS, Hubler WR Jr, Dodson RF, Rudolph A. Mutilating granuloma inguinale. Arch Dermatol 1975; 111: 1464–1465.

263. Dodson RF, Fritz GS, Hubler WR Jr et al. Donovanosis: a morphologic study. J Invest Dermatol 1974; 62: 611–614.

264. Sehgal VN, Shyamprasad AL, Beohar PC. The histopathological diagnosis of donovanosis. Br J Vener Dis 1984; 60: 45–47.

265. Kuberski T, Papadimitriou JM, Phillips P. Ultrastructure of *Calymmatobacterium granulomatis* in lesions of granuloma inguinale. J Infect Dis 1980; 142: 744–749.

266. Margolis RJ, Hood AF. Chancroid: Diagnosis and treatment. J Am Acad Dermatol 1982; 6: 493–499.

266a. Ronald AR, Plummer F. Chancroid. A newly important sexually transmitted disease. Arch Dermatol 1989; 125: 1413–1414.

267. Ronald AR. Chancroid. Recent advances in treatment and control. Int J Dermatol 1986; 25: 31–33.

268. Falk ES, Vorland LH, Bjorvatn B. A case of mixed chancre. Dermatologica 1984; 168: 47–49.

269. Salzman RS, Kraus SJ, Miller RG et al. Chancroidal ulcers that are not chancroid. Cause and epidemiology. Arch Dermatol 1984; 120: 636–639.

270. Werman BS, Herskowitz LJ, Olansky S et al. A clinical variant of chancroid resembling granuloma inguinale. Arch Dermatol 1983; 119: 890–894.

271. Fiumara NJ, Rothman K, Tang S. The diagnosis and treatment of chancroid. J Am Acad Dermatol 1986; 15: 939–943.

272. Hammond GW, Slutchuk M, Scatliff J et al. Epidemiologic, clinical, laboratory, and therapeutic features of an urban outbreak of chancroid in North America. Rev Infect Dis 1980; 2: 867–879.

273. McCarley ME, Cruz PD Jr, Sontheimer RD. Chancroid: Clinical variants and other findings from an epidemic in Dallas County, 1986–1987. J Am Acad Dermatol 1988; 19: 330–337.

274. Kraus SJ, Werman BS, Biddle JW et al. Pseudogranuloma inguinale caused by *Haemophilus ducreyi*. Arch Dermatol 1982; 118: 494–497.

275. Tapia A. Rhinoscleroma: A naso-oral dermatosis. Cutis 1987; 40: 101–103.

276. Convit J, Kerdel-Vegas F, Gordon B. Rhinoscleroma. Review and presentation of a case. Arch Dermatol 1961; 84: 55–62.

277. Hoffmann EO, Loose LD, Harkin JC. The Mikulicz cell in rhinoscleroma. Light, fluorescent and electron microscopic studies. Am J Pathol 1973; 73: 47–58.

278. Fisher ER, Dimling C. Rhinoscleroma. Light and electron microscopic studies. Arch Pathol 1964; 78: 501–512.

279. Pullen RL, Stuart BM. Tularemia. Analysis of 225 cases. JAMA 1945; 129: 495–500.

280. Leggiadro RJ, Kenigsberg K, Annunziato D. Tick-borne ulceroglandular tularemia. N Y State J Med 1983; 83: 1053–1054.

281. Hughes WT. Tularemia in children. J Pediatr 1963; 62: 495–502.

282. Young LS, Bicknell DS, Archer BG et al. Tularemia epidemic: Vermont, 1968. Forty-seven cases linked to contact with Muskrats. N Engl J Med 1969; 280: 1253–1260.

283. Evans ME, Gregory DW, Schaffner W, McGee ZA. Tularemia: a 30-year experience with 88 cases. Medicine (Baltimore) 1985; 64: 251–269.

284. Martin T, Holmes IH, Wobeser GA et al. Tularemia in Canada with a focus on Saskatchewan. Can Med Assoc J 1982; 127: 279–282.

285. Lewis JE. Suppurative inflammatory eruption occurring in septicemic tularemia. Cutis 1982; 30: 92–100.

286. Kalter SS. Cat scratch disease. Int J Dermatol 1978; 17: 656–658.

287. Margileth AW, Wear DJ, Hadfield TL et al. Cat-scratch disease. Bacteria in skin at the primary inoculation site. JAMA 1984; 252: 928–931.

288. Margileth AM. Dermatologic manifestations and update of cat scratch disease. Pediatr Dermatol 1988; 5: 1–9.

289. Shinall EA. Cat-scratch disease: a review of the literature. Pediatr Dermatol 1990; 7: 11–18.

290. Carithers HA. Cat-scratch disease. An overview based on a study of 1,200 patients. Am J Dis Child 1985; 139: 1124–1133.

291. Gregory DW, Decker MD. Case report: cat scratch disease: an infection beyond the lymph node. Am J Med Sci 1986; 292: 389–390.

292. Margileth AM, Wear DJ, English CK. Systemic cat scratch disease: report of 23 patients with prolonged or recurrent severe bacterial infection. J Infect Dis 1987; 155: 390–402.

293. Sundaresh KV, Madjar DD, Camisa C, Carvallo E. Cat scratch disease associated with erythema nodosum. Cutis 1986; 38: 317–319.

294. Miller-Catchpole R, Variakojis D, Vardiman JW et al. Cat scratch disease. Identification of bacteria in seven cases of lymphadenitis. Am J Surg Pathol 1986; 10: 276–281.

295. Cotter B, Maurer R, Hedinger C. Cat scratch disease: evidence for a bacterial etiology. Virchows Arch (A) 1986; 410: 103–106.

296. Wear DJ, Margileth AM, Hadfield TL et al. Cat-scratch disease: a bacterial infection. Science 1983; 221: 1403–1405.

297. Gerber MA, Sedgwick AK, MacAlister TJ et al. The aetiological agent of cat scratch disease. Lancet 1985; 1: 1236–1239.

298. Walford N, van der Wouw PA, Das PK et al.

Epithelioid angiomatosis in the acquired immunodeficiency syndrome: morphology and differential diagnosis. Histopathology 1990; 16: 83–88.

299. Johnson WT, Helwig EB. Cat-scratch disease. Histopathologic changes in the skin. Arch Dermatol 1969; 100: 148–154.
300. McLure J. Malakoplakia. J Pathol 1983; 140: 275–330.
301. Palazzo JP, Ellison DJ, Garcia IE et al. Cutaneous malakoplakia simulating relapsing malignant lymphoma. J Cutan Pathol 1990; 17: 171–175.
302. Sian CS, McCabe RE, Lattes CG. Malacoplakia of skin and subcutaneous tissue in a renal transplant recipient. Arch Dermatol 1981; 117: 654–655.
303. Nieland ML, Borochovitz D, Silverman AR, Saferstein HL. Cutaneous malakoplakia. Am J Dermatopathol 1981; 3: 287–294.
304. Arul KJ, Emmerson RW. Malacoplakia of the skin. Clin Exp Dermatol 1977; 2: 131–135.
305. Almagro UA, Choi H, Caya JG, Norbach DH. Cutaneous malakoplakia. Report of a case and review of the literature. Am J Dermatopathol 1981; 3: 295–301.
306. Singh M, Kaur S, Vijpayee BK, Banerjee AK. Cutaneous malakoplakia with dermatomyositis. Int J Dermatol 1987; 26: 190–191.
307. Sencer O, Sencer H, Uluoglu O et al. Malakoplakia of the skin. Ultrastructure and quantitative x-ray microanalysis of Michaelis-Gutmann bodies. Arch Pathol Lab Med 1979; 103: 446–450.

Chlamydial infections

308. Sarner M, Wilson RJ. Erythema nodosum and psittacosis: report of five cases. Br Med J 1965; 2: 1469–1470.
309. Green ST, Hamlet NW, Willocks L et al. Psittacosis presenting with erythema-marginatum-like lesions — a case report and a historical review. Clin Exp Dermatol 1990; 15: 225–227.
310. Semel JD. Cutaneous findings in a case of psittacosis. Arch Dermatol 1984; 120: 1227–1229.
311. Abrams AJ. Lymphogranuloma venereum. JAMA 1968; 205: 199–202.
312. Schachter J, Osoba AO. Lymphogranuloma venereum. Br Med Bull 1983; 39: 151–154.
313. de la Monte SM, Hutchins GM. Follicular proctocolitis and neuromatous hyperplasia with lymphogranuloma venereum. Hum Pathol 1985; 16: 1025–1032.
314. Becker LE. Lymphogranuloma venereum. Int J Dermatol 1976; 15: 26–33.
315. Hopsu-Havu VK, Sonck CE. Infiltrative, ulcerative, and fistular lesions of the penis due to lymphogranuloma venereum. Br J Vener Dis 1973; 49: 193–202.
316. Smith EB, Custer RP. The histopathology of lymphogranuloma venereum. J Urol 1950; 63: 546–563.
317. Alacoque B, Cloppet H, Dumontel C, Moulin G. Histological, immunofluorescent, and ultrastructural features of lymphogranuloma venereum: a case report. Br J Vener Dis 1984; 60: 390–395.

Rickettsial infections

318. Turner RC, Chaplinski TJ, Adams HG. Rocky Mountain spotted fever presenting as thrombotic thrombocytopenic purpura. Am J Med 1986; 81: 153–157.
319. Helmick CG, Bernard KW, D'Angelo LJ. Rocky Mountain spotted fever: clinical, laboratory, and epidemiological features of 262 cases. J Infect Dis 1984; 150: 480–488.
320. Zaki MH. Selected tickborne infections. A review of Lyme disease, Rocky Mountain spotted fever, and babesiosis. N Y State J Med 1989; 89: 320–335.
321. Woodward TE. Rocky Mountain spotted fever: Epidemiological and early clinical signs are keys to treatment and reduced mortality. J Infect Dis 1984; 150: 465–468.
322. Kaplan JE, Schonberger LB. The sensitivity of various serologic tests in the diagnosis of Rocky Mountain spotted fever. Am J Trop Med Hyg 1986; 35: 840–844.
323. Brettman LR, Lewin S, Holzman RS et al. Rickettsialpox: Report of an outbreak and a contemporary review. Medicine (Baltimore) 1981; 60: 363–372.
324. Walker DH, Gay RM, Valdes-Dapena M. The occurrence of eschars in Rocky Mountain spotted fever. J Am Acad Dermatol 1981; 4: 571–576.
325. Silverman DJ. Rickettsia rickettsii — induced cellular injury of human vascular endothelium in vitro. Infect Immun 1984; 44: 545–553.
326. Brown GW. Recent studies in scrub typhus: a review. J R Soc Med 1978; 71: 507–510.
327. Walker DH, Occhino C, Tringali GR et al. Pathogenesis of Rickettsial eschars: the tache noire of Boutonneuse fever. Hum Pathol 1988; 19: 1449–1454.
328. Raoult D, Jean-Pastor M-J, Xeridat B et al. La fièvre boutonneuse méditerranéenne: à propos de 154 cas récents. Ann Dermatol Venereol 1983; 110: 909–914.
329. Andrew R, Bonnin JM, Williams S. Tick typhus in North Queensland. Med J Aust 1946; 2: 253–258.
330. Herrero-Herrero JI, Walker DH, Ruiz-Beltran R. Immunohistochemical evaluation of the cellular immune response to Rickettsia conorii in taches noires. J Infect Dis 1987; 155: 802–805.
331. Montenegro MR, Mansueto S, Hegarty BC, Walker DH. The histology of "taches noires" of boutonneuse fever and demonstration of Rickettsia conorii in them by immunofluorescence. Virchows Arch (A) 1983; 400: 309–317.
332. Woodward TE, Pedersen CE Jr, Oster CN et al. Prompt confirmation of Rocky Mountain spotted fever: identification of Rickettsiae in skin tissues. J Infect Dis 1976; 134: 297–301.
333. Bradford WD, Hawkins HK. Rocky Mountain spotted fever in childhood. Am J Dis Child 1977; 131: 1228–1232.
334. Walker DH, Cain BG, Olmstead PM. Laboratory diagnosis of Rocky Mountain spotted fever by immunofluorescent demonstration of Rickettsia rickettsii in cutaneous lesions. Am J Clin Pathol 1978; 69: 619–623.

Spirochaetal infections

SYPHILIS

Syphilis is an infectious disease of worldwide distribution, caused by the spirochaete *Treponema pallidum*.[1–4] The mode of infection is almost always by sexual contact and, consequently, seropositivity for human immunodeficiency virus (HIV) is sometimes present in individuals with active syphilis.[5,5a] Congenital infection is now quite rare.[6,7] Acquired syphilis may be considered in four stages: primary, secondary, latent and tertiary.

Primary syphilis

The initial lesion of syphilis — the primary chancre — is an indurated, painless ulcer with a sharply defined edge that often is surrounded by an inflammatory zone. It is usually found on genital or perianal skin, although about 5% of chancres are extragenital.[8] The serous exudate from the ulcer generally contains numerous treponemes which can be identified by dark-ground microscopy.

In time, the ulcer heals, leaving a small, stellate or nondescript scar. The chancre is often accompanied by painless enlargement of the regional lymph nodes.

Secondary syphilis

In untreated cases, the multiplication of the widely dispersed treponemes results in *secondary syphilis*, some four to eight weeks after the chancre. Besides the mucocutaneous lesions, there may be constitutional symptoms which include fever, lymphadenitis, and hepatitis.[9,10] A self-limited febrile reaction (the Jarisch–Herxheimer reaction), accompanied by systemic symptoms, may occur following the commencement of antibiotic therapy for syphilis.[11]

The cutaneous lesions of secondary syphilis[12] are usually maculopapular or erythematosquamous, somewhat psoriasiform lesions, but lichenoid, nodular,[13] corymbose,[14] annular,[15] follicular,[16] pustular, rupial and ulcerative[17–19] lesions may develop. They may mimic a wide variety of skin diseases. Pruritus is only occasionally present.[20] Large, fleshy, somewhat verrucous papules (condylomata lata) may develop in the anogenital region: these should not be confused with viral condylomata acuminata (see p. 690).

Latent syphilis

Even without treatment, the manifestations of secondary syphilis subside spontaneously. During this phase there are no signs or symptoms, although there is a liability for relapses of cutaneous lesions to occur in the first few years after the disappearance of the lesions of secondary syphilis. Serology is positive.

Tertiary syphilis

The manifestations of tertiary syphilis appear many years after the initial infection. They reflect the generalized nature of the disease. They involve predominantly the cardiovascular system, the central nervous system and the skeleton, but lesions also occur in the testes, lymph nodes and skin.

There are two types of cutaneous lesion in tertiary syphilis. One is a nodular lesion and the other a chronic gummatous ulcer.[21] They are usually solitary. The nodular form presents an undulating, advancing border of red-brown, scaly nodules, some of which may become ulcerated. The gummatous form starts as a deep, firm swelling that eventually breaks down to form an ulcer.

Histopathology

Endothelial swelling of blood vessels and an inflammatory infiltrate which includes numerous plasma cells are the histological hallmarks of lesions of primary and secondary syphilis. Although great emphasis is placed on the presence of plasma cells, it should be noted that they are sometimes quite sparse in lesions of secondary syphilis.

Primary syphilis. The epidermis at the periphery of the chancre shows marked acanthosis, but at the centre it becomes thin and eventually is lost. The base of the ulcer is infiltrated with lymphocytes and plasma cells, particularly adjacent to the blood vessels, in which there is prominent endothelial swelling. The treponemes can usually be demonstrated by appropriate silver impregnation techniques, such as the Levaditi or Warthin–Starry stains. On dark-field examination of a wet film from a chancre, *Treponema pallidum* can be seen as a thin, delicate spiral organism 4 to 15 μm in length and 0.25 μm in diameter. Electron microscopy has shown *T. pallidum* to be principally in the intercellular spaces in the vicinity of small blood vessels as well as in macrophages, endothelial cells and even plasma cells.[22] Collagen fibres appear to be damaged by the treponeme.[23]

Secondary syphilis. There is considerable variation in its histological pattern.[10,24,25] Plasma cells may be absent or sparse in up to one-third of all biopsies and the vascular changes may not be prominent. The infiltrate usually involves both the superficial and deep dermis, except in the macular lesions where it is more superficial (Fig. 24.1). Extension of the inflammatory infiltrate into the subcutis is uncommon.[10] Plasma cells are less numerous in macular lesions.[26] The infiltrate is predominantly lymphocytic, with some histiocytes and variable numbers of plasma cells. Early lesions often show a neutrophilic vascular reaction which is presumed to be related to immune complex deposition.[27] A heavy neutrophil infiltrate resembling that in Sweet's syndrome

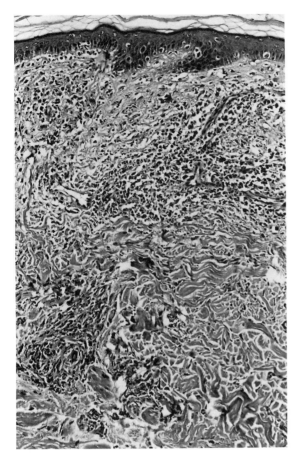

Fig. 24.1 Secondary syphilis. There is a superficial and deep perivascular infiltrate in the dermis.
Haematoxylin — eosin

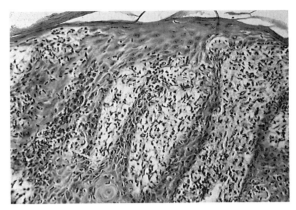

Fig. 24.2 Late secondary syphilis. There is a mixed lichenoid and psoriasiform reaction pattern.
Haematoxylin — eosin

secondary syphilis,[32] particularly after about 16 weeks of the disease.[24] In the rare ulcerative form there is necrosis of the upper dermis,[19] while in the follicular type there is microabscess formation in the outer root sheath of the hair follicle, or a follicular pustule (Fig. 24.3). There may be perifollicular granulomas.[16]

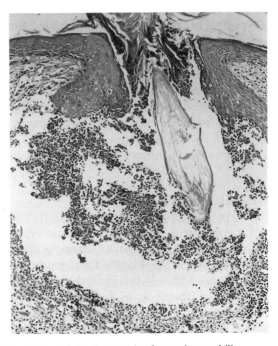

Fig. 24.3 A follicular pustule of secondary syphilis.
Haematoxylin — eosin

has been reported.[28] Follicles and sweat glands may be sleeved by inflammatory cells.[24] Sometimes the dermal infiltrate is dense and diffuse and it has been likened to cutaneous lymphoma,[29,30] although its heterogeneous nature is against lymphoma. Epithelioid granulomas may be found in late secondary syphilis, and there is a report of a palisading granuloma similar to that seen in granuloma annulare.[31] The epidermis is frequently involved. It may show acanthosis with spongiosis, psoriasiform hyperplasia and spongiform pustulation with considerable exocytosis of neutrophils.[25] A lichenoid tissue reaction may be present, particularly in late lesions (Fig. 24.2). A granulomatous pattern may also be seen in

cutaneous lesion is a centrifugally spreading erythematous lesion at the site of the bite of the tick, *Ixodes dammini*, or other species such as *I. ricinus* in Great Britain.[49] Lesions are multiple in about 25% of cases.[44] The spirochaete *Borrelia burgdorferi* has been isolated from the vector and from some patients with Lyme disease,[50] and antibodies to it have been found in the sera of patients with the disease.[51] Antigenic differences exist between the American and European spirochaetes.[52] The organisms may be isolated using modified Kelly's medium.[53] Recent studies suggest that acrodermatitis chronica atrophicans may be a late manifestation of infection with the same spirochaete (see below).[52]

Histopathology

There is a superficial and deep perivascular and interstitial infiltrate of lymphocytes, sometimes with abundant plasma cells and eosinophils. Rarely there are scattered neutrophils. With the Warthin–Starry silver stain a spirochaete can be found in nearly one half of the specimens in the papillary dermis near the dermo–epidermal junction.[54,55] The diagnosis requires an index of suspicion based on the clinical features. The diagnosis has also been confirmed using an indirect immunofluorescence technique with a monoclonal antibody to the axial filaments of several *Borrelia* species.[56]

ACRODERMATITIS CHRONICA ATROPHICANS

Acrodermatitis chronica atrophicans results from infection by a spirochaete of the genus *Borrelia*, transmitted by the tick *Ixodes ricinus*. It is most often reported from Northern, Central and Eastern Europe. There are several reports of this condition being preceded by erythema chron-

icum migrans, suggesting that acrodermatitis chronica atrophicans is a chronic or late manifestation of infection with *Borrelia burgdorferi* or a related species.[52]

Clinically there is an initial inflammatory stage characterized by diffuse or localized erythema which gradually spreads to involve the extensor surfaces of the extremities and areas around joints.[52,57] After some months there is gradual atrophy of the skin with loss of appendages and often hypopigmentation. Areas resembling lichen sclerosus et atrophicus, sclerodermatous patches, and linear fibrotic bands over the ulna and tibia may also be found.

Histopathology

The early stages of the disease show a chronic inflammatory cell infiltrate in the dermis which is moderately heavy and composed predominantly of lymphocytes with some histiocytes and plasma cells. There is often accentuation around blood vessels, which may show telangiectasia, and also around adnexae. Sometimes there is a superficial band-like infiltrate of inflammatory cells with a thin zone of collagen separating the inflammatory cells from the basal layer. Scattered vacuoles or groups of vacuoles which morphologically resemble fat cells (but which do not appear to stain for fat) have been reported in the upper dermis in some cases.[52] As the lesions progress there will be atrophy of the dermis to about one-half its normal thickness or less. This is usually accompanied by loss of elastic fibres and pilosebaceous follicles, atrophy of the subcutis and variable epidermal atrophy with loss of the rete pegs.

Other changes which may be found include diffuse dermal oedema, a subepidermal oedematous or sclerotic zone, basal vacuolar change, hyperkeratosis, and changes resembling lichen sclerosus et atrophicus. Dense dermal sclerosis may be seen in the sclerodermatous patches.

REFERENCES

1. Crissey JT, Denenholz DA. Syphilis — Epidemiology. Clin Dermatol 1984; 2: 24–33.
2. Morbidity and Mortality Report Centers for Disease Control, Atlanta. Continuing increase in infectious syphilis — United States. Arch Dermatol 1988; 124: 509–510.
3. Rolfs RT, Cates W Jr. The perpetual lesions of syphilis. Arch Dermatol 1989; 125: 107–109.
4. Felman YM. Syphilis. From 1945 Naples to 1989 AIDS. Arch Dermatol 1989; 125: 1698–1700.
5. Radolf JD, Kaplan RP. Unusual manifestations of secondary syphilis and abnormal humoral immune response to *Treponema pallidum* antigens in a homosexual man with asymptomatic human immunodeficiency virus infection. J Am Acad Dermatol 1988; 18: 423–428.
5a. Gregory N, Sanchez M, Buchness MR. The spectrum of syphilis in patients with human immunodeficiency virus infection. J Am Acad Dermatol 1990; 22: 1061–1067.
6. Mascola C, Pelosi R, Blount JH et al. Congenital syphilis. Why is it still occurring? JAMA 1984; 252: 1719–1722.
7. Noppakun N, Hendrick SJ, Raimer SS, Sanchez RL. Palmoplantar milia: sequelae of early congenital syphilis. Pediatr Dermatol 1986; 3: 395–398.
8. Chapel T, Prasad P, Chapel J, Lekas N. Extragenital syphilitic chancres. J Am Acad Dermatol 1985; 13: 582–584.
9. Longstreth P, Hoke AW, McElroy C. Hepatitis and bone destruction as uncommon manifestations of early syphilis. Report of a case. Arch Dermatol 1976; 112: 1451–1454.
10. Jordaan HF. Secondary syphilis. A clinicopathological study. Am J Dermatopathol 1988; 10: 399–409.
11. Rosen T, Rubin H, Ellner K et al. Vesicular Jarisch–Herxheimer reaction. Arch Dermatol 1989; 125: 77–81.
12. Rudolph AH. Acquired infectious syphilis. JCE Dermatology 1978; 16(8): 17–33.
13. Sapra S, Weatherhead L. Extensive nodular secondary syphilis. Arch Dermatol 1989; 125: 1666–1669.
14. Kennedy CTC, Sanderson KV. Corymbrose secondary syphilis. Arch Dermatol 1980; 116: 111–112.
15. Jain HC, Fisher BK. Annular syphilid mimicking granuloma annulare. Int J Dermatol 1988; 27: 340–341.
16. Mikhail GR, Chapel TA. Follicular papulopustular syphilid. Arch Dermatol 1969; 100: 471–473.
17. Petrozzi JW, Lockshin NA, Berger BJ. Malignant syphilis. Severe variant of secondary syphilis. Arch Dermatol 1974; 109: 387–389.
18. Pariser H. Precocious noduloulcerative cutaneous syphilis. Arch Dermatol 1975; 111: 76–77.
19. Fisher DA, Chang LW, Tuffanelli DL. Lues maligna. Report of a case and a review of the literature. Arch Dermatol 1969; 99: 70–73.
20. Cole GW, Amon RB, Russell PS. Secondary syphilis presenting as a pruritic dermatosis. Arch Dermatol 1977; 113: 489–490.
21. Pembroke AC, Michell PA, McKee PH. Nodulo-squamous tertiary syphilide. Clin Exp Dermatol 1980; 5: 361–364.
22. Azar HA, Pham TD, Kurban AK. An electron microscopic study of a syphilitic chancre. Arch Pathol 1970; 90: 143–150.
23. Poulsen A, Kobayasi T, Secher L, Weismann K. Treponema pallidum in human chancre tissue: an electron microscopic study. Acta Derm Venereol 1986; 66: 423–430.
24. Abell E, Marks R, Wilson Jones E. Secondary syphilis: a clinico–pathological review. Br J Dermatol 1975; 93: 53–61.
25. Jeerapaet P, Ackerman AB. Histologic patterns of secondary syphilis. Arch Dermatol 1973; 107: 373–377.
26. Alessi E, Innocenti M, Ragusa G. Secondary syphilis. Clinical morphology and histopathology. Am J Dermatopathol 1983; 5: 11–17.
27. McNeely MC, Jorizzo JL, Solomon AR et al. Cutaneous secondary syphilis: preliminary immunohistopathologic support for a role for immune complexes in lesion pathogenesis. J Am Acad Dermatol 1986; 14: 564–571.
28. Jordaan HF, Cilliers J. Secondary syphilis mimicking Sweet's syndrome. Br J Dermatol 1986; 115: 495–496.
29. Cochran REI, Thomson J, Fleming KA, Strong AMM. Histology simulating reticulosis in secondary syphilis. Br J Dermatol 1976; 95: 251–254.
30. Hodak E, David M, Rothem A et al. Nodular secondary syphilis mimicking cutaneous lymphoreticular process. J Am Acad Dermatol 1987; 17: 914–917.
31. Green KM, Heilman E. Secondary syphilis presenting as a palisading granuloma. J Am Acad Dermatol 1985; 12: 957–960.
32. Kahn LB, Gordon WG. Sarcoid-like granulomas in secondary syphilis. Arch Pathol 1971; 92: 334–337.
33. Beckett JH, Bigbee JW. Immunoperoxidase localization of *Treponema pallidum*. Arch Pathol Lab Med 1979; 103: 135–138.
34. Poulsen A, Kobayasi T, Secher L, Weismann K. *Treponema pallidum* in macular and papular secondary syphilitic skin eruptions. Acta Derm Venereol 1986; 66: 251–258.
35. Poulsen A, Kobayasi T, Secher L, Weismann K. Ultrastructural changes of Treponema pallidum isolated from secondary syphilitic skin lesions. Acta Derm Venereol 1987; 67: 289–294.
36. Handsfield HH, Lukehart SA, Sell S et al. Demonstration of *Treponema pallidum* in a cutaneous gumma by indirect immunofluorescence. Arch Dermatol 1983; 119: 677–680.
37. Matsuda-John SS, McElgunn PSJ, Ellis CN. Nodular late syphilis. J Am Acad Dermatol 1983; 9: 269–272.
38. Tanabe JL, Huntley AC. Granulomatous tertiary syphilis. J Am Acad Dermatol 1986; 15: 341–344.
39. Pace JL, Csonka GW. Endemic non-venereal syphilis (bejel) in Saudi Arabia. Br J Vener Dis 1984; 60: 293–297.
40. Browne SG. Yaws. Int J Dermatol 1982; 21: 220–223.
41. Yaws or syphilis? Editorial. Br Med J 1979; 1: 912.
41a. Engelkens HJH, Judanarso J, van der Sluis JJ et al. Disseminated early yaws: report of a child with a remarkable genital lesion mimicking venereal syphilis. Pediatr Dermatol 1990; 7: 60–62.
42. Green CA, Harman RRM. Yaws truly — a survey of patients indexed under "yaws" and a review of the clinical and laboratory problems of diagnosis. Clin Exp Dermatol 1986; 11: 41–48.
43. Binford CH, Connor DH. Pathology of tropical and

microscopy has shown that the majority of the fungal elements are inside the epithelial cells.[95,96]

Chronic mucocutaneous candidosis

The term chronic mucocutaneous candidosis covers a heterogeneous group of disorders characterized by chronic and persistent infections of the mucous membranes, and infections of the skin and nails by various species of *Candida*, usually *C. albicans*.[97–99] The condition ranges in severity from a mild, localized and persistent infection of the mouth, nails or vulva to a severe generalized condition.[92] It may be associated with a spectrum of cellular immunodeficiency states,[100] including several defined syndromes that range from life threatening to subtle.[99,101] Other associations include endocrinopathies and nutritional deficiencies, the latter including disorders of iron metabolism.[92,99,102] Late onset in adults is rare and usually associated with cancer, particularly a thymoma.[99,103,104]

In all clinical groups, vaginitis, paronychia and oral thrush may also be present. The cutaneous lesions are asymptomatic plaques on the dorsum of the hands and feet and periorificial skin.[104] They are brown-red with sharp margins and a soft scale.[104] Sometimes a more extensive scaling eruption is present. Granulomatous lesions have been recorded.[105,106] In 20% of all cases there is a concurrent dermatophyte infection.[102,104]

Histopathology

There is some histological resemblance to the acute form, although the lesions tend to have more epidermal acanthosis, sometimes being vaguely psoriasiform in type (Fig. 25.6). There may be areas of compact orthokeratosis[107] and others of scale crust formation with degenerating neutrophils. This reflects the chronicity of the lesions. Spores and hyphae are usually found without difficulty in PAS preparations.[108]

In granulomatous lesions there are vaguely formed granulomas in the dermis composed of lymphocytes, plasma cells, epithelioid cells and occasional Langhans giant cells.[105,109] Occasional

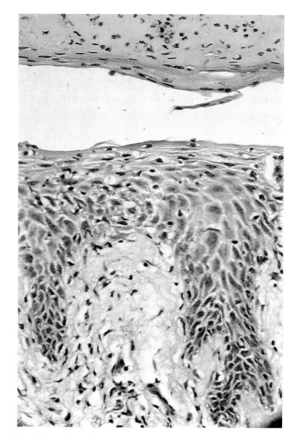

Fig. 25.6 Chronic candidosis. There is mild psoriasiform hyperplasia of the epidermis with overlying scale crust containing degenerate neutrophils. Haematoxylin — eosin

yeast forms and pseudohyphae may be found in the granulomas.

Disseminated candidosis

Disseminated candidosis (systemic candidosis) is increasingly being recognized in immunosuppressed and debilitated patients, particularly those with central venous catheters and those receiving broad spectrum antibiotics.[92,110–111] Multisystem involvement occurs, although cutaneous lesions are present in only 15% of cases.[111] *C. tropicalis* is a frequent isolate from the cutaneous lesions in this type of candidosis.[112]

There is an erythematous, papulonodular rash with multiple lesions on the trunk and proximal parts of the extremities. Sometimes only isolated lesions are present. Another rare clinical presentation mimics that of ecthyma gangrenosum.[113,114]

Systemic candidosis is well recognized in heroin addicts, but only recently have cutaneous lesions, in the form of folliculitis, been reported in some addicts.[115,116]

Histopathology

There are small microabscesses in the upper dermis, sometimes centred on blood vessels.[111] A few budding yeasts may be found in these areas on a PAS stain.[111] At other times the reaction is much milder with only a perivascular mixed inflammatory cell infiltrate. A leucocytoclastic angiitis has been reported.[112] In lesions resembling ecthyma gangrenosum, the papillae are oedematous and distended by numerous pseudohyphae which may extend into vessel walls.[114] Ulceration is also present. In heroin addicts there is a suppurative folliculitis and perifolliculitis. Pseudohyphae are sometimes found within the hair.

Candidosis of the newborn

There are several distinct clinicopathological entities within this group — congenital cutaneous candidosis, neonatal candidosis and infantile gluteal granuloma.[92] Immunity is not impaired.

Congenital cutaneous candidosis presents at birth or in the first days of life with generalized erythematous macules and papulopustules.[117,118] It results from intrauterine infections.[119] Organisms may be demonstrated in the placenta and in the stratum corneum of the neonatal lesions.[117]

Neonatal candidosis presents with oral and perioral lesions in the first two weeks of life.[119] Infection is probably acquired during intravaginal passage at the time of delivery.[119] Sometimes there is involvement of the diaper area.[119]

Infantile gluteal granuloma is an aetiologically controversial entity characterized by discrete granulomatous lesions in the diaper (napkin) area.[120] The role of *Candida* is uncertain.[92,120,121] The use of topical fluorinated steroids and plastic pants in infants with diaper dermatitis has been incriminated.[120,122] Rarely, a similar entity has been reported in this region in adults, possibly as a consequence of *Candida* infection.[123]

Oral candidosis

Oral candidosis (thrush) is found mostly in infants as irregular, white patches and plaques.[92,124] It can also be found as part of chronic mucocutaneous candidosis and in debilitated adults on long-term antibiotics or with a haematological malignancy. Rarely, thrush is related to poor oral hygiene and dentures.[124] Oral candidosis has been reported as an initial manifestation of the acquired immunodeficiency syndrome (AIDS).[125]

Other patterns of mucosal involvement occur on the tongue. These include median rhomboid glossitis[126] and black hairy tongue, although the latter has been attributed to species of *Candida* other than *C. albicans*.[92] A perioral pustular eruption has been ascribed to *Candida*.[127]

Epithelial hyperplasia is a characteristic feature of mucosal infection.[128]

Genital candidosis

Vaginal candidosis is a common gynaecological infection.[129] It tends to occur in the absence of other lesions. A thick creamy vaginal discharge is present. Sexual transmission of the infection sometimes occurs, but balanitis is much less common than vulvovaginitis.[129]

Periungual candidosis

Paronychia may occur as an isolated infection, particularly in females who frequently immerse their hands in water.[130] Minor mechanical trauma, diabetes and circulatory disturbances may also be incriminated.[92] The nail of the middle finger of the dominant hand is most frequently involved.[130] In chronic mucocutaneous candidosis there is usually onychodystrophy with nail bed deformity rather than onycholysis which is more often a manifestation of acute infection.[103]

PITYROSPORUM FOLLICULITIS

This condition presents as erythematous follicular papules and pustules, 2–4 mm in diameter, with a predilection for the upper back, shoulders, chest and upper arms.[154,169] The lesions can be quite pruritic.[170] It is more common in females, and in those over the age of 30.[171] Sometimes there is associated seborrhoeic dermatitis or pityriasis versicolor.[159,169,172] It has been reported in pregnancy,[173] and in immunocompromised patients,[174] in whom it may be confused clinically with more serious infections.[175] *Malassezia furfur* (*P. orbiculare*) can be cultured from lesions in about 75% of cases,[169] and affected individuals have serum antibody titres against this organism.[172] There is some evidence to suggest that follicular occlusion is the primary event in the pathogenesis of this condition, with yeast overgrowth a secondary occurrence.[175a]

Histopathology[176]

Involved follicles are dilated and often plugged with keratinous material and debris. There is a mild chronic inflammatory cell infiltrate around the infundibular portion of the follicle. If serial sections are examined, disruption of the follicular epithelium is sometimes found with basophilic granular debris, keratinous material,

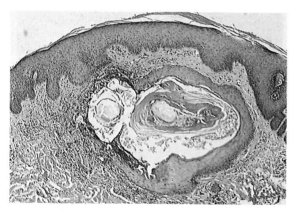

Fig. 25.9 Pityrosporum folliculitis. There are inflammatory cells and basophilic granular debris in the dermis adjacent to the point of rupture of the hair follicle. Haematoxylin — eosin

neutrophils and other inflammatory cells in the perifollicular dermis (Fig. 25.9).[176] A few foreign body giant cells may also be present when rupture of the follicle has occurred. A PAS or silver methenamine stain will reveal spherical to oval yeast-like organisms, 2–4 μm in diameter. These are sometimes budding. They are found most often in the follicle, but following rupture they can also be found in the perifollicular inflammatory exudate.[177] Sometimes a few hyphae can also be seen.[169]

TRICHOSPORONOSIS AND WHITE PIEDRA

The yeast *Trichosporon beigelii* is a rare cause of a generalized blood-borne infection in immunosuppressed patients, particularly those with leukaemia or a lymphoma.[178] Trichosporonosis is frequently fatal in this clinical setting.[178]

This yeast is also responsible for white piedra, a rare superficial infection of the hair resulting in white to tan-coloured gritty nodules, just visible to the naked eye, along the hair shaft.[179,180] The scalp, face or pubic area may be involved. White piedra must be distinguished from black piedra in which tightly adherent black nodules form on the hair, particularly on the scalp.[181] Black piedra is caused by infection with *Piedraia hortae*, which is not a yeast but an ascomycete. Piedra is discussed further in Chapter 15 (p. 454).

Another rare manifestation of *Trichosporon* infection is the formation of a localized deep dermal and subcutaneous granulomatous infection.[182]

Histopathology

In fatal systemic infections, numerous slender hyphae and budding yeasts can be seen in the deep dermis and in the walls of blood vessels.[178,183] The inflammatory response is usually poor because of the underlying neutropenia.[178]

In white piedra, discrete nodules are found at intervals along the hair shaft.[180] High-power light microscopy shows that the nodules consist of numerous spores. Scanning electron microscopy has shown hyphae perpendicular to the surface which are overlaid by budding arthrospores.[184] In black piedra, masses of brown hyphae with ovoid asci containing 2–8 single-celled ascospores are present along the hair shaft (see p. 454).[181]

A granulomatous chronic inflammatory response occurs in the deep dermis and subcutis in the rare localized form of infection with *Trichosporon*, mentioned above.[182]

SYSTEMIC MYCOSES

The term *systemic mycoses* is used here to refer to infections caused by organisms in the following genera — *Blastomyces*, *Coccidioides*, *Paracoccidioides*, *Histoplasma*, and *Cryptococcus*. In most cases the infection develops initially in the lungs; later, the skin and other organs may be involved. All these organisms except *Cryptococcus neoformans* are dimorphic, growing as mycelia in their natural state and assuming a yeast form in tissues. Cryptococcosis has already been considered with the infections caused by yeasts (see p. 648) and will not be considered in this section. The dematiaceous fungi have also been excluded from this group (see p. 653).

NORTH AMERICAN BLASTOMYCOSIS

This infection, caused by *Blastomyces dermatitidis*, occurs on the North American continent and in parts of Africa.[185,185a] There are three clinical forms — pulmonary blastomycosis, disseminated blastomycosis and a primary cutaneous form which results from direct inoculation of organisms into the skin.[185,185b] Most cutaneous lesions occur in the course of disseminated disease (secondary cutaneous blastomycosis); in this form the lesions may be restricted to the lungs, skin and subcutaneous tissue.[186,187] The rare primary inoculation form may be followed by lymphangitic lesions comparable to those of sporotrichosis (see p. 655).[185,188] The more usual lesion is a crusted verrucous nodule, sometimes with central healing and scarring, or an ulcerated plaque.[187] Multiple lesions are sometimes present. A widespread pustular

eruption has been reported.[189] The disease is more frequent in adult males. It shows a predilection for the exposed skin, particularly the face.[186]

Histopathology[185,186]

An established verrucous lesion has many histological features in common with chromomycosis and sporotrichosis. There is pseudoepitheliomatous hyperplasia and a polymorphous dermal inflammatory cell infiltrate with scattered giant cells. Microabscesses are characteristic and occur in the dermis and in acanthotic downgrowths of the epidermis. Poorly formed granulomas and suppurative granulomas may be present.

The thick-walled yeasts measure 7–15 μm in diameter; they are found in the centre of the abscesses and in some of the giant cells. A single bud is sometimes present on the surface of the organism. If organisms are difficult to find in haematoxylin and eosin stained sections, a PAS or silver methenamine stain will usually demonstrate them.

The primary inoculation form shows less epidermal hyperplasia and a mixed dermal infiltrate containing numerous budding organisms.[188] There are usually no giant cells or granulomas.

COCCIDIOIDOMYCOSIS

Infection with *Coccidioides immitis* is most frequently an acute, self-limited pulmonary infection resulting from inhalation of dust-borne arthrospores.[190] The disease is endemic in the south west of the USA, Mexico, and parts of Central and South America. In less than 1% of cases, but particularly in immunocompromised patients,[191,192] dissemination of the infection occurs. The skin may be involved in disseminated disease, the cutaneous manifestations taking the form of a verrucous plaque, usually on the face,[193,194] or subcutaneous abscesses,[195] pustular lesions,[195] or rarely papules and plaques.[196] Primary cutaneous coccidioidomycosis is extremely rare and follows inoculation of the organisms at sites of minor trauma,[197,198] particularly in laboratory[199,200] or agricultural workers.[201] Rarely lymphangitic nodules, similar to those in sporotrichosis, develop.[202] Erythema nodosum occurs in up to 20% of patients with pulmonary infections, and erythema multiforme and a toxic erythema may also occur.[195]

Histopathology

Established lesions show non-caseating granulomas in the upper and mid dermis with overlying pseudoepitheliomatous hyperplasia of the epidermis.[193,202] Thick-walled spherules of *C. immitis*, which usually range from 10–80 μm in diameter, are present within the granulomas, often in multinucleate giant cells.[194] Endospore (sporangiospore) formation is often seen in the largest spherules (sporangia).[194] The spherules can usually be seen without difficulty in haematoxylin and eosin stained preparations. They are sometimes quite sparse.

Early lesions and subcutaneous abscesses show numerous neutrophils with a variable admixture of lymphocytes, histiocytes and eosinophils.[201,202] There are only occasional giant cells. Organisms are usually abundant in these lesions.

Collections of altered red blood cells can rarely mimic the appearances of an endosporulating fungus like *C. immitis*. The term subcutaneous myospherulosis has been applied to this artefact.[202a]

PARACOCCIDIOIDOMYCOSIS

This condition, also known as South American blastomycosis, is a systemic mycosis endemic in rural areas of Latin America.[203] It is caused by the dimorphic fungus *Paracoccidioides brasiliensis*. The respiratory tract is the usual portal of entry from where haematogenous dissemination to other parts of the body occurs.[204] Disseminated paracoccidioidomycosis with skin lesions has been reported in a patient with the acquired immunodeficiency syndrome.[204a] Transcutaneous infection is less common.[205] Oral and mucosal involvement is frequently present in

paracoccidioidomycosis, but cutaneous lesions are less common.[206] There are usually several crusted ulcers when the skin is involved.[207,208] Over 90% of cases occur in males.[204]

Histopathology

Cutaneous lesions often show pseudoepitheliomatous hyperplasia overlying an acute and chronic inflammatory cell infiltrate in the dermis.[209] Granulomas are usually present and there may be foci of suppuration. The characteristic feature is the presence of small and large budding yeasts measuring 5–60 μm in diameter.[209] The buds are distributed on the surface in such a way as to give a 'steering wheel' appearance.[210] The organisms often have a thick wall with a double contour appearance.[207] They can be found in macrophages, foreign body giant cells and lying free in the tissues.[211] They may be overlooked in haematoxylin and eosin stained sections and are best seen with the Grocott silver methenamine stain.[210]

HISTOPLASMOSIS

Histoplasmosis results from infection with *Histoplasma capsulatum*, a dimorphic soil fungus which occurs in parts of America, Africa and Asia. The lung is the most usual primary focus of involvement, except in the African form (see below), and in 99% of cases the pulmonary infection is self-limited and asymptomatic.[212] Immunosuppression, including the acquired immunodeficiency syndrome,[213–219] old age, and chronic disease states predispose to disseminated disease.[220–222] Cutaneous lesions occur in 5% or less of these patients.[212,222,223] This secondary cutaneous form presents as papules,[216] ulcerated nodules, cellulitis-like areas,[214] acneiform lesions,[217] or rarely as an erythroderma.[224] Erythema nodosum is an uncommon manifestation of histoplasmosis.[225] Rarely, a cutaneous lesion is the only manifestation.[226] This primary cutaneous form usually presents as a solitary, self-limited, ulcerated nodule at the site of fungal inoculation.[227,228]

The *African form* of histoplasmosis usually presents with cutaneous granulomas or with skin lesions secondary to underlying osteo-myelitis.[229–231] Disseminated disease can also occur. The causative organism, *H. capsulatum* var. *duboisii*, has much larger yeasts but is otherwise identical in laboratory characteristics to *H. capsulatum*.[230]

The laboratory diagnosis of histoplasmosis can be made by serological testing, positive cultures or histological visualization of organisms in affected tissue. The histoplasmin skin test is no longer considered useful because a positive reaction does not distinguish a current infection from a past one, and negative reactions often occur in disseminated disease.[222]

Histopathology

Usually there is a granulomatous infiltrate in the dermis, and sometimes the subcutis,[232,233] with numerous parasitized macrophages containing small ovoid yeast-like organisms, measuring 2–3 by 3–5 µm in diameter. There is often a surrounding clear halo. Langhans giant cells, lymphocytes and plasma cells are usually present, except in some acute disseminated cases in which parasitized macrophages predominate (Fig. 25.10). Extracellular organisms are some-times found. Transepidermal elimination of macrophages has been reported. Healing lesions show progressive fibrosis.

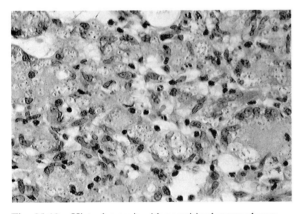

Fig. 25.10 Histoplasmosis with parasitized macrophages and scant lymphocytes.
Haematoxylin — eosin

In the *African form*, the organisms measure from 7–15 µm in diameter.[229,231] Suppuration is sometimes present[230] but the characteristic tissue reaction is the formation of multinucleate giant cells of classic 'foreign body' type, in the cytoplasm of which are usually 5–12 organisms.

Electron microscopy. The organism has a large eccentric nucleus, and a cell wall but no capsule.[231,234] The fungi are present in phagosomes in the cytoplasm of the macro-phages.[234]

INFECTIONS BY DEMATIACEOUS FUNGI

The dematiaceous (pigmented) fungi are a clinically important group.[235] They are world-wide in distribution, although they are partic-ularly prevalent in tropical and subtropical areas.[236] They are found in soil and decaying vegetable matter. The brown pigment of dematiaceous fungi is a melanin, which may be highlighted in tissue sections by the various stains for melanin.[237] They are capable of producing clinical diseases which range from a mild, superficial cutaneous infection to life-threatening visceral disease.[238] Infection usually results from direct inoculation of infected material into the skin, but in some cases of systemic infection inhalation of organisms into the lungs may be the origin.

Various classifications have been proposed for the infections produced by dematiaceous fungi, with a proliferation of nomenclature.[236,239,240] Some of the fungi have been reclassified several times in the last 20 years, resulting in taxonomic confusion. There are two distinct clinico-pathological groups, chromomycosis and phaeohyphomycosis.[240] Pigmented fungi may also produce mycetomas, which are tumefactive lesions with draining sinuses and the presence of grains in the tissue. These cases are best considered with the mycetomas caused by other organisms (see p. 658).[240]

Chromomycosis is characterized by localized cutaneous infection and the presence in the tissues of thick-walled septate bodies (sclerotic

terized by intraepidermal abscesses and often a thick scale crust containing neutrophils. Septate hyphae and spores can be seen in the dermis and the epidermis.[310]

The organisms often show degenerative changes on ultrastructural examination.[311]

MYCETOMA AND MORPHOLOGICALLY SIMILAR CONDITIONS

On a strict aetiological basis, only the eumycetic mycetomas (mycetomas caused by true fungi) should be included in this chapter. As will be seen from the discussions which follow, a similar tissue reaction can be produced by filamentous bacteria of the order Actinomycetales (actinomycetic mycetoma) and certain other bacteria (botryomycosis). This is the rationale for the inclusion here of actinomycosis, nocardiosis and botryomycosis.

MYCETOMA

Mycetoma is an uncommon, chronic infective disease of the skin and subcutaneous tissues, characterized by the triad of tumefaction, draining sinuses and the presence in the exudate of colonial grains.[312,313] The sinuses do not develop until relatively late in the course of the disease, discharging grains which are aggregates of the causal organism embedded in a matrix substance.[314,315] There are two main aetiological groups of mycetoma: actinomycetic mycetomas, which are caused by aerobic filamentous bacteria of the order Actinomycetales, and eumycetic (maduromycotic) mycetomas caused by a number of species of true fungi. The therapy of these two aetiological groups is quite different.[316] Similar clinical lesions can be produced by bacteria (botryomycosis), and rarely by dermatophytes.[313,317,318]

Mycetoma is predominantly a disease of tropical countries, particularly West Africa, parts of India, and Central and South America.[319] There are only sporadic reports of cases in the USA,[320–322] Canada, Europe (including the United Kingdom),[323] and Australia.[324] Different species predominate in different countries.[319–325] Rural workers, particularly males, are most commonly infected. Over 70% of infections occur on the feet (Madura foot), with the hand the next most common site of involvement.

Repeated minor trauma or penetrating injury provides a portal of entry for the organism, which then produces a slowly progressive subcutaneous nodule after an incubation period of several weeks or months.[319] Sinuses develop after 6–12 months. Extension to involve the underlying fascia, muscle and bone is common. Rarely there is lymphatic dissemination to regional lymph nodes.[315] No unequivocal cases of visceral dissemination have been reported. Actinomycetic mycetomas often expand faster, are more invasive, and have more sinuses than eumycetic variants.[319]

Macroscopic features of the grains

The grains which are discharged from the sinuses vary in size, colour and consistency, features which can be used for rapid provisional identification of the aetiological agent.[319] Over 30 species have been identified as causes of mycetoma, and the grains of many of these have overlapping morphological features. Accordingly, culture is required for accurate identification of the causal agent.

The size of the grains varies from microscopic to 1–2 mm in diameter. Large grains are seen with madurellae (particularly *Madurella mycetomatis*) and with *Actinomadura madurae* and

Table 25.1 Colour of the grains (granules) in mycetomas[315,319,328]

EUMYCETOMAS
Black grains: *Madurella mycetomatis, M. grisea, Leptosphaeria senegalensis, Exophiala jeanselmei, Pyrenochaeta romeroi, Curvularia lunata*
Pale grains: *Petriellidium boydii, Aspergillus nidulans, A. flavus, Fusarium* sp., *Acremonium* sp., *Neotestudina rosatii*, dermatophytes

ACTINOMYCETOMAS
Red grains: *Actinomadura pelletieri*
Yellow grains: *Streptomyces somaliensis*
Pale grains: *Nocardia brasiliensis, N. cavae, N. asteroides, Actinomadura madurae*

A. pelletieri while the granules of *Nocardia brasiliensis*, *N. cavae* and *N. asteroides* are small.

The colour of the grains of the most common species is shown in Table 25.1. Dark (black) grain mycetomas are found only among the eumycetic mycetomas.[326] The pigment is a melanoprotein or related substance.[327] The consistency of most grains is soft, but those of *Streptomyces somaliensis* and *Madurella mycetomatis* can be quite hard.[315]

Histopathology[312,315]

The characteristic grains are found in the centre of zones of suppuration and in suppurative granulomas in the subcutis (Fig. 25.16). Neutrophils sometimes invade the grains. Surrounding the areas of suppuration there may be a palisade of histiocytes, beyond which is a mixed inflammatory infiltrate and progressive fibrosis. A few multinucleate giant cells are usually present. An eosinophilic fringe, resembling the Splendore–Hoeppli phenomenon found around some parasites, is sometimes present around the grains.

Several reviews have discussed the morphology of the grains on light microscopy.[315,319] Some of these features are highlighted in Table 25.2. It should be noted that the granules in pale grain eumycetomas are not morphologically distinctive and overlap exists between the various species.

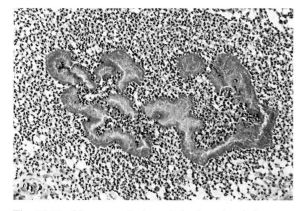

Fig. 25.16 Mycetoma. An irregularly-shaped grain is present in the centre of a zone of suppuration. Haematoxylin — eosin

Table 25.2 Morphology of the grains (granules) in mycetomas

EUMYCETOMAS

Madurella mycetomatis: Large granules (up to 5 mm or more) with interlacing hyphae embedded in interstitial brownish matrix; hyphae at periphery arranged radially with numerous chlamydospores

Petriellidium boydii: Eosinophilic, lighter in the centre; numerous vesicles or swollen hyphae; peripheral eosinophilic fringe; other pale eumycetomas have a minimal fringe and contain a dense mass of intermeshing hyphae[328]

ACTINOMYCETOMAS

Actinomadura madurae: Large (1–5 mm and larger) and multilobulate; peripheral basophilia and central eosinophilia or pale staining; filaments grow from the peripheral zone

Streptomyces somaliensis: Large (0.5–2 mm or more) with dense thin filaments; often stains homogeneously; transverse fracture lines

Nocardia brasiliensis: Small grains (approximately 1 mm); central purple zone; loose clumps of filaments; Gram-positive delicate branching filaments breaking up into bacillary and coccal forms;[329] Gram-negative amorphous matrix (Brown and Benn method)

The large, segmented mycelial filaments (2–4 μm in diameter, with club-shaped hyphal swellings and chlamydospores) that characterize the fungi that cause eumycetomas contrast with the Gram-positive thin filaments (1 μm or less in diameter) of the organisms that cause actinomycetomas.[312,324]

NOCARDIOSIS

Nocardiae are usually Gram-positive, partially acid-fast bacteria which are native to soil and decaying vegetable matter.[330] The common pathogenic species are *N. asteroides*,[331] *N. brasiliensis*[332,333] and *N. caviae*.[334,335] The majority of cases of nocardiosis are septicaemic infections, usually of pulmonary origin, in immunocompromised patients.[331,336] Cutaneous lesions develop in approximately 10% or more of haematogenous infections.[337,337a] Primary cutaneous involvement can be of three different types: mycetoma, lymphocutaneous infection, and superficial cutaneous infections which may take the form of an abscess, an ulcer or cellulitis.[338,339] The lymphocutaneous (sporotrichoid,[340] chancriform) infection,[341]

the order Entomophthorales.[381] Two genera, *Basidiobolus* and *Conidiobolus* (*Entomophthora*) are usually implicated in the infections, which typically are solitary and involve the subcutis of healthy individuals.[382] Spontaneous resolution of the lesions sometimes occurs. These infections have been mainly reported from Africa and South-East Asia.[383]

Phycomycoses have also been reported in animals, particularly horses ('swamp cancer').[384] In addition to fungi from this order, aquatic fungi (particularly *Pythium* sp.) from a totally unrelated 'class' have been incriminated in equine phycomycosis.[385] They are mentioned here because I have seen two cases of a periorbital cellulitis in humans who had contact with horses, which were probably the source of these equine fungi.[385a]

Histopathology[386]

There is granulomatous inflammation in the dermis and subcutis with scattered abscesses, and sometimes areas of necrosis.[387] The most striking feature is the presence of smudgy eosinophilic material surrounding the hyphae.[387,387a] This resembles the Splendore–Hoeppli phenomenon seen in relation to certain metazoan parasites.[388,389] Eosinophils are also present in the inflammatory infiltrate.[389a]

In my human cases of equine phycomycosis,[385a] granulomas and foci resembling the flame figures of eosinophilic cellulitis were present (Fig. 25.17). The fungi were not visualized in H&E and PAS preparations but only with the silver methenamine stain.

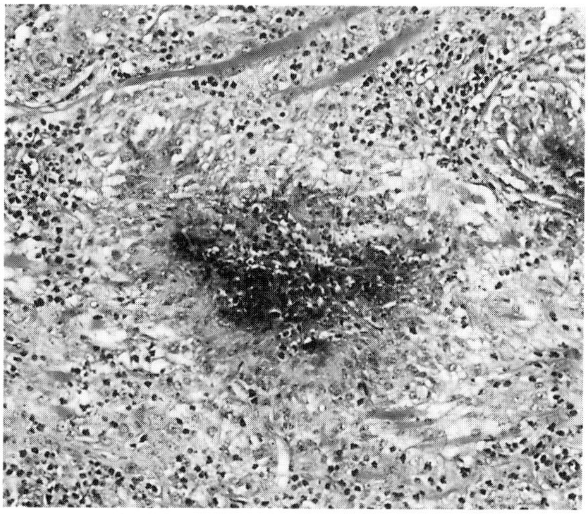

HYALOHYPHOMYCOSES

This term has been applied to a heterogeneous group of opportunistic infections in which the pathogenic fungi grow in tissue in the form of hyphal elements that are unpigmented, septate, and branched or unbranched.[240] Dematiaceous fungi are excluded (see p. 653). Examples of hyalohyphomycoses include infections caused by *Schizophyllum commune* and species of *Acremonium*, *Fusarium*,[390] *Penicillium* and *Scedosporium*.[240] Infections caused by species of *Aspergillus* can also be accommodated in this group.[240] Species of *Fusarium* have been associated with disseminated infection[391] and a facial granuloma.[392] Predisposing immunological disturbances are almost invariably present in individuals with these infections.

Fig. 25.17 Equine phycomycosis in a human. Multinucleate giant cells surround zones of necrosis. There are numerous eosinophils in the infiltrate. Haematoxylin — eosin

ASPERGILLOSIS

Aspergillosis is an opportunistic infection second only to candidosis in frequency among patients with cancer.[393] It usually involves the lungs, and only rarely the skin.[394] Cutaneous lesions are usually part of a systemic infection in immunocompromised patients, although rarely they may be the only manifestation (primary cutaneous aspergillosis).[110a,380a,394,395] Many of the patients with primary cutaneous aspergillosis have leukaemia, and lesions have developed at the sites of intravenous cannulae or of the associated dressings.[396–398] There are one or more violaceous plaques or nodules that rapidly progress to necrotic ulcers with a black eschar.[397,398a] *Aspergillus flavus* is the most common isolate;[396,399] *A. fumigatus* and *A. niger* have also been responsible.[397] Rarely, burns are secondarily infected with *Aspergillus* species.[400]

Histopathology

Depending on the host response, there can be a variety of changes ranging from well-developed granulomas[395] to areas of suppuration and abscess formation,[398] or the presence of masses of fungi with a minimal mixed inflammatory cell response.[394] *Aspergillus* sp. are found as septate hyphae that branch dichotomously.

MISCELLANEOUS MYCOSES

KELOIDAL BLASTOMYCOSIS (LÔBO'S DISEASE)

This is a rare, chronic fungal disease in which slowly growing, keloid-like nodules develop on exposed areas of the body.[401] Lymph node involvement occurs in up to 10% of patients.[402] The infection is caused by the fungus *Loboa loboi*, which is found almost exclusively in Central and South America.[403] Squamous cell carcinoma is a rare complication in chronic lesions.[403a]

Histopathology[403,404]

There is an extensive granulomatous infiltrate in the dermis composed of histiocytes and giant cells of Langhans and foreign body types, together with a few small collections of lymphocytes and plasma cells. There are numerous unstained fungal cells in haematoxylin and eosin stained preparations, both free and in macrophages, giving a characteristic 'sieve-like' appearance (Fig. 25.18). They have a somewhat refractile wall and measure 6–12 μm in diameter. Some budding with the formation of short chains may be present. The organisms are PAS positive; they do not stain with mucicarmine.

RHINOSPORIDIOSIS

Rhinosporidiosis usually presents as polypoid lesions of the nasal and pharyngeal mucosa. Cutaneous lesions are rare, even in India, Ceylon and South America where the fungus, *Rhinosporidium seeberi*, is endemic.[405,406] The skin may be affected by contiguous spread from a mucosal lesion, by autoinoculation, and rarely through haematogenous dissemination.[407,408]

Histopathology[409]

The large spherical sporangia (100 to 400 μm in diameter), containing from hundreds to thousands of endospores, each measuring up to 7 μm in diameter, are characteristic (Fig. 25.19). There is also a mixed inflammatory cell infiltrate, with the formation of some granulomas.

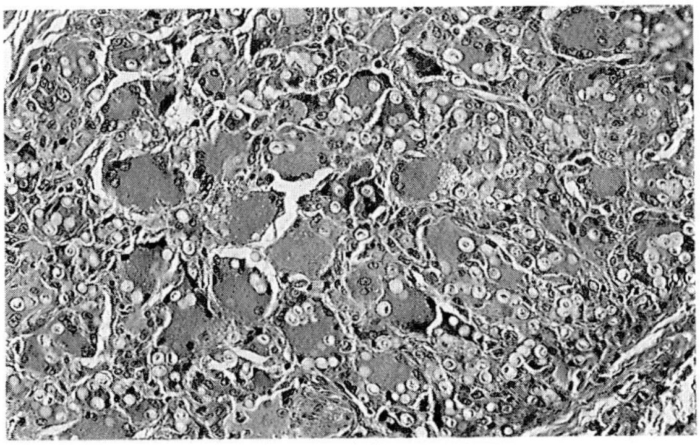

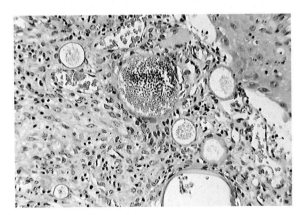

Fig. 25.18 Keloidal blastomycosis. Numerous fungi with slightly refractile cell walls are present in the cytoplasm of macrophages and giant cells. Haematoxylin — eosin

Fig. 25.19 Rhinosporidiosis. There are large spherical sporangia containing numerous endospores. Haematoxylin — eosin

ALGAL INFECTIONS

PROTOTHECOSIS

Protothecosis is a rare infection due to achlorophyllic alga-like organisms of the genus *Prototheca*. There are several species, but *P. wickerhamii* is most often found in man.[410] It can be cultured on Sabouraud's medium, which is the usual medium used for the culture of fungi.[411]

Infection usually results from traumatic inoculation in an immunocompromised host.[412,413] It may involve the skin and subcutaneous tissue.[414] Infection of an olecranon bursa has been recorded.[413] Rarely there is visceral dissemination. Cutaneous lesions are eczematous,[415] herpetiform,[416] or papules[417] and papulonodules which may coalesce, resulting in the formation of slowly progressive plaques.[413,418]

Histopathology[410]

The usual picture is a chronic granulomatous reaction throughout the dermis with a variable admixture of lymphocytes, plasma cells and occasionally eosinophils and even neutrophils. In early lesions there are fewer multinucleate giant cells and the infiltrate shows greater localization to a perivascular and periappendageal position. There is focal necrosis in some lesions, particularly those with subcutaneous involvement. Epidermal changes are variable.[412]

Organisms are found in the cytoplasm of macrophages and multinucleate giant cells as thick-walled spherical bodies, often with a clear halo around them. They may also be free in the dermis, but these are difficult to see in haematoxylin and eosin stained preparations. *Prototheca wickerhamii*, the species usually responsible for the infection in the human, measures from 3–11 μm in diameter. Many show internal septation with endospore formation. They stain with the PAS and silver methenamine stains. Specific identification can be made with a fluorescein-labelled monoclonal antibody.

REFERENCES

Introduction

1. McGinnis MR. Dematiaceous fungi. In: Lennette EH, Balows A, Hausler WJ Jr, Shadomy HJ, eds. Manual of clinical microbiology. 4th ed. Washington, D.C.: American Society for Microbiology, 1985; 561–574.
1a. Elewski BE, Hazen PG. The superficial mycoses and the dermatophytes. J Am Acad Dermatol 1989; 21: 655–673.
2. Mann JL. Autofluorescence of fungi: an aid to detection in tissue sections. Am J Clin Pathol 1983; 79: 587–590.
3. Monheit JE, Cowan DF, Moore DG. Rapid detection of fungi in tissues using calcofluor white and fluorescence microscopy. Arch Pathol Lab Med 1984; 108: 616–618.
4. Anthony PP. A guide to the histological identification of fungi in tissues. J Clin Pathol 1973; 26: 828–831.
5. Graham AR. Fungal autofluorescence with ultraviolet illumination. Am J Clin Pathol 1983; 79: 231–234.
6. Moskowitz LB, Ganjei P, Ziegels-Weissman J et al. Immunohistologic identification of fungi in systemic and cutaneous mycoses. Arch Pathol Lab Med 1986; 110: 433–436.

Superficial filamentous infections

7. Matsumoto T, Ajello L. Current taxonomic concepts pertaining to the dermatophytes and related fungi. Int J Dermatol 1987; 26: 491–499.

8. McGinnis MR, Ajello L, Schell WA. Mycotic diseases. A proposed nomenclature. Int J Dermatol 1985; 24: 9–15.
9. Barlow AJE. Recent advances in fungus diseases. Int J Dermatol 1976; 15: 418–424.
10. Svejgaard E. Epidemiology and clinical features of dermatomycoses and dermatophytoses. Acta Derm Venereol (Suppl) 1986; 121: 19–26.
11. Marks R. Tinea incognito. Int J Dermatol 1978; 17: 301–302.
12. Svejgaard E. Immunologic investigations of dermatophytoses and dermatophytosis. Semin Dermatol 1985; 4: 201–221.
13. Mayou SC, Calderon RA, Goodfellow A, Hay RJ. Deep (subcutaneous) dermatophyte infection presenting with unilateral lymphoedema. Clin Exp Dermatol 1987; 12: 385–388.
14. Kamalam A, Yesudian P, Thambiah AS. An unusual presentation of *Trichophyton violaceum* infection. Br J Dermatol 1977; 96: 205–209.
15. Swart E, Smit FJA. *Trichophyton violaceum* abscesses. Br J Dermatol 1979; 101: 177–184.
15a. Faergemann J, Gisslen H, Dahlberg E et al. *Trichophyton rubrum* abscesses in immunocompromised patients. Acta Derm Venereol 1989; 69: 244–247.
16. Hironaga M, Okazaki N, Saito K, Watanabe S. *Trichophyton mentagrophytes* granulomas. Arch Dermatol 1983; 119: 482–490.
17. Khan KA, Anwar AA. Study of 73 cases of tinea capitis

and tinea favosa in adults and adolescents. J Invest Dermatol 1968; 51: 474–477.

17a. Stephens CJM, Hay RJ, Black MM. Fungal kerion — total scalp involvement due to *Microsporum canis* infection. Clin Exp Dermatol 1989; 14: 442–444.

18. Gamborg Nielsen P. The prevalence of dermatophyte infections in hereditary palmo-plantar keratoderma. Acta Derm Venereol 1983; 63: 439–441.

19. De Vroey C. Epidemiology of ringworm (dermatophytosis). Semin Dermatol 1985; 4: 185–200.

20. Sinski JT, Flouras K. A survey of dermatophytes isolated from human patients in the United States from 1979 to 1981 with chronological listings of worldwide incidence of five dermatophytes often isolated in the United States. Mycopathologia 1984; 85: 97–120.

21. Bhakhtaviziam C, Shafi M, Mehta MC et al. Tinea capitis in Tripoli. Clin Exp Dermatol 1984; 9: 84–88.

22. Onsberg P. Human infections with *Microsporum gypseum* in Denmark. Br J Dermatol 1978; 99: 527–536.

23. Muir DB, Pritchard RC, Gregory JD. Dermatophytes identified at the Australian National Reference Laboratory in Medical Mycology 1966–1982. Pathology 1984; 16: 179–183.

24. McLean T, Levy H, Lue YA. Ecology of dermatophyte infections in South Bronx, New York, 1969 to 1981. J Am Acad Dermatol 1987; 16: 336–340.

25. Vanbreuseghem R. *Trichophyton soudanense* in and outside Africa. Br J Dermatol 1968; 80: 140–148.

26. Harari Z, Sommer B, Feinstein A. *Trichophyton soudanense* infection in two white families. Br J Dermatol 1973; 88: 243–244.

27. Hay RJ, Reid S, Talwat E, Macnamara K. Immune responses of patients with tinea imbricata. Br J Dermatol 1983; 108: 581–586.

28. Hay RJ. Tinea imbricata. The factors affecting persistent dermatophytosis. Int J Dermatol 1985; 24: 562–564.

29. Simpson JR. Tinea barbae caused by *Trichophyton erinacei*. Br J Dermatol 1974; 90: 697–698.

30. Roller JA, Westblom TU. *Microsporum nanum* infection in hog farmers. J Am Acad Dermatol 1986; 15: 935–939.

31. Kelly R, Searls S. *Microsporum nanum* infection in Victoria. Australas J Dermatol 1977; 18: 137–138.

32. Mullins JF, Willis CJ, Bergeron JR et al. *Microsporum nanum*. A review of the literature and a report of two cases. Arch Dermatol 1966; 94: 300–303.

33. Barsky S, Knapp D, McMillen S. *Trichophyton simii* infection in the United States not traceable to India. Arch Dermatol 1978; 114: 118.

34. O'Grady KJ, English MP, Warin RP. *Microsporum equinum* infection of the scalp in an adult. Br J Dermatol 1972; 86: 175–176.

35. Maslen M, Thompson PG. Human infections due to *Trichophyton equinum* var. *autotrophicum* in Victoria. Australas J Dermatol 1984; 25: 29–32.

36. Jones HE, Reinhardt JH, Rinaldi MG. Acquired immunity to dermatophytes. Arch Dermatol 1974; 109: 840–848.

37. Svejgaard E, Christiansen AH, Stahl D, Thomsen K. Clinical and immunological studies in chronic dermatophytosis caused by *Trichophyton rubrum*. Acta Derm Venereol 1984; 64: 493–500.

38. Hay RJ. Chronic dermatophyte infections. I. Clinical and mycological features. Br J Dermatol 1982; 106: 1–7.

39. Ahmed AR. Immunology of human dermatophyte infections. Arch Dermatol 1982; 118: 521–525.

40. Hay RJ, Shennan G. Chronic dermatophyte infections. II. Antibody and cell-mediated immune responses. Br J Dermatol 1982; 106: 191–198.

41. Sherwin WK, Ross TH, Rosenthal CM, Petrozzi JW. An immunosuppressive serum factor in widespread cutaneous dermatophytosis. Arch Dermatol 1979; 115: 600–604.

42. Svejgaard E, Jakobsen B, Svejgaard A. HLA studies in chronic dermatophytosis caused by *Trichophyton rubrum*. Acta Derm Venereol 1983; 63: 254–255.

43. Rasmussen JE, Ahmed AR. Trichophytin reactions in children with tinea capitis. Arch Dermatol 1978; 114: 371–372.

43a. Hebert AA. Tinea capitis. Current concepts. Arch Dermatol 1988; 124: 1554–1557.

44. Bronson DM, Desai DR, Barsky S, Foley SMc. An epidemic of infection with *Trichophyton tonsurans* revealed in a 20-year survey of fungal infections in Chicago. J Am Acad Dermatol 1983; 8: 322–330.

45. Shelley WB, Shelley ES. The infected hairs of tinea capitis due to *Microsporum canis*: Demonstration of uniqueness of the hair cuticle by scanning electron microscopy. J Am Acad Dermatol 1987; 16: 354–361.

46. Rudolph AH. The diagnosis and treatment of tinea capitis due to *Trichophyton tonsurans*. Int J Dermatol 1985; 24: 426–431.

47. Schockman J, Urbach F. Tinea capitis in Philadelphia. Int J Dermatol 1983; 22: 521–524.

48. Suite M, Moore MK, Hay RJ. Leucocyte chemotaxis to antigens of dermatophytes causing scalp ringworm. Clin Exp Dermatol 1987; 12: 171–174.

49. Hebert AA, Head ES, Macdonald EM. Tinea capitis caused by *Trichophyton tonsurans*. Pediatr Dermatol 1985; 2: 219–223.

50. Imamura S, Tanaka M, Watanabe S. Use of immunofluorescence staining in kerion. Arch Dermatol 1975; 111: 906–909.

51. Powell FC, Muller SA. Kerion in the glabrous skin. J Am Acad Dermatol 1982; 7: 490–494.

52. Dvoretzky I, Fisher BK, Movshovitz M, Schewach-Millet M. Favus. Int J Dermatol 1980; 19: 89–93.

53. Joly J, Delage G, Auger P, Ricard P. Favus. Twenty indigenous cases in the Province of Quebec. Arch Dermatol 1978; 114: 1647–1648.

54. Inman P. Favus of scalp with unusual epidemiological features. Br J Dermatol 1954; 66: 409–415.

55. Pravda DJ, Pugliese MM. Tinea faciei. Arch Dermatol 1978; 114: 250–252.

56. Raimer SS, Beightler EL, Hebert AA et al. Tinea faciei in infants caused by *Trichophyton tonsurans*. Pediatr Dermatol 1986; 3: 452–454.

57. Frankel DH, Soltani K, Medenica MM, Rippon JW. Tinea of the face caused by *Trichophyton rubrum* with histologic changes of granuloma faciale. J Am Acad Dermatol 1988; 18: 403–406.

58. Blank H, Taplin D, Zaias N. Cutaneous *Trichophyton mentagrophytes* infections in Vietnam. Arch Dermatol 1969; 99: 135–144.

59. Midgley G, Clayton YM. Distribution of dermatophytes and candida spores in the environment. Br J Dermatol (Suppl) 1972; 86: 69–77.

59a. Logan RA, Kobza-Black A. Tinea imbricata in a British nurse. Clin Exp Dermatol 1988; 13: 232–233.
60. Blank F, Mann SJ. *Trichophyton rubrum* infections according to age, anatomical distribution and sex. Br J Dermatol 1975; 92: 171–174.
61. Leyden JJ, Kligman AM. Interdigital athlete's foot. The interaction of dermatophytes and resident bacteria. Arch Dermatol 1978; 114: 1466–1472.
62. Cooper JL, Mikhail GR. *Trichophyton rubrum.* Perifolliculitis on amputation stump. Arch Dermatol 1966; 94: 56–59.
63. Mikhail GR. *Trichophyton rubrum* granuloma. Int J Dermatol 1970; 9: 41–46.
64. Barson WJ. Granuloma and pseudogranuloma of the skin due to *Microsporum canis.* Arch Dermatol 1985; 121: 895–897.
65. Ravaghi M. Superficial and deep granulomatous lesions caused by *Trichophyton violaceum.* Cutis 1976; 17: 976–977.
66. Ramesh V, Reddy BSN, Singh R. Onychomycosis. Int J Dermatol 1983; 22: 148–152.
67. Andre J, Achten G. Onychomycosis. Int J Dermatol 1987; 26: 481–490.
68. Roberts DT, Tuyp E. Onychomycosis. Semin Dermatol 1985; 4: 222–226.
69. Walshe MM, English MP. Fungi in nails. Br J Dermatol 1966; 78: 198–207.
70. Weismann K, Knudsen EA, Pedersen C. White nails in AIDS/ARC due to *Trichophyton rubrum* infection. Clin Exp Dermatol 1988; 13: 24–25.
71. Hay RJ, Baran R, Moore MK, Wilkinson JD. *Candida* onychomycosis — an evaluation of the role of *Candida* species in nail disease. Br J Dermatol 1988; 118: 47–58.
72. Zaias N. Onychomycosis. Arch Dermatol 1972; 105: 263–274.
73. Lee S, Bang D. Hyphae on the ventral nailplate as a clue to onychomycosis. Am J Dermatopathol 1987; 9: 445–446.
74. Scher RK, Ackerman AB. Histologic differential diagnosis of onychomycosis and psoriasis of the nail unit from cornified cells of the nail bed alone. Am J Dermatopathol 1980; 2: 255–257.
75. Graham JH. Superficial fungus infections. In: Graham JH, Johnson WC, Helwig EB. Dermal pathology. Hagerstown, Md: Harper & Row, 1972; 137–253.
76. Ackerman AB. Neutrophils within the cornified layer as clues to infection by superficial fungi. Am J Dermatopathol 1979; 1: 69–75.
77. Ollague J, Ackerman AB. Compact orthokeratosis as a clue to chronic dermatophytosis and candidiasis. Am J Dermatopathol 1982; 4: 359–363.
78. Gottlieb GJ, Ackerman AB. The "sandwich sign" of dermatophytosis. Am J Dermatopathol 1986; 8: 347–350.
79. Berk SH, Penneys NS, Weinstein GD. Epidermal activity in annular dermatophytosis. Arch Dermatol 1976; 112: 485–488.
80. Carter RL. Majocchi's granuloma. J Am Acad Dermatol 1980; 2: 75.
81. Kuo T-T, Chen S-Y, Chan H-L. Tinea infection histologically simulating eosinophilic pustular folliculitis. J Cutan Pathol 1986; 13: 118–122.
82. Graham JH, Johnson WC, Burgoon CF Jr, Helwig EB. Tinea capitis. A histopathological and histochemical study. Arch Dermatol 1964; 89: 528–543.
83. Greer DL, Gutierrez MM. Tinea pedis caused by *Hendersonula toruloidea.* A new problem in dermatology. J Am Acad Dermatol 1987; 16: 1111–1115.
84. Ho Ping Kong B, Kapica L, Lee R. Keratin invasion by *Hendersonula toruloidea.* A tropical pathogenic fungus resistant to therapy. Int J Dermatol 1984; 23: 65–66.
85. Peiris S, Moore MK, Marten RH. *Scytalidium hyalinum* infection of skin and nails. Br J Dermatol 1979; 100: 579–584.
86. Campbell CK, Kurwa A, Abdel-Aziz A-HM, Hodgson C. Fungal infection of skin and nails by *Hendersonula toruloidea.* Br J Dermatol 1973; 89: 45–52.
87. Hay RJ, Moore MK. Clinical features of superficial fungal infections caused by *Hendersonula toruloidea* and *Scytalidium hyalinum.* Br J Dermatol 1984; 110: 677–683.

Yeast infections

88. Cooper BH, Silva-Hutner M. Yeasts of medical importance. In: Lennette EH, Balows A, Hausler WJ Jr, Shadomy HJ, eds. Manual of clinical microbiology. 4th ed. Washington, D.C.: American Society for Microbiology, 1985; 526–541.
89. Stenderup A. Ecology of yeast and epidemiology of yeast infections. Acta Derm Venereol (Suppl) 1986; 121: 27–37.
89a. Groisser D, Bottone EJ, Lebwohl M. Association of *Pityrosporum orbiculare (Malassezia furfur)* with seborrheic dermatitis in patients with acquired immunodeficiency syndrome (AIDS). J Am Acad Dermatol 1989; 20: 770–773.
90. Faergemann J, Maibach HI. The Pityrosporon yeasts. Their role as pathogens. Int J Dermatol 1984; 23: 463–465.
91. Bergman AG, Kauffman CA. Dermatitis due to *Sporobolomyces* infection. Arch Dermatol 1984; 120: 1059–1060.
92. DeCastro P, Jorizzo JL. Cutaneous aspects of candidosis. Semin Dermatol 1985; 4: 165–172.
92a. Ro BI. Chronic mucocutaneous candidosis. Int J Dermatol 1988; 27: 457–462.
92b. Winton GB. Skin diseases aggravated by pregnancy. J Am Acad Dermatol 1989; 20: 1–13.
93. Ray TL, Wuepper KD. Recent advances in cutaneous candidiasis. Int J Dermatol 1978; 17: 683–690.
94. Dekio S, Imaoka C, Jidoi J. Candida folliculitis associated with hypothyroidism. Br J Dermatol 1987; 117: 663–664.
95. Scherwitz C. Ultrastructure of human cutaneous candidosis. J Invest Dermatol 1982; 78: 200–205.
96. Montes LF, Wilborn WH. Fungus-host relationship in candidiasis. A brief review. Arch Dermatol 1985; 121: 119–124.
97. Rockoff AS. Chronic mucocutaneous candidiasis. Successful treatment with intermittent oral doses of clotrimazole. Arch Dermatol 1979; 115: 322–323.
98. Kirkpatrick CH, Montes LF. Chronic mucocutaneous candidiasis. J Cutan Pathol 1974; 1: 211–229.
99. Jorizzo JL. Chronic mucocutaneous candidosis. An update. Arch Dermatol 1982; 118: 963–965.
100. Horsmanheimo M, Krohn K, Virolainen M, Blomqvist K. Immunologic features of chronic granulomatous

mucocutaneous candidiasis before and after treatment with transfer factor. Arch Dermatol 1979; 115: 180–184.

101. Higgs JM, Wells RS. Chronic muco-cutaneous candidiasis: new approaches to treatment. Br J Dermatol 1973; 89: 179–190.

102. Shama SK, Kirkpatrick CH. Dermatophytosis in patients with chronic mucocutaneous candidiasis. J Am Acad Dermatol 1980; 2: 285–294.

103. Maize JC, Lynch PJ. Chronic mucocutaneous candidiasis of the adult. A report of a patient with an associated thymoma. Arch Dermatol 1972; 105: 96–98.

104. Palestine RF, Su WPD, Liesegang TJ. Late-onset chronic mucocutaneous and ocular candidiasis and malignant thymoma. Arch Dermatol 1983; 119: 580–586.

105. Piamphongsant T, Yavapolkul V. Diffuse chronic granulomatous mucocutaneous candidiasis. Int J Dermatol 1976; 15: 219–224.

106. Montes LF, Cooper MD, Bradford LG et al. Prolonged oral treatment of chronic mucocutaneous candidiasis with amphotericin B. Arch Dermatol 1971; 104: 45–56.

107. Ollague J, Ackerman AB. Compact orthokeratosis as a clue to chronic dermatophytosis and candidiasis. Am J Dermatopathol 1982; 4: 359–363.

108. Imperato PJ, Buckley E III, Callaway JL. Candida granuloma. A clinical and immunologic study. Arch Dermatol 1968; 97: 139–146.

109. Newcomer VD, Landau JW, Lehman R et al. Candida granuloma. Studies of host-parasite relationships. Arch Dermatol 1966; 93: 149–160.

110. Myerowitz RL, Pazin GJ, Allen CM. Disseminated candidiasis. Changes in incidence, underlying diseases, and pathology. Am J Clin Pathol 1977; 68: 29–38.

110a. Radentz WH. Opportunistic fungal infections in immunocompromised hosts. J Am Acad Dermatol 1989; 20: 989–1003.

111. Jacobs MI, Magid MS, Jarowski CI. Disseminated candidiasis. Newer approaches to early recognition and treatment. Arch Dermatol 1980; 116: 1277–1279.

112. Grossman ME, Silvers DN, Walther RR. Cutaneous manifestations of disseminated candidiasis. J Am Acad Dermatol 1980; 2: 111–116.

113. File TM Jr, Marina OA, Flowers FP. Necrotic skin lesions associated with disseminated candidiasis. Arch Dermatol 1979; 115: 214–215.

114. Fine JD, Miller JA, Harrist TJ, Haynes HA. Cutaneous lesions in disseminated candidiasis mimicking ecthyma gangrenosum. Am J Med 1981; 70: 1133–1135.

115. Dupont B, Drouhet E. Cutaneous, ocular, and osteoarticular candidiasis in heroin addicts: new clinical and therapeutic aspects in 38 patients. J Infect Dis 1985; 152: 577–591.

116. Podzamczer D, Ribera M, Gudiol F. Skin abscesses caused by Candida albicans in heroin abusers. J Am Acad Dermatol 1987; 16: 386–387.

117. Kam LA, Giacoia GP. Congenital cutaneous candidiasis. Am J Dis Child 1975; 129: 1215–1218.

118. Rudolph N, Tariq AA, Reale MR et al. Congenital cutaneous candidiasis. Arch Dermatol 1977; 113: 1101–1103.

119. Chapel TA, Gagliardi C, Nichols W. Congenital cutaneous candidiasis. J Am Acad Dermatol 1982; 6: 926–928.

120. Bonifazi E, Garofalo L, Lospalluti M et al. Granuloma gluteale infantum with atrophic scars: clinical and histological observations in eleven cases. Clin Exp Dermatol 1981; 6: 23–29.

121. Montes LF. The histopathology of diaper dermatitis. Historical review. J Cutan Pathol 1978; 5: 1–4.

122. Lovell CR, Atherton DJ. Infantile gluteal granulomata — case report. Clin Exp Dermatol 1984; 9: 522–525.

123. Maekawa Y, Sakazaki Y, Hayashibara T. Diaper area granuloma of the aged. Arch Dermatol 1978; 114: 382–383.

124. Jolly M. White lesions of the mouth. Int J Dermatol 1977; 16: 713–725.

125. Klein RS, Harris CA, Small CB et al. Oral candidiasis in high-risk patients as the initial manifestation of the acquired immunodeficiency syndrome. N Engl J Med 1984; 311: 354–358.

126. Cooke BED. Median rhomboid glossitis. Candidiasis and not a developmental anomaly. Br J Dermatol 1975; 93: 399–405.

127. Brandrup F, Wantzin GL, Thomsen K. Perioral pustular eruption caused by Candida albicans. Br J Dermatol 1981; 105: 327–329.

128. Cawson RA. Induction of epithelial hyperplasia by Candida albicans. Br J Dermatol 1973; 89: 497–503.

129. Odds FC. Genital candidosis. Clin Exp Dermatol 1982; 7: 345–354.

130. Ganor S, Pumpianski R. Chronic Candida albicans paronychia in adult Israeli women. Sources and spread. Br J Dermatol 1974; 90: 77–83.

131. Hay RJ. Cryptococcus neoformans and cutaneous cryptococcosis. Semin Dermatol 1985; 4: 252–259.

132. Sarosi GA, Silberfarb PM, Tosh FE. Cutaneous cryptococcosis. A sentinel of disseminated disease. Arch Dermatol 1971; 104: 1–3.

132a. Barfield L, Iacobelli D, Hashimoto K. Secondary cutaneous cryptococcosis: case report and review of 22 cases. J Cutan Pathol 1988; 15: 385–392.

133. Gordon LA, Gordon DL. Cryptococcal infection simulating varicella. Australas J Dermatol 1987; 28: 24–26.

134. Iacobellis FW, Jacobs MI, Cohen RP. Primary cutaneous cryptococcosis. Arch Dermatol 1979; 115: 984–985.

135. Bee OB, Tan T, Pang R. A case of primary cutaneous cryptococcosis successfully treated with miconazole. Arch Dermatol 1981; 117: 290–291.

136. Sussman EJ, McMahon F, Wright D, Friedman HM. Cutaneous cryptococcosis without evidence of systemic involvement. J Am Acad Dermatol 1984; 11: 371–374.

137. Webling DD'A, Mahajani A. Localized dermal cryptococcosis following a scorpion sting. Australas J Dermatol 1981; 22: 127–128.

138. Gandy WM. Primary cutaneous cryptococcosis. Arch Dermatol 1950; 62: 97–104.

139. Granier F, Kanitakis J, Hermier C et al. Localized cutaneous cryptococcosis successfully treated with ketoconazole. J Am Acad Dermatol 1987; 16: 243–249.

140. Birkett DA, McMurray J. Cutaneous cryptococcosis. Proc R Soc Med 1976; 69: 515–517.

141. Borton LK, Wintroub BU. Disseminated cryptococcosis presenting as herpetiform lesions in a homosexual man with acquired immunodeficiency syndrome. J Am Acad Dermatol 1984; 10: 387–390.

141a. Pierard GE, Pierard-Franchimont C, Estrada JE et al. Cutaneous mixed infections in AIDS. Am J Dermatopathol 1990; 12: 63–66.

142. Rico MJ, Penneys NS. Cutaneous cryptococcosis resembling molluscum contagiosum in a patient with AIDS. Arch Dermatol 1985; 121: 901–902.

142a. Picon L, Vaillant L, Duong T et al. Cutaneous cryptococcosis resembling molluscum contagiosum: a first manifestation of AIDS. Acta Derm Venereol 1989; 69: 365–367.

143. Schupbach CW, Wheeler CE, Briggaman RA et al. Cutaneous manifestations of disseminated cryptococcosis. Arch Dermatol 1976; 112: 1734–1740.

144. Gauder JP. Cryptococcal cellulitis. JAMA 1977; 237: 672–673.

145. Rook A, Woods B. Cutaneous cryptococcosis. Br J Dermatol 1962; 74: 43–49.

146. Hall JC, Brewer JH, Crouch TT, Watson KR. Cryptococcal cellulitis with multiple sites of involvement. J Am Acad Dermatol 1987; 17: 329–332.

147. Carlson KC, Mehlmauer M, Evans S, Chandrasoma P. Cryptococcal cellulitis in renal transplant recipients. J Am Acad Dermatol 1987; 17: 469–472.

148. Massa MC, Doyle JA. Cutaneous cryptococcosis simulating pyoderma gangrenosum. J Am Acad Dermatol 1981; 5: 32–36.

149. Kamalam A, Yesudian P, Thambiah AS. Cutaneous infection by Cryptococcus laurentii. Br J Dermatol 1977; 97: 221–223.

150. Chu AC, Hay RJ, MacDonald DM. Cutaneous cryptococcosis. Br J Dermatol 1980; 103: 95–100.

150a. Leidel GD, Metcalf JS. Formation of palisading granulomas in a patient with chronic cutaneous cryptococcosis. Am J Dermatopathol 1989; 11: 560–562.

151. Gutierrez F, Fu YS, Lurie HI. Cryptococcosis histologically resembling histoplasmosis. A light and electron microscopical study. Arch Pathol 1975; 99: 347–352.

152. Collins DN, Oppenheim IA, Edwards MR. Cryptococcosis associated with systemic lupus erythematosus. Light and electron microscopic observations on a morphologic variant. Arch Pathol 1971; 91: 78–88.

153. Noble RC, Fajardo LF. Primary cutaneous cryptococcosis: review and morphologic study. Am J Clin Pathol 1972; 57: 13–22.

154. Faergemann J. Lipophilic yeasts in skin disease. Semin Dermatol 1985; 4: 173–184.

155. Faergemann J, Fredriksson T. Tinea versicolor with regard to seborrheic dermatitis. An epidemiological investigation. Arch Dermatol 1979; 115: 966–968.

156. Faergemann J. Tinea versicolor and Pityrosporum orbiculare: mycological investigations, experimental infections and epidemiological surveys. Acta Derm Venereol (Suppl) 1979; 86: 5–20.

157. Roberts SOB. Pityriasis versicolor: a clinical and mycological investigation. Br J Dermatol 1969; 81: 315–326.

158. McGinley KJ, Lantis LR, Marples RR. Microbiology of tinea versicolor. Arch Dermatol 1970; 102: 168–171.

159. Ford G. Pityrosporon folliculitis. Int J Dermatol 1984; 23: 320–321.

160. Roberts SOB. Pityrosporum orbiculare: incidence and distribution on clinically normal skin. Br J Dermatol 1969; 81: 264–269.

161. Weary PE. Pityrosporum ovale. Observations on some aspects of host-parasite interrelationship. Arch Dermatol 1968; 98: 408–422.

162. Borgers M, Cauwenbergh G, Van de Ven M-A et al. Pityriasis versicolor and Pityrosporum ovale. Morphogenetic and ultrastructural considerations. Int J Dermatol 1987; 26: 586–589.

163. Faergemann J, Fredriksson T. Tinea versicolor: some new aspects on etiology, pathogenesis, and treatment. Int J Dermatol 1982; 21: 8–11.

164. Allen HB, Charles CR, Johnson BL. Hyperpigmented tinea versicolor. Arch Dermatol 1976; 112: 1110–1112.

165. Karaoui R, Bou-Resli M, Al-Zaid NS, Mousa A. Tinea versicolor: ultrastructural studies on hypopigmented and hyperpigmented skin. Dermatologica 1981; 162: 69–85.

166. Dotz WI, Henrikson DM, Yu GSM, Galey CI. Tinea versicolor: A light and electron microscopic study of hyperpigmented skin. J Am Acad Dermatol 1985; 12: 37–44.

167. Scheynius A, Faergemann J, Forsum U, Sjoberg O. Phenotypic characterization in situ of inflammatory cells in pityriasis (tinea) versicolor. Acta Derm Venereol 1984: 64: 473–479.

168. Marinaro RE, Gershenbaum MR, Roisen FJ, Papa CM. Tinea versicolor: a scanning electron microscopic view. J Cutan Pathol 1978; 5: 15–22.

169. Back O, Faergemann J, Hornqvist R. Pityrosporum folliculitis: A common disease of the young and middle-aged. J Am Acad Dermatol 1985; 12: 56–61.

170. Berretty PJM, Neumann HAM, Hulsebosch HJ. Pityrosporum folliculitis: is it a real entity? Br J Dermatol 1980; 103: 565.

171. Ford GP, Ive FA, Midgley G. Pityrosporum folliculitis and ketoconazole. Br J Dermatol 1982; 107: 691–695.

172. Faergemann J, Johansson S, Back O, Scheynius A. An immunologic and cultural study of Pityrosporum folliculitis. J Am Acad Dermatol 1986; 14: 429–433.

173. Heymann WR, Wolf DJ. Malassezia (Pityrosporon) folliculitis occurring during pregnancy. Int J Dermatol 1986; 25: 49–51.

174. Bufill JA, Lum LG, Caya JG et al. Pityrosporum folliculitis after bone marrow transplantation. Clinical observations in five patients. Ann Intern Med 1988; 108: 560–563.

175. Klotz SA, Drutz DJ, Huppert M, Johnson JE. Pityrosporum folliculitis. Its potential for confusion with skin lesions of systemic candidiasis. Arch Intern Med 1982; 142: 2126–2129.

175a. Hill MK, Goodfield MJD, Rodgers FG et al. Skin surface electron microscopy in Pityrosporum folliculitis. Arch Dermatol 1990; 126: 181–184.

176. Potter BS, Burgoon CF, Johnson WC. Pityrosporum folliculitis. Arch Dermatol 1973; 107: 388–391.

177. Hanna JM, Johnson WT, Wyre HW. Malassezia

(Pityrosporum) folliculitis occurring with granuloma annulare and alopecia areata. Arch Dermatol 1983; 119: 869–871.

178. Walsh TJ, Newman KR, Moody M et al. Trichosporonosis in patients with neoplastic disease. Medicine (Baltimore) 1986; 65: 268–279.

179. Steinman HK, Pappenfort RB. White piedra — a case report and review of the literature. Clin Exp Dermatol 1984; 9: 591–598.

180. Smith JD, Murtishaw WA, McBride ME. White piedra (trichosporosis). Arch Dermatol 1973; 107: 439–442.

181. Benson PM, Lapins NA, Odom RB. White piedra. Arch Dermatol 1983; 119: 602–604.

182. Otsuka F, Seki Y, Takizawa K et al. Facial granuloma associated with *Trichosporon cutaneum* infection. Arch Dermatol 1986; 122: 1176–1179.

183. Manzella JP, Berman IJ, Kukrika MD. *Trichosporon beigelii* fungemia and cutaneous dissemination. Arch Dermatol 1982; 118: 343–345.

184. Lassus A, Kanerva L, Stubb S. White piedra. Report of a case evaluated by scanning electron microscopy. Arch Dermatol 1982; 118: 208–211.

Systemic mycoses

185. Harrell ER, Curtis AC. North American blastomycosis. Am J Med 1959; 27: 750–766.

185a. Malak JA, Farah FS. Blastomycosis in the Middle East. Report of a suspected case of North American blastomycosis. Br J Dermatol 1971; 84: 161–166.

185b. Landay ME, Schwarz J. Primary cutaneous blastomycosis. Arch Dermatol 1971; 104: 408–411.

186. Klapman MH, Superfon NP, Solomon LM. North American blastomycosis. Arch Dermatol 1970; 101: 653–658.

187. Witorsch P, Utz JP. North American blastomycosis: a study of 40 patients. Medicine (Baltimore) 1968; 47: 169–200.

188. Wilson JW, Cawley EP, Weidman FD, Gilmer WS. Primary cutaneous North American blastomycosis. Arch Dermatol 1955; 71: 39–45.

189. Hashimoto K, Kaplan RJ, Daman LA et al. Pustular blastomycosis. Int J Dermatol 1977; 16: 277–280.

190. Basler RSW, Lagomarsino SL. Coccidioidomycosis: clinical review and treatment update. Int J Dermatol 1979; 18: 104–110.

191. Deresinski SC, Stevens DA. Coccidioidomycosis in compromised hosts. Medicine (Baltimore) 1975; 54: 377–395.

192. Lynch PJ, Rather EP, Rutala PJ. Pemphigus and coccidioidomycosis. Cutis 1978; 22: 581–583.

193. Schwartz RA, Lamberts RJ. Isolated nodular cutaneous coccidioidomycosis. The initial manifestation of disseminated disease. J Am Acad Dermatol 1981; 4: 38–46.

194. Hamner RW, Baum EW, Pritchett PS. Coccidioidal meningitis diagnosed by skin biopsy. Cutis 1982; 29: 603–610.

195. Bayer AS, Yoshikawa TT, Galpin JE, Guze LB. Unusual syndromes of coccidioidomycosis: diagnostic and therapeutic considerations. A report of 10 cases and review of the English literature. Medicine (Baltimore) 1976; 55: 131–152.

196. Hobbs ER, Hempstead RW. Cutaneous coccidioidomycosis simulating lepromatous leprosy. Int J Dermatol 1984; 23: 334–336.

197. Winn WA. Primary cutaneous coccidioidomycosis. Reevaluation of its potentiality based on study of three new cases. Arch Dermatol 1965; 92: 221–228.

198. Harrell ER, Honeycutt WM. Coccidioidomycosis: a traveling fungus disease. Arch Dermatol 1963; 87: 188–196.

199. Overholt EL, Hornick RB. Primary cutaneous coccidioidomycosis. Arch Intern Med 1964; 114: 149–153.

200. Carroll GF, Haley LD, Brown JM. Primary cutaneous coccidioidomycosis. A review of the literature and a report of a new case. Arch Dermatol 1977; 113: 933–936.

201. Levan NE, Huntington RW. Primary cutaneous coccidioidomycosis in agricultural workers. Arch Dermatol 1965; 92: 215–220.

202. Trimble JR, Doucette J. Primary cutaneous coccidioidomycosis. Report of a case of a laboratory infection. Arch Dermatol 1956; 74: 405–410.

202a. Waldman JS, Barr RJ, Espinoza FP, Simmons GE. Subcutaneous myospherulosis. J Am Acad Dermatol 1989; 21: 400–403.

203. Teixeira F, Gayotto LC, de Brito T. Morphological patterns of the liver in South American blastomycosis. Histopathology 1978; 2: 231–237.

204. Murray HW, Littman ML, Roberts RB. Disseminated paracoccidioidomycosis (South American blastomycosis) in the United States. Am J Med 1974; 56: 209–220.

204a. Bakos L, Kronfeld M, Hampse S et al. Disseminated paracoccidioidomycosis with skin lesions in a patient with acquired immunodeficiency syndrome. J Am Acad Dermatol 1989; 20: 854–855.

205. Gimenez MF, Tausk F, Gimenez MM, Gigli I. Langerhans' cells in paracoccidioidomycosis. Arch Dermatol 1987; 123: 479–481.

206. Londero AT, Ramos CD. Paracoccidioidomycosis. A clinical and morphological study of forty-one cases observed in Santa Maria, RS, Brazil. Am J Med 1972; 52: 771–775.

207. Perry HO, Weed LA, Kierland RA. South American blastomycosis. Report of case and review of laboratory features. Arch Dermatol 1954; 70: 477–482.

208. Kroll JJ, Walzer RA. Paracoccidioidomycosis in the United States. Arch Pathol 1972; 106: 543–546.

209. Hernandez-Perez E, Orellana-Diaz O. Paracoccidioidomycosis. Report of the first autochthonous case in El Salvador. Int J Dermatol 1984; 23: 617–618.

210. Salfelder K, Doehnert G, Doehnert H-R. Paracoccidioidomycosis. Anatomic study with complete autopsies. Virchows Arch Path Anat 1969; 348: 51–76.

211. de Brito T, Furtado JS, Castro RM, Manini M. Intraepithelial parasitism as an infection mechanism in human paracoccidioidomycosis (South American blastomycosis). Virchows Arch Path Anat 1973; 361: 129–138.

212. Goodwin RA, Shapiro JL, Thurman GH et al. Disseminated histoplasmosis: clinical and pathologic correlations. Medicine (Baltimore) 1980; 59: 1–33.

213. Peterson PK, Dahl MV, Howard RJ et al. Mucormycosis and cutaneous histoplasmosis in a

renal transplant recipient. Arch Dermatol 1982; 118: 275–277.

214. Giessel M, Rau JM. Primary cutaneous histoplasmosis. A new presentation. Cutis 1980; 25: 152–154.

215. Bonner JR, Alexander WJ, Dismukes WE et al. Disseminated histoplasmosis in patients with the acquired immune deficiency syndrome. Arch Intern Med 1984; 144: 2178–2181.

216. Mayoral F, Penneys NS. Disseminated histoplasmosis presenting as a transepidermal elimination disorder in an AIDS victim. J Am Acad Dermatol 1985; 13: 842–844.

217. Hazelhurst JA, Vismer HF. Histoplasmosis presenting with unusual skin lesions in acquired immunodeficiency syndrome (AIDS). Br J Dermatol 1985; 113: 345–348.

218. Hernandez DE, Morgenstern J, Weiss E et al. Cutaneous lesions of disseminated histoplasmosis in a Haitian man with the acquired immunodeficiency syndrome. Int J Dermatol 1986; 25: 117–118.

219. Taylor MN, Baddour LM, Alexander JR. Disseminated histoplasmosis associated with the acquired immune deficiency syndrome. Am J Med 1984; 77: 579–580.

220. Paya CV, Roberts GD, Cockerill FR. Laboratory methods for the diagnosis of disseminated histoplasmosis: clinical importance of the lysis – centrifugation blood culture technique. Mayo Clin Proc 1987; 62: 480–485.

221. Wheat LJ, Slama TG, Zeckel ML. Histoplasmosis in the acquired immune deficiency syndrome. Am J Med 1985; 78: 203–210.

222. Sathapatayavongs B, Batteiger BE, Wheat J et al. Clinical and laboratory features of disseminated histoplasmosis during two large urban outbreaks. Medicine (Baltimore) 1983; 62: 263–270.

223. Studdard J, Sneed WF, Taylor MR et al. Cutaneous histoplasmosis. Am Rev Respir Dis 1976; 113: 689–693.

224. Samovitz M, Dillon TK. Disseminated histoplasmosis presenting as exfoliative erythroderma. Arch Dermatol 1970; 101: 216–219.

225. Ozols II, Wheat LJ. Erythema nodosum in an epidemic of histoplasmosis in Indianapolis. Arch Dermatol 1981; 117: 709–712.

226. Soo-Hoo TS, Adam BA, Yusof D. Disseminated primary cutaneous histoplasmosis. Australas J Dermatol 1980; 21: 105–107.

227. Chanda JJ, Callen JP. Isolated nodular cutaneous histoplasmosis. Arch Dermatol 1978; 114: 1197–1198.

228. Tesh RB, Schneidau JD. Primary cutaneous histoplasmosis. N Engl J Med 1966; 275: 597–599.

229. Lucas AO. Cutaneous manifestations of African histoplasmosis. Br J Dermatol 1970; 82: 435–447.

230. Nethercott JR, Schachter RK, Givan KF, Ryder DE. Histoplasmosis due to *Histoplasma capsulatum* var *duboisii* in a Canadian immigrant. Arch Dermatol 1978; 114: 595–598.

231. Williams AO, Lawson EA, Lucas AO. African histoplasmosis due to *Histoplasma duboisii*. Arch Pathol 1971; 92: 306–318.

232. Abildgaard WH, Hargrove RH, Kalivas J. *Histoplasma* panniculitis. Arch Dermatol 1985; 121: 914–916.

233. Johnston CA, Tang C-K, Jiji RM. Histoplasmosis of skin and lymph nodes and chronic lymphocytic leukemia. Arch Dermatol 1979; 115: 336–337.

234. Dumont A, Piché C. Electron microscopic study of human histoplasmosis. Arch Pathol 1969; 87: 168–178.

Infections by dematiaceous fungi

235. McGinnis MR, Hilger AE. Infections caused by black fungi. Arch Dermatol 1987; 123: 1300–1302.

236. Vollum DI. Chromomycosis: a review. Br J Dermatol 1977; 96: 454–458.

237. Wood C, Russel-Bell B. Characterization of pigmented fungi by melanin staining. Am J Dermatopathol 1983; 5: 77–81.

238. Fukushiro R. Chromomycosis in Japan. Int J Dermatol 1983; 22: 221–229.

239. Sindhuphak W, MacDonald E, Head E, Hudson RD. *Exophiala jeanselmei* infection in a postrenal transplant patient. J Am Acad Dermatol 1985; 13: 877–881.

240. McGinnis MR. Chromoblastomycosis and phaeohyphomycosis: New concepts, diagnosis, and mycology. J Am Acad Dermatol 1983; 8: 1–16.

241. Matsumoto T, Matsuda T. Chromoblastomycosis and phaeohyphomycosis. Semin Dermatol 1985; 4: 240–251.

242. Ajello L, Georg LK, Steigbigel RT, Wang CJK. A case of phaeohyphomycosis caused by a new species of *Phialophora*. Mycologia 1974; 66: 490–498.

243. Zaias N. Chromomycosis. J Cutan Pathol 1978; 5: 155–164.

244. Leslie DF, Beardmore GL. Chromoblastomycosis in Queensland: a retrospective study of 13 cases at the Royal Brisbane Hospital. Australas J Dermatol 1979; 20: 23–30.

245. Azulay RD, Serruya J. Hematogenous dissemination in chromoblastomycosis. Report of a generalized case. Arch Dermatol 1967; 95: 57–60.

245a. Tomecki KJ, Steck WD, Hall GS, Dijkstra JWE. Subcutaneous mycoses. J Am Acad Dermatol 1989; 21: 785–790.

246. Iwatsu T, Takano M, Okamoto S. Auricular chromomycosis. Arch Dermatol 1983; 119: 88–89.

247. Bayles MAH. Chromomycosis. Treatment with thiabendazole. Arch Dermatol 1971; 104: 476–485.

248. Carrion AL. Chromoblastomycosis and related infections. New concepts, differential diagnosis and nomenclatorial implications. Int J Dermatol 1975; 14: 27–32.

249. Ajello L. Phaeohyphomycosis: definition and etiology. In: Mycoses. Pan American Health Organization Scientific Publication No. 304. Washington, D.C.: Pan American Health Organization, 1975; 126–130.

250. Zaias N, Rebell G. A simple and accurate diagnostic method in chromoblastomycosis. Arch Dermatol 1973; 108: 545–546.

251. Walter P, Garin Y, Richard-Lenoble D. Chromoblastomycosis. A morphological investigation of the host-parasite interaction. Virchows Arch (Pathol Anat) 1982; 397: 203–214.

252. Rosen T, Gyorkey F, Joseph LM, Batres E. Ultrastructural features of chromoblastomycosis. Int J Dermatol 1980; 19: 461–468.

252a. Blakely FA, Rao BK, Wiley EL et al. Chromoblastomycosis with unusual histological features. J Cutan Pathol 1988; 15: 298 (abstract).

253. Batres E, Wolf JE, Rudolph AH, Knox LM. Transepithelial elimination of cutaneous chromomycosis. Arch Dermatol 1978; 114: 1231–1232.

254. Goette DK, Robertson D. Transepithelial elimination in chromomycosis. Arch Dermatol 1984; 120: 400–401.

255. Uitto J, Santa–Cruz DJ, Eisen AZ, Kobayashi GS. Chromomycosis. Successful treatment with 5-fluorocytosine. J Cutan Pathol 1979; 6: 77–84.

256. Caplan RM. Epidermoid carcinoma arising in extensive chromoblastomycosis. Arch Dermatol 1968; 97: 38–41.

256a. Kotylo PK, Israel KS, Cohen JS, Bartlett MS. Subcutaneous phaeohyphomycosis of the finger caused by Exophiala spinifera. Am J Clin Pathol 1989; 91: 624–627.

257. Adam RD, Paquin ML, Petersen EA et al. Phaeohyphomycosis caused by the fungal genera Bipolaris and Exserohilum. A report of 9 cases and review of the literature. Medicine (Baltimore) 1986; 65: 203–217.

257a. Straka BF, Cooper PH, Body BA. Cutaneous Bipolaris spicifera infection. Arch Dermatol 1989; 125: 1383–1386.

257b. Ikai K, Tomono H, Watanabe S. Phaeohyphomycosis caused by Phialophora richardsiae. J Am Acad Dermatol 1988; 19: 478–481.

258. Burges GE, Walls CT, Maize JC. Subcutaneous phaeohyphomycosis caused by Exserohilum rostratum in an immunocompetent host. Arch Dermatol 1987; 123: 1346–1350.

259. Symmers W St C. A case of cerebral chromoblastomycosis (cladosporiosis) occurring in Britain as a complication of polyarteritis treated with cortisone. Brain 1960; 83: 37–51.

260. Fathizadeh A, Rippon JW, Rosenfeld SI et al. Pheomycotic cyst in an immunosuppressed host. J Am Acad Dermatol 1981; 5: 423–427.

260a. Hachisuka H, Matsumoto T, Kusuhara M et al. Cutaneous phaeohyphomycosis caused by Exophiala jeanselmei after renal transplantation. Int J Dermatol 1990; 29: 198–200.

261. Cains GD, Krivanek JFC, Paver K. Subcutaneous chromoblastomycosis occurring in a patient with systemic lupus erythematosus. Australas J Dermatol 1977; 18: 84–85.

262. Greer KE, Gross GP, Cooper PH, Harding SA. Cystic chromomycosis due to Wangiella dermatitidis. Arch Dermatol 1979; 115: 1433–1434.

263. Weedon D, Ritchie G. Cystic chromomycosis of the skin. Pathology 1979; 11: 389–392.

264. Kempson RL, Sternberg WH. Chronic subcutaneous abscesses caused by pigmented fungi, a lesion distinguishable from cutaneous chromoblastomycosis. Am J Clin Pathol 1963; 39: 598–606.

264a. Noel SB, Greer DL, Abadie SM et al. Primary cutaneous phaeohyphomycosis. Report of three cases. J Am Acad Dermatol 1988; 18: 1023–1030.

265. Schwartz IS, Emmons CW. Subcutaneous cystic granuloma caused by a fungus of wood pulp (Phialophora richardsiae). Am J Clin Pathol 1968; 49: 500–505.

265a. Zackheim HS, Halde C, Goodman RS et al. Phaeohyphomycotic cyst of the skin caused by Exophiala jeanselmei. J Am Acad Dermatol 1985; 12: 207–212.

266. Tschen JA, Knox JM, McGavran MH, Duncan WC. Chromomycosis. The association of fungal elements and wood splinters. Arch Dermatol 1984; 120: 107–108.

266a. Iwatsu T, Miyaji M. Phaeomycotic cyst. A case with a lesion containing a wood splinter. Arch Dermatol 1984; 120: 1209–1211.

267. Estes SA, Merz WG, Maxwell LG. Primary cutaneous phaeohyphomycosis caused by Drechslera spicifera. Arch Dermatol 1977; 113: 813–815.

268. Grotte M, Younger B. Sporotrichosis associated with sphagnum moss exposure. Arch Pathol Lab Med 1981; 105: 50–51.

269. Auld JC, Beardmore GL. Sporotrichosis in Queensland: a review of 37 cases at the Royal Brisbane Hospital. Australas J Dermatol 1979; 20: 14–22.

270. Nusbaum BP, Gulbas N, Horwitz SN. Sporotrichosis acquired from a cat. J Am Acad Dermatol 1983; 8: 386–391.

271. Dunstan RW, Langham RF, Reimann KA, Wakenell PS. Feline sporotrichosis: A report of five cases with transmission to humans. J Am Acad Dermatol 1986; 15: 37–45.

272. Lurie HI. Histopathology of sporotrichosis. Notes on the nature of the asteroid body. Arch Pathol 1963; 75: 421–437.

273. Dolezal JF. Blastomycoid sporotrichosis. Response to low-dose amphotericin B. J Am Acad Dermatol 1981; 4: 523–527.

274. Orr ER, Riley HD. Sporotrichosis in childhood: Report of ten cases. J Pediatr 1971; 78: 951–957.

275. Prose NS, Milburn PB, Papayanopulos DM. Facial sporotrichosis in children. Pediatr Dermatol 1986; 3: 311–314.

276. Rudolph RI. Facial sporotrichosis in an infant. Cutis 1984; 33: 171–176.

277. Robertson D. Report of two cases of sporotrichosis on the face. Aust J Dermatol 1967; 9: 76–82.

278. Cox RL, Reller LB. Auricular sporotrichosis in a brick mason. Arch Dermatol 1979; 115: 1229–1230.

279. Dellatorre DL, Lattanand A, Buckley HR, Urbach F. Fixed cutaneous sporotrichosis of the face. J Am Acad Dermatol 1982; 6: 97–100.

280. Kwon-Chung KJ. Comparison of isolates of Sporothrix schenckii obtained from fixed cutaneous lesions with isolates from other types of lesions. J Infect Dis 1979; 139: 424–431.

281. Bargman H. Sporotrichosis of the skin with spontaneous cure — report of a second case. J Am Acad Dermatol 1983; 8: 261–262.

282. Grekin RH. Sporotrichosis. Two cases of exogenous second infection. J Am Acad Dermatol 1984; 10: 233–234.

283. Schamroth JM, Grieve TP, Kellen P. Disseminated sporotrichosis. Int J Dermatol 1988; 27: 28–30.

284. Smith PW, Loomis GW, Luckasen JL, Osterholm RK. Disseminated cutaneous sporotrichosis. Three illustrative cases. Arch Dermatol 1981; 117: 143–144.

285. Lynch PJ, Voorhees JJ, Harrell ER. Systemic sporotrichosis. Ann Intern Med 1970; 73: 23–30.

286. Stroud JD. Sporotrichosis presenting as pyoderma gangrenosum. Arch Dermatol 1968; 97: 667–670.

372. Edwards JE. Clinical aspects of mucormycosis. In: Lehrer RI, Moderator. Mucormycosis. Ann Intern Med 1980; 93: 96–99.

372a. Clark R, Greer DL, Carlisle T, Carroll B. Cutaneous zygomycosis in a diabetic HTLV-1-seropositive man. J Am Acad Dermatol 1990; 22: 956–959.

373. Gartenberg G, Bottone EJ, Keusch GT, Weitzman I. Hospital-acquired mucormycosis (*Rhizopus rhizopodiformis*) of skin and subcutaneous tissue. N Engl J Med 1978; 299: 1115–1118.

374. Sheldon DL, Johnson WC. Cutaneous mucormycosis. Two documented cases of suspected nosocomial cause. JAMA 1979; 241: 1032–1034.

375. Hammond DE, Winkelmann RK. Cutaneous phycomycosis. Report of three cases with identification of *Rhizopus*. Arch Dermatol 1979; 115: 990–992.

376. Veliath AJ, Rao R, Prabhu MR, Aurora AL. Cutaneous phycomycosis (mucormycosis) with fatal pulmonary dissemination. Arch Dermatol 1976; 112: 509–512.

377. Maliwan N, Reyes CV, Rippon JW. Osteomyelitis secondary to cutaneous mucormycosis. Am J Dermatopathol 1984; 6: 479–481.

378. Myskowski PL, Brown AE, Dinsmore R et al. Mucormycosis following bone marrow transplantation. J Am Acad Dermatol 1983; 9: 111–115.

379. Meyer RD, Kaplan MH, Ong M, Armstrong D. Cutaneous lesions in disseminated mucormycosis. JAMA 1973; 225: 737–738.

380. Kramer BS, Hernandez AD, Reddick RL, Levine AS. Cutaneous infarction. Manifestation of disseminated mucormycosis. Arch Dermatol 1977; 113: 1075–1076.

380a. Khardori N, Hayat S, Rolston K, Bodey GP. Cutaneous *Rhizopus* and *Aspergillus* infections in five patients with cancer. Arch Dermatol 1989; 125: 952–956.

380b. Umbert IJ, Su WPD. Cutaneous mucormycosis. J Am Acad Dermatol 1989; 21: 1232–1234.

381. Tio TH, Djojopranoto M, Eng N-IT. Subcutaneous phycomycosis. Arch Dermatol 1966; 93: 550–553.

382. Harman RRM, Jackson H, Willis AJP. Subcutaneous phycomycosis in Nigeria. Br J Dermatol 1964; 76: 408–420.

383. Mugerwa JW. Subcutaneous phycomycosis in Uganda. Br J Dermatol 1976; 94: 539–544.

384. Miller RI, Campbell RSF. The comparative pathology of equine cutaneous phycomycosis. Vet Pathol 1984; 21: 325–332.

385. Miller RI, Olcott BM, Archer M. Cutaneous pythiosis in beef calves. JAVMA 1985; 186: 984–985.

385a. Weedon D. Unpublished observations.

386. Symmers W St C. Histopathologic aspects of the pathogenesis of some opportunistic fungal infections, as exemplified in the pathology of aspergillosis and the phycomycetoses. Lab Invest 1962; 11: 1073–1090.

387. Herstoff JK, Bogaars H, McDonald CJ. Rhinophycomycosis entomophthorae. Arch Dermatol 1978; 114: 1674–1678.

387a. Towersey L, Wanke B, Ribeiro Estrella R et al. *Conidiobolus coronatus* infection treated with ketoconazole. Arch Dermatol 1988; 124: 1392–1396.

388. Williams AO. Pathology of phycomycosis due to *Entomophthora* and *Basidiobolus* species. Arch Pathol 1969; 87: 13–20.

389. Williams AO, von Lichtenberg F, Smith JH, Martinson FD. Ultrastructure of phycomycosis due to *Entomophthora*, *Basidiobolus*, and associated "Splendore–Hoeppli" phenomenon. Arch Pathol 1969; 87: 459–468.

389a. de Leon-Bojorge B, Ruiz-Maldonado R, Lopez-Martinez R. Subcutaneous phycomycosis caused by *Basidiobolus haptosporus*: A clinicopathologic and mycologic study in a child. Pediatr Dermatol 1988; 5: 33–36.

Hyalohyphomycoses

390. English MP. Invasion of the skin by filamentous non-dermatophyte fungi. Br J Dermatol 1968; 80: 282–286.

391. Veglia KS, Marks VJ. *Fusarium* as a pathogen. A case report of *Fusarium* sepsis and review of the literature. J Am Acad Dermatol 1987; 16: 260–263.

392. Benjamin RP, Callaway JL, Conant NF. Facial granuloma associated with *Fusarium* infection. Arch Dermatol 1970; 101: 598–600.

393. Young RC, Bennett JE, Vogel CL et al. Aspergillosis. The spectrum of the disease in 98 patients. Medicine (Baltimore) 1970; 49: 147–173.

394. Caro I, Dogliotti M. Aspergillosis of the skin. Report of a case. Dermatologica 1973; 146: 244–248.

395. Cahill KM, El Mofty AM, Kawaguchi TP. Primary cutaneous aspergillosis. Arch Dermatol 1967; 96: 545–547.

396. Estes SA, Hendricks AA, Merz WG, Prystowsky SD. Primary cutaneous aspergillosis. J Am Acad Dermatol 1980; 3: 397–400.

397. Grossman ME, Fithian EC, Behrens C et al. Primary cutaneous aspergillosis in six leukemic children. J Am Acad Dermatol 1985; 12: 313–318.

398. Carlile JR, Millet RE, Cho CT, Vats TS. Primary cutaneous aspergillosis in a leukemic child. Arch Dermatol 1978; 114: 78–80.

398a. Googe PB, DeCoste SD, Herold WH, Mihm MC Jr. Primary cutaneous aspergillosis mimicking dermatophytosis. Arch Pathol Lab Med 1989; 113: 1284–1286.

399. Granstein RD, First LR, Sober AJ. Primary cutaneous aspergillosis in a premature neonate. Br J Dermatol 1980; 103: 681–684.

400. Panke TW, McManus AT, Spebar MJ. Infection of a burn wound by *Aspergillus niger*. Gross appearance simulating ecthyma gangrenosa. Am J Clin Pathol 1979; 72: 230–232.

Miscellaneous mycoses

401. Tapia A, Torres-Calcindo A, Arosemena R. Keloidal blastomycosis (Lobo's disease) in Panama. Int J Dermatol 1978; 17: 572–574.

402. Azulay RD, Carneiro JA, Da Graca M et al. Keloidal blastomycosis (Lobo's disease) with lymphatic involvement. A case report. Int J Dermatol 1976; 15: 40–44.

403. Bhawan J, Bain RW, Purtilo DT et al. Lobomycosis. An electronmicroscopic, histochemical and

immunologic study. J Cutan Pathol 1976; 3: 5–16.

403a. Baruzzi RG, Rodriques DA, Michalany NS, Salomao R. Squamous-cell carcinoma and lobomycosis (Jorge Lobo's disease). Int J Dermatol 1989; 28: 183–185.

404. Jaramillo D, Cortés A, Restrepo A et al. Lobomycosis. Report of the eighth Colombian case and review of the literature. J Cutan Pathol 1976; 3: 180–189.

405. Mikat DM. Unusual fungal conditions of the skin. Int J Dermatol 1980; 19: 18–22.

406. Sahoo S, Das S. Rhinosporidiosis of subcutaneous tissue. J Indian Med Assoc 1982; 78: 114–116.

407. Mahakrisnan A, Rajasekaram V, Pandian PI. Disseminated cutaneous rhinosporidiosis treated with dapsone. Trop Geogr Med 1981; 33: 189–192.

408. Agrawal S, Sharma KD, Shrivastava JB. Generalized rhinosporidiosis with visceral involvement. Report of a case. Arch Dermatol 1959; 80: 22–26.

409. Yesudian P. Cutaneous rhinosporidiosis mimicking verruca vulgaris. Int J Dermatol 1988; 27: 47–48.

Algal infections

410. Venezio FR, Lavoo E, Williams JE et al. Progressive cutaneous protothecosis. Am J Clin Pathol 1982; 77: 485–493.

411. Sudman MS. Protothecosis. A critical review. Am J Clin Pathol 1974; 61: 10–19.

412. Tindall JP, Fetter BF. Infections caused by achloric algae (protothecosis). Arch Dermatol 1971; 104: 490–500.

413. McAnally T, Parry EL. Cutaneous protothecosis presenting as recurrent chromomycosis. Arch Dermatol 1985; 121: 1066–1069.

414. Mars PW, Rabson AR, Rippey JJ, Ajello L. Cutaneous protothecosis. Br J Dermatol (Suppl) 1971; 7: 76–84.

415. Kuo T-t, Hsueh S, Wu J-L, Wang A-M. Cutaneous protothecosis. A clinicopathologic study. Arch Pathol Lab Med 1987; 111: 737–740.

416. Goldstein GD, Bhatia P, Kalivas J. Herpetiform protothecosis. Int J Dermatol 1986; 25: 54–55.

417. Tyring SK, Lee PC, Walsh P et al. Papular protothecosis of the chest. Arch Dermatol 1989; 125: 1249–1252.

418. Mayhall CG, Miller CW, Eisen AZ et al. Cutaneous protothecosis. Successful treatment with amphotericin B. Arch Dermatol 1976; 112: 1749–1752.

Viral infections

INTRODUCTION

Viral infections of the skin are of increasing clinical importance, particularly in patients who are immunocompromised. Viruses may reach the skin by direct inoculation, as in warts, milker's nodule and orf, or by spread from other locations as in herpes zoster. Many viral exanthems result from a generalized infection with localization of the virus in the epidermis or dermis or in the endothelium of blood vessels.[1] The usual clinical appearance of this group is an erythematous maculopapular rash, but sometimes macular, vesicular, petechial, purpuric or urticarial reactions may be seen. Some of the varied manifestations of viral diseases may result from an immune reaction to the virus. This is the probable explanation for the erythema multiforme and erythema nodosum that occasionally follow viral infections.

Viruses are separated into families on the basis of the type and form of the nucleic acid genome, of the morphological features of the virus particle, and of the mode of replication. There are four important families involved in cutaneous diseases: the DNA families of Poxviridae, Herpesviridae and Papovaviridae, and the RNA family, Picornaviridae. In addition to these four families, exanthems can occur in the course of infections with the following families — Adenoviridae, Reoviridae,[2] Togaviridae, Paramyxoviridae, Arenaviridae, and an unclassified group which includes hepatitis B virus and Marburg virus.[1] The three major DNA families produce lesions which are histologically diagnostic for a disease or group of diseases, whereas the other viruses produce lesions which are often histologically non-specific. These non-specific features include a superficial perivascular infiltrate of lymphocytes, mild epidermal spongiosis, occasional Civatte bodies and sometimes urticarial oedema or mild haemorrhage. Inclusion bodies, which represent sites of virus replication, are uncommon in skin lesions produced by viruses outside the four major families.

Various laboratory techniques can be used to assist in the specific diagnosis of a suspected viral disease.[3] These include light and electron microscopy of a biopsy or smear, serology, viral culture and immunomorphological methods. Although viral isolation in tissue culture remains the paramount diagnostic method, the development of monoclonal antibodies to various viruses, for use with fluorescent, immunoperoxidase and ELISA (enzyme-linked immunosorbent assay) techniques has made possible the rapid diagnosis of many viral infections with a high degree of specificity.[3a] Serology is still the preferred method of diagnosis for certain viral infections such as rubella and infectious mononucleosis. Brief mention must be made of the Tzanck smear, which was traditionally used by clinicians, especially dermatologists, in the diagnosis of certain vesicular lesions, especially those caused by the herpes simplex and varicella-zoster viruses. A smear is made by scraping the lesion. It is then stained by the Giemsa or Papanicolaou methods and examined for the presence of viral inclusion bodies. Its use is declining with the advent of the more specific immunomorphological techniques.

The various virus families, and the cutaneous diseases they produce, will be considered in turn.

POXVIRIDAE

Poxvirus infections of humans include cowpox, vaccinia, variola (smallpox), molluscum contagiosum, milker's nodule (paravaccinia) and orf (ecthyma contagiosum). The causative viruses are large, with a DNA core and a surrounding capsid. There are two subgroups, based on the morphological features of the virus. The viruses of molluscum contagiosum and orf are oval or cylindrical in shape and measure approximately 150 × 300 nm. The remaining viruses are brick-shaped and range in size from 250–300 nm × 200–250 nm. Clusters of these poxviruses can be identified in haematoxylin and eosin stained sections as intracytoplasmic eosinophilic inclusions.

COWPOX

Cowpox is a viral disease of cattle which may be contracted by milkers, who develop a pustular eruption on the hands, forearms or face, accompanied by slight fever and lymphadenitis. The disease is of historical interest, because it was the immunity to smallpox of those who had had cowpox that led Jenner to substitute inoculation with cowpox for the more dangerous procedure of variolation. Recently doubt has been cast on the role of cattle as a reservoir of infection in cowpox.[4] It appears that the domestic cat has an important role in the transmission of cowpox virus.[4]

VACCINIA

Vaccination against smallpox was carried out with the vaccinia virus, a laboratory-developed member of the poxvirus group.[5] In previously unvaccinated individuals, a papule developed on about the fifth day at the site of inoculation of vaccinia virus. This quickly became vesicular and gradually dried up, producing a crust which fell away, leaving a scar.

With the eradication of smallpox, vaccination is no longer recommended. As a result, generalized vaccinia infection (eczema vaccinatum), a serious complication of vaccination, is now of historical interest only. Eczema vaccinatum has many similarities to eczema herpeticum, an infection by the herpes simplex virus seen also in predisposed patients, such as those with an atopic diathesis.

Histopathology

The appearances are similar to those of herpes simplex, zoster and varicella, except that intracytoplasmic rather than intranuclear inclusion bodies are seen in vaccinia.

Complications of vaccination

Many cutaneous and systemic complications of smallpox vaccination have been reported.[6,7] Generalized complications have included toxic erythema, erythema multiforme, erythema nodosum, pityriasis rosea, and eczema vaccinatum. Local complications have included pyogenic granuloma,[8] secondary infection with pyogenic or acid-fast bacilli, and vaccinia gangrenosa.[9] The latter complication occurred in children with hypogammaglobulinaemia and consisted of a spreading blister which rapidly ulcerated.

Late sequelae are much less common and have included keloid formation, basal and squamous cell carcinoma,[10] malignant melanoma, dermatofibrosarcoma protuberans, and malignant fibrous histiocytoma.[11] Dermatoses have also developed, including discoid lupus erythematosus,[12] lichen sclerosus et atrophicus,[13] contact dermatitis and 'localized eczema'.[7] It is possible that some of the late complications represent the chance localization of a particular lesion at the site of previous vaccination.

VARIOLA (SMALLPOX)

Variola has now been eradicated.[14] Two types were encountered: variola major, a severe form with a significant fatality rate, and variola minor (alastrim), a mild form with a fatality rate of less than 1%. Variola begins with generalized papules after contact with or inhalation of the virus. After several days the papules become umbilicated vesicles and later they develop into crusted pustules. The lesions heal with scarring.

Histopathology

Variola results in vesicular lesions which resemble those of herpes simplex, zoster and varicella except, usually, for the absence of multinucleate epidermal cells and for the localization of the inclusion bodies.[15] In variola, intracytoplasmic inclusions (Guarnieri bodies) are present. These are eosinophilic and Feulgen positive. Basophilic cytoplasmic inclusions and eosinophilic intranuclear bodies have been described. Reticular degeneration is usually prominent and ballooning less so.

MOLLUSCUM CONTAGIOSUM

Molluscum contagiosum occurs as solitary or multiple dome-shaped, umbilicated, waxy papules with a predilection for flexural areas or the genitalia of children and adolescents. Sexual transmission may occur. Papules range from 2–8mm in diameter, although solitary lesions may be slightly larger. Spontaneous regression often occurs within a year, although more persistent lesions are encountered. Extensive lesions can occur in immunocompromised patients.[16,16a]

The disease is caused by a large, brick-shaped, DNA poxvirus with an ultrastructural resemblance to vaccinia virus.[17] There is a well-defined sac enclosing the virion colony of each infected keratinocyte.[18]

Histopathology

A lesion consists of several inverted lobules of hyperplastic squamous epithelium which expand into the underlying dermis (Fig. 26.1).[17] The lobules are separated by fine septa of compressed dermis. Eosinophilic inclusion bodies form in the cytoplasm of keratinocytes just above the basal

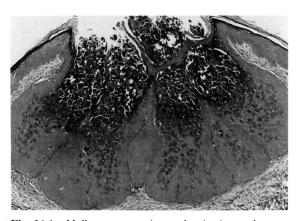

Fig. 26.1 Molluscum contagiosum showing inverted lobules of squamous epithelium with molluscum bodies. Haematoxylin — eosin

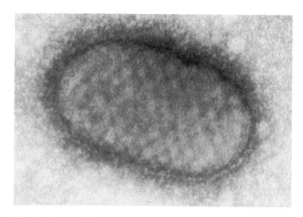

Fig. 26.5 Orf. Ultrastructural features of the orf virus with its laminated capsule and internal cross-hatched appearance. Electron micrograph × 20 000

although full-thickness epidermal necrosis seems to be more common in orf. Immunoperoxidase techniques using orf-specific monoclonal antibodies can be used to confirm the diagnosis, if necessary.[42a]

Electron microscopy. This shows an oval virus with an electron-dense core, surrounded by a laminated capsule similar to the virus of milker's nodule (Fig. 26.5).[43a,44] Rapid diagnosis may be made by electron microscopy of negatively stained suspensions from the lesion. The number of virus-containing cells is greatest in the first 2 weeks of the disease and they may be absent by the fourth week.[44a]

HERPESVIRIDAE

There are three subfamilies within the family Herpesviridae. The first includes the herpes simplex virus (types 1 and 2) and the varicella-zoster virus. The second subfamily contains cytomegalovirus, while the third includes the Epstein–Barr virus.[45]

HERPES SIMPLEX

There are two types of herpes simplex virus, type 1 (HSV-1) and type 2 (HSV-2).[46] Primary infection with HSV-1 is usually in childhood and is mild. Recurrent lesions occur most commonly around the lips (herpes labialis — 'cold sores'). Other sites of infection include the oral cavity, pharynx, oesophagus, eye, lung and brain.

Infection with HSV-2 generally involves the genitalia and surrounding areas after puberty; it is usually sexually transmitted.[47] The incubation period for genital lesions averages five days. HSV-2 may also result in generalized infections of the newborn.[48] The relationship between the site of infection and HSV type is not absolute.

Once infected, a person will usually harbour the virus for life. The virus can travel along sensory nerves to infect the neurons in the sensory ganglia. Recurrent disease follows this latency in the sensory ganglia and can be stimulated by ultraviolet light,[49] trauma, fever, menstruation and stress, to name the most common factors. Prostaglandins may play a role in the reactivation of infections.[50]

The usual lesions of herpes simplex consist of a group of clear vesicles. They heal without scarring except in those cases where secondary bacterial infection supervenes. Special clinical variants[51] include herpes folliculitis of the beard or scalp, herpetic whitlow[52] (usually in medical or nursing personnel), necrotizing balanitis[53] (a very rare HSV-2 complication), a varicella-like eruption,[54] infection localized to sites of atopic dermatitis[55] and eczema herpeticum (see p. 684).[56] Severe primary or secondary infection with systemic involvement may occur in immunocompromised patients. Disseminated herpes simplex infection is a rare complication of pregnancy.[57]

HSV-1 and HSV-2 are biologically and serologically distinct. They are usually isolated using human embryonic fibroblast cell cultures.[58] Characteristic cytopathic changes can be seen after one or two days.

Histopathology

The histological appearances of herpes simplex, varicella and herpes zoster are very similar. The earliest changes involve the epidermal cell nuclei, which develop peripheral clumping of chromatin and a homogeneous ground glass appearance, combined with ballooning of the nucleus[59]. Vacuolization is the earliest cytoplasmic alteration. These changes begin focally along the basal layer, but soon involve the entire epidermis.[59] By the time lesions are biopsied, there is usually an established intraepidermal vesicle (Fig. 26.6). This results from two types of degenerative change, ballooning degeneration and reticular degeneration. *Ballooning degeneration* is peculiar to viral vesicles. The affected cells swell and lose their attachment to adjacent cells, thus separating from them (secondary acantholysis). The cytoplasm of these cells becomes homogeneous and intensely eosinophilic, while some are also multinucleate (Tzanck cells). At times the basal layer of the epidermis is also destroyed in this way, leading to the formation of a subepidermal vesicle. The change known as *reticular degeneration* is characterized by progressive hydropic swelling of epidermal cells, which become large and clear with only fine cytoplasmic strands remaining at the edge of the cells. These eventually rupture, contributing further to the formation of a vesicle. This change is not specific for viral infection and can be seen also in allergic contact dermatitis. Whereas ballooning degeneration is found mainly at the base of the vesicle, reticular degeneration is seen on its superficial aspect and margin.

Eosinophilic intranuclear inclusion bodies are found, particularly in ballooned cells. They are more common in multinucleate cells of lesions that have been present for several days. Neutrophils are present within established vesicles. There are also moderate numbers in the underlying dermis, as well as lymphocytes. Neutrophils are prominent in the lesions of herpetic whitlow. Marked inflammation and even vasculitis have been noted in some lesions.[60] As a rule, the dermal inflammation is less severe in herpes simplex than in zoster. Atypical lymphoid cells may be present in the infiltrate when herpes simplex complicates an underlying haematological malignancy.[60a]

Uncommonly, erythema-multiforme-like changes may be seen in the adjacent skin, concurrent with a vesicle of herpes simplex. A related reaction pattern is so-called lichenoid lymphocytic vasculitis, a term coined for the changes seen in presumptive cases of herpes simplex with an immunological response.[60b] There is an upper dermal infiltrate of lymphocytes and histiocytes with lichenoid changes in the epidermis and a dermal lymphocytic vasculitis.

Focal involvement of pilosebaceous units is not uncommon in recurrent lesions.[59] In the variant known as herpes folliculitis, pilosebaceous involvement is the dominant lesion (Fig. 26.7). Ballooning degeneration may involve cells of the outer root sheath of the deep portion of the follicle. A dermal inflammatory infiltrate is often present in these cases; it is heaviest in the deep reticular dermis — a so-called 'bottom-heavy' infiltrate.

In late lesions of herpes simplex, ulceration is often present. Ghosts of acantholytic, multinucleate epithelial cells with slate grey nuclei on routine staining may still be seen in the overlying crust.

Recently, attention has been drawn to the histological appearance of the lesions which recur

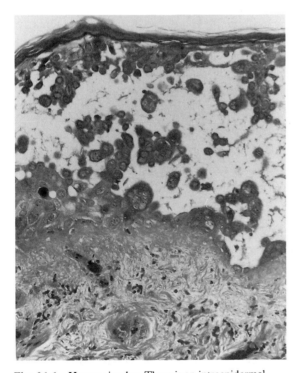

Fig. 26.6 Herpes simplex. There is an intraepidermal vesicle containing ballooned, acantholytic keratinocytes in which there are intranuclear inclusion bodies. Haematoxylin — eosin

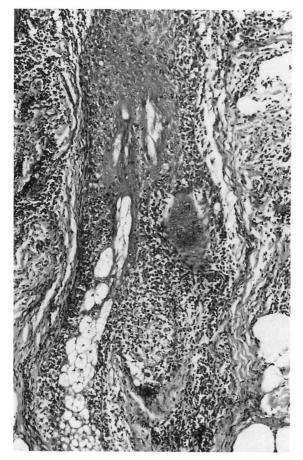

Fig. 26.7 Herpes folliculitis. The 'bottom-heavy' infiltrate and the cuffing and infiltration of the pilosebaceous follicle are characteristic. There are usually no inclusion bodies in the cells of the pilosebaceous follicle. There may be the typical changes of herpes simplex in the overlying dermis. Haematoxylin — eosin

at the site of previous surgery. These vesicles are subepidermal with an inflammatory response, complete with multinucleate giant cells,[61] in the uppermost dermis.

A rapid cytological diagnosis of a vesicular lesion can be made by making a smear from the base of a freshly opened vesicle and staining it with the Giemsa stain. Ballooned cells, some of which are multinucleate, will be seen in herpes simplex, varicella and zoster.

Electron microscopy. Virus particles of *Herpesvirus hominis*, measuring between 90 and 130 nm, can be seen in the nuclei of the basal cells. Cells in the malpighian layer often contain other viral-related material such as nuclear granules and capsules. Viral capsids have also been seen within the nuclei of monocytes, young histiocytes and lymphocytes in the epidermal vesicles.[62] Large lymphocytes are sometimes seen adjacent to keratinocytes exhibiting lytic changes, suggesting that cell-mediated immunity may be responsible, in part, for the epidermal damage that occurs.[62a]

Eczema herpeticum

This is a generalized infection of the skin with the herpes simplex virus.[62b] A similar condition (eczema vaccinatum) occurs with the vaccinia virus.[9] Both lesions have been grouped together as Kaposi's varicelliform eruption. This condition occurs most commonly in association with atopic dermatitis, but it has also been reported in Darier's disease, benign familial pemphigus, pemphigus foliaceus, seborrhoeic dermatitis, ichthyosiform erythroderma, the Sézary syndrome and mycosis fungoides,[56] and following thermal injury.[63] Separation of eczema herpeticum from eczema vaccinatum depends partly on the history and partly on laboratory studies. Histopathology may occasionally assist in their differentiation.

Histopathology

Although eczema herpeticum is characterized by the presence of multinucleate epidermal cells and intranuclear inclusions, rather than the intracytoplasmic inclusions of eczema vaccinatum, these features are often obscured by the heavy inflammatory cell infiltrate of neutrophils and early breakdown of the vesicles. Recently formed lesions usually show the typical features of a vesicle of herpes simplex.

VARICELLA

Varicella (chickenpox) is characterized by an acute vesicular eruption. It is predominantly a disease of childhood. The lesions develop in successive crops, so that the rash typically consists of pocks at different stages of development. Thus, papules, vesicles, pustules, crusted lesions and healing lesions may all be present. Varicella pneumonia may be seen in adults as a primary infection. In immunocompromised hosts dissemination may occur, or large ulcerated and necrotic lesions (varicella gangrenosa) may develop. An interesting observation is the finding of marked intensification of the varicella eruption in areas of skin which are normally covered but which become sunburnt just before the eruption commences.[64] Varicella has also been reported largely restricted to an area covered by a plaster cast.[65]

Histopathology

The appearances are virtually indistinguishable from those of herpes simplex although the degree of inflammation is said to be greater in herpes simplex than in varicella-zoster lesions.[66] Direct immunofluorescence, using a monoclonal antibody specific for varicella-zoster virus,[67] and the Tzanck smear are superior to culture techniques in the diagnosis of varicella-zoster;[68] direct immunofluorescence has the advantage of specificity over the Tzanck smear.[67]

Electron microscopy. The ultrastructural features of *Herpesvirus varicellae* are similar to those of *Herpesvirus hominis*. However, colloidal gold immunoelectron microscopy using monoclonal antibodies can distinguish between these two viruses.[68a]

HERPES ZOSTER

Herpes zoster is caused by the same virus as varicella.[69] It occurs in individuals with partial immunity resulting from a prior varicella infection. With few exceptions, zoster appears to represent reactivation of latent virus in sensory ganglia, often in an immunocompromised host.[70] The virus travels through the sensory nerves to reach the skin, where it replicates in the epidermal keratinocytes.

Zoster is not highly infectious. When children are infected by adults suffering from zoster they develop varicella and not zoster. An attack of either disease leaves the patient with some measure of immunity against both. Recurrent attacks of zoster can occur,[69] although many cases diagnosed as recurrent herpes zoster are probably recurrent herpes simplex.[71] Disseminated herpes zoster is a rare complication of AIDS.[71a]

Clinically, herpes zoster (shingles) is an acute disease that occurs almost exclusively in adults. The illness is febrile and begins with pain in the area innervated by the affected sensory ganglia. The skin in this area becomes red, and papules soon develop. These quickly transform into vesicles and then pustules. Crusts then form and, later, healing takes place. Sometimes there is residual scarring, particularly if there has been secondary bacterial infection of the vesicles. Granuloma annulare has been reported at sites of healing herpes zoster.[72]

The ganglia most usually involved are those of the lumbar and thoracic nerves. Severe ocular damage may result when the ophthalmic division of a trigeminal nerve is involved.

Histopathology

The appearances resemble those described for herpes simplex. Despite the comment made earlier that lesions of herpes simplex are usually more inflammatory than those due to varicella-zoster infection,[66] dermal inflammation may be prominent in some cases of herpes zoster, and there may occasionally be a vasculitis. These factors, as well as secondary infection, contribute to the scarring which sometimes ensues. Eccrine duct involvement has been reported, but it is quite uncommon.[73]

CYTOMEGALOVIRUS

There are few reports of cutaneous involvement with cytomegalovirus.[74–75a] A maculopapular eruption is the most common clinical presentation and this is seen most often in patients with cytomegalovirus infection who are treated with ampicillin. This is analogous to the situation in infectious mononucleosis.[75] Urticaria,[76] vesiculobullous lesions,[77] ulceration, keratotic lesions[78]

cases are familial. There may be disturbed cellular immune function.[133-135] There is no tendency to malignant transformation in this form. Regression of the lesions has been reported.[132]

The second form of EV is related to HPV-5 and sometimes HPV-8,9,10,12,14,17,19,22,24 and others.[136,137] There is often a familial history with an autosomal recessive inheritance, or a history of parental consanguinity.[130] X-linked recessive inheritance has also been reported.[138] In addition to the plane warts, reddish-brown patches and scaling pityriasis-versicolor-like lesions develop, with the eventual complication of Bowen's disease or invasive squamous cell carcinoma. Malignant transformation, which occurs in about 25% of patients with EV, depends on the oncogenic potential of the infecting virus.[94] This is highest for HPV-5, followed by HPV-8. Carcinomas develop mainly in light-exposed lesions. Such tumours have a very low rate of metastasis.[136] Patients with this form of EV have an altered natural killer cell cytotoxic response.[136]

Histopathology

The cases induced by HPV-3 resemble plane warts. In the other form, there is some variability in the changes seen. Some lesions may resemble plane warts, while others consist of thickened epidermis with swollen cells in the upper epidermis, some with vacuolated nuclei. Dysplastic epidermal cells may be seen. Changes of Bowen's disease or squamous cell carcinoma may ultimately supervene.

CONDYLOMA ACUMINATUM

Although traditionally defined as fleshy exophytic lesions of the anogenital region, it is now known that small inconspicuous lesions may occur on the penis,[139] vulva and cervix.[140-142] They are usually sexually transmitted and spread rapidly.[104] The incubation period is variable but averages 2–3 months.[143] Children occasionally develop lesions, raising the issue of sexual abuse.[144,145] Condylomas are recurrent in up to one-third of cases.[146] Although malignant trans-

formation of condylomas of the anogenital region is rare, it is more common than in other types of warts, with the exception of epidermodysplasia verruciformis.[147,148] Giant condyloma acuminatum of Buschke–Lowenstein is now regarded as a variant of verrucous carcinoma.[149-151]

As only small amounts of virus are present, characterization of the aetiological subtype of HPV involved was made only recently. HPV-6 and 11 are the most commonly identified but other unclassified types have been implicated.[94,152] HPV-16 has oncogenic properties and is sometimes isolated from condylomas, although more usually it is seen in association with bowenoid papulosis. The concurrence of condyloma acuminatum and bowenoid papulosis has been reported.[153]

Histopathology[104]

There is marked acanthosis with some papillomatosis and hyperkeratosis (Fig. 26.12). Vacuolization of granular cells is not as prominent as in other varieties of warts, although there are usually some vacuolated koilocytes in the upper malpighian layer. Coarse keratohyaline granules may also be present. Langerhans cells are sometimes prominent.[154]

If the lesions are treated with podophyllum resin (podophyllin) 48 hours or so prior to

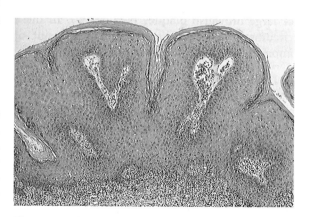

Fig. 26.12 Condyloma acuminatum. This small lesion from the penis is characterized by an underlying lichenoid inflammatory infiltrate.
Haematoxylin — eosin

removal, there are striking histological changes. These include pallor of the epidermis, numerous degenerate keratinocytes in the lower half of the epidermis, and a marked increase in this region in the number of mitotic figures.[155]

Papilloma virus common antigen can be detected in about 60% of lesions by immunoperoxidase techniques.[156] Its presence correlates with that of coarse keratohyaline granules and koilocytes.[156]

FOCAL EPITHELIAL HYPERPLASIA

This condition, also known as Heck's disease, is characterized by multiple, soft, pink or white papules and confluent plaques, particularly on the mucosa of the lips and cheeks. There is a high incidence among Innuits (Eskimos) and American Indians, but there are isolated reports of involvement of other races.[157–159] HPV-13 and 32 have been implicated in the aetiology of this condition.[105,160]

Histopathology

The involved mucosa is hyperplastic, with acanthosis and some clubbing of rete pegs. There is a characteristic pallor of epidermal cells, particularly in the upper layers.[161] There are often binucleate cells but inclusion bodies are not found.

BOWENOID PAPULOSIS

Bowenoid papulosis refers to the presence on the genitalia of solitary or multiple verruca-like papules or plaques having a close histological resemblance to Bowen's disease.[162,163] It has a predilection for sexually active young adults. If children develop lesions, the possibility of child sexual abuse should be considered.[164] In males it tends to involve the glans penis and also the foreskin, while in females the vulval lesions are often bilateral and pigmented.[165] This condition was first described as multicentric pigmented Bowen's disease,[166] and several other terms were used before acceptance of the term bowenoid papulosis.[167–169] Although increasing in inci-

dence, it is still a relatively uncommon condition.

Lesions are often resistant to treatment and may have a protracted course, particularly in those persons with depressed immunity.[170] Spontaneous regression is uncommon. Sometimes there is a history of a previous condyloma. In a small number of cases, invasive carcinoma develops. This risk is greatest in females over the age of 40.[165,171] It has been suggested that a cocarcinogenic factor, as yet undetected, may be implicated in this malignant transformation.[172]

Most cases of bowenoid papulosis are due to HPV-16, but in a small number HPV-18, 35 and 39, or mixed infections, have been present.[165,173–176] The HPV-16 strain has also been implicated in the pathogenesis of vulvar carcinomas and cervical intraepithelial neoplasia.[177] The latter condition is occasionally present in the sexual partner of patients with bowenoid papulosis of the penis.[165]

Histopathology

The histological differentiation of bowenoid papulosis and Bowen's disease is difficult, and may be impossible. Bowenoid papulosis is char-

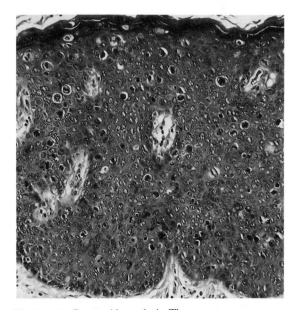

Fig. 26.13 Bowenoid papulosis. There are numerous mitoses in metaphase.

acterized by full-thickness epidermal atypia and loss of architecture. The basement membrane is intact. Mitoses are frequent, sometimes with abnormal forms. They are often in metaphase. Dyskeratotic cells are also present. True koilocytes are uncommon,[178] although partly vacuolated cells with a 'koilocytotic aura' are sometimes present (Fig. 26.13). The stratum corneum and granular cell layer often contain small inclusion-like bodies which are deeply basophilic, rounded and sometimes surrounded by a halo. These bodies, together with the numerous metaphase mitoses, are the features which suggest a diagnosis of bowenoid papulosis rather than Bowen's disease itself.

Bowenoid papulosis is commonly classified by gynaecological pathologists as vulvar intraepithelial neoplasia (VIN) III.[171]

PICORNAVIRIDAE

This is an important family of RNA viruses which includes the Coxsackievirus and ECHO virus. They are now the commonest cause of exanthems in children.[1] As most of the cutaneous manifestations are transient macular or maculopapular lesions in the course of an obvious viral illness, biopsies are rarely taken. As a result very little is known of the histology. Urticarial and vesicular lesions have also been reported.[179] The most important of the vesicular group is so-called hand-foot-and-mouth disease, caused mostly by Coxsackievirus A-16. This virus has also been associated with an eruption resembling that of the Gianotti–Crosti syndrome,[180] although this condition is more usually associated with hepatitis B infection (see below).[181]

HAND-FOOT-AND-MOUTH DISEASE

Most cases are caused by Coxsackievirus A-16, although other types have also been implicated.[182] The disease is a febrile illness characterized by vesicles in the anterior parts of the mouth and on the hands and feet.[183] The vesicles are usually small and they may be sparse.

Histopathology

There are intraepidermal vesicles with prominent reticular degeneration and sometimes a few ballooned cells in the base. There are no multinucleate cells or inclusion bodies. Similar changes, usually without ballooning, are seen in the vesicular lesions of other viruses in this family. There is sometimes the additional feature of papillary dermal oedema and a mild perivascular inflammatory infiltrate.

OTHER VIRUSES

PARVOVIRUS

Human parvovirus is a member of the family Parvoviridae, a group of single-stranded DNA viruses. It can produce an influenza-like illness, symmetrical polyarthritis, aplastic crises, purpura and erythema infectiosum (fifth disease), an exanthem which may be difficult to distinguish from rubella.[184–187]

MEASLES

A biopsy from the rash of measles shows epidermal spongiosis and mild vesiculation with scattered shrunken and degenerate keratinocytes.[188] Occasional multinucleate epithelial giant cells may be seen in the upper dermis.

TOGAVIRUSES

This group includes the viruses that cause rubella and dengue,[189] as well as the Sindbis, Ross River, West Nile, Chikungunya, and O'nyong-nyong viruses.[1,190] The rashes are usually maculopapular but petechial or purpuric lesions are not uncommon. In the latter instance there is a lymphocytic perivasculitis with haemorrhage.

HEPATITIS B VIRUS

The dermatological manifestations of this virus include

1. a serum-sickness-like prodrome with urticarial or vasculitic lesions and, rarely, an erythema multiforme or lichenoid picture;[191]
2. polyarteritis nodosa;[192,193]
3. essential mixed cryoglobulinaemia; and
4. papular acrodermatitis of childhood (Gianotti–Crosti syndrome).[181,194]

Gianotti–Crosti syndrome is characterized by a non-relapsing erythematopapular rash, lasting about 3 weeks and localized to the face and limbs, with the addition sometimes of lymphadenopathy and acute hepatitis, usually anicteric (see p. 112).[195] It has also been associated with many other viruses including hepatitis A,[196] cytomegalovirus,[196a] Epstein–Barr virus, adenovirus[196a] and Coxsackievirus.[197,198] The histology can show a characteristic mixture of three tissue reactions — spongiotic, lichenoid and lymphocytic vasculitis.

Recently, a recurrent, erythematous, asymptomatic papular rash on the trunk and proximal extremities has been reported in hepatitis B carriers.[199] Histopathological study showed a superficial and deep perivascular mononuclear infiltrate in the dermis.[199]

ACQUIRED IMMUNODEFICIENCY SYNDROME (AIDS)

AIDS is one manifestation of a variety of disorders caused by infection with the human T-cell lymphotropic virus type III (HTLV III), now known as human immunodeficiency virus (HIV). It is a retrovirus which infects and destroys helper T lymphocytes with resulting disturbances in cellular immune function[200, 201]. It also infects cells of the central nervous system, producing dementia and motor disturbances. Lymphadenopathy is another manifestation of HIV infection. AIDS is found most commonly in male homosexuals, in haemophiliacs who have received infected blood, in intravenous drug users and in parts of Africa where heterosexual transmission is important. Viraemia is lifelong.

Kaposi's sarcoma was the first cutaneous manifestation of AIDS to be reported (see p. 964). It is found in up to one-third of patients,

Table 26.1 Cutaneous manifestations of AIDS

Infections
Viral — molluscum contagiosum, herpes simplex, herpes zoster, verruca vulgaris, condylomas, cytomegalovirus, oral hairy leucoplakia.

Bacterial — mycobacterial infections, more usual bacterial infections, bacillary angiomatosis.

Fungal — candidosis, dermatophytosis, histoplasmosis, cryptococcosis, tinea versicolor.

Protozoa — acanthamoebiasis.

Arthropod — scabies.

Neoplasms
Kaposi's sarcoma, cutaneous lymphomas,[202] squamous and basal cell carcinomas (?).

Dermatoses
Seborrhoeic dermatitis,[202] acquired ichthyosis,[222] asteatosis,[222] vasculitis,[222] folliculitis,[223] vitiligo,[224] yellow nail syndrome, papular eruption,[225] idiopathic pruritus,[226] a chronic diffuse dermatitis[227] and palmoplantar keratoderma.[228]

and it is an adverse prognostic factor. Many other cutaneous effects have been described in recent years. These fall into three broad categories — infections, usually of an opportunistic nature, neoplasms, and non-infectious dermatoses. They are detailed in Table 26.1. Detailed references can be found in a number of reviews of this subject.[202–210]

Early signs of AIDS may be a roseola-like rash associated with recent infection and seroconversion,[211] or the development of seborrhoeic dermatitis,[212] pruritic lesions,[213,214] a chronic acneiform folliculitis, fungal infection or impetigo of the neck and beard region.[215] Infections in immunocompromised patients may differ in severity and other clinical features from those in normal hosts.[216]

A unique manifestation of HIV infection is oral 'hairy' leucoplakia which is characterized by raised, poorly demarcated projections on the lateral borders of the tongue, resulting in a corrugated or 'hairy' surface.[217–221] Human papilloma virus and Epstein–Barr virus have been identified in biopsy specimens.[217] *Candida* is frequently observed in the keratin projections. There is also some parakeratosis and acanthosis, and large pale-staining cells resembling koilocytes are present in the upper stratum malpighii.[217]

REFERENCES

Introduction

1. Cherry J D. Viral exanthems. DM 1982; 28 (8): 1–56.
2. Ruzicka T, Rosendahl C, Braun-Falco O. A probable case of rotavirus exanthem. Arch Dermatol 1985; 121: 253–254.
3. Drew WL. Laboratory diagnosis of viral skin disease. Semin Dermatol 1984; 3: 146–153.
3a. Solomon AR. New diagnostic tests for herpes simplex and varicella zoster infections. J Am Acad Dermatol 1988; 18: 218–221.

Poxviridae

4. Casemore DP, Emslie ES, Whyler DK et al. Cowpox in a child, acquired from a cat. Clin Exp Dermatol 1987; 12: 286–287.
5. Kempe CH. Studies on smallpox and complications of smallpox vaccination. Pediatrics 1960; 26: 176–189.
6. Lane JM, Ruben FL, Neff JM, Millar JD. Complications of smallpox vaccination, 1968; national surveillance in the United States. N Engl J Med 1968; 281: 1201–1208.
7. Sarkany I, Caron GA. Cutaneous complications of smallpox vaccination. Trans St John's Hosp Dermatol Soc 1962; 48: 163–170.
8. Zayid I, Farraj S. Granuloma pyogenicum — a hitherto unrecognized complication of smallpox vaccination. Br J Dermatol 1974; 90: 293–299.
9. Keane JT, James K, Blankenship ML, Pearson RW. Progressive vaccinia associated with combined variable immunodeficiency. Arch Dermatol 1983; 119: 404–408.
10. Marmelzat WL. Malignant tumors in smallpox vaccination scars. A report of 24 cases. Arch Dermatol 1968; 97: 400–406.
11. Slater DN, Parsons MA, Fussey IV. Malignant fibrous histiocytoma arising in a smallpox vaccination scar. Br J Dermatol 1981; 105: 215–217.
12. Lupton GP. Discoid lupus erythematosus occurring in a smallpox vaccination scar. J Am Acad Dermatol 1987; 17: 688–690.
13. Anderton RL, Abele DC. Lichen sclerosus et atrophicus in a vaccination site. Arch Dermatol 1976; 112: 1787.
14. Breman JG, Arita I. The confirmation and maintenance of smallpox eradication. N Engl J Med 1980; 303: 1263–1273.
15. Michelson HE, Ikeda K. Microscopic changes in variola. Arch Dermatol Syph 1927; 15: 138–164.
16. Cotton DWK, Cooper C, Barrett DF, Leppard BJ. Severe atypical molluscum contagiosum infection in an immunocompromised host. Br J Dermatol 1987; 116: 871–876.
16a. Katzman M, Carey JT, Elmets CA et al. Molluscum contagiosum and the acquired immunodeficiency syndrome: clinical and immunological details of two cases. Br J Dermatol 1987; 116: 131–138.
17. Kwittken J. Molluscum contagiosum: some new histologic observations. Mt Sinai J Med 1980; 47: 583–588.
18. Shelley WB, Burmeister V. Demonstration of a unique viral structure: the molluscum viral colony sac. Br J Dermatol 1986; 115: 557–562.
19. Reed RJ, Parkinson RP. The histogenesis of molluscum contagiosum. Am J Surg Pathol 1977; 1: 161–166.
20. Uehara M, Danno K. Central pitting of molluscum contagiosum. J Cutan Pathol 1980; 7: 149–153.
21. Steigleder G-K. Histology of benign virus induced tumors of the skin. J Cutan Pathol 1978; 5: 45–52.
22. Fellner MJ, Osowsky MJ. Molluscum contagiosum in an epidermal inclusion cyst on the eyelid. Int J Dermatol 1979; 18: 160–161.
23. Hodge SJ, Fliegelman MT, Schrodt GR, Owen LG. Molluscum contagiosum occurring in epidermal inclusion cysts. Arch Dermatol 1973; 108: 257–258.
24. Aloi FG, Pippione M. *Molluscum contagiosum* occurring in an epidermoid cyst. J Cutan Pathol 1985; 12: 163–165.
25. Ackerman AB. Epidermal inclusion cysts. Arch Dermatol 1974; 109: 736.
25a. Brandrup F, Asschenfeldt P. Molluscum contagiosum-induced comedo and secondary abscess formation. Pediatr Dermatol 1989; 6: 118–121.
26. Steffen C, Markman J-A. Spontaneous disappearance of molluscum contagiosum. Report of a case. Arch Dermatol 1980; 116: 923–924.
26a. Heng MCY, Steuer ME, Levy A et al. Lack of host cellular immune response in eruptive molluscum contagiosum. Am J Dermatopathol 1989; 11: 248–254.
27. Ackerman AB, Tanski EV. Pseudoleukaemia cutis. Report of a case in association with molluscum contagiosum. Cancer 1977; 40: 813–817.
28. Marks JG Jr, White JW Jr. Molluscum contagiosum in a halo nevus. Int J Dermatol 1980; 19: 258–259.
29. Hanau D, Grosshans E. Response to molluscum contagiosum in a halo nevus. Int J Dermatol 1981; 20: 218–220.
30. Charley MR, Sontheimer RD. Clearing of subacute cutaneous lupus erythematosus around molluscum contagiosum lesions. J Am Acad Dermatol 1982; 6: 529–533.
30a. Naert F, Lachapelle JM. Multiple lesions of molluscum contagiosum with metaplastic ossification. Am J Dermatopathol 1989; 11: 238–241.
31. Schuler G, Hönigsmann H, Wolff K. The syndrome of milker's nodules in burn injury. Evidence for indirect viral transmission. J Am Acad Dermatol 1982; 6: 334–339.
32. Leavell UW Jr, Phillips IA. Milker's nodules. Pathogenesis, tissue culture, electron microscopy, and calf inoculation. Arch Dermatol 1975; 111: 1307–1311.
33. Kuokkanen K, Launis J, Morttinen A. Erythema nodosum and erythema multiforme associated with milker's nodules. Acta Derm Venereol 1976; 56: 69–72.
33a. Labeille B, Duverlie G, Daniel P, Denoeux J-P. Bullous eruption complicating a milker's nodule. Int J Dermatol 1988; 27: 115–116.
34. Evins S, Leavell UW Jr, Phillips IA. Intranuclear inclusions in milker's nodules. Arch Dermatol 1971; 103: 91–93.
35. Davis CM, Musil G. Milker's nodule. A clinical and

electron microscopic report. Arch Dermatol 1970; 101: 305–311.

36. Leavell UW Jr, McNamara MJ, Muelling R et al. Orf, report of 19 human cases with clinical and pathological observations. JAMA 1968; 204: 657–664.

37. Johannessen JV, Krogh H-K, Solberg I et al. Human orf. J Cutan Pathol 1975; 2: 265–283

38. Hunskaar S. Giant orf in a patient with chronic lymphocytic leukaemia. Br J Dermatol 1986; 114: 631–634.

39. Pether JVS, Guerrier CJW, Jones SM et al. Giant orf in a normal individual. Br J Dermatol 1986; 115: 497–499.

40. Kennedy CTC, Lyell A. Perianal orf. J Am Acad Dermatol 1984; 11: 72–74.

40a. Rees J, Marks JM. Two unusual cases of orf following trauma to the scalp. Br J Dermatol 1988; 118: 445–447.

41. Wilkinson JD. Orf: a family with unusual complications. Br J Dermatol 1977; 97: 447–450.

42. Kahn D, Hutchinson EA. Generalized bullous orf. Int J Dermatol 1980; 19: 340–341.

42a. Groves RW, Wilson-Jones E, MacDonald DM. Human orf: morphologic characteristics and immunohistochemical diagnosis. J Cutan Pathol 1989; 16: 305 (abstract).

43. Sanchez RL, Hebert A, Lucia H, Swedo J. Orf. A case report with histologic, electron microscopic, and immunoperoxidase studies. Arch Pathol Lab Med 1985; 109: 166–170.

43a. Gill MJ, Arlette J, Buchan KA, Barber K. Human orf. A diagnostic consideration? Arch Dermatol 1990; 126: 356–358.

44. Yeh H-P, Soltani K. Ultrastructural studies in human orf. Arch Dermatol 1974; 109: 390–392.

44a. Taieb A, Guillot M, Carlotti D, Maleville J. Orf and pregnancy. Int J Dermatol 1988; 27: 31–33.

Herpesviridae

45. Chang T-W. Herpes simplex virus infection. Int J Dermatol 1983; 22: 1–7.

46. Rawls WE, Hammerberg O. Epidemiology of the herpes simplex viruses. Clin Dermatol 1984; 2 (2): 29–45.

47. Corey L, Vontver LA, Brown ZA. Genital herpes simplex virus infections: clinical manifestations, course, and complications. Semin Dermatol 1984; 3: 89–101.

48. Meissner HV. Herpes simplex virus infections in the newborn. Clin Dermatol 1984; 2(2): 23–28.

49. Perna JJ, Mannix ML, Rooney JF et al. Reactivation of latent herpes simplex virus infection by ultraviolet light: A human model. J Am Acad Dermatol 1987; 17: 473–478.

50. Hill TJ, Altman DM, Blyth WA et al. Herpes simplex virus latency. Clin Dermatol 1984; 2(2): 46–55.

51. Snavely SR, Liu C. Clinical spectrum of herpes simplex virus infections. Clin Dermatol 1984; 2(2): 8–22.

52. Giacobetti R. Herpetic whitlow. Int J Dermatol 1979; 18: 55–58.

53. Peutherer JF, Smith IW, Robertson DH. Necrotising balanitis due to a generalised primary infection with herpes simplex virus type 2. Br J Vener Dis 1979; 55: 48–51.

54. Long JC, Wheeler CE Jr, Briggaman RA. Varicella-like infection due to herpes simplex. Arch Dermatol 1978; 114: 406–409.

55. Leyden JJ, Baker DA. Localized herpes simplex infections in atopic dermatitis. Arch Dermatol 1979; 115: 311–312.

56. Toole JWP, Hofstader SL, Ramsay CA. Darier's disease and Kaposi's varicelliform eruption. J Am Acad Dermatol 1979; 1: 321–324.

57. Hillard P, Seeds J, Cefalo R. Disseminated herpes simplex in pregnancy: two cases and a review. Obstet Gynecol Surv 1982; 37: 449–453.

58. Hsiung GD, Landry ML, Mayo DR, Fong CKY. Laboratory diagnosis of herpes simplex virus type 1 and type 2 infections. Clin Dermatol 1984; 2 (2): 67–82.

59. Huff JC, Krueger GG, Overall JC Jr et al. The histopathologic evolution of recurrent herpes simplex labialis. J Am Acad Dermatol 1981; 5: 550–557.

60. Cohen C, Trapuckd S. Leukocytoclastic vasculitis associated with cutaneous infection by herpesvirus. Am J Dermatopathol 1984; 6: 561–565.

60a. Hassel MH, Lesher JL Jr. Herpes simplex mimicking leukemia cutis. J Am Acad Dermatol 1989; 21: 367–371.

60b. Ferguson DL, Hawk RJ, Covington NM, Reed RJ. Lichenoid lymphocytic vasculitis with a high component of histiocytes. Histogenetic implications in a specified clinical setting. Am J Dermatopathol 1989; 11: 259–269.

61. Shelley WB, Wood MG. Surgical conversion of herpes simplex from an epidermal to a dermal disease. Br J Dermatol 1979; 100: 649–655.

62. Boddingius J, Dijkman H, Hendriksen E et al. HSV-2 replication sites, monocyte and lymphocytic cell infection and virion phagocytosis by neutrophils, in vesicular lesions on penile skin. J Cutan Pathol 1987; 14: 165–175.

62a. Heng MCY, Allen SG, Heng SY et al. An electron microscopic study of the epidermal infiltrate in recurrent herpes simplex. Clin Exp Dermatol 1989; 14: 199–202.

62b. Vestey JP, Howie SEM, Norval M et al. Immune responses to herpes simplex virus in patients with facial herpes simplex and those with eczema herpeticum. Br J Dermatol 1988; 118: 775–782.

63. Nishimura M, Maekawa M, Hino Y et al. Kaposi's varicelliform eruption. Development in a patient with a healing second-degree burn. Arch Dermatol 1984; 120: 799–800.

64. Findlay GH, Forman L, Hull PR. Actinic chickenpox. Light-distributed varicella eruption. S Afr Med J 1979; 55: 989–991.

65. Wilkin JK, Ribble JC, Wilkin OC. Vascular factors and the localization of varicella lesions. J Am Acad Dermatol 1981; 4: 665–666.

66. McSorley J, Shapiro L, Brownstein MH, Hsu KC. Herpes simplex and varicella-zoster: comparative histopathology of 77 cases. Int J Dermatol 1974; 13: 69–75.

67. Sadick NS, Swenson PD, Kaufman RL, Kaplan MH. Comparison of detection of varicella-zoster virus by the Tzanck smear, direct immunofluorescence with a monoclonal antibody, and virus isolation. J Am Acad Dermatol 1987; 17: 64–69.

68. Solomon AR, Rasmussen JE, Weiss JS. A comparison of the Tzanck smear and viral isolation in varicella and herpes zoster. Arch Dermatol 1986; 122: 282–285.

68a. Folkers E, Vreeswijk J, Oranje AP, Duivenvoorden JN. Rapid diagnosis in varicella and herpes zoster: re-evaluation of direct smear (Tzanck test) and electron microscopy including colloidal gold immuno-electron microscopy in comparison with virus isolation. Br J Dermatol 1989; 121: 287–296.

69. Liesegang TJ. The varicella-zoster virus: Systemic and ocular features. J Am Acad Dermatol 1984; 11: 165–191.

70. Nagashima K, Nakazawa M, Endo H. Pathology of the human spinal ganglia in varicella-zoster virus infection. Acta Neuropathol 1975; 33: 105–117.

71. Heskel NS, Hanifin JM. "Recurrent herpes zoster": An unproved entity? J Am Acad Dermatol 1984; 10: 486–490.

71a. Cohen PR, Grossman ME. Clinical features of human immunodeficiency virus-associated disseminated herpes zoster virus infection — a review of the literature. Clin Exp Dermatol 1989; 14: 273–276.

72. Guill MA, Goette DK. Granuloma annulare at sites of healing herpes zoster. Arch Dermatol 1978; 114: 1383.

73. Rinder HM, Murphy GF. Eccrine duct involvement by herpes zoster. Arch Dermatol 1984; 120: 261–262.

74. Minars N, Silverman JF, Escobar MR, Martinez AJ. Fatal cytomegalic inclusion disease. Associated skin manifestations in a renal transplant patient. Arch Dermatol 1977; 113: 1569–1571.

74a. Lesher JL Jr. Cytomegalovirus infections and the skin. J Am Acad Dermatol 1988; 18: 1333–1338.

75. Walker JD, Chesney TMcC. Cytomegalovirus infection of the skin. Am J Dermatopathol 1982; 4: 263–265.

75a. Feldman PS, Walker AN, Baker R. Cutaneous lesions heralding disseminated cytomegalovirus infection. J Am Acad Dermatol 1982; 7: 545–548.

76. Doeglas HMG, Rijnten WJ, Schroder FP, Schirm J. Cold urticaria and virus infections: a clinical and serological study in 39 patients. Br J Dermatol 1986; 114: 311–318.

77. Bhawan J, Gellis S, Ucci A, Chang T-W. Vesiculobullous lesions caused by cytomegalovirus infection in an immunocompromised adult. J Am Acad Dermatol 1984; 11: 743–747.

78. Bournerias I, Boisnic S, Patey O et al. Unusual cutaneous cytomegalovirus involvement in patients with acquired immunodeficiency syndrome. Arch Dermatol 1989; 125: 1243–1246.

79. Horn TD, Hood AF. Clinically occult cytomegalovirus present in skin biopsy specimens in immunosuppressed hosts. J Am Acad Dermatol 1989; 21: 781–784.

80. Lee JY-Y, Peel R. Concurrent cytomegalovirus and herpes simplex virus infections in skin biopsy specimens from two AIDS patients with fatal CMV infection. Am J Dermatopathol 1989; 11: 136–143.

81. Boudreau S, Hines HC, Hood AF. Dermal abscesses with Staphylococcus aureus, cytomegalovirus and acid-fast bacilli in a patient with acquired immunodeficiency syndrome (AIDS). J Cutan Pathol 1988; 15: 53–57.

82. Abel EA. Cutaneous manifestations of immunosuppression in organ transplant recipients. J Am Acad Dermatol 1989; 21: 167–179.

83. Fine J-D, Arndt KA. The TORCH syndrome: A clinical review. J Am Acad Dermatol 1985; 12: 697–706.

84. Pariser RJ. Histologically specific skin lesions in disseminated cytomegalovirus infection. J Am Acad Dermatol 1983; 9: 937–946.

85. Curtis JL, Egbert BM. Cutaneous cytomegalovirus vasculitis: an unusual clinical presentation of a common opportunistic pathogen. Hum Pathol 1982; 13: 1138–1141.

86. Patterson JW, Broecker AH, Kornstein MJ, Mills AS. Cutaneous cytomegalovirus infection in a liver transplant patient. Diagnosis by in situ DNA hybridization. Am J Dermatopathol 1988; 10: 524–530.

87. Coskey RJ, Paul L. Ampicillin sensitivity in infectious mononucleosis. Arch Dermatol 1969; 100: 717–719.

88. Spencer SA, Fenske NA, Espinoza CG et al. Granuloma annulare-like eruption due to chronic Epstein–Barr virus infection. Arch Dermatol 1988; 124: 250–255.

89. Lowe L, Hebert AA, Duvic M. Gianotti–Crosti syndrome associated with Epstein–Barr virus infection. J Am Acad Dermatol 1989; 20: 336–338.

Papovaviridae

90. Orth G, Favre M. Human papillomaviruses. Biochemical and biologic properties. Clin Dermatol 1985; 3: 27–42.

91. Androphy EJ. Human papillomavirus. Current concepts. Arch Dermatol 1989; 125: 683–685.

92. Highet AS. Viral warts. Semin Dermatol 1988; 7: 53–57.

92a. Cobb MW. Human papillomavirus infection. J Am Acad Dermatol 1990; 22: 547-566.

93. Gross G, Pfister H, Hagedorn M, Gissmann L. Correlation between human papillomavirus (HPV) type and histology of warts. J Invest Dermatol 1982; 78: 160–164.

94. Jablonska S. Wart viruses: human papillomaviruses. Semin Dermatol 1984; 3: 120–129.

95. Jablonska S, Orth G, Obalek S, Croissant O. Cutaneous warts. Clinical, histologic, and virologic correlations. Clin Dermatol 1985; 3: 71–82.

96. Laurent R, Kienzler JL, Croissant O, Orth G. Two anatomoclinical types of warts with plantar localization: specific cytopathogenic effects of papillomavirus. Type 1 (HPV-1) and type 2 (HPV-2). Arch Dermatol Res 1982; 274: 101–111.

97. Jenson AB, Lim LY, Singer E. Comparison of human papillomavirus Type I serotyping by monoclonal antibodies with genotyping by in situ hybridization of plantar warts. J Cutan Pathol 1989; 16: 54–59.

98. Eversole LR, Laipis PJ, Green TL. Human papillomavirus Type 2 DNA in oral and labial verruca vulgaris. J Cutan Pathol 1987; 14: 319–325.

99. Ostrow R, Zachow K, Watts S et al. Characterization of two HPV-3 related papillomaviruses from common warts that are distinct clinically from flat warts or epidermodysplasia verruciformis. J Invest Dermatol 1983; 80: 436–440.

100. Finkel ML, Finkel DJ. Warts among meat handlers. Arch Dermatol 1984; 120: 1314–1317.

101. de Villiers E-M, Neumann C, Olsterdorf T et al. Butcher's wart virus (HPV 7) infections in non-

butchers. J Invest Dermatol 1986; 87: 236–238.

102. De Peuter M, De Clercq B, Minette A, Lachapelle JM. An epidemiological survey of virus warts of the hands among butchers. Br J Dermatol 1977; 96: 427–431.

103. Rudlinger R, Bunney MH, Grob R, Hunter JAA. Warts in fish handlers. Br J Dermatol 1989; 120: 375–381.

104. von Krogh G. Condyloma acuminata 1983: an updated review. Semin Dermatol 1983; 2: 109–129.

105. Beaudenon S, Praetorius F, Kremsdorf D et al. A new type of human papillomavirus associated with oral focal epithelial hyperplasia. J Invest Dermatol 1987; 88: 130–135.

106. von Krogh G, Syrjanen SM, Syrjanen KJ. Advantage of human papillomavirus typing in the clinical evaluation of genitoanal warts. J Am Acad Dermatol 1988; 18: 495–503.

107. Ostrow RS, Shaver MK, Turnquist S et al. Human papillomavirus-16 DNA in a cutaneous invasive cancer. Arch Dermatol 1989; 125: 666–669.

108. van der Leest RJ, Zachow KR, Ostrow RS et al. Human papillomavirus heterogeneity in 36 renal transplant recipients. Arch Dermatol 1987; 123: 354–357.

109. Obalek S, Favre M, Jablonska S et al. Human papillomavirus type 2-associated basal cell carcinoma in two immunosuppressed patients. Arch Dermatol 1988; 124: 930–934.

110. Guillet GY, del Grande P, Thivolet J. Cutaneous and mucosal warts. Clinical and histopathological criteria for classification. Int J Dermatol 1982; 21: 89–93.

111. Laurent R, Kienzler J-L. Epidemiology of HPV infections. Clin Dermatol 1985; 3: 64–70.

112. Barnett N, Mak H, Winkelstein JA. Extensive verrucosis in primary immunodeficiency diseases. Arch Dermatol 1983; 119: 5–7.

113. Milburn PB, Brandsma JL, Goldsman CI et al. Disseminated warts and evolving squamous cell carcinoma in a patient with acquired immunodeficiency syndrome. J Am Acad Dermatol 1988; 19: 401–405.

114. Phillips ME, Ackerman AB. "Benign" and "malignant" neoplasms associated with verrucae vulgares. Am J Dermatopathol 1982; 4: 61–84.

115. Kimura S, Komatsu T, Ohyama K. Common and plantar warts with trichilemmal keratinization-like keratinizing process: a possible existence of pseudo-trichilemmal keratinization. J Cutan Pathol 1982; 9: 391–395.

116. Eng AM, Jin Y-T, Matsuoka LY et al. Correlative studies of *verruca vulgaris* by H&E, PAP immunostaining, and electronmicroscopy. J Cutan Pathol 1985; 12: 46–54.

117. Kossard S, Xenias SJ, Palestine RF et al. Inflammatory changes in verruca vulgaris. J Cutan Pathol 1980; 7: 217–221.

118. Berman A, Winkelmann RK. Involuting common warts. Clinical and histopathologic findings. J Am Acad Dermatol 1980; 3: 356–362.

119. Goette DK. Carcinoma in situ in verruca vulgaris. Int J Dermatol 1980; 19: 98–101.

120. Shelley WB, Wood MG. Transformation of the common wart into squamous cell carcinoma in a patient with primary lymphedema. Cancer 1981; 48: 820–824.

121. Berman A, Domnitz JM, Winkelmann RK. Plantar warts recently turned black. Clinical and histopathologic findings. Arch Dermatol 1982; 118: 47–51.

122. Tagami H, Takigawa M, Ogino A et al. Spontaneous regression of plane warts after inflammation: clinical and histologic studies in 25 cases. Arch Dermatol 1977; 113: 1209–1213.

123. Berman A. Depigmented haloes associated with the involution of flat warts. Br J Dermatol 1977; 97: 263–265.

124. Berman A, Berman JE. Efflorescence of new warts: a sign of onset of involution in flat warts. Br J Dermatol 1978; 99: 179–182.

125. Tagami H, Oguchi M, Ofuji S. The phenomenon of spontaneous regression of numerous flat warts: immunohistological studies. Cancer 1980; 45: 2557–2563.

126. Iwatsuki K, Tagami H, Takigawa M, Yamada M. Plane warts under spontaneous regression. Arch Dermatol 1986; 122: 655–659.

127. Bender ME. Concepts of wart regression. Arch Dermatol 1986; 122: 645–647.

128. Berman A, Winkelmann RK. Flat warts undergoing involution: histopathological findings. Arch Dermatol 1977; 113: 1219–1221.

129. Weedon D, Robertson I. Regressing plane warts — an ultrastructural study. Australas J Dermatol 1978; 19: 65–68.

130. Lutzner MA. Epidermodysplasia verruciformis. An autosomal recessive disease characterized by viral warts and skin cancer. A model for viral oncogenesis. Bull Cancer 1978; 65: 169–182.

131. Jablonska S, Orth G. Epidermodysplasia verruciformis. Clin Dermatol 1985; 3: 83–96.

132. Jablonska S, Obalek S, Orth G et al. Regression of the lesions of epidermodysplasia verruciformis. Br J Dermatol 1982; 107: 109–115.

133. Majewski S, Skopinska-Rozewska E, Jablonska S et al. Partial defects of cell-mediated immunity in patients with epidermodysplasia verruciformis. J Am Acad Dermatol 1986; 15: 966–973.

134. Ostrow RS, Manias D, Mitchell AJ et al. Epidermodysplasia verruciformis. A case associated with primary lymphatic dysplasia, depressed cell-mediated immunity, and Bowen's disease containing human papillomavirus 16 DNA. Arch Dermatol 1987; 123: 1511–1516.

134a. Majewski S, Malejczyk J, Jablonska S et al. Natural cell-mediated cytotoxicity against various target cells in patients with epidermodysplasia verruciformis. J Am Acad Dermatol 1990; 22: 423–427.

135. Aizawa H, Abo T, Aiba S et al. Epidermodysplasia verruciformis accompanied by large granular lymphocytosis. Report of a case and immunological studies. Arch Dermatol 1989; 125: 660–665.

136. Kaminski M, Pawinska M, Jablonska S et al. Increased natural killer cell activity in patients with epidermodysplasia verruciformis. Arch Dermatol 1985; 121: 84–86.

137. van Voorst Vader PC, Orth G, Dutronquay V et al. Epidermodysplasia verruciformis. Acta Derm Venereol 1986; 66: 231–236.

138. Androphy EJ, Dvoretzky I, Lowy DR. X-linked inheritance of epidermodysplasia verruciformis. Genetic and virologic studies of a kindred. Arch

Dermatol 1985; 121: 864–868.

139. Comite SL, Castadot M-J. Colposcopic evaluation of men with genital warts. J Am Acad Dermatol 1988; 18: 1274–1278.

140. Chuang T-Y. Condylomata acuminata (genital warts). An epidemiologic view. J Am Acad Dermatol 1987; 16: 376–384.

141. Oriel JD. Genital papillomavirus infection. Semin Dermatol 1989; 8: 48–53.

142. Sehgal VN, Koranne RV, Srivastava SB. Genital warts. Current status. Int J Dermatol 1989; 28: 75–85.

143. Grussendorf-Conen E-I. Condyloma acuminata. Clin Dermatol 1985; 3: 97–103.

144. Rock B, Naghashfar Z, Barnett N et al. Genital tract papillomavirus infection in children. Arch Dermatol 1986; 122: 1129–1132.

145. Bender ME. New concepts of condyloma acuminata in children. Arch Dermatol 1986; 122: 1121–1124.

146. Chuang T-Y, Perry HO, Kurland LT, Ilstrup DM. Condyloma acuminatum in Rochester, Minn, 1950–1978. I. Epidemiology and clinical features. Arch Dermatol 1984; 120: 469–475.

147. Boxer RJ, Skinner DG. Condylomata acuminata and squamous cell carcinoma. Urology 1977; 9: 72–78.

148. Lee SH, McGregor DH, Kuziez MN. Malignant transformation of perianal condyloma acuminatum: a case report with review of the literature. Dis Colon Rectum 1981; 24: 462–467.

149. Bogomoletz WV, Potet F, Molas G. Condylomata acuminata, giant condyloma acuminatum (Buschke–Loewenstein tumour) and verrucous squamous carcinoma of the perianal and anorectal region: a continuous precancerous spectrum? Histopathology 1985; 9: 1155–1169.

150. Alexander RM, Kaminsky DB. Giant condyloma acuminatum (Buschke–Loewenstein tumor) of the anus: case report and review of the literature. Dis Colon Rectum 1979; 22: 561–565.

151. Norris CS. Giant condyloma acuminatum (Buschke–Lowenstein tumor) involving a pilonidal sinus: a case report and review of the literature. J Surg Oncol 1983; 22: 47–50.

152. Gross G, Ikenberg H, Gissmann L, Hagedorn M. Papillomavirus infection of the anogenital region: correlation between histology, clinical picture, and virus type. Proposal of a new nomenclature. J Invest Dermatol 1985; 85: 147–152.

153. Steffen C. Concurrence of condylomata acuminata and bowenoid papulosis. Am J Dermatopathol 1982; 4: 5–8.

154. Bhawan J, Dayal Y, Bhan AK. Langerhans cells in molluscum contagiosum, verruca vulgaris, plantar wart, and condyloma acuminatum. J Am Acad Dermatol 1986; 15: 645–649.

155. Wade TR, Ackerman AB. The effects of resin of podophyllin on condyloma acuminatum. Am J Dermatopathol 1984; 6: 109–122.

156. Kimura S, Masuda M. A comparative immunoperoxidase and histopathologic study of condylomata acuminata. J Cutan Pathol 1985; 12: 142–146.

157. Goodfellow A, Calvert H. Focal epithelial hyperplasia of the oral mucosa. Br J Dermatol 1979; 101: 341–344.

158. Starink TM, Woerdeman MJ. Focal epithelial hyperplasia of the oral mucosa. Br J Dermatol 1977; 96: 375–380.

159. van Wyk CW. Focal epithelial hyperplasia of the mouth: recently discovered in South Africa. Br J Dermatol 1977; 96: 381–388.

160. Lutzner M, Kuffer R, Blanchet-Bardon C, Croissant O. Different papillomaviruses as the causes of oral warts. Arch Dermatol 1982; 118: 393–399.

161. Stiefler RE, Solomon MP, Shalita AR. Heck's disease (focal epithelial hyperplasia). J Am Acad Dermatol 1979; 1: 499–502.

162. Kimura S. Bowenoid papulosis of the genitalia. Int J Dermatol 1982; 21: 432–436.

163. Hodl S. [Bowenoid papulosis of the genitals.] Z Hautkr 1981; 56: 368–377.

164. Halasz C, Silvers D, Crum CP. Bowenoid papulosis in three-year-old girl. J Am Acad Dermatol 1986; 14: 326–330.

165. Obalek S, Jablonska S, Baudenon S et al. Bowenoid papulosis of the male and female genitalia: Risk of cervical neoplasia. J Am Acad Dermatol 1986; 14: 433–444.

166. Lloyd KM. Multicentric pigmented Bowen's disease of the groin. Arch Dermatol 1970; 101: 48–51.

167. Kopf AW, Bart RS. Multiple bowenoid papules of the penis: a new entity? J Dermatol Surg Oncol 1977; 3: 265–269.

168. Wade TR, Kopf AW, Ackerman AB. Bowenoid papulosis of the penis. Cancer 1978; 42: 1890–1903.

169. Wade TR, Kopf AW, Ackerman AB. Bowenoid papulosis of the genitalia. Arch Dermatol 1979; 115: 306–308.

170. Feldman SB, Sexton FM, Glenn JD, Lookingbill DP. Immunosuppression in men with bowenoid papulosis. Arch Dermatol 1989; 125: 651–654.

171. Crum CP, Liskow A, Petras P et al. Vulvar intraepithelial neoplasia (severe atypia and carcinoma in situ). A clinicopathologic analysis of 41 cases. Cancer 1984; 54: 1429–1434.

172. Guillet GY, Braun L, Masse R et al. Bowenoid papulosis. Demonstration of human papillomavirus (HPV) with anti-HPV immune serum. Arch Dermatol 1984; 120: 514–516.

173. Penneys NS, Mogollon RJ, Nadji M, Gould E. Papillomavirus common antigens. Arch Dermatol 1984; 120: 859–861.

174. Lookingbill DP, Kreider JW, Howett MK et al. Human papillomavirus type 16 in bowenoid papulosis, intraoral papillomas, and squamous cell carcinoma of the tongue. Arch Dermatol 1987; 123: 363–368.

175. Abdennader S, Lessana-Leibowitch M, Pelisse M. An atypical case of penile carcinoma in situ associated with human papillomavirus DNA type 18. J Am Acad Dermatol 1989; 20: 887–889.

176. Rudlinger R, Grob R, Yu YX, Schnyder UW. Human papillomavirus-35-positive bowenoid papulosis of the anogenital area and concurrent human papillomavirus-35-positive verruca with bowenoid dysplasia of the periungual area. Arch Dermatol 1989; 125: 655–659.

177. Gupta J, Pilotti S, Shah KV et al. Human papillomavirus-associated early vulvar neoplasia investigated by in situ hybridization. Am J Surg Pathol 1987; 11: 430–434.

178. Gross G, Hagedorn M, Ikenberg H et al. Bowenoid papulosis. Presence of human papillomavirus (HPV)

structural antigens and of HPV 16-related DNA sequences. Arch Dermatol 1985; 121: 858–863.

Picornaviridae

179. Deseda-Tous J, Byatt PH, Cherry JD. Vesicular lesions in adults due to Echovirus 11 infections. Arch Dermatol 1977; 113: 1705–1706.
180. James WD, Odom RB, Hatch MH. Gianotti–Crosti-like eruption associated with coxsackievirus A-16 infection. J Am Acad Dermatol 1982; 6: 862–866.
181. McElgunn PSJ. Dermatologic manifestations of hepatitis B virus infection. J Am Acad Dermatol 1983; 8: 539–548.
182. Ellis AW, Kennett ML, Lewis FA, Gust ID. Hand, foot and mouth disease: an outbreak with interesting virological features. Pathology 1973; 5: 189–196.
183. Fields JP, Mihm MC Jr, Hellreich PD, Danoff SS. Hand, foot and mouth disease. Arch Dermatol 1969; 99: 243–246.

Other viruses

184. Lefrere J-J, Courouce A-M, Muller J-Y et al. Human parvovirus and purpura. Lancet 1985; 2: 730–731.
185. Listernick R. Parvovirus infections in childhood. Pediatr Dermatol 1986; 3: 435–438.
186. Plummer FA, Hammond GW, Forward K et al. An erythema infectiosum-like illness caused by human parvovirus infection. N Engl J Med 1985; 313: 74–79.
187. Bialecki C, Feder HM Jr, Grant-Kels JM. The six classic childhood exanthems: A review and update. J Am Acad Dermatol 1989; 21: 891–903.
188. Ackerman AB, Suringa DWR. Multinucleate epidermal cells in measles. A histologic study. Arch Dermatol 1971; 103: 180–184.
189. de Andino RM, Vazquez Botet M, Gubler DJ et al. The absence of dengue virus in the skin lesions of dengue fever. Int J Dermatol 1985; 24: 48–51.
190. Hart CA. Viral redskins. Semin Dermatol 1988; 7: 48–52.
191. Rosen LB, Rywlin AM, Resnick L. Hepatitis B surface antigen positive skin lesions. Two case reports with an immunoperoxidase study. Am J Dermatopathol 1985; 7: 507–514.
192. Whittaker SJ, Dover JS, Greaves MW. Cutaneous polyarteritis nodosa associated with hepatitis B surface antigen. J Am Acad Dermatol 1986; 15: 1142–1145.
193. van de Pette JEW, Jarvis JM, Wilton JMA, MacDonald DM. Cutaneous periarteritis nodosa. Arch Dermatol 1984; 120: 109–111.
194. Lee S, Kim KY, Hahn CS et al. Gianotti–Crosti syndrome associated with hepatitis B surface antigen (subtype adr). J Am Acad Dermatol 1985; 12: 629–633.
195. Gianotti F. Papular acrodermatitis of childhood and other papulo-vesicular acro-located syndromes. Br J Dermatol 1979; 100: 49–59.
196. Sagi EF, Linder N, Shouval D. Papular acrodermatitis of childhood associated with hepatitis A virus infection. Pediatr Dermatol 1985; 3: 31–33.
196a. Patrizi A, Di Lernia V, Ricci G et al. Papular and papulovesicular acrolocated eruptions and viral

infections. Pediatr Dermatol 1990; 7: 22–26.
197. Taieb A, Plantin P, Du Pasquier P et al. Gianotti–Crosti syndrome: a study of 26 cases. Br J Dermatol 1986; 115: 49–59.
198. Spear KL, Winkelmann RK. Gianotti–Crosti syndrome. A review of ten cases not associated with hepatitis B. Arch Dermatol 1984; 120: 891–896.
199. Martinez MI, Sánchez JL, López-Malpica F. Peculiar papular skin lesions occurring in hepatitis B carriers. J Am Acad Dermatol 1987; 16: 31–34.
200. Nutting WB, Beerman H, Parish LC, Witkowski JA. Retrovirus (HIV). Transfer, potential vectors, and biomedical concerns. Int J Dermatol 1987; 26: 426–433.
201. Lisby G, Lisby S, Wantzin GL. Retroviruses in dermatology. Int J Dermatol 1988; 27: 463–467.
202. Matis WL, Triana A, Shapiro R et al. Dermatologic findings associated with human immunodeficiency virus infection. J Am Acad Dermatol 1987; 17: 746–751.
203. Goodman DS, Teplitz ED, Wishner A et al. Prevalence of cutaneous disease in patients with acquired immunodeficiency syndrome (AIDS) or AIDS-related complex. J Am Acad Dermatol 1987; 17: 210–220.
204. Kaplan MH, Sadick N, McNutt NS et al. Dermatologic findings and manifestations of acquired immunodeficiency syndrome (AIDS). J Am Acad Dermatol 1987; 16: 485–506.
205. Warner LC, Fisher BK. Cutaneous manifestations of the acquired immunodeficiency syndrome. Int J Dermatol 1986; 25: 337–350.
206. Fisher BK, Warner LC. Cutaneous manifestations of the acquired immunodeficiency syndrome. Update 1987. Int J Dermatol 1987; 26: 615–630.
207. Straka BF, Whitaker DL, Morrison SH et al. Cutaneous manifestations of the acquired immunodeficiency syndrome in children. J Am Acad Dermatol 1988; 18: 1089–1102.
208. Hira SK, Wadhawan D, Kamanga J et al. Cutaneous manifestations of human immunodeficiency virus in Lusaka, Zambia. J Am Acad Dermatol 1988; 19: 451–457.
209. Alessi E, Cusini M, Zerboni R. Mucocutaneous manifestations in patients infected with human immunodeficiency virus. J Am Acad Dermatol 1988; 19: 290–297.
209a. Cockerell CJ. Cutaneous manifestations of HIV infection other than Kaposi's sarcoma: Clinical and histologic aspects. J Am Acad Dermatol 1990; 22: 1260–1269.
210. Coldiron BM, Bergstresser PR. Prevalence and clinical spectrum of skin disease in patients infected with human immunodeficiency virus. Arch Dermatol 1989; 125: 357–361.
211. Wantzin GRL, Lindhardt BO, Weismann K, Ulrich K. Acute HTLV III infection associated with exanthema, diagnosed by seroconversion. Br J Dermatol 1986; 115: 601–606.
212. Berger RS, Stoner MF, Hobbs ER et al. Cutaneous manifestations of early human immunodeficiency virus exposure. J Am Acad Dermatol 1988; 19: 298–303.
213. Liautaud B, Pape JW, DeHovitz JA et al. Pruritic skin lesions. A common initial presentation of acquired

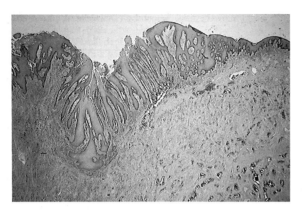

Fig. 27.1 Amoebiasis of the penis. This case was misdiagnosed on biopsy as a squamous cell carcinoma because of the marked pseudoepitheliomatous hyperplasia. Haematoxylin — eosin

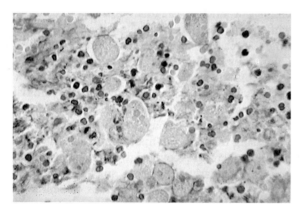

Fig. 27.2 Amoebiasis. Organisms are present in the ulcer base.
Haematoxylin — eosin

prominent central karyosome and occasional phagocytosed red blood cells in the cytoplasm.[3] In sections of fixed tissue, their diameters are usually within the range 12–20 μm.

ACANTHAMOEBIASIS

The free-living amoebae of soil and water, *Acanthamoeba* and *Naegleria*, are facultative parasites of man.[6] Although meningoencephalitis is the major clinical feature, there have been several reports of chronic ulcerating or nodular lesions in the skin.[7–8]

Histopathology

Sections have shown tuberculoid granulomatous lesions in the deep dermis and subcutaneous tissue with accompanying vasculitis.[7] Amoebae, 15–40 μm in width, can often be seen lying free in the tissues.[9] There may be overlying ulceration.

TRYPANOSOMIASIS

African trypanosomiasis is caused by the protozoa *Trypanosoma gambiense* and *Trypanosoma rhodesiense*, which are transmitted by the bite of the tsetse fly (*Glossina* species).[10] Although the major clinical manifestations are fever and neurological signs, cutaneous lesions develop in about one-half of the patients.[11] These consist of an indurated, erythematous 'chancre' at the site of the bite and a fleeting erythematous, maculopapular rash, often with circinate lesions.[12] The diagnosis is made by finding haemoflagellates in thick, peripheral blood smears.

There are usually no significant skin lesions in American trypanosomiasis (Chagas's disease), caused by *T. cruzi*, although a macular and ulcerative eruption due to parasitosis of the skin by amastigotes of this organism has been reported in an immunosuppressed patient.[12a]

Histopathology

Sections of the chancre show a superficial and deep, predominantly perivascular infiltrate with lymphocytes and prominent plasma cells, with some resemblance to lesions of secondary syphilis.[11] Organisms can be seen in Giemsa-stained smears taken from the exudate of a chancre, but they are not usually seen in tissue sections.[11] Amastigotes of *T. cruzi* were present in the walls of blood vessels, in arrector pili muscles, and in the cytoplasm of inflammatory cells in the immunosuppressed patient referred to above.[12a]

LEISHMANIASIS

Leishmaniasis can be classified into three types, each caused by a different species of *Leishmania*:

1. cutaneous (oriental) leishmaniasis caused by *L. tropica* in Asia and Africa, and by *L. mexicana* in Central and South America;[13]

2. mucocutaneous (American) leishmaniasis caused by *L. brasiliensis*; and

3. visceral leishmaniasis (kala-azar) caused by *L. donovani.*

This classification is an oversimplification as a great deal of clinical overlap exists between the various forms.[14] The diagnosis can be made by identifying parasites on histological section, or in smears,[15] by culture on specialized media, by the leishmanin intradermal skin test (Montenegro test), or by fluorescent antibody tests using the patient's serum.[16]

Cutaneous leishmaniasis

This chronic, self-limited granulomatous disease of the skin is usually caused by *L. tropica*. It is endemic in the Middle East, around the Eastern Mediterranean, in North Africa and in parts of Asia.[17–19] Sandflies of the genus *Phlebotomus* are the usual vectors. The incubation period following the sandfly bite is weeks to months and depends on the size of the inoculum.[20] In Central and South America *L. mexicana* is the species involved.

Acute, chronic, recidivous and disseminated forms are recognized.[20] The acute lesions are usually single papules which become nodules, ulcerate, and heal, leaving a scar.[17,21,22] Chronic lesions which persist for 1–2 years are single, or occasionally multiple, raised, non-ulcerated plaques. The recidivous form consists of erythematous papules, often circinate, near the scars of previously healed lesions.[23] The disseminated form develops in anergic individuals as widespread nodules and macules, without ulceration or visceral involvement. It is quite rare in *L. tropica* infections, but less so with *L. brasiliensis*. Sporotrichoid[24] and satellite lesions[25] are very uncommon clinical manifestations of cutaneous leishmaniasis, reported recently from Saudi Arabia.

Histopathology

In acute lesions there is a massive dermal infil-

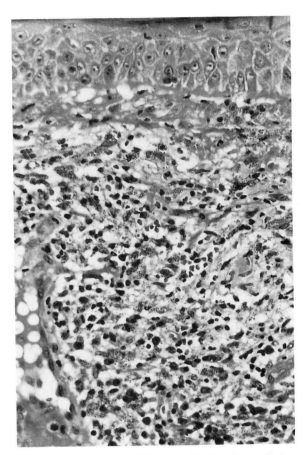

Fig. 27.3   Leishmaniasis. The dermal infiltrate is composed of lymphocytes, some plasma cells and parasitized macrophages.
Haematoxylin — eosin

trate of lymphocytes, parasitized macrophages, epithelioid cells, and occasional giant cells, plasma cells, and sometimes a few eosinophils (Fig. 27.3).[26] Variable numbers of neutrophils are present in the upper dermis. Granulated, calcific Michaelis–Gutmann bodies have been reported in the cytoplasm of macrophages in two cases.[27] Rarely, the inflammatory infiltrate extends around small nerves in the deep dermis in a manner similar to leprosy.[28] The parasites are round to oval basophilic structures, 2–4 μm in size. They have an eccentrically located kinetoplast. Their lack of a capsule is helpful in distinguishing them from *Histoplasma capsulatum*. Although organisms can be seen in macrophages in haematoxylin and eosin stained sections (Fig. 27.4), the morpho-

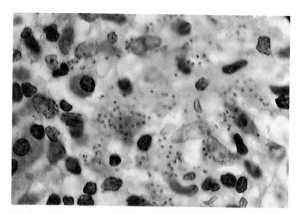

Fig. 27.4 Leishmaniasis. Numerous organisms are present in the cytoplasm of macrophages.
Haematoxylin — eosin

logical details are better seen with a Giemsa stain, preferably on a slit-skin smear.[29] The epidermis shows hyperkeratosis and acanthosis, but sometimes atrophy, ulceration or intraepidermal abscesses.[24,30] Pseudoepitheliomatous hyperplasia is present in some longstanding lesions.

With increasing chronicity, there is a reduction in the number of parasitized macrophages, and the appearance of small tuberculoid granulomas which consist predominantly of epithelioid cells and histiocytes with occasional giant cells.[30] There is an intervening mild to moderate mononuclear cell infiltrate.

In the recidivous form, the appearances resemble those seen in lupus vulgaris with tubercles surrounded by lymphocytes and histiocytes with some giant cells.[30] However there is no necrosis, and only sparse plasma cells. Occasional organisms may be found on careful search.

In the disseminated anergic lesions, the infiltrate is almost entirely composed of parasitized macrophages with scant lymphocytes.[31]

Mucocutaneous leishmaniasis

The initial lesions of mucocutaneous (American) leishmaniasis, caused by *L. brasiliensis*, resemble those seen in the cutaneous form.[32] Vegetating, verrucous and sporotrichoid[33] lesions may also occur. In up to 20% of cases, destructive, ulcerative lesions of mucous membranes develop, par-

ticularly in the nasopharynx and at body orifices.[34] This complication, known as espundia, may develop up to 25 years after the apparent clinical cure of the primary lesion.[32] Mucocutaneous leishmaniasis is found in Central and South America, or in travellers from those areas. The disseminated anergic form is a rare complication.[31]

Histopathology

The appearances resemble those seen in the acute cutaneous form, although the number of organisms is considerably smaller, and occasional tuberculoid granulomas may be seen. Suppurative granulomas have been described.[32] The mucosal lesions show non-specific chronic inflammation with only a few parasitized macrophages. Pseudoepitheliomatous hyperplasia may be prominent in some lesions, particularly at the periphery. There may be fibrosis in the dermis. A favourable prognostic feature is the presence of necrosis with a reactive response.[35]

Visceral leishmaniasis

Visceral leishmaniasis (kala-azar), caused by *L. donovani*, results in fever, anaemia, and hepatosplenomegaly.[31] It is endemic in many tropical countries. Cutaneous involvement (post-kala-azar dermal leishmaniasis) develops in about 5% of cases, some 1–5 years after the original infection.[36] The lesions comprise areas of erythema (usually on the face), macules which may be hyper- or hypopigmented (usually on the trunk), and nodules (usually on the face but not infrequently on the limbs).[36] Lesions may clinically resemble leprosy, but differ by having normal sensation.

Histopathology

Lesions are composed of a variable admixture of histiocytes, lymphocytes, plasma cells, and epithelioid cells.[37] There may be an occasional tuberculoid granuloma. Organisms (Leishman–Donovan bodies) are nearly always present, but their number varies from case to case and from lesion to lesion.

TOXOPLASMOSIS

There are two clinical forms of toxoplasmosis, congenital and acquired.[38] The acquired form is seen most often in immunocompromised patients.[39] Skin changes in both are rare and not clinically distinctive. Macular, haemorrhagic and even exfoliative lesions have been reported in congenital toxoplasmosis,[40] while in the acquired form the lesions have been described as maculopapular, haemorrhagic, lichenoid,[41] nodular and erythema-multiforme-like.[40,42] There have been several reports of a dermatomyositis-like syndrome.[43,44]

Histopathology

There is a superficial and mid-dermal perivascular lymphohistiocytic infiltrate. In about half the cases, parasites can be seen in the cytoplasm of macrophages, in the form of pseudocysts, or lying free in the dermis,[42] or rarely the epidermis,[39] in the form of trophozoites. Pseudo-epitheliomatous hyperplasia may develop in a few cases.[42] The histology has resembled dermatomyositis in those cases presenting with a dermatomyositis-like syndrome. Some of the rare histological expressions of the disease have recently been reviewed.[45]

PNEUMOCYSTOSIS

One case of cutaneous pneumocystosis has been reported, in a patient with the acquired immunodeficiency syndrome.[46] There were polypoid lesions in both external auditory canals.

Histopathology

Sections showed perivascular mantles of amphophilic, foamy to finely stippled material similar to that seen in pulmonary pneumocystosis.[46] The methenamine-silver stain showed large numbers of small cysts typical of *Pneumocystis carinii*.

REFERENCES

1. El-Zawahry M, El-Komy M. Amoebiasis cutis. Int J Dermatol 1973; 12: 305–307.
2. Binford CH, Connor DH. Amebiasis. In: Pathology of tropical and extraordinary diseases. Vol 1. Washington, D.C.: Armed Forces Institute of Pathology, 1976; 308–316.
3. Fujita WH, Barr RJ, Gottschalk HR. Cutaneous amebiasis. Arch Dermatol 1981; 117: 309–310.
4. Elsahy NI. Cutaneous amoebiasis. Br J Plast Surg 1978; 31: 48–49.
5. Majmudar B, Chaiken ML, Lee KU. Amebiasis of clitoris mimicking carcinoma. JAMA 1976; 236: 1145–1146.
6. Beaver PC, Jung RC, Cupp EW. Clinical parasitology. 9th ed. Philadelphia: Lea & Febiger, 1984.
7. Bhagwandeen SB, Carter RF, Naik KG, Levitt D. A case of Hartmannellid amebic meningoencephalitis in Zambia. Am J Clin Pathol 1975; 63: 483–492.
7a. Bass J, Karrs T, Pomeranz J. Disseminated cutaneous acanthamoeba associated with the acquired immunodeficiency syndrome: histopathologic electron microscopic and immunofluorescent studies. J Cutan Pathol 1989; 16: 296 (abstract).
8. Gullett J, Mills J, Hadley K et al. Disseminated granulomatous acanthamoeba infection presenting as an unusual skin lesion. Am J Med 1979; 67: 891–896.
9. Ringsted J, Jager BV, Suk D, Visvesvara GS. Probable acanthamoeba meningoencephalitis in a Korean child.

Am J Clin Pathol 1976; 66: 723–730.
10. Robinson B, Clark RM, King JF et al. Chronic Gambian trypanosomiasis. South Med J 1980; 73: 516–518.
11. Cochran R, Rosen T. African trypanosomiasis in the United States. Arch Dermatol 1983; 119: 670–674.
12. Spencer HC Jr, Gibson JJ Jr, Brodsky RE, Schultz MG. Imported African trypanosomiasis in the United States. Ann Intern Med 1975; 82: 633–638.
12a. McNutt NS, von Kreuter BF, Santos-Buch CA et al. Cutaneous manifestations of Chagas' disease in an immunosuppressed patient. J Cutan Pathol 1988; 15: 329 (abstract).
13. Nelson DA, Gustafson TL, Spielvogel RL. Clinical aspects of cutaneous leishmaniasis acquired in Texas. J Am Acad Dermatol 1985; 12: 985–992.
14. Dowlati Y. Cutaneous leishmaniasis. Int J Dermatol 1979; 18: 362–368.
15. Berger RS, Perez-Figaredo RA, Spielvogel RL. Leishmaniasis: The touch preparation as a rapid means of diagnosis. J Am Acad Dermatol 1987; 16: 1096–1105.
16. Moriearty PL, Pereira C. Diagnosis and prognosis of new world leishmaniasis. Arch Dermatol 1978; 114: 962–963.
17. Azab AS, Kamal MS, El Haggar MS et al. Early surgical treatment of cutaneous leishmaniasis. J Dermatol Surg Oncol 1983; 9: 1007–1012.

18. Marsden PD. Current concepts in parasitology: Leishmaniasis. N Engl J Med 1979; 300: 350–352.
19. Farah FS, Malak JA. Cutaneous leishmaniasis. Arch Dermatol 1971; 103: 467–474.
20. Barsky S, Storino W, Salgea K, Knapp DP. Cutaneous leishmaniasis. Arch Dermatol 1978; 114: 1354–1355.
21. Kubba R, Al-Gindan Y, El-Hassan AM, Omer AHS. Clinical diagnosis of cutaneous leishmaniasis (oriental sore). J Am Acad Dermatol 1987; 16: 1183–1189.
22. Albanese G, Giorgetti P, Santagostino L et al. Cutaneous leishmaniasis. Treatment with itraconazole. Arch Dermatol 1989; 125: 1540–1542.
23. Stratigos J, Tosca A, Nicolis G et al. Epidemiology of cutaneous leishmaniasis in Greece. Int J Dermatol 1980; 19: 86–88.
24. Kibbi A-G, Karam PG, Kurban AK. Sporotrichoid leishmaniasis in patients from Saudi Arabia: Clinical and histologic features. J Am Acad Dermatol 1987; 17: 759–764.
25. Kubba R, Al-Gindan Y, El-Hassan AM et al. Dissemination in cutaneous leishmaniasis. II. Satellite papules and subcutaneous induration. Int J Dermatol 1988; 27: 702–706.
26. Kurban AK, Malak JA, Farah FS, Chaglassian HT. Histopathology of cutaneous leishmaniasis. Arch Dermatol 1966; 93: 396–401.
27. Sandbank M. Michaelis–Gutmann bodies in macrophages of cutaneous leishmaniasis. J Cutan Pathol 1976; 3: 263–268.
28. Satti MB, El-Hassan AM, Al-Gindan Y et al. Peripheral neural involvement in cutaneous leishmaniasis. Int J Dermatol 1989; 28: 243–247.
29. Bryceson A. Tropical dermatology. Cutaneous leishmaniasis. Br J Dermatol 1976; 94: 223–226.
30. Nicolis GD, Tosca AD, Stratigos JD, Capetanakis JA. A clinical and histological study of cutaneous leishmaniasis. Acta Derm Venereol 1978; 58: 521–525.
31. Rau RC, Dubin HV, Taylor WB. *Leishmania tropica* infections in travellers. Arch Dermatol 1976; 112: 197–201.
32. Price SM, Silvers DN. New world leishmaniasis.
33. Spier S, Medenica M, McMillan S, Virtue C. Sporotrichoid leishmaniasis. Arch Dermatol 1977; 113: 1104–1105.
34. Farge D, Frances C, Vouldoukis I et al. Chronic destructive ulcerative lesion of the midface and nasal cavity due to leishmaniasis contracted in Djibouti. Clin Exp Dermatol 1987; 12: 211–213.
35. Ridley DS, Marsden PD, Cuba CC, Barreto AC. A histological classification of mucocutaneous leishmaniasis in Brazil and its clinical evaluation. Trans R Soc Trop Med Hyg 1980; 74: 508–514.
36. Girgla HS, Marsden RA, Singh GM, Ryan TJ. Post-kala-azar dermal leishmaniasis. Br J Dermatol 1977; 97: 307–311.
37. Yesudian P, Thambiah AS. Amphotericin B therapy in dermal leishmaniasis. Arch Dermatol 1974; 109: 720–722.
38. Justus J. Cutaneous manifestations of toxoplasmosis. Curr Probl Dermatol 1971; 4: 24–47.
39. Leyva WH, Santa Cruz DJ. Cutaneous toxoplasmosis. J Am Acad Dermatol 1986; 14: 600–605.
40. Andreev VC, Angelov N, Zlatkov NB. Skin manifestations in toxoplasmosis. Arch Dermatol 1969; 100: 196–199.
41. Menter MA, Morrison JGL. Lichen verrucosus et reticularis of Kaposi (porokeratosis striata of Nekam): a manifestation of acquired adult toxoplasmosis. Br J Dermatol 1976; 94: 645–654.
42. Binazzi M, Papini M. Cutaneous toxoplasmosis. Int J Dermatol 1980; 19: 332–335.
43. Topi GC, D'Alessandro L, Catricala C, Zardi O. Dermatomyositis-like syndrome due to toxoplasma. Br J Dermatol 1979; 101: 589–591.
44. Pollock JL. Toxoplasmosis appearing to be dermatomyositis. Arch Dermatol 1979; 115: 736–737.
45. Binazzi M. Profile of cutaneous toxoplasmosis. Int J Dermatol 1986; 25: 357–363.
46. Coulman CU, Greene I, Archibald RWR. Cutaneous pneumocystosis. Ann Intern Med 1987; 106: 396–398.

Serologic aids to diagnosis. Arch Dermatol 1977; 113: 1415–1416.

Marine injuries

INTRODUCTION

Cutaneous injuries from various forms of marine life are uncommon recreational and occupational hazards. In most instances a localized urticarial and inflammatory lesion results at the point of injury but this may be accompanied by a laceration if a sharp dorsal spine is involved. Severe systemic reactions and even fatality may result from the toxins of some marine organisms.

There have been several reviews of the cutaneous manifestations of marine animal injuries,[1–4] including Fisher's 'Atlas of Aquatic Dermatology'.[5] Although of great dermatological and medical interest, these cutaneous lesions are of little dermatopathological importance. Biopsies are rarely taken, and, if they are, the findings, with several exceptions, are not diagnostically or aetiologically specific.

In the brief account which follows, various categories of marine organisms will be considered.

COELENTERATES

Although the phylum Coelenterata has over 9000 species, fewer than 80 are of clinical significance.[2–5] The toxic effects of coelenterates result from contact with the nematocyst, a coiled thread-like tube, found particularly on the tentacles, which pierces the skin on contact. The toxin contained in the nematocysts of some species is capable of producing such diverse reactions as erythema, urticaria, a burning sensation or, rarely, fatal anaphylaxis and cardio-respiratory arrest. The coelenterates of dermato-

fatal jellyfish stinging. Trans Roy Soc Trop Med Hyg 1960; 54: 373–384.
14. Yaffee HS. A delayed cutaneous reaction following contact with jellyfish. Derm Int 1968; 7: 75–77.
15. Strutton G, Lumley J. Cutaneous light microscopic and ultrastructural changes in a fatal case of jellyfish envenomation. J Cutan Pathol 1988; 15: 249–255.
16. Drury JK, Noonan JD, Pollock JG, Reid WH. Jelly fish sting with serious hand complications. Injury 1980; 12: 66–68.

Molluscs

17. Sutherland SK, Lane WR. Toxins and mode of envenomation of the common ringed or blue-banded octopus. Med J Aust 1969; 1: 893–898.
18. Edmonds C. A non-fatal case of blue-ringed octopus bite. Med J Aust 1969; 2: 601.

Echinoderms

19. Kinmont PDC. Sea-urchin sarcoidal granuloma. Br J Dermatol 1965; 77: 335–343.
20. Rocha G, Fraga S. Sea urchin granuloma of the skin. Arch Dermatol 1962; 85: 406–408.
21. Strauss MB, MacDonald RI. Hand injuries from sea urchin spines. Clin Orthop 1976; 114: 216–218.

Sponges

22. Yaffee HS, Stargardter F. Erythema multiforme from *Tedania ignis*. Arch Dermatol 1963; 87: 601–604.

Seaweed

23. Grauer FH, Arnold HL Jr. Seaweed dermatitis. Arch Dermatol 1961; 84: 720–730.
24. Seville RH. Dogger Bank itch. Br J Dermatol 1957; 69: 92–93.

Venomous fish

25. Wiener S. A case of stone-fish sting treated with antivenene. Med J Aust 1965; 1: 191.
26. Russell FE. Stingray injuries: a review and discussion of their treatment. Am J Med Sci 1953; 226: 611–622.
27. Russell FE, Panos TC, Kang LW et al. Studies on the mechanism of death from stingray venoms. A report of two fatal cases. Am J Med Sci 1958; 235: 566–583.
28. Barss P. Wound necrosis caused by the venom of stingrays. Pathological findings and surgical management. Med J Aust 1984; 141: 854–855.

Helminth infestations

INTRODUCTION

Helminthic parasites are responsible for a number of important diseases of tropical countries. These include schistosomiasis caused by the trematode flukes, cysticercosis and sparganosis resulting from the larvae of certain tapeworms (cestodes), and onchocerciasis, dirofilariasis and larva migrans occurring as a consequence of nematode infestations.[1]

TREMATODE INFESTATIONS

SCHISTOSOMIASIS

It has been estimated that 200 million people are infested with one or other of the three major species of schistosome fluke.[2] *Schistosoma haematobium* (found in most of Africa and in the Near East) has a predilection for the bladder, *S. japonicum* (common in parts of the Orient) for the gut, and *S. mansoni* (found in parts of the Caribbean region and the north east part of South America) for the portal circulation. Four types of skin lesions have been described:[3–11]

1. a pruritic, erythematous and urticarial papular rash (cercarial dermatitis, 'swimmer's itch') associated with the penetration of the cercariae through the skin en route to the various venous plexuses to mature;

2. urticarial lesions associated with the dissemination of the cercariae or the laying of eggs by the adult flukes;

3. papular, granulomatous and even warty,

vegetating lesions of the genital and perineal skin secondary to the deposition of ova in dermal vessels;[10] and

4. extragenital cutaneous lesions secondary to lodgement of ova and, rarely, worms.[11]

Urticarial lesions are more common with *S. japonicum*,[5] and perineal lesions with *S. haematobium*,[6] while extragenital cutaneous manifestations are usually a complication of *S. japonicum* and *S. haematobium* but are quite rare with *S. mansoni*. The late development of squamous cell carcinoma has been reported in the verrucous genital lesions.[7]

Cercarial dermatitis may also be seen, rarely, as a result of penetration of the skin by cercariae of species of schistosome that are unable to develop further in man, being destroyed before they reach the venous plexus.[7]

Histopathology

The cercarial dermatitis shows intraepidermal spongiosis with exocytosis of eosinophils and neutrophils, sometimes forming microabscesses.[5] Cercariae are not usually seen. The dermal reaction is mild, with oedema, vascular dilatation and a mild perivascular inflammatory cell infiltrate and some interstitial eosinophils.

Genital and perineal lesions show hyperkeratosis and acanthosis. There may be prominent pseudoepitheliomatous hyperplasia, and at times focal ulceration or draining sinuses with accompanying acute inflammation.[4,10] The dermis contains numerous ova, some associated with a granulomatous reaction, including foreign body giant cells. Other eggs are in microabscesses, often containing numerous eosinophils. Flukes may be seen in cutaneous vessels.

Extragenital lesions show numerous ova in the superficial dermis associated with palisading granulomas.[8,9] Eosinophils, neutrophils and foreign body giant cells are found in most lesions, while in later lesions there may be degenerating or calcified ova, plasma cells and fibroblasts, with variable fibrosis.

The ova of the three major species have characteristic features. The ova of *S. haematobium* have an apical spine, those of *S. mansoni* a lateral spine, while the ova of *S. japonicum* have no spine.[5] The ova of *S. mansoni* and of *S. japonicum* may be acid fast.

OTHER TREMATODES

A larval trematode, identified as a mesocercaria of an undescribed species belonging to the subfamily Alariinae, has been removed from an intradermal swelling.[12] The lung fluke *Paragonimus westermani* can also produce a cutaneous inflammatory lesion which includes eosinophils and plasma cells.[13]

CESTODE INFESTATIONS

CYSTICERCOSIS

The larval phase of *Taenia solium*, the pork tapeworm, may infect man as an accidental intermediate host, with the formation of multiple asymptomatic subcutaneous nodules 1–3 cm in diameter.[14–16] They have a predilection for the chest wall, upper arms and thighs.[17] The nodules are composed of a white cystic structure with an outer membrane containing clear fluid and a cysticercus larva attached to one edge. Surrounding the gelatinous cyst is a host response of fibrous tissue.

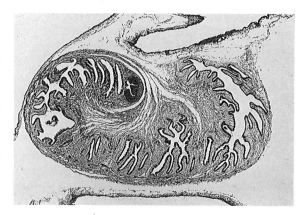

Fig. 29.1 Cysticercus larva removed from a subcutaneous 'cyst' of the skin.

Histopathology

The diagnosis is made by the characteristic appearance of the scolex of the cysticercus larva (Fig. 29.1). The fibrous tissue reaction in the subcutaneous tissue contains a moderate chronic inflammatory cell infiltrate which includes variable numbers of eosinophils.

SPARGANOSIS

This is a rare infestation caused by the larval form of a tapeworm of the genus *Spirometra*.[18,19] It occurs in many parts of the world, mainly within the tropics. Man is a second intermediate host. Infestation may result in a subcutaneous nodule which slowly migrates. Bisection of the nodule after excision will reveal a white thread-like worm about 1 mm in width and from a few centimetres to 50 cm in length.[20]

Histopathology

There is a subcutaneous, partly granulomatous, inflammatory mass composed of lymphocytes, plasma cells, neutrophils and variable numbers of eosinophils. Portions of worm are usually seen within the mass[18] or there may be a cavity where the larva has been. The larva has a flattened structure with both longitudinal and horizontal muscle bundles, giving a 'checker board' appearance. A longitudinal excretory canal is also present and basophilic calcareous corpuscles, a characteristic feature of cestodes, may also be seen scattered in varying numbers throughout the matrix.[19]

NEMATODE INFESTATIONS

ONCHOCERCIASIS

Onchocerciasis, which is common in tropical Africa, the Yemen and Central and South America, is caused by the nematode *Onchocerca volvulus*.[21–23] The larvae are transmitted by several species of flies of the genus *Simulium*. The larvae mature into adult worms in the subcutaneous tissue where they form non-tender subcutaneous nodules 2.5–10 cm in diameter. The nodules, which may occur anywhere on the body, are either isolated or grouped in large conglomerations. They may contain one or several tightly coiled worms which may live for many years.

The adult worms produce microfilariae which are found in the neighbouring lymphatics. The microfilariae may migrate to the dermis and eye. Onchocercal dermatitis, which results from infiltration of the skin by these microfilariae, is a pruritic papular rash with altered pigmentation.[22] The dermatitis is typically generalized, but an eruption localized to one limb, usually a leg, is found in the northern Sudan and also in the Yemen, where it is known as sowda.[24]

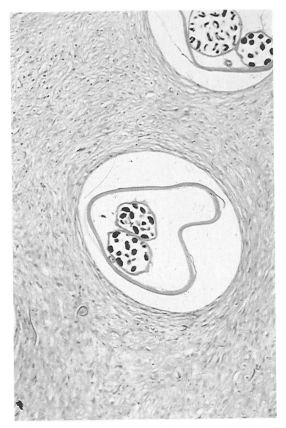

Fig. 29.2 Onchocerciasis. Several fine, coiled microfilariae are present in the fibrous tissue that surrounds the worm. Haematoxylin — eosin

Histopathology[25,26]

The subcutaneous nodules have an outer wall of dense fibrous tissue which usually extends between the worms (Fig. 29.2).[25] Centrally there is granulation tissue and a mixed inflammatory cell infiltrate in early lesions, although in longstanding lesions in which the worms are dead there is only dense fibrous tissue with some calcification and foreign body giant cells and a chronic inflammatory cell infiltrate. Eosinophils are usually present at all stages. Microfilariae may be seen in lymphatics in this region.

In onchocercal dermatitis there is a light superficial and deep infiltrate of chronic inflammatory cells and eosinophils in the dermis. Microfilariae may be seen in slits between collagen bundles in the upper dermis.[26,27] Eosinophils and eosinophil major basic protein are usually present around degenerating microfilariae.[24,25] There is progressive fibrosis of the dermis. The epidermis shows acanthosis and hyperkeratosis.

DIROFILARIASIS

Human infection with *Dirofilaria immitis* (the dog heartworm) is rare.[28] It may cause symptomatic subcutaneous nodules or pulmonary lesions which are usually asymptomatic.[29] Skin lesions are usually solitary, erythematous and tender subcutaneous nodules. Other species of *Dirofilaria* may rarely produce similar lesions.[30]

Histopathology

The centre of the nodule contains a degenerating filaria with a thick laminated cuticle, distinct longitudinal ridges, and large lateral chords as well as typical musculature.[31] There is an intense surrounding inflammatory reaction of lymphocytes, plasma cells, histiocytes, eosinophils and sometimes giant cells. There is usually central suppuration and neutrophils may extend out into the adjacent inflammatory zone.[31] The diagnostic histological features of various zoonotic filariae in tissue sections have been reviewed by Gutierrez.[30]

LARVA MIGRANS

Cutaneous larva migrans is caused by the intracutaneous wanderings of hookworm and certain other nematode larvae.[32] The creeping eruption caused by fly larvae is usually considered separately. In larva migrans there are pruritic papules which form serpiginous tunnels which are at first erythematous but soon become elevated and vesicular. The lesion may extend several millimetres per day. Older parts of the track may become crusted.

Larva migrans is most commonly caused by larvae of *Ancylostoma braziliense*, a hookworm of dogs and cats, but *Necator americanus* may give a creeping eruption of shorter duration.[1] Other hookworms which may produce cutaneous larva migrans include *Ancylostoma caninum*, *Uncinaria stenocephala* and *Bunostomum phlebotomum*.

A deep subcutaneous form of larva migrans may be seen with *Gnathostoma spinigerum*.[33-35]

The larvae of *Strongyloides stercoralis* usually provoke little reaction as they migrate through the skin to reach vessels for their passage to the lung. In some individuals with strongyloidiasis, a variant of larva migrans is found with a rapidly progressing linear urticarial lesion, which may extend at up to 10 cm per hour.[36,37] The term larva currens (racing larva) has been used for these cases.[37-39] There is still a high incidence of *Strongyloides stercoralis* infestation in former prisoners of war interned many years ago in South-East Asia.[40] In one series, almost one-third had suffered episodes of larva currens.[41] Another cutaneous manifestation of strongyloidiasis is the presence of widespread petechiae and purpura. These features are seen in immunosuppressed patients with disseminated infections.[37,42]

Histopathology

In larva migrans there are small cavities in the epidermis corresponding to the track of the larva, although the parasite itself is uncommonly seen in section. There may be a diffuse spongiotic dermatitis with intraepidermal vesicles containing some eosinophils.[43] There is usually no inflammatory reaction around the larva (when it can be found), whereas there is a mixed inflammatory reaction behind the migrating larva with a superficial dermal infiltrate of neutrophils, lymphocytes, plasma cells and usually abundant eosinophils.[43] An eosinophilic folliculitis has been recorded.[44]

Reports of larva currens have mentioned a perivascular round cell infiltrate with interstitial eosinophils, a picture common to many parasitic infestations.[45] In disseminated strongyloidiasis there are numerous larvae, 9–15 μm in diameter, in the dermal collagen and rarely in the lumina of small blood vessels.[37,42]

OTHER NEMATODES

There are various other nematodes that are sometimes of dermatopathological interest.[1] *Mansonella streptocerca* is found in West Africa. The adult worm lives in the dermis and microfilariae may also be seen. It usually presents with hypopigmented macules and itching. The adult worms of *Loa loa* live in the subcutaneous tissue and migrate, producing fugitive swellings and temporary inflammation. The elevated outline of the subcutaneous worms may be visible on the skin surface.[46] There is high eosinophilia. Liberation of the microfilariae may produce urticarial lesions. *Wuchereria bancrofti* and *Brugia malayi* produce lymphangitis and lymphadenopathy, with the later development of elephantiasis. Further discussion is beyond the scope of this chapter.

Dracunculus medinensis may produce a blistering lesion due to the migration of the worm, which will eventually be extruded through rupture of the bleb. The female worm measures 70–120 cm in length and is coiled through the subcutaneous tissues. The anterior end is surrounded by granulation tissue containing a mixed inflammatory infiltrate while there is fibrosis and some inflammation in the deeper parts.

Trichinella spiralis may produce variable clinical lesions ranging from urticaria to maculopapular lesions following its development in striated muscle.[47] The changes are not diagnostic.

Gnathostoma spinigerum is endemic in South-East Asia and Japan. Human infestation occurs from eating uncooked infested meat from the second intermediate host, such as pigs, chickens, and freshwater fish of the genus *Ophicephalus*.[35] It may produce migratory cutaneous swellings with localized erythema, or a true creeping eruption.[33,35] Excoriation of a pruritic patch may reveal the worm, which measures up to 3 cm in length.

There are rare reports of larvae of the soil nematode *Pelodera (Rhabditis) strongyloides* producing nodular lesions associated with a heavy mixed dermal inflammatory infiltrate and the presence of larvae in tissue sections.[48,49]

Larvae of *Dioctophyme renale*, the giant kidney worm which occurs naturally in several fish-eating mammals throughout the world, have been recovered from the subcutaneous tissues of humans on several occasions.[50]

REFERENCES

Introduction

1. Beaver PC, Jung RC, Cupp EW. Clinical parasitology. 9th ed. Philadelphia: Lea & Febiger, 1984.

Trematode infestations

2. Mahmoud AA. Schistosomiasis. N Engl J Med 1977; 297: 1329–1331.
3. Obasi OE. Cutaneous schistosomiasis in Nigeria. An update. Br J Dermatol 1986; 114: 597–602.
4. Amer M. Cutaneous schistosomiasis. Int J Dermatol 1982; 21: 44–46.
5. Wood MG, Srolovitz H, Schetman D. Schistosomiasis. Paraplegia and ectopic skin lesions as admission symptoms. Arch Dermatol 1976; 112: 690–695.
6. Torres VM. Dermatologic manifestations of Schistosomiasis mansoni. Arch Dermatol 1976; 112: 1539–1542.
7. Walther RR. Chronic papular dermatitis of the scrotum due to *Schistosoma mansoni*. Arch Dermatol 1979; 115: 869–870.
8. Jacyk WK, Lawande RV, Tulpule SS. Unusual presentation of extragenital cutaneous Schistosomiasis mansoni. Br J Dermatol 1980; 103: 205–208.
9. Findlay GH, Whiting DA. Disseminated and zosteriform cutaneous schistosomiasis. Br J Dermatol (Suppl) 1971; 7: 98–101.
10. McKee PH, Wright E, Hutt MSR. Vulval schistosomiasis. Clin Exp Dermatol 1983; 8: 189–194.

There are five major classes of arthropods.[1,2] The Class Insecta is the largest group, although the Class Arachnida, which includes ticks, spiders and mites, is probably of greater dermatopathological interest. The Class Crustacea, which includes lobsters, crabs and shrimps, and the Classes Diplopoda and Chilopoda, which include millipedes and centipedes respectively, are not of major dermatopathological importance and will not be considered in detail. They may produce local reactions at the site of contact. These include erythema, urticaria and purpura in the case of millipedes and centipedes. A brief classification of the arthropods is given in Table 30.1. Mention should also be made of the comprehensive monograph on arthropods and the skin by Alexander.[3]

ARACHNIDS

SCORPION AND SPIDER BITES

Scorpion venom may produce throbbing indurated lesions at the site of attack, usually on acral parts. Lymphadenitis and systemic symptoms usually develop.[1]

Local necrosis may be produced at the site of spider bites; in some cases, e.g. following the bite of a black-widow spider (usually *Latrodectus mactans*), severe systemic symptoms and even death may result. The genus *Loxosceles* (which includes the brown recluse spider, *Loxosceles reclusa*), may produce a local lesion with quite extensive necrosis, haemorrhage, blistering and ulceration.[4,5] A chronic pyoderma-gangrenosum -like reaction has also been reported.[6] Less severe reactions, such as erythema and oedema, are more usual with other species of spiders.[6a] An excellent review of spider bites has been published by Wong and colleagues.[7]

Histopathology

The appearances change from a neutrophilic vasculitis with haemorrhage, through a phase with arterial wall necrosis, to eschar-covered ulceration and subcutaneous necrosis.[4] There are usually eosinophils in the accompanying inflammatory infiltrate.

TICK BITES

Ticks are important as hosts and transmitters of a wide range of diseases.[8] Their salivary secretions may produce systemic toxaemia and their embedded mouthparts may produce a local erythematous lesion or a more persistent granulomatous or nodular response.[9] Unusual reactions include papular urticaria, bullae and haemorrhage. There are two major families of ticks, soft ticks (Argasidae) and hard ticks (Ixodidae). Soft ticks (*Ornithodoros* species) are generally not perceived by the victim, although hard ticks — of which there are several genera, including *Ixodes* and *Dermacentor* — are eventually noticed because they remain attached for days and slowly engorge with blood. Attempts to remove the tick may lead to the embedded mouthparts separating and remaining in the tissue.

Histopathology

In acute lesions there is an intradermal cavity, below which the mouthparts may be seen (Fig. 30.1). There is often a tract of 'necrosis' on either side, and in the first few days intense extravasation of fibrin may be seen in relation to vessels.[9] A moderately dense, predominantly perivascular infiltrate of neutrophils, lympho-

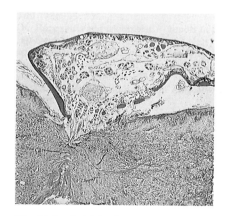

Fig. 30.1 A tick in-situ.
Haematoxylin — eosin

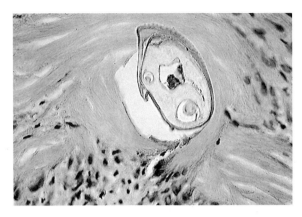

Fig. 30.2 A tick-bite reaction. Mouth parts are present in the dermis.
Haematoxylin — eosin

cytes, plasma cells and histiocytes is present, with a considerable admixture of eosinophils.[10] The diagnosis may be difficult if tick mouthparts are not seen (Fig. 30.2).

In chronic persistent lesions there is a diffuse superficial and deep infiltrate which includes all the cells found in acute lesions but usually with many fewer neutrophils and more lymphocytes. There may be occasional giant cells, dermal fibrosis and even granuloma formation.[11] The epidermis may show acanthosis or pseudo-epitheliomatous hyperplasia.

Erythema chronicum migrans (Lyme disease), which follows the bite of *Ixodes*, has recently been shown to be due to a spirochaete transmitted by the tick.[12] It is considered with other spirochaetal diseases in Chapter 24 (page 635).

DEMODICOSIS

Two species of follicle mites are found as normal inhabitants of human skin:[13–22] *Demodex folliculorum* lives mainly in the hair follicles and *Demodex brevis* in the sebaceous glands. *Demodex folliculorum*, the larger of the two mites, measures about 0.4 mm in length. Mites of this species are often aggregated in a follicle whereas *D. brevis* is usually solitary.[15] The mites have been found in 10% of routine skin biopsies (from all sites), and in 12% of all follicles examined in these same biopsies.[16] The face is most often involved,

although *D. brevis* has a wider distribution.[22] Although increased numbers of mites are found in sections of rosacea, this does not prove a causal relationship. It is generally accepted that demodex mites are not aetiologically involved in the usual form of rosacea, although they may possibly play a role in the granulomatous form, in which extrafollicular mites are sometimes seen. *Demodex* may produce a blepharitis[17] and so-called rosacea-like demodicosis.[17a,21] It has been incriminated as a cause of localized pustular folliculitis of the face[18] and of a more widespread, papular, pruritic eruption in patients with acquired immunodeficiency syndrome.[18a] Facial erythema with follicular plugging (pityriasis folliculorum) is another manifestation of *Demodex* infestation.[18b]

Histopathology

The effects of *Demodex* infestation include follicular dilatation, the presence of dense homogeneous, eosinophilic material surrounding the mites, folliculitis, and perifollicular chronic

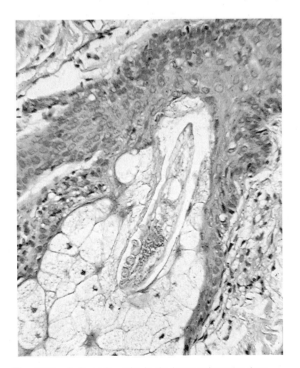

Fig. 30.3 A demodex mite in the lower sebaceous duct.
Haematoxylin — eosin

inflammation (Fig. 30.3). There are several reports of a granulomatous reaction to extra-follicular *Demodex*, usually in granulomatous or pustular rosacea.[19,20]

In rosacea-like demodicosis up to 10–15 *D. folliculorum* may be found in individual follicles.[21] Telangiectasia of superficial vessels, perifollicular granulomas and mild perivascular chronic inflammation may also be seen in this condition.

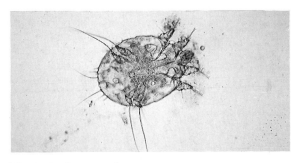

Fig. 30.4 *Sarcoptes* mite. × 100

SCABIES

Scabies is a contagious disease caused by the mite *Sarcoptes scabiei* var. *hominis*. It is acquired particularly under conditions of overcrowding and poor personal hygiene or during sexual contact. Patients with both minimal disease and only a few mites[23] and exaggerated atypical lesions complicating AIDS[24,24a] are now being seen. The disease tends to appear in epidemics which have a cyclical character, recurring at intervals of about 30 years and lasting for about 15 years.[25] The reasons for these cyclic fluctuations are not understood. Based on this observation, a new cycle can be expected in about 1994.

Three clinical forms are found — papulovesicular lesions, persistent nodules, and Norwegian (crusted) scabies. The usual lesions are papules and papulovesicles which are intensely pruritic. The vesicles are usually found at the end of very fine wavy dark lines, best seen with the help of a hand lens or by applying a small amount of ink to the surface and removing the excess.[26] These lines represent the excreta-soiled burrows in the horny layer in which the female travels to deposit her eggs.

The female mite measures up to 0.4 mm in length and rather less in breadth, while the adult male, which dies after copulation, is much smaller (Fig. 30.4). The sites most commonly affected are the interdigital skin folds, the palmar surfaces of the hands and fingers, the wrists, the nipples, the inframammary regions and the male genitals. In addition to the burrows, there is nearly always a secondary rash of small urticarial papules with no mites, which may result from autosensitization.[27]

In about 7% of patients, particularly children and young adults, reddish-brown pruritic nodules develop with a predilection for the lower trunk, scrotum and thighs.[25] These lesions may persist for a year, despite treatment. Mites are rarely found and this form (persistent nodular scabies) is thought to represent a delayed hypersensitivity reaction similar to that found following some other arthropod bites.

Norwegian (crusted) scabies is a rare, contagious form consisting of widespread crusted and secondarily infected hyperkeratotic lesions, found in the mentally and physically debilitated[28] as well as in immunosuppressed patients.[29–32a] There is an extremely heavy infestation with mites.

Human infestation with varieties of *Sarcoptes scabiei* of animal origin is not uncommon. They produce a self-limiting disease without the presence of burrows.[33,34] These animal variants are morphologically indistinguishable from the human variant of *Sarcoptes scabiei*.

Immunological features. There is some evidence that immunological phenomena are involved in scabies.[35,36] Immediate hypersensitivity may result in the primary lesions, and delayed hypersensitivity in the persistent nodular lesions. Elevated levels of IgE have been found in the serum of some patients with scabies but the serum IgA is reduced in many with the Norwegian form.[37] IgE has been demonstrated by immunofluorescence in vessel walls in the dermis,[38] IgA and C3 in the stratum corneum, and IgM and/or C3 along the basement

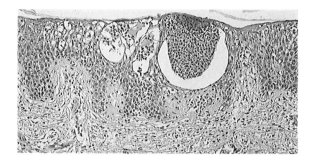

Fig. 30.5 Scabies. There are spongiotic vesicles containing many eosinophils.
Haematoxylin — eosin

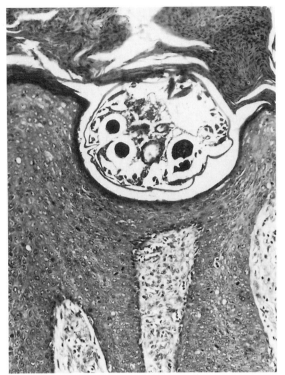

Fig. 30.6 Scabies. A mite is present in the stratum corneum. The epidermis shows coincidental Bowen's disease.
Haematoxylin — eosin

membrane in some cases.[39] IgE-containing plasma cells have been found in nodular lesions.[40]

Histopathology

The histological changes are sufficiently distinctive at least to suggest the diagnosis.[41] There is a superficial and deep infiltrate of lymphocytes, histiocytes and eosinophils, together with some interstitial eosinophils. These features are common to many arthropod reactions. In addition, there are spongiotic foci and spongiotic vesicles within the epidermis with exocytosis of variable numbers of eosinophils and sometimes neutrophils (Fig. 30.5). Eggs, larvae, mites and excreta may be seen in the stratum corneum if an obvious burrow is excised (Fig. 30.6).[42] If the secondary (autosensitization) lesions are biopsied, the picture may not be diagnostic; no mites will be seen, and there is a report which suggests that even eosinophils may be absent.[27] Older lesions may simply show excoriation and overlying scale crusts.[41]

The lesions of *persistent nodular scabies* resemble those of other persistent bite reactions, with a more dense superficial and deep inflammatory cell infiltrate which includes lymphocytes, macrophages, plasma cells, eosinophils and sometimes atypical mononuclear cells (Fig. 30.7).[42] Lymphoid follicles are sometimes present, and the infiltrate may even extend into the subcutaneous fat. Pseudoepitheliomatous hyperplasia is not a feature. Cases have been pub-

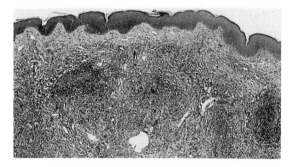

Fig. 30.7 Persistent nodular scabies. There is a superficial and deep infiltrate within the dermis. The interstitial eosinophils are not obvious at this magnification.
Haematoxylin — eosin

lished that purportedly resembled cutaneous lymphoma, but the descriptions provided in those instances are not those of lymphoma.[43]

In *Norwegian scabies*, there is a massive

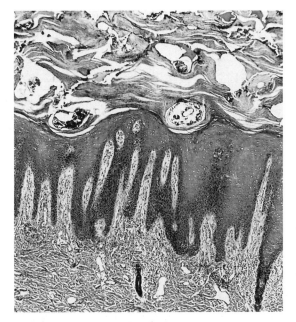

Fig. 30.8 Norwegian scabies. The thick keratin layer
contains several mites.
Haematoxylin — eosin

orthokeratosis and parakeratosis containing
mites in all stages of development (Fig. 30.8).
The underlying epidermis shows psoriasiform
hyperplasia with focal spongiosis and exocytosis
of eosinophils and neutrophils, sometimes producing intraepidermal microabscesses. The
dermis contains a superficial and deep infiltrate
of chronic inflammatory cells and usually some
interstitial eosinophils.

CHEYLETIELLA DERMATITIS

Several species of *Cheyletiella*, a mite found on
dogs, rabbits and cats, can produce an intensely
pruritic dermatitis in humans.[44-46] There are
erythematous papules and papulovesicles, sometimes grouped, with a predilection for the chest,
abdomen and proximal extremities.[47] The mite
is almost never found on man and the diagnosis
may be confirmed by examining fur brushings of
the patient's pet for the mite.[48,49] This condition
may be synonymous with so-called 'itchy red
bump' disease, a papular, pruritic disorder of
uncertain histogenesis which has been reported
from Florida, USA.[45,50] Delayed hypersensitivity mechanisms are thought to play a role in
the pathogenesis of the eruption.[51]

Histopathology

Sections show focal epidermal spongiosis at the
site of the bite. There is a superficial and mid-
dermal, predominantly perivascular infiltrate
composed of lymphocytes, macrophages and
some eosinophils. There are usually some interstitial eosinophils, suggesting an arthropod bite.
However, the reaction is more superficial and
less inflammatory than the usual arthropod reaction.

OTHER MITE LESIONS

There are four other families of mites that have
been incriminated in the production of cutaneous lesions. They are Tyroglyphoidea (food
mites), Pyemotidae (predacious or grain itch
mites), Dermanyssidae (parasitoid or rat mites)
and Trombiculidae (trombiculid or harvest
mites, chiggers).[1,2]

Food mites and predacious mites produce
erythematous papules, papulovesicles or urticaria
in workers handling certain foods and grain. The
lesions may be mistaken for scabies, but there
are no burrows.[9] The genera involved include
Glycophagus (grocery mite), *Acarus* (cheese
mite), *Tyrophagus* (copra mite), *Pyemotes* (grain
itch mite) and *Tyroglyphus*.[9,33] The house dust
mite, *Dermatophagoides pteronyssinus*, and related
species are widely distributed in bedding and
clothing, and may play a role in producing or
exacerbating chronic dermatitis.[52,53] Paper mites
may also produce a mild pruritic rash in persons
handling stored paper or old books.

The parasitoid mites may produce papular
urticaria in people employed in grain stores or
living in places harbouring rats.[54] Pet rabbits
may be infected by the mite *Listrophorus gibbus*
which can produce a papular urticaria in the
handler.[55]

The trombiculid mites may produce a severe
dermatitis with intensely pruritic, minute, red
elevations. They have a predilection for the
lower legs, groin and waistline.

Histopathology

The lesions produced by mites other than chiggers resemble those generally seen in mild arthropod reactions with a superficial and mid-dermal perivascular infiltrate, some interstitial eosinophils and mild epidermal spongiosis.[9] The mite is almost never found. Some neutrophils are usually present in lesions produced by *Pyemotes* species.[9]

Bites by chiggers (*Trombicula* species) may be centred on hair follicles or in skin with a thin epidermis. A tissue canal or 'stylostome' sur-rounded by a mass of hyaline tissue runs into the malpighian layer.[9] There is usually epidermal spongiosis, dermal oedema with some neutro-phils and later a more mixed dermal inflamm-atory infiltrate as in other arthropod lesions. A chronic granulomatous response has been described.[9]

INSECTS

HUMAN LICE (PEDICULOSIS)

Pediculosis is caused by three types of lice, each having a separate microenvironment. The head louse (*Pediculus humanus capitis*) infests the hairs of the scalp. It is an increasing problem in many urban communities, with outbreaks particularly in schools.[55a]

The pubic louse (*Phthirius pubis*) infests pubic and axillary hair in particular, although there may be colonization of any heavy growth of hair on the trunk and limbs.[56] Occasionally the eye-brows are infested and very rarely the scalp.[57] Both the pubic louse and the head louse cement their eggs to hair, forming the minute, gritty projection that is known as a nit. Multiple bluish spots (maculae caeruleae) may be found, partic-ularly on the trunk, in persons infested with the pubic louse.[58]

The body louse (*Pediculus humanus corporis*) divides its existence between the host and the host's clothing, in the seams of which it deposits its eggs.

The lice are blood-suckers and the injected saliva produces an allergic reaction. The result-ing itching may lead to excoriation or secondary bacterial infection.

Histopathology

A louse may be removed from the body and examined microscopically for confirmation (Fig. 30.9). Nits may also be identified by examining involved hairs (Fig. 30.10).

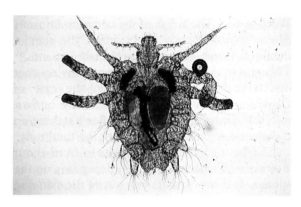

Fig. 30.9   Crab louse (*Phthirius pubis*). × 25

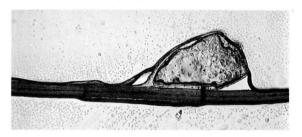

Fig. 30.10   Hair shaft with an attached egg (nit) of the head louse. × 40

BEDBUGS

Bedbugs (*Cimicidae*), found usually in dirty and dilapidated housing and associated with un-washed bed linen, produce urticarial or indurat-ed lesions.[59] Persistent nodular lesions are also found in some individuals.

the deep dermis, in some persistent insect bites; rarely the appearances may simulate a plasmacytoma.

Focal epidermal necrosis is seen with some gnat bites.[77,83] Bullous lesions seen in some hosts susceptible to mosquitoes have large intraepidermal vesicles with thin strands of epidermis between the vesicles and prominent oedema of the papillary dermis. Intraepidermal vesicles containing eosinophils may be seen in caterpillar dermatitis and in some other bite reactions, particularly at the point of entry of any mouthparts. Moths of the genus *Hylesia* produce a spongiotic epidermal reaction related to a fine hair shaft implanted by the moth; there is some exocytosis of neutrophils and lymphocytes.

Other findings which may be seen in persistent insect bite reactions include pseudo-epitheliomatous hyperplasia, sometimes quite severe, and atypical dermal infiltrates which may be mistaken for malignant lymphoma.[84,85] The presence of a heterogeneous cell population with interstitial eosinophils is a reassuring sign in these rare atypical lesions.

It should be noted that the coelenterates can produce lesions which mimic both clinically and histologically those produced by arthropods (see p. 708), including the development of persistent nodular lesions.[86,87]

REFERENCES

Introduction

1. Beaver PC, Jung RC, Cupp EW. Clinical parasitology. 9th ed. Philadelphia: Lea & Febiger, 1984.
2. Southcott RV. Some harmful Australian arthropods. Med J Aust 1986; 145: 590–595.
3. Alexander JO'D. Arthropods and human skin. Berlin: Springer Verlag, 1984.

Arachnids

4. Pucevich MV, Chesney TMcC. Histopathologic analysis of human bites by the brown recluse spider. Arch Dermatol 1983; 119: 851 (abstract).
5. Hillis TJ, Grant-Kels JM, Jacoby LM. Presumed arachnidism. Int J Dermatol 1986; 25: 44–48.
6. King LE. Spider bites. Arch Dermatol 1987; 123: 41–43.
6a. White J, Hirst D, Hender E. 36 cases of bites by spiders, including the white-tailed spider, *Lampona cylindrata*. Med J Aust 1989; 150: 401–403.
7. Wong RC, Hughes SE, Voorhees JJ. Spider bites. Arch Dermatol 1987; 123: 98–104.
8. Marshall J. Ticks and the human skin. Dermatologica 1967; 135: 60–65.
9. Krinsky WL. Dermatoses associated with the bites of mites and ticks (Arthropoda:Acari). Int J Dermatol 1983; 22: 75–91.
10. Patterson JW, Fitzwater JE, Connell J. Localized tick bite reaction. Cutis 1979; 24: 168–172.
11. Russell FE. Dermatitis due to imbedded tick parts. JAMA 1974; 228: 1581.
12. Berger BW. Erythema chronicum migrans of Lyme disease. Arch Dermatol 1984; 120: 1017–1021.
13. Nutting WB. Hair follicle mites (Acari:Demodicidae) of man. Int J Dermatol 1976; 15: 79–98.
14. Nutting WB, Beerman H. Demodicosis and symbiophobia: status, terminology and treatments. Int J Dermatol 1983; 22: 13–17.

15. Nutting WB, Green AC. Pathogenesis associated with hair follicle mites (*Demodex* spp.) in Australian Aborigines. Br J Dermatol 1976; 94: 307–312.
16. Aylesworth R, Vance JC. *Demodex folliculorum* and *Demodex brevis* in cutaneous biopsies. J Am Acad Dermatol 1982; 7: 583–589.
17. English FP, Nutting WB, Cohn D. Demodectic oviposition in the eyelid. Aust NZ J Ophthalmol 1985; 13: 71–73.
17a. Shelley WB, Shelley ED, Burmeister V. Unilateral demodectic rosacea. J Am Acad Dermatol 1989; 20: 915–917.
18. Purcell SM, Hayes TJ, Dixon SL. Pustular folliculitis associated with *Demodex folliculorum*. J Am Acad Dermatol 1986; 15: 1159–1162.
18a. Ashack RJ, Frost ML, Norins AL. Papular pruritic eruption of *Demodex* folliculitis in patients with acquired immunodeficiency syndrome. J Am Acad Dermatol 1989; 21: 306–307.
18b. Dominey A, Tschen J, Rosen T et al. Pityriasis folliculorum revisited. J Am Acad Dermatol 1989; 21: 81–84.
19. Ecker RI, Winkelmann RK. *Demodex* granuloma. Arch Dermatol 1979; 115: 343–344.
20. Grosshans EM, Kremer M, Maleville J. Demodex folliculorum und die Histogenese der granulomatosen Rosacea. Hautarzt 1974; 25: 166–177.
21. Ayres S Jr, Mihan R. *Demodex* granuloma. Arch Dermatol 1979; 115: 1285–1286.
22. Crosti C, Menni S, Sala F, Piccinno R J. Demodectic infestation of the pilosebaceous follicle. J Cutan Pathol 1983; 10: 257–261.
23. Orkin M, Maibach HI. Current concepts in parasitology: This scabies pandemic. N Engl J Med 1978; 298: 496–498.
24. Sadick N, Kaplan MH, Pahwra SG, Sarngadharan MG. Unusual features of scabies complicating human T-lymphotropic virus type III infection. J Am Acad Dermatol 1986; 15: 482–486.

24a. Jucowics P, Ramon ME, Don PC et al. Norwegian scabies in an infant with acquired immunodeficiency syndrome. Arch Dermatol 1989; 125: 1670–1671.

25. Orkin M. Today's scabies. Arch Dermatol 1975; 111: 1431–1432.

26. Woodley D, Saurat JH. The Burrow Ink Test and the scabies mites. J Am Acad Dermatol 1981; 4: 715–722.

27. Falk ES, Eide TJ. Histologic and clinical findings in human scabies. Int J Dermatol 1981; 20: 600–605.

28. Wolf R, Krakowski A. Atypical crusted scabies. J Am Acad Dermatol 1987; 17: 434–436.

29. Hubler WR Jr, Clabaugh W. Epidemic Norwegian scabies. Arch Dermatol 1976; 112: 179–181.

30. Dick GF, Burgdorf WHC, Gentry WC Jr. Norwegian scabies in Bloom's syndrome. Arch Dermatol 1979; 115: 212–213.

31. Espy PD, Jolly HW Jr. Norwegian scabies. Occurrence in a patient undergoing immunosuppression. Arch Dermatol 1976; 112: 193–196.

32. Anolik MA, Rudolph RI. Scabies simulating Darier disease in an immunosuppressed host. Arch Dermatol 1976; 112: 73–74.

32a. Barnes L, McCallister RE, Lucky AW. Crusted (Norwegian) scabies. Occurrence in a child undergoing a bone marrow transplant. Arch Dermatol 1987; 123: 95–97.

33. Fain A. Epidemiological problems of scabies. Int J Dermatol 1978; 17: 20–30.

34. Arlian LG, Runyan RA, Estes SA. Cross infestivity of *Sarcoptes scabei*. J Am Acad Dermatol 1984; 10: 979–986.

35. van Neste D, Lachapelle JM. Host-parasite relationships in hyperkeratotic (Norwegian) scabies: pathological and immunological findings. Br J Dermatol 1981; 105: 667–678.

36. Falk ES, Bolle R. *In vitro* demonstration of specific immunological hypersensitivity to scabies mite. Br J Dermatol 1980; 103: 367–373.

37. Van Neste DJJ. Human scabies in perspective. Int J Dermatol 1988; 27: 10–15.

38. Frentz G, Keien NK, Eriksen K. Immunofluorescence studies in scabies. J Cutan Pathol 1977; 4: 191–193.

39. Hoefling KK, Schroeter AL. Dermatoimmunopathology of scabies. J Am Acad Dermatol 1980; 3: 237–240.

40. Reunala T, Ranki A, Rantanen T, Salo OP. Inflammatory cells in skin lesions of scabies. Clin Exp Dermatol 1984; 9: 70–77.

41. Hejazi N, Mehregan AH. Scabies. Histological study of inflammatory lesions. Arch Dermatol 1975; 111: 37–39.

42. Fernandez N, Torres A, Ackerman AB. Pathologic findings in human scabies. Arch Dermatol 1977; 113: 320–324.

43. Thomson J, Cochrane T, Cochran R, McQueen A. Histology simulating reticulosis in persistent nodular scabies. Br J Dermatol 1974; 90: 421–429.

44. Fox JG, Reed C. *Cheyletiella* infestation of cats and their owners. Arch Dermatol 1978; 114: 1233–1234.

45. Lee BW. *Cheyletiella* dermatitis. Arch Dermatol 1981; 117: 677–678.

46. Hewitt M, Walton GS, Waterhouse M. Pet animal infestations and human skin lesions. Br J Dermatol 1971; 85: 215–225.

47. Cohen SR. *Cheyletiella* dermatitis. A mite infestation of rabbit, cat, dog, and man. Arch Dermatol 1980; 116: 435–437.

48. Powell RF, Palmer SM, Palmer CH, Smith EB. Cheyletiella dermatitis. Int J Dermatol 1977; 16: 679–682.

49. Rivers JK, Martin J, Pukay B. Walking dandruff and *Cheyletiella* dermatitis. J Am Acad Dermatol 1986; 15: 1130–1133.

50. Ackerman AB. Histologic diagnosis of inflammatory skin diseases. Philadelphia: Lea & Febiger, 1978; 184.

51. Maurice PDL, Schofield O, Griffiths WAD. Cheyletiella dermatitis: a case report and the role of specific immunological hypersensitivity in its pathogenesis. Clin Exp Dermatol 1987; 12: 381–384.

52. Hewitt M, Barrow GI, Miller DC et al. Mites in the personal environment and their role in skin disorders. Br J Dermatol 1973; 89: 401–409.

53. Aylesworth R. Feather pillow dermatitis caused by an unusual mite, *Dermatophagoides scheremetewskyi*. J Am Acad Dermatol 1982; 13: 680–681.

54. Theis J, Lavoipierre MM, La Perriere R, Kroese H. Tropical rat mite dermatitis. Arch Dermatol 1981; 117: 341–343.

55. Burns DA. Papular urticaria produced by the mite *Listrophorus gibbus*. Clin Exp Dermatol 1987; 12: 200–201.

Insects

55a. Gillis D, Slepon R, Karsenty E, Green M. Seasonality and long-term trends of pediculosis capitis and pubis in a young adult population. Arch Dermatol 1990; 126: 638–641.

56. Burns DA, Sims TA. A closer look at *Pthirus pubis*. Br J Dermatol 1988; 118: 497–503.

57. Gartmann H, Dickmans-Burmeister D. Phthiri im Bereich der Kopfhaare. Hautarzt 1970; 21: 279–281.

58. Miller RAW. Maculae ceruleae. Int J Dermatol 1986; 25: 383–384.

59. Crissey JT. Bedbugs. An old problem with a new dimension. Int J Dermatol 1981; 20: 411–414.

60. Grogan TM, Payne CM, Payne TB et al. Cutaneous myiasis. Am J Dermatopathol 1987; 9: 232–239.

61. Lane RP, Lovell CR, Griffiths WAD, Sonnex TS. Human cutaneous myiasis — a review and report of three cases due to *Dermatobia hominis*. Clin Exp Dermatol 1987; 12: 40–45.

62. Lukin LG. Human cutaneous myiasis in Brisbane: a prospective study. Med J Aust 1989; 150: 237–240.

63. Dondero TJ Jr, Schaffner W, Athanasiou R, Maguire W. Cutaneous myiasis in visitors to Central America. South Med J 1979; 72: 1508–1511.

64. Sauder DN, Hall RP, Wurster CF. Dermal myiasis: the porcine lipid cure. Arch Dermatol 1981; 117: 681–682.

65. Poindexter HA. Cutaneous myiasis. Arch Dermatol 1979; 115: 235.

66. Gunther S. Furuncular Tumbu fly myiasis of man in Gabon, Equatorial Africa. J Trop Med Hyg 1967; 70: 169–174.

66a. Ockenhouse CF, Samlaska CP, Benson PM et al. Cutaneous myiasis caused by the African tumbu fly (*Cordylobia anthropophaga*). Arch Dermatol 1990; 126: 199–202.

67. Newell GB. Dermal myiasis caused by the rabbit botfly (*Cuterebra* sp). Arch Dermatol 1979; 115: 101.
68. Baird JK, Baird CR, Sabrosky CW. North American cuterebrid myiasis. Report of seventeen new infections of human beings and review of the disease. J Am Acad Dermatol 1989; 21: 763–772.
69. Logan JCP, Walkey M. A case of endemic cutaneous myiasis. Br J Dermatol 1964; 76: 218–222.
70. Guillozet N. Erosive myiasis. Arch Dermatol 1981; 117: 59–60.
71. File TM, Thomson RB, Tan JS. *Dermatobia hominis* dermal myiasis. Arch Dermatol 1985; 121: 1195–1196.
72. Goldman L. Tungiasis in travelers from tropical Africa. JAMA 1976; 236: 1386.
73. Sanusi ID, Brown EB, Shepard TG, Grafton WD. Tungiasis: Report of one case and review of the 14 reported cases in the United States. J Am Acad Dermatol 1989; 20: 941–944.
74. Zalar GL, Walther RR. Infestation by *Tunga penetrans*. Arch Dermatol 1980; 116: 80–81.
75. Wentzell JM, Schwartz BK, Pesce JR. Tungiasis. J Am Acad Dermatol 1986; 15: 117–119.
76. Tokura Y, Tamura Y, Takigawa M et al. Severe hypersensitivity to mosquito bites associated with natural killer cell lymphocytosis. Arch Dermatol 1990; 126: 362–368.
77. Steffen C. Clinical and histopathologic correlation of midge bites. Arch Dermatol 1981; 117: 785–787.
78. Rustin MHA, Munro DD. Papular urticaria caused by *Dermestes maculatus Degeer*. Clin Exp Dermatol 1984; 9: 317–321.
79. Kerdel-Vegas F, Goihman-Yahr M. *Paederus* dermatitis. Arch Dermatol 1966; 94: 175–185.
80. Henwood BP, MacDonald DM. Caterpillar dermatitis. Clin Exp Dermatol 1983; 8: 77–93.
81. Garty BZ, Danon YL. Processionary caterpillar dermatitis. Pediatr Dermatol 1985; 2: 194–196.
82. Dinehart SM, Archer ME, Wolf JE et al. Caripito itch: Dermatitis from contact with *Hyselia* moths. J Am Acad Dermatol 1985; 13: 743–747.
83. Altchek DD, Kurtin SB. An unusual histopathologic response to an insect bite. Cutis 1980; 25: 169–170.
84. Allen AC. Persistent "insect bites" (dermal eosinophilic granulomas) simulating lymphoblastomas, histiocytoses, and squamous cell carcinomas. Am J Pathol 1948; 24: 367–387.
85. Kolbusz RV, Micetich K, Armin A-R, Massa MC. Exaggerated response to insect bites. An unusual cutaneous manifestation of chronic lymphocytic leukemia. Int J Dermatol 1989; 28: 186–187.
86. Weedon D, Hart V, Beardmore G, Dickson P. Coral dermatitis. Australas J Dermatol 1981; 22: 104–105.
87. Reed KM, Bronstein BR, Baden HP. Delayed and persistent cutaneous reactions to coelenterates. J Am Acad Dermatol 1984; 10: 462–466.

Tumours of the epidermis

INTRODUCTION

Tumours of the epidermis are a histopathologically diverse group of entities which have in common a localized proliferation of keratinocytes resulting in a clinically discrete lesion. They may be divided into a number of categories reflecting their different biological behaviour. The various categories include hamartomas (epidermal naevi), reactive hyperplasias (pseudoepitheliomatous hyperplasia), benign tumours (acanthomas), as well as premalignant, in situ, and invasive carcinomas.

EPIDERMAL AND OTHER NAEVI

Some authors use the term epithelial or epidermal naevus as a group generic term to cover malformations of adnexal epithelium, as well as those involving the epidermis alone.[1,2] The term epidermal naevus is used here in a restricted sense and does not include organoid, sebaceous, eccrine and pilar naevi. They are considered with the appendageal tumours in Chapter 33. An exception has been made for naevus comedonicus, an abnormality of the infundibulum of the hair follicle. It is considered here because its histological appearance suggests an abnormality of the epidermis rather than of appendages. Furthermore, the recent report of the coexistence of naevus comedonicus and an epidermal naevus suggests that the two entities are closely related.[2a]

EPIDERMAL NAEVUS

An epidermal naevus is a developmental mal-formation of the epidermis in which an excess of keratinocytes, sometimes showing abnormal maturation, results in a visible lesion with a variety of clinical and histological patterns.[3] Such lesions are of early onset, with a predilection for the neck, trunk and extremities. There may be one only, or a few small, warty, brown or pale plaques may be present. At other times the naevus takes the form of a linear or zosteriform lesion, or just a slightly scaly area of discol-oration.[3–5] Various terms have been applied, not always in a consistent manner, to the different clinical patterns.[5] The term *naevus verrucosus* has been used for localized, wart-like variants, and *naevus unius lateris* for long, linear, usually unilateral lesions on the extremities. *Ichthyosis hystrix* refers to large, often disfiguring naevi with a bilateral distribution on the trunk.[6,7]

Various tumours have been reported arising in epidermal naevi, as a rare complication. These include basal cell[8] and squamous cell carcino-mas[9–11] as well as a keratoacanthoma.[12]

The term *epidermal naevus syndrome* refers to the association of epidermal naevi with neuro-logical, ocular and skeletal abnormalities such as epilepsy, mental retardation, cataracts, kyphoscoliosis and limb hypertrophy; there may also be cutaneous haemangiomas.[2,13–15] Sys-temic cancers of various types may arise at a young age in those with the syndrome.[16,17] The epidermal naevi, which are often particularly extensive in patients with the syndrome, may be of any histological type.[18,19] Epidermal naevi have also been reported in association with polyostotic fibrous dysplasia[19a] and the Proteus syndrome, a very rare disorder with various mesodermal malformations.[19b]

Histopathology

At least 10 different histological patterns have been found in epidermal naevi (Fig. 31.1).[3,5] More than one such pattern may be present in a given example. In over 60% of cases the pattern is that of hyperkeratosis, with papillomatosis of relatively flat and broad type, together with acan-

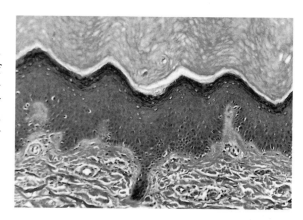

Fig. 31.1   Epidermal naevus. There is mild papillomatosis and acanthosis with overlying laminated hyperkeratosis. Haematoxylin — eosin

thosis. There is thickening of the granular layer and often a slight increase in basal melanin pig-ment. This is the so-called 'common type' of epidermal naevus.

Less frequently, the histological pattern resem-bles acrokeratosis verruciformis, epidermolytic hyperkeratosis or seborrhoeic keratosis.[3,5] Rare patterns include the verrucoid, porokeratotic, focal acantholytic dyskeratotic,[20–23] acanthosis-nigricans-like,[24] Hailey–Hailey-disease-like[25] and the incontinentia-pigmenti-like (verrucous phase) variants.[26] A lichenoid inflammatory infiltrate has also been reported in an epidermal naevus, although usually the dermis is devoid of inflamm-atory cells.[27] Inflammatory linear verrucous epi-dermal naevus and naevus comedonicus are regarded as distinct entities, although they are sometimes included as histological patterns of epidermal naevus.

Frequently the epidermis overlying an organoid naevus (see p. 856) will show the his-tological picture of an epidermal naevus. In such cases this is usually of the common type.

INFLAMMATORY LINEAR VERRUCOUS EPIDERMAL NAEVUS

This entity, also known by the acronym of ILVEN, is a specific clinicopathological sub-group of epidermal naevi which most often presents as a pruritic, linear eruption on the lower extremities.[2,28–30] It is of early onset. Asymptomatic variants and widespread bilateral distribution have been reported.[31,32] ILVEN has been described in association with the epidermal naevus syndrome (see above).[33]

The lesions resemble linear psoriasis both clinically and histologically; in this context it must be noted that the existence of a linear form of psoriasis has been questioned.[34] Interestingly, the epidermal fibrous protein isolated from the scale in ILVEN is different from that found in psoriasis.[35,36]

Histopathology

There is psoriasiform epidermal hyperplasia with overlying areas of parakeratosis, alternating with orthokeratosis. Beneath the orthokeratotic areas of hyperkeratosis there is hypergranulosis, often with a depressed, cup-like appearance; the parakeratosis overlies areas of agranulosis of the upper epidermis.[37] The zones of parakeratosis are usually much broader than in psoriasis. Focal mild spongiosis with some exocytosis and even vesiculation may be seen in some lesions.[38,39] There is also a mild perivascular lymphocytic infiltrate in the upper dermis. A dense lichenoid infiltrate was present in one case, perhaps representing the attempted immunological regression of the lesion.[40]

NAEVUS COMEDONICUS

Naevus comedonicus (comedo naevus) is a rare abnormality of the infundibulum of the hair follicle in which grouped or linear comedonal papules develop at any time from birth to middle age. They are usually restricted to one side of the body, particularly the face, trunk and neck.[41] Rare clinical presentations have included penile,[42] palmar,[43–45] bilateral[46] and verrucous lesions.[43] Rarely, abnormalities of other systems are present, indicating that a naevus comedonicus syndrome, akin to the epidermal naevus syndrome, may occur.[47,48] Inflammation of the lesions is an important complication, resulting in scarring.[46,49]

Histopathology [50]

There are dilated, keratin-filled invaginations of the epidermis. An atrophic sebaceous or pilar structure sometimes opens into the lower pole of the invagination.[50] A small lanugo hair is occasionally present in the keratinous material.

Inflammation and subsequent dermal scarring are a feature in some cases. A tricholemmal cyst has also been reported arising in a comedo naevus.[51]

The epithelial invagination in some cases of palmar involvement has opened into a recognizable eccrine duct.[44,52] Cornoid lamellae have also been present.[53–55] It has been suggested that these are cases of eccrine hamartomas, akin to naevus comedonicus and unrelated to porokeratosis.[56]

Rare histological patterns associated with comedo-naevus-like lesions have included a basal cell naevus,[57] a linear variant with underlying tumours of sweat gland origin,[58] and a variant with epidermolytic hyperkeratosis in the wall of the invaginations.[59] A form with dyskeratosis, accompanied often by acantholysis in the wall, is regarded as a distinct entity, familial dyskeratotic comedones (see below).

FAMILIAL DYSKERATOTIC COMEDONES

This is a rare autosomal dominant condition in which multiple comedones develop in childhood or adolescence, sometimes associated with acne.[60–62] Sites of involvement include the trunk and extremities and, uncommonly, the palms and soles, the scrotum and the penis.[60,63] This entity appears to be distinct from naevus comedonicus, and also from the rare condition of familial comedones.[64,65]

Histopathology [61,63]

There is a follicle-like invagination in the epidermis which is filled with laminated keratinous material. Dyskeratotic cells are present in the wall of the invagination, particularly in the base. This is associated with acantholysis, which may however be mild or inapparent.[61]

Dermatosis papulosa nigra
Melanoacanthoma
Clear cell acanthoma
Large cell acanthoma.

EPIDERMOLYTIC ACANTHOMA

This is an uncommon lesion which may be solitary, resembling a wart, or multiple. It shows the histopathological changes of epidermolytic hyperkeratosis and is therefore considered in Chapter 9 with other lesions showing this disorder of epidermal maturation and keratinization (see p. 279).

WARTY DYSKERATOMA

Warty dyskeratomas are rare, usually solitary, papulonodular lesions with a predilection for the head and neck of middle-aged and elderly individuals (see p. 284). They show suprabasilar clefting with numerous acantholytic and dyskeratotic cells within the cleft and an overlying keratinous plug.

ACANTHOLYTIC ACANTHOMA

Acantholytic acanthoma is a newly recognized solitary tumour with a predilection for the trunk of older individuals.[87] It usually presents as an asymptomatic keratotic papule or nodule.

Histopathology [87]

The features include variable hyperkeratosis, papillomatosis and acanthosis, together with prominent acantholysis, most often involving multiple levels of the epidermis (Fig. 31.3). There is sometimes suprabasilar or subcorneal cleft formation but there is no dyskeratosis. The pattern resembles that seen in pemphigus or Hailey–Hailey disease but there has been no evidence of these diseases in the cases reported.

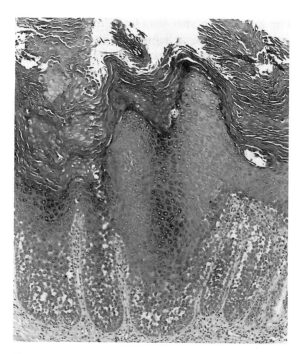

Fig. 31.3   Acantholytic acanthoma. Acantholysis involves the lower layers of the hyperplastic epidermis. There is a thick, orthokeratotic stratum corneum. Haematoxylin — eosin

SEBORRHOEIC KERATOSIS

Seborrhoeic keratoses (senile warts, basal cell papillomas) are common, often multiple, benign tumours which usually first appear in middle life. They may occur on any part of the body except the palms and soles, although there is a predilection for the chest, interscapular region, waistline and forehead. Seborrhoeic keratoses are sharply demarcated, grey-brown to black lesions, which are slightly raised. They may be covered with greasy scales. Most lesions are no more than a centimetre or so in diameter, but larger variants, sometimes even pedunculated, have been reported.[88,89] A flat, plaque-like form is sometimes found on the buttocks or thighs.

Rare clinical variants include a familial form, which may be of early or late onset,[90,91] and a halo variant with a depigmented halo around each lesion.[92] Multiple seborrhoeic keratoses may sometimes assume a patterned arrangement along lines of cleavage.[93] The eruptive form associated with internal cancer (sign of Leser and Trélat) is discussed below.

The nature of seborrhoeic keratoses is still disputed. A follicular origin has been proposed. They have also been regarded as a late onset naevoid disturbance, or the result of a local arrest of maturation of keratinocytes.[94] Human papillomavirus (HPV) has been detected in a very small number of cases.[94a] The basosquamous cell acanthoma of Lund, the inverted follicular keratosis and the stucco keratosis have all been regarded, at some time, as variants of seborrhoeic keratosis.[86,95]

Histopathology [86,96]

Seborrhoeic keratoses are sharply defined tumours which may be endophytic or exophytic.[96] They are composed of basaloid cells with a varying admixture of squamoid cells. Keratin-filled invaginations and small cysts (horn cysts) are a characteristic feature. Nests of squamous cells (squamous eddies) may be present, particularly in the irritated type. Approximately one-third of seborrhoeic keratoses appear hyper-pigmented in haematoxylin and eosin stained sections.[89]

At least five distinct histological patterns have been recognized — acanthotic (solid), reti-culated (adenoid), hyperkeratotic (papillo-matous), clonal and irritated.[96] Overlapping features are quite common. The *acanthotic type* is composed of broad columns or sheets of basaloid cells with intervening horn cysts. The *reticulated type* has interlacing thin strands of basaloid cells, often pigmented, enclosing small horn cysts. This variant often evolves from a solar lentigo.[96] The *hyperkeratotic type* is exophytic with varying degrees of hyperkeratosis, papillomatosis and acanthosis (Fig. 31.4). There are both basaloid and squamous cells. *Clonal seborrhoeic keratoses* have intraepidermal nests of basaloid cells resembling the Borst–Jadassohn phenomenon (see p. 744). In the *irritated variant*, there is a heavy inflammatory cell infiltrate, with lichenoid features, in the upper dermis (Fig. 31.5). Apoptotic cells are present in the base of the lesion. This represents the attempted immunological regression of a

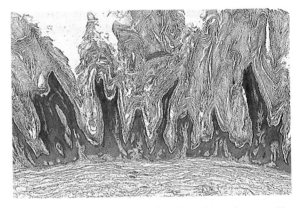

Fig. 31.4 Seborrhoeic keratosis of hyperkeratotic type with marked papillomatosis and hyperkeratosis. Haematoxylin — eosin

seborrhoeic keratosis.[97,98] Sometimes there is a heavy inflammatory cell infiltrate without lichenoid qualities;[99] rarely neutrophils are abundant in the infiltrate.[89] This may be regarded as a true inflammatory variant, although often lesions with features overlapping with those of the irritated type are found.[99]

Tricholemmal differentiation with glycogen-rich cells is an uncommon, usually focal, change.[100,101] Acantholysis is another uncommon histological feature.[102,102a] Trichostasis

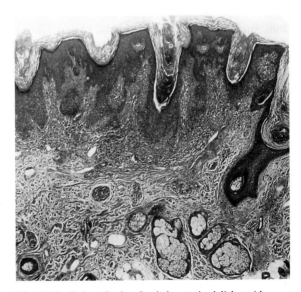

Fig. 31.5 Irritated seborrhoeic keratosis. A lichenoid infiltrate is present in the underlying dermis. Haematoxylin — eosin

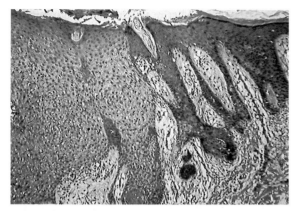

Fig. 31.7   Clear cell acanthoma. The lesion is acanthotic with pale-staining keratinocytes except at the periphery of the lesion where they appear normal.
Haematoxylin — eosin

atinocytes: it is often devoid of melanin pigment, although melanocytes are present.[153a]

The dermal papillae are oedematous, with increased vascularity and a mixed inflammatory cell infiltrate which includes a variable proportion of lymphocytes, plasma cells and neutrophils. In several cases the sweat ducts have been dilated, and rarely they may be hyperplastic.

A PAS stain, with and without diastase, will confirm the presence of abundant glycogen in the pale cells. Electron microscopy has also confirmed that the keratinocytes contain glycogen.[154,155] Langerhans cells are also abundant.[148,156] Immunohistochemistry shows that the cells contain keratin and involucrin but not carcinoembryonic antigen.[157]

It has recently been proposed that there is a distinct tissue reaction, pale cell acanthosis (clear cell acanthosis), characterized by the presence of pale cells in an acanthotic epidermis.[158] This histological pattern can be seen not only in clear cell acanthoma but also in some seborrhoeic keratoses, usually the clonal subtype, and rarely in verruca vulgaris.

LARGE CELL ACANTHOMA

Large cell acanthoma occurs as a sharply demarcated, scaly, often lightly pigmented patch, approximately 3–10 mm in diameter, on the sun-exposed skin of middle-aged and elderly individuals.[159,160] It is usually solitary. Clinically, it resembles a seborrhoeic or actinic keratosis. Large cell acanthoma is thought to comprise sunlight-induced clones of abnormal cells, without a tendency to malignancy.[159]

Histopathology[159,160]

There is epidermal thickening, due to the enlargement of keratinocytes to about twice their normal size (Fig. 31.8). There is also a proportional increase in nuclear size. The lesions are sharply demarcated from the adjacent normal keratinocytes; the adnexal epithelium within a lesion is usually spared. Other features include orthokeratosis, a prominent granular layer, mild papillomatosis, mild basal pigmentation, and some downward budding of the rete ridges. Occasionally, there is a focal lichenoid inflammatory cell infiltrate.

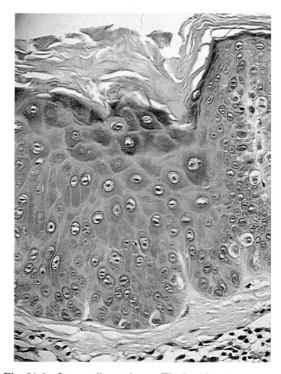

Fig. 31.8   Large cell acanthoma. The keratinocytes are larger than usual and the granular layer is thickened. Normal epidermis is present at the edge of the photograph.
Haematoxylin — eosin

It has been suggested, on the basis of the disordered arrangement of malpighian cells, the nuclear variability and the occasional finding of dyskeratoses and suprabasal mitoses, that large cell acanthoma is a cytological variant of Bowen's disease.[161] There is no evidence to support this view.

EPIDERMAL DYSPLASIAS

This group of epidermal tumours has the potential for malignant transformation. It includes actinic (solar) keratosis, actinic cheilitis and arsenical keratoses.

ACTINIC KERATOSIS

Actinic (solar) keratoses present clinically as circumscribed, scaly, erythematous lesions, usually less than 1 cm in diameter, on the sun-exposed skin of older individuals.[162] The face, ears, scalp, hands and forearms are sites of predilection. In Australia, actinic keratoses are found in 40–50% of people aged 40 years and over.[163] They develop most often in those with a fair complexion, who do not tan readily.

Actinic keratoses may remit, or remain unchanged for many years. It has been stated that 10–20% gradually transform into squamous cell carcinoma, if untreated.[162] In one study the annual incidence rate of malignant transformation of a solar keratosis was less than 0.25% for each keratosis,[164] but this study has been criticized on several grounds.[165]

Several clinical variants of actinic keratosis have been described. In the *hyperplastic (hypertrophic) form*, found almost exclusively on the dorsum of the hands and the forearms, individual lesions are quite thick.[166,167] The changes probably result, in part, from the superadded effects of rubbing and scratching. They may be overdiagnosed clinically as squamous cell carcinoma.[166] The *spreading pigmented actinic keratosis* is a brown patch or plaque, usually greater than 1 cm in diameter, that tends to spread centrifugally.[168,169] Some cases appear to represent the collision of a solar keratosis and solar lentigo.[170] The cheeks and forehead are sites of predilection. The *lichenoid actinic keratosis* (not to be confused with the lichen-planus-like keratosis) is not usually distinctive, although sometimes local irritation is noted.[171] The large cell acanthoma (see above) has been regarded as another variant of actinic keratosis.[162]

Cumulative exposure to sunlight appears to be important in the aetiology. Abnormalities in DNA synthesis in keratinocytes in the skin around the lesion suggest that there is a gradual stepwise progression from sun-damaged epidermis to clinically obvious keratoses and eventually to squamous cell carcinoma.[172] The keratinocytes in solar keratoses, like those in squamous cell carcinomas, lose various surface carbohydrates.[173]

Histopathology[173a]

Diagnostic biopsy is undertaken in only a small percentage of actinic keratoses diagnosed clinically.[163] The usual actinic keratosis is characterized by focal parakeratosis with loss of the underlying granular layer and a slightly thickened epidermis with some irregular downward buds. Uncommonly the epidermis is thinner than normal. In all cases, there is variable loss of the normal orderly stratified arrangement of the epidermis; this is associated with cytological atypia of keratinocytes which varies from slight to extreme. The term bowenoid keratosis may be used when the atypia is close to full thickness.[168] Sometimes, the dysplastic epithelium shows suprabasal cleft formation.[162,174] There is often a sharp slanting border between the normal epidermis of the acrotrichia and acrosyringia and the parakeratotic atypical epithelium of the keratosis.[175] However, dysplastic epithelium may involve the infundibular portion of the hair follicle.[175] The parakeratotic scale may sometimes pile up to form a cutaneous horn.[162]

The dermal changes include actinic elastosis, which is usually quite severe, and a variable, but usually mild, chronic inflammatory cell infiltrate.[162] Histological studies have not been reported on the inflammatory keratoses which may develop during chemotherapy of malignant disease with fluorouracil,[176] but in the one case that I have studied there was vascular telangiectasia and a moderately heavy mixed inflammatory cell infiltrate in the upper dermis.

In the hyperplastic (hypertrophic) form there is prominent orthokeratosis with alternating parakeratosis.[166] The epidermis usually shows irregular psoriasiform hyperplasia, and sometimes there is mild papillomatosis. Dysplastic changes are sometimes minimal and confined to the basal layer.[167] The presence of vertical collagen bundles and of some dilated vessels in the papillary dermis is evidence that these lesions represent actinic keratoses with superimposed changes of rubbing or scratching (lichen simplex chronicus).[166]

In the pigmented variant there is excess melanin in the lower epidermis, usually both in keratinocytes and melanocytes, but sometimes only in one or the other.[168] Melanophages are usually found in the papillary dermis.[168]

In lichenoid actinic keratoses there is a superficial, often band-like, chronic inflammatory cell infiltrate with occasional apoptotic keratinocytes in the basal layer and some basal vacuolar change.[171]

In all types of actinic keratoses in immunosuppressed patients there is usually marked atypia of the keratinocytes;[177] multinucleate forms may be present.[177]

It is sometimes a matter of personal judgement whether a lesion is considered to show early squamous cell carcinomatous change or not.[178] The protrusion of atypical cells into the reticular dermis and the detachment of individual nests of keratinocytes from the lower layers of the epidermis are criteria used to diagnose invasive transformation.[178]

Electron microscopy. Ultrastructural studies suggest that the hyperpigmentation in the pigmented variant is due to enhanced melanosome formation and distribution and not to a block in the transfer of melanosomes to keratinocytes.[169]

ACTINIC CHEILITIS

Actinic cheilitis (solar cheilosis, actinic keratosis of the lip) is a premalignant condition seen predominantly on the vermilion part of the lower lip. It results from chronic exposure to sunlight,[179] although smoking and chronic irritation may also contribute.[180] There are dry, whitish-grey scaly plaques in which areas of erythema, erosions and ulceration may develop.[179] The whitish areas were known in the past as leucoplakia.[181] Large areas of the lower lip may be affected. Squamous cell carcinoma may develop after a latent period of 20–30 years,[182,183] although the incidence of this transformation is difficult to quantify.[180]

An acute form of actinic cheilitis, characterized by oedema, erythema and erosions has been recognized.[181] It is an uncommon response to prolonged exposure to sunlight.

Histopathology[181,184]

The lesions show alternating areas of orthokeratosis and parakeratosis. The epidermis may be hyperplastic or atrophic. Other features are disordered maturation of epidermal cells, increased mitotic activity and variable cytological atypia.[182] Squamous cell carcinoma may develop in areas of marked atypia.

There is prominent solar elastosis of the submucosal connective tissue, some vascular telangiectasia, and a mild to moderate infiltrate of chronic inflammatory cells. Plasma cells are usually prominent, particularly beneath areas of ulceration.[184]

ARSENICAL KERATOSES

Inorganic arsenic was used for more than a century in the treatment of many diverse conditions. The recognition of its adverse effects, and its replacement by more effective therapeutic agents have led to a marked reduction in the incidence of arsenic-related conditions. However, there is a high arsenic content in some drinking waters and naturopathic medicines.[185,186]

The best-known effect of chronic arsenicism is cutaneous pigmentation which may be diffuse or of 'rain-drop' type.[187] More than 40% of affected individuals develop keratoses on the palms and soles, and sometimes this is associated with a mild diffuse keratoderma.[187] There is an increased incidence of multiple skin cancers which include Bowen's disease, basal cell carcinomas and squamous cell carcinomas.[188] The lesions are sometimes quite exophytic in appearance. Visceral cancers, particularly involving the lung and genitourinary system, may also be found.[189]

Histopathology[185,186]

Arsenical keratoses are of the hyperkeratotic type. Sometimes there is prominent hyperkeratosis and papillomatosis but no atypia. These lesions have a superficial resemblance to the hyperkeratotic type of seborrhoeic keratosis. Similar lesions follow exposure to tar (Fig. 31.9). In other cases there is mild atypia resembling the hyperkeratotic variant of actinic keratosis.

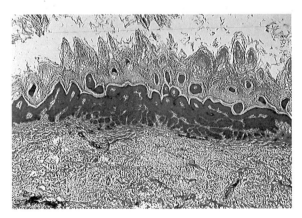

Fig. 31.9   Tar keratosis. There is pronounced hyperkeratosis, papillomatosis and acanthosis. Haematoxylin — eosin

In some lesions of Bowen's disease related to exposure to arsenic, there may be areas resembling seborrhoeic keratosis, superficial basal cell carcinoma or intraepidermal epithelioma of Jadassohn. Invasive carcinomas arising in Bowen's disease show the non-keratinizing pattern of squamous cell carcinoma, sometimes with areas of appendageal differentiation (see below).

The basal cell carcinomas which develop may be of solid or multifocal superficial type.

INTRAEPIDERMAL CARCINOMAS

Although the term intraepidermal carcinoma is often used synonymously with Bowen's disease, it is used here in a broader sense to include not only carcinoma in situ of the skin (Bowen's disease) and penis (erythroplasia of Queyrat), but also intraepidermal epithelioma of Jadassohn, a controversial entity of disputed histogenesis. Paget's disease is sometimes included in this category because of the presence of cytologically malignant cells within the epidermis. Paget's disease is discussed with the appendageal tumours on page 837.

BOWEN'S DISEASE

Bowen's disease is a clinical expression of squamous cell carcinoma in situ of the skin.[190] It presents as an asymptomatic, well-defined, erythematous, scaly plaque which expands centrifugally. Verrucous, nodular, eroded and pigmented[191–193] variants occur. Many of the pigmented lesions reported in the anogenital area as Bowen's disease[194–196] would be regarded by some authorities as examples of bowenoid papulosis[197] (see p. 691).

Bowen's disease has a predilection for the sun-exposed areas of fair-skinned, older individuals.[198] It is uncommon in black people,[199] in whom it is found more often on areas of the skin that are not exposed to the sun.[200] Lesions may also develop on the trunk and the vulva, and rarely on the nail bed,[201–203] palm,[204–206] sole,[207] and margin of an eyelid.[208] Bowen's disease has been reported in the wall of an epidermoid cyst,[209] in a lesion of porokeratosis of Mibelli,[210] in erythema ab igne[211] and in seborrhoeic keratoses (see p. 736).

Several investigators have proposed that Bowen's disease should be considered to be a skin marker for internal malignant disease,[212–215] although recent studies have shown no evidence for this association.[216–218]

Invasive carcinoma develops in up to 8% of untreated cases.[219–220] This complication, which is not well recognized, is characterized by the development of a rapidly growing tumour, 1–15 cm in diameter, in a pre-existing scaly lesion.[220] The invasive tumour has metastatic potential which has been stated to be as high as 13%,[220] although this would appear to be an overestimation of the risk.[219,221]

Several factors have been implicated in the aetiology of Bowen's disease. These include prolonged exposure to solar radiation, the ingestion of arsenic,[187,212] and infection with the human papilloma virus (HPV). Whereas HPV type 16 (HPV-16) and HPV-18 have been repeatedly detected in Bowen's disease of the genital region and its precursors,[222] there are now several reports of non-genital Bowen's disease related to infections with HPV-2,[223] HPV-16,[224] and HPV-34.[225] Bowen's disease is a rare complication of the treatment of psoriasis with psoralens and ultraviolet-A radiation (PUVA).[226,227]

Histopathology[162,228]

Bowen's disease is a form of carcinoma in situ, and accordingly shows full-thickness involvement of the epidermis, and sometimes the pilosebaceous epithelium, by atypical keratinocytes.[229,230] This is associated with disorderly maturation of the epidermis, mitoses at different levels, multinucleate keratinocytes and dyskeratotic cells. Usually there is loss of the granular layer, with overlying parakeratosis and sometimes hyperkeratosis.

Several histological variants have been described, and more than one of these patterns may be present in different areas of the same lesion.[228] In the *psoriasiform* pattern, there is regular acanthosis with thickening of the rete ridges and overlying parakeratosis (Fig. 31.10).[228] In the *atrophic* form, there is thinning of the epidermis which shows full-thickness atypia and disorganization.[228] There is usually overlying hyperkeratosis and parakeratosis. The *verrucous-hyperkeratotic* type is characterized by hyperkeratosis, papillomatosis, and sometimes intervening pit-like invagination.[228] The *irregular* variant shows irregular acanthosis, and often extensive chronic inflammation in the underlying dermis.[228] In the *pigmented* type there is melanin in individual tumour cells and melanophages in the underlying dermis.[197] The *pagetoid* variant

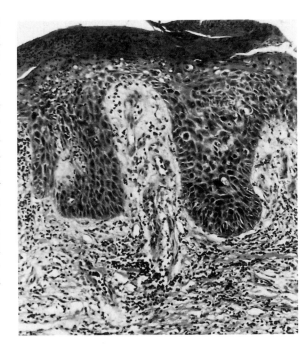

Fig. 31.10 Bowen's disease. There is full thickness atypia of the epidermis which also shows psoriasiform hyperplasia. Haematoxylin — eosin

has nests of cells with pale cytoplasm and thin strands of relatively normal keratinocytes intervening; the basal layer may also be spared (Fig. 31.11). Sometimes this is associated with psoriasiform hyperplasia of the epidermis. Mucinous and sebaceous metaplasia characterize two other rare histological patterns.[231]

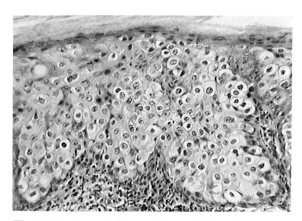

Fig. 31.11 Bowen's disease. The atypical keratinocytes are pale with a pagetoid appearance. Haematoxylin — eosin

As already mentioned, the atypical epithelium may also involve the pilosebaceous units. This may lead to treatment failure when superficial methods of destruction are used.[232,233] Involvement of the eccrine ducts is uncommon[234,234a] and in my experience it has usually been confined to cases of Bowen's disease of the temple region.[235]

Changes in the underlying dermis include increased vascularity, and a variable inflammatory response, which is usually composed of lymphocytes. Occasionally this has lichenoid features. Small deposits of amyloid may be found in the papillary dermis, particularly in lesions of long standing.[228]

The pagetoid variant of Bowen's disease is sometimes difficult to distinguish from Paget's disease and from in situ superficial spreading melanoma, particularly if only a small biopsy is available. In these instances, immunoperoxidase markers may be of assistance. Melanoma cells are positive for S100 protein, while Paget cells usually demonstrate carcinoembryonic antigen (CEA).[236] Melanoma cells do not contain cytokeratins while Paget cells are positive for cytokeratins with a molecular weight of 54 kilodaltons (kd) and negative for those of 66 kd; the reverse applies with the cells in Bowen's disease.[237]

In the invasive form, there are large islands of non-keratinizing squamoid cells throughout the dermis.[220] The cells usually have pale cytoplasm. Basaloid and adnexal differentiation are common patterns.[220,238,238a] The invasive tumour which supervenes is best regarded as a variant of squamous cell carcinoma.

The term Bowen's disease is no longer used in gynaecological pathology, having been replaced by the concept of vulvar intraepithelial neoplasia (VIN).[239–241] Progressive atypia of the epithelium is semi-quantified, VIN I representing atypia confined to the basal one-third of the epidermis, and VIN II corresponding to involvement of from one-third to two-thirds of the epithelium. In VIN III, the atypical cells involve more than two-thirds of the thickness of the epidermis. Bowen's disease therefore corresponds to severe VIN III. There has been an attempt to apply this concept, in part, to other areas of the skin.[242] The term 'squamous intraepidermal neoplasia, Bowen's type' has been suggested for ful-thickness atypia of the epidermis and 'squamous intraepidermal neoplasia, non-Bowen's type' when the atypia is limited to the lower two-thirds of the epidermis.[242] This categorization has not received wide acceptance.

Bowen's disease differs from actinic (solar) keratosis in the full-thickness atypia of the epithelium and in usually sparing the acrosyringium. In arsenical keratoses, in situ carcinoma indistinguishable from Bowen's disease may develop. Bowenoid papulosis of the genitalia is regarded by some as a variant of Bowen's disease of the genitalia; although the two conditions may be histologically indistinguishable, features which favour a diagnosis of bowenoid papulosis include numerous mitoses in metaphase, small basophilic inclusions in the cytoplasm of the granular layer, and the presence sometimes of cells with a vague resemblance to koilocytes.

Electron microscopy.[243] The keratinocytes have large nuclei and nucleoli, and a reduced number of desmosomal attachments.[244] The dyskeratotic cells show an aggregation of cytoplasmic tonofilaments. Occasional apoptotic bodies are present in the intercellular spaces, while others have been phagocytosed by neighbouring keratinocytes.[245,246] Cytoplasmic projections of keratinocytes may extend through gaps in the basement membrane.[243]

ERYTHROPLASIA OF QUEYRAT

Erythroplasia of Queyrat is a clinical expression of carcinoma in situ of the penis.[247–249] It is found most commonly on the glans penis of uncircumcised males as a sharply circumscribed, asymptomatic, bright red, shiny plaque.[249] It may also arise on the coronal sulcus or the inner surface of the prepuce. As in Bowen's disease, invasive carcinoma may develop in up to 10% of cases of erythroplasia of Queyrat, and such tumours have metastatic potential.[247]

Histopathology [247,248]

The changes are those of a carcinoma in situ, as

stromal dependence of basal cell carcinomas, which presupposes that only large tumour emboli with attached stroma are successful in implanting.[395] Accordingly, it is not surprising that lesions which give origin to metastases are large, ulcerated and neglected. Metatypical features and/or squamous differentiation have also been regarded as important,[357] although these changes were present in only 15% of the primary lesions in one review of metastasizing basal cell carcinomas.[393]

Metastases occur most commonly in the regional lymph nodes; bones, lungs[396,397] and liver are less frequent sites of involvement.[398] Other organs and the subcutis are rarely affected.[357] Aspiration metastasis to the lung has been recorded.[399] The median interval between the diagnosis of the primary lesion and signs of metastasis is approximately nine years, while the interval between the appearance of the metastases and the death of the patient is approximately one year.[393] Long survivals have occasionally been reported.[400] Systemic amyloidosis[401,402] and a myelophthisic anaemia secondary to marrow infiltration[403] have been documented in patients with metastatic basal cell carcinomas.

NAEVOID BASAL CELL CARCINOMA SYNDROME

This syndrome is a multisystem disorder characterized by multiple basal cell carcinomas with an early age of onset, odontogenic keratocysts, pits on the palms and/or soles, cutaneous cysts,[404] skeletal and neurological anomalies and ectopic calcifications.[405] Often there is a characteristic facies with hypertelorism and an enlarged calvaria.[406] Less common manifestations include lipomas and fibromas of various organs,[407] ovarian cysts, and medulloblastomas.[405] The inheritance is autosomal dominant with high gene penetrance and variable expressivity.[408]

Only 15% of affected individuals have basal cell carcinomas before puberty and these may take the form of pigmented macules resembling naevi.[405] Tumours are usually harmless before puberty and only a small percentage become aggressive in later life.[406,409] The tumours may develop anywhere, including within the palmar pits,[410] but there is a predilection for the face, neck and upper part of the trunk. They may vary in number from few to hundreds of lesions. A defective in-vitro cellular response to X-irradiation has been found in the syndrome[411] and this may help to explain the development of skin tumours in these patients at sites of X-irradiation.[410,412]

The unilateral linear basal cell naevus is an unrelated condition which may be associated with comedones and, rarely, osteoma cutis[413] (see p. 822).

Histopathology [414]

The whole spectrum of histological variants of basal cell carcinoma is found in the naevoid basal cell carcinoma syndrome.[415] Calcification, keratinizing cysts, pigmentation and osteoid tissue have all been said to occur more frequently in basal cell carcinomas occurring in the syndrome than in sporadic cases, although some studies have failed to confirm this.[415]

The cutaneous cysts usually take the form of epidermal cysts.[404] Occasionally, they may have a festooned lining of squamous cells that form keratin without the presence of a granular layer, thus resembling the keratocysts of the jaws.[416]

The palmar and plantar pits show marked thinning of the stratum corneum with a thin parakeratotic or orthokeratotic layer in the base overlying a mildly acanthotic epidermis.[417] Basal cell hyperplasia, and rarely basal cell carcinomas, may be found in the base of the pits.[418,419]

SQUAMOUS CELL CARCINOMA

Squamous cell carcinoma is the second most common form of skin cancer in Caucasians. Its incidence in a recent Australian study was 166 cases per 100 000 of the population, the highest in the world.[420] There is a predisposition for it to arise in the sun-damaged skin of fair-skinned people who tan poorly.[420] It is relatively uncommon in black people, in whom the tumours often arise in association with scarring processes.[421]

Most squamous cell carcinomas arise in areas of direct exposure to the sun, such as the forehead, face, neck and dorsum of the hands.[422] The ears, scalp and vermilion part of the lower lip are also involved, particularly in males.[422] Non-exposed areas such as the buttocks, genitalia[423] and subungual regions[424-425a] are occasionally affected. Uncommonly, squamous cell carcinomas may develop at sites of chronic ulceration, trauma, burns, frost bite,[426] vaccination scars,[427] fistula tracts,[428] pilonidal sinuses of long standing,[429,430] hidradenitis suppurativa and acne conglobata.[431,432] The term Marjolin's ulcer has been used for cancers arising in sites of chronic injury or irritation such as scars, ulcers and sinuses,[433,434] although Marjolin did not describe the condition with which he is eponymously credited.[435] Tumours arising in these circumstances are sometimes aggressive, and local recurrences are common.[434]

There are isolated reports of the occurrence of squamous cell carcinomas in various conditions such as dystrophic epidermolysis bullosa, Hailey–Hailey disease,[436] porokeratosis, discoid lupus erythematosus,[437] lichen planus,[438,439] erythema ab igne, lupus vulgaris, lichen sclerosus et atrophicus, balanitis xerotica obliterans, acrodermatitis chronica atrophicans, organoid and epidermal naevi,[440] granuloma inguinale, lymphogranuloma venereum, poikiloderma,[441] epidermodysplasia verruciformis, acrokeratosis verruciformis and the Jadassohn phenomenon. A squamous cell carcinoma has been recognized in association with a condyloma acuminatum of the perineum accompanying infection by human papilloma virus (HPV) Types 6 and 11.[442] Several cases have been associated with hypercalcaemia.[443,444] Squamous cell carcinomas are also increased in frequency among patients with xeroderma pigmentosum and albinism.

Patients whose immune status is deficient,[445] particularly renal transplant recipients,[446-448] are also predisposed to develop these tumours. It has been estimated that renal transplant recipients have a risk of developing squamous cell carcinoma of the skin which is 18 times that of the general population. They also develop warts with varying dysplasia, and verrucous keratoses with a putative viral contribution.[309] In a significant number of these tumours HPV-5 or HPV-8 is found, suggesting a role for the virus in the aetiology of the skin cancers which result.[309] In genital lesions HPV-16 and/or HPV-18 have been detected.[447a] The tumours often infiltrate widely, indicating their aggressive nature. Most of the fatal cases have been reported from Australia, suggesting that sunlight plays a role in the formation of these aggressive lesions.[448]

Squamous cell carcinomas are found predominantly in older people; they are rare in adolescence and childhood.[449] Clinically, they present as shallow ulcers, often with a keratinous crust and elevated, indurated surrounds. The adjacent skin usually shows features of actinic damage. The acantholytic variant is usually a nodular tumour on the head or neck. It is almost invariably misdiagnosed clinically as a basal cell carcinoma. It tends to be more aggressive than the conventional squamous cell carcinoma.[450] The metastatic potential of this tumour will be considered after the discussion of the histopathology.

Ultraviolet-B radiation appears to be the most important aetiological factor; ultraviolet-A plays a minor role.[451,452] Ultraviolet radiation is known to damage the DNA of epidermal cells, but there appear to be other complex mechanisms involved in UV-induced carcinogenesis. Squamous cell carcinomas can be produced in various animals with ultraviolet radiation, almost to the exclusion of other types of tumours.[452,453] Less important aetiological agents include radiation therapy,[279] arsenic, coal tar and various hydrocarbons.[454] Human papilloma virus may play a role in immunosuppressed patients (see above).[309,447a]

Histopathology

The usual squamous cell carcinoma consists of nests of squamous epithelial cells which arise from the epidermis and extend into the dermis for a variable distance. The cells have abundant, eosinophilic cytoplasm and a large, often vesicular nucleus. There is variable central keratinization and horn pearl formation depending on the differentiation of the tumour. Individual cell keratinization is often present. The degree of anaplasia in the tumour nests has been used to grade squamous cell carcinomas. Usually a rather subjective assessment of differentiation is made using the categories of 'well', 'moderately' and 'poorly' differentiated, rather than Broder's classic grading of 1–4, where Grade 4 applies to the most poorly differentiated lesions (Fig. 31.16).

Most squamous cell carcinomas arise in solar keratoses or sun-damaged skin.[317] The borderline between a thick solar keratosis and a superficial squamous cell carcinoma is somewhat arbitrary (see p. 740). Squamous cell carcinomas sometimes arise in Bowen's disease and in these cases the cells are usually non-keratinizing; they may show variable tricholemmal or even sebaceous-like differentiation.[220] These tumours should not be confused with the rare clear cell[455] and 'signet-ring'[456] variants of squamous cell carcinoma, both of which have cells with pale cytoplasm; in the case of the 'signet-ring' variant the nucleus is eccentric.

Squamous cell carcinomas occasionally infiltrate along nerve sheaths, the adventitia of blood vessels, lymphatics, fascial planes, and embryological fusion planes.[457] They may evoke

a stromal desmoplastic response. There is often a mild to moderate chronic inflammatory cell infiltrate at the periphery of the tumour. Eosinophils are occasionally prominent in the infiltrate and sometimes extend into the tumour islands.[458] Melanin pigment is only rarely present in tumour cells or in the stroma.

Immunoperoxidase studies are sometimes helpful if the tumour is poorly differentiated or of spindle cell type. The cells are positive for epithelial membrane antigen[459] and cytokeratin.[460,461] Squamous cell carcinomas contain keratins of higher molecular weight than those in basal cell carcinomas.[462] Involucrin is present in larger keratinized cells.[342] Stains for lysozyme, S100 protein and desmin are negative.

Spindle cell squamous carcinoma. This uncommon variant usually arises in sun-damaged or irradiated skin. It may be composed entirely of spindle cells, or have a variable component of more conventional squamous cell carcinoma.[463] The spindle cells have a large vesicular nucleus and scanty eosinophilic cytoplasm, often with indistinct cell borders. There is variable pleomorphism, usually with many mitoses. The presence of squamous differentiation, dyskeratotic cells and continuity with the epidermis may assist in making the diagnosis. Electron microscopy and immunoperoxidase markers may be necessary in some circumstances to differentiate this variant from malignant melanoma and atypical fibroxanthoma.[464–465]

Adenoid squamous cell carcinoma. The adenoid (acantholytic, pseudoglandular) variant, which is found most often on the head and neck, accounts for 2–4% of all squamous cell carcinomas.[466–468] It consists of nests of squamous cells with central acantholysis leading to an impression of gland formation,[466] although the peripheral cells are cohesive (Fig. 31.17). Acantholysis is sometimes minimal. Mucin has been reported in some,[467] but these tumours may have been variants of adenosquamous carcinoma (see p. 754). Adenoid variants often arise from an acantholytic solar keratosis. Sometimes this is in the vicinity of the pilosebaceous follicle.[467]

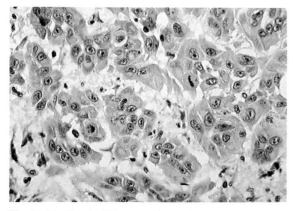

Fig. 31.16   Poorly differentiated squamous cell carcinoma composed of nests of non-keratinizing cells. Mitoses are present.
Haematoxylin — eosin

with aggressive histological features such as deep invasion,[472] poor differentiation, perineural invasion and acantholytic features.[392,473] Narrow surgical margins also contribute to local recurrence. Squamous cell carcinomas developing in patients who are immunosuppressed or who have an underlying malignant lymphoma or leukaemia are often more aggressive.[474–476] The majority of squamous cell carcinomas are only locally aggressive and are cured by several different methods of treatment. The recurrence rate is approximately double that for basal cell carcinomas.[477]

The risk of metastasis varies with the clinical setting in which the lesion arises.[478] The lowest risk is for tumours arising in sun-damaged skin.[479,480] The usually quoted figure of 0.5%[479] has been challenged as being too low on the basis of several hospital series which might be expected to be weighted in favour of more aggressive and deeply invasive lesions.[452] In this regard it appears that vertical tumour thickness is a prognostic variable, just as it is for melanomas,[472,481] although further studies are required to ascertain the critical tumour thickness required for metastasis. Acantholytic variants arising in sun-damaged skin have a slightly greater risk of metastasis, of the order of 2%,[478] although in one study it was as high as 19%.[467a] Invasive lesions arising in Bowen's disease metastasize in 2–5% of cases.[220]

For lesions arising in skin not exposed to the sun, the incidence of metastasis is approximately 2–3%.[481a,482] There is a further increase in this risk for lesions of the lip, although the quoted range (2–16%) is quite wide.[481–483] Tumours of the lips are more likely to metastasize if there is perineural invasion, if the tumour is of high grade with a dispersed pattern, and if the tumour thickness exceeds 6 mm.[481] Muscle invasion is not useful in predicting the development of lymph node metastases, as once was thought. For squamous cell carcinomas arising in Marjolin's ulcers, the incidence of metastasis is thought to be 10–30%,[482] while for perineal tumours it may be as high as 30–60%.[478]

Metastases usually occur in the regional lymph nodes in the first instance. Uncommonly the lung is involved, and then it is usually a

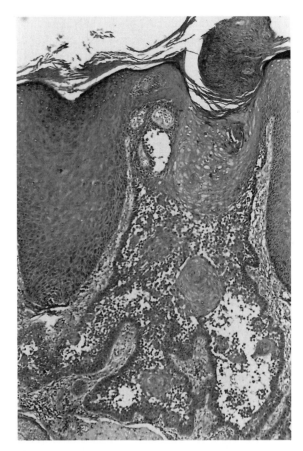

Fig. 31.17 Squamous cell carcinoma of acantholytic type. The cells at the periphery of the tumour nests are still cohesive.
Haematoxylin — eosin

Electron microscopy. The tumour cells in conventional lesions have tonofilaments and well-developed desmosomes and some interdigitating microvilli. In some studies of spindle cell lesions, the cells have shown the features of squamous epithelium with well-developed desmosomes and tonofilaments.[469,470] In other cases there have been cells resembling fibroblasts as well as cells exhibiting both mesenchymal and epithelial features.[471] This mixed pattern of differentiation may result from cell fusion rather than metaplasia.[471]

Recurrences and metastases

Recurrences are more likely in those tumours

terminal phenomenon associated with metastasis to other organs. Cutaneous metastases are exceedingly rare.[484] A circulating tumour antigen, thought to be specific for squamous cell carcinoma, has been detected in patients with metastatic disease;[485] however, this antigen has been reported recently in patients with inflammatory dermatoses.[485a]

VERRUCOUS CARCINOMA

Verrucous carcinoma is a distinctive clinico-pathological variant of squamous cell carcinoma which may involve the oral cavity,[486] larynx, oesophagus and skin.[487,488] It is a slow-growing, often large, warty tumour which invades contiguous structures, but rarely metastasizes.[489] Cutaneous lesions are usually in the genitocrural area[490] or on the plantar surface of the foot (epithelioma cuniculatum), although exceptionally it can arise in any part of the skin surface.[491–494]

Plantar lesions are the most common form of verrucous carcinoma.[495–499] They are usually exophytic, pale lesions, sometimes with draining sinuses.[500] They are often painful and tender. Similar lesions have rarely been reported on the palm or thumb.[501,502] Occasionally explosive growth occurs after a prolonged period of slow progression. The mean duration of lesions at the time of diagnosis is 13–16 years.[503]

Various factors have been implicated in the aetiology of verrucous carcinomas. The chewing of tobacco or betel may predispose to oral lesions, while viruses have been implicated in the aetiology of genitocrural lesions.[491] A case of plantar verrucous carcinoma has been reported contiguous with a plantar wart, and this may have been of aetiological significance.[504] Trauma and chronic irritation have also been implicated in the aetiology.[505]

Histopathology [491,495,499,506]

Often multiple biopsies are required for the diagnosis of verrucous carcinoma. Lesions are both exophytic, with papillomatosis and a covering of hyperkeratosis and parakeratosis, and endophytic.[499] The rete pegs have a bulbous appearance and are composed of large, well-differentiated, squamous epithelial cells with a deceptively benign appearance.[506] These acanthotic downgrowths sometimes extend into the deep reticular dermis. They are blunted projections in contrast to the uneven, sharply pointed and jagged downgrowths seen in pseudoepitheliomatous hyperplasia.[506] There is usually only very low mitotic activity and this is confined to the basal layer.[507] The downgrowths are mostly contained by an intact basement membrane although frankly invasive features are sometimes present. A more aggressive, cytologically malignant squamous cell carcinoma may sometimes arise in a verrucous carcinoma, either de novo, or following X-irradiation of the lesion.[508]

Other features include the presence of burrows in the surface filled with parakeratotic horn as well as draining sinuses containing inflammatory and keratinous debris. Keratin-filled cysts may develop within the tumour mass.[506] The fibrous stroma surrounding the epithelial downgrowths contains ectatic vessels and a variable inflammatory infiltrate in which eosinophils are sometimes prominent.[495] Intraepidermal abscesses are often present in lesions of long standing.

A rare entity affecting the glans penis and known as 'pseudoepitheliomatous keratotic and micaceous balanitis' may present with the histological features of a verrucous carcinoma; in other instances it has features of a hyperplastic dystrophy akin to vulval dystrophy.[509–511]

Verrucous carcinoma should be distinguished from the exceedingly rare papillary variant of squamous cell carcinoma which is a purely exophytic lesion in contrast to the mixed endophytic and exophytic character of verrucous carcinoma.[512]

ADENOSQUAMOUS CARCINOMA

Primary adenosquamous carcinoma of the skin is a rare, usually aggressive tumour with a potential for local recurrence and metastasis.[513–514] Most cases in the literature have been reported as mucoepidermoid carcinomas,[513a] but this term is best reserved for morphologically related tumours arising in the salivary glands and lungs.[513]

Histopathology [513,514]

Adenosquamous carcinomas are usually deeply invasive tumours composed of islands and strands of squamous cell carcinoma admixed with glandular structures containing mucin. The mucin, which is of epithelial type (sialomucin), is present in the lumen and the cytoplasm of the lining cells. It stains with mucicarmine, alcian blue at pH 2.5 and the PAS method, and it is digested by sialidase. The cells are positive for epithelial membrane antigen and cytokeratin, while those lining the glandular spaces stain for carcinoembryonic antigen.

Adenosquamous carcinoma has been confused with adenoid (acantholytic) squamous cell carcinoma, but in the latter tumour there is no mucin and the glandular spaces contain acantholytic squamous cells.[515] Adenosquamous carcinoma also differs from the case reported as 'squamous cell carcinoma with mucinous metaplasia' which was composed of mucin-containing, vacuolated cells, resembling 'signet-ring' cells; there were no gland spaces.[513]

CARCINOSARCOMA

Carcinosarcoma of the skin is an exceedingly rare entity with only a few cases reported to date.[516–518] This tumour has metastatic potential.[519]

Histopathology

For this diagnosis, the tumour must contain an intimate admixture of epithelial and mesenchymal elements, both of which are malignant.[517] In the cases so far reported the epithelial component has been a basal cell carcinoma, sometimes with squamous differentiation,[516] while the mesenchymal component has included fibrosarcoma, osteogenic sarcoma and sometimes other elements.[517]

LYMPHOEPITHELIOMA-LIKE CARCINOMA

Lymphoepithelioma-like carcinoma of the skin is a rare tumour which resembles histologically the nasopharyngeal tumour of the same name.[519a–519c] It presents clinically as a papulonodular lesion, usually on the face or scalp. Metastasis may occur.

Histopathology [519a]

The tumour may arise in the dermis or subcutis. It is composed of islands of large epithelial cells surrounded by a dense infiltrate of lymphocytes and some plasmacytoid cells. The epithelial cells have a vesicular nucleus and a large nucleolus. There is no squamous or glandular differentiation and no connection with the epidermis.

The epithelial cells contain cytokeratin and express epithelial membrane antigen but not S100 protein, while the stromal lymphocytes express CD45 (leucocyte common antigen).

MISCELLANEOUS 'TUMOURS'

CUTANEOUS HORN

A cutaneous horn is a hard, yellowish-brown keratotic excrescence: to earn the designation of 'horn' its height conventionally must exceed at least one-half its greatest diameter.[520] It may be straight or curved, and up to several centimetres in length.[521] Cutaneous horns are usually solitary. They have a predilection for the face, the ears, and the dorsum of the hands of older individuals.[522] A rare site is the penis.[523] It is a clinical entity which may be associated with many different pathological lesions. Most commonly, a horn overlies an actinic keratosis, seborrhoeic keratosis, inverted follicular keratosis,[522] tricholemmoma, verruca vulgaris or squamous cell carcinoma.[520,524] Rarely, there may be an underlying keratoacanthoma, epidermal naevus, epidermal cyst, angiokeratoma or basal cell carcinoma.[525] There is one report of underlying Kaposi's sarcoma,[526] and one of psoriasis.[527]

area of the body,[566] and a *secondary type* in which the lesions develop at sites of trauma,[549] treatment, or an underlying dermatosis. Multiple keratoacanthomas may be associated with internal cancer[574–576] as in Torre's syndrome (Muir–Torre syndrome) in which multiple keratoacanthomas accompany the presence of a primary visceral cancer, particularly of the gastrointestinal tract.[567,577]

The *Ferguson Smith type* is characterized by the development of a succession of lesions, one or a few at a time, on covered as well as exposed areas of the body, and beginning usually in adolescence.[549,568,569] They heal, leaving an atrophic and sometimes disfiguring scar. It seems that the variant found in Scottish kindreds is a more aggressive form with an autosomal dominant inheritance and histological appearances which may resemble those found in a squamous cell carcinoma.[570] The term multiple self-healing squamous carcinomas is still applied to this variant.[570,571]

In the *eruptive type* there are multiple (often several hundred) papules and nodules of varying size, with an onset in the fifth and sixth decades.[572,573] Lesions may develop on the palms and soles and mucous membranes, as well as in the more usual sites. They may exemplify the Koebner phenomenon. The lesions may be intensely pruritic.[572]

Although viruses have long been suggested as an aetiological agent, there is still no proof of this hypothesis.[578] In animals, chemical carcinogens can produce lesions resembling keratoacanthomas; such tumours develop from the hair follicles.[578] Exposure to tars, either industrial or therapeutic, will induce lesions in man. Exposure to excessive sunlight is the most frequently incriminated factor in the aetiology of keratoacanthomas. Other factors include trauma,[549] immunosuppressed states (in which the keratoacanthomas are prone to aggressive growth, early recurrence, and even transformation into squamous cell carcinoma)[446,579] and xeroderma pigmentosum.[545] They have rarely followed bites, vaccinations,[580] arterial puncture[581] and PUVA therapy.[582] They have been known to develop in linear epidermal naevi,[583] at the site of treated psoriatic lesions[584] and in association with several dermatoses.[585]

Histopathology

As there is no consistent, single histological feature that characterizes a keratoacanthoma,[586] the diagnosis may cause difficulty for the inexperienced pathologist, particularly if only a snippet biopsy is submitted. However, there should be no difficulty in making a correct diagnosis on excision specimens and in fusiform biopsies which extend across the central diameter of the lesion for its full width or at least well into its centre. A constellation of histological features needs to be assessed.

Keratoacanthomas are exo-endophytic lesions with an invaginating mass of keratinizing, well-differentiated squamous epithelium at the sides and bottom of the lesion. There is a central keratin-filled crater which enlarges with the maturation and evolution of the lesion. Another key feature is the lipping (also known as buttressing) of the edges of the lesion which overlap the central crater, giving it a symmetrical appearance (Figs 31.19 and 31.20). In some lesions a

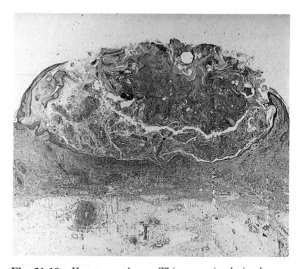

Fig. 31.19   Keratoacanthoma. This regressing lesion has a large keratin plug and shows characteristic overhanging shoulders ('marginal buttressing').
Haematoxylin — eosin

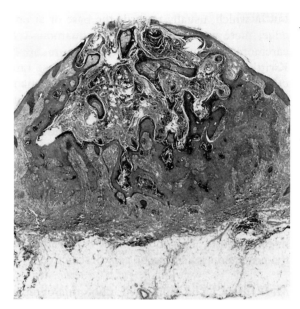

Fig. 31.20   Keratoacanthoma in the late proliferative phase. Haematoxylin — eosin

keratotic plug overlies discrete infundibula and a central horn-filled crater is not formed.

The component cells have a distinctive eosinophilic hue to their cytoplasm and, as they mature, towards the centre of the islands of squamous epithelium, they can become quite large (Fig. 31.21). Epithelial atypia and mitoses are not a usual feature. There is a mixed infil-

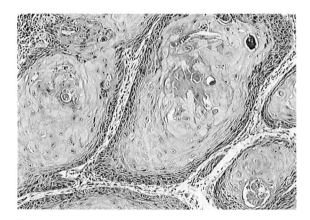

Fig. 31.21   Keratoacanthoma. The keratinocytes are large, particularly towards the centre of the tumour-cell nests. Haematoxylin — eosin

trate of inflammatory cells in the adjacent dermis, and this is sometimes moderately heavy. Eosinophils and neutrophils may be prominent, and these may extend into the epithelial nests to form small microabscesses. There is no stromal desmoplasia except in late involuting lesions. Extension below the level of the sweat glands is unusual,[587] and if present necessitates particularly careful assessment of the other histological features. Atypical hyperplasia of the sweat duct epithelium may be present in some cases.[588] Perineural invasion is an incidental and infrequent finding which does not usually affect the prognosis or behaviour of the lesion,[589,590] although local recurrence has been reported in two perioral keratoacanthomas with extensive perineural invasion and intravenous growth.[591]

In *keratoacanthoma centrifugum marginatum* there is progressive involution and fibrosis towards the centre of the lesion, although the advancing edge will show the typical overhanging lip with nests of squamous epithelium in the underlying dermis.

Subungual keratoacanthomas contain more dyskeratotic cells and fewer neutrophils and eosinophils than the usual keratoacanthoma, and their orientation is more vertical.[559] Some of the smaller lesions in the various syndromes of multiple keratoacanthomas may show a dilated follicle or cup-shaped depression filled with keratin and showing only limited proliferation of squamous epithelium in the base. Keratoacanthomas developing in the Muir–Torre syndrome may have an accompanying sebaceous proliferation.[592]

Some authorities believe that the Ferguson Smith type of lesion should be separated from keratoacanthoma.[571] There is histological support for this view. The Ferguson Smith tumour may have an indefinite edge, some pleomorphism of cells and the production of only a small amount of keratin. The infiltrate is usually lymphocytic rather than composed of polymorphs.[571]

Distinction of keratoacanthoma from squamous cell carcinoma. Histological features which favour a diagnosis of keratoacanthoma

38. Skoven I. Inflammatory linear verrucous epidermal nevus (ILVEN). Acta Derm Venereol 1979; 59: 364–366.
39. Hodge SJ, Barr JM, Owen LG. Inflammatory linear verrucose epidermal nevus. Arch Dermatol 1978; 114: 436–438.
40. Ahrens EM, Hodge SJ. Lichen planus arising in an inflammatory linear verrucous epidermal nevus. Int J Dermatol 1986; 25: 527–528.
41. Beck MH, Dave VK. Extensive nevus comedonicus. Arch Dermatol 1980; 116: 1048–1050.
42. Abdel-Aal H, Abdel-Aziz AHM. Nevus comedonicus. Report of three cases localized on the glans penis. Acta Derm Venereol 1975; 55: 78–80.
43. Cripps DJ, Bertram JR. Nevus comedonicus bilateralis et verruciformis. J Cutan Pathol 1976; 3: 273–281.
44. Wood MG, Thew MA. Nevus comedonicus. A case with palmar involvement and review of the literature. Arch Dermatol 1968; 98: 111–116.
45. Harper KE, Spielvogel RL. Nevus comedonicus of the palm and wrist. J Am Acad Dermatol 1985; 12: 185–188.
46. Paige TN, Mendelson CG. Bilateral nevus comedonicus. Arch Dermatol 1967; 96: 172–175.
47. Engber PB. The nevus comedonicus syndrome: a case report with emphasis on associated internal manifestations. Int J Dermatol 1978; 17: 745–749.
48. Whyte HJ. Unilateral comedo nevus and cataract. Arch Dermatol 1968; 97: 533–535.
49. Rodriguez JM. Nevus comedonicus. Arch Dermatol 1975; 111: 1363–1364.
50. Nabai H, Mehregan AH. Nevus comedonicus. A review of the literature and report of twelve cases. Acta Derm Venereol 1973; 53: 71–74.
51. Leppard BJ. Trichilemmal cysts arising in an extensive comedo naevus. Br J Dermatol 1977; 96: 545–548.
52. Marsden RA, Fleming K, Dawber RPR. Comedo naevus of the palm — a sweat duct naevus? Br J Dermatol 1979; 101: 717–722.
53. Abell E, Read SI. Porokeratotic eccrine ostial and dermal duct naevus. Br J Dermatol 1980; 103: 435–441.
54. Coskey RJ, Mehregan AH. Porokeratotic eccrine duct and hair follicle nevus. J Am Acad Dermatol 1982; 6: 940–943.
55. Aloi FG, Pippione M. Porokeratotic eccrine ostial and dermal duct nevus. Arch Dermatol 1986; 122: 892–895.
56. Moreno A, Pujol RM, Salvatella N et al. Porokeratotic eccrine ostial and dermal duct nevus. J Cutan Pathol 1988; 15: 43–48.
57. Horio T, Komura J. Linear unilateral basal cell nevus with comedo-like lesions. Arch Dermatol 1978; 114: 95–97.
58. Blanchard L, Hodge SJ, Owen LG. Linear eccrine nevus with comedones. Arch Dermatol 1981; 117: 357–359.
59. Plewig G, Christophers E. Nevoid follicular epidermolytic hyperkeratosis. Arch Dermatol 1975; 111: 223–226.
60. Price M, Russell Jones R. Familial dyskeratotic comedones. Clin Exp Dermatol 1985; 10: 147–153.
61. Hall JR, Holder W, Knox JM et al. Familial dyskeratotic comedones. J Am Acad Dermatol 1987; 17: 808–814.
62. Carneiro SJC, Dickson JE, Knox JM. Familial dyskeratotic comedones. Arch Dermatol 1972; 105: 249–251.
63. Leppard BJ. Familial dyskeratotic comedones. Clin Exp Dermatol 1982; 7: 329–332.
64. Cantú JM, Gómez-Bustamente MO, González-Mendoza A, Sánchez-Corona J. Familial comedones. Evidence for autosomal dominant inheritance. Arch Dermatol 1978; 114: 1807–1809.
65. Rodin HH, Blankenship ML, Bernstein G. Diffuse familial comedones. Arch Dermatol 1967; 95: 145–146.

Pseudoepitheliomatous hyperplasia

66. Grumwald MH, Lee J Y-Y, Ackerman AB. Pseudocarcinomatous hyperplasia. Am J Dermatopathol 1988; 10: 95–103.
67. Civatte J. Pseudo-carcinomatous hyperplasia. J Cutan Pathol 1985; 12: 214–223.
68. Ju DMC. Pseudoepitheliomatous hyperplasia of the skin. Dermatol Int 1967; 6: 82–92.
69. Freeman RG. On the pathogenesis of pseudoepitheliomatous hyperplasia. J Cutan Pathol 1974; 1: 231–237.
70. Hurwitz RM. Pseudocarcinomatous or infundibular hyperplasia. Am J Dermatopathol 1989; 11: 189–191.
71. Weber PJ, Johnson BL, Dzubow LM. Pseudoepitheliomatous hyperplasia following Mohs micrographic surgery. J Dermatol Surg Oncol 1989; 15: 557–560.
72. Epstein E. Granuloma fissuratum of the ears. Arch Dermatol 1965; 91: 621–622.
73. Cerroni L, Soyer HP, Chimenti S. Acanthoma fissuratum. J Dermatol Surg Oncol 1988; 14: 1003–1005.
74. MacDonald DM, Martin SJ. Acanthoma fissuratum — spectacle frame acanthoma. Acta Derm Venereol 1975; 55: 485–487.
75. Farrell WJ, Wilson JW. Granuloma fissuratum of the nose. Arch Dermatol 1968; 97: 34–37.
76. Delaney TJ, Stewart TW. Granuloma fissuratum. Br J Dermatol 1971; 84: 373–375.
77. Rowland Payne CME, Wilkinson JD, McKee PH. Nodular prurigo — a clinicopathological study of 46 patients. Br J Dermatol 1985; 113: 431–439.
78. Boer J, Smeenk G. Nodular prurigo-like eruptions induced by etretinate. Br J Dermatol 1987; 116: 271–274.
79. Doyle JA, Connolly SM, Hunziker N, Winkelmann RK. Prurigo nodularis: a reappraisal of the clinical and histologic features. J Cutan Pathol 1979; 6: 392–403.
80. Miyauchi H, Uehara M. Follicular occurrence of prurigo nodularis. J Cutan Pathol 1988; 15: 208–211.
81. Cowan MA. Neurohistological changes in prurigo nodularis. Arch Dermatol 1964; 89: 754–758.
82. Lindley RP, Rowland Payne CME. Neural hyperplasia is not a diagnostic prerequisite in nodular prurigo. J Cutan Pathol 1989; 16: 14–18.
83. Feuerman EJ, Sandbank M. Prurigo nodularis. Histological and electron microscopical study. Arch Dermatol 1975; 111: 1472–1477.
84. Runne U, Orfanos CE. Cutaneous neural proliferation in highly pruritic lesions of chronic prurigo. Arch Dermatol 1977; 113: 787–791.
85. Sandbank M. Cutaneous nerve lesions in prurigo nodularis. Electron microscopic study of two patients. J Cutan Pathol 1976; 3: 125–132.

Acanthomas

86. Brownstein MH. The benign acanthomas. J Cutan Pathol 1985; 12: 172–188.

87. Brownstein MH. Acantholytic acanthoma. J Am Acad Dermatol 1988; 19: 783–786.

88. Baer RL. Giant pedunculated seborrheic keratosis. Arch Dermatol 1979; 115: 627.

89. Becker SW. Seborrheic keratosis and verruca, with special reference to the melanotic variety. Arch Dermatol 1951; 63: 358–372.

90. Bedi TR. Familial congenital multiple seborrheic verrucae. Arch Dermatol 1977; 113: 1441–1442.

91. Reiches AJ. Seborrheic keratoses. Are they delayed hereditary nevi? Arch Dermatol 1952; 65: 596–600.

92. Migally M, Migally N. Halo seborrheic keratosis. Int J Dermatol 1983; 22: 307–309.

93. Kaminsky CA, De Kaminsky AR, Sanguinetti O, Shaw M. Acquired pigmentation of skin folds with the histological picture of seborrhoeic wart. Br J Dermatol 1975; 93: 713–716.

94. Sanderson KV. The structure of seborrhoeic keratoses. Br J Dermatol 1968; 80: 588–593.

94a. Zhao Y, Lin Y, Luo R et al. Human papillomavirus (HPV) infection in seborrheic keratosis. Am J Dermatopathol 1989; 11: 209–212.

95. Morales A, Hu F. Seborrheic verruca and intraepidermal basal cell epithelioma of Jadassohn. Arch Dermatol 1965; 91: 342–344.

96. Wade TR, Ackerman AB. The many faces of seborrheic keratoses. J Dermatol Surg Oncol 1979; 5: 378–382.

97. Berman A, Winkelmann RK. Seborrheic keratoses. Appearance in course of exfoliative erythroderma and regression associated with histologic mononuclear cell inflammation. Arch Dermatol 1982; 118: 615–618.

98. Berman A, Winkelmann RK. Histologic changes in seborrheic keratoses after rubbing. J Cutan Pathol 1980; 7: 32–38.

99. Berman A, Winkelmann RK. Inflammatory seborrheic keratoses with mononuclear cell infiltration. J Cutan Pathol 1978; 5: 353–360.

100. Nakayasu K, Nishimura A, Maruo M, Wakabayashi S. Trichilemmal differentiation in seborrheic keratosis. J Cutan Pathol 1981; 8: 256–262.

101. Masuda M, Kimura S. Trichilemmal keratinization in seborrheic keratoses. J Cutan Pathol 1984; 11: 12–17.

102. Tagami H, Yamada M. Seborrheic keratosis: an acantholytic variant. J Cutan Pathol 1978; 5: 145–149.

102a. Chen M, Shinmori H, Takemiya M, Miki Y. Acantholytic variant of seborrheic keratosis. J Cutan Pathol 1990; 17: 27–31.

103. Kossard S, Berman A, Winkelmann RK. Seborrheic keratoses and trichostasis spinulosa. J Cutan Pathol 1979; 6: 492–496.

104. Kwittken J. The changing seborrheic keratosis. Int J Dermatol 1974; 13: 129–134.

105. Kwittken J. Squamous cell carcinoma arising in seborrheic keratosis. Mt Sinai J Med 1981; 48: 61–62.

106. Kwittken J. Keratoacanthoma arising in seborrheic keratosis. Cutis 1974; 14: 546–547.

107. Mikhail GR, Mehregan AH. Basal cell carcinoma in seborrheic keratosis. J Am Acad Dermatol 1982; 6: 500–506.

108. Baer RL, Garcia RL, Partsalidou V, Ackerman AB. Papillated squamous cell carcinoma in situ arising in a seborrheic keratosis. J Am Acad Dermatol 1981; 5: 561–565.

109. Bloch PH. Transformation of seborrheic keratosis into Bowen's disease. J Cutan Pathol 1978; 5: 361–367.

110. Cooper Booth J. Atypical seborrhoeic keratosis. Aust J Dermatol 1977; 18: 10–14.

111. Rahbari H. Bowenoid transformation of seborrhoeic verrucae (keratoses). Br J Dermatol 1979; 101: 459–463.

111a. Monteagudo JC, Jorda E, Terencio C, Llombart-Bosch A. Squamous cell carcinoma in situ (Bowen's disease) arising in seborrheic keratosis: three lesions in two patients. J Cutan Pathol 1989; 16: 348–352.

112. Kwittken J. Malignant changes in seborrheic keratoses. Mt Sinai J Med (NY) 1974; 41: 792–801.

113. Shelley WB, Shelley ED, Burmeister V. Melanosome macrocomplex: An ultrastructural component of patterned and nonpatterned seborrheic keratoses. J Am Acad Dermatol 1987; 16: 124–128.

114. Nyfors A, Kruger PG. Langerhans' cells in seborrheic keratosis. A clinical and ultrastructural study. Acta Derm Venereol 1985; 65: 333–335.

115. Wilborn WH, Dismukes DE, Montes LF. Ultrastructural identification of Langerhans cells in seborrheic keratoses. J Cutan Pathol 1978; 5: 368–372.

116. Dantzig PI. Sign of Leser-Trélat. Arch Dermatol 1973; 108: 700–701.

117. Holdiness MR. The sign of Leser-Trélat. Int J Dermatol 1986; 25: 564–572.

118. Holdiness MR. On the classification of the sign of Leser-Trélat. J Am Acad Dermatol 1988; 19: 754–757.

118a. Rampen FHJ, Schwengle LEM. The sign of Leser-Trélat: does it exist? J Am Acad Dermatol 1989; 21: 50–55.

119. Czarnecki DB, Rotstein H, O'Brien TJ et al. The sign of Leser-Trélat. Australas J Dermatol 1983; 24: 93–99.

120. Venencie PY, Perry HO. Sign of Leser-Trélat: Report of two cases and review of the literature. J Am Acad Dermatol 1984; 10: 83–88.

121. Elewski BE, Gilgor RS. Eruptive lesions and malignancy. Int J Dermatol 1985; 24: 617–629.

122. Sperry K, Wall J. Adenocarcinoma of the stomach with eruptive seborrheic keratoses. The sign of Leser-Trélat. Cancer 1980; 45: 2434–2437.

123. Curry SS, King LE. The sign of Leser-Trélat. Report of a case with adenocarcinoma of the duodenum. Arch Dermatol 1980; 116: 1059–1060.

124. Wagner RF Jr, Wagner KD. Malignant neoplasms and the Leser-Trélat sign. Arch Dermatol 1981; 117: 598–599.

125. Safai B, Grant JM, Good RA. Cutaneous manifestations of internal malignancies (II): the sign of Leser-Trélat. Int J Dermatol 1978; 17: 494–495.

126. Liddell D, White JE, Caldwell IW. Seborrhoeic keratoses and carcinoma of the large bowel. Br J Dermatol 1975; 92: 449–452.

microscopic, autoradiographic, and immuno-fluorescence study. Cancer 1980; 45: 2849–2857.

508. Youngberg GA, Thornthwaite JT, Inoshita T, Franzus D. Cytologically malignant squamous-cell carcinoma arising in a verrucous carcinoma of the penis. J Dermatol Surg Oncol 1983; 9: 474–479.

509. Read SI, Abell E. Pseudoepitheliomatous, keratotic, and micaceous balanitis. Arch Dermatol 1981; 117: 435–437.

510. Jenkins D Jr, Jakubovic HR. Pseudoepitheliomatous, keratotic, micaceous balanitis. A clinical lesion with two histologic subsets: hyperplastic dystrophy and verrucous carcinoma. J Am Acad Dermatol 1988; 18: 419–422.

511. Beljaards RC, Van Dijk E, Hausman R. Is pseudoepitheliomatous, micaceous and keratotic balanitis synonymous with verrucous carcinoma? Br J Dermatol 1987; 117: 641–646.

512. Landman G, Taylor RM, Friedman KJ. Cutaneous papillary squamous cell carcinoma. A report of two cases. J Cutan Pathol 1988; 15: 323 (abstract).

513. Friedman KJ, Hood AF, Farmer ER. Cutaneous squamous cell carcinoma with mucinous metaplasia. J Cutan Pathol 1988; 15: 176–182.

513a. Landman G, Farmer ER. Primary cutaneous mucoepidermoid carcinoma: report of a case. J Cutan Pathol 1991; 18: 56–59.

514. Weidner N, Foucar E. Adenosquamous carcinoma of the skin. Arch Dermatol 1985; 121: 775–779.

515. Underwood JW, Adcock LL, Okagaki T. Adenosquamous carcinoma of skin appendages (adenoid squamous cell carcinoma, pseudoglandular squamous cell carcinoma, adenoacanthoma of sweat gland of Lever) of the vulva. Cancer 1978; 42: 1851–1858.

516. Dawson EK. Carcinosarcoma of the skin. J R Coll Surg Edinb 1972; 17: 242–246.

517. Quay SC, Harrist TJ, Mihm MC Jr. Carcinosarcoma of the skin. Case report and review. J Cutan Pathol 1981; 8: 241–246.

518. Tschen JA, Goldberg LH, McGavran MH. Carcinosarcoma of the skin. J Cutan Pathol 1988; 15: 31–35.

519. Harrist TJ, Hassell LA, Bronstein BR, Mihm MC Jr. Follow-up of a previously reported carcinosarcoma of the skin. J Cutan Pathol 1983; 10: 359–360.

519a. Swanson SA, Cooper PH, Mills SE, Wick JR. Lymphoepithelioma-like carcinoma of the skin. Mod Pathol 1988; 1: 359–365.

519b. Malhotra R, Woda B, Bhawan J. Lymphoepithelial-like carcinoma of the skin. The microscopic and immunohistochemical findings of two patients. J Cutan Pathol 1989; 16: 317 (abstract).

519c. Walker AN, Kent D, Mitchell AR. Lymphoepithelioma-like carcinoma in the skin. J Am Acad Dermatol 1990; 22: 691–693.

Miscellaneous 'tumours'

520. Bart RS, Andrade R, Kopf AW. Cutaneous horns. A clinical and histopathologic study. Acta Derm Venereol 1968; 48: 507–515.

521. Ingram NP. Cutaneous horns: a review and case history. Ann R Coll Surg Engl 1978; 60: 128–129.

522. Mehregan AH. Cutaneous horn: A clinicopathologic study. Dermatol Digest 1965; 4: 45–54.

523. Lowe FC, McCullough AR. Cutaneous horns of the penis: An approach to management. J Am Acad Dermatol 1985; 13: 369–373.

524. Hubler WR. Horrendous cutaneous horns. Cutis 1978; 22: 592–593.

525. Sandbank M. Basal cell carcinoma at the base of cutaneous horn (cornu cutaneum). Arch Dermatol 1971; 104: 97–98.

526. Gibbs RC, Hyman AB. Kaposi's sarcoma at the base of cutaneous horn. Arch Dermatol 1968; 98: 37–40.

527. Lucky PA, Carter DM. Psoriasis presenting as cutaneous horns. J Am Acad Dermatol 1981; 5: 681–683.

528. Brownstein MH. Trichilemmal horn: cutaneous horn showing trichilemmal keratinization. Br J Dermatol 1979; 100: 303–309.

529. Nakamura K. Two cases of trichilemmal-like horn. Arch Dermatol 1984; 120: 386–387.

530. Peteiro MC, Toribio J, Caeiro JL. Trichilemmal horn. J Cutan Pathol 1984; 11: 326–328.

531. Kimura S. Trichilemmal keratosis (horn): a light and electron microscopic study. J Cutan Pathol 1983; 10: 59–68.

532. Brownstein MH, Shapiro EE. Trichilemmomal horn: cutaneous horn overlying trichilemmoma. Clin Exp Dermatol 1979; 4: 59–63.

533. Haneke E. 'Onycholemmal' horn. Dermatologica 1983; 167: 155–158.

534. Kuokkanen K, Niemi K-M, Reunala T. Parakeratotic horns in a patient with myeloma. J Cutan Pathol 1987; 14: 54–58.

535. Kocsard E, Ofner F. Keratoelastoidosis verrucosa of the extremities (stucco keratoses of the extremities). Dermatologica 1966; 133: 225–235.

536. Kocsard E, Carter JJ. The papillomatous keratoses. The nature and differential diagnosis of stucco keratosis. Aust J Dermatol 1971; 12: 80–88.

537. Scott O, Ward J. Stucco keratosis. Br J Dermatol 1971; 84: 376–379.

538. Willoughby C, Soter NA. Stucco keratosis. Arch Dermatol 1972; 105: 859–861.

539. Hutchinson J. The crateriform ulcer of the face: a form of epithelial cancer. Trans Pathol Soc London 1889; 40: 275–281.

540. Cohen N, Plaschkes Y, Pevzner S, Loewenthal M. Review of 57 cases of keratoacanthoma. Plast Reconstr Surg 1972; 49: 138–142.

541. Sullivan JJ, Colditz GA. Keratoacanthoma in a sub-tropical climate. Australas J Dermatol 1979; 20: 34–40.

542. Rank BK, Dixon PL. Another look at keratoacanthoma. Aust NZ J Surg 1979; 49: 654–658.

543. Friedman RP, Morales A, Burnham TK. Multiple cutaneous and conjunctival keratoacanthomata. Arch Dermatol 1965; 92: 162–165.

544. Silberberg I, Kopf AW, Baer RL. Recurrent keratoacanthoma of the lip. Arch Dermatol 1962; 86: 92–101.

545. Azaz B, Lustmann J. Keratoacanthoma of the lower lip. Oral Surg 1974; 38: 918–927.

546. Svirsky JA, Freedman PD, Lumerman H. Solitary intraoral keratoacanthoma. Oral Surg 1977; 43: 116–119.

547. Tkach JR, Thorne EG. Keratoacanhoma of the glans penis. Cutis 1979; 24: 615–616.

548. Drut R. Solitary keratoacanthoma of the nipple in a male. Case report. J Cutan Pathol 1976; 3: 195–198.

549. Sullivan JJ, Donoghue MF, Kynaston B, McCaffrey JF. Multiple keratoacanthomas: report of four cases. Australas J Dermatol 1980; 21: 16–24.

550. Schwartz RA. The keratoacanthoma: a review. J Surg Oncol 1979; 12: 305–317.

551. Rapaport J. Giant keratoacanthoma of the nose. Arch Dermatol 1975; 111: 73–75.

552. Wolinsky S, Silvers DN, Kohn SR. Spontaneous regression of a giant keratoacanthoma. J Dermatol Surg Oncol 1981; 7: 897–900.

553. Kopf AW, Bart RS. Giant keratoacanthoma. J Dermatol Surg Oncol 1978; 4: 444–445.

554. Weedon D, Barnett L. Keratoacanthoma centrifugum marginatum. Arch Dermatol 1975; 111: 1024–1026.

555. Eliezri YD, Libow L. Multinodular keratoacanthoma. J Am Acad Dermatol 1988; 19: 826–830.

556. Stevanovic DV. Keratoacanthoma dyskeratoticum and segregans. Arch Dermatol 1965; 92: 666–669.

557. Macaulay WL. Subungual keratoacanthoma. Arch Dermatol 1976; 112: 1004–1005.

558. Keeney GL, Banks PM, Linscheid RL. Subungual keratoacanthoma. Report of a case and review of the literature. Arch Dermatol 1988; 124: 1074–1076.

559. Stoll DM, Ackerman AB. Subungual keratoacanthoma. Am J Dermatopathol 1980; 2: 265–271.

560. Shapiro L, Baraf CS. Subungual epidermoid carcinoma and keratoacanthoma. Cancer 1970; 25: 141–152.

561. Ahmed AR. Multiple keratoacanthoma. Int J Dermatol 1980; 19: 496–499.

562. Jolly HW Jr, Carpenter CL Jr. Multiple keratoacanthomata. A report of two cases. Arch Dermatol 1966; 93: 348–353.

563. Ferguson Smith J. A case of multiple primary squamous-celled carcinomata of the skin in a young man, with spontaneous healing. Br J Dermatol 1934; 46: 267–272.

564. Grzybowski M. A case of peculiar generalized epithelial tumours of the skin. Br J Dermatol 1950; 62: 310–313.

564a. Lloyd KM, Madsen DK, Lin PY. Grzybowski's eruptive keratoacanthoma. J Am Acad Dermatol 1989; 21: 1023–1024.

565. Sohn D, Chin TCM, Fellner MJ. Multiple keratoacanthomas associated with steatocystoma multiplex and rheumatoid arthritis. A case report. Arch Dermatol 1980; 116: 913–914.

566. Rook A, Moffatt JL. Multiple self-healing epithelioma of Ferguson Smith type. Report of a case of unilateral distribution. Arch Dermatol 1956; 74: 525–532.

567. Schwartz RA, Flieger DN, Saied NK. The Torre syndrome with gastrointestinal polyposis. Arch Dermatol 1980; 116: 312–314.

568. Benoldi D, Alinovi A. Multiple persistent keratoacanthomas: Treatment with oral etretinate. J Am Acad Dermatol 1984; 10: 1035–1038.

569. Tarnowski WM. Multiple keratoacanthomata. Response of a case to systemic chemotherapy. Arch Dermatol 1966; 94: 74–80.

570. Alexander J O'D, Lyell A. Multiple kerato-acanthomas. J Am Acad Dermatol 1985; 12: 376.

571. Jackson IT, Alexander JO'D, Verheyden CN. Self-healing squamous epithelioma: a family affair. Br J Plast Surg 1983; 36: 22–28.

572. Winkelmann RK, Brown J. Generalized eruptive keratoacanthoma. Arch Dermatol 1968; 97: 615–623.

573. Reid BJ, Cheesbrough MJ. Multiple keratoacanthomata. A unique case and review of the current classification. Acta Derm Venereol 1978; 58: 169–173.

574. Fathizadeh A, Medenica MM, Soltani K et al. Aggressive keratoacanthoma and internal malignant neoplasm. Arch Dermatol 1982; 118: 112–114.

575. Inoshita T, Youngberg GA. Keratoacanthomas associated with cervical squamous cell carcinoma. Arch Dermatol 1984; 120: 123–124.

576. Snider BL, Benjamin DR. Eruptive keratoacanthoma and internal malignant neoplasm. Arch Dermatol 1981; 117: 788–790.

577. Housholder MS, Zeligman I. Sebaceous neoplasms associated with visceral carcinomas. Arch Dermatol 1980; 116: 61–64.

578. Ghadially FN, Barton BW, Kerridge DF. The etiology of keratoacanthoma. Cancer 1963; 16: 603–610.

579. Claudy A, Thivolet J. Multiple keratoacanthomas: association with deficient cell mediated immunity. Br J Dermatol 1975; 93: 593–595.

580. Bart RS, Lagin S. Keratoacanthoma following pneumococcal vaccination: a case report. J Dermatol Surg Oncol 1983; 9: 381–382.

581. Shellito JE, Samet JM. Keratoacanthoma as a complication of arterial puncture for blood gases. Int J Dermatol 1982; 21: 349.

582. Sina B, Adrian RM. Multiple keratoacanthomas possibly induced by psoralens and ultraviolet A photochemotherapy. J Am Acad Dermatol 1983; 9: 686–688.

583. Rosen T. Keratoacanthoma arising within a linear epidermal nevus. J Dermatol Surg Oncol 1982; 8: 878–880.

584. Maddin WS, Wood WS. Multiple keratoacanthomas and squamous cell carcinomas occurring at psoriatic treatment sites. J Cutan Pathol 1979; 6: 96–100.

585. Allen JV, Callen JP. Keratoacanthomas arising in hypertrophic lichen planus. Arch Dermatol 1981; 117: 519–521.

586. Fisher ER, McCoy MM, Wechsler HL. Analysis of histopathologic and electron microscopic determinants of keratoacanthoma and squamous cell carcinoma. Cancer 1972; 29: 1387–1397.

587. Mikhail GR. Squamous cell carcinoma diagnosed as keratoacanthoma. Cutis 1974; 13: 378–382.

588. Santa Cruz DJ, Clausen K. Atypical sweat duct hyperplasia accompanying keratoacanthoma. Dermatologica 1977; 154: 156–160.

589. Lapins NA, Helwig EB. Perineural invasion by keratoacanthoma. Arch Dermatol 1980; 116: 791–793.

590. Janecka IP, Wolff M, Crikelair GF, Cosman B. Aggressive histological features of keratoacanthoma. J Cutan Pathol 1978; 4: 342–348.

591. Cooper PH, Wolfe JT III. Perioral keratoacanthomas with extensive perineural invasion and intravenous growth. Arch Dermatol 1988; 124: 1397–1401.

592. Burgdorf WHC, Pitha J, Fahmy A. Muir-Torre syndrome. Histologic spectrums of sebaceous proliferations. Am J Dermatopathol 1986; 8: 202–208.

593. Kern WH, McCray MK. The histopathologic differentiation of keratoacanthoma and squamous cell carcinoma of the skin. J Cutan Pathol 1980; 7: 318–325.

594. King DF, Barr RJ. Intraepithelial elastic fibers and intracytoplasmic glycogen: diagnostic aids in differentiating keratoacanthoma from squamous cell carcinoma. J Cutan Pathol 1980; 7: 140–148.

595. Smoller BR, Kwan TH, Said JW, Banks-Schlegel S. Keratoacanthoma and squamous cell carcinoma of the skin. Immunohistochemical localization of involucrin and keratin proteins. J Am Acad Dermatol 1986; 14: 226–234.

595a. Jambrosic J, Albrecht S, Hradsky N. Involucrin — a possible diagnostic aid in differentiating keratoacanthoma and squamous cell carcinoma. J Cutan Pathol 1989; 16: 309 (abstract).

595b. Kannon G, Park HK. Utility of peanut agglutinin (PNA) in the diagnosis of squamous cell carcinoma and keratoacanthoma. Am J Dermatopathol 1990; 12: 31–36.

596. Goldenhersh MA, Olsen TG. Invasive squamous cell carcinoma initially diagnosed as a giant keratoacanthoma. J Am Acad Dermatol 1984; 10: 372–378.

597. Rook A, Whimster I. Keratoacanthoma — a thirty year retrospect. Br J Dermatol 1979; 100: 41–47.

597a. Requena L, Romero E, Sanchez M et al. Aggressive keratoacanthoma of the eyelid: "malignant" keratoacanthoma or squamous cell carcinoma? J Dermatol Surg Oncol 1990; 16: 564–568.

598. Kwittken J. Histologic chronology of the clinical course of the keratocarcinoma (so-called keratoacanthoma). Mt Sinai J Med (NY) 1975; 42: 127–135.

599. Kligman LH, Kligman AM. Histogenesis and progression of ultraviolet light-induced tumors in hairless mice. JNCI 1981; 67: 1289–1293.

600. Kingman J, Callen JP. Keratoacanthoma. A clinical study. Arch Dermatol 1984; 120: 736–740.

601. Piscioli F, Zumiani G, Boi S, Christofolini M. A gigantic, metastasizing keratoacanthoma. Report of a case and discussion on classification. Am J Dermatopathol 1984; 6: 123–129.

602. Flannery GR, Muller HK. Immune response to human keratoacanthoma. Br J Dermatol 1979; 101: 625–632.

603. Ramselaar CG, van der Meer JB. The spontaneous regression of keratoacanthoma in man. Acta Derm Venereol 1976; 56: 245–251.

604. Korenberg R, Penneys NS, Kowalczyk A, Nadji M. Quantitation of S100 protein-positive cells in inflamed and non-inflamed keratoacanthoma and squamous cell carcinoma. J Cutan Pathol 1988; 15: 104–108.

605. Rook A, Champion RH. Keratoacanthoma. Natl Cancer Inst Monogr 1963; 10: 257–273.

Lentigines, naevi and melanomas

INTRODUCTION

The histopathological diagnosis of pigmented skin tumours is an important area of dermatopathology. It should be noted that melanin pigment may also be present in skin tumours other than naevocellular naevi and malignant melanomas. For instance, seborrhoeic keratoses, basal cell carcinomas and, rarely, squamous cell carcinomas, schwannomas and dermatofibrosarcoma protuberans may contain melanin. Furthermore, there is a group of dermatoses characterized by variable patterns of hyperpigmentation covering, at times, significant areas of the body.[1]

This chapter is devoted to proliferative disturbances of the melanocyte–naevus-cell system. Other disorders of pigmentation are considered in Chapter 10 (pages 303–324).

LESIONS WITH BASAL MELANOCYTE PROLIFERATION

This group is characterized by basal hyperpigmentation and an increase in melanocytes in the basal layer. The melanocytes are usually single and cytologically normal. Small junctional nests are sometimes seen. Epidermal acanthosis and the presence of melanophages in the papillary dermis are additional histological features that are usually seen in entities within this group.

LENTIGO SIMPLEX (SIMPLE LENTIGO)

The simple lentigo is a brown to black, sharply circumscribed and usually uniformly pigmented macule, measuring a few millimetres in diameter. It may be found anywhere on the body surface. A lentigo occurring on the lip is often referred to as a *labial melanotic macule*.[2,3] The term *genital lentiginosis* has been suggested for the pigmented macules, up to 2 cm in diameter, which develop uncommonly on the penis and vulva.[4-6] Genital lesions differ from those on other sites by their size, irregular outline, variegated pigmentation and a tendency to be multifocal.[4] The oral melanoacanthoma (mucosal melanotic macule — reactive type, oral melanoacanthosis) is sometimes included in this group of lesions.[7-10] It is regarded as a reactive lesion, unlike its cutaneous counterpart (see p. 737) which is a benign tumour.

Histopathology

There is variable basal hyperpigmentation with an increased number of single melanocytes in the basal layer. There is usually acanthosis with regular elongation of the rete ridges. The papillary dermis may contain a sparse lymphohistiocytic infiltrate, including scattered melanophages. Some lesions evolve with the formation of nests of melanocytes in the junctional zone,[11] but it is best to designate these lesions with mixed features of a lentigo and a junctional or compound naevus as lentiginous naevi (see below).

Labial and genital lentigines show a moderate amount of epithelial hyperplasia but, usually, there is no elongation of the rete ridges as seen in a lentigo occurring at other sites.[2,4] The melanocytes usually have prominent dendrites. Hyperplasia of melanocytes is usually present, despite reports to the contrary. Lesions judged not to have an increase in basal melanocytes have been referred to in some reports as 'melanotic macules' and 'melanosis'.[4,6]

The oral melanoacanthoma is characterized by dendritic melanocytes of benign morphology at all levels of the acanthotic epithelium, in contrast to their basal location in the lentigo. Spongiosis is sometimes present.[10]

MULTIPLE LENTIGINES

Various syndromes characterized by the presence of numerous lentigines developing in childhood or adolescence have been described.[1] The pigmented macules may be unilateral in distribution,[12] or generalized,[13,14] the latter form sometimes being a marker of an underlying developmental defect (see below).[15] The term lentiginous mosaicism has been used for cases with regional or segmental lesions,[1] while the older term lentiginosis profusa is still used sometimes for cases of multiple lentigines with or without associated abnormalities.[16] Multiple lentigines are associated with internal manifestations in several rare syndromes — the LEOPARD syndrome, the NAME and LAMB syndromes and centrofacial lentiginosis. In the Peutz–Jeghers syndrome (see p. 314) there are conflicting views as to whether the lesions are lentiginous (with an increased number of melanocytes) on histological examination.

The LEOPARD syndrome is inherited as an autosomal dominant trait.[17] It is characterized by lentigines (L), electrocardiographic conduction defects (E), ocular hypertelorism (O), pulmonary stenosis (P), gonadal hypoplasia (A), retarded growth (R), and nerve deafness (D). These features are not all present in every case.

The NAME syndrome is another rare cardiocutaneous syndrome.[18] Its features include naevi (N), as well as lentigines, ephelides and blue naevi, atrial myxoma (A), myxoid tumours of the skin (M), and endocrine abnormalities (E). A similar syndrome has been reported as the LAMB syndrome — mucocutaneous lentigines (L), atrial myxoma (A), mucocutaneous myxomas (M) and blue naevi (B).[19] The NAME and LAMB syndromes are sometimes referred to collectively as Carney's syndrome.[20] Lentigines have been reported in association with an atrial myxoma only.[15]

SOLAR (SENILE) LENTIGO

Solar lentigos are dark brown to black macules, 3–12 mm or more in diameter, which develop on the sun-exposed skin of middle-aged to elderly patients. They are often multiple. Lesions may increase slowly in size over many years. Solar lentigos may evolve into the reticulated form of seborrhoeic keratosis, such lesions developing a slightly verrucose surface.[21]

Histopathology

The solar lentigo is characterized by elongation of the rete ridges, which are usually short and bulb-like (Fig. 32.1). As they extend more deeply into the dermis, finger-like projections form which connect with adjacent rete ridges to form a reticulate pattern resembling that seen in the reticulate type of seborrhoeic keratosis.[21,22] In addition, there is basal hyperpigmentation which is sometimes quite heavy. There is an increased number of melanocytes, particularly at the bases of the clubbed and budding rete ridges;[22] sometimes the increase is not appreciated on casual examination. Variable numbers of melanophages are present in the papillary dermis.

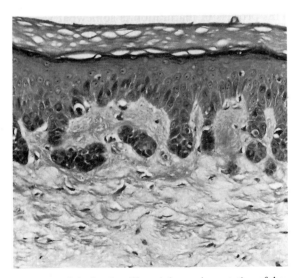

Fig. 32.1 Solar lentigo. There is hyperpigmentation of the bulbous rete ridges.
Haematoxylin — eosin

On electron microscopy the melanosome complexes are much larger than those found in non-involved skin.[22]

LENTIGINOUS NAEVUS

This is a neglected entity which appears to represent the evolution of a lentigo simplex into a junctional and sometimes a compound naevus.[11] It has also been called naevoid lentigo and naevus incipiens.[23] They are well-circumscribed, sometimes deeply pigmented, often quite small lesions found most frequently on the trunk of adults between the ages of 20 and 40 years.

Histopathology

At the advancing edge there is a lentiginous proliferation of melanocytes resembling that seen in a simple lentigo while in the more central areas there is junctional nest formation and sometimes a small number of mature intradermal naevus cell nests as well. There is usually elongation of the rete pegs and some melanophages in the papillary dermis.

SPECKLED LENTIGINOUS NAEVUS (NAEVUS SPILUS)

Speckled lentiginous naevus is the preferred term for a lesion composed of small dark hyperpigmented speckles, superimposed on a tan-brown macular background.[23] Lesions are present at birth or appear in childhood. They may have a zosteriform or regional distribution. Similar cases have been reported as naevus spilus,[24] but this does not accord with the original use of this term. The term zosteriform lentiginous naevus has also been used synonymously, but it is sometimes used for speckled lesions without the background macular pigmentation.[25-28] Finally, the term spotted grouped pigmented naevus has been used for a closely related lesion.[29,30] Malignant melanoma has been reported as a very rare complication.[31-33]

INTRADERMAL NAEVUS

Intradermal naevi are the most common type of melanocytic naevi. The vast majority are found in adults. They are usually dome-shaped, nodular or polypoid lesions which are flesh-coloured or only lightly pigmented. Coarse hairs may protrude from the surface.

Histopathology

Naevus cells are confined to the dermis where they are arranged in nests and cords. Multinucleate naevus cells may be present. In the deeper parts of the lesion, the naevus cells may assume a neuroid appearance ('neural naevus', neurotized melanocytic naevus) with spindle-shaped cells and structures resembling Meissner's tactile bodies (Fig. 32.4). However, these cells are quite distinct with electron microscopy and immunohistochemistry from those seen in a neurofibroma.[65,66] The cells in a neurofibroma show focal staining for Leu 7, glial fibrillary acid protein (GFAP) and myelin basic protein (MBP), antigens not expressed in neurotized melanocytic naevi.[65] With increasing age of the lesion there may also be replacement of naevus cells within the dermis by collagen, fat, elastin and ground substance (Fig. 32.5).[55]

Electron microscopy. The ultrastructural features of naevus cells are similar to those of

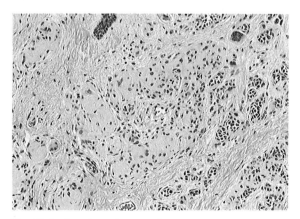

Fig. 32.4 Intradermal naevus. Some naevus cell nests have a neuroid appearance.
Haematoxylin — eosin

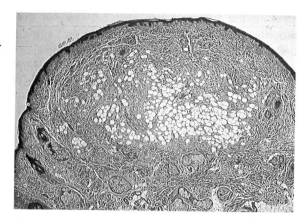

Fig. 32.5 Intradermal naevus from a male of 45 years. There is partial replacement of the lesion by fat.
Haematoxylin — eosin

melanocytes although they lack the long dendritic processes of the melanocyte. Instead they have microvillous processes. The cells contain abundant cytoplasmic organelles including melanosomes.[57,67]

Secondary changes in naevi

Many interesting changes may be found in naevi.[68] They include: the incidental finding of amyloid[69] or of bone (osteonaevus of Nanta);[70,71] epidermal spongiosis producing a clinical eczematous halo — Meyerson's naevus (Fig. 32.6);[72–75] increased amounts of elastic tissue;[76] cystic dilatation of related hair follicles,[77] folliculitis,[78] epidermal or tricholemmal cyst formation,[79,79a] sometimes with rupture, producing sudden clinical enlargement; psammoma body formation;[80] perinaevoid alopecia;[81] focal epidermal necrosis;[82] an incidental molluscum contagiosum;[83] and an associated trichoepithelioma,[84] basal cell carcinoma,[85] syringoma[86] or sweat duct proliferation.[68] Artefacts may be caused by paraffin-processing or by the injection of local anaesthetic.[87] In the latter instance, there is separation of naevus cells into parallel rows. Changes associated with tissue processing include the formation of clefts and spaces resembling vascular or lymphatic channels. The cells lining these pseudovascular spaces have been identified as naevus cells by immunoperoxidase studies using various markers.[88]

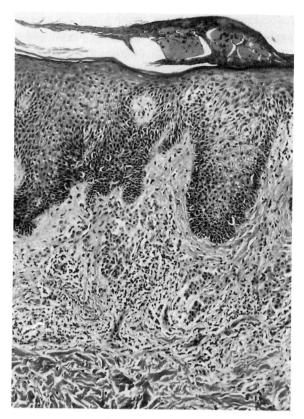

Fig. 32.6 Spongiotic (eczematous) changes superimposed on a benign compound naevus. Clinically, the lesion had recently developed an 'eczematous halo'. Haematoxylin — eosin

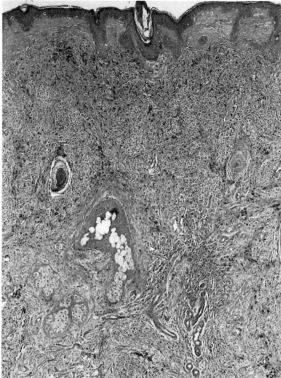

Fig. 32.7 Deep penetrating naevus. Nests of naevus cells extend into the deep reticular dermis. Haematoxylin — eosin

DEEP PENETRATING NAEVUS

The deep penetrating naevus is a recently described variant of melanocytic naevus found on the face, the upper part of the trunk and the proximal part of the limbs of young adults.[89] It is often deeply pigmented, leading to a mistaken clinical diagnosis of blue naevus or malignant melanoma. There are also histological features which overlap with these two entities and with the Spitz naevus.

Histopathology [89]

The deep penetrating naevus is usually of compound type but the junctional nests are only small in most cases. It is composed of loosely arranged nests and fascicles of pigmented naevus cells, interspersed with melanophages. The nests extend into the deep reticular dermis and often into the subcutaneous fat (Fig. 32.7). They surround hair follicles, sweat glands and nerves. Pilar muscles are sometimes infiltrated.

Although there is some pleomorphism of the nuclei of the naevus cells, nucleoli are generally inconspicuous and mitoses are absent. Nuclear vacuoles and smudging of the chromatin pattern are additional features.

Only a few cases have been studied by immunohistochemistry: in these, the cells expressed S100 protein and HMB-45.

BALLOON CELL NAEVUS

This is a rare lesion which is clinically indistinguishable from an ordinary melanocytic naevus. A depigmented halo has rarely been described.[90]

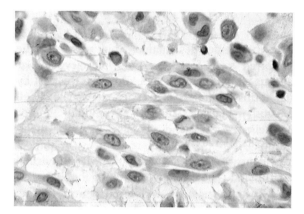

Fig. 32.9   Spitz naevus. It is composed of plump, spindle-shaped cells.
Haematoxylin — eosin

cells only were found in 45% of lesions, spindle and epithelioid cells in 34%, and epithelioid cells only in 21%.[135] Sometimes the spindle cells are quite plump (Fig. 32.9). On low power magnification, Spitz naevi are usually quite symmetrical in appearance with no lateral extension of junctional activity beyond the limits of the dermal component (Fig. 32.10). There is usually 'maturation' of naevus cells in depth; this refers to the presence of cells in the deeper parts of the lesion which are smaller and resemble ordinary naevus cells. It has been suggested, on the basis of ultrastructural studies, that the process of 'maturation' of naevus cells is really one of atrophy.[136] Single melanocytes extending upwards within the epidermis are quite uncommon in Spitz naevi, although clusters of three or more cells may be found within the epidermis, in places appearing to be undergoing trans-epidermal elimination (Fig. 32.11). Solitary or coalescent eosinophilic globules (Kamino bodies) may be found at the dermo–epidermal junction.[137,138] The presence of coalescent globules is an important diagnostic sign, but multiple step sections may be needed to demonstrate them (Fig. 32.12). They are usually PAS positive and trichrome positive.[120] On immuno-histochemistry they contain various components of the basement membrane including laminin and types IV and VII collagen.[139] Electron microscopy shows them to be composed of

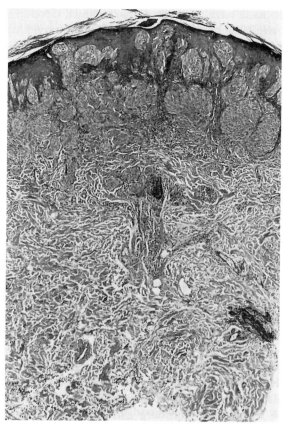

Fig. 32.10   Spitz naevus. There is irregular epidermal hyperplasia.
Haematoxylin — eosin

bundles of filaments, situated extracellularly.[137,138]

Minor diagnostic criteria include the presence of junctional cleavage (separation of the epidermis from nests of naevus cells at the junctional zone — Fig. 32.13), pseudoepitheliomatous hyperplasia,[140] superficial dermal oedema and telangiectasia, giant naevus cells (both multinucleate and uninucleate), and absence of nuclear pleomorphism.[120] Mitoses may be quite frequent in some actively growing lesions, but extreme caution should be adopted in making a diagnosis of Spitz naevus if mitoses, particularly atypical ones, are present in the deeper portion of a lesion. There may be an inflammatory infiltrate which shows perivascular localization.[124] Not infrequently, individual naevus cells may be

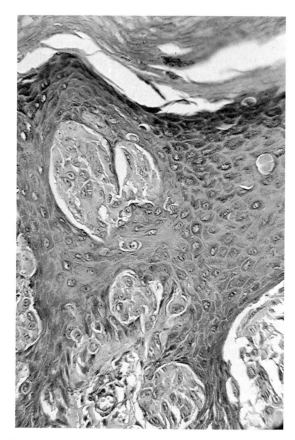

Fig. 32.11 Spitz naevus. There is some upward spread of melanocytes within the epidermis, but most of the cells are in small nests and not solitary
Haematoxylin — eosin

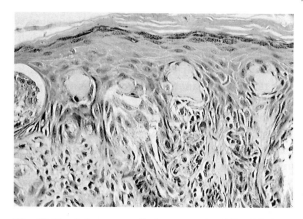

Fig. 32.12 Spitz naevus. Coalescent eosinophilic globules (Kamino bodies) are present in the junctional zone.
Haematoxylin — eosin

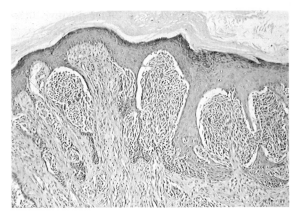

Fig. 32.13 Spitz naevus. There is conspicuous 'cleavage' at the junctional zone resulting from the artefactual separation of naevus cells from the basal layer of the epidermis.
Haematoxylin — eosin

found at a depth of up to one high power field or more below the deep aspect of the tumour. In some Spitz naevi of epithelioid cell type a distinct component of smaller naevus cells is present, usually at the periphery of the lesion.[141] This 'combined Spitz naevus' represents the association of a common melanocytic naevus with a Spitz naevus.

In a histological review of Spitz naevi and melanomas of childhood and adolescence, Peters and Goellner found that pagetoid spread, cellular pleomorphism, nuclear hyperchromatism and mitotic activity were greater in melanomas than in Spitz naevi.[142] These nuclear differences can be quantitated using image analysis cytometry, but this is still at the experimental stage.[143]

Other techniques which may be applied in the diagnosis of Spitz naevi are immunohistochemistry[144,145] and the measurement of nucleolar organizer regions[146] (loops of DNA that transcribe ribosomal RNA and which are easily identified in paraffin-embedded sections using a silver stain). Unfortunately neither method gives unequivocal results in borderline lesions. With immunohistochemistry the cells express S100 protein; the results are inconsistent with HMB-45. This latter marker is usually expressed weakly in the superficial cells, but sometimes there is staining throughout the tumour in a pattern near to that seen in malignant mela-

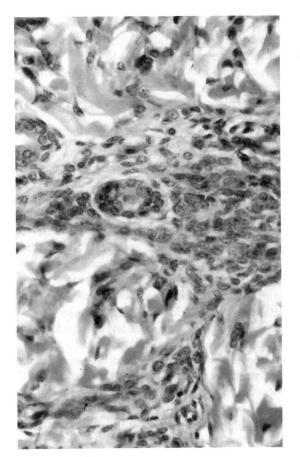

Fig. 32.15 Congenital naevus. Nests of naevus cells extend deeply in the dermis and surround a sweat gland. The cells also show some angiocentricity. The lesion was a large one. It was removed at the age of 10 years.
Haematoxylin — eosin

the melanomas are often non-epidermal in origin.[179] Patterns described include spindle and round cell differentiation, malignant blue naevus[180] and heterologous malignant mesenchymal differentiation including neurosarcoma,[181] rhabdomyosarcoma, liposarcoma and undifferentiated spindle cell carcinoma.[182] Sometimes a cellular 'nodule' of naevus cells develops in a congenital naevus; it should not be misdiagnosed as a melanoma. Features that favour a diagnosis of malignancy include the presence of atypical mitoses or focal necrosis within the 'nodule' or a lack of circumscription, with nests of cells infiltrating into the adjacent naevus.

DERMAL MELANOCYTIC LESIONS

In this group, dendritic melanocytes are present in the dermis. These melanocytes may be derived from precursor cells which did not complete their migration from the neural crest to the epidermis during embryogenesis.

MONGOLIAN SPOT

Mongolian spots are slate-coloured patches of discoloration with a predilection for the sacral region of certain races, particularly Orientals.[183–185] They are present at birth or soon afterwards, but tend to disappear with increasing age, except in the Japanese among whom persistent lesions may be found in approximately 3% of middle-aged adults.[186,187]

Histopathology

There are widely scattered, melanin-containing melanocytes in the lower half of the dermis. The cells are elongated and slender. Occasional melanophages are also present.

NAEVUS OF OTA AND NAEVUS OF ITO

The naevus of Ota is a diffuse, although sometimes slightly speckled, macular area of blue to dark brown pigmentation of skin in the region of the ophthalmic and maxillary divisions of the trigeminal nerve. There is often conjunctival involvement as well. Lesions are bilateral in a small number of cases.[188] There is a predilection for certain races and for females.[189] The naevus of Ito is a similar condition located in the supraclavicular and deltoid regions and sometimes in the scapular area.[190] Both lesions are occasionally present in the same patient.[188] Pigmentation is often present at birth, but it may not become apparent until early childhood. Malignant change is exceptionally rare.[191,192]

Histopathology

There are often nodular collections of

melanocytes which resemble those of blue naevi (see below). The intervening macular areas are composed of a more diffuse infiltrate of elongated melanocytes situated in the upper dermis.[193]

BLUE NAEVUS

The common or classic blue naevus is a small slate-blue to blue-black macule or papule found most commonly on the extremities. It is almost invariably acquired after infancy.[194] The cellular variant is a much larger nodular lesion, often found on the buttocks, but sometimes on the extremities.[195,196] Eruptive,[197] plaque[198] and target[199] forms have been described.

Histopathology

The *common blue naevus* is composed of elongate, sometimes finely branching melanocytes in the interstices of the dermal collagen of the mid and upper dermis (Fig. 32.16). There are some melanophages. Some lesions show dermal fibrosis (sclerosing blue naevus). Occasionally an overlying intradermal naevus is present: such lesions are called combined[200,201] or 'true and blue' naevi.

The *cellular blue naevus* is composed of dendritic melanocytes, as in the common type,

together with islands of epithelioid and plump spindle cells with abundant pale cytoplasm and usually little pigment (Fig. 32.17). Melanophages are found between the cellular islands. The tumour often bulges into the subcutaneous fat as a nodular downgrowth which has a rather characteristic appearance.

Rare variants include the association of a blue naevus with a trichoepithelioma,[202] and a bizarre blue naevus with striking cytological atypia, but without any other features of malignancy.[203]

The melanocytes in blue naevi of both types express S100 protein and HMB-45.[203a]

Electron microscopy. Melanosomes are present in both the dendritic melanocytes and the

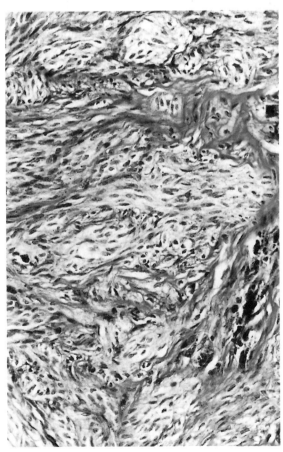

Fig. 32.17 Cellular blue naevus. There are nests and fascicles of melanocytes, some with a spindle shape. The cytoplasm of the cells is pale staining.
Haematoxylin — eosin

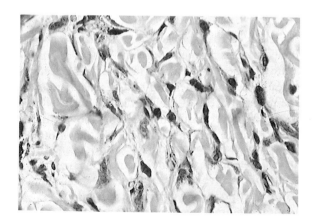

Fig. 32.16 Blue naevus. Melanocytes with long dendritic processes and cytoplasmic melanin are present between the collagen bundles in the dermis.
Haematoxylin — eosin

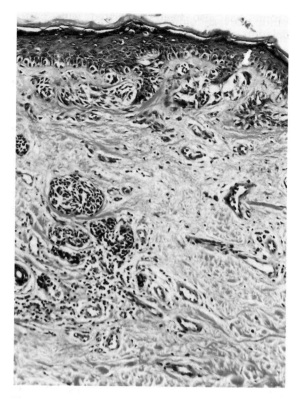

Fig. 32.19 Dysplastic naevus. There is a lentiginous proliferation of melanocytes in the basal layer with some nests of naevo-melanocytes in the junctional zone and in the upper dermis. Only mild cytological atypia is present. There is mild fibroplasia involving the papillary dermis.
Haematoxylin — eosin

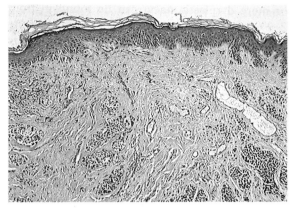

Fig. 32.20 Dysplastic naevus of compound type. There is fibrosis of the superficial dermis and an absence of naevo-melanocytes in the overlying junctional zone, suggesting focal regression. Focal scarring of this type is not uncommon in dysplastic naevi.
Haematoxylin — eosin

often a progression of cytological atypia with increasing age of the patient.[254] Furthermore, increasing atypia has been found to correlate with increasing darkness and confluence of pigmentation clinically.[255] Several reports have inferred that severe atypia is associated with an increased risk of melanoma change, but this was not confirmed in one study.[256–258] Atypia may also be present in naevi that do not otherwise fulfil the criteria for the diagnosis of a dysplastic naevus.[259,260]

The *stromal response* consists of lamellar and concentric fibroplasia of the papillary dermis, associated with a proliferation of dermal dendrocytes.[261] Sometimes there is fibrosis in the upper reticular dermis resulting in more widely spaced nests, often of larger size than usual. Such cases can be worrisome; they are often received in consultation (Fig. 32.20). There is also a patchy superficial lymphocytic infiltrate.[229] There is sometimes new vessel formation.

A dermal naevus cell component is usually present in the central part of the lesion, consisting of small cells or epithelioid cells, but showing only slight evidence of maturation and with impairment of pigment synthesis. In other words, dysplastic naevi are usually compound naevi with peripheral lentiginous and junctional activity and random cytological atypia in the epidermal component.

Ackerman and others have placed emphasis on architectural rather than cytological atypia in defining a dysplastic naevus. They stress the importance of the 'shoulder phenomenon' (peripheral extension of the junctional component beyond the dermal component) in making the diagnosis.[257,262,263] This approach leads to the misdiagnosis of lentiginous naevi (see p. 779) as dysplastic naevi. Lentiginous naevi are not uncommon in patients with the dysplastic naevus syndrome.

Dysplastic naevi have been reported in contiguity with up to one-third or more of superficial spreading melanomas.[264–267] In determining whether a dysplastic naevus is present it has been proposed that the atypical lentiginous melanocytic hyperplasia should extend three or more rete pegs beyond the most lateral margin of the in situ or invasive melanoma.[265] Critics of this definition would argue that the diagnosis of dysplastic naevus is being applied indiscriminately in this and other situations.[268,269] Dysplastic (atypical) melanocytes in an evolving melanoma in situ should not be regarded as indicative of a precursor dysplastic naevus.

The AgNOR rating (see p. 801) of dysplastic naevi is not significantly different from that of common naevi.[270–273] With immunoperoxidase techniques, S100 protein can be detected in the cells. However, the expression of HMB-45 is limited to epidermal melanocytes and cells in the papillary dermis.[274,275]

Electron microscopy. The melanosomes in epidermal melanocytes in dysplastic naevi are abnormal, with incompletely developed lamellae and uneven melanization.[276,277] The melanosomes are spherical. These abnormal melanosomes are transferred to keratinocytes before being completely melanized, and they reveal marked degradation.[276]

MALIGNANT MELANOMA

The incidence of malignant melanoma varies in different parts of the world. Several studies have examined the sun exposure habits of patients with melanoma and found evidence that they have increased light sensitivity.[278,279] A history of painful or blistering sunburn during childhood or adolescence is sometimes obtained.[280] The role of chronic sun exposure is more controversial.[281,282] However, evidence from recent case-control studies suggests that both total accumulated exposure to sunlight and intermittent intense exposure increase the risk of developing malignant melanoma.[283]

The subtropical state of Queensland in northern Australia has the highest incidence of melanoma in the world — 32 new cases annually per 100 000 of the population.[284,285] The incidence in Scotland is 4.9/100 000, in Scandinavia it is 10/100 000, and in Arizona 27/100 000.[286] There appears to have been a doubling in the incidence of melanoma in the last decade or so.[286] Despite this alarming trend, the prognosis has continued to improve because patients are presenting at an earlier stage with smaller and, therefore, potentially curable lesions.[287]

There is increasing interest in identifying other risk factors for the development of malignant melanoma, in particular precursor melanocytic lesions.[288,289] The role of dysplastic and congenital naevi has been described already (see pp. 793 and 789). A more diffuse form of melanocytic dysplasia associated clinically with diffuse mottling or freckling around a melanoma has been described.[290] To date, this finding has been retrospective and its full significance remains to be evaluated.

There is also evidence that the presence of large numbers of common (banal, non-dysplastic) acquired naevi is a strong risk factor for the development of melanoma.[291–293] In turn, proneness to develop naevi correlates with skin complexion, hair colour and tanning ability.[294–297] Xeroderma pigmentosum (see p. 288),[298] Cowden's disease (see p. 826)[299] and infection with the human immunodeficiency virus[300] have been associated with the development of melanoma.

Classification

The clinicopathological classification of malignant melanoma has evolved into six groups, based on proposals by Clark[301] and McGovern[302,303] 20 years ago. The relative incidence of each type of melanoma varies considerably in different areas — for example, there is a higher proportion of lentigo maligna melanomas in Caucasians living in subtropical and tropical areas[291,304] and of acral lentiginous melanomas in Japanese.[305] The figures quoted in parentheses are therefore only a guide to the relative incidence of each type.

1. Lentigo maligna melanoma (5–15%)
2. Superficial spreading melanoma (50–75%)
3. Nodular melanoma (15–35%)
4. Acral lentiginous melanoma (5–10%)
5. Desmoplastic (and neurotropic) melanoma (rare)
6. Miscellaneous group (rare)

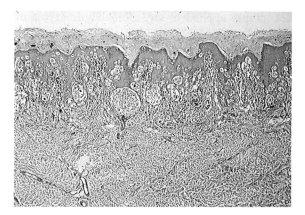

Fig. 32.22   Superficial spreading melanoma. This lesion is level 1 (in situ). Atypical melanocytes show 'buckshot scatter' within the epidermis.
Haematoxylin — eosin

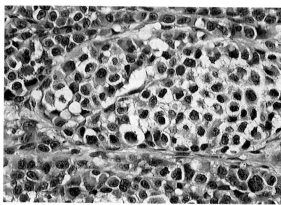

Fig. 32.23   Nodular melanoma. The tumour cells in the dermis have large, hyperchromatic nuclei. There is no melanin present in the cells. They were positive for S100 protein.
Haematoxylin — eosin

and resemble those of normal melanocytes, unlike the spheroidal and abnormal appearance of the melanosomes in superficial spreading and nodular melanomas.[357]

Superficial spreading melanoma is characterized by a proliferation of atypical melanocytes, singly and in nests, at all levels within the epidermis. This pagetoid spread within the epidermis is sometimes known as 'buckshot scatter' (Fig. 32.22). Superficial adnexal epithelium may also be involved. The infiltrative component may be arranged in solid masses or may have a fascicular arrangement. The cells may be epithelioid, naevus cell-like, or even spindle-shaped without evidence of maturation during their descent into the dermis.[358] Again the degree of cytological atypia varies from case to case.[359]

A rare variant of melanoma, usually of the superficial spreading type, is the *verrucous melanoma*.[360] It is characterized by marked epidermal hyperplasia, elongation of the rete ridges and overlying hyperkeratosis.[360a] It is often misdiagnosed clinically as a seborrhoeic keratosis.[360]

Nodular melanoma has no adjacent intraepidermal component of atypical melanocytes, although there is usually epidermal invasion by malignant cells directly overlying the dermal mass. The dermal component is usually composed of oval to round epithelioid cells but, as in

other types of melanoma, this can be quite variable (Fig. 32.23).

Acral lentiginous melanomas have a radial growth phase which is characterized by a lentiginous pattern of atypical melanocytes, with some nesting (Fig. 32.24).[330] There may be some 'buckshot scatter' of melanocytes, but this is never as marked as in superficial spreading melanoma.

The melanocytes may be plump with a surrounding clear halo giving a lacunar appearance, or they may have heavily pigmented dendritic

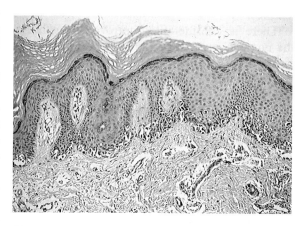

Fig. 32.24   Acral lentiginous melanoma (radial growth phase). There are atypical melanocytes within the basal layer. They show only slight upward spread.
Haematoxylin — eosin

processes. The epidermal component may look misleadingly benign. The epidermis is usually hyperplastic; focal ulceration may occur. The invasive component may consist of epithelioid cells or spindle cells or resemble naevus cells. There may be a desmoplastic stromal response. Osteosarcomatous change has been reported in the stroma in one case.[361] It is not uncommon for tumour cells to have infiltrated the deep dermis or subcutaneous tissue by the time of diagnosis.[362]

Desmoplastic melanomas are composed of strands of elongated, spindle-shaped cells surrounded by mature collagen bundles (Fig. 32.25). These cells resemble fibroblasts but there are scattered cells with hyperchromatic and even bizarre nuclei.[363] Multinucleate cells are often present. Small foci of neurotropism may be seen.[364] The tumour infiltrates deeply. There may be scattered collections of lymphocytes within the tumour. Heterotopic bone and cartilage may form.[365,366] There is often a lentigo maligna epidermal component overlying or towards one edge of the lesion.[350] The tumour cells are nearly always amelanotic, but they are positive for vimentin in all cases and for S100 protein in approximately 95% of cases.[363,367] HMB-45, which has more specificity for melanoma cells than S100 protein, is not expressed in most of the cases (see p. 801).

Sometimes only a minority of the malignant cells (10–20%) express S100 protein or HMB-45. In these instances, clusters and nests of cells stain positively. Sometimes, occasional scattered tumour cells stain positively with these markers in immunoperoxidase preparations of non-melanocytic lesions. This is a false-positive reaction. The cells in a desmoplastic melanoma have abundant rough endoplasmic reticulum, and sometimes intracytoplasmic collagen and macular desmosomes. Non-membrane-bound melanin granules and premelanosomes have been noted in some cases[347,368] although they have been specifically excluded in others.[367] The most accepted view is that the desmoplastic component is derived from melanocytes that have undergone adaptive fibroplasia,[363] although contrary views favour a fibroblastic stromal response[346] or neurosarcomatous differentiation.[369]

In the *neurotropic variant* (Fig. 32.26) there are spindle-shaped cells with neuroma-like patterns and a tendency to adopt a circumferential arrangement around small nerves in the deep dermis and subcutaneous tissue (neurotropism).[370,371] Interlacing bundles of cells are seen. Often desmoplastic and neurotropic patterns occur together in the same neoplasm.[372] The cells vary in size and nuclear staining. The absence of S100 protein using immunoperoxidase techniques does not exclude the

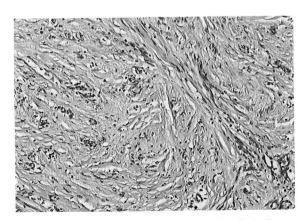

Fig. 32.25 Desmoplastic melanoma. Bundles of spindle shaped cells are present in the dermis admixed with collagen and blood vessels. This case was initially misdiagnosed as 'scar tissue'.
Haematoxylin — eosin

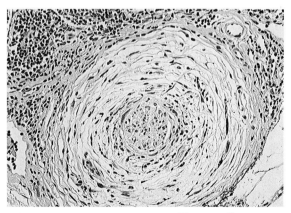

Fig. 32.26 Neurotropic melanoma. Tumour cells are loosely arranged in a concentric fashion around a small nerve in the subcutis. Lymphocytes are present in the surrounding tissue.
Haematoxylin — eosin

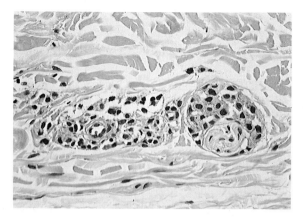

Fig. 32.27   Melanoma composed of small naevus-like cells. Tumour cells surround a small nerve in the deep dermis. The patient developed metastases one year after the removal of this lesion.
Haematoxylin — eosin

diagnosis, as this antigen may be absent in up to 20% of cases;[373] this figure seems unusually high in my experience.

Minimal deviation melanoma is the term applied to melanomas in which the vertical growth phase is composed of a uniform population of cells whose cytological features deviate only minimally from naevus cells.[306,374-376] Epithelioid or spindle cell features may be present. Included in this group by some pathologists is the melanoma composed of cells resembling small naevus cells (Fig. 32.27). The concept of minimal deviation melanoma has not gained universal acceptance.[377,378] There is some evidence that this diagnosis has been applied indiscriminately to difficult and borderline lesions.

Level and thickness. In any report on a malignant melanoma the anatomical level of invasion (Clark's level) and the thickness of the tumour (Breslow thickness)[379,380] should be stated. Five anatomical levels are recognized:[303]

1 — confined to the epidermis (in situ melanoma)
2 — invasion of the papillary dermis
3 — invasion to the papillary/reticular dermal interface
4 — invasion into the reticular dermis
5 — invasion into subcutaneous fat.

The thickness of a melanoma is measured from the top of the granular layer (undersurface of the stratum corneum) to the deepest tumour cell. Melanomas less than 0.76 mm in thickness are regarded as being 'thin melanomas'. They generally have an excellent prognosis. It has been suggested that 0.85 mm is a better break-point than 0.76 mm for defining a prognostically favourable group of melanomas.[381] Numerous clinical and histological features are related to the tumour thickness.[382]

Regression. Partial regression may be found in up to one-third of melanomas;[383,384] the figure is higher in thin melanomas.[385-388] Active regression is recognized by the presence of a heavy lymphocytic infiltrate in the dermis with loss or degeneration of tumour cells.[389] It seems likely that tumour cells are removed by lymphocyte-mediated apoptosis.[390] Previous (old) regression is characterized by the presence of vascular fibrous tissue with or without melanophages, and perhaps a scanty lymphocytic infiltrate.[389] The prognostic significance of partial regression will be considered later (see p. 801).

Approximately 5% of patients with melanoma present with metastatic disease in the absence of a recognized primary tumour. In many of these cases of so-called 'occult primary melanoma' it is probable that the primary lesion underwent spontaneous regression.[391,392] Other possibilities include origin of the tumour in lymph nodes or in visceral organs, or a primary cutaneous lesion which is initially undetectable.[391,393]

Metastases

Metastases in cases of malignant melanoma are usually to regional lymph nodes in the first instance. The probability of nodal metastases is related to the Clark level[394] and the Breslow tumour thickness (see above).[395,396] Nodal metastases are quite uncommon in lesions less than 1 mm in thickness; their frequency exceeds 50% among lesions greater than 4 mm in thickness.[394,396,397] Metastases also take place to the skin and subcutaneous tissue, lungs, brain and dura, gastrointestinal tract, heart, liver and adrenal glands.[398,399] Rarely, dermal lymphatic invasion associated with cutaneous metastatic disease may give a picture resembling that of so-called 'inflammatory' carcinoma of the breast.[400]

The development of generalized melanosis in patients with malignant melanoma has been attributed by some to an unlimited spread of single melanoma cells throughout the dermis,[401] but others have specifically excluded the presence of tumour cells and have found numerous perivascular melanophages in the dermis.[402,403]

Multiple primary lesions

Additional primary lesions may develop in approximately 5% of patients with malignant melanoma.[404] Sometimes it is difficult to distinguish between a new primary lesion and an epidermotropic metastasis.[405] Furthermore, the whole subject of multiple primary lesions needs re-evaluation in the light of the dysplastic naevus syndrome (see p. 792), the recognition of which post-dates the studies on multiple primary lesions.[82]

Special techniques

In suspected cases of melanoma which are amelanotic or oligomelanotic, a number of special stains and techniques may be used to establish a diagnosis.[308,406] These include the Masson–Fontana, Schmorl's and modified Warthin–Starry stains for melanin,[407] the identification of premelanosomes on electron microscopy, and the demonstration of S100 protein, HMB-45 and NKI/C-3 using immunoperoxidase techniques.[408–413] S100 protein is also found in naevi and Langerhans cells as well as cutaneous neural tumours.[414,415] HMB-45, a monoclonal antibody with putative specificity for melanoma cells, stains stimulated melanocytes such as junctional melanocytes in naevi, some cells in the papillary dermis in dysplastic naevi, melanocytes in blue naevi and some cells in Spitz naevi (see p. 787). It is a highly sensitive marker for melanoma cells although it does not stain the cells of spindle cell melanomas.[411–413] Neuron-specific enolase[416] and vimentin[417] have also been found in melanomas, but myelin basic protein has not.[410] Melanoma cells and some naevi will show positive fluorescence when unstained sections from formalin-fixed, paraffin-embedded tissue is examined.[418,419] To date, this method has not been used in routine diagnosis.

A recently developed technique which shows considerable promise in the assessment of borderline lesions is the measurement of silver-positive nucleolar organizer regions (AgNOR count) in a representative number of tumour cells. The mean AgNOR count for melanoma cells is significantly higher than for benign naeval cells although some overlap occurs. However, an AgNOR count of more than 2.0 per cell is very suggestive of a malignant melanoma.[270–273,420]

Frozen sections are now used infrequently in the surgical management of melanoma. The technique is reliable in experienced hands.[421,422]

Surface microscopy is the most recent method to have been suggested in the assessment of pigmented lesions.[423] Currently it has little practical application to routine diagnosis.

Prognostic factors in melanoma

The comparatively recent introduction of sophisticated statistical techniques, such as multivariate analyses, has led to the delineation of histological criteria with independent predictive value with respect to prognosis.[82]

Survival rates for malignant melanoma continue to improve because patients are now presenting earlier with thinner (and therefore low risk) melanomas.[424,425] 5-year survival rates of 85% or better for females and 75% for males are being reported.[426]

It is now accepted that the *maximum tumour thickness* (Breslow thickness) is the most important single predictor of survival in clinical stage 1 melanomas.[427,428] A possible caveat is for thin melanomas where the level may be a more reliable predictor of low risk status,[426] and for thin melanomas with regression where several reports,[385,429,430] but not the majority,[386,431–434] have suggested that the presence of regression may carry a significant risk of metastasis. Put in another way, the 5-year survival rate for thin melanomas in some series has been 100%,[425,435] although some studies have recorded a small number of deaths, particularly in patients whose tumours were more than level 2, or for those with regression.[436–440]

Most authors now agree that the prognostic significance of the *Clark level* is derived from its secondary correlation with tumour thickness.[441,442] The level of invasion may have independent prognostic significance in certain circumstances, particularly as a predictor of low risk status in thin melanomas.[426,437]

Ulceration, particularly where its width is greater than 3 mm, has adverse prognostic significance.[443–446] Ulcerated melanomas also have significantly more mitoses.[447]

In some studies the *anatomical site* has been shown to be a prognostic predictive variable.[448,449] High risk sites include the so-called BANS areas of the body — B (back), A (posterior upper arm), N (posterior neck), S (scalp) — and the feet and genitalia.[387,448] Subsequent studies have been unable to confirm a site-dependent difference in mortality for the BANS area,[437,450] except for melanomas of intermediate thickness (0.76–1.69 mm).[451] In one study, lesions of the upper trunk had a worse prognosis than those of the lower trunk, for the same thickness.[452] The *mitotic rate*, particularly if greater than 6/mm^2, has prognostic significance.[453,454] The product of the thickness in mm and the number of mitoses per mm^2 (the prognostic index) may give prognostic information.[455,456] The presence of *microscopic satellite deposits* separated from the main body of the tumour has an adverse influence.[443,457,458] The presence of satellites has been shown to be a better indicator of occult regional lymph node metastases in clinical stage 1 melanoma than the tumour thickness.[459]

It is generally agreed that there is no survival difference between superficial spreading, nodular and acral lentiginous melanomas when these are corrected for thickness.[337,384,426,460] Although McGovern and his colleagues presented evidence that lentigo maligna melanoma, particularly in women, has a more favourable prognosis, independent of thickness,[461] this has not been confirmed in subsequent studies.[462]

Increased nuclear area and *deviation from diploidy* are two further parameters which have an adverse prognostic significance.[463]

The clinical[464,465] and pathological stages[441] of the disease obviously have a bearing on the survival of the patient. The probability of lymph nodal metastases is directly related to the Clark level[394] and the thickness of the tumour.[395,396] The presence of plasma cells in the primary lesion is a recently delineated criterion for the occurrence of lymph node metastases.[466,467] Tumour cells which are not apparent in haematoxylin and eosin stained preparations of regional lymph nodes may be detected using immunoperoxidase methods and antibodies to S100 protein or HMB-45. The presence of these so-called 'occult metastases' is of adverse prognostic significance.[468]

The following factors have not been shown to have independent prognostic significance, according to various studies: the presence of a lymphocytic infiltrate (see below),[453] angioinvasion,[427,469] regression[383] (except possibly in thin melanomas), size and shape of the lesion,[470,470a] cell type,[471] pigmentation,[302] age of the patient,[426] and incisional biopsy prior to excision,[472–474] although in the latter circumstance, one group has found an adverse effect.[475] The prognostic significance of a coexisting intradermal naevus has been controversial.[82,476] Naevi have been found in approximately 10–30% of melanomas, depending on the diligence with which a search is made and the criteria used for accepting a naevus.[477,478] It has been suggested that this feature may be associated with a more favourable prognosis,[165,479] but it needs to be reconsidered in the light of the recognition of sporadic dysplastic naevi (see p. 792).[265]

Various clinical aspects have been studied for prognostic significance. It is well established that females with clinical stage 1 and stage 2 melanoma have superior survival rates to males.[480–483] This may result from the occurrence of lesions in prognostically more favourable sites than in males (lower extremities rather than the trunk) and the presence of thinner tumours at the time of removal.[426] However, other factors may lead to a more favourable prognosis in premenopausal[447,484] and, in some circumstances, postmenopausal women.[485,486] There are conflicting results regarding the influence of pregnancy on survival rates.[487] An intercurrent melanoma arising during pregnancy may[488] or may not[489] lead to a worse prognosis than in control groups. However, pregnancy seems to have no effect on patients who have had a melanoma diagnosed and treated prior to the pregnancy.[488]

The presence of vitiligo, usually commencing after the diagnosis of melanoma, appears to be prognostically favourable in patients with secondary melanoma.[490–492]

Controlled studies suggest that arbitrary wide margins of excision are not justified.[458,493–496] Local recurrence rates for thick melanomas are increased when the surgical margin is less than 3 cm, although the overall survival rates do not appear to be affected.[493,497] With subungual melanomas, the survival rate is reasonably good provided a radical surgical approach is adopted initially.[498]

A pooled study of 15 798 stage 1 and 2116 stage 2 melanomas recorded a 5-year survival of 79% for stage 1 lesions and 34% for stage 2.[499] The pooled 5-year survival for thin melanomas was 96%. Multifactorial analyses using the data from eight centres found that the most significant prognostic variables were tumour thickness, the presence of ulceration, the anatomical site, the patient's sex and the tumour growth pattern.[499] This compares with a study by Clark's group that found that the favourable prognostic features in a stage 1 melanoma were low mitotic rate, tumour-infiltrating lymphocytes, a thin lesion, location on the extremities, female sex and absence of regression.[317a]

Finally, recent hazard rate analyses suggest that the peak hazard rate for death in clinical stage 1 cutaneous melanoma is the 48th month of follow-up and that after 120 months' survival the risk of dying from melanoma is virtually zero.[500] Although rare, late recurrences (beyond 10 years) are recorded.[501,502]

REFERENCES

Introduction

1. Fulk CS. Primary disorders of hyperpigmentation. J Am Acad Dermatol 1984; 10: 1–16.

Lesions with basal melanocyte proliferation

2. Sexton FM, Maize JC. Melanotic macules and melanoacanthomas of the lip. Am J Dermatopathol 1987; 9: 438–444.
3. Spann CR, Owen LG, Hodge SJ. The labial melanotic macule. Arch Dermatol 1987; 123: 1029–1031.
4. Barnhill RL, Albert LS, Shama SK et al. Genital lentiginosis: A clinical and histopathologic study. J Am Acad Dermatol 1990; 22: 453–460.
5. Leicht S, Youngberg G, Diaz-Miranda C. Atypical pigmented penile macules. Arch Dermatol 1988; 124: 1267–1270.
6. Revuz J, Clerici T. Penile melanosis. J Am Acad Dermatol 1989; 20: 567–570.
7. Lambert WC, Lambert MW, Mesa ML et al. Melanoacanthoma and related disorders. Simulants of acral-lentiginous (P-P-S-M) melanoma. Int J Dermatol 1987; 26: 508–510.
8. Tomich CE, Zunt SL. Melanoacanthosis (melanoacanthoma) of the oral mucosa. J Dermatol Surg Oncol 1990; 16: 231–236.
9. Horlick HP, Walther RR, Zegarelli DJ et al. Mucosal melanotic macule, reactive type: A simulation of melanoma. J Am Acad Dermatol 1988; 19: 786–791.
10. Zemtsov A, Bergfeld WF. Oral melanoacanthoma with prominent spongiotic intraepithelial vesicles. J Cutan Pathol 1989; 16: 365–369.
11. Ackerman AB, Ragaz A. The lives of lesions. Chronology in dermatology. New York: Masson Publishing USA; 1984: 203–209.
12. Thompson GW, Diehl AK. Partial unilateral lentiginosis. Arch Dermatol 1980; 116: 356.
13. O'Neill JF, James WD. Inherited patterned lentiginosis in blacks. Arch Dermatol 1989; 125: 1231–1235.
14. Uhle P, Norvell SS Jr. Generalized lentiginosis. J Am Acad Dermatol 1988; 18: 444–447.
15. Peterson LL, Serrill WS. Lentiginosis associated with left atrial myxoma. J Am Acad Dermatol 1984; 10: 337–340.
16. Selmanowitz VJ, Orentreich N, Felsenstein JM. Lentiginosis profusa syndrome (multiple lentigines syndrome). Arch Dermatol 1971; 104: 393–401.
17. Gorlin RJ, Anderson RC, Blaw M. Multiple lentigenes syndrome. Am J Dis Child 1969; 117: 652–662.
18. Atherton DJ, Pitcher DW, Wells RS, MacDonald DM. A syndrome of various cutaneous pigmented lesions, myxoid neurofibromata and atrial myxoma: the NAME syndrome. Br J Dermatol 1980; 103: 421–429.
19. Rhodes AR, Silverman RA, Harrist TJ, Perez-Atayde AR. Mucocutaneous lentigines, cardiocutaneous myxomas, and multiple blue nevi: The 'LAMB' syndrome. J Am Acad Dermatol 1984; 10: 72–82.
20. Carney JA, Gordon H, Carpenter PG et al. The complex of myxomas, spotty pigmentation, and

Ultrastructure of halo nevi. J Cutan Pathol 1975; 2: 71–81.

111. Mehregan AH, King JR. Multiple target-like pigmented nevi. Arch Dermatol 1972; 105: 129–130.

112. Happle R. Kokardennaevus. Hautarzt 1974; 25: 594–596.

113. Warin AP. Cockarde naevus. Clin Exp Dermatol 1976; 1: 221–224.

114. James MP, Wells RS. Cockade naevus: An unusual variant of the benign cellular naevus. Acta Derm Venereol 1980; 60: 360–363.

115. Guzzo C, Johnson B, Honig P. Cockarde nevus: a case report and review of the literature. Pediatr Dermatol 1988; 5: 250–253.

116. Mishima Y. Eccrine-centered nevus. Arch Dermatol 1973; 107: 59–61.

117. Kornberg R, Ackerman AB. Pseudomelanoma. Recurrent melanocytic nevus following partial surgical removal. Arch Dermatol 1975; 111: 1588–1590.

118. Park HK, Leonard DD, Arrington JH, Lund HZ. Recurrent melanocytic nevi: Clinical and histologic review of 175 cases. J Am Acad Dermatol 1987; 17: 285–292.

118a. Estrada JA, Pierard-Franchimont C, Pierard GE. Histogenesis of recurrent nevus. Am J Dermatopathol 1990; 12: 370–372.

118b. Ho VC, Sober AJ. Pigmented streaks in melanoma scars. J Dermatol Surg Oncol 1990; 16: 663–666.

119. Weedon D, Little JH. Spindle and epithelioid cell nevi in children and adults. A review of 211 cases of the Spitz nevus. Cancer 1977; 40: 217–225.

120. Weedon D. The Spitz naevus. Clin Oncol 1984; 3: 493–507.

121. Spitz S. Melanomas of childhood. Am J Pathol 1948; 24: 591–609.

122. Allen AC. Juvenile melanomas. Ann NY Acad Sci 1963; 100: 29–46.

123. Coskey RJ, Mehregan A. Spindle cell nevi in adults and children. Arch Dermatol 1973; 108: 535–536.

124. Paniago-Pereira C, Maize JC, Ackerman AB. Nevus of large spindle and/or epithelioid cells (Spitz's nevus). Arch Dermatol 1978; 114: 1811–1823.

125. Capetanakis J. Juvenile melanoma disseminatum. Br J Dermatol 1975; 92: 207–211.

126. Gould DJ, Bleehen SS. Multiple agminate juvenile melanoma. Clin Exp Dermatol 1980; 5: 63–65.

127. Lancer HA, Muhlbauer JE, Sober AJ. Multiple agminated spindle cell nevi. Unique clinical presentation and review. J Am Acad Dermatol 1983; 8: 707–711.

128. Krakowski A, Tur E, Brenner S. Multiple agminated juvenile melanoma: A case with a sunburn history, and a review. Dermatologica 1981; 163: 270–275.

129. Smith SA, Day CL. Eruptive widespread Spitz nevi. J Am Acad Dermatol 1986; 15: 1155–1159.

130. Paties CT, Borroni G, Rosso R, Vassalo G. Relapsing eruptive multiple Spitz nevi or metastatic Spitzoid malignant melanoma? Am J Dermatopathol 1987; 9: 520–527.

131. Hamm H, Happle R, Brocker E-B. Multiple agminate Spitz naevi: review of the literature and report of a case with distinctive immunohistological features. Br J Dermatol 1987; 117: 511–522.

132. Palazzo JP, Duray PH. Congenital agminated Spitz nevi: immunoreactivity with a melanoma-associated

133. Renfro L, Grant-Kels JM, Brown SA. Multiple agminate Spitz nevi. Pediatr Dermatol 1989; 6: 114–117.

134. Kopf A, Andrade R. Benign juvenile melanoma. In: Baer R, Kopf A, eds. Yearbook of dermatology (1965–1966). Chicago: Yearbook Medical Publishers, 1966; 7–52.

135. Gartmann H, Ganser M. Der Spitz-Naevus. Z Hautkr 1985; 60: 22–28.

136. Goovaerts G, Buyssens N. Nevus cell maturation or atrophy? Am J Dermatopathol 1988; 10: 20–27.

137. Kamino H, Flotte TJ, Misheloff E. Eosinophilic globules in Spitz's nevi. New findings and a diagnostic sign. Am J Dermatopathol 1979; 1: 319–324.

138. Arbuckle S, Weedon D. Eosinophilic globules in the Spitz nevus. J Am Acad Dermatol 1982; 7: 324–327.

139. Schmoeckel C, Stolz W, Burgeson R, Krieg T. Identification of basement membrane components in eosinophilic globules in a case of Spitz's nevus. Am J Dermatopathol 1990; 12: 272–274.

140. Scott G, Chen KTK, Rosai J. Pseudoepitheliomatous hyperplasia in Spitz nevi. Arch Pathol Lab Med 1989; 113: 61–63.

141. Rogers G, Advani H, Ackerman AB. Combined Spitz's nevus: a histologic simulator of malignant melanoma. Arch Dermatol 1984; 120: 1607 (abstract).

142. Peters MS, Goellner JR. Spitz naevi and malignant melanomas of childhood and adolescence. Histopathology 1986; 10: 1289–1302.

143. LeBoit PE, van Fletcher H. A comparative study of Spitz nevus and nodular malignant melanoma using image analysis cytometry. J Invest Dermatol 1987; 88: 753–757.

144. Argenyi ZB, Wick MR, Kemp JD, Baldwin MM. Comparative immunohistochemical evaluation of benign and malignant spindle cell melanocytic lesions. J Cutan Pathol 1988; 15: 294 (abstract).

145. Palazzo J, Duray PH. Typical, dysplastic, congenital, and Spitz nevi: a comparative histochemical study. Hum Pathol 1989; 20: 341–346.

146. Howat AJ, Giri DD, Cotton DWK, Slater DN. Nucleolar organizer regions in Spitz nevi and malignant melanomas. Cancer 1989; 63: 474–478.

147. Barr RJ, Morales RV, Graham JH. Desmoplastic nevus. A distinct histologic variant of mixed spindle cell and epithelioid cell nevus. Cancer 1980; 46: 557–564.

148. Reed RJ, Ichinose H, Clark WH, Mihm MC. Common and uncommon melanocytic nevi and borderline melanomas. Semin Oncol 1975; 2: 119–147.

149. Barnhill RL, Barnhill MA, Berwick M, Mihm MC. The histologic spectrum of pigmented spindle cell nevus. Hum Pathol 1991; 22: 52–58.

150. Smith NP. The pigmented spindle cell tumor of Reed: an underdiagnosed lesion. Semin Diagn Pathol 1987; 4: 75–87.

151. Sau P, Graham JH, Helwig EB. Pigmented spindle cell nevus. Arch Dermatol 1984; 120: 1615 (abstract).

152. Barnhill RL, Mihm MC Jr. Pigmented spindle cell naevus and its variants: distinction from melanoma. Br J Dermatol 1989; 121: 717–726.

153. Wistuba I, Gonzalez S. Eosinophilic globules in

monoclonal antibody. J Cutan Pathol 1988; 15: 166–170.

pigmented spindle cell nevus. Am J Dermatopathol 1990; 12: 268–271.

154. Smith KJ, Barrett TL, Skelton HG III et al. Spindle cell and epithelioid cell nevi with atypia and metastasis (malignant Spitz nevus). Am J Surg Pathol 1989; 13: 931–939.

155. Walton RG, Jacobs AH, Cox AJ. Pigmented lesions in newborn infants. Br J Dermatol 1976; 95: 389–396.

156. Kroon S, Clemmensen OJ. Incidence of congenital melanocytic nevi in newborn babies in Denmark. J Am Acad Dermatol 1987; 17: 422–426.

157. Castilla EE, Dutra MDG, Orioli-Parreiras IM. Epidemiology of congenital pigmented naevi: 1. Incidence rates and relative frequencies. Br J Dermatol 1981; 104: 307–315.

158. Kopf AW, Bart RS, Hennessey P. Congenital nevocytic nevi and malignant melanoma. J Am Acad Dermatol 1979; 1: 123–130.

159. Alper JC. Congenital nevi. The controversy rages on. Arch Dermatol 1985; 121: 734–735.

160. Illig L, Weidner F, Hundeiker M et al. Congenital nevi ≤ 10cm as precursors to melanoma. 52 cases, a review, and a new conception. Arch Dermatol 1985; 121: 1274–1281.

161. Elder DE. The blind men and the elephant. Different views of small congenital nevi. Arch Dermatol 1985; 121: 1263–1265.

162. Clemmensen O, Ackerman AB. All small congenital nevi need not be removed. Am J Dermatopathol (Suppl) 1984; 1: 189–194.

163. Keipert JA. Giant pigmented naevus: the frequency of malignant change and indications for treatment in prepubertal children. Australas J Dermatol 1985; 26: 81–85.

164. Rhodes AR, Melski JW. Small congenital nevocellular nevi and the risk of cutaneous melanoma. J Pediatr 1982; 100: 219–224.

165. Rhodes AR, Sober AJ, Day CL et al. The malignant potential of small congenital nevocellular nevi. An estimate of association based on a histologic study of 234 primary cutaneous melanomas. J Am Acad Dermatol 1982; 6: 230–241.

166. Rhodes AR, Silverman RA, Harrist TJ, Melski JW. A histologic comparison of congenital and acquired nevomelanocytic nevi. Arch Dermatol 1985; 121: 1266–1273.

167. Schneiderman H, Wu A Y-Y, Campbell WA et al. Congenital melanoma with multiple prenatal metastases. Cancer 1987; 60: 1371–1377.

168. Silvers DN, Helwig EB. Melanocytic nevi in neonates. J Am Acad Dermatol 4: 166–175.

169. Kuehnl-Petzoldt C, Volk B, Kunze J et al. Histology of congenital nevi during the first year of life. Am J Dermatopathol (Suppl) 1984; 1: 81–88.

170. Mark GJ, Mihm MC, Liteplo MG et al. Congenital melanocytic nevi of the small and garment type. Clinical, histologic, and ultrastructural studies. Hum Pathol 1973; 4: 395–418.

171. Stenn KS, Arons M, Hurwitz S. Patterns of congenital nevocellular nevi. A histologic study of thirty-eight cases. J Am Acad Dermatol 1983; 9: 388–393.

172. Nickoloff BJ, Walton R, Pregerson-Rodan K et al. Immunohistologic patterns of congenital nevocellular nevi. Arch Dermatol 1986; 122: 1263–1268.

173. Rhodes AR. Congenital nevomelanocytic nevi. Histologic patterns in the first year of life and evolution during childhood. Arch Dermatol 1986; 122: 1257–1262.

174. Zitelli JA, Grant MG, Abell E, Boyd JB. Histologic patterns of congenital nevocytic nevi and implications for treatment. J Am Acad Dermatol 1984; 11: 402–409.

175. Kirschenbaum MB. Congenital melanocytic nevi. Arch Dermatol 1981; 117: 379–380.

176. Everett MA. Histopathology of congenital pigmented nevi. Am J Dermatopathol 1989; 11: 11–12.

177. Clemmensen OJ, Kroon S. The histology of "congenital features" in early acquired melanocytic nevi. J Am Acad Dermatol 1988; 19: 742–746.

178. Walsh MY, Mackie RM. Histological features of value in differentiating small congenital melanocytic naevi from acquired naevi. Histopathology 1988; 12: 145–154.

179. Padilla RS, McConnell TS, Gribble JT, Smoot C. Malignant melanoma arising in a giant congenital melanocytic nevus. A case report with cytogenetic and histopathologic analyses. Cancer 1988; 62: 2589–2594.

180. Kaplan EN. The risk of malignancy in large congenital nevi. Plast Reconstr Surg 1974; 53: 421–428.

181. Weidner N, Flanders DJ, Jochimsen PR, Stamler FW. Neurosarcomatous malignant melanoma arising in a neuroid giant congenital melanocytic nevus. Arch Dermatol 1985; 121: 1302–1306.

182. Hendrickson MR, Ross JC. Neoplasms arising in congenital giant nevi. Morphologic study of seven cases and a review of the literature. Am J Surg Pathol 1981; 5: 109–135.

Dermal melanocytic lesions

183. Uribe MGA. The Mongoloid spot. Australas J Dermatol 1976; 17: 61–64.

184. Hidano A. Persistent Mongolian spot in the adult. Arch Dermatol 1971; 103: 680–681.

185. Leung AKC. Mongolian spots in Chinese children. Int J Dermatol 1988; 27: 106–108.

186. Kikuchi I. What is a Mongolian spot? Int J Dermatol 1982; 21: 131–133.

187. Kikuchi I, Inoue S. Natural history of the Mongolian spot. J Dermatol 1980; 7: 449–450.

188. Hidano A, Kajima H, Endo Y. Bilateral nevus Ota associated with nevus Ito. A case of pigmentation on the lips. Arch Dermatol 1965; 91: 357–359.

189. Hidano A, Kajima H, Ikeda S et al. Natural history of nevus of Ota. Arch Dermatol 1967; 95: 187–195.

190. Mishima Y, Mevorah B. Nevus Ota and nevus Ito in American negroes. J Invest Dermatol 1961; 36: 133–154.

191. Kopf AW, Bart RS. Malignant blue (Ota's?) nevus. J Dermatol Surg Oncol 1982; 8: 442–445.

192. van Krieken JHJM, Boom BW, Scheffer E. Malignant transformation in a naevus of Ito. A case report. Histopathology 1988; 12: 100–102.

193. Burkhart CG, Gohara A. Dermal melanocyte hamartoma. A distinctive new form of dermal melanocytosis. Arch Dermatol 1981; 117: 102–104.

194. Radentz WH. Congenital common blue nevus. Arch Dermatol 1990; 126: 124–125.

195. Rodriguez HA, Ackerman LV. Cellular blue nevus. Clinicopathologic study of forty-five cases. Cancer 1968; 21: 393–405.
196. Temple-Camp CRE, Saxe N, King H. Benign and malignant cellular blue nevus. A clinicopathological study of 30 cases. Am J Dermatopathol 1988; 10: 289–296.
197. Hendricks WM. Eruptive blue nevi. J Am Acad Dermatol 1981; 4: 50–53.
198. Pittman JL, Fisher BK. Plaque-type blue nevus. Arch Dermatol 1976; 112: 1127–1128.
199. Bondi EE, Elder D, Guerry D, Clark WH. Target blue nevus. Arch Dermatol 1983; 119: 919–920.
200. Leopold JG, Richards DB. The interrelationship of blue and common naevi. J Pathol 1968; 95: 37–46.
201. Gartmann H, Muller HD. Über das gemeinsame Vorkommen von blauem Naevus und Naevuszellnaevus in em und derselbem Geschwulst ("combined nevus"). Z Hautkr 1977; 52: 389–398.
202. Newton JA, McGibbon DH. Blue naevus associated with trichoepithelioma: a report of two cases. J Cutan Pathol 1984; 11: 549–552.
203. Youngberg GA, Rasch EM, Douglas HL. Bizarre blue nevus: A case report with deoxyribonucleic acid content analysis. J Am Acad Dermatol 1986; 15: 336–341.
203a. Sun J, Morton TH Jr, Gown AM. Antibody HMB-45 identifies the cells of blue nevi. Am J Surg Pathol 1990; 14: 748–751.
204. Bhawan J, Chang WH, Edelstein LM. Cellular blue nevus. An ultrastructural study. J Cutan Pathol 1980; 7: 109–122.
205. Lambert WC, Brodkin RH. Nodal and subcutaneous cellular blue nevi. A pseudometastasizing pseudomelanoma. Arch Dermatol 1984; 120: 367–370.
206. Lamovec J. Blue nevus of the lymph node capsule. Report of a new case with review of the literature. Am J Clin Pathol 1984; 81: 367–372.
207. Merkow LP, Burt RC, Hayeslip DW et al. A cellular and malignant blue nevus: a light and electron microscopic study. Cancer 1969; 24: 888–896.
208. Goldenhersh MA, Savin RC, Barnhill RL, Stenn KS. Malignant blue nevus. Case report and literature review. J Am Acad Dermatol 1988; 19: 712–722.
209. Gartmann H, Lischka G. Maligner blauer naevus (Malignes dermales Melanozytom). Hautarzt 1972; 23: 175–178.
210. Kwittken J, Negri L. Malignant blue nevus. Case report of a negro woman. Arch Dermatol 1966; 94: 64–69.
211. Mishima Y. Cellular blue nevus. Melanogenic activity and malignant transformation. Arch Dermatol 1970; 101: 104–110.
212. Hernandez FJ. Malignant blue nevus. A light and electron microscopic study. Arch Dermatol 1973; 107: 741–744.
213. Kuhn A, Groth W, Gartmann H, Steigleder GK. Malignant blue nevus with metastases to the lung. Am J Dermatopathol 1988; 10: 436–441.
214. Levene A. Disseminated dermal melanocytosis terminating in melanoma. Br J Dermatol 1979; 101: 197–205.
215. Mevorah B, Frenk E, Delacretaz J. Dermal melanocytosis. Report of an unusual case.

Dermatologica 1977; 154: 107–114.
216. Tuthill RJ, Clark WH Jr, Levene A. Pilar neurocristic hamartoma. Its relationship to blue nevus and equine melanotic disease. Arch Dermatol 1982; 118: 592–596.
217. Hasegawa Y, Yasuhara M. Phakomatosis pigmentovascularis type IVa. Arch Dermatol 1985;121: 651–655.
218. Ruiz-Maldonado R, Tamayo L, Laterza AM. Phacomatis pigmentovascularis: a new syndrome? Report of four cases. Pediatr Dermatol 1987; 4: 189–196.

Dysplastic naevus

219. Sagebiel RW. The dysplastic melanocytic nevus. J Am Acad Dermatol 1989; 20: 496–501.
220. Rigel DS, Rivers JK, Kopf AW et al. Dysplastic nevi. Markers for increased risk for melanoma. Cancer 1989; 63: 386–389.
221. Greene MH. Dysplastic nevus syndrome. Hosp Pract 1984; 19: 91–103, 107–108.
222. Cooke KR, Spears GFS, Elder DE, Greene MH. Dysplastic nevi in a population-based survey. Cancer 1989; 63: 1240–1244.
223. Barnhill RL, Kiryu H, Sober AJ, Mihm MC JR. Frequency of dysplastic nevi among nevomelanocytic lesions submitted for histopathologic examination. Time trends over a 37-year period. Arch Dermatol 1990; 126: 463–465.
224. Elder DE, Goldman LI, Goldman SC et al. Dysplastic nevus syndrome. A phenotypic association of sporadic cutaneous melanoma. Cancer 1980; 46: 1787–1794.
225. Clark WH, Reimer RR, Greene M et al. Origin of familial malignant melanomas from heritable melanocytic lesions. 'The B-K mole syndrome'. Arch Dermatol 1978; 114: 732–738.
226. Lynch HT, Frichot BC, Lynch JF. Familial atypical multiple mole-melanoma syndrome. J Med Genet 1978; 15: 352–356.
227. Kopf AW, Friedman RJ, Rigel DS. Atypical mole syndrome. J Am Acad Dermatol 1990; 22: 117–118.
228. Greene MH, Clark WH Jr, Tucker MA et al. Acquired precursors of cutaneous malignant melanoma. The familial dysplastic nevus syndrome. N Engl J Med 1985; 312: 91–97.
229. Elder DE, Kraemer KH, Greene MH et al. The dysplastic nevus syndrome. Our definition. Am J Dermatopathol 1982; 4: 455–460.
230. Grob JJ, Andrac L, Romano MH et al. Dysplastic naevus in non-familial melanoma. A clinicopathological study of 101 cases. Br J Dermatol 1988; 118: 745–752.
231. Black WC, Hunt WC. Histologic correlations with the clinical diagnosis of dysplastic nevus. Am J Surg Pathol 1990; 14: 44–52.
232. Barnes LM, Nordlund JJ. The natural history of dysplastic nevi. A case history illustrating their evolution. Arch Dermatol 1987; 123: 1059–1061.
233. Clark WH Jr. The dysplastic nevus syndrome. Arch Dermatol 1988; 124: 1207–1210.
234. Mehregan AH. Dysplastic nevi: a histopathological investigation. J Cutan Pathol 1988; 15: 276–281.
235. Kopf AW, Lindsay AC, Rogers GS et al. Relationship of nevocytic nevi to sun exposure in dysplastic nevus

syndrome. J Am Acad Dermatol 1985; 12: 656–662.

236. Kopf AW, Gold RS, Rogers GS et al. Relationship of lumbosacral nevocytic nevi to sun exposure in dysplastic nevus syndrome. Arch Dermatol 1986; 122: 1003–1006.

237. Rampen FHJ, Fleuren BAM, de Boo TM, Lemmens WAJG. Prevalence of common "acquired" nevocytic nevi and dysplastic nevi is not related to ultraviolet exposure. J Am Acad Dermatol 1988; 18: 679–683.

238. Greene MH, Goldin LR, Clark WH et al. Familial cutaneous malignant melanoma: Autosomal dominant trait possibly linked to the Rh locus. Proc Natl Acad Sci USA 1983; 80: 6071–6075.

239. Bale SJ, Dracopoli NC, Tucker MA et al. Mapping the gene for hereditary cutaneous malignant melanoma-dysplastic nevus to chromosome 1_p. N Engl J Med 1989; 320: 1367–1372.

240. McDonagh AJG, Wright AL, Messenger AG. Dysplastic naevi in association with partial deletion of chromosome 11. Clin Exp Dermatol 1990; 15: 44–45.

241. Lynch HT, Fusaro RM, Pester J et al. Tumour spectrum in the FAMMM syndrome. Br J Cancer 1981; 44: 553–560.

242. Adams SJ, Rustin MHA, Robinson TWE, Munro DD. The dysplastic naevus syndrome and endocrine disease. Br Med J 1984; 288: 1790–1791.

243. Greene MH, Tucker MA, Clark WH et al. Hereditary melanoma and the dysplastic nevus syndrome: The risk of cancers other than melanoma. J Am Acad Dermatol 1987; 16: 792–797.

244. National Institutes of Health Consensus Development Conference. Precursors to malignant melanoma, 1983; volume 4, number 9.

245. Albert LS, Rhodes AR, Sober AJ. Dysplastic melanocytic nevi and cutaneous melanoma: Markers of increased melanoma risk for affected persons and blood relatives. J Am Acad Dermatol 1990; 22: 69–75.

246. Duvic M, Lowe L, Rapini RP et al. Eruptive dysplastic nevi associated with human immunodeficiency virus infection. Arch Dermatol 1989; 125: 397–401.

247. Barker JNWN, MacDonald DM. Eruptive dysplastic naevi following renal transplantation. Clin Exp Dermatol 1988; 13: 123–125.

248. Sterry W, Christophers E. Quadrant distribution of dysplastic nevus syndrome. Arch Dermatol 1988; 124: 926–929.

249. Cook MG, Fallowfield ME. Dysplastic naevi — an alternative view. Histopathology 1990; 16: 29–35.

250. Clemente C, Cochran AJ, Elder DE et al. Histopathologic diagnosis of dysplastic nevi: concordance among pathologists convened by the W.H.O. melanoma programme. (in press).

251. Rivers JK, Cockerell CJ, McBride A, Kopf AW. Quantification of histologic features of dysplastic nevi. Am J Dermatopathol 1990; 12: 42–50.

252. Barnhill RL, Roush GC, Duray PH. Correlation of histologic architectural and cytoplasmic features with nuclear atypia in atypical (dysplastic) nevomelanocytic nevi. Hum Pathol 1990; 21: 51–58.

253. Steijlen PM, Bergman W, Hermans J et al. The efficacy of histopathological criteria required for diagnosing dysplastic naevi. Histopathology 1988; 12: 289–300.

254. Sagebiel RW, Banda PW, Schneider JS, Crutcher WA. Age distribution and histologic patterns of dysplastic nevi. J Am Acad Dermatol 1985; 13: 975–982.

255. Kelly JW, Crutcher WA, Sagebiel RW. Clinical diagnosis of dysplastic melanocytic nevi. A clinicopathologic correlation. J Am Acad Dermatol 1986; 14: 1044–1052.

256. Bergman W, Ruiter DJ, Scheffer E, van Vloten WA. Melanocytic atypia in dysplastic nevi. Immunohistochemical and cytophotometrical analysis. Cancer 1988; 61: 1660–1666.

257. Murphy GF, Halpern A. Dysplastic melanocytic nevi. Normal variants or melanoma precursors? Arch Dermatol 1990; 126: 519–522.

258. Ahmed I, Piepkorn MW, Rabkin MS et al. Histopathologic characteristics of dysplastic nevi. Limited association of conventional histologic criteria with melanoma risk group. J Am Acad Dermatol 1990; 22: 727–733.

259. Klein LJ, Barr RJ. Histologic atypia in clinically benign nevi. A prospective study. J Am Acad Dermatol 1990; 22: 275–282.

260. Piepkorn M, Meyer LJ, Goldgar D et al. The dysplastic melanocytic nevus: A prevalent lesion that correlates poorly with clinical phenotype. J Am Acad Dermatol 1989; 20: 407–415.

261. Cerio R, Deal P, Headington JT, Wilson Jones E. Lamellar fibrosis in dysplastic naevi, a misconception! J Cutan Pathol 1989; 16: 299 (abstract).

262. Ackerman AB. What naevus is dysplastic, a syndrome and the commonest precursor of malignant melanoma? A riddle and an answer. Histopathology 1988; 13: 241–256.

263. Clark WH Jr, Ackerman AB. An exchange of views regarding the dysplastic nevus controversy. Semin Dermatol 1989; 8: 229–250.

264. McGovern VJ, Shaw HM, Milton GW. Histogenesis of malignant melanoma with an adjacent component of superficial spreading type. Pathology 1985; 17: 251–254.

265. Rhodes AR, Harrist TJ, Day CL et al. Dysplastic melanocytic nevi in histologic association with 234 primary cutaneous melanomas. J Am Acad Dermatol 1983; 9: 563–574.

266. Duray PH, Ernstoff MS. Dysplastic nevus in histologic contiguity with acquired nonfamilial melanoma. Clinicopathologic experience in a 100-bed hospital. Arch Dermatol 1987; 123: 80–84.

267. Black WC. Residual dysplastic and other nevi in superficial spreading melanoma. Clinical correlations and association with sun damage. Cancer 1988; 62: 163–173.

268. Maize JC. Dysplastic melanocytic nevi in histologic association with primary cutaneous melanomas. J Am Acad Dermatol 1984; 10: 831–835.

269. Ackerman AB. Critical commentary on statements in "Precursors to Malignant Melanoma". Am J Dermatopathol (Suppl) 1984; 1: 181–183.

270. Fallowfield ME, Dodson AR, Cook MG. Nucleolar organizer regions in melanocytic dysplasia and melanoma. Histopathology 1988; 13: 95–99.

271. Fallowfield ME, Cook MG. The value of nucleolar organizer region staining in the differential diagnosis of borderline melanocytic lesions. Histopathology 1989; 14: 299–304.

272. Mackie RM, White SI, Seywright MM, Young H. An assessment of the value of Ag NOR staining in the identification of dysplastic and other borderline

melanocytic naevi. Br J Dermatol 1989; 120: 511–516.

273. Howat AJ, Wright AL, Cotton DWK et al. AgNORs in benign, dysplastic, and malignant melanocytic skin lesions. Am J Dermatopathol 1990; 12: 156–161.

274. Smoller BR, McNutt NS, Hsu A. HMB-45 recognizes stimulated melanocytes. J Cutan Pathol 1989; 16: 49–53.

275. Smoller BR, McNutt NS, Hsu A. HMB-45 staining of dysplastic nevi. Support for a spectrum of progression toward melanoma. Am J Surg Pathol 1989; 13: 680–684.

276. Takahashi H, Yamana K, Maeda K et al. Dysplastic melanocytic nevus. Electron-microscopic observation as a diagnostic tool. Am J Dermatopathol 1987; 9: 189–197.

277. Rhodes AR, Seki Y, Fitzpatrick TB, Stern RS. Melanosomal alterations in dysplastic melanocytic nevi. A quantitative, ultrastructural investigation. Cancer 1988; 61: 358–369.

Malignant melanoma

278. Beitner H, Ringborg U, Wennersten G, Lagerlof B. Further evidence for increased light sensitivity in patients with malignant melanoma. Br J Dermatol 1981; 104: 289–294.

279. Beral V, Evans S, Shaw H, Milton G. Cutaneous factors related to the risk of melanoma. Br J Dermatol 1983; 109: 165–172.

280. Lew RA, Sober AJ, Cook N et al. Sun exposure habits in patients with cutaneous melanoma: a case control study. J Dermatol Surg Oncol 1983; 9: 981–986.

281. Schreiber MM, Moon TE, Bozzo PD. Chronic solar ultraviolet damage associated with malignant melanoma of the skin. J Am Acad Dermatol 1984; 10: 755–759.

282. Kopf AW, Kripke ML, Stern RS. Sun and malignant melanoma. J Am Acad Dermatol 1984; 11: 674–684.

283. Armstrong BK. Epidemiology of malignant melanoma: intermittent or total accumulated exposure to the sun? J Dermatol Surg Oncol 1988; 14: 835–849.

284. Little JH, Holt J, Davis N. Changing epidemiology of malignant melanoma in Queensland. Med J Aust 1980; 1: 66–69.

285. Green A, Little JH, Weedon D. The diagnosis of Hutchinson's melanotic freckle (lentigo maligna) in Queensland. Pathology 1983; 15: 33–35.

286. MacKie RM. The changing face of melanoma. Clin Exp Dermatol 1982; 7: 231–246.

287. Shafir R, Hiss J, Tsur H, Bubis JJ. The thin malignant melanoma: Changing patterns of epidemiology and treatment. Cancer 1982; 50: 817–819.

288. Rhodes AR. Melanocytic precursors of cutaneous melanoma. Estimated risks and guidelines for management. Med Clin North Am 1986; 70: 3–37.

289. Greene MH, Clark WH, Tucker MA et al. High risk of malignant melanoma in melanoma-prone families with dysplastic nevi. Ann Intern Med 1985; 102: 458–465.

290. Robertson I, Cook MG. Multiple melanomas associated with diffuse melanocytic dysplasia. Histopathology 1987; 11: 395–402.

291. Green A, MacLennan R, Siskind V. Common acquired naevi and the risk of malignant melanoma. Int J Cancer 1985; 35: 297–300.

292. Swerdlow AJ, English J, MacKie RM et al. Benign melanocytic naevi as a risk factor for malignant melanoma. Br Med J 1986; 292: 1555–1559.

293. Holly EA, Kelly JW, Shpall SN, Chiu S-H. Number of melanocytic nevi as a major risk factor for malignant melanoma. J Am Acad Dermatol 1987; 17: 459–468.

294. English JSC, Swerdlow AJ, MacKie RM et al. Relation between phenotype and banal melanocytic naevi. Br Med J 1987; 294: 152–154.

295. Rampen FHJ, van der Meeren HLM, Boezeman JBM. Frequency of moles as a key to melanoma incidence? J Am Acad Dermatol 1986; 15: 1200–1203.

296. Evans RD, Kopf AW, Lew RA et al. Risk factors for the development of malignant melanoma — I: Review of case-control studies. J Dermatol Surg Oncol 1988; 14: 393–408.

297. Beitner H, Norell SE, Ringborg U et al. Malignant melanoma: aetiological importance of individual pigmentation and sun exposure. Br J Dermatol 1990; 122: 43–51.

298. Tullis GD, Lynde CW, McLean DI, Stewart WD. Multiple melanomas occurring in a patient with xeroderma pigmentosum. J Am Acad Dermatol 1984; 11: 364–367.

299. Greene SL, Thomas JR, Doyle JA. Cowden's disease with associated malignant melanoma. Int J Dermatol 1984; 23: 466–467.

300. Tindall B, Finlayson R, Mutimer K et al. Malignant melanoma associated with human immunodeficiency virus infection in three homosexual men. J Am Acad Dermatol 1989; 20: 587–591.

301. Clark WH, From L, Bernadino EA, Mihm MC. The histogenesis and biologic behavior of primary human malignant melanomas of the skin. Cancer Res 1969; 29: 705–727.

302. McGovern VJ. The classification of melanoma and its relationship with prognosis. Pathology 1970; 2: 85–98.

303. McGovern VJ, Mihm MC, Bailly C et al. The classification of malignant melanoma and its histologic reporting. Cancer 1973; 32: 1446–1457.

304. Roberts G, Martyn AL, Dobson AJ, McCarthy WH. Tumour thickness and histological type in malignant melanoma in New South Wales, Australia, 1970–76. Pathology 1981; 13: 763–770.

305. Kukita A, Ishihara K. Clinical features and distribution of malignant melanoma and pigmented nevi on the soles of the feet in Japan. J Invest Dermatol 1989; 92: 210s–213s.

306. Reed RJ. Consultation case. Am J Surg Pathol 1978; 2: 215–220.

307. Bhawan J. Amelanotic melanoma or poorly differentiated melanoma? J Cutan Pathol 1980; 7: 55–56.

308. Gibson LE, Goellner JR. Amelanotic melanoma: cases studied by Fontana stain, S-100 immunostain, and ultrastructural examination. Mayo Clin Proc 1988; 63: 777–782.

309. Sheibani K, Battifora H. Signet-ring cell melanoma. A rare morphologic variant of malignant melanoma. Am J Surg Pathol 1988; 12: 28–34.

310. Bonetti F, Colombari R, Zamboni G et al. Signet ring melanoma, S-100 negative. Am J Surg Pathol 1989; 13: 522–526.

311. Urso C, Giannotti B, Bondi R. Myxoid melanoma of the skin. Arch Pathol Lab Med 1990; 114: 527–528.

311a. Nottingham JF, Slater DN. Malignant melanoma: a new mimic of colloid adenocarcinoma. Histopathology 1988; 13: 576–578.

312. Ackerman AB. Malignant melanoma: a unifying concept. Hum Pathol 1980; 11: 591–595.

313. Ackerman AB, David KM. A unifying concept of malignant melanoma: biologic aspects. Hum Pathol 1986; 17: 438–440.

314. Flotte TJ, Mihm MC. Melanoma: the art versus the science of dermatopathology. Hum Pathol 1986; 17: 441–442.

315. Clark WH, Ainsworth AM, Bernardino EA et al. The developmental biology of primary human malignant melanoma. Semin Oncol 1975; 2: 83–103.

316. Clark WH, Elder DE, van Horn M. The biologic forms of malignant melanoma. Hum Pathol 1986; 17: 443–450.

317. Elder DE, Lusk E, Guerry D IV et al. Invasive malignant melanomas lacking competence for metastasis. Am J Dermatopathol (Suppl) 1984; 1: 55–61.

317a. Clark WH, Elder DE, Guerry DIV et al. Model for predicting survival in Stage 1 melanoma based on tumor progression. J Natl Cancer Inst 1989; 81: 1893–1904.

318. Sober AJ, Fitzpatrick TB, Mihm MC. Primary melanoma of the skin: Recognition and management. J Am Acad Dermatol 1980; 2: 179–197.

319. Flemming AFS, Ruggins N. Malignant melanoma in childhood. Br J Plast Surg 1985; 38: 432–434.

320. Pratt CB, Palmer MK, Thatcher N, Crowther D. Malignant melanoma in children and adolescents. Cancer 1981; 47: 392–397.

321. Roth ME, Grant-Kels JM, Kuhn K et al. Melanoma in children. J Am Acad Dermatol 1990; 22: 265–274.

322. Wagner RF, Nathanson L. Paraneoplastic syndromes, tumor markers, and other unusual features of malignant melanoma. J Am Acad Dermatol 1986; 14: 249–256.

323. Borkovic SP, Schwartz RA. Amelanotic lentigo maligna melanoma manifesting as a dermatitislike plaque. Arch Dermatol 1983; 119: 423–425.

324. Weinstock MA, Sober AJ. The risk of progression of lentigo maligna to lentigo maligna melanoma. Br J Dermatol 1987; 116: 303–310.

325. Michalik EE, Fitzpatrick TB, Sober AJ. Rapid progression of lentigo maligna to deeply invasive lentigo maligna melanoma. Report of two cases. Arch Dermatol 1983; 119: 831–835.

326. Goldberg DJ. Amelanotic melanoma presenting as Bowen's disease. J Dermatol Surg Oncol 1983; 9: 902–904.

327. Kossard S, Commens C. Hypopigmented malignant melanoma simulating vitiligo. J Am Acad Dermatol 1990; 22: 840–842.

328. McGovern VJ, Shaw HM, Milton GW. Prognostic significance of a polypoid configuration in malignant melanoma. Histopathology 1983; 7: 663–672.

329. Rosenberg L, Goldstein J, Ben-Yakar Y, Mahler D. The pedunculated malignant melanoma: A misunderstood and neglected variant. J Dermatol Surg Oncol 1981; 7: 123–126.

330. Arrington JH, Reed RJ, Ichinose H, Krementz ET. Plantar lentiginous melanoma: A distinctive variant of human cutaneous malignant melanoma. Am J Surg Pathol 1977; 1: 131–143.

331. Vazquez M, Ramos FA, Sanchez JL. Melanomas of volar and subungual skin in Puerto Ricans. A clinicopathologic study. J Am Acad Dermatol 1984; 10: 39–45.

332. Papachristou DN, Fortner JG. Melanoma arising under the nail. J Surg Oncol 1982; 21: 219–222.

333. Patterson RH, Helwig EB. Subungual malignant melanoma: A clinical-pathologic study. Cancer 1980; 46: 2074–2087.

334. Lin C-S, Wang W-J, Wong C-K. Acral melanoma. A clinicopathologic study of 28 patients. Int J Dermatol 1990; 29: 107–112.

335. Coleman WP, Loria PR, Reed RJ, Krementz ET. Acral lentiginous melanoma. Arch Dermatol 1980; 116: 773–776.

336. Seiji M, Takematsu H, Hosokawa M et al. Acral melanoma in Japan. J Invest Dermatol 1983; 80: 56s–60s.

337. Jimbow K, Ikeda S, Takahashi H et al. Biological behavior and natural course of acral malignant melanoma. Am J Dermatopathol (Suppl) 1984; 1: 43–53.

338. Saida T. Malignant melanoma in situ on the sole of the foot. Its clinical and histopathologic characteristics. Am J Dermatopathol 1989; 11: 124–130.

338a. Saida T, Yoshida N, Ikegawa S et al. Clinical guidelines for the early detection of plantar malignant melanoma. J Am Acad Dermatol 1990; 23: 37–40.

339. Krementz ET, Reed RJ, Coleman WP et al. Acral lentiginous melanoma. A clinicopathologic entity. Ann Surg 1982; 195: 632–645.

340. Paladugu RR, Winberg CD, Yonemoto RH. Acral lentiginous melanoma. A clinicopathologic study of 36 patients. Cancer 1983; 52: 161–168.

341. Scrivner D, Oxenhandler RW, Lopez M, Perez-Mesa C. Plantar lentiginous melanoma. A clinicopathologic study. Cancer 1987; 60: 2502–2509.

342. McDonald JS, Miller RL, Wagner W, Giammara B. Acral lentiginous melanoma of the oral cavity. Head Neck Surg 1983; 5: 257–262.

343. Ronan SG, Eng AM, Briele HA et al. Malignant melanoma of the female genitalia. J Am Acad Dermatol 1990; 22: 428–435.

344. Kato T, Takematsu H, Tomita Y et al. Malignant melanoma of mucous membranes. A clinicopathologic study of 13 cases in Japanese patients. Arch Dermatol 1987; 123: 216–220.

345. Conley J, Lattes R, Orr W. Desmoplastic malignant melanoma. Cancer 1971; 28: 914–936.

346. Man D, Weiner LJ, Reiman HM. Desmoplastic malignant melanoma: a case report. Br J Plast Surg 1981; 34: 79–82.

347. Berry RB, Subbuswamy SG, Hackett MEJ. Desmoplastic malignant melanoma: the first British report. Br J Plast Surg 1982; 35: 324–327.

348. Reiman HM, Goellner JR, Woods JE, Mixter RC. Desmoplastic melanoma of the head and neck. Cancer 1987; 60: 2269–2274.

349. Jain S, Allen PW. Desmoplastic malignant melanoma and its variants. A study of 45 cases. Am J Dermatopathol 1989; 13: 358–373.

350. Egbert B, Kempson R, Sagebiel R. Desmoplastic

melanoma. Am J Dermatopathol (Suppl) 1984; 1: 109–111.

496. Urist MM, Balch CM, Soong S-J et al. The influence of surgical margins and prognostic factors predicting the risk of local recurrence in 3445 patients with primary cutaneous melanoma. Cancer 1985; 55: 1398–1402.

497. Day CL, Lew RA. Malignant melanoma prognostic factors 3: Surgical margins. J Dermatol Surg Oncol 1983; 9: 797–801.

498. Milton GW, Shaw HM, McCarthy WH. Subungual malignant melanoma: a disease entity separate from other forms of cutaneous melanoma. Australas J Dermatol 1985; 26: 61–64.

499. Balch CM, Soong S-J, Shaw HM. A comparison of worldwide melanoma data. In: Balch CM, Milton GW, eds. Cutaneous melanoma. Clinical management and treatment results worldwide. Philadelphia: J.B. Lippincott, 1985; 507–518.

500. Rogers GS, Kopf AW, Rigel DS et al. Hazard-rate analysis in Stage I malignant melanoma. Arch Dermatol 1986; 122; 999–1002.

501. Steiner A, Wolf C, Pehamberger H, Wolff K. Late metastases of cutaneous malignant melanoma. Br J Dermatol 1986; 114: 737–740.

502. Raderman D, Giler S, Rothem A, Ben-Bassat M. Late metastases (beyond ten years) of cutaneous malignant melanoma. Literature review and case report. J Am Acad Dermatol 1986; 15: 374–378.

Tumours of cutaneous appendages

INTRODUCTION

The cutaneous appendages give rise to a bewildering number of neoplasms — more than 60 at a recent count. Various classifications have been

completely recapitulated.[17,39–43] They have been likened to the odontogenic tumours which may also be epithelial and/or mesenchymal.[1] They are regarded by some as a giant solitary variant of trichoepithelioma.[17] The terms immature trichoepithelioma[43a,43b] and hair matrix adenoma[43c] have been used for trichogenic tumours composed of epithelial elements. Trichogenic tumours are usually greater than 1 cm in diameter and involve the deep dermis and subcutis. Multiple lesions have been reported.[44]

Histopathology[1,43]

The tumours show irregular nests of basaloid cells resembling a basal cell carcinoma but with variable stromal condensation and pilar differentiation. Keratinous cysts are not usually present. Stromal amyloid is not uncommon.[17] The following variants have been proposed by Headington[1] in his review:

Trichoblastoma: a pure epithelial neoplasm
Trichogenic myxoma: a tumour resembling the dermal papilla
Trichogenic trichoblastoma: a mixed epithelial-mesenchymal tumour with follicular differentiation[44a]
Trichoblastic fibroma: a mixed tumour without follicular differentiation.[44b]

This complicated nomenclature makes it tempting to use the simpler term 'trichogenic tumour' for them all.

GENERALIZED HAIR FOLLICLE HAMARTOMA

There are now several reports of patients with papules and plaques on the face, progressive alopecia and myasthenia gravis.[45–48] Involved skin shows lesions resembling trichoepithelioma, while uninvolved skin may show small islands of basaloid cells.[48]

BASALOID FOLLICULAR HAMARTOMA

This term was coined by Mehregan and Baker for three patients with localized or systematized lesions in which individual hair follicles were replaced or were associated with solid strands and branching cords of undifferentiated basaloid cells with some intervening fibrous stroma.[49] Although they regarded the condition as a localized variant of generalized hair follicle hamartoma, there was less resemblance to trichoepithelioma and more to premalignant fibroepithelial tumour of Pinkus (see p. 748) in their cases.[49]

BASAL CELL HAMARTOMA WITH FOLLICULAR DIFFERENTIATION

This tumour has features intermediate between the tumour of the follicular infundibulum, basal follicular hamartoma and multifocal superficial basal cell carcinoma.[50] The patient reported had multiple periorbital papules.[50] The lesions showed basal cell proliferation resembling multifocal basal cell carcinoma, but with the formation of follicular structures with varying degrees of differentiation.

LINEAR UNILATERAL BASAL CELL NAEVUS WITH COMEDONES

This entity is characterized by the presence of linear or zosteriform lesions, some with comedone plugs, at birth or soon after.[51–54] Although there is some clinical resemblance to naevus comedonicus (see p. 731), the histology resembles a basal cell carcinoma. Some cases have had a lattice-like growth of basaloid cells attached to the undersurface of the epidermis and vague follicular differentiation.[52]

INFUNDIBULAR TUMOURS

At least four varieties of tumour arise from the infundibulum, the uppermost portion of the hair follicle, above the opening of the sebaceous duct. These include the tumour of the follicular infundibulum, the dilated pore, pilar sheath acanthoma and inverted follicular keratosis. All are characterized by a superficial location, connection with the epidermis and pilar structures, and infundibular (epidermoid) keratinization. The epidermal cyst could be included here, but for convenience is considered with other cysts (see Ch. 16, p. 483). The tricholemmoma is included in Mehregan's review as an infundibular tumour,[55] but it is best discussed with other tumours showing tricholemmal differentiation (see p. 825).

TUMOUR OF THE FOLLICULAR INFUNDIBULUM

This is a rare tumour which usually occurs as a solitary, asymptomatic, smooth or slightly keratotic papule on the head and neck or upper chest.[55-57] Multiple lesions, including a mantle distribution on the upper trunk (infundibulomatosis, eruptive infundibulomas),[58,58a] have been reported.[56,59]

Histopathology[55]

The growth pattern resembles that of a superficial basal cell carcinoma and the basal cell hamartoma with follicular differentiation.[1] There is a plate-like, fenestrated, subepidermal tumour composed of pale-staining, glycogen-containing cells, with a peripheral palisade of basal cells. The tumour connects at intervals with the undersurface of the epidermis by slender pedicles. Hair follicles entering the tumour from below lose their identity and merge with it. The surrounding loose connective tissue stroma contains a network of elastic fibres.[55,58] The histological features sometimes overlap those of tricholemmoma.[60]

The tumour of the follicular infundibulum is histologically dissimilar to the cases reported as *multiple infundibular tumours of the head and neck*.[60a] In these latter cases there were clusters of enlarged follicular infundibula making up each lesion, somewhat similar to the appearances of prurigo nodularis (see p. 732). The illustrations in the recent report of a tumour called an *infundibular keratosis* showed some features of the multiple infundibular tumour referred to above and others of an inverted follicular keratosis (see below) but without squamous eddies.[60b]

DILATED PORE OF WINER

The dilated pore of Winer[61] is a relatively common adnexal lesion which occurs predominantly on the head and neck, but also on the upper trunk of elderly individuals.[62] Clinically and histologically it is a comedo-like structure. Dilated pores may be acquired as a sequel of inflammatory cystic acne, or of actinic damage.[1,62]

Histopathology[55,62]

There is a markedly dilated follicular pore which may extend to the mid or lower dermis. The follicle is lined by outer root sheath epithelium in which there is infundibular keratinization with the formation of keratohyaline granules. The epithelium shows acanthosis and finger-like projections which radiate into the surrounding dermis (Fig. 33.5). There is sometimes heavy melanin pigmentation of the follicular wall; pigmentation may also involve the central horny plug. The pilary unit of the involved follicle and the sebaceous gland are absent or rudimentary.

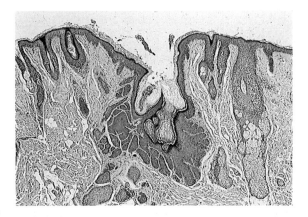

Fig. 33.5 Dilated pore of Winer. Acanthotic projections extend from the base of a dilated follicular pore. Haematoxylin — eosin

PILAR SHEATH ACANTHOMA

Pilar sheath acanthoma is a rare, benign follicular tumour found almost exclusively on the upper lip of older individuals.[63-65] The tumours, which measure 5 to 10 mm in diameter, have a central pore-like opening plugged with keratin.

Histopathology[63-65]

There is a central, cystically dilated follicle, containing keratinous material, which opens on to the surface (Fig. 33.6). Tumour lobules composed of outer root sheath epithelium extend from the wall of the cystic cavity into the adjacent dermis (Fig. 33.7). Lobules sometimes

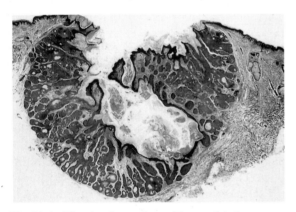

Fig. 33.6 Pilar sheath acanthoma. Tumour lobules, composed of outer root-sheath epithelium, radiate from a central cystic cavity.
Haematoxylin — eosin

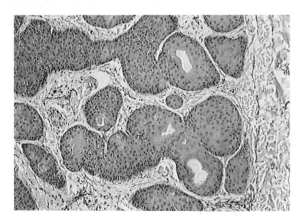

Fig. 33.7 Pilar sheath acanthoma. The tumour lobules are composed of outer root sheath epithelium.
Haematoxylin — eosin

reach the subcutis. Occasional abortive hair follicles may be present. The tumour epithelium shows infundibular keratinization. There may be abundant glycogen in some of the tumour cells.

The condition may be distinguished from the dilated pore of Winer, in which there is a patulous follicle with only small projections of epithelium extending into the surrounding connective tissue. In trichofolliculoma, well-formed follicles radiate from the central keratin-filled sinus and there is a well-formed stroma which is absent in pilar sheath acanthoma.

INVERTED FOLLICULAR KERATOSIS

This benign tumour of the follicular infundibulum was first described by Helwig in 1954.[66] It is a somewhat controversial entity, having been regarded by some as a variant of seborrhoeic keratosis or verruca vulgaris.[66-69] It occurs as a solitary, flesh-coloured, nodular or filiform lesion which measures from 0.3–1 cm in diameter.[55] In about 90% of cases the tumour occurs on the head and neck, with the cheeks and upper lip the sites of predilection.[69] The eyelids may be involved.[70] It is more common in males and older individuals. Human papilloma virus has not been detected, suggesting that the inverted follicular keratosis is not a variant of verruca vulgaris, as has been claimed.[71]

Histopathology[55,72-74]

Inverted follicular keratoses are predominantly endophytic tumours with large lobules or finger-like projections of tumour cells extending into the dermis. An exophytic growth pattern is present in some lesions, and it is occasionally the dominant feature. Mehregan has described four growth patterns:

1. a papillomatous wart-like variant which is largely exophytic with overlying hyperkeratosis and parakeratosis;
2. a keratoacanthoma-like pattern with marginal buttress formation and a central exo-endophytic mass of solid epithelium;
3. a solid-nodular form which is largely endo-

phytic with solid, lobulated masses of epithelium; and

4. an uncommon cystic type with irregular clefts within the tumour and the formation of small cysts.[55]

Each tumour lobule is composed of basaloid and squamous cells with the basaloid cells at the periphery and larger keratinizing cells towards the centre. Mitoses are not uncommon in the basaloid cells.

A characteristic feature is the presence of squamous eddies which are formed by concentric layers of squamous cells with a whorled pattern and which may become keratinized with the formation of keratohyaline and sometimes keratin at the centre of these islands (Fig. 33.8). There is sometimes clefting at the periphery of the squamous eddies and even focal acantholysis.

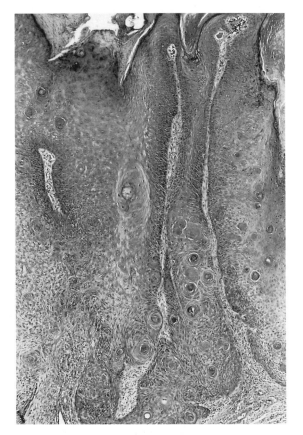

Fig. 33.8 Inverted follicular keratosis. Squamous eddies are seen towards the base of the tumour.
Haematoxylin — eosin

Melanin pigment is usually inconspicuous. The surrounding dermis sometimes contains a mild inflammatory cell infiltrate which is predominantly lymphohistiocytic. Telangiectatic vessels may be found in the dermal papillae in the filiform lesions.

Overlying the tumour there is variable hyperkeratosis and parakeratosis. Funnel-shaped keratinous plugs may form. Occasionally, a prominent cutaneous horn is present.

TRICHOLEMMAL (EXTERNAL SHEATH) TUMOURS

This group of tumours is characterized by cells which differentiate towards those of the outer sheath of the hair follicle.[1] As such, they show a variable extent of clear cell change resulting from cytoplasmic accumulation of glycogen. There are also cells which are intermediate between those of the outer sheath and infundibular keratinocytes. These cells may have anisotropic tonofibrils, a characteristic feature of tricholemmal keratinization, and also seen in both tricholemmal cysts (see p. 484) and proliferating tricholemmal cysts (see p. 485).

TRICHOLEMMOMA

Tricholemmomas (trichilemmomas) are small, solitary, asymptomatic, papular lesions found almost exclusively on the face.[1,39,55,75,76] Multiple tricholemmomas are a cutaneous marker of Cowden's syndrome (see below).

Although they appear to arise from the follicular infundibulum, they differentiate towards the outer root sheath. Ackerman regarded tricholemmomas as old viral warts,[77,78] a view not supported by most dermatopathologists[79,80] or by immunoperoxidase studies to detect viral antigens.[81]

Histopathology[82,83]

Tricholemmomas are sharply circumscribed tumours composed of one or more lobules which extend into the upper dermis and which are in

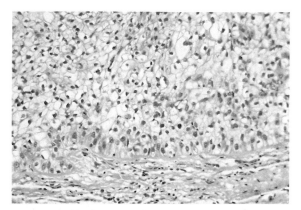

Fig. 33.9   Tricholemmoma. Vacuolation of the tumour cells near the base of the lesion is marked. Haematoxylin — eosin

continuity with the epidermis or follicular epithelium at several points. In small lesions, follicular concentricity is apparent.[84] The tumour is composed of squamoid cells showing variable glycogen vacuolation, this change being most marked deeply (Fig. 33.9). Centrally there may be foci of epidermal keratinization and occasionally small squamous eddies. Keratinous microcysts may form in large lesions. There is a peripheral layer of columnar cells with nuclear palisading resembling the outer root sheath of hair follicles. A thickened glassy basement membrane surrounds the tumour in part. This is PAS positive, diastase resistant. The stroma is occasionally hyalinized or desmoplastic.[76]

The overlying epidermis shows hyperkeratosis, mild acanthosis and sometimes a prominent granular layer. Uncommonly, a cutaneous horn will form (tricholemmomal horn).[85] Warts, basal and squamous cell carcinomas, and inverted follicular keratoses and seborrhoeic keratoses sometimes contain small areas of tricholemmal differentiation.[78,86]

COWDEN'S DISEASE

Cowden's disease (multiple hamartoma and neoplasia syndrome) is a rare multisystem condition with autosomal dominant inheritance.[87–90] The eponym is the surname of the propositus of the report by Lloyd and Dennis in 1963.[91] The

mucocutaneous features are the most constant findings. These include multiple tricholemmomas,[92,93] which usually are on the face, acral keratoses, palmar pits and oral fibromas.[88] They usually appear in late adolescence. There is also a high incidence of visceral hamartomas and tumours, including fibrocystic disease of the breast,[94] thyroid adenomas, ovarian cysts, subcutaneous lipomas and neuromas, gastrointestinal polyps,[95,96] and carcinomas of the breast and thyroid.[90] Also documented are eye changes,[97,98] skeletal abnormalities,[99] acromelanosis,[97] non-Hodgkin's lymphoma,[92] and carcinomas of the skin,[95] tongue[100] and cervix.[98] Impaired T-cell function has been reported in this syndrome.[99]

Histopathology[101–104]

Most of the facial lesions are tricholemmomas or tumours of the follicular infundibulum. The tricholemmomas are cylindrical or lobular in configuration.[101] Sometimes the lesions keratinize with squamous eddies, resembling an inverted follicular keratosis (see p. 825). Non-specific verrucous acanthomas and lesions resembling digitate warts may also be present.[101]

The extrafacial lesions are mostly hyperkeratotic papillomas that resemble either verruca vulgaris, acrokeratosis verruciformis or a nondescript hyperkeratotic acanthoma.[102,105] This latter change may take the form of hyperplasia of the follicular infundibulum.[102] No evidence of a viral aetiology has been found on electron microscopy[99,106] or with immunoperoxidase studies.

Distinctive dermal fibromas with interwoven fascicles of coarse collagen, sometimes showing marked hyalinization, are not uncommon in Cowden's disease.[102,107] They may have a plywood-like appearance histologically.

TRICHOLEMMAL CARCINOMA

Headington has defined tricholemmal carcinoma (tricholemmocarcinoma)[108] as a 'histologically invasive, cytologically atypical clear cell neoplasm of adnexal keratinocytes which is in continuity with the epidermis and/or follicular epithelium'.[1] Only a small number of cases, purporting to be this entity, have been reported.[1,108–109] Some of the illustrations in the case reported by Ten Seldam resemble intraepidermal carcinoma with follicular extension, a tumour which often shows adnexal differentiation in its invasive form.[108]

The tumour reported as 'clear cell pilar sheath tumor of scalp' had some histological similarities to the tricholemmal carcinoma. The reported case was composed of small nests of glycogen-containing clear cells infiltrating the dermis and subcutis.[109a] There was no underlying cyst or evidence of tricholemmal keratinization.[109a]

TUMOURS WITH MATRICAL DIFFERENTIATION

In this group, there is differentiation towards cells of the hair matrix and hair cortex and cells of the inner sheath. The prototype tumour is the pilomatrixoma. A rare malignant variant, the pilomatrix carcinoma, has also been described. Rarely, a limited amount of matrical differentiation is seen in epidermal cysts[110] and other appendageal tumours such as trichoepitheliomas, chondroid syringomas, complex appendageal tumours and the rare trichoblastic hamartomas found in some organoid naevi.[1,111] Basal cell carcinomas may also show focal matrical differentiation.

PILOMATRIXOMA AND PILOMATRIX CARCINOMA

Pilomatrixoma (pilomatricoma, calcifying epithelioma of Malherbe), which accounts for almost 20% of pilar tumours, is a benign lesion with differentiation towards the matrix of the hair follicle.[60] It is found particularly on the head and neck and upper extremities.[2] About 60% develop in the first two decades of life.[112] They are mostly solitary, but multiple lesions, usually less than five in all, are sometimes found.[113–116] Some patients with multiple lesions have myotonic dystrophy.[2,117,118] A familial occurrence is rarely noted. A pilomatrixoma-like change is not uncommon in the epidermal cysts found in Gardner's syndrome (see p. 483).[119,120]

Pilomatrixomas are firm nodules, approximately 0.5–3.0 cm in diameter. They are usually slowly growing, but rapid enlargement due to haemorrhage has been reported.[121] Rarely, there is sufficient melanin pigment in the lesion to be visible clinically.[122] They have a variegated appearance macroscopically with grey, white and brown areas on the cut surface. Small spicules of bone and minute thorny fragments may be discernible.[123] The consistency of the nodules depends on the amount of calcification and ossification.

Most tumours, even if inadequately excised, will not recur. However, local recurrence and aggressive forms have been documented.[124,125] About 20 examples of a presumed malignant variant, pilomatrix carcinoma, have been reported.[126–133a] This diagnosis has been based on cytological atypia and local aggressive behaviour. In only three of these cases have metastases developed.[127,132,133a]

Histopathology[1,124,134]

The appearances vary according to the age of the lesion. Established lesions are sharply demarcated tumours in the lower dermis, extending quite often into the subcutis. There are masses of epithelial cells of various shapes with an intervening connective tissue stroma containing blood vessels, a mixed inflammatory cell infiltrate, foreign body giant cells and sometimes haemosiderin, melanin, bone and rarely amyloid.[1,134a]

There are two basic cell types, basophilic cells and eosinophilic shadow cells (Fig. 33.10). The basophilic cells tend to be at the periphery of the cell islands and have little cytoplasm, indistinct cell borders, hyperchromatic nuclei and plentiful mitoses. They resemble the cells of a basal cell carcinoma. The eosinophilic shadow cells are found towards the central areas of the cell masses. They have more cytoplasm and distinct cell borders, but no nuclear staining. These shadow (mummified) cells form from the basophilic cells and the transition may be relatively abrupt or take place over several layers

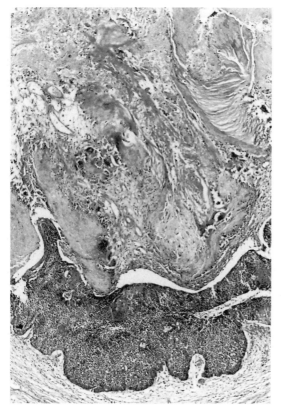

Fig. 33.10   Pilomatrixoma. There are two cell types present — nests of basaloid cells and shadow cells. Haematoxylin-eosin

of cells. The intermediary cells develop progressively more eosinophilic cytoplasm and the nucleus becomes pyknotic. Hyalinization of the cells, squamous change or disruption into amorphous debris may result.[124]

Calcification occurs in more than two-thirds of the tumours and is usually in the shadow cells. Ossification of the stroma occurs in about 13%;[135] haemosiderin is found in about 25% of cases;[112] melanin is present in nearly 20% of lesions and may be in the shadow cells as well as in the stroma.[112] Dendritic cells are sometimes seen among the basophilic cells in the cases with pigmentation.[136]

In early lesions there is often a small cyst with basophilic cells in the wall.[134] Rarely, a pilomatrixoma appears to arise in an established epidermal cyst.[137,137a] Pilomatrixoma-like changes can also develop in the epidermal cysts

in Gardner's syndrome (see above). As the lesion ages, the number of basophilic cells decreases as the process of mummification outstrips the proliferation of the basophilic cells. About 20% of lesions are fully keratinized (mummified) at the time of removal and have no basophilic cells remaining.[112] Transepidermal elimination of the tumour is a rare outcome.[138–139a]

Pilomatrix carcinoma (pilomatrical carcinoma, malignant pilomatrixoma) is a somewhat subjective diagnosis. The usual criteria listed for its diagnosis are high mitotic activity, cytological atypia, locally aggressive behaviour and, rarely, vascular or lymphatic invasion.[126,131,132]

Electron microscopy. The cells differentiate and keratinize in a manner analogous to the cells that form the cortex of the hair.[140] The fully developed shadow cells contain interlacing sworls of keratin that form a mantle around the nuclear remnants.[140]

TUMOURS OF PERIFOLLICULAR MESENCHYME

The connective tissue sheath of the hair follicle plays an important role in the differentiation of the latter. Three distinct, but extremely rare, tumours can arise from this perifollicular mesenchyme — the perifollicular fibroma, the fibrofolliculoma and the trichodiscoma.[141,142] Leiomyomas derived from the arrectores pilorum are sometimes included in this category.[1] They are considered with the tumours of smooth muscle (see p. 915). Fibrofolliculomas and trichodiscomas may occur in the same patient, usually in association with acrochordons (skin tags — see page 877).[143] This clinical triad, known as the Birt–Hogg–Dubé syndrome, is inherited as an autosomal dominant trait.[143–145] Perifollicular fibromas and individual lesions with overlap features between acrochordons and fibrofolliculomas have also been reported in patients with this syndrome, testimony to the close relationship of tumours derived from the perifollicular mesenchyme.[144]

TRICHODISCOMA

Trichodiscomas are rare hamartomas of the dermal portion of the hair disc (*Haarscheibe*), a specialized component of the perifollicular mesenchyme which serves as a slowly adapting mechanoreceptor.[141,142,146] The hair disc is a richly vascularized dermal pad, supplied by a myelinated nerve and covered by an epidermis which contains Merkel cells.[146]

Trichodiscomas are found as asymptomatic, skin-coloured papules, 1–3 mm in diameter, usually on the face, arms, trunk and sometimes the thighs.[142,147] Hundreds of lesions may be present. A hair follicle usually opens just inside the rim of the papule.[148] Multiple trichodiscomas may be found in pure form, sometimes with early onset and autosomal dominant inheritance,[141,149] or they may be associated with fibrofolliculomas.[143–145] A solitary variant also occurs.[150]

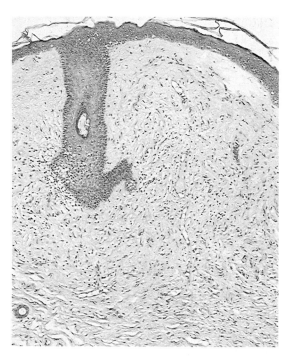

Fig. 33.11   Trichodiscoma. A poorly defined angiofibroma-like proliferation is present on one side of a hair follicle.
Haematoxylin — eosin

Histopathology[142,148]

Trichodiscomas are well-demarcated, non-encapsulated, dome-shaped, fibrovascular tumours of the dermis. They are covered by a flattened epidermis. A hair follicle will usually be found at one margin of the tumour if sufficient sections are examined. Trichodiscomas are composed of fascicles of loose, finely fibrillar connective tissue with intervening mucinous ground substance (Fig. 33.11). Elastic fibres are sparse or absent. There are prominent small vessels, some of which are telangiectatic. Sometimes, blood vessels with a concentric arrangement of PAS-positive collagen, forming a thickened wall, have been present towards the lower edge of the tumour. There is a moderate increase in fibroblasts, with occasional stellate forms. Nerve fibres have been described at the periphery of the lesions and also extending into the base.

Electron microscopy. Deposits of fibrillar-amorphous material have been shown between the collagen bundles.[142] The significance of this material is uncertain. Banded structures and a Merkel-cell–neurite complex in the basal layer of the epidermis have also been noted, although Merkel cells are not seen in the dermis.[142]

FIBROFOLLICULOMA

This rare tumour of the perifollicular connective tissue also has an epithelial component involving a proliferation of the epithelium of the infundibular portion of the hair follicle.

Fibrofolliculomas may be solitary[151,152] or multiple.[153] When multiple they are often associated with trichodiscomas and skin tags, and there is an autosomal dominant inheritance.[143–145] They have also been reported in association with a connective tissue naevus.[154] Fibrofolliculomas are small papules, 2–4 mm in diameter, involving the head and neck, the upper trunk and arms. Their onset is usually in the third or fourth decades of life. A central hair follicle is sometimes discernible.

The recently described *neurofollicular hamartoma* has a similar clinical presentation.[154a]

Histopathology[143,145,151]

Centrally, there is a reasonably well-formed hair which has a dilated infundibulum containing keratin debris. Around this, there is a well-circumscribed proliferation of loose connective tissue composed of fine fibres with intervening hyaluronic acid. Elastic fibres are scant or absent. Epithelial strands, two to four cells thick, radiate from the upper follicle into the surrounding connective tissue. These strands may anastomose or rejoin the infundibulum at several points. In patients with both fibrofolliculomas and trichodiscomas, the two lesions have been seen in close apposition.[145]

The *neurofollicular hamartoma* consists of hyperplastic pilosebaceous units with an intervening stroma of spindle cells arranged in broad, haphazard fascicles.[154a] The stroma has features of both an angiofibroma and a neurofibroma. The stromal cells are S100-positive.[154a]

PERIFOLLICULAR FIBROMA

This is a rather controversial entity which is regarded by some as a primary hyperplasia of the perifollicular dermis[155,156] and by others as a variant of angiofibroma.[157,158] Furthermore, a number of earlier reports mention epithelial proliferation, suggesting that some of the lesions reported as perifollicular fibromas may have been fibrofolliculomas.[144]

Perifollicular fibromas may be solitary[159] or multiple lesions,[160] clinically resembling fibrofolliculomas. They have been reported in patients with fibrofolliculomas and trichodiscomas[161] and also in association with colonic polyps.[162]

Histopathology[144,156]

There are concentric layers of cellular fibrous tissue in a perifollicular arrangement. There is no proliferation of the epithelium of the follicle.

SEBACEOUS TUMOURS

Sebaceous glands are usually found in association with hair follicles, the so-called pilosebaceous unit. Sebaceous glands without attached follicles may be found not uncommonly near mucocutaneous junctions, particularly the upper lip, as tiny yellow papules (Fordyce's spots).[60] They may also be found in the buccal mucosa, nipple, labia minora and in rare sites such as the oesophagus and vagina.[163] By far the most common 'tumour' of the sebaceous gland is sebaceous hyperplasia. This entity and the sebaceous gland neoplasms were reviewed in 1984.[164]

SEBACEOUS HYPERPLASIA

Sebaceous hyperplasia occurs as asymptomatic, solitary or multiple yellowish papules, often umbilicated, on the forehead and cheeks of elderly, and sometimes younger individuals.[165,166] Clinically, it may mimic basal cell carcinoma. Rare variants include a 'giant' form,[166a,166b] a linear or zosteriform arrangement,[167] a familial occurrence[168] and involvement of the areola[169,169a] or the vulva.[169b]

The aetiopathogenesis of sebaceous hyperplasia is unknown. Interestingly, sebaceous hyperplasia can be produced in rats by the topical application of Citrol (3,7-dimethyl-2,6-octadienol), a chemical used in foods as a flavouring agent.[169c]

Histopathology

There are large mature sebaceous lobules, grouped around a central dilated duct which is usually filled with debris, bacteria and occasionally a vellus hair. The lobules usually lack the indentations by fibrous septa which characterize the normal gland (Fig. 33.12). The sebocytes are smaller than usual and there are more basal cells per unit basement membrane length than in normal glands.[170] Autoradiographic studies have shown a lower labelling index.[170,170a]

Although sebaceous glands are prominent in rhinophyma (see p. 469), the sebaceous lobules are not as well defined and grouped as in sebaceous hyperplasia.

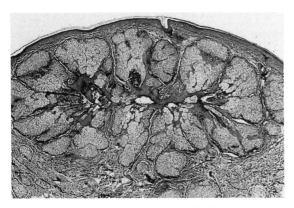

Fig. 33.12 Sebaceous gland hyperplasia. There are lobules of enlarged, mature sebaceous glands attached to a central hair follicle.
Haematoxylin–eosin

SEBACEOUS ADENOMA

The sebaceous adenoma is an uncommon benign tumour which usually presents as a slowly growing, pink or flesh-coloured, solitary nodule, predominantly on the head and neck of older individuals.[171] Rarely, it may involve the buccal mucosa.[172] Sebaceous adenomas are usually about 0.5 cm in diameter but larger variants, up to 9 cm in diameter, can develop. Occasionally they ulcerate and bleed or become tender. Sebaceous adenomas, either solitary or multiple, may be associated with visceral cancer, usually of the gastrointestinal tract — the Muir–Torre syndrome (see below).

Histopathology[171]

The tumour is composed of multiple, sharply circumscribed, sebaceous lobules separated by compressed connective tissue septa. It is usually centred on the mid dermis, but it may adjoin the epidermis or exhibit multiple openings on to the skin surface with partial replacement of the epidermis by basaloid epithelium showing sebaceous differentiation (Fig. 33.13). The sebaceous lobules have a peripheral germinative layer of small cells with mature sebaceous cells centrally, and transitional forms in between. This maturation is not as orderly or as well developed as in normal sebaceous glands.

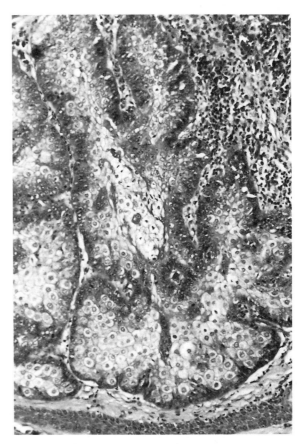

Fig. 33.13 Sebaceous adenoma. The sebaceous lobules have a peripheral layer of smaller basaloid cells.
Haematoxylin — eosin

Nevertheless, mature cells still outnumber the darker germinative cells.[60] There is variable central holocrine degeneration with granular debris scattered in the area of cystic change. The connective tissue stroma may contain a patchy chronic inflammatory cell infiltrate.

MUIR–TORRE SYNDROME

This syndrome, the first examples of which were reported in 1967,[173] is characterized by the development of sebaceous tumours, often multiple, in association with visceral neoplasms, usually gastrointestinal carcinomas.[174–176] Keratoacanthomas, epidermal cysts and colonic polyps may also be present. The sebaceous tumours are sometimes difficult to classify,[177] but they most resemble either sebaceous adenoma or sebaceoma, and occasionally sebaceous carcinomas.[178] The cutaneous tumours may precede or follow the first direct manifestation of the visceral cancer and they may occur sporadically in other family members.[179] The visceral tumour is usually of the gastrointestinal tract, particularly adenocarcinoma or polyps of the large bowel, but other sites such as larynx, ovary and uterus may be involved.[180,181] Lymphoma has been reported. The visceral tumours may behave in a less aggressive fashion than would be expected from the histology.[174] There may be a family history of internal cancer,[181] a trait which is autosomal dominant in inheritance.[174]

Histopathology[174,177]

The sebaceous tumours resemble to a varying degree those already described. Often they appear 'unique' and difficult to classify.[177] There may be solid sheets of basaloid cells in some lobules or an intermingling of these cells and sebaceous cells without any orderly maturation. Mucinous and cystic areas may be present. Other tumours may connect with the surface and have a central debris-filled crater resembling, in part, a keratoacanthoma.

SEBACEOMA

This term was coined by Ackerman for a distinctive sebaceous tumour,[182] examples of which have been reported in the past as basal cell carcinoma with sebaceous differentiation[171,183] or sebaceous epithelioma.[60] These tumours are usually solitary, yellowish papulonodules on the face or scalp, but they are sometimes multiple, particularly in the Muir–Torre syndrome (see above), or associated with organoid naevi.[171] They grow slowly and do not usually recur after treatment.

Histopathology[171,182]

There are multiple nests of basaloid cells with a random admixture of sebaceous cells, either solitary or in clusters (Fig. 33.14). The tumour is centred on the upper and mid dermis, but some nests may be continuous with the basal layer of the epidermis. The small basaloid cells of the tumour outnumber the mature sebaceous component. Cysts and duct-like structures containing the debris of holocrine degeneration may be present. There are scattered mitoses, but

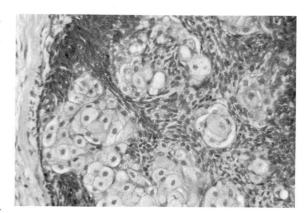

Fig. 33.14 Sebaceoma. There is a nest of basaloid cells randomly admixed with small clusters of sebaceous cells. Haematoxylin — eosin

Table 33.1 Histological features of sebaceous tumours

Sebaceous hyperplasia	Large sebaceous lobules clustered around dilated ducts; normal maturation pattern
Sebaceous adenoma	Lobules of basaloid and sebaceous cells with less orderly maturation; majority of cells mature; may open on to epidermal surface
Sebaceoma	Nests of basaloid cells with randomly admixed sebaceous cells; majority of cells are basaloid
Superficial epithelioma with sebaceous differentiation	Superficial plate-like proliferation with broad attachments to epidermis; clusters of mature sebaceous cells
Sebaceous carcinoma	Poorly defined lobules and sheets; infiltrating border; lack of differentiation with variable sebaceous changes

the tumour lacks the atypia of sebaceous carcinoma.

There exist tumours with close morphological resemblance to basal cell carcinoma which may show focal sebaceous differentiation. Such tumours are best classified as basal cell carcinomas with sebaceous differentiation. It is acknowledged that there is some overlap of this tumour with what has been designated sebaceoma.[182]

SUPERFICIAL EPITHELIOMA WITH SEBACEOUS DIFFERENTIATION

This term has been applied to a rare tumour with a predilection for the face of elderly individuals. It is usually solitary,[184] but multiple papules have been recorded.[185] It behaves in a benign fashion.

Histopathology

The tumour is characterized by a superficial plate-like proliferation of basaloid to squamoid cells with broad attachments to the overlying epidermis.[184] Clusters of mature sebaceous cells are present within the tumour.

SEBACEOUS CARCINOMA

Sebaceous carcinomas have traditionally been considered in two groups: those arising in the ocular adnexa, particularly the meibomian glands and glands of Zeis; and tumours arising in extra-ocular sites.[186] The latter are rare, and usually found as yellow-tan firm tumour nodules, often ulcerated, and measuring 1–4 cm or more in diameter. They are found particularly on the head and neck of elderly patients. Rare sites include the foot,[187] labia[171,188] and penis.[189]

Those arising in the ocular adnexa are more common and comprise 1% of all eyelid neoplasms. They have a slight female preponderance and tend to involve the upper eyelid more than the lower.[190–192] They often masquerade clinically as a chalazion, delaying effective treatment. Rarely, there is a history of radiation to the area.[191,193] Up to one-third develop lymph node metastases, usually to the pre-auricular and cervical nodes, and there is a 20% 5–year mortality. Recently, extra-ocular cases with nodal and even visceral metastases have been reported, leading the authors to question the notion that extra-ocular tumours are less aggressive than sebaceous carcinomas of the eyelid.[189,194–195]

Rarely, sebaceous carcinomas are associated with the Muir–Torre syndrome (see above).[186]

Histopathology[171,191,196]

The tumour is composed of lobules or sheets of cells separated by a fibrovascular stroma. The cells extend deeply and often involve the subcutaneous tissue and even the underlying muscle. There is infiltration at the edges. The cells show variable sebaceous differentiation, manifest as finely vacuolated or foamy rather than clear cytoplasm. There is usually more differentiation at the centre of the nests. The nuclei are large with large nucleoli. There are scattered mitoses. Smaller basaloid cells and cells resembling those in a squamous cell carcinoma may be present; even focal keratinization does not negate the diagnosis. Focal necrosis is not uncommon. The vacuolated cells show abundant lipid if a frozen section is stained with oil red O or Sudan black. There may be a very small amount of PAS-positive, diastase-resistant material in some cells.

The periocular lesions often show a pagetoid or less commonly a carcinoma in situ change in the overlying conjunctiva or epidermis of the eyelid.[190,191,197,198] Such changes are not usually seen in extra-ocular cases.

Adverse prognostic features for tumours of the ocular adnexa include vascular and lymphatic invasion, orbital extension, poor differentiation, an infiltrative growth pattern and large tumour size.[191]

Electron microscopy. The tumour cells contain cytoplasmic lipid droplets and tonofilaments which insert into well-formed desmosomes.[189,190]

APOCRINE TUMOURS

Apocrine tumours were reviewed, in some detail, in 1984 by Warkel.[199]

APOCRINE NAEVUS

This is a rare tumour composed of increased numbers of mature apocrine glands.[200,200a] It usually occurs as an element of an organoid naevus (naevus sebaceus) — see page 856.

APOCRINE CYSTADENOMA (HIDROCYSTOMA)

This tumour is regarded as an adenomatous cystic proliferation of apocrine glands, and not as a simple retention cyst. It has a predilection for the head and neck and is uncommon in the usual sites where apocrine glands are found. It may clinically have a bluish colour. Apocrine cystadenoma is considered further with other cutaneous cysts (see p. 488).

Histopathology

The cysts are lined by two layers of cells, an inner lining of large columnar cells with eosinophilic cytoplasm often showing luminal decapitation secretion, and an outer flattened layer of myoepithelial cells. Papillary projections of epithelium into the lumen are found in about one-half of the cases.

HIDRADENOMA PAPILLIFERUM

This is a variant of apocrine adenoma with specific morphology. It is almost always found in the vulval and perianal regions.[201,202] There are reports of eyelid[203] and auditory canal[204] involvement. It presents usually as a solitary nodule, usually less than 1 cm in diameter and usually in middle-aged women.

Histopathology[201,205]

The tumour is usually partly cystic and has both papillary and glandular areas (Fig. 33.15). The papillae often have an arborizing trabecular pattern; the glandular structures vary in size. Two types of epithelium are noted in both the papillary and glandular areas. Usually, the cells are tall and columnar with pale eosinophilic cytoplasm and nipple-like cytoplasmic projections on the surface. An underlying thin myoepithelial layer is often present. In about one-third of lesions, cuboidal cells with eosinophilic cytoplasm and small round nuclei, resembling apocrine metaplasia as seen in the breast, are present in some areas of the tumour.

PAS-positive, diastase-resistant granules are present in the apices of the large cells, while material in the glandular spaces stains with the colloidal iron method for acid mucopolysaccharides.

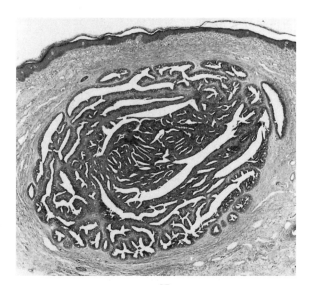

Fig. 33.15   Hidradenoma papilliferum with papillary and glandular areas.
Haematoxylin — eosin

Electron microscopy. This has shown characteristic secretory granules and 'decapitation' secretion.[206]

SYRINGOCYSTADENOMA PAPILLIFERUM

This is an uncommon, benign tumour of disputed histogenesis,[199] with a predilection for the scalp and forehead.[207] Less common sites of involvement are the chest,[208] upper arms[209] and thighs. There is an associated organoid naevus in approximately one-third of cases[207] and for this reason it is not always possible to be certain at what age the syringocystadenoma (syringoadenoma) papilliferum component developed. Probably one-half are present at birth or develop in childhood. A coexisting basal cell carcinoma is noted in 10% of cases,[207] and there is one report of an associated verrucous carcinoma.[210] Other congenital lesions have been associated with the presence of the tumour.[211]

The tumour has a varied clinical appearance, most often presenting as a raised warty plaque or as an irregular, flat, grey or reddened area. Linear papules and nodules are occasionally present.[209] The lesions measure from 1–3 cm in diameter. They are usually solitary. Alopecia accompanies those on the scalp.

There is increasing evidence for an apocrine histogenesis,[212,213] but the possibility of an eccrine origin for some cases cannot be excluded.[214]

Several examples of a malignant variant, *syringadenocarcinoma papilliferum* have been reported.[215–218] Some have been present for many years, suggesting the possibility of malignant transformation of a benign lesion.

Histopathology[207,214]

The tumour is composed of duct-like structures which extend as invaginations from the surface epithelium into the underlying dermis (Fig. 33.16). These may be lined by squamous epithelium near the epidermal surface, with a transition to double-layered cuboidal and columnar epithelium below. Sometimes this latter epithelium replaces, in part, the overlying epidermis. At other times, the surface is composed of irregular papillary projections covered by stratified squamous epithelium. The dilated and contorted ducts may lead into cystic spaces into which villous projections of diverse size and

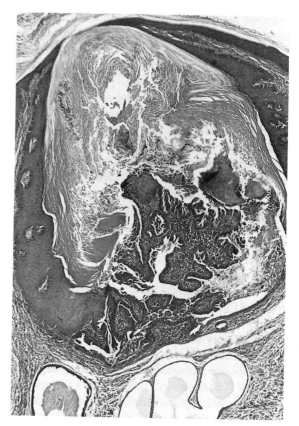

Fig. 33.16 Syringocystadenoma papilliferum. Irregular papillary projections protrude into the lumen of the invagination of surface epithelium. The stroma contains numerous plasma cells.
Haematoxylin — eosin

shape protrude. The ducts and papillary projections are usually covered by an inner layer of columnar epithelium and an outer layer of cuboidal or flattened cells.

The stroma of the papillary processes contains connective tissue, dilated vessels and, characteristically, numerous plasma cells admixed with a few lymphocytes. The underlying dermis contains a few inflammatory cells also.

There may be underlying dilated sweat glands and, occasionally, dilated apocrine glands.[219] In those cases associated with an organoid naevus, apocrine glands are said to be always present.[220]

Carcinoembryonic antigen is usually present in the epithelial cells.[221,222] Gross cystic disease fluid protein-15 (GCDFP-15), an apocrine marker, is variably positive in the tumour

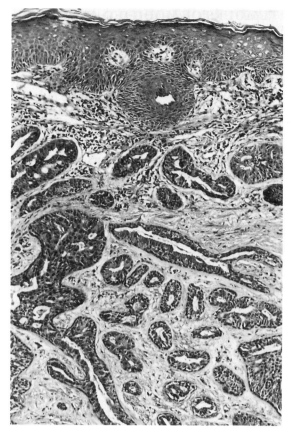

Fig. 33.19 Papillary adenoma of the nipple composed of duct-like structures of varying size. Haematoxylin — eosin

CERUMINOUS ADENOMA AND ADENOCARCINOMA

The ceruminous glands are modified apocrine glands in the external auditory canal. They give rise to rare tumours in which the distinction between adenoma and adenocarcinoma may be difficult on histological grounds.[287-291] The term 'ceruminoma' has been used in the past not only for the ceruminous adenoma and adenocarcinoma, but also for adenoid cystic carcinomas and mixed tumours of the auditory canal. The term is best abandoned. These tumours are discussed in Volume 1, pages 323–327.

ECCRINE TUMOURS

In the past, there has been some debate as to the eccrine or apocrine origin and differentiation of certain adnexal tumours. Histochemistry and electron microscopy sometimes gave conflicting results, with features suggestive of both apocrine and eccrine differentiation in some tumours. The recent development of various monoclonal antibodies, for use with immunoperoxidase techniques, has assisted in the classification of the various adnexal tumours.[221-223,292] The first of these to have diagnostic value was the finding of carcinoembryonic antigen (CEA) in sweat gland tumours. However, the rare finding of combined adnexal tumours with differentiation towards more than one adnexal structure indicates that the pluripotential cells that give rise to adnexal tumours may have the capacity to differentiate along more than one line. Other monoclonal antibodies have been developed recently with variable specificity and sensitivity for eccrine-related antigens. They include:

1. SKH1, which reacts with the secretory portion and coiled duct of the eccrine gland and the secretory portion of apocrine glands;[293]

2. ferritin antibody, which demonstrates ferritin in the outermost layer of the eccrine duct;[294]

3. antibodies to IgA and secretory component which detect antigen in the lumen and on the surface of the epithelium of sweat glands;[295] and

4. Dako-CK1 and Cam 5.2 (both commercially available) which react with two cytokeratins of different molecular weight.[296]

Whereas Dako-CK1 detects a cytokeratin in the intraepidermal eccrine duct and the inner layer of the intradermal portion of the duct but not other structures, Cam 5.2 reacts with the apocrine gland and duct and the eccrine secretory coils but not the eccrine duct.[296]

The eccrine hamartomas will be considered first, followed by a discussion of the benign eccrine tumours and the eccrine carcinomas. Hyperplastic and metaplastic lesions of the eccrine glands are discussed in Chapter 15 (pp. 470–471).

ECCRINE HAMARTOMAS

This term is used to cover the diverse group of naevoid conditions involving the eccrine sweat glands. The simplest lesion is an *eccrine naevus*,[297–299] a rare abnormality in which there is an increased number of normal-appearing eccrine coils or an increase in the size of the coils.

In *eccrine angiomatous hamartoma*,[300–302] there is an increase in the number of small blood vessels, and sometimes of nerve fibres or of fat, in addition to the increase in eccrine glands.

The *acrosyringeal naevus* consists of a proliferation of PAS-positive, acrosyringeal keratinocytes which extend down into the dermis as thin anastomosing cords from the undersurface of the epidermis (Fig. 33.20).[303] Some of these structures are recognizable as eccrine ducts. Stromal plasma cells may be prominent. Lesions may be linear,[303a] plaque-like or multiple.[303] Diffuse lesions have been observed in ectodermal dysplasia.[303b] Although regarded by some as an identical lesion,[304,305] the solitary tumour reported as a syringo-fibroadenoma[306] does have clinicopathological differences and will be considered with the benign tumours (see p. 849).[307,308] However, a recent report seems to indicate that cases with features overlapping both these conditions occur.[308a]

There are three somewhat-related lesions characterized by comedonal dilatation of eccrine ostia, with or without cornoid lamellae. These lesions are comedo naevus of the palm, linear eccrine naevus with comedones and porokeratotic eccrine ostial naevus. In *comedo naevus of the palm*,[309] there are keratotic pits formed by parakeratotic plugs within dilated eccrine ostia. The lesion reported as *linear eccrine naevus with comedones*[310] resembles naevus comedonicus (see p. 731) with the addition of basaloid nests in the dermis resembling eccrine spiradenoma in some areas and eccrine acro-spiroma in others. In *porokeratotic eccrine ostial naevus* there are cornoid lamellae associated with eccrine ducts.[311–312b]

In *eccrine-centred naevus* there are naevus cells intimately associated with eccrine sweat ducts.[313,314]

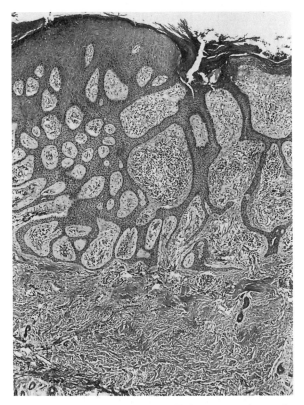

Fig. 33.20 Acrosyringeal naevus. Thin anastomosing cords of cells extend from the undersurface of the epidermis. Haematoxylin — eosin

ECCRINE HIDROCYSTOMA

This cystic lesion is usually solitary, but multiple lesions may occur. There is a predilection for the periorbital area.[315,316] It is discussed further with the other cystic lesions in Chapter 16 (p. 488).

Histopathology

The cysts are unilocular and lined by two layers of cuboidal epithelium.

PAPILLARY ECCRINE ADENOMA

This benign eccrine tumour was first described by Rulon and Helwig in 1977.[317] It presents as a slowly growing firm nodule with a predilection for the extremities of black people.[317–320] There was some controversy as to whether this is the same as the entity reported as tubular apocrine adenoma (see p. 836), or whether it is simply the eccrine equivalent;[318,321] most authors now regard it as a distinct eccrine tumour.[318a]

Histopathology[317,318]

Papillary eccrine adenoma is a circumscribed dermal tumour composed of multiple, variably dilated, duct-like structures lined by two or more layers of cells.[318a] The inner layer often forms intraluminal papillations of variable complexity (Fig. 33.21).[318] This latter feature is not always prominent in all areas of the tumour. The epithelial cells may show focal clear cell change and even focal squamous differentiation. Some of the lumina contain an amorphous, eosinophilic material.[321] Immunoperoxidase studies have demonstrated the presence of CEA, cytokeratins and S100 protein.[318a,320] The stromal connective tissue may show hyalinized collagen and a focal increase in fibroblasts. Inflammatory cells are usually sparse.

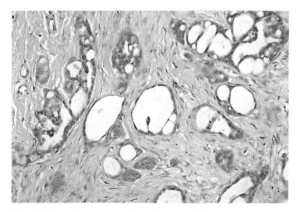

Fig. 33.21 Papillary eccrine adenoma. A few intraluminal papillations arise from the wall of the duct-like structures in the dermis.
Haematoxylin — eosin

Electron microscopy. The duct-like structures are composed of basal and luminal cells, the latter containing intracytoplasmic cavities but not secretory granules.[319a]

AGGRESSIVE DIGITAL PAPILLARY ADENOMA

This recently described entity occurs as a solitary painless mass, almost exclusively on the fingers, toes and adjacent parts of the palms and soles.[322] Most tumours are nodular growths, less than 2 cm in diameter. Over 90% are grossly cystic. There is a high rate of local recurrence.

A malignant variant — *aggressive digital papillary adenocarcinoma* — also occurs. It is characterized by aggressive local growth; there are distant metastases in nearly half of the cases, particularly to the lungs.[322]

Histopathology[322-323a]

The tumour involves the dermis and subcutis; it is usually poorly circumscribed. There are tubuloalveolar and ductal structures with areas of papillary projections protruding into cystic lumina (Fig. 33.22). The ductal structures are usually larger and more dilated than those in the papillary eccrine adenoma (see above). A cribriform pattern without obvious epithelial papillations is seen in about 20% of cases. The glandular lumina may contain eosinophilic secretory material. Scattered mitoses are present. The stroma varies from thin fibrous septa to areas of dense hyalinized collagen.

The malignant variant is characterized by

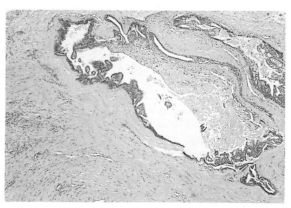

Fig. 33.22 Aggressive digital papillary adenoma. There are large dilated ductal structures with papillary projections into the lumen.
Haematoxylin — eosin

poor glandular differentiation, focal necrosis, cellular atypia and pleomorphism, and invasion of soft tissues, blood vessels and sometimes the underlying bone.

Immunoperoxidase studies have shown positivity for S100 protein, CEA and cytokeratins suggesting an origin from, or differentiation towards, the eccrine secretory coil.[322,323a] Staining has been more intense in the benign variants. Electron microscopy has shown eccrine glandular differentiation.

SYRINGOMA

Syringomas are usually found as multiple small papules on the lower eyelids and cheeks of adolescent females.[323] Other variants include solitary lesions, a plaque form, milia-like lesions,[324] tumours limited to the vulva,[325,326] penis[327,327a] or scalp,[328] and acral,[329,330] linear[331] or bathing trunk distributions.[332] Eruptive[333] and disseminated forms,[334] some of which may be familial,[335] have also been described. The clear cell variant of syringoma has been associated clinically with diabetes mellitus in many instances.[336]

Histopathology[323]

Syringomas are dermal tumours composed of multiple small ducts of eccrine type, lined usually by two layers of cuboidal epithelium (Fig. 33.23). Sometimes the ducts have a comma-like tail resembling those seen in desmoplastic trichoepithelioma (see p. 821). Solid nests and strands of cells, sometimes having a basaloid appearance, may be present. Some ducts are dilated and contain eosinophilic material. There is usually a dense fibrous stroma.

In the clear cell variant, the ducts are lined by larger epithelial cells with pale or clear cytoplasm (Fig. 33.24).[336–338] This clear cell change may involve only part of the tumour or be limited to the cells adjacent to the duct lumina. The clear cells contain abundant glycogen.

Rare variants include the presence of numerous mast cells in the stroma[339] or of naevus cells admixed with the syringomatous ele-

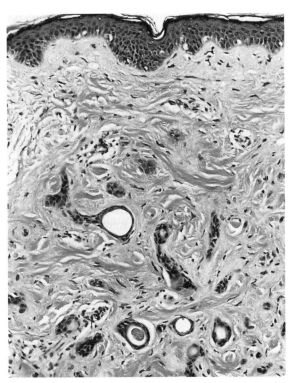

Fig. 33.23 Syringoma. Multiple small ductal structures, lined by two layers of cuboidal epithelium, are present in a fibrous stroma.
Haematoxylin — eosin

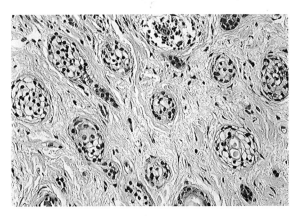

Fig. 33.24 Syringoma (clear cell variant). The ductal structures are lined by epithelium having pale cytoplasm.
Haematoxylin — eosin

ments.[323,340] Malignant degeneration is very rare and the tumours designated as malignant syringoma (syringoid eccrine carcinoma) are probably malignant ab initio.

in the tumour. Between the strands, there is a rich fibrovascular stroma. The tumour does not have the strong PAS positivity or the abundant stromal plasma cells of the acrosyringeal naevus.[303] Furthermore, the intervening stroma is not a prominent feature of the acrosyringeal naevus. However, they share many features in common.[308a]

HIDRADENOMA (ACROSPIROMA)

Considerable confusion exists in the literature as to the most appropriate designation for this tumour. Wilson Jones has called it a 'nosological jungle'.[410] Terms used have included 'solid-cystic hidradenoma',[411] 'eccrine acrospiroma',[381] 'clear cell hidradenoma',[412] 'eccrine sweat gland adenoma'[413] and 'clear cell myoepithelioma'.[414] Further difficulties are encountered in selecting the most appropriate term for those tumours which have a dermal component resembling a hidradenoma and a superficial component of eccrine poroma or, rarely, hidroacanthoma simplex.

HIDRADENOMA (ECCRINE ACROSPIROMA)

Hidradenoma, qualified if desired by the adjectives 'solid' or 'cystic', as appropriate, is the most suitable designation for this tumour of eccrine duct origin. It usually presents as a solitary, solid or partially cystic nodule with a slight preponderance in females of middle age,[412] but with no site predilection. It averages 1–2 cm in diameter, but larger variants up to 6 cm or more in diameter have been recorded.[415] Serous fluid occasionally drains from them.[381] Local recurrences are not uncommon, particularly if the lesion is inadequately excised. Malignant transformation or ab initio malignant variants are rare.[416–418]

Histopathology[381]

Hidradenomas are usually circumscribed, non-encapsulated, multilobular tumours, centred on the dermis but sometimes extending into the subcutis. Epidermal connections are present in up to one-quarter of cases,[411] and this superficial component may resemble an eccrine poroma. Hidradenomas may be solid or cystic in varying proportions. Sometimes large cystic spaces are present and the cystic spaces may contain sialomucin attached to the surface of the lining cells. The closely arranged tumour cells, which may be round, fusiform or polygonal in shape, are biphasic in cytoplasmic architecture, with one type having clear and the other eosinophilic cytoplasm (Fig. 33.33). There are variable proportions of each cell type in different tumours, but clear cells predominate in less than one-third of tumours.[411] Sometimes only a few clear cells can be seen. The clear cells contain glycogen and some PAS-positive, diastase-resistant material, but no lipid. The nuclei of the clear cells tend to be smaller than those in the eosinophilic cells. Mitoses are variable in number; their presence does not necessarily indicate malignancy.[419] However, in one study mitoses and atypical nuclear changes were associated with an increased local recurrence rate and even subsequent malignant transformation.[420] Other cellular variations include an epidermoid variant[421,421a] with large polyhedral cells having a squamous appearance, and a pigmented variant with some melanocytes and

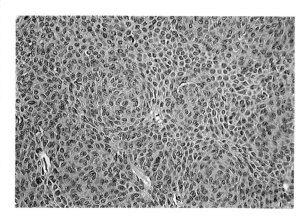

Fig. 33.33 Solid hidradenoma. It is composed of nests of tumour cells having eosinophilic cytoplasm. The cells have a subtle whorled arrangement in some areas. Haematoxylin — eosin

melanin pigment in cells and macrophages.[410,422]

Duct-like structures are often present in the tumour. Some resemble eccrine ducts, while others consist of several layers of concentric squamous cells with slit-like lumina. The stroma between the lobules varies from thin, delicate, vascularized cords of fibrous tissue to abundant, focally hyalinized collagen. A myxoid or chondroid stroma is rarely present.

The malignant variant has an infiltrative growth pattern, frequent mitoses (although some overlap exists in the mitotic rate between benign and malignant variants),[419] and sometimes angiolymphatic invasion.[417]

Electron microscopy.[423] The cells composing the tumour are connected by desmosomes. The clear cells have abundant glycogen and few tonofilaments, while the other cell type has abundant tonofilaments and small amounts of glycogen.

MALIGNANT ECCRINE TUMOURS

The classification of malignant eccrine tumours is the most confusing area of dermatopathology, with identical tumours reported in the literature under three or more designations. Furthermore, tumours with heterogeneous histological features that defy classification are common. Some earlier reports give scant histological details, precluding reassessment.[424] It is tempting to suggest that the term 'eccrine carcinoma' be applied to all malignant eccrine tumours, in much the same way that the term 'basal cell carcinoma' has proved adequate for a histologically diverse group of tumours. However, because there is a wide range of biological behaviour among the different eccrine tumours it seems justified to continue the search for an appropriate classification.

In his recent major review of sweat gland carcinomas, Santa Cruz lists the synonyms and related terms used for each of the tumours he describes.[218] He also suggests a classification based on the malignant potential as currently understood. For the most part, the eccrine tumours with the highest malignant potential are the malignant counterparts of the benign eccrine tumours (malignant acrospiroma, malignant mixed tumour, malignant spiradenoma and malignant cylindroma, as well as some of the ductal adenocarcinomas). The malignant eccrine poroma is of intermediate malignancy. The group of low malignancy includes sclerosing sweat duct carcinoma, eccrine epithelioma, adenoid cystic carcinoma and mucinous carcinoma.[218]

There has been much interest recently in assessing the various immunohistochemical markers of the eccrine carcinomas. In a study of 32 cases, epithelial membrane antigen and cytokeratin were present in all cases, while carcinoembryonic antigen (CEA) was detected in 25 and S100 in 19 cases.[425] Diffuse staining for ferritin is another marker of eccrine carcinomas.[294]

SCLEROSING SWEAT DUCT CARCINOMA

This tumour was first reported in 1982 by Goldstein and colleagues as *microcystic adnexal carcinoma*.[426] It has also been referred to as malignant syringoma,[427] and sweat gland carcinoma with syringomatous features.[428] One of the cases reported as a combined adnexal tumour[429] is also thought to be a sclerosing sweat duct carcinoma.[430] *Syringomatous adenoma of the nipple* is a closely related entity.[430a]

Sclerosing sweat duct carcinoma is a slowly growing, locally aggressive tumour, which presents as an indurated plaque or nodule, usually on the upper lip or elsewhere on the face.[431] It may also be found in the axilla[431a] and on the trunk and scalp.[431b] It affects adults of all ages. In two cases, the patient had previously received radiotherapy for adolescent acne.[432,433]

Local recurrence occurs in nearly 50% of cases,[433] but this is less likely if the excision margins are free of tumour in the initial excision. Only one case has had histological evidence of lymph node involvement, and this was almost certainly due to in-continuity extension.[433]

slowly growing tumour arising on the face (particularly the eyelids),[456] scalp,[215] axilla and trunk of middle-aged and older individuals.[457] The tumour nodules are often reddish, painless nodules measuring 0.5–7 cm in diameter. Late recurrences are common. Metastasis to regional nodes and widespread dissemination occur in about 15% of cases.[453,458,459]

Histopathology[457]

Mucinous carcinomas are dermal tumours which sometimes extend into the subcutis and deeper tissues. There are large pools of basophilic mucin, separated by thin fibrovascular septa. Small islands of epithelial cells appear to float in these mucinous pools (Fig. 33.38). The epithelial component is denser at the periphery of the lesion. The tumour cells are small and cuboidal and some have vacuolated cytoplasm. The cell nests in some areas have a cribriform appearance,[460] while other cells form small glandular or tubular spaces containing mucin.

The mucin is PAS positive, and stains with mucicarmine and colloidal iron. It is hyaluronidase resistant and sialidase labile, indicating that it is a sialomucin. This feature assists in differentiating this tumour from a metastatic mucinous carcinoma, which it may closely mimic on histological examination.[461]

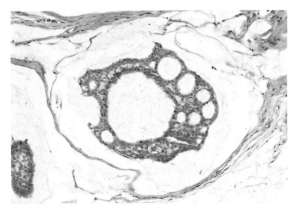

Fig. 33.38   Mucinous carcinoma. Islands of epithelial tumour cells are set in a mucinous stroma. Haematoxylin — eosin

Electron microscopy. The tumour is composed of peripheral dark cells, some of which contain mucin-like material, and inner pale cells which are less well differentiated.[462]

MALIGNANT CHONDROID SYRINGOMA

This rare eccrine tumour is most often found on the trunk and extremities, which are not the usual sites of the benign variant.[218,344-348] Sometimes juxtaposed areas of benign and malignant tumour are found, evidence for malignant transformation of a benign chondroid syringoma, at least in some cases.[218] Local or distant metastases are common, although there is usually a prolonged course.

Histopathology

The tumours have a lobulated appearance. They are composed of an epithelial and mesenchyme-like component, the latter consisting of myxomatous and cartilaginous areas.[344,345,348] The epithelial component predominates at the periphery of the tumour where there are cords and nests of cuboidal or polygonal cells with some glandular structures.[345] There is variable pleomorphism. Scattered mitoses are present. Mesenchymal elements are progressively more abundant towards the centre.[346] Ossification is occasionally present.[344] The histological appearance may be a poor indicator of the biological behaviour of a particular tumour in this category.[218,463]

MALIGNANT CYLINDROMA

This is a very rare tumour which usually arises in a cylindroma of the scalp of long standing.[362-364] Ab-initio variants probably also occur.[218] The tumours are aggressive, although subsequent metastasis is rare.[364a]

Histopathology

The tumour is composed of nests and cords of basaloid cells showing frequent mitoses, focal necrosis, and loss of the PAS-positive hyaline membrane. Foci of squamous differentiation occur. A contiguous benign cylindroma is usually present.

MALIGNANT ECCRINE SPIRADENOMA

The malignant transformation of eccrine spiradenoma is a rare event, heralded by the rapid enlargement of a cutaneous nodule of long standing.[364,368,374-376] Many different sites have been involved, with several occurring on the digits.[218] The tumours are quite aggressive, with fatal metastasis developing in at least 20% of cases.[218]

Histopathology

There are solid islands of tumour cells which may show either a squamous or a basaloid pattern. Glandular and sarcomatous areas have also been reported.[218,374a] The diagnosis depends on finding a contiguous eccrine spiradenoma, as the malignant component usually lacks any distinguishing features.

MALIGNANT ECCRINE POROMA

Malignant eccrine poroma (porocarcinoma) was first described by Pinkus and Mehregan as 'epidermotropic eccrine carcinoma'.[464] Since that time over 70 cases have been reported; there have been two large series.[440,465] The tumour occurs at all ages, although there is a predilection for older individuals. Acral locations are favoured. Malignant eccrine poromas present as verrucous plaques or polypoid growths which sometimes bleed with minor trauma.[465,466]

Some tumours are of long duration suggesting malignant transformation of an eccrine poroma or hidroacanthoma simplex.[467,468] Rarely, a malignant eccrine poroma arises in an organoid naevus.[469] Local recurrences and metastasis, particularly to regional nodes, occur.[470] Distant metastases are less common than in some of the other malignant counterparts of benign eccrine tumours. An unusual pattern of metastasis is the development of multiple cutaneous deposits with a lymphangitic pattern and microscopic epidermotropic deposits.

Histopathology[218,440,465]

The intraepidermal component is composed of nests and islands of small basaloid cells, sharply demarcated from the adjacent keratinocytes.[440] Broad anastomosing cords and solid columns and nests of large cells extend into the dermis to varying levels. Clear cell areas and focal necrosis may be present in the dermal nests.[471] Ductal structures are also found. A benign component of eccrine poroma or hidroacanthoma simplex may be present.[364,399,400]

The cells contain variable amounts of PAS-positive material, much of which is diastase labile. They stain positively for CEA, cytokeratin and epithelial membrane antigen.[425] There is an absence of cell membrane B2-microglobulin.[472]

Electron microscopy. The tumour cells contain a variable amount of glycogen, rare tonofilaments and intracellular lumina. The cell membranes have complex interdigitating microvilli-like cell processes.[218] Crystalline membrane-bound granules have also been reported.[473]

HIDRADENOCARCINOMA

Although the term malignant acrospiroma is sometimes used for these tumours, it has also been applied to a heterogeneous group of eccrine carcinomas. For this reason the term hidradenocarcinoma is preferred. This is a rare tumour with a predilection for the face and extremities.[455] It usually presents as an ulcerated reddish nodule[474] in older individuals, but cases have been recorded in children[475] and at birth.[416] The tumours have an aggressive course with eventual distant metastasis to bones and lungs.[418,455]

Histopathology[416,455]

The tumour is composed of sheets of cells with

COMBINED ADNEXAL TUMOUR

This term has been used for a tumour with differentiation towards the formation of sebaceous glands and pilar and sweat duct structures.[429] It has also been applied to a tumour showing only pilar and sweat duct structures, but the case was probably a sclerosing sweat duct carcinoma.[435] Apocrine, sebaceous and pilar differentiation have been reported in mixed tumours of the skin.[495] It should also be noted that divergent differentiation is sometimes seen in various eccrine carcinomas. The term 'cutaneous adnexal carcinoma with divergent differentiation' has been used in these circumstances.[496]

POROMA-LIKE ADNEXAL ADENOMA

This tumour, at first glance, resembles an eccrine poroma, but the epithelial proliferations show apocrine and sebaceous, rather than eccrine, differentiation.[483] The term *sebocrine adenoma* has also been proposed for such cases.[484]

HEMIFACIAL MIXED APPENDAGEAL TUMOUR

The condition to which this name was given was an erythematous papulonodular eruption confined to one side of the face of an infant.[485] It had a linear array on the cheek. The lesion was composed of islands of cells with eccrine, apocrine and basaloid features. Similar cases in the literature, usually with comedones, have been classed as linear basal cell naevi (see p. 822).

REFERENCES

HAIR FOLLICLE TUMOURS

1. Headington JT. Tumors of the hair follicle. A review. Am J Pathol 1976; 85: 480–505.
2. Mehregan AH. Hair follicle tumors of the skin. J Cutan Pathol 1985; 12: 189–195.
2a. Rosen LB. A review and proposed new classification of benign acquired neoplasms with hair follicle differentiation. Am J Dermatopathol 1990; 12: 496–516.

Hamartomas and tumours of hair germ

3. Pippione M, Aloi F, Depaoli MA. Hair-follicle nevus. Am J Dermatopathol 1984; 6: 245–247.
4. Weir TW. Hair-follicle nevus. Am J Dermatopathol 1985; 7: 304.
5. Bass J, Pomeranz JR. Linear hair follicle naevus. Presentation American Society of Dermatopathology Meeting, San Antonio; 1987.
5a. Jackson CE, Callies QC, Krull EA, Mehregan A. Hairy cutaneous malformations of palms and soles. Arch Dermatol 1975; 111: 1146–1149.
6. Gray HR, Helwig EB. Trichofolliculoma. Arch Dermatol 1962; 86: 619–625.
7. Pinkus H, Sutton RL. Trichofolliculoma. Arch Dermatol 1965; 91: 46–49.
8. Kligman AM, Pinkus H. The histogenesis of nevoid tumors of the skin. The folliculoma — a hair-follicle tumor. Arch Dermatol 1960; 81: 922–930.
9. Hyman AB, Clayman SJ. Hair-follicle nevus. Arch Dermatol 1957; 75: 678–684.

10. Plewig G. Sebaceous trichofolliculoma. J Cutan Pathol 1980; 7: 394–403.
11. Nikolowski W. Tricho-Adenom (Organoides Follikel-Hamartoma). Arch Klin Exp Dermatol 1958; 207: 34–45.
12. Rahbari H, Mehregan A, Pinkus H. Trichoadenoma of Nikolowski. J Cutan Pathol 1977; 4: 90–98.
13. Rahbari H, Mehregan AH. Benign follicular neoplasias. J Dermatol Surg Oncol 1979; 5: 295–298.
13a. Jaqueti G, Requena L, Sanchez Yus E. Verrucous trichoadenoma. J Cutan Pathol 1989; 16: 145–148.
14. Gray HR, Helwig EB. Epithelioma adenoides cysticum and solitary trichoepithelioma. Arch Dermatol 1963; 87: 102–114.
15. Filho GB, Toppa NH, Miranda D et al. Giant solitary trichoepithelioma. Arch Dermatol 1984; 120: 797–798.
16. Czernobilsky B. Giant solitary trichoepithelioma. Arch Dermatol 1972; 105: 587–588.
16a. Beck S, Cotton DWK. Recurrent solitary giant trichoepithelioma located in the perianal area; a case report. Br J Dermatol 1988; 118: 563–566.
17. Tatnall FM, Wilson Jones E. Giant solitary trichoepitheliomas located in the perianal area: a report of three cases. Br J Dermatol 1986; 115: 91–99.
18. Anderson DE, Howell JB. Epithelioma adenoides cysticum: genetic update. Br J Dermatol 1976; 95: 225–232.
19. Geffner RE, Goslen JB, Santa Cruz DJ. Linear and dermatomal trichoepitheliomas. J Am Acad Dermatol 1986; 14: 927–930.

20. Lambert WC, Bilinski DL, Khan MY, Brodkin RH. Trichoepithelioma in a systematized epidermal nevus with acantholytic dyskeratosis. Arch Dermatol 1984; 120: 227–230.

21. Rasmussen JE. A syndrome of trichoepitheliomas, milia, and cylindromas. Arch Dermatol 1975; 111: 610–614.

22. Magnin PH, Duhm G, Casas JG. Espiroadenoma, cilindroma cutaneo y tricoepitelioma multiple y familiar. Med Cut ILA 1977; 3: 179–187.

23. Parhizgar B, Leppard BJ. Epithelioma adenoides cysticum. A condition mimicking tuberose sclerosis. Clin Exp Dermatol 1977; 2: 145–152.

24. Cramers M. Trichoepithelioma multiplex and dystrophia unguis congenita: a new syndrome? Acta Derm Venereol 1981; 61: 364–365.

25. Michaelsson G, Olsson E, Westermark P. The ROMBO syndrome: a familial disorder with vermiculate atrophoderma, milia, hypotrichosis, trichoepitheliomas, basal cell carcinomas and peripheral vasodilation with cyanosis. Acta Derm Venereol 1981; 61: 497–503.

26. Sandbank M, Bashan D. Multiple trichoepithelioma and breast carcinoma. Arch Dermatol 1978; 114: 1230.

27. Pariser RJ. Multiple hereditary trichoepitheliomas and basal cell carcinomas. J Cutan Pathol 1986; 13: 111–117.

28. Howell JB, Anderson DE. Transformation of epithelioma adenoides cysticum into multiple rodent ulcers: fact or fallacy. A historical vignette. Br J Dermatol 1976; 95: 233–242.

28a. Lee Y-S, Fong P-H. Secondary localized amyloidosis in trichoepithelioma. A light microscopic and ultrastructural study. Am J Dermatopathol 1990; 12: 469–478.

28b. Brooke JD, Fitzpatrick JE, Golitz LE. Papillary mesenchymal bodies: A histologic finding useful in differentiating trichoepitheliomas from basal cell carcinomas. J Am Acad Dermatol 1989; 21: 523–528.

29. Ueda K, Komori Y, Maruo M, Kusaba K. Ultrastructure of trichoepithelioma papulosum multiplex. J Cutan Pathol 1981; 8: 188–198.

30. MacDonald DM, Wilson Jones E, Marks R. Sclerosing epithelial hamartoma. Clin Exp Dermatol 1977; 2: 153–160.

31. Brownstein MH, Shapiro L. Desmoplastic trichoepithelioma. Cancer 1977; 40: 2979–2986.

32. Dervan PA, O'Loughlin S, O'Hegarty M, Corrigan T. Solitary familial desmoplastic trichoepithelioma. Am J Dermatopathol 1985; 7: 277–282.

33. Lazorik FC, Wood MG. Multiple desmoplastic trichoepitheliomas. Arch Dermatol 1982; 118: 361–362.

34. Rahbari H, Mehregan AH. Trichoepithelioma and pigmented nevus. A combined malformation. J Cutan Pathol 1975; 2: 225–231.

35. Brownstein MH, Starink TM. Desmoplastic trichoepithelioma and intradermal nevus: A combined malformation. J Am Acad Dermatol 1987; 17: 489–492.

36. Landau-Price D, Barnhill RL, Kowalcyzk AP et al. The value of carcinoembryonic antigen in differentiating sclerosing epithelial hamartoma from syringoma. J Cutan Pathol 1985; 12: 8–12.

36a. Hashimoto T, Inamoto N, Nakamura K, Harada R. Involucrin expression in skin appendage tumours. Br J Dermatol 1987; 117: 325–332.

37. Bondi R, Donati E, Santucci M et al. An ultrastructural study of a sclerosing epithelial hamartoma. Am J Dermatopathol 1985; 7: 223–229.

38. Takei Y, Fukushiro S, Ackerman AB. Criteria for histologic differentiation of desmoplastic trichoepithelioma (sclerosing epithelial hamartoma) from morphea-like basal-cell carcinoma. Am J Dermatopathol 1985; 7: 207–221.

38a. Hashimoto K, Prince C, Kato I et al. Rippled-pattern trichomatricoma. J Cutan Pathol 1989; 16: 19–30.

39. Headington JT, French AJ. Primary neoplasms of the hair follicle. Histogenesis and classification. Arch Dermatol 1962; 86: 430–441.

40. Headington JT. Differentiating neoplasms of hair germ. J Clin Pathol 1970; 23: 464–471.

41. Arata J. An unusual hair follicle tumor, an intimate relative of trichogenic adnexal tumor (Headington and French). J Dermatol 1976; 3: 221–229.

42. Grouls V, Hey A. Trichoblastic fibroma. Pathol Res Pract 1988; 183: 462–468.

43. Slater DN. Trichoblastic fibroma: hair germ (trichogenic) tumours revisited. Histopathology 1987; 11: 327–331.

43a. Long SA, Hurt MA, Santa Cruz DJ. Immature trichoepithelioma: report of six cases. J Cutan Pathol 1988; 15: 353–358.

43b. Zaim MT. "Immature" trichoepithelioma. J Cutan Pathol 1989; 16: 287–289.

43c. Martin PC, Pulitzer DR, Reed RJ. Hair matrix adenoma. A clinicopathologic study of 11 cases. Am J Surg Pathol (in press).

44. Cohen C, Davis TS. Multiple trichogenic adnexal tumors. Am J Dermatopathol 1986; 8: 241–246.

44a. Requena L, Requena I, Romero E et al. Trichogenic trichoblastoma. An unusual neoplasm of hair germ. Am J Dermatopathol 1990; 12: 175–181.

44b. Gilks CB, Clement PB, Wood WS. Trichoblastic fibroma. A clinicopathologic study of three cases. Am J Dermatopathol 1989; 11: 397–402.

45. Brown AC, Crounse RG, Winkelmann RK. Generalized hair-follicle hamartoma: associated with alopecia, aminoaciduria, and myasthenia gravis. Arch Dermatol 1969; 99: 478–492.

46. Ridley CM, Smith N. Generalized hair follicle hamartoma associated with alopecia and myasthenia gravis: report of a second case. Clin Exp Dermatol 1981; 6: 283–289.

47. Starink TM, Lane EB, Meijer CJLM. Generalized trichoepitheliomas with alopecia and myasthenia gravis: Clinicopathologic and immunohistochemical study and comparison with classic and desmoplastic trichoepithelioma. J Am Acad Dermatol 1986; 15: 1104–1112.

48. Weltfriend S, David M, Ginzburg A, Sandbank M. Generalized hair follicle hamartoma: The third case reported in association with myasthenia gravis. Am J Dermatopathol 1987; 9: 428–432.

49. Mehregan AH, Baker S. Basaloid follicular hamartoma: three cases with localized and systematized unilateral lesions. J Cutan Pathol 1985; 12: 55–65.

50. Johnson WC, Hookerman BJ. Basal cell hamartoma

with follicular differentiation. Arch Dermatol 1972; 105: 105–106.

51. Carney RG. Linear unilateral basal-cell nevus with comedones. Report of a case. Arch Dermatol 1952; 65: 471–476.

52. Anderson TE, Best PV. Linear basal-cell naevus. Br J Dermatol 1962; 74: 20–23.

53. Bleiberg J, Brodkin RH. Linear unilateral basal cell nevus with comedones. Arch Dermatol 1969; 100: 187–190.

54. Horio T, Komura J. Linear unilateral basal cell nevus with comedo-like lesions. Arch Dermatol 1978; 114: 95–97.

Infundibular tumours

55. Mehregan AH. Infundibular tumors of the skin. J Cutan Pathol 1984; 11: 387–395.

56. Mehregan AH, Butler JD. A tumor of follicular infundibulum. Arch Dermatol 1961; 83: 924–927.

57. Mehregan AH. Tumor of follicular infundibulum. Dermatologica 1971; 142: 177–183.

58. Kossard S, Kocsard E, Poyzer KG. Infundibulomatosis. Arch Dermatol 1983; 119: 267–268.

58a. Kossard S, Finley AG, Poyzer K, Kocsard E. Eruptive infundibulomas. A distinctive presentation of the tumor of follicular infundibulum. J Am Acad Dermatol 1989; 21: 361–366.

59. Trunnell TN, Waisman M. Tumor of the follicular infundibulum. Cutis 1979; 24: 317–318.

60. Brownstein MH, Shapiro L. The pilosebaceous tumors. Int J Dermatol 1977; 16: 340–352.

60a. Findlay GH. Multiple infundibular tumours of the head and neck. Br J Dermatol 1989; 120: 633–638.

60b. Ishida-Yamamoto A, Iizuka H. Infundibular keratosis — a prototype of benign infundibular tumours. Clin Exp Dermatol 1989; 14: 145–149.

61. Winer LH. The dilated pore, a trichoepithelioma. J Invest Dermatol 1954; 23: 181–188.

62. Klövekorn G, Klövekorn W, Plewig G, Pinkus H. Riesenpore und Haarscheidenakanthom. Klinische und histologische Diagnose. Hautarzt 1983; 34: 209–216.

63. Smolle J, Kerl H. Das Pilar Sheath Acanthoma — ein gutartiges follikuläres Hamartom. Dermatologica 1983; 167: 335–338.

64. Mehregan AH, Brownstein MH. Pilar sheath acanthoma. Arch Dermatol 1978; 114: 1495–1497.

65. Bhawan J. Pilar sheath acanthoma. A new benign follicular tumor. J Cutan Pathol 1979; 6: 438–440.

66. Spielvogel RL, Austin C, Ackerman AB. Inverted follicular keratosis is not a specific keratosis but a verruca vulgaris (or seborrheic keratosis) with squamous eddies. Am J Dermatopathol 1983; 5: 427–445.

67. Reed RJ, Pulitzer DR. Inverted follicular keratosis and human papillomaviruses. Am J Dermatopathol 1983; 5: 453–465.

68. Mascaro JM. Inverted follicular keratoses are acrotrichomas. Am J Dermatopathol 1983; 5: 447–451.

69. Mehregan AH. Inverted follicular keratosis is a distinct follicular tumor. Am J Dermatopathol 1983; 5: 467–470.

70. Sassani JW, Yanoff M. Inverted follicular keratosis. Am J Ophthalmol 1979; 87: 810–813.

71. Mehregan AH, Nadji M. Inverted follicular keratosis and Verruca vulgaris. An investigation for the papillomavirus common antigen. J Cutan Pathol 1984; 11: 99–102.

72. Azzopardi JG, Laurini R. Inverted follicular keratosis. J Clin Pathol 1975; 28: 465–471.

73. Sim-Davis D, Marks R, Wilson Jones E. The inverted follicular keratosis. A surprising variant of seborrheic wart. Acta Derm Venereol 1976; 56: 337–344.

74. Mehregan AH. Inverted follicular keratosis. Arch Dermatol 1964; 89: 229–235.

Tricholemmal (external sheath) tumours

75. Goldman L, Richfield DF. Tricholemmoma clinical lesions. Arch Dermatol 1977; 113: 107–108.

76. Hunt SJ, Kilzer B, Santa Cruz DJ. Desmoplastic trichilemmoma: histologic variant resembling invasive carcinoma. J Cutan Pathol 1990; 17: 45–52.

77. Ackerman AB. Trichilemmoma. Arch Dermatol 1978; 114: 286.

78. Ackerman AB, Wade TR. Tricholemmoma. Am J Dermatopathol 1980; 2: 207–224.

79. Headington JT. Tricholemmoma. To be or not to be? Am J Dermatopathol 1980; 2: 225–228.

80. Brownstein MH. Trichilemmoma. Benign follicular tumor or viral wart? Am J Dermatopathol 1980; 2: 229–231.

81. Penneys NS, Mogollon RJ, Nadji M, Gould E. Survey of verruca, benign verrucous lesions, trichilemmoma, and bowenoid papulosis for the presence of papilloma common antigen: an immunoperoxidase study. Arch Dermatol 1983; 119: 848–849 (abstract).

82. Brownstein MH, Shapiro L. Trichilemmoma. Analysis of 40 new cases. Arch Dermatol 1973; 107: 866–869.

83. Ingrish FM, Reed RJ. Tricholemmoma. Dermatol Int 1968; 7: 182–190.

84. Reed RJ. Tricholemmoma. A cutaneous hamartoma. Am J Dermatopathol 1980; 2: 227–228.

85. Brownstein MH, Shapiro EE. Trichilemmomal horn: cutaneous horn overlying trichilemmoma. Clin Exp Dermatol 1979; 4: 59–63.

86. Richfield DF. Tricholemmoma. True and false types. Am J Dermatopathol 1980; 2: 233–234.

87. Gentry WC Jr. Autosomal dominant genodermatoses associated with internal malignant disease. Semin Dermatol 1984; 3: 273–281.

88. Salem OS, Steck WD. Cowden's disease (multiple hamartoma and neoplasia syndrome). A case report and review of the English literature. J Am Acad Dermatol 1983; 8: 686–696.

88a. Shapiro SD, Lambert WC, Schwartz RA. Cowden's disease. A marker for malignancy. Int J Dermatol 1988; 27: 232–237.

89. Weary PE, Gorlin RJ, Gentry WC Jr et al. Multiple hamartoma syndrome (Cowden's disease). Arch Dermatol 1972; 106: 682–690.

90. Starink TM. Cowden's disease: Analysis of fourteen new cases. J Am Acad Dermatol 1984; 11: 1127–1141.

91. Lloyd KM, Dennis M. Cowden's disease. A possible new symptom complex with multiple system involvement. Ann Intern Med 1963; 58: 136–142.

92. Elston DM, James WD, Rodman OG, Graham GF. Multiple hamartoma syndrome (Cowden's disease)

associated with non-Hodgkin's lymphoma. Arch Dermatol 1986; 122: 572–575.

93. Brownstein MH, Mehregan AH, Bikowski JB. Trichilemmomas in Cowden's disease. JAMA 1977; 238: 26.

94. Grattan CEH, Hamburger J. Cowden's disease in two sisters, one showing partial expression. Clin Exp Dermatol 1987; 12: 360–363.

95. Nuss DD, Aeling JL, Clemons DE, Weber WN. Multiple hamartoma syndrome (Cowden's disease). Arch Dermatol 1978; 114: 743–746.

96. Ortonne JP, Lambert R, Daudet J et al. Involvement of the digestive tract in Cowden's disease. Int J Dermatol 1980; 19: 570–576.

97. Aram H, Zidenbaum M. Multiple hamartoma syndrome (Cowden's disease). J Am Acad Dermatol 1983; 9: 774–776.

98. Allen BS, Fitch MH, Smith JG Jr. Multiple hamartoma syndrome. A report of a new case with associated carcinoma of the uterine cervix and angioid streaks of the eyes. J Am Acad Dermatol 1980; 2: 303–308.

99. Halevy S, Sandbank M, Pick AI, Feuerman EJ. Cowden's disease in three siblings: electron-microscope and immunological studies. Acta Derm Venereol 1985; 65: 126–131.

100. Camisa C, Bikowski JB, McDonald SG. Cowden's disease. Association with squamous cell carcinoma of the tongue and perianal basal cell carcinoma. Arch Dermatol 1984; 120: 677–678.

101. Starink TM, Hausman R. The cutaneous pathology of facial lesions in Cowden's disease. J Cutan Pathol 1984; 11: 331–337.

102. Starink TM, Hausman R. The cutaneous pathology of extrafacial lesions in Cowden's disease. J Cutan Pathol 1984; 11: 338–344.

103. Starink TM, Meijer CJLM, Brownstein MH. The cutaneous pathology of Cowden's disease: new findings. J Cutan Pathol 1985; 12: 83–93.

104. Brownstein MH, Mehregan AH, Bikowski JB et al. The dermatopathology of Cowden's syndrome. Br J Dermatol 1979; 100: 667–673.

105. Gentry WC, Eskritt NR, Gorlin RJ. Multiple hamartoma syndrome (Cowden disease). Arch Dermatol 1974; 109: 521–525.

106. Johnson BL, Kramer EM, Lavker RM. The keratotic tumors of Cowden's disease: an electronmicroscopic study. J Cutan Pathol 1987; 14: 291–298.

107. Barax CN, Lebwohl M, Phelps RG. Multiple hamartoma syndrome. J Am Acad Dermatol 1987; 17: 342–346.

108. Ten Seldam REJ. Tricholemmocarcinoma. Australas J Dermatol 1977; 18: 62–72.

108a. Lee JY, Tank CK, Leung YS. Clear cell carcinoma of the skin: a tricholemmal carcinoma. J Cutan Pathol 1989; 16: 31–39.

109. Swanson PE, Cherwitz DL, Wick MR. Tricholemmal carcinoma: a clinicopathologic study of 6 cases (poster display). American Society of Dermatopathology, Annual Meeting: San Antonio; 1987.

109a. Mehregan AH, Medenica M, Whitney D, Kato I. A clear cell pilar sheath tumor of scalp: case report. J Cutan Pathol 1988; 15: 380–384.

Tumours with matrical differentiation

110. LeBoit PE, Parslow TG, Choy S-H. Hair matrix differentiation. Occurrence in lesions other than pilomatricoma. Am J Dermatopathol 1987; 9: 399–405.

111. Jacobson M, Ackerman AB. "Shadow" cells as clues to follicular differentiation. Am J Dermatopathol 1987; 9: 51–57.

112. Moehlenbeck FW. Pilomatrixoma (calcifying epithelioma). A statistical study. Arch Dermatol 1973; 108: 532–534.

113. Schlechter R, Hartsough NA, Guttman FM. Multiple pilomatricomas (calcifying epitheliomas of Malherbe). Pediatr Dermatol 1984; 2: 23–25.

114. Wong WK, Somburanasin R, Wood MG. Eruptive, multicentric pilomatricoma (calcifying epithelioma). Arch Dermatol 1972; 106: 76–78.

114a. Taaffe A, Wyatt EH, Bury HPR. Pilomatricoma (Malherbe). A clinical and histopathologic survey of 78 cases. Int J Dermatol 1988; 27: 477–480.

115. Olivo M, Damm S. Multiple pilomatrixomas. Arch Dermatol 1977; 113: 977.

116. Hernandez-Perez E, Cestoni-Parducci RF. Pilomatricoma (calcifying epithelioma). A study of 100 cases in El Salvador. Int J Dermatol 1981; 20: 491–494.

117. Chiaramonti A, Gilgor RS. Pilomatricomas associated with myotonic dystrophy. Arch Dermatol 1978; 114: 1363–1365.

118. Schwartz BK, Peraza JE. Pilomatricomas associated with myotonic dystrophy. J Am Acad Dermatol 1987; 16: 887–888.

119. Leppard BJ, Bussey HJR. Gardner's syndrome with epidermoid cysts showing features of pilomatrixomas. Clin Exp Dermatol 1976; 1: 75–82.

120. Cooper PH, Fechner RE. Pilomatricoma-like changes in the epidermal cysts of Gardner's syndrome. J Am Acad Dermatol 1983; 8: 639–644.

121. Swerlick RA, Cooper PH, Mackel SE. Rapid enlargement of pilomatricoma. J Am Acad Dermatol 1982; 7: 54–56.

122. Spitz D, Fisher D, Friedman RJ, Kopf AW. Pigmented pilomatricoma. A clinical simulator of malignant melanoma. J Dermatol Surg Oncol 1981; 7: 903–906.

123. Zina AM, Bundino S, Torre C. Gross pathology and scanning electron microscopy of pilomatricoma. J Cutan Pathol 1985; 12: 33–36.

124. Forbis R, Helwig EB. Pilomatrixoma (calcifying epithelioma). Arch Dermatol 1961; 83: 606–618.

125. Rothman D, Kendall AB, Baldi A. Giant pilomatrixoma (Malherbe calcifying epithelioma). Arch Surg 1976; 111: 86–87.

126. Manivel C, Wick MR, Mukai K. Pilomatrix carcinoma: an immunohistochemical comparison with benign pilomatrixoma and other benign cutaneous lesions of pilar origin. J Cutan Pathol 1986; 13: 22–29.

127. Gould E, Kurzon R, Kowalczyk AP, Saldana M. Pilomatrix carcinoma with pulmonary metastasis. Report of a case. Cancer 1984; 54: 370–372.

128. Lopansri S, Mihm MC. Pilomatrix carcinoma or calcifying epitheliocarcinoma of Malherbe. A case report and review of literature. Cancer 1980; 45: 2368–2373.

129. Weedon D, Bell J, Mayze J. Matrical carcinoma of the skin. J Cutan Pathol 1980; 7: 39–42.
130. Wood MG, Parhizgar B, Beerman H. Malignant pilomatricoma. Arch Dermatol 1984; 120: 770–773.
130a. Rabkin M, Wittwer CT, Soong VY. Flow cytometric DNA content analysis of a case of pilomatrix carcinoma showing multiple recurrences and invasion of the cranial vault. J Am Acad Dermatol 1990; 23: 104–108.
131. van der Walt JD, Rohlova B. Carcinomatous transformation in a pilomatrixoma. Am J Dermatopathol 1984; 6: 63–69.
132. Mir R, Cortes E, Papantoniou PA et al. Metastatic trichomatricial carcinoma. Arch Pathol Lab Med 1986; 110: 660–663.
133. Green DE, Sanusi ID, Fowler MR. Pilomatrix carcinoma. J Am Acad Dermatol 1987; 17: 264–270.
133a. Miller K, Lechner W, Burg G. Malignant pilomatricoma with distant metastasis. J Cutan Pathol 1989; 16: 318 (abstract).
134. Booth JC, Kramer H, Taylor KB. Pilomatrixoma — calcifying epithelioma (Malherbe). Pathology 1969; 1: 119–127.
134a. Sano Y, Mihara M, Miyamoto T, Shimao S. Simultaneous occurrence of calcification and amyloid deposit in pilomatricoma. Acta Derm Venereol 1990; 70: 256–259.
135. Kumasa S, Mori H, Tsujimura T, Mori M. Calcifying epithelioma of Malherbe with ossification. Special reference to lectin binding and immunohistochemistry of ossified sites. J Cutan Pathol 1987; 14: 181–187.
136. Cazers JS, Okun MR, Pearson SH. Pigmented calcifying epithelioma. Review and presentation of a case with unusual features. Arch Dermatol 1974; 110: 773–774.
137. Kanitakis J, Hermier C, Chouvet B, Thivolet J. [Calcifying epithelioma (of Malherbe) of unusual histological type]. Dermatologica 1984; 168: 259–262.
137a. Benharroch D, Sacks MI. Pilomatricoma associated with epidermoid cyst. J Cutan Pathol 1989; 16: 40–43.
138. Uchiyama N, Shindo Y, Saida T. Perforating pilomatricoma. J Cutan Pathol 1986; 13: 312–318.
138a. Zulaica A, Peteiro C, Quintas C et al. Perforating pilomatricoma. J Cutan Pathol 1988; 15: 409–411.
139. Tsoitis G, Mandinaos C, Kanitakis JC. Perforating calcifying epithelioma of Malherbe with a rapid evolution. Dermatologica 1984; 168: 233–237.
139a. Arnold M, McGuire LJ. Perforating pilomatricoma — difficulty in diagnosis. J Am Acad Dermatol 1988; 18: 754–755.
140. McGavran MH. Ultrastructure of pilomatrixoma (calcifying epithelioma). Cancer 1965; 18: 1445–1456.

Tumours of perifollicular mesenchyme

141. Camarasa JG, Calderon P, Moreno A. Familial multiple trichodiscomas. Acta Derm Venereol 1988; 68: 163–165.
142. Balus L, Crovato F, Breathnach AS. Familial multiple trichodiscomas. J Am Acad Dermatol 1986; 15: 603–607.
143. Birt AR, Hogg GR, Dubé WJ. Hereditary multiple fibrofolliculomas with trichodiscomas and acrochordons. Arch Dermatol 1977; 113: 1674–1677.
144. Ubogy-Rainey Z, James WD, Lupton GP, Rodman OG. Fibrofolliculomas, trichodiscomas, and acrochordons: The Birt-Hogg-Dubé syndrome. J Am Acad Dermatol 1987; 16: 452–457.
144a. Rongioletti F, Hazini R, Gianotti G, Rebora A. Fibrofolliculomas, tricodiscomas and acrochordons (Birt-Hogg-Dubé) associated with intestinal polyposis. Clin Exp Dermatol 1989; 14: 72–74.
145. Fujita WH, Barr RJ, Headley JL. Multiple fibrofolliculomas with trichodiscomas and acrochordons. Arch Dermatol 1981; 117: 32–35.
146. Pinkus H, Coskey R, Burgess GH. Trichodiscoma. A benign tumor related to Haarscheibe (hair disk). J Invest Dermatol 1974; 63: 212–218.
147. Wells M, Golitz LE. Multiple trichodiscomas. Arch Dermatol 1979; 115: 1348.
148. Coskey RJ, Pinkus H. Trichodiscoma. Int J Dermatol 1976; 15: 600–601.
149. Starink TM, Kisch LS, Meijer CJLM. Familial multiple trichodiscomas. A clinicopathologic study. Arch Dermatol 1985; 121: 888–891.
150. Weedon D. Unpublished observation.
151. Scully K, Bargman H, Assaad D. Solitary fibrofolliculoma. J Am Acad Dermatol 1984; 11: 361–363.
152. Starink TM, Brownstein MH. Fibrofolliculoma: Solitary and multiple types. J Am Acad Dermatol 1987; 17: 493–496.
153. Foucar K, Rosen T, Foucar E, Cochran RJ. Fibrofolliculoma: a clinicopathologic study. Cutis 1981; 28: 429–432.
154. Weintraub R, Pinkus H. Multiple fibrofolliculomas (Birt–Hogg–Dubé) associated with a large connective tissue nevus. J Cutan Pathol 1977; 4: 289–299.
154a. Barr RJ, Goodman MM. Neurofollicular hamartoma: a light microscopic and immunohistochemical study. J Cutan Pathol 1989; 16: 336–341.
155. Pinkus H. Perifollicular fibromas. Pure periadnexal adventitial tumors. Am J Dermatopathol 1979; 1: 341–342.
156. Zackheim HS, Pinkus H. Perifollicular fibromas. Arch Dermatol 1960; 82: 913–917.
157. Reed RJ, Ackerman AB. Pathology of the adventitial dermis. Anatomic observations and biologic speculations. Hum Pathol 1973; 4: 207–217.
158. Meigel WN, Ackerman AB. Fibrous papule of the face. Am J Dermatopathol 1979; 1: 329–340.
159. Freeman RG, Chernosky ME. Perifollicular fibroma. Arch Dermatol 1969; 100: 66–69.
160. Smith LR, Heaton CL. Perifollicular fibroma. Cutis 1979; 23: 354–355.
161. Chemaly PH, Cavelier B, Civatte J. Syndrome de Birt, Hogg et Dubé. Ann Dermatol Venereol 1983; 110: 699–700.
162. Hornstein OP, Knickenberg M. Perifollicular fibromatosis cutis with polyps of the colon: a cutaneo-intestinal syndrome sui generis. Arch Dermatol Res 1975; 253: 161–175.

SEBACEOUS TUMOURS

163. Zak FG, Lawson W. Sebaceous glands in the esophagus. Arch Dermatol 1976; 112: 1153–1154.

164. Prioleau PG, Santa Cruz DJ. Sebaceous gland neoplasia. J Cutan Pathol 1984; 11: 396–414.
165. Burton CS, Sawchuk WS. Premature sebaceous gland hyperplasia. Successful treatment with isotretinoin. J Am Acad Dermatol 1985; 12: 182–184.
166. De Villez RL, Roberts LC. Premature sebaceous gland hyperplasia. J Am Acad Dermatol 1982; 6: 933–935.
166a. Kudoh K, Hosokawa M, Miyazawa T, Tagami H. Giant solitary sebaceous gland hyperplasia clinically simulating epidermoid cyst. J Cutan Pathol 1988; 15: 396–398.
166b. Czarnecki DB, Dorevitch AP. Giant senile sebaceous hyperplasia. Arch Dermatol 1986; 122: 1101.
167. Fernandez N, Torres A. Hyperplasia of sebaceous glands in a linear pattern of papules. Report of four cases. Am J Dermatopathol 1984; 6: 237–243.
168. Dupre A, Bonafe JL, Lamon R. Functional familial sebaceous hyperplasia of the face. Clin Exp Dermatol 1980; 5: 203–207.
169. Catalano PM, Ioannides G. Areolar sebaceous hyperplasia. J Am Acad Dermatol 1985; 13: 867–868.
169a. Sanchez Yus E, Montull C, Valcayo A, Robledo A. Areolar sebaceous hyperplasia: a new entity? J Cutan Pathol 1988; 15: 62–63.
169b. Rocamora A, Santonja C, Vives R, Varona C. Sebaceous gland hyperplasia of the vulva: a case report. Obstet Gynecol (Suppl) 1986; 68: 63s–65s.
169c. Sandbank M, Abramovici A, Wolf R, David EB. Sebaceous gland hyperplasia following topical application of citral. An ultrastructural study. Am J Dermatopathol 1988; 10: 415–418.
170. Luderschmidt C, Plewig G. Circumscribed sebaceous gland hyperplasia: autoradiographic and histoplanimetric studies. J Invest Dermatol 1978; 70: 207–209.
170a. Kumar P, Barton SP, Marks R. Tissue measurements in senile sebaceous gland hyperplasia. Br J Dermatol 1988; 118: 397–402.
171. Rulon DB, Helwig EB. Cutaneous sebaceous neoplasms. Cancer 1974; 33: 82–102.
172. Ferguson JW, Geary CP, MacAlister AD. Sebaceous cell adenoma. Rare intra-oral occurrence of a tumour which is a frequent marker of Torre's syndrome. Pathology 1987; 19: 204–208.
173. Torre D. Multiple sebaceous tumors. Arch Dermatol 1968; 98: 549–551.
174. Banse-Kupin L, Morales A, Barlow M. Torre's syndrome: Report of two cases and review of the literature. J Am Acad Dermatol 1984; 10: 803–817.
175. Housholder MS, Zeligman I. Sebaceous neoplasms associated with visceral carcinomas. Arch Dermatol 1980; 116: 61–64.
176. Sciallis GF, Winkelmann RK. Multiple sebaceous adenomas and gastrointestinal carcinoma. Arch Dermatol 1974; 110: 913–916.
177. Burgdorf WHC, Pitha J, Fahmy A. Muir-Torre syndrome. Histologic spectrum of sebaceous proliferations. Am J Dermatopathol 1986; 8: 202–208.
178. Graham R, McKee P, McGibbon D, Heyderman E. Torre-Muir syndrome. An association with isolated sebaceous carcinoma. Cancer 1985; 55: 2868–2873.
179. Rulon DB, Helwig EB. Multiple sebaceous neoplasms of the skin. An association with multiple visceral

carcinomas, especially of the colon. Am J Clin Pathol 1973; 60: 745–752.
180. Leonard DD, Deaton WR. Multiple sebaceous gland tumors and visceral carcinomas. Arch Dermatol 1974; 110: 917–920.
181. Finan MC, Connolly SM. Sebaceous gland tumors and systemic disease: a clinicopathologic analysis. Medicine (Baltimore) 1984; 63: 232–242.
182. Troy JL, Ackerman AB. Sebaceoma. A distinctive benign neoplasm of adnexal epithelium differentiating toward sebaceous cells. Am J Dermatopathol 1984; 6: 7–13.
183. Lasser A, Carter DM. Multiple basal cell epitheliomas with sebaceous differentiation. Arch Dermatol 1973; 107: 91–93.
184. Friedman KJ, Boudreau S, Farmer ER. Superficial epithelioma with sebaceous differentiation. J Cutan Pathol 1987; 14: 193–197.
185. Rothko K, Farmer ER, Zeligman I. Superficial epithelioma with sebaceous differentiation. Arch Dermatol 1980; 116: 329–331.
186. Graham RM, McKee PH, McGibbon D. Sebaceous carcinoma. Clin Exp Dermatol 1984; 9: 466–471.
187. Pricolo VE, Rodil JV, Vezeridis MP. Extraorbital sebaceous carcinoma. Arch Surg 1985; 120: 853–855.
188. Jacobs DM, Sandles LG, LeBoit PE. Sebaceous carcinoma arising from Bowen's disease of the vulva. Arch Dermatol 1986; 122: 1191–1193.
189. Wick MR, Goellner JR, Wolfe JT, Su WPD. Adnexal carcinomas of the skin. II. Extraocular sebaceous carcinomas. Cancer 1985; 56: 1163–1172.
190. Wolfe JT, Campbell RJ, Yeatts RP et al. Sebaceous carcinoma of the eyelid. Errors in clinical and pathologic diagnosis. Am J Surg Pathol 1984; 8: 597–606.
191. Rao NA, Hidayat A, McLean IW, Zimmerman LE. Sebaceous carcinomas of the ocular adnexa: A clinicopathologic study of 104 cases with five-year follow-up data. Hum Pathol 1982; 13: 113–122.
192. Ni C, Searl SS, Kuo PK et al. Sebaceous cell carcinomas of the ocular adnexa. Int Ophthalmol Clin 1982; 22: 23–61.
193. Lemos LB, Santa Cruz DJ, Baba N. Sebaceous carcinoma of the eyelid following radiation therapy. Am J Surg Pathol 1978; 2: 305–311.
194. Mellette JR, Amonette RA, Gardner JH, Chesney TMcC. Carcinoma of sebaceous glands on the head and neck. A report of four cases. J Dermatol Surg Oncol 1981; 7: 404–406.
194a. Jensen ML. Extraocular sebaceous carcinoma of the skin with visceral metastases: case report. J Cutan Pathol 1990; 17: 117–121.
195. King DT, Hirose FM, Gurevitch AW. Sebaceous carcinoma of the skin with visceral metastases. Arch Dermatol 1979; 115: 862–863.
196. Urban FH, Winkelmann RK. Sebaceous malignancy. Arch Dermatol 1961; 84: 63–72.
197. Russell WG, Page DL, Hough AJ, Rogers LW. Sebaceous carcinoma of Meiobomian gland origin. Am J Clin Pathol 1980; 73: 504–511.
198. Lee SC, Roth LM. Sebaceous carcinoma of the eyelid with pagetoid involvement of the bulbar and palpebral conjunctiva. J Cutan Pathol 1977; 4: 134–145.

275. Kariniemi A-L, Ramaekers F, Lehto V-P, Virtanen I.Paget cells express cytokeratins typical of glandular epithelia. Br J Dermatol 1985; 112: 179–183.

276. Tazawa T, Ito M, Fujiwara H et al. Immunologic characteristics of keratins in extramammary Paget's disease. Arch Dermatol 1988; 124: 1063–1068.

277. Russell Jones R, Spaull J, Gusterson B. The histogenesis of mammary and extramammary Paget's disease. Histopathology 1989; 14: 409–416.

277a. Reed W, Oppedal BR, Eeg Larsen T. Immunohistology is valuable in distinguishing between Paget's disease, Bowen's disease and superficial spreading malignant melanoma. Histopathology 1990; 16: 583–588.

278. Demopoulos RI. Fine structure of the extramammary Paget's cell. Cancer 1971; 27: 1202–1210.

279. Belcher RW. Extramammary Paget's disease. Enzyme histochemical and electron microscopic study. Arch Pathol 1972; 94: 59–64.

280. Mitchell RE. Mammary and extramammary Paget's disease. Aust J Dermatol 1974; 15: 51–63.

Tumours of modified apocrine glands

281. Futrell JW, Krueger GR, Chretien PB, Ketcham AS. Multiple primary sweat gland carcinomas. Cancer 1971; 28: 686–691.

282. Aurora AL, Luxenberg MN. Case report of adenocarcinoma of glands of Moll. Am J Ophthalmol 1970; 70: 984–990.

283. Lewis HM, Ovitz ML, Golitz LE. Erosive adenomatosis of the nipple. Arch Dermatol 1976; 112: 1427–1428.

284. Smith EJ, Kron SD, Gross PR. Erosive adenomatosis of the nipple. Arch Dermatol 1970; 102: 330–332.

285. Shapiro L, Karpas CM. Florid papillomatosis of the nipple. Am J Clin Pathol 1965; 44: 155–159.

286. Smith NP, Wilson Jones E. Erosive adenomatosis of the nipple. Clin Exp Dermatol 1977; 2: 79–84.

287. Neldner KH. Ceruminoma. Arch Dermatol 1968; 98: 344–348.

288. Michel RG, Woodard BH, Shelburne JD, Bossen EH. Ceruminous gland adenocarcinoma. A light and electron microscopic study. Cancer 1978; 41: 545–553.

289. Lynde CW, McLean DI, Wood WS. Tumors of ceruminous glands. J Am Acad Dermatol 1984; 11: 841–847.

290. Wetli CV, Pardo V, Millard M, Gerston K. Tumors of ceruminous glands. Cancer 1972; 29: 1169–1178.

291. Wassef M, Kanavaros P, Polivka M et al. Middle ear adenoma. A tumor displaying mucinous and neuroendocrine differentiation. Am J Surg Pathol 1989; 13: 838–847.

ECCRINE TUMOURS

292. Kanitakis J, Schmitt D, Bernard A et al. Anti-D47: a monoclonal antibody reacting with the secretory cells of human eccrine sweat glands. Br J Dermatol 1983; 109: 509–513.

293. Suzuki Y, Hashimoto K, Kato I et al. A monoclonal antibody, SKHI, reacts with 40 Kd sweat gland-associated antigen. J Cutan Pathol 1989; 16: 66–71.

294. Penneys NS, Zlatkiss I. Immunohistochemical demonstration of ferritin in sweat gland and sweat gland neoplasms. J Cutan Pathol 1990; 17: 32–36.

295. Metze D, Jurecka W, Gebhart W, Schuller-Petrovic S. Secretory immunoglobulin A in sweat gland tumors. J Cutan Pathol 1989; 16: 126–132.

296. Zuk JA, West KP, Fletcher A. Immunohistochemical staining patterns of sweat glands and their neoplasms using two monoclonal antibodies to keratins. J Cutan Pathol 1988; 15: 8–17.

297. Mayou SC, Black MM, Russell Jones R. Sudoriferous hamartoma. Clin Exp Dermatol 1988; 13: 107–108.

298. Pippione M, Depaoli MA, Sartoris S. Naevus eccrine. Dermatologica 1976; 152: 40–46.

299. Goldstein N. Ephidrosis (local hyperhidrosis). Nevus sudoriferous. Arch Dermatol 1967; 96: 67–68.

300. Donati P, Amantea A, Balus L. Eccrine angiomatous hamartoma: a lipomatous variant. J Cutan Pathol 1989; 16: 227–229.

301. Hyman AB, Harris H, Brownstein MH. Eccrine angiomatous hamartoma. NY State J Med 1968; 68: 2803–2806.

302. Challa VR, Jona J. Eccrine angiomatous hamartoma: a rare skin lesion with diverse histological features. Dermatologica 1977; 155: 206–209.

303. Weedon D, Lewis J. Acrosyringeal nevus. J Cutan Pathol 1977; 4: 166–168.

303a. Ogino A. Linear eccrine poroma. Arch Dermatol 1976; 112: 841–844.

303b. Aloi FG, Torre C. Hidrotic ectodermal dysplasia with diffuse eccrine syringofibroadenomatosis. Arch Dermatol 1989; 125: 1715.

304. Mehregan AH, Marufi M, Medenica M. Eccrine syringofibroadenoma (Mascaro). Report of two cases. J Am Acad Dermatol 1985; 13: 433–436.

305. Civatte J, Jeanmougin M, Barrandon Y, Jimenez de Franch A. Syringofibroadenoma ecrino de Mascaro. Med Cutan Iber Lat Am 1981; 9: 193–196.

306. Mascaro JM. Considérations sur les tumeurs fibro-épithéliales: Le syringofibroadénome eccrine. Ann Dermatol Syphil 1963; 90: 146–153.

307. Kanitakis J, Zambruno G, Euvrard S et al. Eccrine syringofibroadenoma. Immunohistological study of a new case. Am J Dermatopathol 1987; 9: 37–40.

308. Weedon D. Eccrine syringofibroadenoma versus acrosyringeal nevus. J Am Acad Dermatol 1987; 16: 622.

308a. Hurt MA, Igra-Serfaty H, Stevens CS. Eccrine syringofibroadenoma (Mascaro). An acrosyringeal hamartoma. Arch Dermatol 1990; 126: 945–949.

309. Marsden RA, Fleming K, Dauber RPR. Comedo naevus of the palm — a sweat duct naevus? Br J Dermatol 1979; 101: 717–722.

310. Blanchard L, Hodge SJ, Owen LG. Linear eccrine nevus with comedones. Arch Dermatol 1981; 117: 357–359.

311. Abell E, Read SI. Porokeratotic eccrine ostial and dermal duct naevus. Br J Dermatol 1980; 103: 435–441.

312. Driban NE, Cavicchia JC. Porokeratotic eccrine ostial and dermal duct nevus. J Cutan Pathol 1987; 14: 118–121.

312a. Fernandez-Redondo V, Toribio J. Porokeratotic eccrine ostial and dermal duct nevus. J Cutan Pathol 1988; 15: 393–395.

312b. Stoof TJ, Starink TM, Nieboer C. Porokeratotic

eccrine ostial and dermal duct nevus. Report of a case of adult onset. J Am Acad Dermatol 1989; 20: 924–927.

313. Mishima Y. Eccrine-centered nevus. Arch Dermatol 1973; 107: 59–61.
314. Hollander A. Eccrine-centered nevus. Arch Dermatol 1973; 108: 177.
315. Smith JD, Chernosky ME. Hidrocystomas. Arch Dermatol 1973; 108: 676–679.
316. Sperling LE, Sakas EL. Eccrine hidrocystomas. J Am Acad Dermatol 1982; 7: 763–770.
317. Rulon DB, Helwig EB. Papillary eccrine adenoma. Arch Dermatol 1977; 113: 596–598.
318. Cooper PH, Frierson HF. Papillary eccrine adenoma. Arch Pathol Lab Med 1984; 108: 55–57.
318a. Sexton M, Maize JC. Papillary eccrine adenoma. A light microscopic and immunohistochemical study. J Am Acad Dermatol 1988; 18: 1114–1120.
319. Sina B, Dilaimy M, Kallayee D. Papillary eccrine adenoma. Arch Dermatol 1980; 116: 719–720.
319a. Jerasutus S, Suvanprakorn P, Wongchinchai M. Papillary eccrine adenoma: an electron microscopic study. J Am Acad Dermatol 1989; 20: 1111–1114.
320. Urmacher C, Lieberman PH. Papillary eccrine adenoma. Light-microscopic, histochemical, and immunohistochemical studies. Am J Dermatopathol 1987; 9: 243–249.
321. Falck VG, Jordaan HF. Papillary eccrine adenoma. A tubulopapillary hidradenoma with eccrine differentiation. Am J Dermatopathol 1986; 8: 64–72.
322. Kao GF, Helwig EB, Graham JH. Aggressive digital papillary adenoma and adenocarcinoma. A clinicopathological study of 57 patients, with histochemical, immunopathological, and ultrastructural observations. J Cutan Pathol 1987; 14: 129–146.
323. Weedon D. Eccrine tumors: a selective review. J Cutan Pathol 1984; 11: 421–436.
323a. Ceballos PI, Penneys NS, Acosta R. Aggressive digital papillary adenocarcinoma is a tumor of eccrine coil. J Cutan Pathol 1988; 15: 299 (abstract).
324. Friedman SJ, Butler DF. Syringoma presenting as milia. J Am Acad Dermatol 1987; 16: 310–314.
325. Carneiro SJC, Gardner HL, Knox JM. Syringoma of the vulva. Arch Dermatol 1971; 103: 494–496.
326. Isaacson D, Turner ML. Localized vulvar syringomas. J Am Acad Dermatol 1979; 1: 352–356.
327. Zalla JA, Perry HO. An unusual case of syringoma. Arch Dermatol 1971; 103: 215–217.
327a. Lo JS, Dijkstra JW, Bergfeld WF. Syringomas on the penis. Int J Dermatol 1990; 29: 309–310.
328. Shelley WB, Wood MG. Occult syringomas of scalp associated with progressive hair loss. Arch Dermatol 1980; 116: 843–844.
329. Hughes PSH, Apisarnthanarax P. Acral syringoma. Arch Dermatol 1977; 113: 1435–1436.
330. Port M, Farmer ER. Syringoma of the ankle. J Am Acad Dermatol 1984; 10: 291–293.
331. Yung CW, Soltani K, Bernstein JE, Lorincz AL. Unilateral linear nevoidal syringoma. J Am Acad Dermatol 1981; 4: 412–416.
332. Holden CA, MacDonald DM. Syringomata: a bathing trunk distribution. Clin Exp Dermatol 1981; 6: 555–559.
333. Urban CD, Cannon JR, Cole RD. Eruptive

334. Haneke E, Gutschmidt E. Generalisierte Syringome. Hautarzt 1978; 29: 222–223.
335. Hashimoto K, Blum D, Fukaya T, Eto H. Familial syringoma. Case history and application of monoclonal anti-eccrine gland antibodies. Arch Dermatol 1985; 121: 756–760.
336. Furue M, Hori Y, Nakabayashi Y. Clear-cell syringoma. Association with diabetes mellitus. Am J Dermatopathol 1984; 6: 131–138.
337. Kitamura K, Muraki R, Tamura N. Clear cell syringoma. Cutis 1983; 32: 169–172.
338. Feibelman CE, Maize JC. Clear-cell syringoma. A study by conventional and electron microscopy. Am J Dermatopathol 1984; 6: 139–150.
339. Seifert HW. Multiple Syringome mit Vermehrung von Mastzellen unter dem klinischen Bild einer Urticaria pigmentosa. Z Hautkr 1981; 56: 303–306.
340. Schellander F, Marks R, Wilson Jones E. Basal cell hamartoma and cellular naevus: an unusual combined malformation. Br J Dermatol 1974; 90: 413–419.
341. Hashimoto K, Gross BG, Lever WF. Syringoma. Histochemical and electron microscopic studies. J Invest Dermatol 1966; 46: 150–166.
342. Hashimoto K, Lever WF. Histogenesis of skin appendage tumors. Arch Dermatol 1969; 100: 356–369.
343. Hirsch P, Helwig EB. Chondroid syringoma: mixed tumor of skin, salivary gland type. Arch Dermatol 1961; 84: 835–847.
343a. Hassab-El-Naby HM, Tam S, White WL, Ackerman AB. Mixed tumors of the skin. A histological and immunohistochemical study. Am J Dermatopathol 1989; 11: 413–428.
344. Harrist TJ, Aretz TH, Mihm MC Jr. Cutaneous malignant mixed tumor. Arch Dermatol 1981; 117: 719–724.
345. Matz LR, McCully DJ, Stokes BAR. Metastasizing chondroid syringoma: case report. Pathology 1969; 1: 77–81.
345a. Scott A, Metcalf JS. Cutaneous malignant mixed tumor. Report of a case and review of the literature. Am J Dermatopathol 1988; 10: 335–342.
346. Redono C, Rocamora A, Villoria F, Garcia M. Malignant mixed tumor of the skin. Malignant chondroid syringoma. Cancer 1982; 49: 1690–1696.
346a. Sanchez Yus E, Aguilar A, Urbina F et al. Malignant cutaneous mixed tumor. A new case with unusual clinical features. Am J Dermatopathol 1988; 10: 330–334.
347. Webb JN, Stott WG. Malignant chondroid syringoma of the thigh: Report of a case with electron microscopy of the tumour. J Pathol 1975; 116: 43–46.
348. Shvili D, Rothem A. Fulminant metastasizing chondroid syringoma of the skin. Am J Dermatopathol 1986; 8: 321–325.
349. Hernandez FJ. Mixed tumors of the skin of the salivary gland type: a light and electron microscopic study. J Invest Dermatol 1976; 66: 49–52.
349a. Argenyi ZB, Balogh K. Collagenous spherulosis in chondroid syringomas. Am J Dermatopathol 1991; 13: 115–121.
350. Rapini RP, Kennedy LJ, Golitz LE. Hair matrix differentiation in chondroid syringoma. J Cutan Pathol 1984; 11: 318–321.

418. Keasbey LE, Hadley GG. Clear-cell hidradenoma. Report of three cases with widespread metastases. Cancer 1954; 7: 934–952.

419. Cooper PH. Mitotic figures in sweat gland adenomas. J Cutan Pathol 1987; 14: 10–14.

420. Mambo NC. The significance of atypical nuclear changes in benign eccrine acrospiromas: a clinical and pathological study of 18 cases. J Cutan Pathol 1984; 11: 35–44.

421. Stanley RJ, Sanchez NP, Massa MC et al. Epidermoid hidradenoma. A clinicopathologic study. J Cutan Pathol 1982; 9: 293–302.

421a. Satoh T, Katsumata M, Tokura Y et al. Clear cell hidradenoma with whorl formation of squamoid cells: Immunohistochemical and electron microscopic studies. J Am Acad Dermatol 1989; 21: 271–277.

422. Fathizadeh A, Miller-Catchpole R, Medenica MM, Lorincz AL. Pigmented eccrine acrospiroma. Report of a case. Arch Dermatol 1981; 117: 599–600.

423. Hashimoto K, DiBella RJ, Lever WF. Clear cell hidradenoma. Histological, histochemical, and electron microscopic studies. Arch Dermatol 1967; 96: 18–38.

Malignant eccrine tumours

424. El-Domeiri AA, Brasfield RD, Huvos AG, Strong EW. Sweat gland carcinoma: a clinico-pathologic study of 83 patients. Ann Surg 1971; 173: 270–274.

425. Swanson PE, Cherwitz DL, Neumann MP, Wick MR. Eccrine sweat gland carcinoma: an histologic and immunohistochemical study of 32 cases. J Cutan Pathol 1987; 14: 65–86.

426. Goldstein DJ, Barr RJ, Santa Cruz DJ. Microcystic adnexal carcinoma. A distinct clinicopathologic entity. Cancer 1982; 50: 566–572.

427. Glatt HJ, Proia AD, Tsoy EA et al. Malignant syringoma of the eyelid. Ophthalmology 1984; 91: 987–990.

428. Lipper S, Peiper SC. Sweat gland carcinoma with syringomatous features. A light microscopic and ultrastructural study. Cancer 1979; 44: 157–163.

429. Apisarnthanarax P, Bovenmyer DA, Mehregan AH. Combined adnexal tumor of the skin. Arch Dermatol 1984; 120: 231–233.

430. Cooper PH. Sclerosing carcinomas of sweat ducts (microcystic adnexal carcinoma). Arch Dermatol 1986; 122: 261–264.

430a. Jones MW, Norris HJ, Snyder RC. Infiltrating syringomatous adenoma of the nipple. A clinical and pathological study of 11 cases. Am J Surg Pathol 1989; 13: 197–201.

431. Lupton GP, McMarlin SL. Microcystic adnexal carcinoma. Report of a case with 30-year follow-up. Arch Dermatol 1986; 122: 286–289.

431a. Ceballos PI, Penneys NS, Cohen BH. Microcystic adnexal carcinoma: a case showing eccrine duct differentiation. J Dermatol Surg Oncol 1988; 14: 1236–1239.

431b. Chow WC, Cockerell CJ, Geronemus RG. Microcystic adnexal carcinoma of the scalp. J Dermatol Surg Oncol 1989; 15: 768–771.

432. Cooper PH, Mills SE. Microcystic adnexal carcinoma. J Am Acad Dermatol 1984; 10: 908–914.

433. Cooper PH, Headington JT, Mills SE et al. Sclerosing sweat duct (syringomatous) carcinoma. Am J Surg Pathol 1985; 9: 422–433.

434. Cooper PH, Robinson CR, Greer KE. Low-grade clear cell eccrine carcinoma. Arch Dermatol 1984; 120: 1076–1078.

434a. Birkby CS, Argenyi ZB, Whitaker DC. Microcystic adnexal carcinoma with mandibular invasion and bone marrow replacement. J Dermatol Surg Oncol 1989; 15: 308–312.

435. Nickoloff BJ, Fleischmann HE, Carmel J et al. Microcystic adnexal carcinoma. Immunohistologic observations suggesting dual (pilar and eccrine) differentiation. Arch Dermatol 1986; 122: 290–294.

435a. Wick MR, Cooper PH, Swanson PE et al. Microcystic adnexal carcinoma. An immunohistochemical comparison with other cutaneous appendage tumors. Arch Dermatol 1990; 126: 189–194.

436. Rongioletti F, Grosshans E, Rebora A. Microcystic adnexal carcinoma. Br J Dermatol 1986; 115: 101–104.

436a. Requena L, Marquina A, Alegre V et al. Sclerosing-sweat-duct (microcystic adnexal) carcinoma — a tumour from a single eccrine origin. Clin Exp Dermatol 1990; 15: 222–224.

436b. Kato H, Mizuno N, Nakagawa K et al. Microcystic adnexal carcinoma: a light microscopic, immunohistochemical and ultrastructural study. J Cutan Pathol 1990; 17: 87–95.

437. Freeman RG, Winkelmann RK. Basal cell tumor with eccrine differentiation (eccrine epithelioma). Arch Dermatol 1969; 100: 234–242.

438. Sanchez NP, Winkelmann RK. Basal cell tumor with eccrine differentiation (eccrine epithelioma). J Am Acad Dermatol 1982; 6: 514–518.

439. Sequeira J, Wright S, Baker H. Basal cell tumour with eccrine differentiation (eccrine epithelioma) — a histochemical and immunocytochemical analysis of a case. Clin Exp Dermatol 1987; 12: 58–60.

440. Mehregan AH, Hashimoto K, Rahbari H. Eccrine adenocarcinoma. A clinicopathologic study of 35 cases. Arch Dermatol 1983; 119: 104–114.

441. Weber PJ, Gretzula JC, Garland LD et al. Syringoid eccrine carcinoma. J Dermatol Surg Oncol 1987; 13: 64–67.

442. Hanke CW, Temofeew RK. Basal cell carcinoma with eccrine differentiation (eccrine epithelioma). J Dermatol Surg Oncol 1986; 12: 820–824.

443. Serrano G, Aliaga A, Bonillo J et al. Basal cell tumor with eccrine differentiation (eccrine epithelioma). J Cutan Pathol 1984; 11: 553–557.

444. Sanchez Yus E, Caballero LR, Salazar IG, Menchero SC. Clear cell syringoid eccrine carcinoma. Am J Dermatopathol 1987; 9: 225–231.

445. Boggio R. Adenoid cystic carcinoma of the scalp. Arch Dermatol 1975; 111: 793–794.

445a. Van der Kwast TH, Vuzevski VD, Ramaekers F et al. Primary cutaneous adenoid cystic carcinoma: case report, immunohistochemistry, and review of the literature. Br J Dermatol 1988; 118: 567–578.

446. Meyrick Thomas RH, Lowe DG, Munro DD. Primary adenoid cystic carcinoma of the skin. Clin Exp Dermatol 1987; 12: 378–380.

446a. Kuramoto Y, Tagami H. Primary adenoid cystic carcinoma masquerading as syringoma of the scalp. Am J Dermatopathol 1990; 12: 169–174.

447. Seab JA, Graham JH. Primary cutaneous adenoid cystic carcinoma. J Am Acad Dermatol 1987; 17: 113–118.

448. Perzin KH, Gullane P, Conley J. Adenoid cystic carcinoma involving the external auditory canal. A clinicopathologic study of 16 cases. Cancer 1982; 50: 2873–2883.

449. Cooper PH, Adelson GL, Holthaus WH. Primary cutaneous adenoid cystic carcinoma. Arch Dermatol 1984; 120: 774–777.

450. Headington JT, Teears R, Niederhuber JE, Slinger RP. Primary adenoid cystic carcinoma of skin. Arch Dermatol 1978; 114: 421–424.

451. Sanderson KV, Batten JC. Adenoid cystic carcinoma of the scalp with pulmonary metastases. Proc R Soc Med 1975; 68: 649–650.

452. Wick MR, Swanson PE. Primary adenoid cystic carcinoma of the skin. Am J Dermatopathol 1986; 8: 2–13.

453. Pilgrim JP, Wolfish PS, Kloss SG, Heng MCY. Primary mucinous carcinoma of the skin with metastases to the lymph nodes. Am J Dermatopathol 1985; 7: 461–469.

453a. Balin AK, Fine RM, Golitz LE. Mucinous carcinoma. J Dermatol Surg Oncol 1988; 14: 521–524.

454. Wick MR, Goellner JR, Wolfe JT, Su WPD. Adnexal carcinomas of the skin. I. Eccrine carcinomas. Cancer 1985; 56: 1147–1162.

454a. Weber PJ, Hevia O, Gretzula JC, Rabinovitz HC. Primary mucinous carcinoma. J Dermatol Surg Oncol 1988; 14: 170–172.

455. Berg JW, McDivitt RW. Pathology of sweat gland carcinoma. Pathol Annu 1968; 3: 123–144.

456. Wright JD, Font RL. Mucinous sweat gland adenocarcinoma of eyelid. A clinicopathologic study of 21 cases with histochemical and electron microscopic observations. Cancer 1979; 44: 1757–1768.

457. Mendoza S, Helwig EB. Mucinous (adenocystic) carcinoma of the skin. Arch Dermatol 1971; 103: 68–78.

458. Santa-Cruz DJ, Meyers JH, Gnepp DR, Perez BM. Primary mucinous carcinoma of the skin. Br J Dermatol 1978; 98: 645–653.

459. Yeung K-Y, Stinson JC. Mucinous (adenocystic) carcinoma of sweat glands with widespread metastasis. Case report with ultrastructural study. Cancer 1977; 39: 2556–2562.

460. Grossman JR, Izuno GT. Primary mucinous (adenocystic) carcinoma of the skin. Arch Dermatol 1974; 110: 274–276.

461. Baandrup U, Sogaard H. Mucinous (adenocystic) carcinoma of the skin. Dermatologica 1982; 164: 338–342.

462. Headington JT. Primary mucinous carcinoma of skin. Histochemistry and electron microscopy. Cancer 1977; 39: 1055–1063.

463. Ishimura E, Iwamoto H, Kobashi Y et al. Malignant chondroid syringoma. Report of a case with widespread metastasis and review of pertinent literature. Cancer 1983; 52: 1966–1973.

464. Pinkus H, Mehregan AH. Epidermotropic eccrine carcinoma. A case combining features of eccrine poroma and Paget's dermatosis. Arch Dermatol 1963; 88: 597–606.

465. Shaw M, McKee PH, Lowe D, Black MM. Malignant eccrine poroma: a study of twenty-seven cases. Br J Dermatol 1982; 107: 675–680.

466. Pylyser K, De Wolf-Peeters C, Marien K. The histology of eccrine poromas: a study of 14 cases. Dermatologica 1983; 167: 243–249.

467. Ishikawa K. Malignant hidroacanthoma simplex. Arch Dermatol 1971; 104: 529–532.

468. Puttick L, Ince P, Comaish JS. Three cases of eccrine porocarcinoma. Br J Dermatol 1986; 115: 111–116.

469. Tarkhan II, Domingo J. Metastasizing eccrine porocarcinoma developing in a sebaceous nevus of Jadassohn. Report of a case. Arch Dermatol 1985; 121: 413–415.

470. Ryan JF, Darley CR, Pollock DJ. Malignant eccrine poroma: report of three cases. J Clin Pathol 1986; 39: 1099–1104.

471. Gschnait F, Horn F, Lindlbauer R, Sponer D. Eccrine porocarcinoma. J Cutan Pathol 1980; 7: 349–353.

472. Holden CA, Shaw M, McKee PH et al. Loss of membrane B2 microglobulin in eccrine porocarcinoma. Its association with the histopathologic and clinical criteria of malignancy. Arch Dermatol 1984; 120: 732–735.

473. Bottles K, Sagebiel RW, McNutt NS et al. Malignant eccrine poroma. Case report and review of the literature. Cancer 1984; 53: 1579–1585.

474. Chung CK, Heffernan AH. Clear cell hidradenoma with metastasis. Case report with a review of the literature. Plast Reconstr Surg 1971; 48: 177–179.

475. Chow CW, Campbell PE, Burry AF. Sweat gland carcinomas in children. Cancer 1984; 53: 1222–1227.

476. Czarnecki DB, Aarons I, Dowling JP et al. Malignant clear cell hidradenoma: A case report. Acta Derm Venereol 1982; 62: 173–176.

477. Wick MR, Goellner JR, Wolfe JT, Su WPD. Vulvar sweat gland carcinomas. Arch Pathol Lab Med 1985; 109: 43–47.

478. Friedman KJ. Low-grade primary cutaneous adenosquamous (mucoepidermoid) carcinoma. Report of a case and review of the literature. Am J Dermatopathol 1989; 11: 43–50.

479. Santa Cruz DJ, Prioleau PG. Adnexal carcinomas of the skin. J Cutan Pathol 1984; 11: 450–456.

480. Rosen Y, Kim B, Yermakov VA. Eccrine sweat gland tumor of clear cell origin involving the eyelids. Cancer 1975; 36: 1034–1041.

481. Collina G, Quarto F, Eusebi V. Trabecular carcinoid of the skin with cellular stroma. Am J Dermatopathol 1988; 10: 430–435.

COMPLEX ADNEXAL TUMOURS

482. Hidano A, Kobayashi T. Adnexal polyp of neonatal skin. Br J Dermatol 1975; 92: 659–662.

483. Hanau D, Grosshans E, Laplanche G. A complex poroma-like adnexal adenoma. Am J Dermatopathol 1984; 6: 567–572.

484. Zaim MT. Sebocrine adenoma. An adnexal adenoma with sebaceous and apocrine poroma-like differentiation. Am J Dermatopathol 1988; 10: 311–318.

485. Robinson HN, Barnett NK. Hemifacial mixed appendageal tumor in an infant. Pediatr Dermatol 1986; 3: 406–409.

486. Alessi E, Wong SN, Advani HH, Ackerman AB. Nevus sebaceus is associated with unusual neoplasms. An atlas. Am J Dermatopathol 1988; 10: 116–127.

487. Alessi E, Sala F. Nevus sebaceus. A clinicopathologic study of its evolution. Am J Dermatopathol 1986; 8: 27–31.

488. Wilson Jones E, Heyl T. Naevus sebaceus. A report of 140 cases with special regard to the development of secondary malignant tumours. Br J Dermatol 1970; 82: 99–117.

489. Mehregan AH, Pinkus H. Life history of organoid nevi. Arch Dermatol 1965; 91: 574–588.

490. Moskowitz R, Honig PJ. Nevus sebaceus in association with an intracranial mass. J Am Acad Dermatol 1982; 6: 1078–1080.

491. Kang WH, Koh YJ, Chun SI. Nevus sebaceus syndrome associated with intracranial arteriovenous malformation. Int J Dermatol 1987; 26: 382–384.

492. Diven DG, Solomon AR, McNeely MC, Font RL. Nevus sebaceus associated with major ophthalmologic abnormalities. Arch Dermatol 1987; 123: 383–386.

493. Burden PA, Gentry RH, Fitzpatrick JE. Piloleiomyoma arising in an organoid nevus: a case report and review of the literature. J Dermatol Surg Oncol 1987; 13: 1213–1218.

494. Morioka S. The natural history of *nevus sebaceus*. J Cutan Pathol 1985; 12: 200–213.

495. Poomeechaiwong S, Bonelli JE, Golitz LE. Mixed tumor of the pilosebaceous type: mixed tumor of the skin with apocrine, follicular and sebaceous differentiation. J Cutan Pathol 1988; 15: 338 (abstract).

496. Nakhleh RE, Swanson PE, Wick MR. Cutaneous adnexal carcinomas with divergent differentiation. Am J Dermatopathol 1990; 12: 325–334.

Tumours and tumour-like proliferations of fibrous and related tissues

INTRODUCTION

Recent immunohistochemical and ultrastructural findings have placed in doubt the histogenesis of some of the tumours included in this chapter, particularly those that have traditionally been regarded as 'fibrohistiocytic' in origin. In the circumstances, there is no accurate and concise designation for the heterogeneous group of tumours whose descriptions follow. This chapter includes those entities that have traditionally been grouped together on the basis of collagen production and/or the presence of fibroblasts or fibroblast-like cells forming an integral component of the tumour.

ACRAL ANGIOFIBROMAS

Acral angiofibromas are a clinically diverse group of entities that share distinctive histological features.[1,2] They are thought by some to represent hyperplasias of the papillary and/or periadnexal dermis (the adventitial dermis).[3] Recent immunohistochemical studies have shown that the large stellate fibroblast-like cells that characterize these tumours express factor XIIIa, a cell marker for a specific population of bone-marrow-derived cells which are dendritic but distinct from Langerhans cells.[4,5] These cells, also known as dermal dendrocytes, share some features with macrophages.[4,5] Factor XIIIa appears to be important in the promulgation of fibroplasia.[6]

Tumours derived from the perifollicular mesenchyme — the perifollicular fibroma, trichodiscoma, and fibrofolliculoma — are usual-

fibroma, develops in adolescents, in the form of papules or plaques.[62] The tumour cells are arranged in lobules or fascicles that resemble smooth muscle cells; immunohistochemistry and ultrastructural studies have supported their fibroblastic origin.[62]

KNUCKLE PADS

Knuckle pads (discrete keratodermas over the knuckle and finger articulations) are well-formed, skin-coloured nodules overlying the interphalangeal and metacarpophalangeal joints of the hands.[63,64] They are usually multiple. There are several clinical variants including a familial group, an occupational or recreation-related group and an acquired idiopathic group. An association with pseudoxanthoma elasticum has been reported.[65] Of historical interest is the prominent knuckle pad on the right thumb of Michelangelo's statue of David.[66]

Histopathology[66]

The usual lesions show prominent hyper-keratosis and epidermal acanthosis. There is minimal thickening of the papillary dermis. A variant with prominent subcutaneous fibrosis, belonging to the fibromatoses, has been docu-mented.[66]

NODULAR FASCIITIS

Nodular fasciitis is a reactive proliferation of fibroblast-like cells with a predilection for the subcutaneous tissues of the forearm, upper arm and thigh of young and middle-aged adults.[67] It usually grows quite quickly to reach a median diameter of 1.5 cm. Multiple lesions have been reported.[68] Recurrences are rare, even after incomplete surgical removal, and their occur-rence should lead to a reappraisal of the original histological diagnosis.[69]

Cranial fasciitis of childhood is a distinct clinical variant arising in the deep soft tissues of the scalp with involvement of the underlying cranium.[70,71]

Histopathology[67,72,73]

Nodular fasciitis is composed of a proliferation of spindle-shaped to plump fibroblasts which may be arranged in haphazard array ('tissue culture appearance'), or in bundles which form S-shaped curves (Fig. 34.5).[73] A vague storiform pattern is sometimes present focally. Mitoses are frequent, but atypical forms are rare. Cleft-like spaces may be seen between the fibroblasts. There is a variable amount of myxoid stroma and extravasated erythrocytes. Collagen is usual-ly sparse. Capillaries with plump endothelial cells are common. Scattered lymphocytes are dispersed throughout the lesion.

Less common findings include the presence of bone and cartilage;[73–75] osteoid is not un-

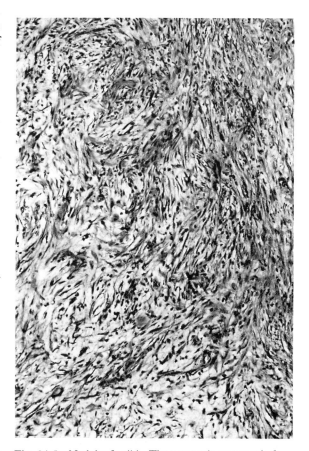

Fig. 34.5 Nodular fasciitis. The tumour is composed of swirling bundles of spindle-shaped cells set in a myxoid stroma.
Haematoxylin — eosin

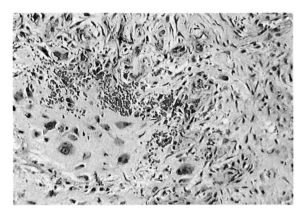

Fig. 34.6   Proliferative fasciitis. Ganglion-like cells are present within a spindle-cell tumour. Haematoxylin — eosin

common in the variant known as cranial fasciitis.[70] Scattered multinucleate fibroblasts and osteoclast-like giant cells are often present and, rarely, the latter cells are quite common.[69,73] A variant with numerous cells resembling ganglion cells, akin to those seen in proliferative myositis, may be separated off as a distinct entity — *proliferative fasciitis* (Fig. 34.6).[76,77]

Various histological subtypes of nodular fasciitis have been proposed, based on the cellularity, the amount of myxoid stroma, the presence of collagen or other histological features such as osteoclast-like cells, ganglion-like cells or bone. Some of the proposed subtypes merely reflect changes in the histological composition during the evolution of the lesion.[67]

Electron microscopy. Few ultrastructural studies have been carried out, but in one study of eight cases, myofibroblasts were the predominant cell present.[78] Myofibroblasts and fibroblasts are also present in cranial fasciitis.[71]

FIBROUS HAMARTOMA OF INFANCY

This uncommon fibroproliferative lesion of the subcutaneous tissue is present at birth, or develops in the first two years of life.[79-81] It most commonly occurs around the shoulder, axilla and upper arms, but cases involving the scalp,[82] inguinal region, scrotum,[83] perianal area[84] and

lower extremities[85] have been reported. There is a male predominance of 3:1.[80] The clinical course is benign, despite its infiltrative appearance and tendency to local recurrence.[81]

The subcutaneous tissue of excised lesions has a glistening grey-white appearance interspersed with fatty tissue. The involved area measures 2–8 cm in maximum diameter.

Histopathology[80,86]

Fibrous hamartoma of infancy has poorly defined margins. It is centred on the subcutis. There are three different tissue components[80,87] — interlacing trabeculae of fibrocollagenous tissue, small nests of loosely arranged mesenchymal cells, and interspersed mature fat (Fig. 34.7). The fibrous trabeculae vary in thickness and arrangement and contain spindle-shaped cells; they do not contain S100 protein.[81] The myxoid areas are more cellular with immature oval or stellate cells, sometimes having a whorled pattern. Sparse lymphocytes may be present in the stroma.

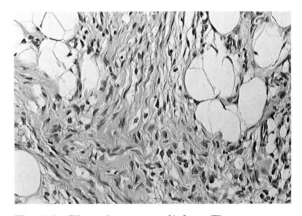

Fig. 34.7   Fibrous hamartoma of infancy. There are bundles of fibrous tissue, some mesenchymal cells and interspersed mature fat. Haematoxylin — eosin

Electron microscopy. The constituent cells have the features of myofibroblasts, although some fibroblasts are also present.[82,88] Fibroblasts alone were present in a case reported recently.[88a]

DIGITAL FIBROMATOSIS OF CHILDHOOD

Digital fibromatosis of childhood (infantile digital fibromatosis,[89] recurring digital fibrous tumour of childhood,[90] inclusion body fibromatosis[90a]) is a rare benign tumour of myofibroblasts with characteristic cytoplasmic inclusion bodies. It presents as a dome-shaped, firm nodule, up to 1 cm in diameter, usually on the digits.[91] The thumbs and great toes are spared.[92] Lesions are usually solitary, but a second tumour is sometimes noted at the time of presentation, or develops subsequently.[91] The tumours may be present at birth, or appear in the first year of life. Onset in late childhood or adult life is rare.[90a,93] A history of preceding trauma has been reported.[94] The tumour often recurs after local excision; very occasionally it may regress spontaneously.[93a]

Because of the characteristic inclusion bodies, a viral aetiology was originally suspected, but all cultures have been negative, excluding this hypothesis.[95,96]

Histopathology[91,92,97]

The tumour is non-encapsulated and extends from beneath the epidermis, through the dermis and usually into the subcutis. It is composed of interlacing bundles of spindle-shaped cells and collagen bundles. There may be some vertical orientation of the cells and fibres superficially (Fig. 34.8). The appendages become incorporated within the tumour. The nuclei of the cells are oval or spindle-shaped and some stellate forms may be present. There are only occasional mitoses. The cytoplasm of the cells merges imperceptibly with the collagen. There are characteristic, small, eosinophilic inclusion bodies within the cytoplasm of the tumour cells, often in a paranuclear position. A clear halo is sometimes discernible in well-stained sections. These bodies measure 2–10 μm in diameter, and may be mistaken for red blood cells. They stain red with the Masson trichrome stain, and deep purple with the PTAH method. They are PAS negative.[98]

There are small capillaries and a few scattered

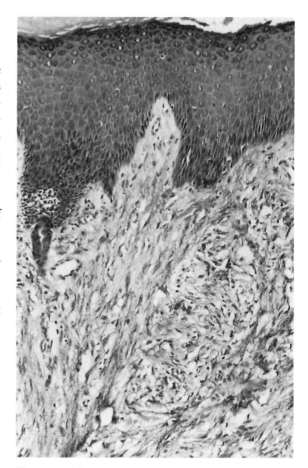

Fig. 34.8 Digital fibromatosis of childhood. The spindle-shaped cells and some collagen bundles have a vertical orientation within the dermis.
Haematoxylin–eosin

elastic fibres in the stroma. The overlying epidermis usually shows flattening of the rete ridges. Ulceration is rare.

The immunocytochemical localization of vimentin and muscle-specific actin in the proliferating cells confirms their myofibroblastic nature.[90a]

Electron microscopy. The spindle cells are myofibroblasts[94,99] and the inclusion bodies are compact masses of amorphous and granular material with some discernible microfilaments, but with no limiting membrane. Actin has been demonstrated within the myofibroblasts, and it has been suggested that the inclusions are masses of actin[89] or, more likely, degradation products of it.[100] This viewpoint has recently been challenged.[101] Cultured tumour cells also develop inclusion bodies.[89]

INFANTILE MYOFIBROMATOSIS

This entity, which is regarded as a proliferative disorder of myofibroblasts, was established by Chung and Enzinger in 1981, with their report of 61 cases.[102] Previous reports had appeared under several designations including congenital fibrosarcoma,[103] congenital generalized fibromatosis,[86,104,105] and congenital mesenchymal hamartoma.[106] Recently Fletcher and colleagues presented evidence that the spindle cell component shows true smooth muscle differentiation rather than being of a myofibroblastic nature.[107] They suggested that the current name may be incorrect.

The lesions are solitary in approximately 70% of cases.[102] Almost half of these are situated in the deep soft tissues, while the remainder are located in the skin and/or subcutaneous tissue. The head, neck and trunk are the usual sites of involvement.[102] There is a male predominance. Most lesions are present at birth, or appear in the first two years of life; onset in adult life has been recorded.[107a,107b] The prognosis is excellent, with recurrence unlikely after excision; aggressive variants are rare.[107c]

In approximately 30% of cases the lesions are multicentric and involve the skin, soft tissues, bones and, uncommonly, the viscera.[102] They are usually present at birth, and there is a female predominance. Spontaneous regression of soft tissue and osseous lesions sometimes occurs,[102,108] but cases with visceral involvement are usually fatal.[102] Recurrence after a long period of quiescence has been documented.[109] Central nervous system abnormalities were present in one case.[110] Both an autosomal recessive[111] and dominant inheritance with reduced penetrance have been proposed.[109]

Macroscopically the tumours measure 0.5 – 7 cm or more in diameter. They are greyish-white in colour, and fibrous in consistency.

Histopathology[102,107]

The nodules are reasonably well circumscribed, although there may be an infiltrative border in the subcutis. There are plump to elongate spindle cells with features of myofibroblasts. They are grouped in short fascicles. Delicate bundles of collagen separate or enclose the cellular aggregates (Fig. 34.9). Mitoses are variable in number, but they are not atypical.

Vascular spaces resembling those of haemangiopericytoma are often found in the centre of the tumour.[102] Sometimes there is an intravascular pattern of growth. Necrosis, hyalinization, calcification and focal haemorrhage may be present centrally.[107]

Immunoperoxidase studies have shown that the tumour cells are positive for vimentin and actin but negative for S100 protein, myoglobin and cytokeratin.[107,107a] Conflicting results have been reported for desmin.[107,107a]

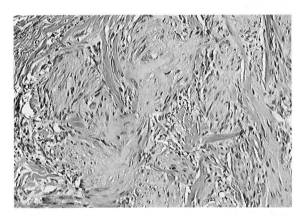

Fig. 34.9 Infantile myofibroma. Short fascicles of plump, spindle-shaped cells are separated by thin bundles of collagen.
Haematoxylin — eosin

Electron microscopy. The cells have the ultrastructural features of myofibroblasts.[106]

JUVENILE HYALINE FIBROMATOSIS

This exceedingly rare autosomal recessive condition is characterized by large tumours, especially on the scalp, whitish cutaneous nodules, hypertrophy of the gingiva, flexural contractures and often focal bone erosion.[112–114b] The onset is in infancy and childhood. Spontaneous regression of tumours sometimes occurs. Recurrent infections may lead to death. Uncommonly, there is widespread visceral involvement; this is known as infantile systemic hyalinosis.[114b]

Histopathology[112–114b]

The tumour nodules are composed of markedly thickened dermis with a vaguely chondroid appearance. They are composed of fibroblast-like cells, with abundant granular cytoplasm, embedded in an amorphous eosinophilic ground substance that is PAS positive. The ground substance is abundant in older lesions; it presumably represents a collagen precursor produced by the fibroblast-like tumour cells.

Electron microscopy. The spindle-shaped cells are fibroblasts with dilated rough endoplasmic reticulum and vesicles in their cytoplasm. There are plentiful collagen fibrils in the stroma.[114b]

GIANT CELL FIBROBLASTOMA

This is a rare, benign soft tissue tumour occurring predominantly in childhood.[115] The back, thigh and chest are the favoured sites. There is a male predominance. Macroscopically the tumour appears grey-pink with a partly gelatinous consistency.[116] Local recurrence is common, following incomplete surgical removal.[116a]

Histopathology[115–117c]

The dermis and subcutis are involved by an infiltrating spindle cell tumour in which the tumour cells are embedded in a loose connective tissue matrix showing areas of mucinous change. Scattered through the tumour are uninucleate and multinucleate giant cells. A characteristic feature is the presence of branching sinusoidal spaces lined by cytoplasmic extensions of the spindle and giant cells.[117] These cells are negative for S100 protein and factor VIII, but show scattered positivity for α_1-anti-

trypsin.[117,117a] Both the spindle cells and the giant cells consistently stain for vimentin.[117c]

Electron microscopy. Ultrastructural examination of this tumour has shown the cells to be fibroblasts, some of which have cytoplasmic extensions.[116]

FIBROSARCOMA

Enzinger and Weiss have defined a fibrosarcoma as a malignant tumour of fibroblasts that shows no evidence of other cellular differentiation.[118] There has been a marked decline in the diagnosis of fibrosarcoma in the last 10–15 years as a result of the delineation of the fibromatoses as a diagnostic entity and the recognition of the malignant fibrous histiocytoma. Furthermore, other spindle cell tumours, which were in the past sometimes misdiagnosed as fibrosarcoma, such as spindle cell melanoma (see p. 799) and spindle cell squamous carcinoma (see p. 752), as well as malignant peripheral nerve sheath tumours (see p. 932), can now be more confidently diagnosed with the assistance of various monoclonal antibodies and immunoperoxidase techniques.

Very little has been written about fibrosarcoma in recent years. However, as it is primarily a tumour of the deep soft tissues which only rarely develops in the skin and superficial subcutis, only brief mention will be made of it. Cutaneous fibrosarcomas may follow thermal burns and radiation therapy, or result from extension of a tumour arising in deeper tissues. The tumour affects predominantly middle-aged adults, although there is an uncommon clinical subset involving neonates and young children.[119–121] Despite their rapid growth and sometimes large size, infantile fibrosarcomas have a much better prognosis than those arising in adults.

Histopathology[118,122]

Typically, fibrosarcomas are composed of interlacing fascicles of spindle cells forming a so-called 'herring-bone' pattern. Mitoses are common. There is a variable meshwork of collagen and reticulin between the individual cells, the amount depending on the differentiation of the tumour.

The infantile variant is usually more cellular and composed of smaller cells with prominent mitotic activity.

FIBROHISTIOCYTIC TUMOURS

The term 'fibrous histiocytoma' was introduced for a group of tumours which share certain morphological features, such as the presence of fibroblast-like spindle cells and presumptive histiocytes, cells that were assumed to arise from a tissue histiocyte that could function as, or transform into, a fibroblast. Although the histiocytic origin of these tumours is now considered unlikely, it is still convenient to retain the term 'fibrohistiocytic' in a morphologically descriptive sense for tumours which show features of fibroblastic and histiocytic differentiation. Some of these tumours appear to be derived from the recently delineated dermal dendrocyte.

DERMATOFIBROMA

The large number of terms that have been used for this entity (histiocytoma,[123,124] fibrous histiocytoma,[125–127] sclerosing haemangioma,[128] nodular subepidermal fibrosis[129,130]) reflects the remarkable variation in its histological features, and continuing controversy regarding its histogenesis.[130a] However, the presence of transitional patterns and different morphological components in the same lesion is strong evidence in favour of its basically common nature and histogenesis.[125]

Fibroblasts, non-lysozyme-containing histiocytes,[130] and endothelial cells have all been regarded at some time as the cell of origin.[123] Dermatofibromas have been regarded by some authors as a benign tumour, and by others as a fibrosing inflammatory or reactive process.[131] In support of the latter concept is the history of trauma, blunt or piercing, recorded in up to 20% of cases.[129] An insect bite has preceded the development of a dermatofibroma.[123] Recently, on the basis of the immunoreactivity of 30–70% of the constituent cells with factor XIIIa, an origin from the 'dermal dendrocyte' has been proposed.[132,132a] The term 'dermal dendrocytoma' has even been suggested in place of dermatofibroma.[132]

Dermatofibromas are common, accounting for almost 3% of specimens received by one dermatopathology laboratory.[133] There is a predilection for the extremities, particularly the lower, of young adults.[123,133] There is a female preponderance.[133] Rare sites of involvement have included the fingers,[129] palms and soles,[134] the scalp,[129] the face,[134a] and a vaccination scar.[135]

Dermatofibromas are round or ovoid, firm dermal nodules, usually less than 1 cm in diameter. Polypoid, flat and depressed configurations occur. Lesions with a preponderance of histiocytes are often larger, and the aneurysmal (angiomatoid) variants may measure up to 10 cm in diameter.[136,137] Dermatofibromas are usually a dusky brown in colour but aneurysmal variants may be red, and tumours with abundant lipid can be cream/yellow, particularly on the cut surface of the excised lesion. Dermatofibromas are most often solitary, but two to five lesions are present in 10% or so of individuals.[123] Multiple lesions have been reported as a rare complication of immunosuppressive therapy.[134,138] There are only a few reports of patients with large numbers of tumours;[127,139,140] one such case was reported recently as 'disseminated dermal dendrocytomas'.[140a] Clinical variants include the aneurysmal type, already referred to,[136] and the rare annular haemosiderotic histiocytoma in which multiple brown papules in annular configurations were present on the buttocks.[141]

Histopathology[123,125,126]

Dermatofibromas are poorly demarcated tumours centred on the dermis. There is sometimes extension into the superficial subcutis. A grenz zone of variable thickness is present in about 70% of cases.[123] Sometimes this contains dilated vessels.[123] Dermatofibromas are composed of a variable admixture of fibroblast-

rudimentary pilar structures, to undoubted basal cell carcinoma.[124,149,153] Sebaceous structures are uncommonly present.[124] Unequivocal basal cell carcinoma is uncommon[143,154] and some of the cases reported as this are examples of exuberant basaloid hyperplasia;[155] the distinction is not always easy. It has been suggested that the hair-follicle-like structures represent regressive changes in pre-existing follicles and not the induction of new pilar units.[133]

A small percentage of cells, usually at the periphery, are S100 positive.[142] α_1-antitrypsin and macrophage markers such as EMB11 and HAM-56 have been reported in the tumour cells.[156,157] The recent finding of factor XIIIa in many dermatofibromas provides a useful marker for this tumour,[132] although it is also present in acral angiofibromas, scars, keloids and atypical fibroxanthoma but not in dermatofibrosarcoma protuberans.[132a]

Electron microscopy. Ultrastructural studies have given conflicting results, with the cells variously reported as resembling fibroblasts, histiocytes and even myofibroblasts.[158,159] Endothelial cells with Weibel–Palade bodies were the prominent cell noted in one study.[128] Vessels are conspicuous in the angiomatoid variant.[145] There is a need for a reappraisal of the ultrastructural findings in the light of the immunoperoxidase studies implicating the dermal dendrocyte as the cell of origin (see above).

DERMATOFIBROSARCOMA PROTUBERANS

Dermatofibrosarcoma protuberans (DFSP) is a slowly growing, locally aggressive tumour of disputed histogenesis, with a marked tendency to local recurrence, but which rarely metastasizes.[160] It has a predilection for the trunk and proximal extremities of young and middle-aged adults[160] but other sites are rarely involved.[160a,160b] The lesions are solitary or multiple polypoid nodules, often arising in an indurated plaque of tumour.[161–162a] The involved area of skin measures from 0.5–10 cm or more in greatest diameter. A violaceous or red colour is sometimes present, but at other times the nodules are flesh coloured.[162] A history of previous trauma at the site is sometimes given.[160,160b,163] Previous arsenic exposure was present in one case.[164]

Local recurrence occurs in up to one-third of all cases.[160,162] Haematogenous metastases, although rare,[165] are more common than those to regional lymph nodes.[166–169] It has been suggested that some of the reported cases of DFSP with metastases may really be malignant fibrous histiocytomas or tumours with overlap features of these two entities.[170] Progression of a recurrent DFSP to a malignant fibrous histiocytoma[171] and the development of fibrosarcomatous areas in a DFSP[171a] have been reported.

The *pigmented storiform neurofibroma of Bednar (Bednar tumour)* is now regarded as a variant of DFSP.[172–177] It is an exceedingly rare tumour which accounts for only 1–5% of all cases of DFSP.[177] The Bednar tumour occurs in a similar clinical setting to DFSP but, as yet, no metastases have been recorded. It is thought to represent the colonization of a DFSP by melanocytes.[177a]

Although DFSP is traditionally regarded as a fibrohistiocytic tumour, several ultrastructural and immunohistochemical studies have questioned this viewpoint;[178] a neuroectodermal origin has also been suggested. Fletcher and colleagues have recently commented that 'the most pragmatic solution at this time may be to regard these tumours as a heterogeneous group, in line with the pluripotentiality of mesenchyme'.[170]

Macroscopically, the cut surface of the tumour nodules appears firm, and grey-white in colour. Recurrent lesions with abundant mucin may have a more glistening appearance. The pigmented variant may appear slate grey or black if sufficient melanin is present within the tumour.[177]

Histopathology[160]

Dermatofibrosarcoma protuberans is a dermal tumour which almost invariably extends into the

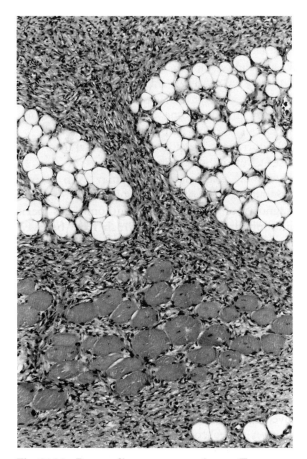

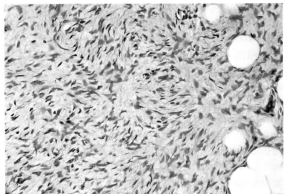

Fig. 34.15 Dermatofibrosarcoma protuberans. The spindle-shaped cells have a storiform or cart-wheel arrangement.
Haematoxylin — eosin

Fig. 34.14 Dermatofibrosarcoma protuberans. Tumour cells insinuate between fat cells in the subcutis and extend into the underlying muscle.
Haematoxylin — eosin

subcutis where it infiltrates around small groups of fat cells in a characteristic manner (Fig. 34.14).[161] Deeper extension to underlying muscle is rare.[179] A superficial grenz zone is often present, but extension to the epidermis, with ulceration, is sometimes seen.[170] Dermal appendages are surrounded but not invaded.

DFSP is a spindle cell tumour composed of interwoven bundles of rather uniform, small spindle cells with plump nuclei. There are small amounts of intermingled collagen. At points of intersection of the fascicles there may be an acellular collagenous focus from which the fascicles appear to radiate (Fig. 34.15).[165] This is referred to as a storiform or cartwheel pattern.

Scattered mitoses are present, but atypical forms are rare. Increased cellularity of the tumour, and more than eight mitoses per 10 high power fields appear to be associated with a predisposition to metastasis.[165]

Other histological features include an occasional histiocyte and multinucleate giant cell.[178] Thin-walled capillaries are randomly distributed. Myxoid areas may be present, particularly in recurrences.[160] A myxoid variant of DFSP has also been proposed.[180] Although usually inconspicuous, the stromal collagen will stain with the trichrome method, but unlike the collagen in a dermatofibroma it is not polarizable.[181] Unlike dermatofibromas, haemosiderin is rarely present in a DFSP.[160] Furthermore, a dermatofibroma is usually smaller and less cellular, with fewer mitoses than DFSP.

The pigmented variants have melanin-containing dendritic cells (melanocytes) scattered throughout the tumour.[177] The amount of melanin pigment is quite variable. Although Bednar reported three cases in which this pigmented variant was present in the core of a naevocellular naevus,[173] no further examples of this phenomenon have been reported.

Immunohistochemical studies have shown that the tumour cells in DFSP contain vimentin[181a] but they are negative for S100 protein. A few scattered cells may stain for lysozyme and α_1-antichymotrypsin.[170] The pigment-laden

Histopathology[209a]

Plexiform fibrohistiocytic tumours are characterized by a multinodular or plexiform proliferation of histiocyte-like and fibroblast-like cells associated with multinucleate giant cells resembling osteoclasts. In some tumours, the pattern is more fibroblastic than fibrohistiocytic and these tumours have some resemblance to a fibromatosis. Immunohistochemistry has given variable results.[209a]

MALIGNANT FIBROUS HISTIOCYTOMA

Malignant fibrous histiocytoma is the commonest soft tissue sarcoma of late adult life.[178] It usually involves the deep soft tissues and striated muscles of the proximal part of the extremities, particularly the lower. The retroperitoneum is another favoured site.[178,210] Up to 25% of cases may arise in the subcutaneous tissues, although less than 10% are confined to the subcutis without underlying fascial involvement.[210,211] Cutaneous tumours are even rarer.[212,212a] Adults between the ages of 50 and 70 years are most often affected, although the angiomatoid variant involves primarily children and adolescents.[213] There are usually no predisposing factors, but rarely cases have followed radiotherapy,[211,213a] or developed at the site of a chronic ulcer,[214] vaccination scar[215] or burn scar.[216]

The tumours are multilobulated, often circumscribed, grey-white fleshy masses.[211] The majority are 5 cm or more in diameter. Focal areas of haemorrhage and necrosis are quite common. The myxoid variant has a somewhat gelatinous appearance and the inflammatory variant may be yellow in colour.

The prognosis is generally poor, with 5-year survivals ranging from 15–30%.[217] Tumours which are small and superficially located have a better prognosis than large, deep tumours.[210,218] Proximal deep tumours and those in the retroperitoneum have a poor prognosis. Local recurrence and metastases are common, with the lungs and regional lymph nodes most often affected.[210]

The histogenesis of this tumour has been controversial. The tumour cells show partial fibroblastic and histiocytic differentiation as reflected by collagen production and the presence of cells which may be immunoreactive for the histiocytic markers as well as showing occasional phagocytosis.[219] It is now believed that the progenitor cell is not the mononuclear phagocyte but rather a poorly defined mesenchymal cell which may differentiate along histiocytic and fibroblastic lines.[220,221]

Histopathology

Five histological subtypes of malignant fibrous histiocytoma have been recognized — pleomorphic, angiomatoid, myxoid, giant cell, and inflammatory.[178,211] Overlap features occur between the various types.[217] All tumours usually have an infiltrative margin. They may show areas of haemorrhage and necrosis, particularly the larger tumours. Chronic inflammatory cells are usually present throughout the tumour, particularly at the periphery. The various types will be considered in further detail.

Pleomorphic. This is the commonest variant.[210,211] It is composed of an admixture of plump spindle-shaped cells, clusters or sheets of histiocytes, and scattered, pleomorphic, multinucleate giant cells (Fig. 34.17). Mitoses are common. The spindle cells may be arranged in whorls or have a storiform appearance. There is usually a delicate collagenous stroma; in some areas this may be more prominent. Focal myxoid change is quite common. Rarely, metaplastic osteoid or chondroid material is formed.[222] Xanthoma cells and siderophages are sometimes present.

Angiomatoid. This variant tends to involve the subcutis.[213] There are large blood-filled cystic spaces and areas of haemorrhage in addition to the solid nests of fibroblast-like and histiocyte-like cells.[213,223] Xanthoma cells, siderophages and giant cells are often present.

Myxoid. Approximately 10% of all malignant fibrous histiocytomas are of this type.[224,224a] It

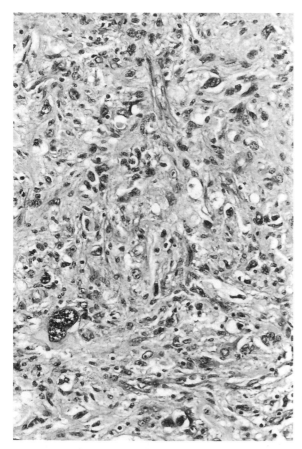

Fig. 34.17 Malignant fibrous histiocytoma. It is composed of spindle-shaped and polygonal cells and scattered pleomorphic giant cells, some of which are multinucleate. Haematoxylin — eosin

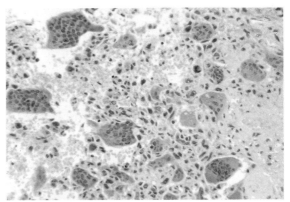

Fig. 34.18 Malignant fibrous histiocytoma composed of numerous osteoclast-like giant cells. Haematoxylin — eosin

has a better prognosis than most other types. Prominent myxoid foci comprise nearly 50% of the tumour.[224] Other areas resemble the pleomorphic variant.

Giant cell. Formerly known as giant cell tumour of soft parts, this variant has numerous osteoclast-like giant cells in addition to the spindle and histiocytic cells (Fig. 34.18).[225]

Inflammatory. This rare variant, which is most frequently retroperitoneal, has a grave prognosis. A diffuse and at times intense neutrophilic infiltrate, unassociated with tissue necrosis, is present not only in the primary tumour, but also in recurrences and metastases.[226,227] Xanthoma

cells, both bland and anaplastic, are also present. A storiform fibrous pattern is usually seen in some areas of the tumour.[226]

The tumour cells contain vimentin; cytokeratin has also been present in a few tumours.[228] Various histiocyte markers can be demonstrated, using immunoperoxidase techniques, in from 60–80% of malignant fibrous histiocytomas. Those used have included α_1-antitrypsin and α_1-antichymotrypsin.[156] Recently, a higher incidence of positivity has been attained using the lectin *Ricinus communis*,[229] although a small percentage of fibrosarcomas was also positive.[229]

Electron microscopy. Studies have consistently shown cells with fibroblastic and histiocytic morphology, as well as undifferentiated mesenchymal cells with a narrow rim of cytoplasm and scattered ribosomes.[220,230] Myofibroblasts were said to be the predominant cell in one case.[230a]

PRESUMPTIVE SYNOVIAL AND TENDON SHEATH TUMOURS

FIBROMA OF TENDON SHEATH

Chung and Enzinger formally documented this entity in 1979 with a report of 138 cases.[231] It is a solitary, slowly growing subcutaneous tumour with a predilection for the fingers, hands and wrists of middle-aged adults, particularly males.[232,232a] Recurrences occur in approximately 20% of cases.

The fibromas are well-circumscribed, often lobulated, grey to white tumours which measure 1–2 cm in diameter. They are usually attached to a tendon sheath.

Histopathology[231,233]

These tumours are situated in the subcutaneous tissue, sometimes with dermal extension. There are relatively sparse spindle or stellate cells embedded in a dense fibrocollagenous stroma. Cellular areas are present and these are sometimes located towards the periphery. The stroma shows variable hyalinization and sometimes has a whorled pattern with associated artefactual clefting. Myxoid degeneration and, rarely, focal calcification of the stroma may be present. A characteristic feature is the presence of dilated or slit-like vascular channels. A sparse mononuclear cell infiltrate is sometimes present at the periphery.

Electron microscopy. Ultrastructural examination has shown the spindle cells to be myofibroblasts[234] with some fibroblasts.[232a,235]

GIANT CELL TUMOUR OF TENDON SHEATH

This not uncommon benign tumour has a predilection for the dorsal surface of the fingers, in the vicinity of the distal interphalangeal joint.[236,236a] It occurs particularly in young and middle-aged adults. It is a slowly growing, usually asymptomatic lesion which may measure up to 3 cm in diameter at the time of removal. Local recurrence, usually a result of incomplete removal, occurs in 15% of cases.[236]

Giant cell tumours are lobulated, and grey-brown in colour with yellowish areas. They are usually attached to a tendon sheath or joint capsule but cutaneous involvement can occur.[237,238] The histogenesis of giant cell tumours has been controversial. They have been regarded as a variant of fibrous histiocytoma, and as a tumour derived from mesenchymal cells.[239] A recent study concluded that the cells are of monocyte/macrophage lineage and that they closely resemble osteoclasts.[239a]

Histopathology[236,240]

The lesion has an eosinophilic collagenous stroma with variable cellularity. In the sparsely cellular areas the cells are plump and spindle-shaped, set in a partly hyalinized stroma, whereas in the more cellular areas the cells are usually polygonal. Small clusters of lipid-laden histiocytes are often present. Multinucleate giant cells with up to 60 or more nuclei are a characteristic feature. They are variable in number and haphazardly distributed. Haemosiderin is invariably present, and sometimes there are cholesterol clefts.

In one study, the cells were positive for leucocyte common antigen (CD45), Leu-M3 (CD14) and Leu-3 (CD4).[239a]

Electron microscopy. Ultrastructural studies have usually supported a synovial or fibrohistiocytic origin,[241] although another report documented a pleomorphic cell population in which the giant cells had some similarity to osteoclasts and the stromal cells similarities to primitive mesenchymal cells, osteoblasts, fibroblasts and histiocytes.[239]

EPITHELIOID SARCOMA

Epithelioid sarcoma, first delineated by Enzinger,[242] is a rare malignant tumour which usually involves the deep subcutis and underlying soft tissues. Infrequently, it arises in the dermis and superficial subcutis where it may be confused both clinically[243] and histologically[244] with various benign cutaneous diseases, including granuloma annulare.[245] It has a predilection for the extremities, particularly the hands, of young adult males.[244,246] Lesions of the vulva[247] and penis[248] have also been described. A history of trauma is sometimes given.[246]

It presents as one or more, slowly growing

tan-white nodules with an indistinct infiltrating margin. Ulceration develops late, if at all. Local recurrence occurs in nearly 80% of cases, and metastases in 30–40%.[246,249] The regional lymph nodes and lungs are the most common initial sites of metastases. The skin of the scalp represents another site of distant metastasis.[250] Adverse prognostic features are a proximal or axial location, deep extension, vascular invasion, metastases, and numerous mitotic figures.[246]

Epithelioid sarcoma is of disputed histogenesis, with a synovial origin most favoured.[251,252] A histiocytic, fibroblastic,[253] myofibroblastic[254] and mesenchymal reserve cell[255] origin have all been suggested.

Histopathology[244–246]

The low power appearance often resembles a necrobiotic or granulomatous process, or an epithelial tumour. Epithelioid sarcoma is an ill-defined cellular lesion forming vague nodules in the dermis and subcutis. There is subtle extension into the contiguous fascial and tendinous structures. It is composed of oval to polygonal cells with abundant, often eosinophilic, cytoplasm and a gradual transition to plump spindle cells (Fig. 34.19).[256] Nuclear pleomorphism and scattered mitoses are present. Multinucleate giant cells are rare or absent.

A characteristic feature is the presence of central necrosis or fibrosis. Collagen also extends between the cells. Calcification is present in approximately 20% of cases, and osseous metaplasia in 10%.[246] Haemosiderin is often present. A perinodular inflammatory cell infiltrate of lymphocytes and histiocytes is a usual feature.[257]

Immunoperoxidase studies show that many tumour cells contain cytokeratin, epithelial membrane antigen and vimentin but not leucocyte common antigen or S100 protein.[258–261] Histiocytic markers have usually been negative.[260]

Electron microscopy. Light and dark cells are present within the tumour cell population. There are many filopodia-like surface extensions of cytoplasm[244,251] and there are bundles of intermediate filaments in the cytoplasm.[260] Occasional pseudoglandular spaces have been present in some tumours.[252]

MISCELLANEOUS ENTITIES

This group of disorders includes several very rare entities in which fibrous tissue forms a significant component and another group with a myxoid stroma.

FIBRO-OSSEOUS PSEUDOTUMOUR OF THE DIGITS

This is a rare tumour of the subcutaneous and soft tissues of the digits, usually in young adults.[262] There is a close histological resemblance to myositis ossificans, with osteoid formation and a background stroma of fibroblasts,

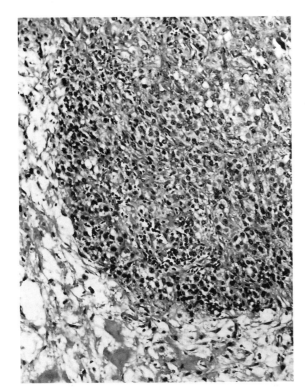

Fig. 34.19 Epithelioid cell sarcoma. The sheets of epithelioid and polygonal cells are arranged irregularly in a partly necrotic and myxoid zone.
Haematoxylin — eosin

collagen and myxoid material.[262] Unlike myositis ossificans, the lesion usually involves the subcutis and has an irregular multinodular growth pattern.[262]

FIBROADENOMA

Fibroadenomas resembling those seen in the breast may arise along the embryonic milkline and elsewhere.[263]

NODULAR FIBROSIS IN ELEPHANTIASIS

Multiple nodules, sometimes large, are a common complication of non-filarial elephantiasis of the lower legs.[264] This idiopathic condition is endemic in Ethiopia.[264] Microscopy shows bundles of collagen in the dermis, in irregular whorls, with a variable number of fibroblasts depending on the age of the lesion.[264] A few small blood vessels, some with a surrounding cuff of lymphocytes, are also present.

MULTIFOCAL FIBROSCLEROSIS

Subcutaneous fibrosis is an uncommon complication of multifocal fibrosclerosis, a condition in which progressive fibrosis of several discrete regions of the body, particularly the retroperitoneum and mediastinum, occurs.[265] Ulceration and vasculitic lesions may also develop in the skin.

COLLAGENOUS PAPULES OF THE EAR

There have been several reports of patients with papules, 1–4 mm in size, on the inner surfaces of the aural conchae and characterized histologically by sclerotic, hyalinized and focally clefted masses of collagen in the upper dermis.[266] The material abutted against the epidermis and contained scattered spindle, stellate and binucleate fibroblasts. Superficial telangiectatic vessels were present. Earlier reports of the same entity have been included with lichen amyloidosus (see p. 410) on the basis of positive histochemical staining for amyloid.[267] However, a recent publication has confirmed the presence of amyloid by electron microscopy and the use of the monoclonal antikeratin antibody EKH4.[268]

CUTANEOUS MYXOMA

Cutaneous myxomas are rare tumours which may be associated with a systemic syndrome, which includes cardiac myxomas as one of its manifestations. At other times they are a solitary tumour, usually on the digits, and unassociated with any systemic abnormalities.[269,270] Because of their close resemblance to digital mucous

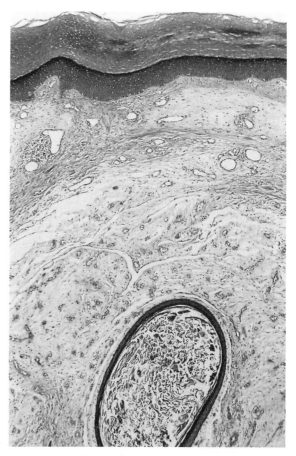

Fig. 34.20 Superficial angiomyxoma. There is a keratinous cyst in the centre of the tumour which has a vascular and myxoid stroma.
Haematoxylin — eosin

cysts, cutaneous myxomas are discussed in further detail with the mucinoses (see Ch. 13, p. 392).

Histopathology[269,270]

Cutaneous myxomas are composed of stellate and spindle-shaped cells set in a loose myxoid stroma.

SUPERFICIAL ANGIOMYXOMA

Angiomyxomas are a distinct variant of myxoma which may also contain epithelial elements (see p. 392).[271] They present as slowly growing, painless nodules which may involve the dermis and subcutis of any part of the body. They usually measure 1–5 cm in diameter but larger variants have been recorded.[271] Local recurrence may occur after surgical removal but not metastasis.

Histopathology[271]

Angiomyxomas are usually centred on the subcutis but extension into the dermis is almost invariable. They are composed of spindle-shaped and stellate cells set in a copious basophilic matrix (Fig. 34.20). Another distinguishing feature of these lesions is the presence, in more than half the lesions, of an epithelial component which takes the form of epithelial strands or a keratin-filled cyst.[271]

REFERENCES

Acral angiofibromas

1. Ackerman AB, Kornberg R. Pearly penile papules. Acral angiofibromas. Arch Dermatol 1973; 108: 673–675.
2. Meigel WN, Ackerman AB. Fibrous papule of the face. Am J Dermatopathol 1979; 1: 329–340.
3. Reed RJ, Ackerman AB. Pathology of the adventitial dermis. Anatomic observations and biologic speculations. Hum Pathol 1973; 4: 207–217.
4. Nemeth AJ, Penneys NS. Factor XIIIa is expressed by fibroblasts in fibrovascular tumors. J Cutan Pathol 1989; 16: 266–271.
5. Cerio R, Griffiths CEM, Cooper KD et al. Characterization of factor XIIIa positive dermal dendritic cells in normal and inflamed skin. Br J Dermatol 1989; 121: 421–431.
6. Penneys NS. Factor XIII expression in the skin: Observations and a hypothesis. J Am Acad Dermatol 1990; 22: 484–488.
7. Pinkus H. Perifollicular fibromas. Pure periadnexal adventitial tumors. Am J Dermatopathol 1979; 1: 341–342.
8. Butterworth T, Graham JH. Linear papular ectodermal-mesodermal hamartoma (hamartoma moniliformis). Arch Dermatol 1970; 101: 191–204.
9. Reed RJ. Cutaneous manifestations of neural crest disorders (neurocristopathies). Int J Dermatol 1977; 16: 807–826.
10. Sanchez NP, Wick MR, Perry HO. Adenoma sebaceum of Pringle: A clinicopathologic review, with a discussion of related pathologic entities. J Cutan Pathol 1981; 8: 395–403.
11. Nickel WR, Reed WB. Tuberous sclerosis; special reference to the microscopic alterations in the cutaneous hamartomas. Arch Dermatol 1962; 85: 209–224.
12. Willis WF, Garcia RL. Giant angiofibroma in tuberous sclerosis. Arch Dermatol 1978; 114: 1843–1844.
13. Park Y–K, Hann SK. Cluster growths in adenoma sebaceum associated with tuberous sclerosis. J Am Acad Dermatol 1989; 20: 918–920.
14. Reed RJ, Hairston MA, Palomeque FE. The histologic identity of adenoma sebaceum and solitary melanocytic angiofibroma. Dermatol Int 1966; 5: 3–11.
15. Reed RJ. Fibrous papule of the face. Melanocytic angiofibroma. Am J Dermatopathol 1979; 1: 343–344.
16. Bhawan J, Edelstein L. Angiofibromas in tuberous sclerosis: a light and electron microscopic study. J Cutan Pathol 1977; 4: 300–307.
17. Graham JH, Sanders JB, Johnson WC, Helwig EB. Fibrous papule of the nose; a clinicopathological study. J Invest Dermatol 1965; 45: 194–203.
18. Saylan T, Marks R, Wilson Jones E. Fibrous papule of the nose. Br J Dermatol 1971; 85: 111–118.
19. McGibbon DH, Wilson Jones E. Fibrous papule of the face (nose). Fibrosing nevocytic nevus. Am J Dermatopathol 1979; 1: 345–348.
20. Santa Cruz DJ, Prioleau PG. Fibrous papule of the face. An electron-microscopic study of two cases. Am J Dermatopathol 1979; 1: 349–352.
21. Ragaz A, Berezowsky V. Fibrous papule of the face. A study of five cases by electron microscopy. Am J Dermatopathol 1979; 1: 353–355.
22. Nemeth AJ, Penneys NS, Bernstein HB. Fibrous papule: A tumour of fibrohistiocytic cells that contain factor XIIIa. J Am Acad Dermatol 1988; 19: 1102–1106.
23. Cerio R, Rao BK, Spaull J, Wilson Jones E. An immunohistochemical study of fibrous papule of the nose: 25 cases. J Cutan Pathol 1989; 16: 194–198.
24. Cerio R, Wilson Jones E. Factor XIIIa positivity in

109. Jennings TA, Sabetta J, Duray PH et al. Infantile myofibromatosis. Evidence for an autosomal–dominant disorder. Am J Surg Pathol 1984; 8: 529–538.

110. Spraker MK, Stack C, Esterly NB. Congenital generalized fibromatosis: A review of the literature and report of a case associated with porencephaly, hemiatrophy, and cutis marmorata telangiectatica congenita. J Am Acad Dermatol 1984; 10: 365–371.

111. Venencie PY, Bigel P, Desgruelles C et al. Infantile myofibromatosis. Report of two cases in one family. Br J Dermatol 1987; 117: 255–259.

112. Puretic S, Puretic B, Fiser-Herman M, Adamcic M. A unique form of mesenchymal dysplasia. Br J Dermatol 1962; 74: 8–19.

113. Kitano Y. Juvenile hyalin fibromatosis. Arch Dermatol 1976; 112: 86–88.

114. Kitano Y, Horiki M, Aoki T, Sagami S. Two cases of juvenile hyalin fibromatosis. Arch Dermatol 1972; 106: 877–883.

114a. Mayer-da-Silva A, Poiares-Baptista A, Guerra Rodrigo F, Teresa-Lopes M. Juvenile hyaline fibromatosis. A histologic and histochemical study. Arch Pathol Lab Med 1988; 112: 928–931.

114b. Kan AE, Rogers M. Juvenile hyaline fibromatosis: an expanded clinicopathologic spectrum. Pediatr Dermatol 1989; 6: 68–75.

115. Shmookler BM, Enzinger FM. Giant cell fibroblastoma: a peculiar childhood tumor. Lab Invest 1982; 46: 76A (abstract).

116. Abdul-Karim FW, Evans HL, Silva EG. Giant cell fibroblastoma: a report of three cases. Am J Clin Pathol 1985; 83: 165–170.

116a. Dymock RB, Allen PW, Stirling JW et al. Giant cell fibroblastoma. A distinctive, recurrent tumor of childhood. Am J Surg Pathol 1987; 11: 263–272.

117. Barr RJ, Young EM Jr, Liao S-Y. Giant cell fibroblastoma: an immunohistochemical study. J Cutan Pathol 1986; 13: 301–307.

117a. Chou P, Gonzalez-Crussi F, Mangkornkanok M. Giant cell fibroblastoma. Cancer 1989; 63: 756–762.

117b. Rosen LB, Amazon K, Weitzner J, Resnick L. Giant cell fibroblastoma. A report of a case and review of the literature. Am J Dermatopathol 1989; 11: 242–247.

117c. Fletcher CDM. Giant cell fibroblastoma of soft tissue: a clinicopathological and immunohistochemical study. Histopathology 1988; 13: 499–508.

118. Enzinger FM, Weiss SW. Soft tissue tumours. St. Louis: C.V. Mosby, 1983; 103–124.

119. Gonzalez-Crussi F, Wiederhold MD, Sotelo-Avila C. Congenital fibrosarcoma. Presence of a histiocytic component. Cancer 1980; 46: 77–86.

120. Soule EH, Pritchard DJ. Fibrosarcoma in infants and children. A review of 110 cases. Cancer 1977; 40: 1711–1721.

121. Chung EB, Enzinger FM. Infantile fibrosarcoma. Cancer 1976; 38: 729–739.

122. Pritchard DJ, Soule EH, Taylor WF, Ivins JC. Fibrosarcoma — a clinicopathologic and statistical study of 199 tumors of the soft tissues of the extremities and trunk. Cancer 1974; 33: 888–897.

Fibrohistiocytic tumours

123. Niemi KM. The benign fibrohistiocytic tumours of the skin. Acta Derm Venereol (Suppl) 1970; 63: 1–60.

124. Dalziel K, Marks R. Hair follicle-like change over histiocytomas. Am J Dermatopathol 1986; 8: 462–466.

125. Vilanova JR, Flint A. The morphological variations of fibrous histiocytomas. J Cutan Pathol 1974; 1: 155–164.

126. Gonzalez S, Duarte I. Benign fibrous histiocytoma of the skin. A morphologic study of 290 cases. Pathol Res Pract 1982; 174: 379–391.

127. Baraf CS, Shapiro L. Multiple histiocytomas. Report of a case. Arch Dermatol 1970; 101: 588–590.

128. Carstens PHB, Schrodt GR. Ultrastructure of sclerosing hemangioma. Am J Pathol 1974; 77: 377–386.

129. Rentiers PL, Montgomery H. Nodular subepidermal fibrosis (dermatofibroma versus histiocytoma). Arch Dermatol 1949; 59: 568–583.

130. Burgdorf W, Moreland A, Wasik R. Negative immunoperoxidase staining for lysozyme in nodular subepidermal fibrosis. Arch Dermatol 1982; 118: 241–243.

130a. Sanchez RL. The elusive dermatofibromas. Arch Dermatol 1990; 126: 522–523.

131. Tamada S, Ackerman AB. Dermatofibroma with monster cells. Am J Dermatopathol 1987; 9: 380–387.

132. Cerio R, Spaull J, Wilson Jones E. Histiocytoma cutis: a tumour of dermal dendrocytes (dermal dendrocytoma). Br J Dermatol 1989; 120: 197–206.

132a. Cerio R, Spaull J, Oliver GF, Wilson Jones E. A study of factor XIIIa and MAC 387 immunolabeling in normal and pathological skin. Am J Dermatopathol 1990; 12: 221–233.

133. Rahbari H, Mehregan AH. Adnexal displacement and regression in association with histiocytoma (dermatofibroma). J Cutan Pathol 1985; 12: 94–102.

134. Bargman HB, Fefferman I. Multiple dermatofibromas in a patient with myasthenia gravis treated with prednisone and cyclophosphamide. J Am Acad Dermatol 1986; 14: 351–352.

134a. Gray MH, Smoller BR, McNutt NS et al. Giant dermal dendrocytoma of the face: a distinct clinicopathologic entity. Arch Dermatol 1990; 126: 689–690.

135. Hendricks WM. Dermatofibroma occurring in a smallpox vaccination scar. J Am Acad Dermatol 1987; 16: 146–147.

136. Santa Cruz DJ, Kyriakos M. Aneurysmal ("angiomatoid") fibrous histiocytoma of the skin. Cancer 1981; 47: 2053–2061.

137. Hairston MA Jr, Reed RJ. Aneurysmal sclerosing hemangioma of skin. Arch Dermatol 1966; 93: 439–442.

138. Newman DM, Walter JB. Multiple dermatofibromas in patients with systemic lupus erythematosus on immunosuppressive therapy. N Engl J Med 1973; 289: 842–843.

139. Gelfarb M, Hyman AB. Multiple noduli cutanei. Arch Dermatol 1962; 85: 89–94.

140. Bedi TR, Pandhi RK, Bhutani LK. Multiple

palmoplantar histiocytomas. Arch Dermatol 1976; 112: 1001–1003.

140a. Nickoloff BJ, Wood GS, Chu M et al. Disseminated dermal dendrocytomas. A new cutaneous fibrohistiocytic proliferative disorder? Am J Surg Pathol 1990; 14: 867–871.

141. Saga K. Annular hemosiderotic histiocytoma. J Cutan Pathol 1981; 8: 251–255.

142. Schwob VS, Santa Cruz DJ. Palisading cutaneous fibrous histiocytoma. J Cutan Pathol 1986; 13: 403–407.

143. Buselmeier TJ, Uecker JH. Invasive basal cell carcinoma with metaplastic bone formation associated with a long-standing dermatofibroma. J Cutan Pathol 1979; 6: 496–500.

143a. Franquemont DW, Cooper PH, Shmookler BM, Wick MR. Benign fibrous histiocytoma of the skin with potential for recurrence. J Cutan Pathol 1989; 16: 303 (abstract).

143b. Hunt SJ, Santa Cruz DJ, Miller CW. Cholesterotic fibrous histiocytoma. Its association with hyperlipoproteinemia. Arch Dermatol 1990; 126: 506–508.

144. Sood U, Mehregan AH. Aneurysmal (angiomatoid) fibrous histiocytoma. J Cutan Pathol 1985; 12: 157–162.

145. Sun C-CJ, Toker C, Breitenecker R. An ultrastructural study of angiomatoid fibrous histiocytoma. Cancer 1982; 49: 2103–2111.

145a. Cerio R, McGibbon D, Wilson Jones E. Angiomatoid fibrous histiocytoma. J Cutan Pathol 1989; 16: 298 (abstract).

146. Barker SM, Winkelmann RK. Inflammatory lymphadenoid reactions with dermatofibroma/histiocytoma. J Cutan Pathol 1986; 13: 222–226.

147. Leyva WH, Santa Cruz DJ. Atypical cutaneous fibrous histiocytoma. Am J Dermatopathol 1986; 8: 467–471.

148. Fukamizu H, Oku T, Inoue K et al. Atypical ("pseudosarcomatous") cutaneous histiocytoma. J Cutan Pathol 1983; 10: 327–333.

148a. Wilson Jones E, Cerio R, Smith NP. Epithelioid cell histiocytoma: a new entity. Br J Dermatol 1989; 120: 185–195.

149. Goette DK, Helwig EB. Basal cell carcinomas and basal cell carcinoma-like changes overlying dermatofibromas. Arch Dermatol 1975; 111: 589–592.

150. Schoenfeld RJ. Epidermal proliferations overlying histiocytomas. Arch Dermatol 1964; 90: 266–270.

151. Halpryn HJ, Allen AC. Epidermal changes associated with sclerosing hemangiomas. Arch Dermatol 1959; 80: 160–166.

152. Ackerman AB, Capland L, Rywlin AM. Focal keratosis folicularis overlying dermatofibroma. Br J Dermatol 1971; 84: 167–168.

153. Caron GA, Clink HM. Clinical association of basal cell epithelioma with histiocytoma. Arch Dermatol 1964; 90: 271–273.

154. Rotteleur G, Chevallier JM, Piette F, Bergoend H. Basal cell carcinoma overlying histiocytofibroma. Acta Derm Venereol 1983; 63: 567–569.

155. Bryant J. Basal cell carcinoma overlying long-standing dermatofibromas. Arch Dermatol 1977; 113: 1445–1446.

156. du Boulay CEH. Demonstration of alpha-1-antitrypsin and alpha-1-antichymotrypsin in fibrous histiocytomas using the immunoperoxidase technique. Am J Surg Pathol 1982; 6: 559–564.

157. Soini Y. Cell differentiation in benign cutaneous fibrous histiocytomas. An immunohistochemical study with antibodies to histiomonocytic cells and intermediate filament proteins. Am J Dermatopathol 1990; 12: 134–140.

158. Carrington SG, Winkelmann RK. Electron microscopy of the histiocytic diseases of the skin. Acta Derm Venereol 1972; 52: 161–178.

159. Katenkamp D, Stiller D. Cellular composition of the so-called dermatofibroma (histiocytoma cutis). Virchows Arch (A) 1975; 367: 325–336.

160. Taylor HB, Helwig EB. Dermatofibrosarcoma protuberans. A study of 115 cases. Cancer 1962; 15: 717–725.

160a. Rockley PF, Robinson JK, Magid M, Goldblatt D. Dermatofibrosarcoma protuberans of the scalp: A series of cases. J Am Acad Dermatol 1989; 21: 278–283.

160b. McLelland J, Chu T. Dermatofibrosarcoma protuberans arising in a BCG vaccination scar. Arch Dermatol 1988; 124: 496–497.

161. Hawk JLM. Dermatofibrosarcoma protuberans. Clin Exp Dermatol 1977; 2: 85–89.

162. Burkhardt BR, Soule EH, Winkelmann RK, Ivins JC. Dermatofibrosarcoma protuberans. Study of fifty-six cases. Am J Surg 1966; 111: 638–644.

162a. Weber PJ, Gretzula JC, Hevia O et al. Dermatofibrosarcoma protuberans. J Dermatol Surg Oncol 1988; 14: 555–558.

163. Morman MR, Lin R-Y, Petrozzi JW. Dermatofibrosarcoma protuberans arising in a site of multiple immunizations. Arch Dermatol 1979; 115: 1453.

164. Shneidman D, Belizaire R. Arsenic exposure followed by the development of dermatofibrosarcoma protuberans. Cancer 1986; 58: 1585–1587.

165. McPeak CJ, Cruz T, Nicastri AD. Dermatofibrosarcoma protuberans: an analysis of 86 cases — five with metastasis. Ann Surg 1967; 166: 803–816.

166. Kahn LB, Saxe N, Gordon W. Dermatofibrosarcoma protuberans with lymph node and pulmonary metastases. Arch Dermatol 1978; 114: 599–601.

167. Hausner RJ, Vargas-Cortes F, Alexander RW. Dermatofibrosarcoma protuberans with lymph node involvement. A case report of simultaneous occurrence with an atypical fibroxanthoma of the skin. Arch Dermatol 1978; 114: 88–91.

168. Brenner W, Schaefler K, Chhabra H, Postel A. Dermatofibrosarcoma protuberans metastatic to a regional lymph node. Report of a case and review. Cancer 1975; 36: 1897–1902.

169. Volpe R, Carbone A. Dermatofibrosarcoma protuberans metastatic to lymph nodes and showing a dominant histiocytic component. Am J Dermatopathol 1983; 5: 327–334.

170. Fletcher CDM, Evans BJ, Macartney JC et al. Dermatofibrosarcoma protuberans: a clinicopathological and immunohistochemical study with a review of the literature. Histopathology 1985; 9: 921–938.

171. O'Dowd J, Laidler P. Progression of dermatofibrosarcoma protuberans to malignant fibrous histiocytoma: Report of a case with implications for tumor histogenesis. Hum Pathol 1988; 19: 368–370.

171a. Wrotnowski U, Cooper PH, Shmookler BM. Fibrosarcomatous change in dermatofibrosarcoma protuberans. Am J Surg Pathol 1988; 12: 287–293.

172. Bednar B. Storiform neurofibromas of the skin, pigmented and nonpigmented. Cancer 1957; 10: 368–376.

173. Bednar B. Storiform neurofibroma in the core of naevocellular naevi. J Pathol 1970; 101: 199–201.

174. Santa Cruz DJ, Yates AJ. Pigmented storiform neurofibroma. J Cutan Pathol 1977; 4: 9–13.

175. Nakamura T, Ogata H, Katsuyama T. Pigmented dermatofibrosarcoma protuberans. Am J Dermatopathol 1987; 9: 18–25.

176. Miyamoto Y, Morimatsu M, Nakashima T. Pigmented storiform neurofibroma. Acta Pathol Jpn 1984; 34: 821–826.

177. Dupree WB, Langloss JM, Weiss SW. Pigmented dermatofibrosarcoma protuberans (Bednar tumor). A pathologic, ultrastructural, and immunohistochemical study. Am J Surg Pathol 1985; 9: 630–639.

177a. Fletcher CDM, Theaker JM, Flanagan A, Krausz T. Pigmented dermatofibrosarcoma protuberans (Bednar tumour): melanocytic colonization or neuroectodermal differentiation? A clinicopathological and immunohistochemical study. Histopathology 1988; 13: 631–643.

178. Fletcher CDM, McKee PH. Sarcomas — a clinicopathological guide with particular reference to cutaneous manifestation I. Dermatofibrosarcoma protuberans, malignant fibrous histiocytoma and the epithelioid sarcoma of Enzinger. Clin Exp Dermatol 1984; 9: 451–465.

179. Sauter LS, De Feo CP. Dermatofibrosarcoma protuberans of the face. Arch Dermatol 1971; 104: 671–673.

180. Frierson HF, Cooper PH. Myxoid variant of dermatofibrosarcoma protuberans. Am J Surg Pathol 1983; 7: 445–450.

181. Barr RJ, Young EM Jr, King DF. Non-polarizable collagen in dermatofibrosarcoma protuberans: a useful diagnostic aid. J Cutan Pathol 1986; 13: 339–346.

181a. Lautier R, Wolff HH, Jones RE. An immunohistochemical study of dermatofibrosarcoma protuberans supports its fibroblastic character and contradicts neuroectodermal or histiocytic components. Am J Dermatopathol 1990; 12: 25–30.

182. Hashimoto K, Brownstein MH, Jakobiec FA. Dermatofibrosarcoma protuberans. A tumor with perineural and endoneural cell features. Arch Dermatol 1974; 110: 874–885.

183. Alguacil-Garcia A, Unni KK, Goellner RJ. Histogenesis of dermatofibrosarcoma protuberans. An ultrastructural study. Am J Clin Pathol 1978; 69: 427–434.

184. Escalona-Zapata J, Fernandez EA, Escuin FL. The fibroblastic nature of dermatofibrosarcoma protuberans. A tissue culture and ultrastructural study. Virchows Arch (A) 1981; 391: 165–175.

185. Zina AM, Bundino S. Dermatofibrosarcoma protuberans. An ultrastructural study of five cases. J Cutan Pathol 1979; 6: 265–271.

186. Ozzello L, Hamels J. The histiocytic nature of dermatofibrosarcoma protuberans. Tissue culture and electron microscopic study. Am J Clin Pathol 1976; 65: 136–148.

187. Helwig EB. Atypical fibroxanthoma. Texas J Med 1963; 59: 664–667.

188. Connors RC, Ackerman AB. Histologic pseudomalignancies of the skin. Arch Dermatol 1976; 112: 1767–1780.

189. Finlay-Jones LR, Nicoll P, Ten Seldam REJ. Pseudosarcoma of the skin. Pathology 1971; 3: 215–222.

190. Bourne RG. Paradoxical fibrosarcoma of skin (pseudosarcoma): a review of 13 cases. Med J Aust 1963; 1: 504–510.

191. Vargas-Cortes F, Winkelmann RK, Soule EH. Atypical fibroxanthomas of the skin. Further observations with 19 additional cases. Mayo Clin Proc 1973; 48: 211–218.

192. Fretzin DF, Helwig EB. Atypical fibroxanthoma of the skin. A clinicopathologic study of 140 cases. Cancer 1973; 31: 1541–1552.

193. Kempson RL, McGavran MH. Atypical fibroxanthomas of the skin. Cancer 1964; 17: 1463–1471.

194. Leong AS-Y, Milios J. Atypical fibroxanthoma of the skin: a clinicopathological and immunohistochemical study and a discussion of its histogenesis. Histopathology 1987; 11: 463–475.

194a. Patterson JW, Jordan WP Jr. Atypical fibroxanthoma in a patient with xeroderma pigmentosum. Arch Dermatol 1987; 123: 1066–1070.

195. Helwig EB, May D. Atypical fibroxanthoma of the skin with metastases. Cancer 1986; 57: 368–376.

195a. Kemmett D, Gawkrodger DJ, Mclaren KM, Hunter JAA. Two atypical fibroxanthomas arising separately in X-irradiated skin. Clin Exp Dermatol 1988; 13: 382–384.

196. Enzinger FM. Questions to the Editorial Board and other authorities. Am J Dermatopathol 1979; 1: 185.

197. Starink TM, Hausman R, Van Delden L, Neering H. Atypical fibroxanthoma of the skin. Presentation of 5 cases and a review of the literature. Br J Dermatol 1977; 97: 167–177.

198. Dahl I. Atypical fibroxanthoma of the skin. A clinico-pathological study of 57 cases. Acta Pathol Microbiol Immunol Scand (A) 1976; 84: 183–197.

199. Hudson AW, Winkelmann RK. Atypical fibroxanthoma of the skin: a reappraisal of 19 cases in which the original diagnosis was spindle-cell squamous carcinoma. Cancer 1972; 29: 413–422.

200. Kemp JD, Stenn KS, Arons M, Fischer J. Metastasizing atypical fibroxanthoma. Coexistence with chronic lymphocytic leukemia. Arch Dermatol 1978; 114: 1533–1535.

201. Glavin FL, Cornwell ML. Atypical fibroxanthoma of the skin metastatic to a lung. Am J Dermatopathol 1985; 7: 57–63.

202. Patterson JW, Konerding H, Kramer WM. "Clear cell" atypical fibroxanthoma. J Dermatol Surg Oncol 1987; 13: 1109–1114.

203. Chen KTK. Atypical fibroxanthoma of the skin with osteoid production. Arch Dermatol 1980; 116: 113–114.

203a. Wilson PR, Strutton GM, Stewart MR. Atypical fibroxanthoma: two unusual variants. J Cutan Pathol 1989; 16: 93–98.

204. Kuwano H, Hashimoto H, Enjoji M. Atypical fibroxanthoma distinguishable from spindle cell carcinoma in sarcoma-like skin lesions. A clinicopathologic and immunohistochemical study of 21 cases. Cancer 1985; 55: 172–180.

205. Winkelmann RK, Peters MS. Atypical fibroxanthoma. A study with antibody to S–100 protein. Arch Dermatol 1985; 121: 753–755.

205a. Ricci A Jr, Cartun RW, Zakowski MF. Atypical fibroxanthoma. A study of 14 cases emphasizing the presence of Langerhans' histiocytes with implications for differential diagnosis by antibody panels. Am J Surg Pathol 1988; 12: 591–598.

206. Silvis NG, Swanson PE, Manivel JC et al. Spindle-cell and pleomorphic neoplasms of the skin. A clinicopathologic and immunohistochemical study of 30 cases, with emphasis on "atypical fibroxanthomas". Am J Dermatopathol 1988; 10: 9–19.

207. Weedon D, Kerr JFR. Atypical fibroxanthoma of skin: an electron microscope study. Pathology 1975; 7: 173–177.

208. Barr RJ, Wuerker RB, Graham JH. Ultrastructure of atypical fibroxanthoma. Cancer 1977; 40: 736–743.

209. Carson JW, Schwartz RA, McCandless CM, French SW. Atypical fibroxanthoma of the skin. Report of a case with Langerhans-like granules. Arch Dermatol 1984; 120: 234–239.

209a. Enzinger FM, Zhang R. Plexiform fibrohistiocytic tumor presenting in children and young adults. An analysis of 65 cases. Am J Surg Pathol 1988; 12: 818–826.

210. Weiss SW, Enzinger FM. Malignant fibrous histiocytoma. An analysis of 200 cases. Cancer 1978; 41: 2250–2266.

211. Weiss SW. Malignant fibrous histiocytoma. Am J Surg Pathol 1982; 6: 773–784.

212. Headington JT, Niederhuber JE, Repola DA. Primary malignant fibrous histiocytoma of skin. J Cutan Pathol 1978; 5: 329–338.

212a. Moran CA, Kaneko M. Malignant fibrous histiocytoma of the glans penis. Am J Dermatopathol 1990; 12: 182–187.

213. Enzinger FM. Angiomatoid malignant fibrous histiocytoma. A distinct fibrohistiocytic tumor of children and young adults simulating a vascular neoplasm. Cancer 1979; 44: 2147–2157.

213a. Seo IS, Warner TFCS, Warren JS, Bennett JE. Cutaneous postirradiation sarcoma. Ultrastructural evidence of pluripotential mesenchymal cell derivation. Cancer 1985; 56: 761–767.

214. Routh A, Hickman BT, Johnson WW. Malignant fibrous histiocytoma arising from chronic ulcer. Arch Dermatol 1985; 121: 529–531.

215. Slater DN, Parsons MA, Fussey IV. Malignant fibrous histiocytoma arising in a smallpox vaccination scar. Br J Dermatol 1981; 105: 215–217.

216. Yamamura T, Aozasa K, Honda T et al. Malignant fibrous histiocytoma developing in a burn scar. Br J Dermatol 1984; 110: 725–730.

217. Kearney MM, Soule EH, Ivins JC. Malignant fibrous histiocytoma. A retrospective study of 167 cases. Cancer 1980; 45: 167–178.

218. Bertoni F, Capanna R, Biagini R et al. Malignant fibrous histiocytoma of soft tissue. An analysis of 78 cases located and deeply seated in the extremities. Cancer 1985; 56: 356–367.

219. Oku T, Takigawa M, Fukamizu H, Yamada M. Tissue cultures of benign and malignant fibrous histiocytomas: SEM observations. J Cutan Pathol 1984; 11: 534–540.

220. Lattes R. Malignant fibrous histiocytoma. A review article. Am J Surg Pathol 1982; 6: 761–771.

221. Dehner LP. Malignant fibrous histiocytoma. Nonspecific morphologic pattern, specific pathologic entity, or both? Arch Pathol Lab Med 1988; 112: 236–237.

222. Bhagavan BS, Dorfman HD. The significance of bone and cartilage formation in malignant fibrous histiocytoma of soft tissue. Cancer 1982; 49: 480–488.

223. Argenyi ZB, Van Rybroek JJ, Kemp JD, Soper RT. Congenital angiomatoid malignant fibrous histiocytoma. A light-microscopic immunopathologic, and electron-microscopic study. Am J Dermatopathol 1988; 10: 59–67.

224. Weiss SW, Enzinger FM. Myxoid variant of malignant fibrous histiocytoma. Cancer 1977; 39: 1672–1685.

224a. Lillemoe T, Steeper T, Manivel JC, Wick MR. Myxoid malignant fibrous histiocytoma (MMFH) of the skin. J Cutan Pathol 1988; 15: 324 (abstract).

225. Angervall L, Hagmar B, Kindblom L-G, Merck C. Malignant giant cell tumor of soft tissues; a clinicopathologic, cytologic, ultrastructural, angiographic, and microangiographic study. Cancer 1981; 47: 736–747.

226. Kyriakos M, Kempson RL. Inflammatory fibrous histiocytoma. An aggressive and lethal lesion. Cancer 1976; 37: 1584–1606.

227. Miller R, Kreutner A Jr, Kurtz SM. Malignant inflammatory histiocytoma (inflammatory fibrous histiocytoma). Report of a patient with four lesions. Cancer 1980; 45: 179–187.

228. Miettin M, Soini Y. Malignant fibrous histiocytoma. Heterogeneous patterns of intermediate filament proteins by immunohistochemistry. Arch Pathol Lab Med 1989; 113: 1363–1366.

229. Ueda T, Aozasa K, Yamamura T et al. Lectin histochemistry of malignant fibrohistiocytic tumors. Am J Surg Pathol 1987; 11: 257–262.

230. Alguacil-Garcia A, Unni KK, Goellner JR. Malignant fibrous histiocytoma. An ultrastructural study of six cases. Am J Clin Pathol 1978; 69: 121–129.

230a. Hayashi Y, Kikuchi-Tada A, Jitsukawa K et al. Myofibroblasts in malignant fibrous histiocytoma — histochemical, immunohistochemical, ultrastructural and tissue culture studies. Clin Exp Dermatol 1988; 13: 402–405.

Presumptive synovial and tendon sheath tumours

231. Chung EB, Enzinger FM. Fibroma of tendon sheath. Cancer 1979; 44: 1945–1954.

232. Humphreys S, McKee PH, Fletcher CDM. Fibroma of tendon sheath: a clinicopathologic study. J Cutan Pathol 1986; 13: 331–338.

David Weedon

Tumours of fat

INTRODUCTION

The tumours of fat are a histologically diverse group. Fortunately, most of these tumours have well-established diagnostic criteria and present no difficulty in diagnosis. However, there are two recently delineated fatty tumours — spindle cell lipoma and pleomorphic lipoma — which may cause diagnostic problems, sometimes leading to a mistaken diagnosis of liposarcoma.

NAEVUS LIPOMATOSUS

This entity, also known by the complicated term 'naevus lipomatosus cutaneus superficialis (Hoffmann–Zurhelle)'[1,2] is a rare type of connective tissue naevus characterized by the presence of mature adipose tissue in the dermis. It is found as plaques or solitary lesions, or in an extremely rare generalized form.

The plaque type has aggregations of flesh-coloured or yellow papules and nodules which are present at birth, or develop in the first two decades of life. There is a predilection for the pelvic girdle, particularly the gluteal region. Lesions are usually unilateral, and sometimes in a linear or zosteriform arrangement. The surface of most lesions is smooth, although it may be verrucous or dimpled. Surface comedones have been noted occasionally. Lesions usually develop insidiously, but later become reasonably stable.

The solitary form consists of isolated papules or nodules, anywhere on the body, but with a predilection for the trunk.[3] They may not appear until the fifth decade. They usually have a broad-

collagen. Sometimes this stroma shows focal myxomatous change which stains positively for acid mucopolysaccharides.

The intervening fat cells are mature, and univacuolated, resembling normal fat. There are no lipoblasts present. A few tumours have a prominent vascular pattern,[55] and this may resemble a lymphangioma or haemangiopericytoma in some areas.[50] A few inflammatory cells may be found in the walls of these vessels. Mast cells are usually present throughout the stroma.

In the past, spindle cell lipoma was sometimes confused histologically with liposarcoma and other spindle cell sarcomas. The absence of multivacuolated lipoblasts and lack of significant nuclear atypia excludes liposarcoma.

Electron microscopy. Ultrastructurally the spindle cells resemble fibroblasts. A few have cytoplasmic lipid droplets.[50,51]

PLEOMORPHIC LIPOMA

Pleomorphic (giant cell) lipoma is a benign tumour of adipose tissue with atypical histological features, which may lead to a misdiagnosis of liposarcoma.[56] It presents as a soft, subcutaneous mass, averaging 5 cm in diameter. A case confined to the dermis has been reported.[57] Pleomorphic lipoma has a predilection for the shoulders, back of the neck, back,[56] and less frequently the face and thighs[58] of middle-aged to elderly males.[56] Macroscopically it resembles a lipoma, although gelatinous grey areas may be present on the cut surface. Some of the cases of atypical lipoma reported recently are examples of this entity.[59,60]

Histopathology[56,58]

These circumscribed tumours have an intricate mixture of mature adipose tissue, collagen and myxoid areas interspersed with cellular foci of varying amounts. In addition to lipoblast-like cells the tumour includes spindle and giant cells, the latter being both uninucleate and multinucleate in type (Fig. 35.5). There are variable

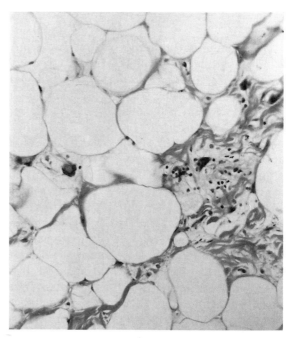

Fig. 35.5 Pleomorphic lipoma. Some fat cells have hyperchromatic nuclei with a smudgy appearance. There are no mitoses.
Haematoxylin — eosin

numbers of giant cells with marginally placed and often overlapping nuclei, the so-called 'floret giant cells'. Sometimes the nuclei of some giant cells are smudgy with indistinct chromatin. Mitoses are rare. Focal collections of lymphocytes and plasma cells are often found within the tumour.

At times, the pleomorphic lipoma is a circumscribed nodule within an otherwise typical lipoma. Areas resembling spindle cell lipoma may sometimes be present within pleomorphic lipomas.

It may be distinguished from liposarcoma by the floret giant cells, the pyknotic or smudgy nuclear features and the absence of mitoses.[61]

HIBERNOMA

Hibernoma is a rare benign tumour of the subcutaneous[62] and deeper soft tissues,[63] generally considered to arise from brown fat. It is found in the scapular area, axilla, lower neck,[62] and less commonly in the thigh,[64,65] abdominal wall[66] and retroperitoneum.[67] It is slowly growing. There may be increased warmth over the area.[68]

Grossly, hibernomas are tan-brown, lobulated tumours, averaging 10 cm in diameter. Several possible malignant variants have been reported, but these have been disputed by others.[62,69]

Histopathology[62,66]

The tumours are thinly encapsulated, and divided into lobules by thin septa. There are usually prominent blood vessels in the septa and lobules, and in one case with possible endocrine activity[64] they assumed a prominent sinusoidal pattern.

There are three cell types with transitional forms.[67] These include large, coarsely vacuolated cells with multiple vacuoles, univacuolated cells and smaller cells with granular cytoplasm (Fig. 35.6). Vacuoles stain with oil red 0 in

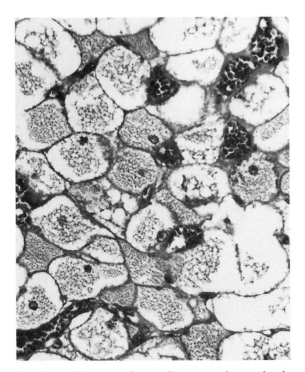

Fig. 35.6 Hibernoma. Some cells are coarsely vacuolated while others have a 'granular' cytoplasm. Haematoxylin — eosin

frozen sections. Lipofuscin pigment is also present.[70] There is often a prominent nucleolus, but there are no mitoses.

Electron microscopy. This shows abundant lipid droplets, numerous pleomorphic mitochondria with transverse cristae, and a well-formed basal lamina.[66,67,70,71]

LIPOSARCOMA

Liposarcomas are uncommon tumours of the deep soft tissues and retroperitoneum which only rarely arise in the subcutis, although they may eventually extend into it from below.[72-74] Accordingly, they will be considered only briefly. They have a predilection for the thighs and buttocks, but may sometimes involve the head and neck[75] or upper extremities. They arise in older adults, and are exceedingly rare in children.[18] Although a few cases have developed in patients with multiple lipomas, they are not thought to arise from pre-existing lipomas.[72,76] They are often large tumours, non-encapsulated, with a colour varying from yellow to grey, to grey-white. There may be some firmer areas and gelatinous foci in the generally soft tissue.

Histopathology[73,77,78]

There are four histological variants, although mixed forms occur. The *well-differentiated (lipoma-like) liposarcoma* resembles normal fat. There is some nuclear pleomorphism and hyperchromatism and rare multivacuolated lipoblasts. The diagnosis is often made in retrospect, after the first recurrence. A sclerosing variant with abundant fibrous tissue is also recognized. This must be distinguished from a spindle cell lipoma. Well-differentiated liposarcomas have a good prognosis. The *myxoid liposarcoma* consists of fusiform or stellate cells, with abundant mucoid stroma, a delicate plexiform network of small capillaries, and a variable number of multivacuolated lipoblasts. The *round cell liposarcoma* has diffuse sheets of closely arranged round or oval cells, frequently with a single small cytoplasmic

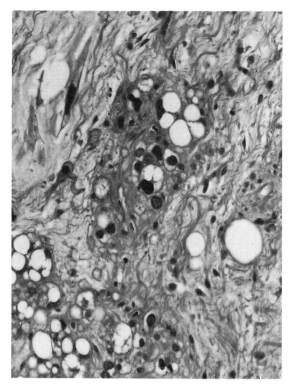

vacuole. Lipoblasts are present, but may be difficult to find. Mitoses are abundant in some areas. Fibrosarcoma-like areas are sometimes present. The *pleomorphic liposarcoma* (Fig. 35.7) is a highly cellular tumour with numerous mitoses and some bizarre and extremely pleomorphic, multivacuolated lipoblasts with one or more hyperchromatic nuclei. Fibrous areas with bizarre tumour cells are also present. Sometimes the cytoplasmic vacuolation is insignificant, making it difficult to differentiate from other pleomorphic sarcomas. A lipid stain sometimes helps in these cases.

Electron microscopy. Liposarcomas are composed of cells showing lipoblastic differentiation with lipid droplets, micropinocytotic vesicles, glycogen, external lamina and intermediate filaments.[79] Most tumours contain lipid-free, poorly differentiated mesenchymal cells and cells resembling early lipoblasts with non-membrane-bound lipid vacuoles.[79]

Fig. 35.7 Pleomorphic liposarcoma. There are many vacuolated lipoblasts present.
Haematoxylin — eosin

REFERENCES

1. Mehregan A, Tavafoghi V, Ghandchi A. Nevus lipomatosus superficialis cutaneus Hoffmann–Zurhelle). J Cutan Pathol 1975; 2: 307–313.
2. Finley AG, Musso LA. Naevus lipomatosus cutaneus superficialis (Hoffmann-Zurhelle). Br J Dermatol 1972; 87: 557–564.
3. Weitzner S. Solitary nevus lipomatosus cutaneus superficialis of scalp. Arch Dermatol 1968; 97: 540–542.
4. Gardner EW, Miller HM, Lowney ED. Folded skin associated with underlying nevus lipomatosus. Arch Dermatol 1979; 115: 978–979.
5. Ross CM. Generalized folded skin with an underlying lipomatous nevus. 'The Michelin tyre baby'. Arch Dermatol 1969; 100: 320–323.
6. Wilson Jones E, Marks R, Pongsehirun D. Naevus superficialis lipomatosus. A clinicopathological report of twenty cases. Br J Dermatol 1975; 93: 121–133.
7. Fergin PE, MacDonald DM. Naevus superficialis lipomatosus. Clin Exp Dermatol 1980; 5: 365–367.
8. Dotz W, Prioleau PG. Nevus lipomatosus cutaneus superficialis. Arch Dermatol 1984; 120: 376–379.
9. Reymond JL, Stoebner P, Amblard P. Nevus lipomatosus cutaneous superficialis. An electron microscopic study of four cases. J Cutan Pathol 1980; 7: 295–301.

10. Shelley WB, Rawnsley HM. Painful feet due to herniation of fat. JAMA 1968; 205: 308–309.
11. Woerdeman MJ, van Dijk E. Piezogenic papules of the feet. Acta Derm Venereol 1972; 52: 411–414.
12. Schlappner OLA, Wood MG, Gerstein W, Gross PR. Painful and nonpainful piezogenic pedal papules. Arch Dermatol 1972; 106: 729–733.
13. Harman RRM, Matthews CNA. Painful piezogenic pedal papules. Br J Dermatol 1974; 90: 573–574.
14. Kahana M, Feinstein A, Tabachnic E et al. Painful piezogenic pedal papules in patients with Ehlers-Danlos syndrome. J Am Acad Dermatol 1987; 17: 205–209.
15. Ronnen M, Suster S, Huszar M, Schewach-Millet M. Solitary painful piezogenic pedal papule in a patient with rheumatoid arthritis. Int J Dermatol 1987; 26: 240–241.
16. Vellios F, Baez J, Shumacker HB. Lipoblastomatosis: a tumor of fetal fat different from hibernoma. Am J Pathol 1958; 34: 1149–1159.
16a. Enghardt MH, Warren RC. Congenital palpebral lipoblastoma. First report of a case. Am J Dermatopathol 1990; 12: 408–411.
17. Chung EB, Enzinger FM. Benign lipoblastomatosis. An analysis of 35 cases. Cancer 1973; 32: 482–492.

18. Kauffman SL, Stout AP. Lipoblastic tumors of children. Cancer 1959; 12: 912–925.

19. Chaudhuri B, Ronan SG, Ghosh L. Benign lipoblastoma. Report of a case. Cancer 1980; 46: 611–614.

20. Greco MA, Garcia RL, Vuletin JC. Benign lipoblastomatosis. Ultrastructure and histogenesis. Cancer 1980; 45: 511–515.

21. Adair FE, Pack GT, Farrior JH. Lipomas. Am J Cancer 1932; 16: 1104–1120.

22. Salasche SJ, McCollough ML, Angeloni VL, Grabski WJ. Frontalis-associated lipoma of the forehead. J Am Acad Dermatol 1989; 20: 462–468.

23. Allen PW. Tumors and proliferations of adipose tissue. A clinicopathologic approach. New York: Masson Publishing USA, 1981.

24. Enzi G. Multiple symmetric lipomatosis: an updated clinical report. Medicine (Baltimore) 1984; 63: 56–64.

25. Uhlin SR. Benign symmetric lipomatosis. Arch Dermatol 1979; 115: 94–95.

26. Ruzicka T, Vieluf D, Landthaler M, Braun–Falco O. Benign symmetric lipomatosis Launois–Bensaude. Report of ten cases and review of the literature. J Am Acad Dermatol 1987; 17: 663–674.

27. Carlin MC, Ratz JL. Multiple symmetric lipomatosis: Treatment with liposuction. J Am Acad Dermatol 1988; 18: 359–362.

28. Findlay GH, Duvenage M. Acquired symmetrical lipomatosis of the hands — a distal form of the Madelung–Launois–Bensaude syndrome. Clin Exp Dermatol 1989; 14: 58–59.

29. Greene ML, Glueck CJ, Fujimoto WY, Seegmiller JE. Benign symmetric lipomatosis (Launois–Bensaude adenolipomatosis) with gout and hyperlipoproteinemia. Am J Med 1970; 48: 239–246.

30. Springer HA, Whitehouse JS. Launois–Bensaude adenolipomatosis. Case report. Plast Reconstr Surg 1972; 50: 291–294.

31. Leffell DJ, Braverman IM. Familial multiple lipomatosis. Report of a case and a review of the literature. J Am Acad Dermatol 1986; 15: 275–279.

32. Rabbiosi G, Borroni G, Scuderi N. Familial multiple lipomatosis. Acta Derm Venereol 1977; 57: 265–267.

33. Mohar N. Familial multiple lipomatosis. Acta Derm Venereol 1980; 60: 509–513.

34. Rubinstein A, Goor Y, Gazit E, Cabili S. Non-symmetric subcutaneous lipomatosis associated with familial combined hyperlipidaemia. Br J Dermatol 1989; 120: 689–694.

35. Blomstrand R, Juhlin L, Nordenstam H et al. Adiposis dolorosa associated with defects of lipid metabolism. Acta Derm Venereol 1971; 51: 243–250.

35a. Held JL, Andrew JA, Kohn SR. Surgical amelioration of Dercum's disease: a report and review. J Dermatol Surg Oncol 1989; 15: 1294–1296.

36. Lynch HT, Harlan WL. Hereditary factors in adiposis dolorosa (Dercum's disease). Am J Hum Genet 1963; 15: 184–190.

37. Klein JA, Barr RJ. Diffuse lipomatosis and tuberous sclerosis. Arch Dermatol 1986; 122: 1298–1302.

38. Nixon HH, Scobie WG. Congenital lipomatosis: a report of four cases. J Pediatr Surg 1971; 6: 742–745.

39. Schlicht D. Recurrent lipomatosis in a child. Med J Aust 1965; 2: 959–962.

40. Slavin SA, Baker DC, McCarthy JG, Mufarrij A. Congenital infiltrating lipomatosis of the face: clinicopathologic evaluation and treatment. Plast Reconstr Surg 1983; 72: 158–164.

41. Howard WR, Helwig EB. Angiolipoma. Arch Dermatol 1960; 82: 924–931.

42. Dixon AY, McGregor DH, Lee SH. Angiolipomas: an ultrastructural and clinicopathological study. Hum Pathol 1981; 12: 739–747.

43. Goodfield MJD, Rowell NR. The clinical presentation of cutaneous angiolipomata and the response to β– blockade. Clin Exp Dermatol 1988; 13: 190–192.

44. Rasanen O, Nohteri H, Dammert K. Angiolipoma and lipoma. Acta Chir Scand 1967; 133: 461–465.

45. Sahl WJ Jr. Mobile encapsulated lipomas. Formerly called encapsulated angiolipomas. Arch Dermatol 1978; 114: 1684–1686.

46. Dionne GP, Seemayer TA. Infiltrating lipomas and angiolipomas revisited. Cancer 1974; 33: 732–738.

47. Lin JJ, Lin F. Two entities in angiolipoma. Cancer 1974; 34: 720–727.

48. Belcher RW, Czarnetzki BM, Carney JF, Gardner E. Multiple (subcutaneous) angiolipomas. Arch Dermatol 1974; 110: 583–585.

49. Rustin GJS. Diffuse intravascular coagulation in association with myocardial infarction and multiple angiolipomata. Postgrad Med J 1977; 53: 228–229.

50. Enzinger FM, Harvey DA. Spindle cell lipoma. Cancer 1975; 36: 1852–1859.

51. Angervall L, Dahl I, Kindblom L-G, Save-Soderbergh J. Spindle cell lipoma. Acta Pathol Microbiol Scand (A) 1976; 84: 477–487.

52. Brody HJ, Meltzer HD, Someren A. Spindle cell lipoma. An unusual dermatologic presentation. Arch Dermatol 1978; 114: 1065–1066.

53. Meister P. Spindle cell lipoma (report of 2 cases and differential diagnosis). Beitr Path 1977; 161: 376–384.

54. Fletcher CDM, Martin-Bates E. Spindle cell lipoma: a clinicopathological study with some original observations. Histopathology 1987; 11: 803–817.

55. Warkel RL, Rehme CG, Thompson WH. Vascular spindle cell lipoma. J Cutan Pathol 1982; 9: 113–118.

56. Shmookler BM, Enzinger FM. Pleomorphic lipoma: a benign tumor simulating liposarcoma. A clinicopathologic analysis of 48 cases. Cancer 1981; 47: 126–133.

57. Nigro MA, Chieregato GC, Querci della Rovere G. Pleomorphic lipoma of the dermis. Br J Dermatol 1987; 116: 713–717.

58. Azzopardi JG, Iocco J, Salm R. Pleomorphic lipoma: a tumour simulating liposarcoma. Histopathology 1983; 7: 511–523.

59. Evans HL, Soule EH, Winkelmann RK. Atypical lipoma, atypical intramuscular lipoma, and well differentiated retroperitoneal liposarcoma. Cancer 1979; 43: 574–584.

60. Kindblom LG, Angervall L, Fassina AS. Atypical lipoma. Acta Pathol Microbiol Immunol Scand (A) 1982; 90: 27–36.

61. Bryant J. A pleomorphic lipoma in the scalp. J Dermatol Surg Oncol 1981; 7: 323–325.

62. Novy FG Jr, Wilson JW. Hibernomas, brown fat tumors. Arch Dermatol 1956; 73: 149–157.

63. Kindblom L-G, Angervall L, Stener B, Wickbom I. Intermuscular and intramuscular lipomas and hibernomas. Cancer 1974; 33: 754–762.

64. Allegra SR, Gmuer C, O'Leary GP Jr. Endocrine activity in a large hibernoma. Hum Pathol 1983; 14: 1044–1052.

65. Angervall L, Nilsson L, Stener B. Microangiographic and histological studies in 2 cases of hibernoma. Cancer 1964; 17: 685–692.

66. Dardick I. Hibernoma: a possible model of brown fat histogenesis. Hum Pathol 1978; 9: 321–329.

67. Rigor VU, Goldstone SE, Jones J et al. Hibernoma. A case report and discussion of a rare tumor. Cancer 1986; 57: 2207–2211.

68. Brines OA, Johnson MH. Hibernoma, a special fatty tumor. Report of a case. Am J Pathol 1949; 25: 467–479.

69. Enterline HT, Lowry LD, Richman AV. Does malignant hibernoma exist? Am J Surg Pathol 1979; 3: 265–271.

70. Levine GD. Hibernoma. An electron microscopic study. Hum Pathol 1972; 3: 351–359.

71. Seemayer TA, Knaack J, Wang N-S, Ahmed MN. On the ultrastructure of hibernoma. Cancer 1975; 36: 1785–1793.

72. Spittle MF, Newton KA, Mackenzie DH. Liposarcoma. A review of 60 cases. Br J Cancer 1970; 24: 696–704.

73. Kindblom L-G, Angervall L, Svendsen P. Liposarcoma. A clinicopathologic, radiographic and prognostic study. Acta Path Microbiol Scand (A) 1975; suppl 253: 1–71.

74. Azumi N, Curtis J, Kempson RL, Hendrickson MR. Atypical and malignant neoplasms showing lipomatous differentiation. A study of 111 cases. Am J Surg Pathol 1987; 11: 161–183.

75. Saunders JR, Jaques DA, Casterline PF et al. Liposarcoma of the head and neck. A review of the literature and addition of four cases. Cancer 1979; 43: 162–168.

76. Kindblom L-G, Angervall L, Jarlstedt J. Liposarcoma of the neck. A clinicopathologic study of 4 cases. Cancer 1978; 42: 774–780.

77. Enterline HT, Culberson JD, Rochlin DB, Brady LW. Liposarcoma. A clinical and pathological study of 53 cases. Cancer 1960; 13: 932–950.

78. Enzinger FM, Winslow DJ. Liposarcoma. A study of 103 cases. Virchows Arch Pathol Anat 1962; 335: 367–388.

79. Rossouw DJ, Cinti S, Dickersin GR. Liposarcoma. An ultrastructural study of 15 cases. Am J Clin Pathol 1986; 85: 649–667.

Tumours of smooth and striated muscle

TUMOURS OF SMOOTH MUSCLE

Smooth muscle is found in the skin in three distinct settings — the arrector pili muscles, the walls of blood vessels, and the specialized muscle of genital skin, which includes the scrotum (dartos muscle), vulva and nipple. Each of these sources of smooth muscle can give rise to benign tumours, resulting in three categories of cutaneous leiomyoma: piloleiomyoma, leiomyoma of genital skin and angioleiomyoma.[1] As the histological features of leiomyomas derived from the arrectores and genital smooth muscle are identical, they will be considered together.

For completeness, it should be noted that smooth muscle has also been reported, rarely, in organoid[2] and blue naevi.[3]

LEIOMYOMA

Leiomyomas derived from the arrector pili muscles (*piloleiomyomas*) are more often multiple than solitary. Multiple lesions usually have their onset in the late second or third decade of life. They present as multiple, firm, reddish-brown papulonodules with a predilection for the face, back and extensor surfaces of the extremities. Several hundred lesions may be present. They may cluster to form plaques,[4-5] which usually involve more than one area of the body.[6,7] Rarely, tumours are symmetrically distributed suggesting a naevoid condition, and these cases have been designated naevus leiomyomatosus systematicus.[8] Some of the multiple cases are familial, with an autosomal dominant inheritance.[9] There is a report of identical twins being involved.[10] Multiple leiomyomas have been associated with uterine leiomyomas in some females.[11–13] Erythropoietic activity in the tumours is a rare finding.[12] Minor trauma or exposure to cold temperatures may lead to severe pain in the tumours.[4]

Solitary piloleiomyomas,[14,15] which are infrequently painful, are usually slightly larger than those found in patients with the multiple form, sometimes reaching 2 cm or more in diameter. Rarely they are present at birth.[16] There has been a female preponderance.

Genital leiomyomas are quite uncommon, with only 20 or so scrotal leiomyomas reported.[6,17,18] They present as firm, solitary, asymptomatic nodules, measuring up to 2.5 cm in diameter. There are only sparse reports of leiomyoma of the nipple[6] and vulva[19] in the dermatological literature.

Histopathology

Leiomyomas are circumscribed, non-encapsulated tumours, centred on the dermis.[6,7] An overlying zone of uninvolved subepidermal tissue (so-called grenz zone) is usually present and there may be some flattening of the epidermis. The tumour is composed of bundles of smooth muscle arranged in an interlacing and sometimes a whorled pattern (Fig. 36.1). The cells have abundant eosinophilic cytoplasm and elongated nuclei with blunt ends. There are usually no mitoses. Tumours of long standing may have fibrous tissue in the stroma and occasionally this shows focal hyalinization. Focal stromal myxoid change and small lymphoid collections have been noted. Hair follicles are sometimes found surviving within the tumour.[6] The smooth muscle nature of the cells can be confirmed with the Masson trichrome stain. A Bodian stain has shown increased numbers of nerve fibres interlacing with the muscle fibres and also in the surrounding tissue.[7]

Smooth muscle hamartoma differs from leiomyoma by having discrete bundles of smooth muscle fibres set in dermal collagen (see below).

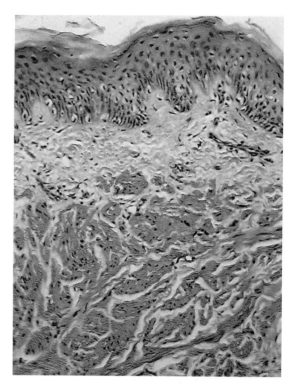

Fig. 36.1 Leiomyoma. The reticular dermis is replaced by interlacing bundles of smooth muscle cells. Haematoxylin — eosin

ANGIOLEIOMYOMA

Angioleiomyoma usually presents as a solitary, slowly growing nodule on the extremities, particularly the lower leg, of middle-aged individuals.[20] There is a female preponderance.[21,22] More than half the lesions are painful or tender, but this feature is usually absent in those found on the face and upper trunk.[20,22a]

The tumours are firm, grey-white, round to oval nodules in the lower dermis and subcutis.[23] They are usually less than 2 cm in diameter. Most authors assume that they arise from veins, although some may be hamartomas.[22]

Histopathology

The tumour is usually well circumscribed with a fibrous capsule of variable thickness and completeness (Fig. 36.2). The main component is

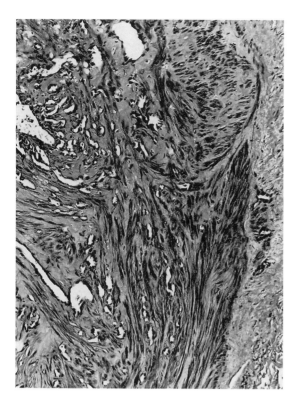

Fig. 36.2 Angioleiomyoma. The smooth muscle bundles are admixed with small blood vessels. Haematoxylin — eosin

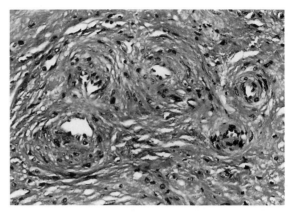

Fig. 36.3 Angioleiomyoma. In this case the individual vessels are thick walled with their outer layers of smooth muscle merging with the intervascular muscle fascicles. Haematoxylin — eosin

haemosiderin and hyalinization of vessel walls. Nerve fibres are only seen occasionally.[1]

In a review of 562 cases, three histological variants were described: a *solid type*, in which smooth muscle bundles surround numerous, small, slit-like channels; a *cavernous type*, with dilated vascular channels, the walls of which are difficult to distinguish from the intervascular smooth muscle; and a *venous type* with thick-walled vessels which are easily distinguished from the intervascular smooth muscle.[22]

SMOOTH MUSCLE HAMARTOMA

This is a rare, usually congenital, hyperplasia of dermal smooth muscle fibres which presents as a flesh-coloured or lightly pigmented plaque up to 10 cm in diameter on the extremities or trunk.[26–32] Within the plaques, small gooseflesh-like papules may be discernible, and these may transiently elevate when rubbed (pseudo-Darier's sign).[33] Hairs are usually more prominent in the skin of the affected site, being slightly longer and thicker than in the adjoining skin.[34] A more generalized variant with prominent skin folds has been reported as a 'Michelin tyre baby'.[35,35a]

Smooth muscle bundles, indistinguishable from those seen in this condition, may also occur in Becker's naevus,[36,37] and this has led to some

smooth muscle which is present as interlacing bundles between the numerous vascular channels.[20,22,23] Most of the vessels have several layers of smooth muscle in the walls which often merges peripherally with the intervascular fascicles (Fig. 36.3). Sometimes there are large sinusoidal vessels with little smooth muscle in their walls. Small, slit-like channels are sometimes present. Most vessels have only scant and scattered elastic fibres in their walls.

The stroma contains varying amounts of fibrous tissue, and in about a third of cases there is a sparse lymphocytic infiltrate. Myxoid change is quite common in the stroma, particularly in the larger tumours.[21] The presence of fat in a few cases has led to suggestions of a hamartomatous origin;[22] a designation of *angiomyolipoma* can be used for these cases which also contain fat.[24,25] Uncommon changes include thrombosis of vascular channels, focal calcification, stromal

controversy about the relationship of these two entities.[33,34] Becker's naevus has an onset in adolescence, with invariable hyperpigmentation and hypertrichosis. The recent report of a patient with clinical features of smooth muscle hamartoma which was said to have developed in late childhood[38] suggests that Becker's naevus and smooth muscle hamartoma belong at different poles of the same developmental spectrum, involving hamartomatous change to the pilar unit and arrectores pilorum.[32,39,40]

Histopathology

There are well-defined smooth muscle bundles in the dermis, oriented in various directions. Some are attached to hair follicles.[32,33] Often there is a thin retraction space around the bundles, separating them from the adjacent dermal collagen. The smooth muscle bundles are clearly seen with the Masson trichrome stain. Bundles of nerve fibres may also be present.[31] There is often slight elongation of the rete ridges of the overlying epidermis, and mild basal hypermelanosis.[39]

Electron microscopy. Ultrastructural examination confirms the presence of normal smooth muscle cells in this lesion.[34,40]

LEIOMYOSARCOMA

Because of their different biological behaviour, leiomyosarcomas of the skin can be divided into three categories — dermal, subcutaneous, and secondary tumours.[41,42]

Over 100 acceptable cases of *dermal leiomyosarcoma* have now been recorded.[41] They have a predilection for the extensor surfaces of the extremities,[41,42] and to a lesser extent the trunk.[43,44] Rare sites include the scrotum,[45,46] a chronic venous stasis ulcer,[47] and the face.[14] There is a male predominance, and the average age of presentation is in the sixth decade. They vary in size from 0.5–3 cm or more in maximum diameter. Subcutaneous extension is present in two-thirds of cases.[41] Pain or tenderness is present in some.[42] Occasionally there is a history

of previous injury to the site.[42,43] These tumours presumably arise from the arrector pili muscles, except for scrotal lesions which derive from the dartos muscle.[41,45] A case apparently arising in an angioleiomyoma has been reported.[48] Dermal leiomyosarcomas may recur locally, but metastases of confirmed cases are unknown.[41]

Subcutaneous leiomyosarcomas tend to be slightly larger tumours at presentation, and more circumscribed in outline.[42] They may also be tender or painful. They presumably arise from the smooth muscle in vessel walls. They have a greater tendency for local recurrence, and metastasis to lung, liver, bone and other sites occurs in about one-third of cases.[42,49] Assessment of the DNA content of the tumour cells by flow cytometry may be used to predict those tumours with metastatic potential.[50]

Secondary leiomyosarcomas are rare in the skin and arise from retroperitoneal and uterine primary lesions.[51] There are usually several dermal or subcutaneous nodules. There has been a predilection for the scalp and back.

Histopathology

Dermal leiomyosarcomas are irregular in outline with tumour cells blending into the collagenous stroma at the periphery.[52] By definition, the major portion of the tumour is in the dermis, although subcutaneous extension occurs in two-thirds.[41] A superficial grenz zone is present in many. Ulceration and pseudoepitheliomatous hyperplasia are rare. There is usually some flattening of the rete ridges of the overlying epidermis.

Leiomyosarcomas are composed of interlacing fascicles of elongated, spindle-shaped cells with eosinophilic cytoplasm and eccentric, blunt-ended (cigar-shaped) nuclei (Fig. 36.4). A rare variant with intracytoplasmic eosinophilic granules (granular cell leiomyosarcoma) has been reported.[53] Sometimes there is a suggestion of nuclear palisading. There is variable nuclear pleomorphism with at least 1 mitosis per 10 high power fields in cellular areas. Pockets of greater mitotic activity (mitotic 'hot spots')[54] are found. Tumour giant cells are usually present in the less well differentiated variants. Perinuclear halos are

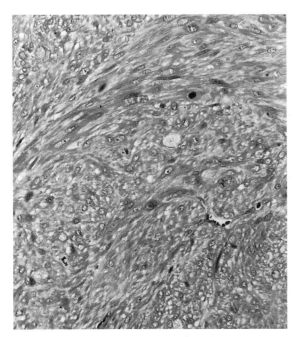

Fig. 36.4 Leiomyosarcoma. The smooth muscle bundles have destroyed the dermal collagen. Scattered mitoses are present within the tumour.
Haematoxylin — eosin

rare. Small lymphoid aggregates are sometimes present within the tumour.[41] Arrector pili muscles are often prominent or hyperplastic, and in some cases transitions from normal to hyperplastic, to benign neoplastic, and to a frankly sarcomatous pattern occur.[41,55]

Subcutaneous leiomyosarcomas often extend into the lower dermis. They frequently have a prominent vascular pattern.[42] There are sometimes small areas of necrosis present.

Secondary leiomyosarcomas are often multiple, spheroidal in outline, and sometimes present in vascular lumina.[41]

Leiomyosarcomas of all three types will have myofilaments, demonstrated by the Masson trichrome stain. Reticulin stains show a fine reticulin network, interspersed between adjacent fibres. A small amount of glycogen is usually present.[56] Immunoperoxidase preparations show the presence of vimentin and, usually, desmin in the cytoplasm.[57] Muscle-specific actin is often present, but not cytokeratin.[58] S100 protein has been demonstrated in a small number of cases.[58]

Reliable criteria for malignancy remain to be established.[54] Usually accepted features include high cellularity, significant nuclear atypia, tumour giant cells, and at least 1 mitosis per 10 high power fields.

Electron microscopy. This confirms the smooth muscle origin of the tumour cells, with numerous fine myofilaments in the cytoplasm, some marginal plaques, pinocytotic vesicles, glycogen, and a basal lamina surrounding individual cells.[45,54] Junctional complexes are uncommon.[54] Some myofibroblasts may also be present.[46]

TUMOURS OF STRIATED MUSCLE

There is an exceedingly rare group of cutaneous tumours which contain either mature striated muscle, or cells differentiating towards striated muscle, as a major component of the lesion. Mature striated muscle is found in the striated muscle hamartoma (see below), the accessory tragus (see p. 549), and in the first arch abnormality reported as dermatorynchus geneae (see p. 550). Rarely, a few striated muscle fibres may be present adjacent to developmental cysts of the head and neck. Malignant cells showing ultrastructural, immunohistochemical and sometimes light microscopic differentiation towards striated muscle are a feature of rhabdomyosarcomas. Brief mention will be made of the malignant rhabdoid tumour, which has some histopathological similarities to a rhabdomyosarcoma, but which is of uncertain histogenesis.

STRIATED MUSCLE HAMARTOMA

This term has been proposed for an exceedingly rare tumour of neonates in which there is a polypoid (skin-tag-like) lesion of the head and neck region which contains striated muscle bundles.[59] A similar tumour has been reported as a *rhabdomyomatous mesenchymal hamartoma*.[60,60a] Striated muscle hamartomas have a midline location whereas accessory tragi, which may also contain striated muscle, are usually found in the preauricular region or in the upper, lateral neck.

Histopathology

The polypoid tumours contain multiple bundles of normal-appearing striated muscle surrounded by fibrofatty tissue containing a few telangiectatic vessels.[59,60] Numerous vellus hair follicles have also been present, a feature noted in accessory tragi.[59]

RHABDOMYOSARCOMA

Rhabdomyosarcoma, a tumour composed of malignant cells showing some differentiation towards striated muscle, has a predilection for the head and neck region, the genitourinary tract, the retroperitoneum and the soft tissues of the extremities. It is the most common soft tissue sarcoma of childhood. Rarely, rhabdomyosarcoma may present as a dermal nodule, particularly on the head or neck, as a result of the dermal extension of a lesion arising in the underlying soft tissues.[61]

Rhabdomyosarcomas have been reported in patients with neurofibromatosis and in the basal cell naevus syndrome.

Histopathology

There are three major histological subtypes of rhabdomyosarcoma: embryonal (including the botryoid variant), alveolar and pleomorphic. They may be composed of small round cells, spindle or polygonal cells or large pleomorphic cells. Cross striations are sometimes seen using the phosphotungstic-acid–haematoxylin stain.

Immunoperoxidase techniques using monoclonal antibodies to vimentin, desmin, myoglobin and muscle-actin may be used to confirm the diagnosis.[61]

MALIGNANT RHABDOID TUMOUR

Malignant rhabdoid tumours were initially regarded as a subset of Wilms' tumour of the kidney showing rhabdomyosarcomatous differentiation. Subsequent studies have not confirmed this and their histogenesis is currently uncertain. Tumours of similar morphology to the renal lesions have been reported in other sites, including facial skin.[62-64]

Histopathology

The tumour is composed of sheets of polygonal cells with abundant, hyaline, eosinophilic cytoplasm and a peripherally displaced, vesicular nucleus. Mitotic activity is prominent and there are usually areas of tumour necrosis.[62]

The cells invariably express vimentin and sometimes there is cytokeratin as well. Other markers are usually negative. Malignant rhabdoid tumour has some morphological and immunohistochemical features in common with epithelioid sarcoma (see p. 892), although the cells in epithelioid sarcoma do not contain rhabdoid filamentous masses.[62,63]

REFERENCES

Tumours of smooth muscle

1. Montgomery H, Winkelmann RK. Smooth-muscle tumors of the skin. Arch Dermatol 1959; 79: 32–39.
2. Burden PA, Gentry RH, Fitzpatrick JE. Piloleiomyoma arising in an organoid nevus: a case report and review of the literature. J Dermatol Surg Oncol 1987; 13: 1213–1218.
3. Pinkus H. Discussion. Arch Dermatol 1959; 79: 40.
4. Abraham Z, Cohen A, Haim S. Muscle relaxing agent in cutaneous leiomyoma. Dermatologica 1983; 166: 255–256.
4a. Tatnall FM, Leigh IM. Facial leiomyomas. Clin Exp Dermatol 1990; 15: 296–297.
5. Thompson JA Jr. Therapy for painful cutaneous leiomyomas. J Am Acad Dermatol 1985; 13: 865–867.
6. Fisher WC, Helwig EB. Leiomyomas of the skin. Arch Dermatol 1963; 88: 510–520.
7. Thyresson HN, Su WPD. Familial cutaneous

leiomyomatosis. J Am Acad Dermatol 1981; 4: 430–434.

8. Peters CW, Hanke CW, Reed JC. Nevus leiomyomatosus systematicus. Cutis 1981; 27: 484–486.

9. Kloepfer HW, Krafchuk J, Derbes V, Burks J. Hereditary multiple leiomyoma of the skin. Am J Hum Genet 1958; 10: 48–52.

10. Rudner EJ, Schwartz OD, Grekin JN. Multiple cutaneous leiomyomata in identical twins. Arch Dermatol 1964; 90: 81–82.

11. Jolliffe DS. Multiple cutaneous leiomyomata. Clin Exp Dermatol 1978; 3: 89–92.

12. Venencie PY, Puissant A, Boffa GA et al. Multiple cutaneous leiomyomata and erythrocytosis with demonstration of erythropoietic activity in the cutaneous leiomyomata. Br J Dermatol 1982; 107: 483–486.

13. Engelke H, Christophers E. Leiomyomatosis cutis et uteri. Acta Derm Venereol (Suppl) 1979; 85: 51–54.

14. Orellana-Diaz O, Hernandez-Perez EJ. Leiomyoma cutis and leiomyosarcoma: a 10-year study and a short review. J Dermatol Surg Oncol 1983; 9: 283–287.

15. Stout AP. Solitary cutaneous and subcutaneous leiomyoma. Am J Cancer 1937; 29: 435–469.

16. Lupton GP, Naik DG, Rodman OG. An unusual congenital leiomyoma. Pediatr Dermatol 1986; 3: 158–160.

17. Livne PM, Nobel M, Savir A et al. Leiomyoma of the scrotum. Arch Dermatol 1983; 119: 358–359.

18. Siegal GP, Gaffey TA. Solitary leiomyomas arising from the tunica dartos scroti. J Urol 1976; 116: 69–71.

19. Jansen LH. Leiomyoma cutis. Acta Derm Venereol 1952; 32: 40–50.

20. Duhig JT, Ayer JP. Vascular leiomyoma. A study of sixty-one cases. Arch Pathol 1959; 68: 424–430.

21. MacDonald DM, Sanderson KV. Angioleiomyoma of the skin. Br J Dermatol 1974; 91: 161–168.

22. Hachisuga T, Hashimoto H, Enjoji M. Angioleiomyoma. A clinicopathologic reappraisal of 562 cases. Cancer 1984; 54: 126–130.

22a. Fox SB, Heryet A, Khong TY. Angioleiomyomas: an immunohistological study. Histopathology 1990; 16: 495–496.

23. Magner D, Hill DP. Encapsulated angiomyoma of the skin and subcutaneous tissues. Am J Clin Pathol 1961; 35: 137–141.

24. Argenyi ZB, Piette WW, Goeken JA. Cutaneous angiomyolipoma: a light-microscopic, immunohistochemical, and electronmicroscopic study. Am J Dermatopathol 1991; 13: 497–502.

25. Fitzpatrick JE, Mellette JR Jr, Zaim MT et al. Cutaneous angiolipoleiomyoma (angiomyolipoma). J Cutan Pathol 1988; 15: 305 (abstract).

26. Tsambaos D, Orfanos CE. Cutaneous smooth muscle hamartoma. J Cutan Pathol 1982; 9: 33–42.

27. Bronson DM, Fretzin DF, Farrell LN. Congenital pilar and smooth muscle nevus. J Am Acad Dermatol 1983; 8: 111–114.

28. Karo KR, Gange RW. Smooth-muscle hamartoma. Possible congenital Becker's nevus. Arch Dermatol 1981; 117: 678–679.

29. Metzker A, Amir J, Rotem A, Merlob P. Congenital smooth muscle hamartoma of the skin. Pediatr Dermatol 1984; 2: 45–48.

30. Plewig G, Schmoeckel C. Naevus musculi arrector pili. Hautarzt 1979; 30: 503–505.

31. Goldman MP, Kaplan RP, Heng MCY. Congenital smooth-muscle hamartoma. Int J Dermatol 1987; 26: 448–452.

32. Johnson MD, Jacobs AH. Congenital smooth muscle hamartoma. A report of six cases and a review of the literature. Arch Dermatol 1989; 125: 820–822.

33. Berberian BJ, Burnett JW. Congenital smooth muscle hamartoma: a case report. Br J Dermatol 1986; 115: 711–714.

34. Berger TG, Levin MW. Congenital smooth muscle hamartoma. J Am Acad Dermatol 1984; 11: 709–712.

35. Wallach D, Sorin M, Saurat JH. Naevus musculaire généralisé avec aspect clinique de "bébé Michelin". Ann Dermatol Venereol 1980; 107: 923–927.

35a. Glover MT, Malone M, Atherton DJ. Michelin-tire baby syndrome resulting from diffuse smooth muscle hamartoma. Pediatr Dermatol 1989; 6: 329–331.

36. Haneke E. The dermal component in melanosis naeviformis Becker. J Cutan Pathol 1979; 6: 53–58.

37. Urbanek RW, Johnson WC. Smooth muscle hamartoma associated with Becker's nevus. Arch Dermatol 1978; 114: 104–106.

38. Wong RC, Solomon AR. Acquired dermal smooth-muscle hamartoma. Cutis 1985; 35: 369–370.

39. Slifman NR, Harrist TJ, Rhodes AR. Congenital arrector pili hamartoma. Arch Dermatol 1985; 121: 1034–1037.

40. Fishman SJ, Phelps RG, Lebwohl M, Lieber C. Immunofluorescence and electron microscopic findings in a congenital arrector pili hamartoma. Am J Dermatopathol 1989; 11: 369–374.

41. Wolff M, Rothenberg J. Dermal leiomyosarcoma: a misnomer? Progress in Surgical Pathology 1986; 6: 147–159.

42. Fields JP, Helwig EB. Leiomyosarcoma of the skin and subcutaneous tissue. Cancer 1981; 47: 156–169.

43. Chow J, Sabet LM, Clark BL, Coire CI. Cutaneous leiomyosarcoma: case reports and review of the literature. Ann Plast Surg 1987; 18: 319–322.

44. Davidson LL, Frost ML, Hanke W, Epinette WW. Primary leiomyosarcoma of the skin. Case report and review of the literature. J Am Acad Dermatol 1989; 21: 1156–1160.

45. Flotte TJ, Bell DA, Sidhu GS, Plair CM. Leiomyosarcoma of the dartos muscle. J Cutan Pathol 1981; 8: 69–74.

46. Johnson S, Rundell M, Platt W. Leiomyosarcoma of the scrotum. A case report with electron microscopy. Cancer 1978; 41: 1830–1835.

47. Nunnery EW, Lipper S, Reddick R, Kahn LB. Leiomyosarcoma arising in a chronic venous stasis ulcer. Hum Pathol 1981; 12: 951–953.

48. White IR, MacDonald DM. Cutaneous leiomyosarcoma with coexistent superficial angioleiomyoma. Clin Exp Dermatol 1981; 6: 333–337.

49. Stout AP, Hill WT. Leiomyosarcoma of the superficial soft tissues. Cancer 1958; 11: 844–854.

50. Oliver GF, Reiman HM, Gonchoroff NJ et al. Cutaneous and subcutaneous leiomyosarcoma: a clinicopathological review of 14 cases with reference to anti-desmin staining and nuclear DNA patterns studied by flow cytometry. Br J Dermatol 1991; 124: 252–257.

51. Alessi E, Innocenti M, Sala F. Leiomyosarcoma metastatic to the back and scalp from a primary neoplasm in the uterus. Am J Dermatopathol 1985; 7: 471–476.

52. Jegasothy BV, Gilgor RS, Hull DM. Leiomyosarcoma of the skin and subcutaneous tissue. Arch Dermatol 1981; 117: 478–481.

53. Suster S, Rosen LB, Sanchez JL. Granular cell leiomyosarcoma of the skin. Am J Dermatopathol 1988; 10: 234–239.

54. Headington JT, Beals TF, Niederhuber JE. Primary leiomyosarcoma of skin: a report and critical appraisal. J Cutan Pathol 1977; 4: 308–317.

55. Dahl I, Angervall L. Cutaneous and subcutaneous leiomyosarcoma: a clinicopathologic study of 47 patients. Pathologia Europaea 1974; 9: 307–315.

56. Fletcher CDM, McKee PH. Sarcomas — a clinicopathological guide with particular reference to cutaneous manifestation II. Malignant nerve sheath tumour, leiomyosarcoma and rhabdomyosarcoma. Clin Exp Dermatol 1985; 10: 201–216.

57. Miettinen M, Lehto V-P, Virtanen I. Antibodies to intermediate filament proteins. The differential diagnosis of cutaneous tumors. Arch Dermatol 1985; 121: 736–741.

58. Swanson PE, Stanley MW, Scheithauer BW, Wick MR. Primary cutaneous leiomyosarcoma. A histological and immunohistochemical study of 9 cases, with ultrastructural correlation. J Cutan Pathol 1988; 15: 129–141.

Tumours of striated muscle

59. Hendrick SJ, Sanchez RL, Blackwell SJ, Raimer SS. Striated muscle hamartoma: description of two cases. Pediatr Dermatol 1986; 3: 153–157.

60. Mills AE. Rhabdomyomatous mesenchymal hamartoma. Am J Dermatopathol 1989; 11: 58–63.

60a. Sahn EE, Garen PD, Pai GS et al. Multiple rhabdomyomatous mesenchymal hamartomas of skin. Am J Dermatopathol 1990; 12: 485–491.

61. Wiss K, Solomon AR, Raimer SS et al. Rhabdomyosarcoma presenting as a cutaneous nodule. Arch Dermatol 1988; 124: 1687–1690.

62. Dabbs DJ, Park HK. Malignant rhabdoid skin tumor: an uncommon primary skin neoplasm. Ultrastructural and immunohistochemical analysis. J Cutan Pathol 1988; 15: 109–115.

63. Perrone T, Swanson PE, Twiggs L et al. Malignant rhabdoid tumor of the vulva: is distinction from epithelioid sarcoma possible? A pathologic and immunohistochemical study. Am J Surg Pathol 1989; 13: 848–858.

64. Dominey A, Paller AS, Gonzalez-Crussi F. Congenital rhabdoid sarcoma with cutaneous metastases. J Am Acad Dermatol 1990; 22: 969–974.

Neural and neuroendocrine tumours

INTRODUCTION

Cutaneous neural tumours arise from, or differentiate towards, one or more elements of the nervous system. Most of these tumours found in the skin and subcutaneous tissue are derived from peripheral nerves or their neurocutaneous end organs. There are three principal cells comprising the sheath of peripheral nerves — the perineurial cell, the Schwann cell and the fibroblast. Perineurial cells differ from Schwann cells by having no basement membrane. These sheath cells give rise to the three main cutaneous neural tumours — neuromas, schwannomas (neurilemmomas) and neurofibromas. The tumours differ from one another by having a different proportion and arrangement of the various constituents of a peripheral nerve — Schwann cells, axons, fibroblasts and supporting stroma. Although Schwann cells are generally viewed as neuroectodermal cells derived from the neural crest, it has been suggested that they may be of mesenchymal origin.[1] The perineurial cell may be of neural crest derivation also.[2]

The other categories to be considered in this chapter are the herniations and heterotopias of glial and meningeal cells giving rise to nasal gliomas, cutaneous meningiomas and related heterotopias, and the neuroendocrine carcinoma (Merkel cell tumour) which may be derived from another neural crest derivative, the Merkel cell. This cell subserves a neurosensory function in the skin.

tortuous hyperplastic nerves with a thickened perineurium.[4]

Hypertrophy of small nerves in the dermis ('dermal hyperneury') has also been noted in the clinically normal skin of patients with this syndrome.[18] Nerve hypertrophy has been reported recently in a patient with striated pigmentation and a marfanoid habitus, a possible forme fruste of this syndrome, but without the endocrine tumours.[19]

Ganglioneuroma

Ganglioneuromas may be found in the skin in patients with neuroblastomas and mature cutaneous secondary deposits, and in von Recklinghausen's disease where ganglion cells have been entrapped by a neurofibroma.[20] Primary cutaneous ganglioneuromas are exceedingly rare.[21,22] They consist of mature ganglion cells which are usually intermixed with fascicles of spindle cells;[22] in one reported case the ganglion cells were separate from the neuromatous elements.[22a]

SCHWANNOMA (NEURILEMMOMA)

Cutaneous schwannomas (neurilemmomas) are uncommon, slowly growing, usually solitary tumours with a propensity for the limbs of adults.[6] Pain, tenderness and paraesthesiae may be present in up to one-third of lesions.[23,24] They measure 2–4 cm in diameter.[6] Multiple tumours are uncommon and can occur in several clinical settings: as multiple, localized (agminate) tumours;[25] in association with neurofibromas in von Recklinghausen's disease;[26] or as the syndrome of schwannomatosis (neurilemmomatosis) in which widespread subcutaneous and intradermal tumours are often associated with tumours of internal organs.[27] This latter syndrome is non-hereditary and not associated with café-au-lait spots or neurofibromas. It has been reported mainly from Japan.[27,27a]

Schwannomas also occur in the deep soft tissues, retroperitoneum, mediastinum, and tongue,[28] and on the vestibulocochlear nerve. Local recurrence and malignant transformation are exceedingly rare. They are of Schwann cell origin.[2,29]

The tumour is grey-white in colour, encapsulated, with a smooth, glistening appearance.[30] Cystic change is sometimes present, particularly in the larger, deeper tumours.

Histopathology[29]

Schwannomas are circumscribed, encapsulated tumours, usually confined to the subcutis. The nerve of origin may sometimes be seen along one border. The agminate tumours and some of those in schwannomatosis are often situated in the dermis.[25] Multiple small tumour nodules may be present in these forms, as well as hypertrophied peripheral nerves.[25,27] The term 'plexiform schwannoma' has been applied to this type.[30a]

Schwannomas are characteristically composed of two tissue types.[29] In the so-called Antoni A areas there are spindle-shaped Schwann cells arranged in interlacing fascicles (Fig. 37.4). The cells have indistinct cytoplasmic borders. The nuclei may be aligned in rows or palisades, between which the cell processes are fused into eosinophilic masses forming Verocay bodies. No axons are present.[4] Antoni B tissue consists of a loose meshwork of gelatinous and microcystic tissue with widely separated Schwann

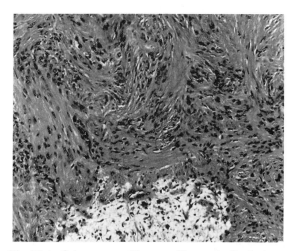

Fig. 37.4 Schwannoma. There are Verocay bodies in the interlacing bundles of spindle-shaped cells (Antoni-A tissue). The loose stroma below is known as Antoni-B tissue. Haematoxylin — eosin

cells. Lipid-laden macrophages, dilated blood vessels with thick hyaline walls, old and recent haemorrhage, lipofuscin and sometimes calcified hyaline areas may also be present in Antoni B areas.[2,29] Sometimes areas with overlap features are found. Mast cells and non-specific cholinesterase may be demonstrated.[6] Immunoperoxidase methods demonstrate S100 protein,[25] vimentin[30b] and myelin basic protein[31] in the tumour cells. Glial fibrillary acidic protein (GFAP) is present in a small number of cases.[30b,31a] Epithelial membrane antigen is found in the perineurial cells in the capsule of schwannomas, as in that of solitary neuromas (see above).[31b]

A cellular variant, mostly found in the deeper tissues, has been described.[32] There are compact spindle-shaped cells with mitoses and some storiform areas, and a near absence of Verocay bodies and Antoni B tissue.[32] A rare variant with multiple glandular elements has also been reported.[33]

A recently delineated type of schwannoma is the psammomatous melanotic schwannoma which contains melanin and scattered psammoma bodies.[33a,33b] This variant of schwannoma is often associated with a familial syndrome in which there are cardiac myxomas, spotty pigmentation and Cushing's syndrome.[33a]

The term congenital neural hamartoma (fascicular schwannoma) was used recently for an unencapsulated dermal tumour composed of fascicles of Schwann cells with frequent Verocay-body-like structures.[33c] Unlike cutaneous neuromas, there were no axons present.

Electron microscopy. There are aggregates of mature Schwann cells with thin, complexly entangled cytoplasmic processes, but only rare cell junctions.[2,34] One report suggested that the Antoni B areas showed features of degeneration,[35] but this finding has not been confirmed by others.[7]

NEUROFIBROMA AND NEUROFIBROMATOSIS

Neurofibromas may occur as a solitary tumour, or as multiple lesions in a segmental or widespread distribution, referred to as neurofibromatosis. The histopathology of the neurofibromas in these different clinical settings is similar and will be considered together.

Solitary neurofibromas are papular, nodular or pedunculated tumours with a predilection for the upper trunk.[6] They are soft and tend to invaginate on pressure (the 'button hole' sign).

Neurofibromatosis, described by von Recklinghausen in 1882, is a clinically heterogeneous disorder with varied manifestations affecting the skin, soft tissues, blood vessels, and the peripheral and central nervous systems.[36] It is said to affect 80 000 individuals in the USA.[37] Riccardi has proposed eight clinical subtypes of neurofibromatosis (NF-1 to NF-8).[38] NF-1 is classic von Recklinghausen's disease, which accounts for 85–90% of all cases. NF-2 is associated with acoustic neuromas and sometimes other intracranial tumours. NF-3 is a mixed form combining features of NF-1 and NF-2. NF-4 is a variant form with diffuse neurofibromas and café-au-lait pigmentation, but without many of the other clinical features that typify NF-1. NF-5 is the segmental form. NF-6 has prominent café-au-lait pigmentation as the sole manifestation. NF-7 is a late onset type, while NF-8 is a miscellaneous group not categorized into the other subtypes.[38,38a] Prenatal diagnosis of neurofibromatosis is not yet possible.[38]

Classic neurofibromatosis (NF-1)

This is the usual form of the disease. It is inherited as an autosomal dominant trait, although spontaneous mutations account for up to 50% of all NF-1 probands. Café-au-lait pigmentation, which varies from small macular areas to large patches of pigmentation, is present in 99% of cases.[37] The pigmentation is present at birth or appears early in childhood before other stigmata of the disease. It may be found in other conditions, but the presence of six or more patches is said to be diagnostic of neurofibromatosis.[39] Axillary freckling is present in about 20% of patients.

The neurofibromas are multiple and sometimes disfiguring. They appear at about puberty. Neurofibromas may develop for the first time in pregnancy; women who already have tumours may experience an increase in the size and number of the lesions during pregnancy.[40] Plexiform neurofibromas,[6] which are diagnostic of neurofibromatosis, may present as large deep tumours, or localized areas of deformity.[41] They are found in about 25% of the cases.[39,42] Schwannomas are sometimes present as well.

Other clinical features of the classic form are pigmented hamartomas of the iris (Lisch nodules),[43] macrocephaly, mental retardation, kyphoscoliosis, bone hypertrophy, pseudo-arthrosis and vascular lesions.[43–45] Elephantiasis neuromatosa, with localized gigantism or thick redundant folds of skin, is rare.[44] Neuro-fibromas, each with a halo of depigmentation, have been reported in one patient with presumptive mild neurofibromatosis.[46]

Malignant degeneration of neurofibromas occurs in 2–3% of patients,[39] although higher figures have been reported in some series.[42] In addition, various other sarcomas,[47] mela-nomas[42,48,49] and visceral carcinomas[42] have been reported, although the latter may not be increased in incidence.[50]

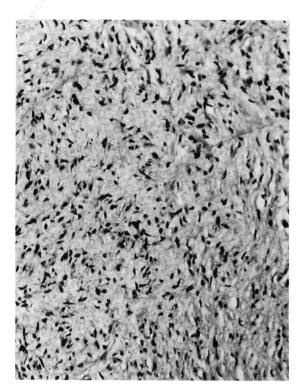

Fig. 37.5 Neurofibroma. It is composed of thin fascicles of cells, each with a 'wavy' spindle-shaped nucleus. Haematoxylin — eosin

Segmental neurofibromatosis (NF-5)

This variant (NF-5) is a heterogeneous group.[51–54a] Café-au-lait pigmentation is present in some cases;[41,55] there are usually no other stigmata of neurofibromatosis and no family history.[56–59] Variants of the segmental form include a unilateral[51,57] and a bilateral[51,60] segmental form, a form associated with deep neural tumours,[61] and a rare hereditary form.[62]

Histopathology

Cutaneous neurofibromas are non-encapsulated, loosely textured tumours, centred on the dermis.[6] There is often extension into the subcutis and an overlying grenz zone beneath the epidermis. The lesion is composed of delicate fascicles, usually only a single cell thick.[4] The cells have an oval or spindle-shaped nucleus and scant, indefinite cytoplasm (Fig. 37.5). There is

sometimes nuclear pleomorphism, but mitoses are rare. The matrix is pale staining with delicate wavy collagen. Solitary neurofibromas are some-times more compact than those in neurofibro-matosis.[29] Blood vessels are increased in number in the stroma. A Bodian stain will demonstrate some axonal material, but not in the 1:1 ratio with Schwann cells, as occurs in neuromas.[4] Mast cells,[63] non-specific cholinesterase,[59] S100 protein, myelin basic protein[31] and factor XIIIa[64] can be demonstrated by the appropriate techniques.

Plexiform neurofibromas are a distinct variant in which there is irregular, cylindrical or fusiform enlargement of a subcutaneous or deep nerve;[6] rarely, they arise in the dermis.[65] There are numerous large nerve fascicles embedded in a cellular matrix containing abundant mucin as well as collagen, fibroblasts and Schwann cells.[4] Initially this proliferation of nerve fibres is confined within the epineurium of the involved nerve.[4]

Other findings in neurofibromatosis are schwannomas (neurilemmomas), tumours with features of both neurofibroma and schwannoma, and neurofibromas containing scattered, possibly entrapped ganglion cells. Pilar dysplasia has been reported overlying a neurofibroma.[66] Vascular changes are rarely found. These include smooth muscle islands in the intima.[45] In elephantiasis neuromatosa there is a diffuse proliferation of Schwann cells and axons in the subcutis.[29] Islands of cartilage are present, rarely, in this tissue.[29] Glandular epithelial structures have been reported in the stroma in segmental neurofibromatosis.[54a]

Giant pigment granules (macromelanosomes) are often present in melanocytes and basal keratinocytes in the café-au-lait spots of neurofibromatosis.[67] The granules can just be seen by the light microscope. They are probably increased in older individuals.[68] Macromelanosomes are not present in all cases of neurofibromatosis; their presence is not pathognomonic as they can also be found in several other conditions.[67,69]

Electron microscopy. Neurofibromas are composed of fusiform or stellate cells which are widely separated by individual collagen bundles and matrix.[7,34] These have usually been interpreted as Schwann cells,[7] but one report has claimed that the principal cell is the perineurial cell although scattered Schwann cell-axon complexes are also present.[2]

PACINIOMA AND PACINIAN NEUROFIBROMA

The term _pacinioma_ has been applied to the rare finding of a hamartomatous overgrowth of mature Vater–Pacini corpuscles (Fig. 37.6). Bale has reported two such lesions in the sacral region associated with spina bifida occulta.[70]

Pacinian neurofibroma (pacinian neuroma) refers to a rare tumour of the digits, hands and feet composed of round or ovoid corpuscles with multiple concentric lamellae.[71-73] They do not

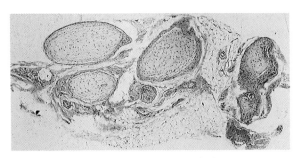

Fig. 37.6 Pacinioma composed of several enlarged Vater–Pacini corpuscles.
Haematoxylin — eosin

have the perfect structure of a Vater–Pacini corpuscle, but the resemblance is close. The recent report of a case with multiple hairy lesions on the buttock composed of rudimentary Vater–Pacini corpuscles suggests that the distinction between the hamartomatous pacinioma and the pacinian neurofibroma is artificial.[74] In another case, multiple tiny lesions were present on the ring finger in one patient, associated with marked vascular changes of the glomus type of arteriovenous anastomoses.[75] Some of the cases reported in the literature as pacinian neurofibromas would now be reclassified as nerve sheath myxomas.[76] These latter tumours have less resemblance to Vater–Pacini corpuscles and they contain more stromal mucin than true pacinian neurofibromas.

NERVE SHEATH MYXOMA

The nomenclature of this tumour has been debated extensively in the literature, and it is not universally agreed that the following terms are all synonymous with nerve sheath myxoma[77] — _pacinian neurofibroma,_[76] _bizarre cutaneous neurofibroma,_[78] _neurothekeoma,_[79] and _cutaneous lobular neuromyxoma._[80] While 'neurothekeoma' has many features in common with nerve sheath myxoma, subtle (and sometimes inconsistent) light and electron microscopic differences, as well as immunohistochemical differences, are starting to emerge.

Nerve sheath myxomas are found mostly on the face and upper extremities.[81] They are not associated with neurofibromatosis. There is a predilection for females and young adults. The tumours usually present as dome-shaped nodules, 1–2 cm in diameter. Rarely, they are recurrent, if inadequately excised. Their histogenesis is in doubt although there is increasing evidence for an origin from the perineural fibroblast.[3a,82,83]

Histopathology[79,81]

The tumour is multilobulated and non-encapsulated. It is centred on the reticular dermis, but it often extends into the superficial subcutis.[84] The lobules are composed of spindle-shaped, stellate and sometimes epithelioid cells arranged in a swirling, lamellar, and often concentric pattern. The cellular elements are embedded in a myxoid stroma which is usually abundant in those tumours in which stellate and bipolar cells predominate, but scanty in those with a predominantly epithelioid pattern.[81] Chondroitin-4 or chondroitin-6 sulphate is the principal heteroglycan present.[77,82] There is variable nuclear hyperchromatism and some-times nuclear atypia. Mitoses are also variable.

In the variant reported as 'neurothekeoma', the mucinous matrix has often been less pronounced and the tumour lobules have sometimes had a poorly differentiated interface between the fascicles and the dermal collagen (Fig. 37.7).[79,85] Low grade cytological atypia and some mitoses are common.[86] Extensive dystrophic calcification has been reported in one case.[87]

Immunohistochemistry has given variable results, with the cells being S100 positive in some tumours,[77,81] but negative in others.[83,85] Myelin basic protein[85] and epithelial membrane antigen[3a] may also be present.

Electron microscopy. There have been conflicting reports of the ultrastructural changes. The tumour cells have had features of Schwann cells in some cases, and of perineural fibroblasts in others.[77,82,88,89] These different ultrastructural findings have not always correlated with the expected immunohistochemistry for that cell.

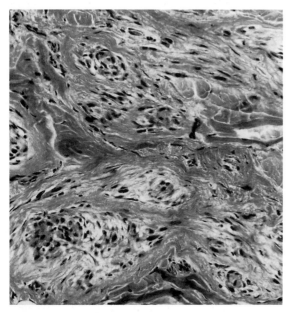

Fig. 37.7 'Neurothekeoma' variant of nerve sheath myxoma. Tumour fascicles merge with the intervening dermal collagen.
Haematoxylin — eosin

PIGMENTED STORIFORM NEUROFIBROMA

This tumour, also known as the Bednar tumour, is now regarded as a variant of dermatofibrosarcoma protuberans which shows some neural differentiation. It is discussed further in Chapter 34 page 886.

The rare pigmented neurofibroma, of which six cases were described by Bird and Willis,[90] is probably a separate entity. It is composed of whorled, fibrillar, ovoid structures.[91] Melanin is present in macrophages and in some of the tumour cells.

GRANULAR CELL TUMOUR

This tumour, previously known as granular cell myoblastoma, is an uncommon, benign tumour of disputed histogenesis, which may develop in many anatomical sites.[92,93] Most are found in the oral cavity, especially the tongue, and in the skin and subcutaneous tissue.[92,94] There is a female predominance, and a predilection for black races. Familiar cases are rare.[95] The average age of presentation is 40–50 years, but they may arise in children.[96] Most lesions are asymptomatic, solitary, skin-coloured nodules, less than 2 cm in diameter. Tumours are multiple in about 10% of cases.[96–100] Sometimes there are associated visceral granular cell tumours.[101]

Morphologically similar tumours are found on the anterior alveolar ridge of neonates, almost exclusively in females.[102] Occasionally they are multiple,[102] or they may involve other areas of the oral cavity.[103] These gingival giant cell tumours (congenital epulis) may regress spontaneously, or following inadequate removal. They are about one-tenth as common as the acquired variant.

Malignant granular cell tumours are exceedingly rare, accounting for only 1–3% of all acquired granular cell tumours.[92] Very few have been reported in the skin.[104–108] They may metastasize to regional lymph nodes or more widely.[95,106] Of interest is the report of a patient with neurofibromatosis in whom a malignant granular cell tumour developed.[109]

Recent immunohistochemical studies have been interpreted as indicating an origin from a 'neural crest-derived peripheral nerve-related cell',[110] rather than a Schwann cell origin as previously thought.[111] Ultrastructural studies of gingival giant cell tumours of the newborn have suggested an origin from undifferentiated mesenchymal cells,[103,112] and by analogy, a similar origin has been proposed for the acquired variant.[103] These theories are not mutually exclusive.[110,113]

Histopathology[92,93,114]

The tumours are non-encapsulated and composed of irregularly arranged sheets of large polyhedral cells with a small, central, hyperchromatic nucleus and abundant fine to coarsely granular, eosinophilic cytoplasm (Fig. 37.8). Dermal tumours often extend into the upper subcutis. Cells infiltrate between collagen bundles, and may displace them. They surround appendages, but may extend into the arrector pili muscles. Cytoplasmic borders are not always distinct. The cytoplasmic granules are PAS positive,

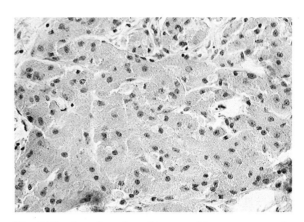

Fig. 37.8 Granular cell myoblastoma. The component cells are finely granular with a comparatively small nucleus. Haematoxylin — eosin

diastase resistant. They are also well seen with Movat's pentachrome technique.[114] The nuclei contain one or two nucleoli. Elastosis is common in the stroma of granular cell tumours.[115]

The overlying epithelium often shows prominent pseudoepitheliomatous hyperplasia, which may be misdiagnosed as squamous cell carcinoma if only a superficial biopsy is available for examination.[92] This epithelial response is usually not present in congenital gingival tumours[103] and is absent in some cutaneous tumours, especially if multiple.[98]

Congenital gingival tumours have a more prominent vascular stroma, often with perivascular collections of lymphocytes and histiocytes.[112] The amount of stromal collagen increases as the lesion ages. Small nerve fibres are sometimes found in and around acquired granular cell tumours.[98]

Immunohistological studies have given conflicting results. Granular cell tumours usually contain S100 protein,[116–118] neuron-specific enolase[110] and the melanoma-associated antigen NKI/C-3.[110] Myelin basic protein has been present in some cases;[119] it was absent in all 25 cases in one series.[110] Granular cell tumours are negative for myoglobin[118,120] and glial fibrillary acidic protein.[31a] Some reports have suggested the presence of carcinoembryonic antigen (CEA),[120] but this appears to be a false positive result, due to a related antigen in the tumour cells.[121,122] The cells are also esterase and acid phosphatase positive.[114]

There are no well-defined criteria for malignancy. Tumour size greater than 5 cm, vascular invasion, and rapid growth are important indicators of malignant behaviour.[101] Mitoses may also be present, but not necessarily so; they are invariably absent in benign variants.

Electron microscopy. The tumour cells are surrounded by a basal lamina.[101] The cytoplasm contains numerous granules of various sizes and shapes; the majority of these are phagolysosomes.[120,123] Microfilaments and microtubules have been reported.[123] Angulate bodies may also be found in acquired tumours,[120] and sometimes these are also found in satellite fibroblasts.[124] Congenital tumours have immature mesenchymal cells as well as forms transitional between these and the granular cells.[103]

MALIGNANT NERVE SHEATH TUMOURS

Malignant (peripheral) nerve sheath tumour[2] is the preferred designation for a tumour which has in the past been called neurosarcoma, neurogenic sarcoma, neurofibrosarcoma[125,126] and malignant schwannoma.[127,128] It is a rare tumour, accounting for approximately 2% of all nerve sheath tumours.[129] Although tumour is sometimes present in the dermis,[130] this usually represents extension of a growth that originated in the deeper soft tissues.[131]

In the past, the diagnosis of a malignant nerve sheath tumour was difficult, particularly in the absence of a clinical history of neurofibromatosis, and in those tumours in which no anatomical relationship to a nerve trunk could be demonstrated. The development of immunoperoxidase techniques has assisted considerably in making a specific diagnosis. These tumours contain S100 protein and myelin basic protein, although sometimes this staining is weak.[3,126] Vimentin may also be present.[31a]

In more than 50% of cases of malignant peripheral nerve sheath tumour, neurofibromatosis is present.[132] There is a predilection for the deep soft tissues of the proximal extremities

of young and middle-aged adults. The mean survival for patients with these tumours is 2–3 years.

Histopathology

There is usually a spindle cell growth pattern with cells arranged in tight wavy or interlacing bundles.[133] There are sometimes densely cellular areas alternating with more loosely textured areas.[134] The cellularity and number of mitoses determine the grading of the tumour. Purely epithelioid variants have been reported.[135,136] Focal divergent differentiation with the formation of foci of osteogenic sarcoma, chondrosarcoma, angiosarcoma, rhabdomyosarcoma or an epithelial element is present in about 15% of tumours.[137] The presence of rhabdomyosarcomatous elements can be confirmed by immunoperoxidase stains for myoglobin.[138] This variant is known as a 'triton tumour'.[138] It should not be confused with the rare neuromuscular hamartoma of infancy composed of nerve fibres admixed with well-differentiated skeletal muscle.[139]

Electron microscopy. This shows undifferentiated cells with some features of Schwann and perineurial cells.[2] Fibroblastic cells have also been identified.[2]

HERNIATIONS AND ECTOPIAS

NASAL GLIOMA AND NEURAL HETEROTOPIAS

The unsatisfactory term 'nasal glioma' refers to the presence of heterotopic neural tissue, predominantly glial in nature, at or near the root of the nose. Approximately 60% of these lesions are confined to the subcutaneous tissue, while 30% are intranasal in location.[140] The remainder have both external and intranasal components. In approximately 20% of cases, intracranial connections are present, sometimes with an associated bony defect in the nasofrontal region,[141,142] but there is no fluid-filled space connecting with the ventricular system, as in an encephalocele.[140,143] Nasal gliomas present at birth, or in early infancy, as a red to blue, firm, smooth tumour near the bridge of the nose. Those confined to the intranasal region may present later with nasal obstruction or epistaxis, or as a nasal polyp. Rarely, similar tissue has been reported in the scalp,[144] either as a midline parietal nodule,[145] or as multiple subcutaneous nodules in the scalp.[146] The term 'heterotopic neural tissue' is the preferred collective term for these lesions, and for nasal gliomas.[145] They are hamartomas which result from sequestration of neural tissue early in embryogenesis.[147]

Histopathology[147,148]

There are islands of neural and fibrovascular tissue in the subcutis. The neural tissue is composed of astrocytes enmeshed in a neurofibrillary stroma (Fig. 37.9). Multinucleate astrocytes are not uncommon but neurons are usually inconspicuous and few in number. They were the predominant element in one case.[149] The nodules are interlaced with vascular fibrous septa. Calcification is rarely present.

Heterotopic neural islands occurring on the scalp may be surrounded by a capsule that structurally resembles the leptomeninges.[145,150]

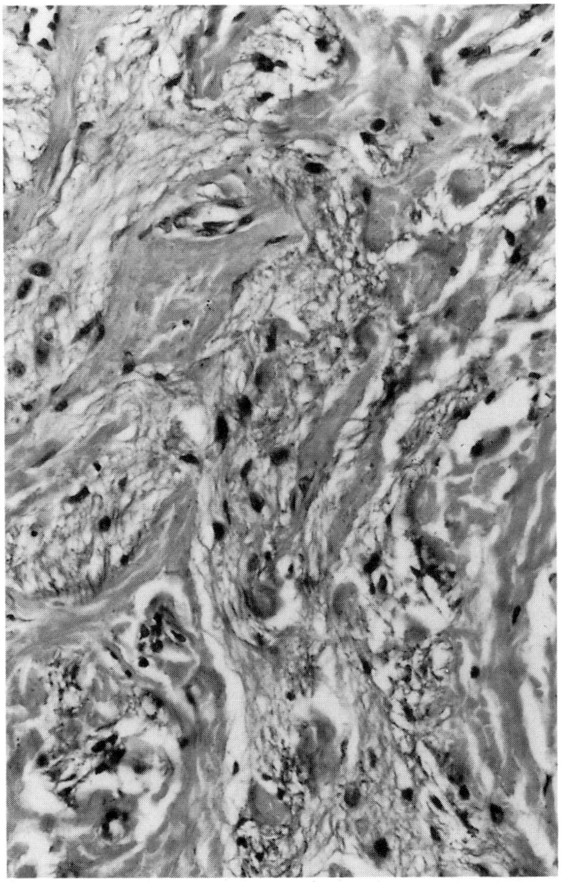

Fig. 37.9 Heterotopic glial tissue admixed with collagen bundles. This lesion was removed from the occipital region. Haematoxylin — eosin

CUTANEOUS MENINGIOMA

Meningiomas (cutaneous meningothelial tumours) are found only rarely in extracranial sites, including the skin.[151–153] The scalp, forehead and paravertebral areas are most commonly involved. Three distinct clinicopathological groups have been recognized.[153] Type I lesions arise in the subcutaneous tissue of the scalp, forehead and paravertebral region. They are usually present at birth, and are thought to be derived from ectopic arachnoid cells misplaced during embryogenesis. This group includes lesions with only scattered meningothelial cells in a collagenous nodule (acelic meningeal hamartoma), lesions with a rudimentary cystic channel (rudimentary meningocele variant) and those with well-circumscribed nodules resem-

bling intracranial meningiomas.[154] Type II lesions are found in adults around sensory organs of the head (periorbital, aural and paranasal), and along the course of cranial and spinal nerves. They are thought to be derived from nests of arachnoid cells which are found along the course of these nerves after they penetrate the dura. Type III lesions represent the direct cutaneous extension or distant metastasis of an intracranial tumour.[153,155]

Histopathology[153]

Whereas type I lesions are usually confined to the subcutis, type II and III tumours may also involve the dermis. Some type I lesions consist merely of irregular strands of meningothelial cells set in a collagenous stroma,[156] while others resemble type II and III tumours in being circumscribed, more cellular tumours akin to intracranial meningiomas and including spindle cell areas and meningothelial whorls. Psammoma bodies are variable in number. Inflammatory cells may be present in type II and III lesions.

Immunoperoxidase studies for S100, vimentin and epithelial membrane antigen have been positive.[151,151a] Ultrastructural studies have shown a similar appearance to intracranial meningiomas.[152,153]

NEUROENDOCRINE CARCINOMAS

NEUROENDOCRINE (MERKEL CELL) CARCINOMA

In 1972, Toker reported five cases of this tumour as *trabecular carcinoma*.[157] Some years later, on the basis of the electron microscopic findings of neurosecretory granules, Tang and Toker suggested that the tumour had a Merkel cell origin.[158] Because a Merkel cell origin is not established beyond doubt,[159] and because a trabecular pattern is not usually a dominant feature, the designation *neuroendocrine carcinoma* is currently favoured.[160,161]

This tumour usually arises on the sun-exposed skin of elderly patients, particularly on the head and neck and extremities.[162] There are two reports[163,164] of its occurrence in young patients with ectodermal dysplasia. There is a slight female preponderance.[165] The tumours are often indistinguishable from other skin cancers. They may have a reddish, nodular appearance which sometimes resembles an angiosarcoma.[166] They average 2 cm in diameter.

Local recurrences occur in about one-third of cases. The tumour spreads to the regional lymph nodes in approximately 50% of cases,[162,167] while distant metastasis with eventual death occurs in one-third or more.[168] Spontaneous regression of the tumour has been reported.[169]

Ectopic peptide production is not uncommon

(see below),[170] but the levels are not high enough to produce a clinical endocrinopathy.[171]

Histopathology[162]

The tumour is composed of small, round to oval cells of uniform size with a vesicular nucleus and multiple small nucleoli (Fig. 37.10). Mitoses and apoptotic bodies are usually numerous.[172] The cytoplasm is scanty and amphophilic and the cell borders are vaguely defined. A few tumours have scattered areas with spindle-shaped nuclei (Fig. 37.11). The cells are present as sheets and solid nests, infiltrating the entire dermis and some-

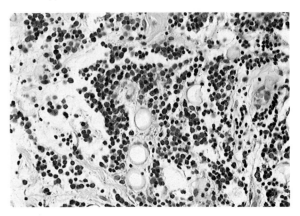

Fig. 37.10 Merkel cell tumour. The cells are small with indistinct cytoplasmic borders and a hyperchromatic nucleus. Haematoxylin — eosin

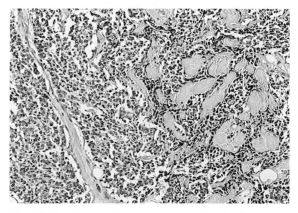

Fig. 37.11 Merkel cell tumour. Some cells are spindle shaped and slightly larger than the others. Haematoxylin — eosin

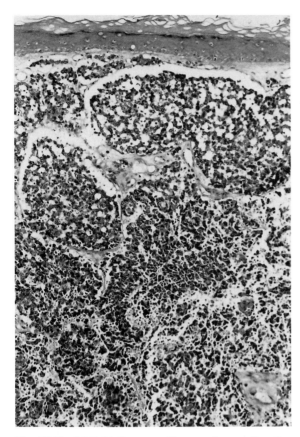

Fig. 37.12 Merkel cell tumour. Sheets and nests of small cells with hyperchromatic nuclei extend throughout the dermis.
Haematoxylin — eosin

hyperplasia. Epidermotropism of tumour cells is rare.[159] Overlying and contiguous Bowen's disease have also been reported,[162,178] as has the admixture of a neuroendocrine and squamous cell carcinoma.[179,180] No transition was seen between the two cell types.[180] Patients with neuroendocrine carcinoma have often had numerous skin cancers in the past.[180] Small swirls of squamoid differentiation[181] and even sweat duct differentiation[178,182] are occasionally seen within the tumour itself. This has led to the suggestion that the tumour arises from a primitive cell that can differentiate in either a neuroendocrine or sudoriferous direction.[178] One case was purported to have arisen in an epidermal cyst.[183]

Because neuroendocrine carcinomas need to be differentiated histologically from anaplastic primary and secondary tumours, there have been numerous immunoperoxidase studies assessing the specificity of various markers.[184,185] The variability in the reported results for the same marker probably reflects the different sensitivity of the techniques used and the level of specificity of the monoclonal antibodies. Most tumours are positive for neuron-specific enolase[181,186] and epithelial membrane antigen.[184] Cytokeratin is usually present as paranuclear globules (Fig. 37.13).[187–190] Neurofilaments,[191] chromogranin,[192] and polypeptides such as calcitonin,[193] gastrin,[194] somatostatin and cortico-

times extending into the subcutis (Fig. 37.12). In many tumours there is a trabecular arrangement of the cells, but this is usually limited to the peripheral areas.[173] Pseudorosettes are quite uncommon.[174] There is a dissociation of tumour cells in poorly fixed areas. Other features include focal necrosis, particularly in large tumours, frequent involvement of dermal lymphatics,[173] and a scattered infiltrate of lymphocytes and sometimes plasma cells. Tumour cells may be larger in recurrences after radiotherapy.[175] Amyloid has been demonstrated in a few tumours.[176,177] Focal argyrophilia is sometimes present, and this is enhanced by fixation in Bouin's solution.[172]

The overlying epidermis is ulcerated in about 20% of cases. Sometimes there is epidermal

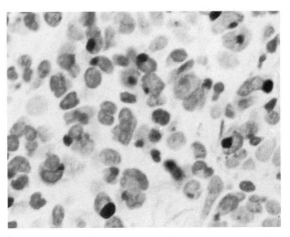

Fig. 37.13 Merkel cell tumour. Paranuclear filaments are seen as small globules ('dots'). Immunoperoxidase preparation for cytokeratin
Photograph provided by Dr A Clouston.

tropin are sometimes present.[160] The tumour cells are negative for S100 protein, laminin, CD45 (leucocyte common antigen)[184] and metenkephalin,[171,188] the latter being a marker for normal Merkel cells. The cells of secondary 'oat cell' carcinomas and carcinoids, some of which are spindle-shaped, usually have more cytoplasm; they may be immunoperoxidase positive for bombesin, leucine enkephalin and β-endorphin, markers which are absent in neuroendocrine carcinomas.[185]

Electron microscopy. The tumour cells contain dense core neurosecretory granules in the cytoplasm,[195] but these tend to be lost in formalin-fixed material.[196] A characteristic feature is the presence of paranuclear aggregates of intermediate-sized filaments.[197] Complex intercellular junctions and cytoplasmic spinous processes are also present.[162,198,199]

MALIGNANT NEUROEPITHELIOMA

The term 'malignant neuroepithelioma' is the most frequently used designation[200] for a rare tumour which has also been called 'peripheral neuroblastoma' and 'peripheral (primitive) neuroectodermal tumour'.[201–204] The malignant small cell tumour of the thoracopulmonary region in childhood (Askin tumour)[205] and even the extraskeletal Ewing's tumour have sometimes been included in this concept.[206,207] Some cases

reported in the past as malignant neuro-epithelioma[208] have now been reclassified as Merkel cell tumours (see above).[209] There are many features in common between these two neurocutaneous tumours.

Most malignant neuroepitheliomas are situated in the deep soft tissues.[200] The subcutis and dermis are involved quite uncommonly.[210] These tumours can usually be distinguished clinically from metastatic neuroblastoma in which multiple cutaneous deposits are present.

Histopathology

Peripheral neuroepitheliomas are composed of sheets of hyperchromatic cells with small amounts of cytoplasm. Rosettes are frequently present and central neurofibrillary material may be seen in the rosettes.[211,212] The tumour cells contain neurosecretory granules and are usually positive for neuron-specific enolase.

Extraskeletal Ewing's tumour has cells which often contain glycogen, but there are no neurosecretory granules or well-developed desmosomes.[213] The cells are negative for S100 protein, desmin and neuron-specific enolase.[214] Merkel cell carcinomas are frequently positive for epithelial membrane antigen and low molecular weight keratin, features not seen usually in peripheral neuroepithelioma.

A final diagnosis can usually be made only after the electron microscopic findings and immunohistochemistry results are correlated.

REFERENCES

Introduction

1. Feigin I. Skin tumors of neural origin. Am J Dermatopathol 1983; 5: 397–399.
2. Erlandson RA, Woodruff JM. Peripheral nerve sheath tumors: an electron microscopic study of 43 cases. Cancer 1982; 49: 273–287.

Nerve sheath tumours

3. Nadji M. Immunoperoxidase techniques II. Application to cutaneous neoplasms. Am J Dermatopathol 1986; 8: 124–129.
3a. Theaker JM, Fletcher CDM. Epithelial membrane antigen expression by the perineurial cell: further studies of peripheral nerve lesions. Histopathology 1989; 14: 581–592.

4. Reed RJ, Fine RM, Meltzer HD. Palisaded, encapsulated neuromas of the skin. Arch Dermatol 1972; 106: 865–870.
5. Mathews GJ, Osterholm JL. Painful traumatic neuromas. Surg Clin North Am 1972; 51: 1313–1324.
6. Reed ML, Jacoby RA. Cutaneous neuroanatomy and neuropathology. Am J Dermatopathol 1983; 5: 335–362.
7. Waggener JD. Ultrastructure of benign peripheral nerve sheath tumors. Cancer 1966; 19: 699–709.
8. Hare PJ. Rudimentary polydactyly. Br J Dermatol 1954; 66: 402–408.
9. Suzuki H, Matsuoka S. Rudimentary polydactyly (cutaneous neuroma) case report with ultrastructural study. J Cutan Pathol 1981; 8: 299–307

10. Shapiro L, Juhlin EA, Brownstein MH. "Rudimentary polydactyly". An amputation neuroma. Arch Dermatol 1973; 108: 223–225.

10a. Fletcher CDM. Solitary circumscribed neuroma of the skin (so-called palisaded, encapsulated neuroma). A clinicopathologic and immunohistochemical study. Am J Surg Pathol 1989; 13: 574–580.

11. Holm TW, Prawer SE, Sahl WJ, Bart BJ. Multiple cutaneous neuromas. Arch Dermatol 1973; 107: 608–610.

11a. Dover JS, From L, Lewis A. Palisaded encapsulated neuromas. A clinicopathologic study. Arch Dermatol 1989; 125: 386–389.

11b. Argenyi ZB. Immunohistochemical characterization of palisading, encapsulated neuroma. J Cutan Pathol 1989; 16: 293 (abstract).

12. Walker DM. Oral mucosal neuroma – medullary thyroid carcinoma syndrome. Br J Dermatol 1973; 88: 599–603.

13. Brown RS, Colle E, Tashjian AH. The syndrome of multiple mucosal neuromas and medullary thyroid carcinoma in childhood. J Pediatr 1975; 86: 77–83.

14. Williams ED, Pollock DJ. Multiple mucosal neuromata with endocrine tumours: a syndrome allied to von Recklinghausen's disease. J Path Bact 1966; 91: 71–80.

15. Ayala F, De Rosa G, Scippa L, Vecchio P. Multiple endocrine neoplasia, type IIb. Report of a case. Dermatologica 1981; 162: 292–299.

16. Gorlin RJ, Sedano HO, Vickers RA, Cervenka J. Multiple mucosal neuromas, pheochromocytoma and medullary carcinoma of the thyroid — a syndrome. Cancer 1968; 22: 293–299.

17. Khairi MRA, Dexter RN, Burzynski NJ, Johnston CC. Mucosal neuroma, pheochromocytoma and medullary thyroid carcinoma: multiple endocrine neoplasia type 3. Medicine (Baltimore) 1975; 54: 89–112.

18. Winkelmann RK, Carney JA. Cutaneous neuropathology in multiple endocrine neoplasia, type 2b. J Invest Dermatol 1982; 79: 307–312.

19. Guillet G, Gauthier Y, Tamisier JM et al. Linear cutaneous neuromas (dermatoneurie en stries): a limited phakomatosis with striated pigmentation corresponding to cutaneous hyperneury (featuring multiple endocrine neoplasia syndrome?). J Cutan Pathol 1987; 14: 43–48.

20. Bolande RP, Towler WF. A possible relationship of neuroblastoma to von Recklinghausen's disease. Cancer 1970; 26: 162–175.

21. Collins J-P, Johnson WC, Burgoon CF. Ganglioneuroma of the skin. Arch Dermatol 1972; 105: 256–258.

22. Geffner RE, Hassell CM. Ganglioneuroma of the skin. Arch Dermatol 1986; 122: 377–378.

22a. Lee JY, Martinez AJ, Abell E. Ganglioneuromatous tumor of the skin: a combined heterotopia of ganglion cells and hamartomatous neuroma: report of a case. J Cutan Pathol 1988; 15: 58–61.

23. White NB. Neurilemomas of the extremities. J Bone Joint Surg 1967; 49-A: 1605–1610.

24. Jacobs RL, Barmada R. Neurilemoma. A review of the literature with six case reports. Arch Surg 1971; 102: 181–186.

25. Berger TG, Lapins NA, Engel ML. Agminated neurilemomas. J Am Acad Dermatol 1987; 17: 891–894.

26. Izumi AK, Rosato FE, Wood MG. Von Recklinghausen's disease associated with multiple neurolemomas. Arch Dermatol 1971; 104: 172–176.

27. Shishiba T, Niimura M, Ohtsuka F, Tsuru N. Multiple cutaneous neurilemmomas as a skin manifestation of neurilemmomatosis. J Am Acad Dermatol 1984; 10: 744–754.

27a. Purcell SM, Dixon SL. Schwannomatosis. An unusual variant of neurofibromatosis or a distinct clinical entity? Arch Dermatol 1989; 125: 390–393.

28. Mercantini ES, Mopper C. Neurilemmoma of the tongue. Arch Dermatol 1959; 79: 542–544.

29. Abell MR, Hart WR, Olson JR. Tumors of the peripheral nervous system. Hum Pathol 1970; 1: 503–551.

30. Phalen GS. Neurilemmomas of the forearm and hand. Clin Orthop 1976; 114: 219–222.

30a. Kao GF, Laskin WB, Olson TG. Solitary cutaneous plexiform neurilemmoma (Schwannoma). J Cutan Pathol 1988; 15: 318 (abstract).

30b. Kawahara E, Oda Y, Ooi A et al. Expression of glial fibrillary acidic protein (GFAP) in peripheral nerve sheath tumors. Am J Surg Pathol 1988; 12: 115–120.

31. Penneys NS, Mogollon R, Kowalczyk A et al. A survey of cutaneous neural lesions for the presence of myelin basic protein. An immunohistochemical study. Arch Dermatol 1984; 120: 210–213.

31a. Gray MH, Rosenberg AE, Dickersin GR, Bhan AK. Glial fibrillary acid protein and keratin expression by benign and malignant nerve sheath tumors. Hum Pathol 1989; 20: 1089–1096.

31b. Theaker JM, Gatter KC, Puddle J. Epithelial membrane antigen expression by the perineurium of peripheral nerve and in peripheral nerve tumours. Histopathology 1988; 13: 171–179.

32. Woodruff JM, Susin M, Godwin TA et al. Cellular schwannoma. A variety of schwannoma sometimes mistaken for a malignant tumor. Am J Surg Pathol 1981; 5: 733–744.

33. Fletcher CDM, Madziwa D, Heyderman E, McKee PH. Benign dermal Schwannoma with glandular elements — true heterology or a local 'organizer' effect? Clin Exp Dermatol 1986; 11: 475–485.

33a. Carney JA. Psammomatous melanotic schwannoma. A distinctive, heritable tumor with special associations, including cardiac myxoma and the Cushing syndrome. Am J Surg Pathol 1990; 14: 206–222.

33b. Killeen RM, Davy CL, Bauserman SC. Melanocytic schwannoma. Cancer 1988; 62: 174–183.

33c. Argenyi ZB, Goodenberger ME, Strauss JS. Congenital neural hamartoma ("fascicular schwannoma"). Am J Dermatopathol 1990; 12: 283–293.

34. Lassmann H, Jurecka W, Lassmann G et al. Different types of benign nerve sheath tumors. Virchows Arch (A) 1977; 375: 197–210.

35. Sian CS, Ryan SF. The ultrastructure of neurilemoma with emphasis on Antoni B tissue. Hum Pathol 1981; 12: 145–160.

36. Riccardi VM. Neurofibromatosis. The importance of localized or otherwise atypical forms. Arch Dermatol 1987; 123: 882–883.

37. Riccardi VM. Von Recklinghausen neurofibromatosis. N Engl J Med 1981; 305: 1617–1627.

38. Riccardi VM. Neurofibromatosis: clinical

heterogeneity. Curr Probl Cancer 1982; 7: 1–35.

38a. Bousema MT, Vuzevski VD, Oranje AP et al. Non-von Recklinghausen's neurofibromatosis resembling a giant pigmented naevus. J Am Acad Dermatol 1989; 20: 358–362.

39. Person JR, Perry HO. Recent advances in the phakomatoses. Int J Dermatol 1978; 17: 1–13.

40. Swapp GH, Main RA. Neurofibromatosis in pregnancy. Br J Dermatol 1973; 80: 431–435.

41. Wasserteil V, Bruce S, Riccardi VM. Non von Recklinghausen's neurofibromatosis presenting as hemifacial neurofibromas and contralateral café au lait spots. J Am Acad Dermatol 1987; 16: 1090–1096.

42. Brasfield RD, Das Gupta TK. Von Recklinghausen's disease: a clinicopathological study. Ann Surg 1972; 175: 86–104.

43. Riccardi VM. Pathophysiology of neurofibromatosis IV. Dermatologic insights into heterogeneity and pathogenesis. J Am Acad Dermatol 1980; 3: 157–166.

44. McCarroll HR. Soft-tissue neoplasms associated with congenital neurofibromatosis. J Bone Joint Surg 1956; 38-A: 717–731.

45. Greene JF Jr, Fitzwater JE, Burgess J. Arterial lesions associated with neurofibromatosis. Am J Clin Pathol 1974; 62: 481–487.

46. Smith WE, Moseley JC. Multiple halo neurofibromas. Arch Dermatol 1976; 112: 987–990.

47. Chaudhuri B, Ronan SG, Manaligod JR. Angiosarcoma arising in a plexiform neurofibroma. A case report. Cancer 1980; 46: 605–610.

48. Knight WA III, Murphy WK, Gottlieb JA. Neurofibromatosis associated with malignant neurofibromas. Arch Dermatol 1973; 107: 747–750.

49. Mastrangelo MJ, Goepp CE, Patel YA, Clark WH Jr. Cutaneous melanoma in a patient with neurofibromatosis. Arch Dermatol 1979; 115: 864–865.

50. Sorensen SA, Mulvihill JJ, Nielsen A. Long-term follow-up of von Recklinghausen neurofibromatosis. Survival and malignant neoplasms. N Engl J Med 1986; 314: 1010–1015.

51. Roth RR, Martines R, James WD. Segmental neurofibromatosis. Arch Dermatol 1987; 123: 917–920.

52. McFadden JP, Logan R, Griffiths WAD. Segmental neurofibromatosis and pruritus. Clin Exp Dermatol 1988; 13: 265–268.

53. Allegue F, Espana A, Fernandez-Garcia JM, Ledo A. Segmental neurofibromatosis with contralateral lentiginosis. Clin Exp Dermatol 1989; 14: 448–450.

54. Sloan JB, Fretzin DF, Boyenmyer DA. Genetic counseling in segmental neurofibromatosis. J Am Acad Dermatol 1990; 22: 461–467.

54a. Jaakkola S, Muona P, James WD et al. Segmental neurofibromatosis: Immunocytochemical analysis of cutaneous lesions. J Am Acad Dermatol 1990; 22: 617–621.

55. Miller RM, Sparkes RS. Segmental neurofibromatosis. Arch Dermatol 1977; 113: 837–838.

56. Oranje AP, Vuzevski VD, Kalis TJ et al. Segmental neurofibromatosis. B J Dermatol 1985; 112: 107–112.

57. Pullara TJ, Greeson JD, Stoker GL, Fenske NA. Cutaneous segmental neurofibromatosis. J Am Acad Dermatol 1985; 13: 999–1003.

58. Garcia RL. Multiple localized neurofibromas. JAMA 1971; 215: 1670.

59. Winkelmann RK, Johnson LA. Cholinesterases in neurofibromas. Arch Dermatol 1962; 85: 106–114.

60. Takiguchi PS, Ratz JL. Bilateral dermatomal neurofibromatosis. J Am Acad Dermatol 1984; 10: 451–453.

61. Nicholls EM. Somatic variation and multiple neurofibromatosis. Hum Hered 1969; 19: 473–479.

62. Rubenstein AE, Bader JL, Aron AA et al. Familial transmission of segmental neurofibromatosis. Neurology 1983; 33 (suppl 2): 76.

63. Johnson MD, Kamso-Pratt J, Federspiel CF, Whetsell WO Jr. Mast cell and lymphoreticular infiltrates in neurofibromas. Comparison with nerve sheath tumors. Arch Pathol Lab Med 1989; 113: 1263–1270.

64. Gray MH, Smoller BR, McNutt NS, Hsu A. Immunohistochemical demonstration of factor XIIIa expression in neurofibromas. Arch Dermatol 1990; 126: 472–476.

65. Jurecka W. Plexiforme neurofibroma of the skin. Am J Dermatopathol 1988; 10: 209–217.

66. Henkes J, Ferrandiz C, Peyri J, Fontarnau R. Pilar dysplasia overlying two neurofibromas of the scalp. J Cutan Pathol 1984; 11: 65–70.

67. Slater C, Hayes M, Saxe N et al. Macromelanosomes in the early diagnosis of neurofibromatosis. Am J Dermatopathol 1986; 8: 284–289.

68. Silvers DN, Greenwood RS, Helwig EB. Café au lait spots without giant pigment granules. Occurrence in suspected neurofibromatosis. Arch Dermatol 1974; 110: 87–88.

69. Jimbow K, Horikoshi T. The nature and significance of macromelanosomes in pigmented skin lesions. Am J Dermatopathol 1982; 4: 413–420.

70. Bale PM. Sacrococcygeal paciniomas. Pathology 1980; 12: 231–235.

71. Prose PH, Gherardi GJ, Coblenz A. Pacinian neurofibroma. Arch Dermatol 1957; 76: 65–69.

72. Fletcher CDM, Theaker JM. Digital Pacinian neuroma: a distinctive hyperplastic lesion. Histopathology 1989; 15: 249–256.

73. Bennin B, Barsky S, Salgia K. Pacinian neurofibroma. Arch Dermatol 1976; 112: 1558.

74. McCormack K, Kaplan D, Murray JC, Fetter BF. Multiple hairy pacinian neurofibromas (nerve-sheath myxomas). J Am Acad Dermatol 1988; 18: 416–419.

75. Levi L, Curri SB. Multiple Pacinian neurofibroma and relationship with the finger-tip arterio-venous anastamoses. Br J Dermatol 1980; 102: 345–349.

76. MacDonald DM, Wilson Jones E. Pacinian neurofibroma. Histopathology 1977; 1: 247–255.

77. Angervall L, Kindblom L-G, Haglid K. Dermal nerve sheath myxoma. A light and electron microscopic, histochemical and immunohistochemical study. Cancer 1984; 53: 1752–1759.

78. King DT, Barr RJ. Bizarre cutaneous neurofibromas. J Cutan Pathol 1980; 7: 21–31.

79. Gallagher RL, Helwig EB. Neurothekeoma — a benign cutaneous tumor of neural origin. Am J Clin Pathol 1980; 74: 759–764.

80. Holden CA, Wilson-Jones E, MacDonald DM. Cutaneous lobular neuromyxoma. Br J Dermatol 1982; 106: 211–215.

81. Pulitzer DR, Reed RJ. Nerve-sheath myxoma (perineurial myxoma). Am J Dermatopathol 1985; 7: 409–421.

82. Fletcher CDM, Chan J K-C, McKee PH. Dermal nerve sheath myxoma: a study of three cases. Histopathology 1986; 10: 135–145.

83. Tuthill RJ. Nerve-sheath myxoma: a case report with immunohistologic evidence of its perineurial cell origin. J Cutan Pathol 1988; 15: 348 (abstract).

84. Goldstein L, Lifshitz T. Myxoma of the nerve sheath. Am J Dermatopathol 1985; 7: 423–429.

85. Aronson PJ, Fretzin DF, Potter BS. Neurothekeoma of Gallager and Helwig (dermal nerve sheath myxoma variant): report of a case with electron microscopic and immunohistochemical studies. J Cutan Pathol 1985; 12: 506–519.

86. Barnhill RL, Mihm MC Jr. Cellular neurothekeoma. A distinctive variant of neurothekeoma mimicking nevomelanocytic tumors. Am J Surg Pathol 1990; 14: 113–120.

87. Goette DK. Calcifying neurothekeoma. J Dermatol Surg Oncol 1986; 12: 958–960.

88. Weiser G. An electron microscope study of "Pacinian neurofibroma". Virchows Arch (A) 1975; 366: 331–340.

89. Webb JN. The histogenesis of nerve sheath myxoma: report of a case with electron microscopy. J Pathol 1979; 127: 35–37.

90. Bird CC, Willis RA. The histogenesis of pigmented neurofibromas. J Pathol 1969; 97: 631–637.

91. Williamson DM, Suggit RIC. Pigmented neurofibroma. Br J Dermatol 1977; 97: 685–688.

92. Apisarnthanarax P. Granular cell tumor. An analysis of 16 cases and review of the literature. J Am Acad Dermatol 1981; 5: 171–182.

93. Lack EE, Worsham GF, Callihan MD et al. Granular cell tumor: a clinicopathologic study of 110 patients. J Surg Oncol 1980; 13: 301–316.

94. Peterson LJ. Granular-cell tumor. Review of the literature and report of a case. Oral Surg 1974; 37: 728–735.

95. Khansur T, Balducci L, Tavassoli M. Granular cell tumor. Clinical spectrum of the benign and malignant entity. Cancer 1987; 60: 220–222.

96. Apted JH. Multiple granular-cell myoblastoma (Schwannoma) in a child. Br J Dermatol 1968; 80: 257–260.

97. Price ML, MacDonald DM. Multiple granular cell tumour. Clin Exp Dermatol 1984; 9: 375–378.

98. Papageorgiou S, Litt JZ, Pomeranz JR. Multiple granular cell myoblastomas in children. Arch Dermatol 1967; 96: 168–171.

99. Goette DK, Olson EG. Multiple cutaneous granular cell tumors. Int J Dermatol 1982; 21: 271–272.

100. Noppakun N, Apisarnthanarax P. Multiple cutaneous granular cell tumors simulating prurigo nodularis. Int J Dermatol 1981; 20: 126–129.

101. Seo IS, Azzarelli B, Warner TF et al. Multiple visceral and cutaneous granular cell tumors. Ultrastructural and immunocytochemical evidence of Schwann cell origin. Cancer 1984; 53: 2104–2110.

102. Lack EE, Crawford BE, Worsham GF et al. Gingival granular cell tumors of the newborn (congenital 'epulis'). Am J Surg Pathol 1981; 5: 37–46.

103. de la Monte SM, Radowsky M, Hood AF. Congenital granular-cell neoplasms. An unusual case report with ultrastructural findings and a review of the literature. Am J Dermatopathol 1986; 8: 57–63.

104. Gamboa LG. Malignant granular-cell myoblastoma.

105. Cadotte M. Malignant granular-cell myoblastoma. Cancer 1974; 33: 1417–1422.

106. Robertson AJ, McIntosh W, Lamont P, Guthrie W. Malignant granular cell tumour (myoblastoma) of the vulva: report of a case and review of the literature. Histopathology 1981; 5: 69–79.

107. Klima M, Peters J. Malignant granular cell tumor. Arch Pathol Lab Med 1987; 111: 1070–1073.

108. Thunold S, von Eyben FE, Maehle B. Malignant granular cell tumour of the neck: immunohistochemical and ultrastructural studies of a case. Histopathology 1989; 14: 655–657.

109. Finkel G, Lane B. Granular cell variant of neurofibromatosis: ultrastructure of benign and malignant tumors. Hum Pathol 1982; 13: 959–963.

110. Buley ID, Gatter KC, Kelly PMA et al. Granular cell tumours revisited. An immunohistological and ultrastructural study. Histopathology 1988; 12: 263–274.

111. Penneys NS, Adachi K, Ziegels-Weissman J, Nadji M. Granular cell tumors of the skin contain myelin basic protein. Arch Pathol Lab Med 1983; 107: 302–303.

112. Lack EE, Perez-Atayde AR, McGill TJ, Vawter GF. Gingival granuloma cell tumor of the newborn (congenital "epulis"): ultrastructural observations relating to histogenesis. Hum Pathol 1982; 13: 686–689.

113. Sobel HJ, Marquet E, Schwarz R. Is schwannoma related to granular cell myoblastoma? Arch Pathol 1973; 95: 396–401.

114. Alkek DS, Johnson WC, Graham JH. Granular cell myoblastoma. A histological and enzymatic study. Arch Dermatol 1968; 98: 543–547.

115. McMahon JN, Rigby HS, Davies JD. Elastosis in granular cell tumours: prevalence and distribution. Histopathology 1990; 16: 37–41.

116. Stefansson K, Wollmann RL. S-100 protein in granular cell tumors (granular cell myoblastomas). Cancer 1982; 49: 1834–1838.

117. Armin A, Connelly EM, Rowden G. An immunoperoxidase investigation of S-100 protein in granular cell myoblastomas: evidence for Schwann cell derivation. Am J Clin Pathol 1983; 79: 37–44.

118. Raju GC, O'Reilly AP. Immunohistochemical study of granular cell tumour. Pathology 1987; 19: 402–406.

119. Kanitakis J, Mauduit G, Viac J, Thivolet J. [Granular cell tumour (Abrikosoff). Immunohistological study of four cases with review of the literature]. Ann Dermatol Venereol 1985; 112: 871–876.

120. Ingram DL, Mossler JA, Snowhite J et al. Granular cell tumors of the breast. Arch Pathol Lab Med 1984; 108: 897–901.

121. Matthews JB, Mason GI. Granular cell myoblastoma: an immunoperoxidase study using a variety of antisera to human carcinoembryonic antigen. Histopathology 1983; 7: 77–82.

122. Kanitakis J, Zambruno G, Viac J, Thivolet J. Granular-cell tumours of the skin do not express carcino-embryonic antigen. J Cutan Pathol 1986; 13: 370–374.

123. Manara GC, De Panfilis G, Bottazzi Bacchi A et al. Fine structure of granular cell tumor of Abrikossoff. J Cutan Pathol 1981; 8: 277–282.

124. Chrestian MA, Gambarelli D, Hassoun J et al. Granular cell myoblastoma. J Cutan Pathol 1977; 4: 80–89.

Arch Pathol 1955; 60: 663–668.

125. Storm FK, Eilber FR, Mirra J, Morton DL. Neurofibrosarcoma. Cancer 1980; 45: 126–129.
126. Dabski C, Reiman HM Jr, Muller SA. Neurofibrosarcoma of skin and subcutaneous tissues. Mayo Clin Proc 1990; 65: 164–172.
127. Das Gupta TK, Brasfield RD. Solitary malignant schwannoma. Ann Surg 1970; 171: 419–428.
128. Robson DK, Ironside JW. Malignant peripheral nerve sheath tumour arising in a schwannoma. Histopathology 1990; 16: 295–308.
129. Trojanowski JQ, Kleinman GM, Proppe KH. Malignant tumors of nerve sheath origin. Cancer 1980; 46: 1202–1212.
130. George E, Swanson PE, Wick MR. Malignant peripheral nerve sheath tumors of the skin. Am J Dermatopathol 1989; 11: 213–221.
131. Mogollon R, Penneys N, Albores-Saavedra J, Nadji M. Malignant schwannoma presenting as a skin mass. Cancer 1984; 53: 1190–1193.
132. Sordillo PP, Helson L, Hadju SI et al. Malignant Schwannoma — clinical characteristics, survival, and response to therapy. Cancer 1981; 47: 2503–2509.
133. Ghosh BC, Ghosh L, Huvos AG, Fortner JG. Malignant schwannoma. A clinicopathologic study. Cancer 1973; 31: 184–190.
134. Taxy JB, Battifora H, Trujillo Y, Dorfman HD. Electron microscopy in the diagnosis of malignant schwannoma. Cancer 1981; 48: 1381–1391.
135. Di Carlo EF, Woodruff JM, Bansal M, Erlandson RA. The purely epithelioid malignant peripheral nerve sheath tumor. Am J Surg Pathol 1986; 10: 478–490.
136. Suster S, Amazon K, Rosen LB, Ollague JM. Malignant epithelioid schwannoma of the skin. A low-grade neurotropic malignant melanoma? Am J Dermatopathol 1989; 11: 338–344.
137. Ducatman BS, Scheithauer BW. Malignant peripheral nerve sheath tumors with divergent differentiation. Cancer 1984; 54: 1049–1057.
138. Daimaru Y, Hashimoto H, Enjoji M. Malignant 'triton' tumors: a clinicopathologic and immunohistochemical study of nine cases. Hum Pathol 1984; 15: 768–778.
139. Markel SF, Enzinger FM. Neuromuscular hamartoma: A benign "Triton tumor" composed of mature neural and striated muscle elements. Cancer 1982; 49: 140–144.

Herniations and ectopias

140. Fletcher CDM, Carpenter G, McKee PH. Nasal glioma. A rarity. Am J Dermatopathol 1986; 8: 341–346.
141. Kopf AW, Bart RS. Nasal glioma. J Dermatol Surg Oncol 1978; 4: 128–130.
142. Lowe RS, Robinson DW, Ketchum LD, Masters FW. Nasal gliomata. Plast Reconstr Surg 1971; 47: 1–5.
143. Berry AD, Patterson JW, Meningoceles, meningomyeloceles and encephaloceles: a neurodermatopathologic study of 132 cases. J Cutan Pathol 1991; 18: 164–177.
144. Commens C, Rogers M, Kan A. Heterotopic brain tissue presenting as bald cysts with a collar of hypertrophic hair. The 'hair collar' sign. Arch Dermatol 1989; 125: 1253–1256.
145. Orkin M, Fisher I. Heterotopic brain tissue (heterotopic neural rest). Arch Dermatol 1966; 94: 699–708.
146. Musser AW, Campbell R. Nasal glioma. Arch Otolaryngol 1961; 73: 732–736.
147. Gebhart W, Hohlbrugger H, Lassmann H, Ramadan W. Nasal glioma. Int J Dermatol 1982; 21: 212–215.
148. Christianson HB. Nasal glioma. Arch Dermatol 1966; 93: 68–70.
149. Mirra SS, Pearl GS, Hoffman JC, Campbell WG. Nasal 'glioma' with prominent neuronal component. Arch Pathol Lab Med 1981; 105: 540–541.
150. Lee CM, McLaurin RL. Heterotopic brain tissue as an isolated embryonic rest. J Neurosurg 1955; 12: 190–195.
151. Theaker JM, Fleming KA. Meningioma of the scalp: a case report with immunohistological features. J Cutan Pathol 1987; 14: 49–53.
151a. Theaker JM, Fletcher CDM, Tudway AJ. Cutaneous heterotopic meningeal nodules. Histopathology 1990; 16: 475–479.
152. Nochomovitz LE, Jannotta F, Orenstein JM. Meningioma of the scalp. Light and electron microscopic observations. Arch Pathol Lab Med 1985; 109: 92–95.
153. Lopez DA, Silvers DN, Helwig EB. Cutaneous meningiomas — a clinicopathologic study. Cancer 1974; 34: 728–744.
154. Sibley DA, Cooper PH. Rudimentary meningocele: a variant of "primary cutaneous meningioma". J Cutan Pathol 1989; 16: 72–80.
155. Umbert I, Nasarre J, Rovira E, Umbert P. Cutaneous meningioma: Report of a case with immunohistochemical study. J Cutan Pathol 1989; 16: 328 (abstract).
156. Suster S, Rosai J. Hamartoma of the scalp with ectopic meningothelial elements. A distinctive benign soft tissue lesion that may simulate angiosarcoma. Am J Surg Pathol 1990; 14: 1–11.

Neuroendocrine carcinomas

157. Toker C. Trabecular carcinoma of the skin. Arch Dermatol 1972; 105: 107–110.
158. Tang C-K, Toker C. Trabecular carcinoma of the skin. An ultrastructural study. Cancer 1978; 42: 2311–2321.
159. Rocamora A, Badia N, Vives R et al. Epidermotropic primary neuroendocrine (Merkel cell) carcinoma of the skin with Pautrier-like microabscesses. Report of three cases and review of the literature. J Am Acad Dermatol 1987; 16: 1163–1168.
160. Hoefler H, Rauch H-J, Kerl H, Denk H. New immunocytochemical observations with diagnostic significance in cutaneous neuroendocrine carcinoma. Am J Dermatopathol 1984; 6: 525–530.
161. Wick MR, Scheithauer BW. In: Wick MR. Pathology of unusual malignant cutaneous tumors. New York: Marcel Dekker, 1985; 107–180.
162. Sibley RK, Dehner LP, Rosai J. Primary neuroendocrine (Merkel cell?) carcinoma of the skin. I. A clinicopathologic and ultrastructural study of 43 cases. Am J Surg Pathol 1985; 9: 95–108.
163. Wick MR, Thomas JR, Scheithauer BW, Jackson IT. Multifocal Merkel's cell tumors associated with a cutaneous dysplasia syndrome. Arch Dermatol 1983; 119: 409–414.

164. Moya CE, Guarda LA, Dyer GA et al. Neuroendocrine carcinoma of the skin in a young adult. Am J Clin Pathol 1982; 78: 783–785.

165. Pilotti S, Rilke F, Lombardi L. Neuroendocrine (Merkel cell) carcinoma of the skin. Am J Dermatopathol 1982; 6: 243–254.

166. Tyring SK, Lee PC, Omura EF et al. Recurrent and metastatic cutaneous neuroendocrine (Merkel cell) carcinoma mimicking angiosarcoma. Arch Dermatol 1987; 123: 1368–1370.

167. Raaf JH, Urmacher C, Knapper WK et al. Trabecular (Merkel cell) carcinoma of the skin. Treatment of primary, recurrent, and metastatic disease. Cancer 1986; 57: 178–182.

168. Hanke CW, Conner AC, Temofeew RK, Lingeman RE. Merkel cell carcinoma. Arch Dermatol 1989; 125: 1096–1100.

169. O'Rourke MGE, Bell JR. Merkel cell tumor with spontaneous regression. J Dermatol Surg Oncol 1986; 12: 994–997.

170. Rustin MHA, Chambers TJ, Levison DA, Munro DD. Merkel cell tumour: report of a case. Br J Dermatol 1983; 108: 711–715.

171. Silva EG, Ordonez NG, Lechago J. Immunohistochemical studies in endocrine carcinoma of the skin. Am J Clin Pathol 1984; 81: 558–562.

172. Frigerio B, Capella C, Eusebi V et al. Merkel cell carcinoma of the skin: the structure and origin of normal Merkel cells. Histopathology 1983; 7: 229–249.

173. Leong A S-Y, Phillips GE, Pieterse AS, Milios J. Criteria for the diagnosis of primary endocrine carcinoma of the skin (Merkel cell carcinoma). A histological, immunohistochemical and ultrastructural study of 13 cases. Pathology 1986; 18: 393–399.

174. Warner TFCS, Uno H, Hafez GR et al. Merkel cells and Merkel cell tumors. Ultrastructure, immunocytochemistry and review of the literature. Cancer 1983; 52: 238–245.

175. Schnitt SJ, Wang H, Dvorak AM. Morphologic changes in primary neuroendocrine carcinoma of the skin following radiation therapy. Hum Pathol 1986; 17: 198–201.

176. Zak FG, Lawson W, Statsinger AL et al. Intracellular amyloid in trabecular (Merkel cell) carcinoma of the skin: ultrastructural study. Mt. Sinai J Med 1982; 49: 46–54.

177. Abaci IF, Zac FG. Multicentric amyloid containing cutaneous trabecular carcinoma. Case report with ultrastructural study. J Cutan Pathol 1979; 6: 292–303.

178. Kroll MH, Toker C. Trabecular carcinoma of the skin. Arch Pathol Lab Med 1982; 106: 404–408.

179. Tang C-K, Nedwich A, Toker C, Zaman ANF. Unusual cutaneous carcinoma with features of small cell (oat cell-like) and squamous cell carcinomas. A variant of malignant Merkel cell neoplasm. Am J Dermatopathol 1982; 4: 537–548.

180. Gomez LG, Silva EG, Di Maio S, Mackay B. Association between neuroendocrine (Merkel cell) carcinoma and squamous carcinoma of the skin. Am J Surg Pathol 1983; 7: 171–177.

181. Layfield L, Ulich T, Liao S et al. Neuroendocrine carcinoma of the skin: an immunohistochemical study of tumor markers and neuroendocrine products. J Cutan Pathol 1986; 13: 268–273.

182. Gould E, Albores-Saavedra J, Dubner B et al. Eccrine and squamous differentiation in Merkel cell carcinoma. An immunohistochemical study. Am J Surg Pathol 1988; 12: 768–772.

183. Perse RM, Klappenbach S, Ragsdale BD. Trabecular (Merkel cell) carcinoma arising in the wall of an epidermal cyst. Am J Dermatopathol 1987; 9: 423–427.

184. Wick MR, Kaye VN, Sibley RK et al. Primary neuroendocrine carcinoma and small-cell malignant lymphoma of the skin. A discriminant immunohistochemical comparison. J Cutan Pathol 1986; 13: 347–358.

185. Wick MR, Millns JL, Sibley RK et al. Secondary neuroendocrine carcinomas of the skin. J Am Acad Dermatol 1985; 13: 134–142.

186. Hall PA, D'Ardenne AJ, Butler MG et al. Cytokeratin and laminin immunostaining in the diagnosis of cutaneous neuroendocrine (Merkel cell) tumours. Histopathology 1986; 10: 1179–1190.

187. Dreno B, Mousset S, Stalder JF et al. A study of intermediate filaments (cytokeratin, vimentin, neurofilament) in two cases of Merkel cell tumor. J Cutan Pathol 1985; 12: 37–45.

188. Tazawa T, Ito M, Okuda C, Sato Y. Immunohistochemical demonstration of simple epithelia-type keratin intermediate filament in a case of Merkel cell carcinoma. Arch Dermatol 1987; 123: 489–492.

189. Szadowska A, Wozniak L, Lasota J et al. Neuroendocrine (Merkel cell) carcinoma of the skin: a clinicomorphological study of 13 cases. Histopathology 1989; 15: 483–493.

190. Heenan PJ, Cole JM, Spagnolo DV. Primary cutaneous neuroendocrine carcinoma (Merkel cell tumor). An adnexal epithelial neoplasm. Am J Dermatopathol 1990; 12: 7–16.

191. Sibley RK, Dahl D. Primary neuroendocrine (Merkel cell?) carcinoma of the skin. II. An immunocytochemical study of 21 cases. Am J Surg Pathol 1985; 9: 109–116.

192. Battifora H, Silva EG. The use of antikeratin antibodies in the immunohistochemical distinction between neuroendocrine (Merkel cell) carcinoma of the skin, lymphoma, and oat cell carcinoma. Cancer 1986; 58: 1040–1046.

193. Johannessen JV, Gould VE. Neuroendocrine skin carcinoma associated with calcitonin production: a Merkel cell carcinoma? Hum Pathol 1980; 11: 586–589.

194. Drijkoningen M, De Wolf-Peeters C, van Limbergen E, Desmet V. Merkel cell tumor of the skin. An immunohistochemical study. Hum Pathol 1986; 17: 301–307.

195. Sibley RK, Rosai J, Foucar E et al. Neuroendocrine (Merkel cell) carcinoma of the skin. A histologic and ultrastructural study of two cases. Am J Surg Pathol 1980; 4: 211–221.

196. Haneke E. Electron microscopy of Merkel cell carcinoma from formalin-fixed tissue. J Am Acad Dermatol 1985; 12: 487–492.

197. Kirkham N, Isaacson P. Merkel cell carcinoma: a report of three cases with neurone-specific enolase activity. Histopathology 1983; 7: 251–259.

TELANGIECTASES

In this group, the vascular channels of which the lesion is composed are predominantly pre-existing blood vessels which have undergone dilatation. The entity known as calibre-persistent artery is included with the telangiectases for convenience.

'PORT WINE' STAIN

This abnormality, also known as naevus flammeus, is present at birth in 0.3% of children.[1a] Although any area may be affected, it occurs most frequently on the face and neck. Single or multiple lesions may be present and they are often sharply unilateral or segmental. Small or extensive areas of skin may be involved. At birth, the lesions are flat and light pink in colour. Unlike the 'salmon' patch (see below), the lesions do not usually fade, but with time become darker and raised, with a rough irregular surface. There is proportional enlargement with the growth of the child.

Histopathology

Initially there is a barely detectable dilatation of the thin-walled vessels of the superficial vascular plexus. Progressive ectasia occurs and there is obvious erythrocyte stasis.[2] There is no significant increase in thickness or number of vessels, with age, in typical superficial lesions. In some cases there is an underlying cavernous haemangioma which may blend with the superficial lesion. Localized exaggeration of the vascular ectasia produces the roughened surface of the older lesions.[3] Secondary angiomatous lesions and pyogenic granulomas may occur within the main lesion.

One study has shown that the lesions are produced by dilatations of post-capillary venules of the superficial horizontal plexus with no evidence of new vessel formation. The walls of the venules are thickened by basement-membrane-like material and reticulin fibres.[4] Progressive dilatation does not appear to be related to decreased fibronectin or type IV collagen in the vessel walls.[5] A decreased nerve density has been demonstrated within affected areas and it has been proposed that abnormal neural control of blood flow may be important in the pathogenesis of this lesion.[6]

Associated clinical syndromes

Sturge–Weber syndrome (encephalotrigeminal angiomatosis). The essential components of this syndrome are:

a) a unilateral facial 'port wine' stain which includes that area of skin supplied by the ophthalmic branch of the trigeminal nerve (forehead and upper eyelid);
b) an ipsilateral vascular abnormality of the leptomeninges; and
c) an ipsilateral vascular abnormality of the choroid of the eye.[7]

The 'port wine' stain may be associated with only one of the other components of the syndrome.

Klippel–Trenaunay–Weber syndrome (angio-osteohypertrophy). The literature on this syndrome is somewhat confusing. However, the major elements are a 'port wine' stain, usually on a limb, associated with varicose veins and limb overgrowth. In some cases, there is a haemodynamically significant arteriovenous fistula.[8] Capillary and cavernous haemangiomas may also be present.[9] There are many incomplete forms of this syndrome and, in one large series, a 'port wine' stain was present in only 32% of cases.[10]

Cobb's syndrome. In this syndrome, there is a 'port wine' stain (or another vascular lesion) on the trunk or limb in a dermatomal distribution, corresponding to a segment of the spinal cord in which there is an arteriovenous or venous haemangioma.[11]

'SALMON' PATCH

The 'salmon' patch (naevus flammeus, erythema

nuchae, naevus simplex) is a pink macular area present at birth in approximately 40% of the population. The nape of the neck, the eyelids or the skin over the glabella may be involved.[12] In the majority of cases the lesions fade in the first year of life.[12] There are usually no associated congenital abnormalities.[13] In a small number of cases, the condition persists for life, particularly a lesion in the nuchal region.

Histopathology

The lesions are characterized by ectatic capillaries in the superficial plexus.

'SPIDER' NAEVUS

One or more 'spider' naevi are present in 10–15% of normal adults.[14] The face, neck, upper part of the trunk and arms are the regions usually involved; it is very uncommon for lesions to occur below the level of the umbilicus. There is a higher incidence in pregnant women and in patients with chronic liver disease. Lesions may regress following the pregnancy. In children, 'spider' naevi tend to arise on the hands and fingers.[15]

'Spider' naevi consist of a central punctum within a generally circular area of erythema. Fine branching vessels or 'legs' radiate from the punctum.

Histopathology

These lesions are rarely biopsied or excised. They consist of a central, ascending, spiral, thick-walled arteriole which ends in a thin-walled ampulla just beneath the epidermis. From the ampulla, thin-walled, branching channels radiate peripherally in the papillary dermis. Glomus cells have been described in the wall of the central arteriole.[14]

VENOUS LAKE

Venous lakes are dark blue, often multiple, papules a few millimetres in diameter, which occur on the ears, face, lips or neck of the elderly.[16] Minor trauma to the lesions may produce persistent bleeding.

The lesions reported as *capillary aneurysms* probably represent venous lakes.[17] The clinical similarity of these lesions to malignant melanomas has been highlighted, particularly if thrombosis of the vascular lumen occurs.

Histopathology

Usually only a single, large, dilated vascular channel is present, in the upper dermis (Fig. 38.1). It has a very thin fibrous wall and a flat endothelial lining. A thrombus is sometimes present in the lumen or part thereof. These lesions appear to represent a dilated segment of a vein or venule.[16]

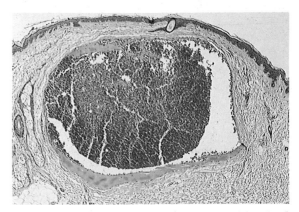

Fig. 38.1 Venous lake. There is a solitary, large, vascular channel in the upper dermis.
Haematoxylin — eosin

ANGIOKERATOMA

The angiokeratoma is characterized by ectasia of superficial dermal blood vessels with associated epidermal changes. Five clinical variants have been recognized: all have similar histopathological features.[18] The variants are discussed below:

1. The *Mibelli type* develops in childhood and adolescence with warty lesions over the bony prominences of the hands, feet, elbows and

knees.[18,19] It is more common in females and it may be associated with pernio.

2. The *Fordyce (scrotal) type* arises as early as the second and third decades but is seen most commonly in elderly men.[20,21] The penis, upper part of the thighs and lower part of the abdomen may also be involved. The lesions are single or multiple, red to black papules, occurring along the course of the superficial scrotal vessels. Scrotal angiokeratomas may be associated with varicoceles, inguinal hernias and thrombophlebitis.[20] Spontaneous regression has been reported following the surgical treatment of an associated varicocele.[22]

An equivalent lesion occurs on the vulva in young adult females. Increased venous pressure associated with pregnancy, vulval varicosities and haemorrhoids has been implicated in the pathogenesis of the vulval lesions.[23] An association with the contraceptive pill has also been suggested.[24]

3. *Solitary and multiple types* occur on any part of the body, but the lower extremities are most commonly affected. In one series, the lesions were solitary in 83% of cases and multiple in 17%.[18]

4. *Angiokeratoma circumscriptum* is the least common variant. It consists either of a plaque composed of small discrete papules or of variable hyperkeratotic papules and nodules with a tendency to confluence.[25] Lesions are almost always unilateral and they occur predominantly on the leg, trunk or arm. They develop in infancy or childhood, predominantly in females.

5. *Angiokeratoma corporis diffusum* consists of multiple papules, frequently in clusters, and usually in a bathing-trunk distribution. Originally thought to be synonymous with Anderson–Fabry disease, it is now evident that this vascular lesion may occur in association with other enzyme disorders and also in people with normal enzyme activity (see p. 521).[26] Anderson–Fabry disease is an X-linked recessive disorder characterized by a deficiency of the lysosomal enzyme α-galactosidase A and the accumulation of the neutral glycolipid ceramide trihexidose in lysosomes in many types of cell. Homozygous male patients generally, but not always, develop the lesions of the disease.[27] The

eruption is usually present by adult life; it is often absent or slight in childhood.[28] Females with the genetic abnormality may also develop the lesion but this occurs in less than 25% of cases.[28] Other enzyme deficiencies associated with angiokeratoma corporis diffusum include α-L-fucosidase deficiency (fucosidosis; see p. 523), β-galactosidase deficiency (see p. 523) and neuraminidase deficiency (see p. 523).[29,30]

Histopathology

In angiokeratomas there is marked dilatation of papillary dermal vessels to form large cavernous channels. There is associated irregular acanthosis of the epidermis with elongation of the rete ridges which partially or completely enclose the vascular channels (Fig. 38.2). A collarette may be formed at the margins of the lesions and there may be thrombosis of the vessels. The surface epidermis may show varying degrees of hyper-

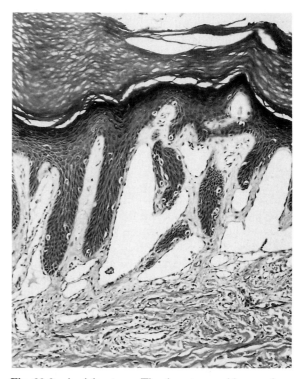

Fig. 38.2 Angiokeratoma. The elongate rete ridges partly surround the vascular channels in the papillary dermis. Haematoxylin — eosin

keratosis. The presence of a deep dermal haem-angioma has been reported in association with angiokeratoma circumscriptum.[25] This combination may represent a verrucous haemangioma. In patients with Anderson–Fabry disease there is vacuolation of smooth muscle in arterioles and arteries and in the arrectores pilorum. Frozen sections of lesions may show PAS-positive and Sudan-black-positive granules in endothelial cells, pericytes, arrectores pilorum and eccrine sweat glands.

Electron microscopy. Examination of lesions or of normal skin from patients with Anderson–Fabry disease shows electron-dense lipid bodies in the cytoplasm which are either membrane-bound or free in the endothelial cells, pericytes, smooth muscle cells and fibroblasts. These bodies may show a characteristic lamellar pattern. They are not seen in the other types of angiokeratoma or in the lesions in cases of angiokeratoma corporis diffusum with normal enzyme activities.[26]

The ultrastructure of the vessels in scrotal angiokeratomas and in Anderson–Fabry disease is similar to that of the small valve-containing collecting veins at the junction of the dermis and subcutaneous fat.[4] The possible role of raised intravenous pressure in the formation of scrotal and vulval angiokeratomas has been mentioned. It has been suggested that the lesions in Anderson–Fabry disease may follow weakening of vessel walls and subsequent dilatation, the result of lysosomal storage of lipid and consequent cellular damage.[31]

'CHERRY' ANGIOMA

'Cherry' angiomas (senile angioma, Campbell de Morgan spots) are very common single or multiple bright red papules, up to a few millimetres in diameter, which occur predominantly on the trunk and proximal parts of the limbs. There is typically a pallid halo surrounding the lesions. Rare before puberty, the incidence rises sharply in the fourth decade, such that they are almost universal in old age.[32]

Histopathology

In small early lesions, one or more dilated inter-connecting thin-walled vascular channels are present in the dermal papillae. In older lesions there is loss of rete ridges and atrophy of the superficial epidermis with formation of a poly-poid lesion composed of a network of dilated communicating channels with scant intervening connective tissue (Fig. 38.3). A collarette may be present at the periphery of the lesions.

These lesions appear to be the dilated and interconnected segments of venous capillaries and post-capillary venules in the dermal papillae. The vessels of the upper horizontal plexus are not involved.[4] The non-replicating nature of the endothelial cells comprising these lesions indicates that they are probably not true neoplasms.[32a] The high incidence of these lesions in old age suggests that their occurrence is an age-related degenerative phenomenon.

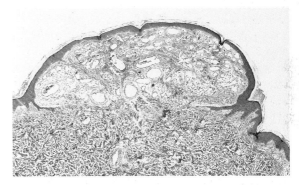

Fig. 38.3 'Cherry angioma'. This polypoid lesion is composed of dilated vascular channels and scant intervening stroma. A collarette is present at the periphery. Haematoxylin — eosin

ANGIOMA SERPIGINOSUM

In this rare condition, multiple pin-sized vascular puncta occur either singly or in clusters on any part of the body except mucous membranes and the palms and soles.[33] The legs are the most common site. Lesions appear before puberty and progress by the development of further puncta at the periphery of the involved area. The lesions do not regress. Females are more commonly affected and a familial grouping of cases has been reported.[34]

Histopathology

Microscopic examination shows single or grouped, ectatic, congested, thin-walled capillaries in the papillary dermis. Thick-walled capillaries and downgrowth of the rete ridges between groups of vessels have also been described.[35,36] The latter lesions resemble angiokeratomas. Although this is generally regarded as a telangiectatic process, an element of vascular proliferation has also been suggested.[35]

HEREDITARY HAEMORRHAGIC TELANGIECTASIA

In this condition, also known as Osler–Rendu–Weber disease, multiple punctate telangiectases occur in the skin and mucous membranes. The respiratory tract, gastrointestinal tract and urinary tract may be involved.[37] Nasal mucosa, lips, mouth and face are frequently affected and epistaxis is the most common presenting symptom. Although lesions may be present in childhood, they do not usually appear until puberty. Fibrovascular abnormalities of the liver, cerebral arteriovenous fistulae and pulmonary arteriovenous fistulae are associated abnormalities.[38-40] Inheritance is by an autosomal dominant trait.

Histopathology

Within the dermal papillae there are dilated thin-walled vessels lined by a single layer of endothelium. Ultrastructural studies have shown these to be venules.[41] Abnormalities in the endothelial lining have also been reported.[42]

GENERALIZED ESSENTIAL TELANGIECTASIA

Telangiectatic macules and diffuse erythematous areas likewise composed of a fine meshwork of ectatic vessels are seen in this condition, which occurs most frequently in women. Lesions appear first on the lower extremities and spread gradually to involve the trunk and arms.[43]

Histopathology

Thin-walled vascular channels are found in the upper dermis. They are produced by dilatation of post-capillary venules of the upper horizontal plexus (Fig. 38.4).[4]

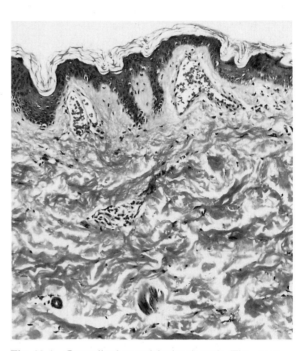

Fig. 38.4 Generalized essential telangiectasia. The upper dermis contains dilated and congested vessels. Haematoxylin — eosin

HEREDITARY BENIGN TELANGIECTASIA

This disorder is inherited as an autosomal dominant trait. It is characterized by widespread cutaneous telangiectases which commonly appear in childhood. Many lesions resemble spider naevi. There are no systemic vascular lesions associated with this form of telangiectasia.[43a,43b]

UNILATERAL DERMATOMAL SUPERFICIAL TELANGIECTASIA

The telangiectases in this condition have a dermatomal distribution and particularly involve the trigeminal and the third and fourth cervical and adjacent dermatomes.[44] The lesions may be present at birth or they may develop at times of physiological or pathological oestrogen excess, including puberty and pregnancy in females, and chronic liver disease.[45] Increased numbers of receptors for oestrogen and progesterone have been reported in the lesional area compared with normal skin.[46]

ATAXIA-TELANGIECTASIA

Telangiectases are a constant but clinically unimportant part of this syndrome, which is also known as Louis-Bar's syndrome.[47] Telangiectases appear in childhood in the bulbar conjunctiva and in the skin of the face, pinnae, neck and limbs. These changes are followed by progressive cerebellar ataxia from cerebellar cortical atrophy. Profound dysfunction of both cell-mediated and humoral immunity results in decreased resistance to viruses and recurrent sinus and pulmonary infections. Thymic aplasia or hypoplasia and a decrease in the lymphoid tissue in lymph nodes, spleen and elsewhere are associated with deficiency of IgA and IgE and abnormal function of T lymphocytes. Chromosomal abnormalities, an increased sensitivity to ionizing radiation and a markedly increased risk of developing cancers, particularly lymphomas and leukaemias, are other facets of this syndrome. Inheritance is autosomal recessive with variable penetrance. The cutaneous and conjunctival telangiectases arise from the superficial vascular plexus.[47]

CUTIS MARMORATA TELANGIECTATICA CONGENITA

This rare condition, also known as congenital generalized phlebectasia, is characterized by a persistent localized or generalized patterning of the skin by a reticulate network of dark violet-blue vessels (cutis marmorata), spider naevus-like telangiectases and venous abnormalities variously described as phlebectasia, venous lakes or venous haemangiomas.[48-50] The skin changes appear in the neonatal period and in many cases have a tendency to improve with time. In addition to atrophy or hypertrophy of the involved tissues, a range of other associated vascular and skeletal abnormalities has been described.[48,50-53] There is no involvement of internal organs by the vascular abnormalities.[48]

Histopathology

Various changes, including dilated capillaries and veins in the dermis and subcutis, have been described in this condition.[48,54]

SECONDARY TELANGIECTASES

Numerous skin disorders are associated with telangiectases. These include such disparate conditions as collagen vascular disease, cutaneous mastocytosis and chronic graft-versus-host disease. Telangiectases may appear following trauma or be associated with skin damage due to solar and other forms of radiation (Fig. 38.5).

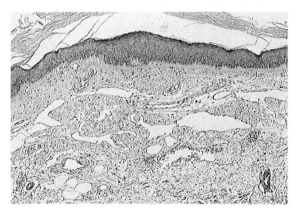

Fig. 38.5 Secondary telangiectasia occurring in sun-damaged skin.
Haematoxylin — eosin

CALIBRE-PERSISTENT ARTERY

Chronic ulceration of the vermilion border of the lips is sometimes associated with the presence of an artery of abnormally large calibre running in a very superficial location beneath the squamous epithelium. These vessels have been called calibre-persistent arteries because of the failure of normal narrowing of the lumen as the vessel approaches the mucosal surface.[55] Some cases have been misdiagnosed clinically as squamous cell carcinoma.[56] The vessel may show fibro-elastotic intimal thickening.[57] Multiple sections may be necessary to demonstrate the vessels.[55]

LYMPHANGIECTASES

Lesions which are clinically and histologically similar to superficial lymphangiomas may develop in areas of skin affected by obstruction or destruction of the lymphatic drainage. The interference with the lymphatics may result from radiotherapy or surgery and has been described in the chest and arm following radical mastectomy and radiotherapy,[58–59a] in the penis and scrotum following surgery for a sacrococcygeal tumour,[60] and on the vulva and on the thigh following surgery and radiotherapy for carcinoma of the cervix.[61–62]

BENIGN BLOOD VESSEL PROLIFERATIONS

This group of vascular tumours includes a variety of lesions in which there is a developmental or acquired proliferation of blood vessels of different types.

CAPILLARY AND CAVERNOUS HAEMANGIOMAS

These lesions arise predominantly in childhood and only rarely in adults.[1,63,64] They appear to be developmental abnormalities although most are not visible at birth. They have also been termed angiomatous naevi. Excluded from this category are the arteriovenous haemangioma (see p. 956) because of distinctive clinicopathological features, the lobular haemangioma (pyogenic granuloma; see p. 953) and the 'cherry' angioma (see p. 947).

It has been suggested that capillary and cavernous haemangiomas either represent an abnormality of differentiation of mesenchymal primordia in embryological development[65] or develop by sprouting from existing capillary endothelium.[66] Although they have traditionally been subdivided into capillary and cavernous, on the basis of poorly defined criteria of luminal size, depth of the lesion or thickness of vessel walls, this division is not clear cut. Many haemangiomas consist of areas with both small and large lumina, and there is evidence to suggest that both types are simply part of a spectrum, with cavernous haemangiomas originating from capillary haemangiomas by way of adaptation of the vessel walls to local changes in blood flow and pressure.[67] Generally, cavernous areas tend to be distributed deeper in the dermis and subcutis and have a lesser tendency to regress with time.

It has been proposed that this group of vascular abnormalities be divided into haemangiomas and vascular malformations.[68] The latter lack a proliferative phase characterized by incorporation of [^{3}H] thymidine, are present at birth, fail to involute, and grow proportionally with the child: they are formed from abnormal vascular elements that often combine capillary, arterial and venous characteristics. Some so-called cavernous haemangiomas probably fit into this group and this would explain in part both the variable rate of involution of cavernous haemangiomas and the differences in histological appearance.

Superficial capillary haemangiomas are commonly known as 'strawberry naevi' and have also been called juvenile haemangiomas and benign haemangioendothelioma of childhood. They commonly involve the dermis and subcutis but they may involve the subcutis only; in some cases they overlie still deeper and more complex vascular malformations. They may be associated with other developmental abnormalities, as in Maffucci's syndrome (see p. 952).

In some series there is a female preponderance of cases.[69,70] One or more lesions may be present on any part of the body, but the head, neck and trunk are the most commonly affected sites.[71] The parotid gland and overlying skin may be involved, this being the most common tumour of the parotid gland in children.[72] Lesions are usually not visible at birth but appear in the first few weeks of life. Rarely, a faint erythematous macule or an area of pallor with telangiectasia is present at birth.[73] The lesions evolve and enlarge over a period of months to become raised and bright red in colour, with a smooth or irregular surface. Most lesions have reached maximum size by the age of 3–6 months.[71,73] Total or partial regression then occurs in the majority of lesions and is usually maximal by 5–7 years of age.[70,71] Hence, most cases require no surgical intervention.[73,74] Periorbital lesions may warrant active therapy because of the association of visual complications.[73] Complete involution is less likely to occur where there is a deep cavernous component.[75]

Superficial cavernous haemangiomas are blue, compressible papules and nodules. Deeper lesions may impart little or no colour to the skin. Multiple cavernous lesions are present in the 'blue rubber bleb' naevus syndrome and Maffucci's syndrome (see below). Occasionally, they have a unilateral dermatomal[76] or zosteriform distribution.[77] Rarely, they enlarge with puberty.[78]

Multiple disseminated cutaneous haemangiomas are sometimes associated with multiple visceral haemangiomas (diffuse neonatal haemangiomatosis). This is usually a fatal disorder (see below).

Histopathology

Early lesions are highly cellular and involve the dermis and/or the subcutis. Vascular lumina are small, often slit-like and inapparent, and lined by plump endothelial cells. Moderate numbers of normal mitotic figures are present and mast cells are frequent in the intervening stroma. It has been suggested that the mast cells may play a role in angiogenesis and therefore in the formation of these lesions.[79] The vascular

proliferation may have a lobular configuration; this is often more obvious in the subcutis. Here fat lobules are partly or completely replaced and the appearance may resemble that of angiolipomas.[71] As the lesions evolve, vascular lumina become more obvious and larger. A central draining lumen may become evident in each lobule. The endothelium lining the vessels becomes flatter. With regression of lesions there is disappearance of vessels, interstitial fibrosis, and fat replacement of vascular tissue in the lobules of the subcutis.[71]

The lesions which have been called *cavernous haemangiomas* are sometimes found in the deep dermis and subcutis and consist of larger dilated vascular channels lined by flat endothelium (Fig. 38.6). The walls of the vessels vary in thickness

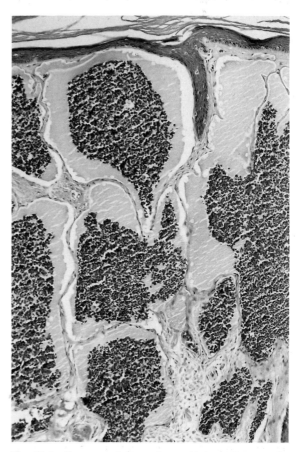

Fig. 38.6 Cavernous haemangioma with large, dilated vascular channels.
Haematoxylin — eosin

but they are generally thin and fibrous. Some vessels may have smooth muscle in their walls and resemble dilated veins. Thrombosis may complicate these lesions. Calcification of the walls and phlebolith-like calcific bodies in the lumina may be found.

Electron microscopy. Ultrastructural studies of *capillary haemangiomas* have shown plump endothelial cells surrounded by a basement membrane and pericytes.[80] Intracytoplasmic vacuoles are present in endothelial cells and they are thought to represent an early stage in lumen formation.[81] Crystalloid inclusions have been identified in endothelial cells in early cellular lesions.[82] Vessels within a haemangioma may have features of capillaries, venules or arterioles.[80] In *cavernous haemangiomas*, the endothelium is flattened and the basal lamina duplicated with interspersed collagen fibrils.[80]

Associated clinical syndromes

There are several, somewhat overlapping syndromes in which multiple cutaneous haemangiomas form the major part of the syndrome. These include diffuse neonatal haemangiomatosis, the 'blue rubber bleb' naevus syndrome and Maffucci's syndrome.

Diffuse neonatal haemangiomatosis. Multiple cutaneous haemangiomas may occur with or without disseminated visceral haemangiomas. The cutaneous lesions are capillary haemangiomas which are present at birth or appear in infancy. In those cases with visceral involvement, any organ may be involved. Visceral involvement is a poor prognostic sign, death occurring in the majority of cases, usually within a few months of birth.[83] Common causes of death include high output congestive cardiac failure associated with arteriovenous shunts (particularly in the liver), central nervous system complications and bleeding associated with the Kasabach–Merritt syndrome.[83–85]

A purely cutaneous form has also been reported and has been called benign neonatal haemangiomatosis.[86] The prognosis in this group is good. In these patients and some survivors of those with visceral haemangiomas, spontaneous regression of lesions occurs.[86,87]

'Blue rubber bleb' naevus syndrome. This syndrome was first named by Bean.[88] It is characterized by multiple, compressible, blue, rubbery, cavernous haemangiomas of the skin and of the gastrointestinal tract and occasionally other organs.[89] The skin lesions may be present at birth or develop in childhood. They do not regress. Some, but not all, of the lesions are characteristically painful or tender on palpation. There may be associated hyperhidrosis in the region of the tumours.[90] Iron-deficiency anaemia sometimes results from gastrointestinal haemorrhage.[91] Most cases are sporadic but there is evidence for an autosomal dominant mode of inheritance.[91] In one family males only were affected.[92]

The cutaneous lesions are composed of irregular cavernous channels in the deep dermis and subcutis. There is smooth muscle in the vessel walls. In some cases vessels may be intimately related to dermal sweat glands.[90]

Maffucci's syndrome. This syndrome is characterized by multiple vascular tumours of the skin and subcutis associated with multiple enchondromas of bones, particularly the long bones. The vascular tumours are usually cavernous haemangiomas, but capillary haemangiomas, phlebectasias (dilated venules and veins) and lymphangiomas also occur. Phlebolith-like bodies may develop in vascular channels. In one case lymphangiomas only were present.[93] The vascular tumours are present at birth or appear during childhood; they do not regress.[94,95] Mucous membrane and visceral haemangiomas have also been reported.[95]

Enchondromatosis results in variable shortening and deformity of the extremities. Skeletal lesions are predominantly unilateral in approximately half the reported cases.[95] There is no anatomical relationship between the osseous and vascular components.

There is probably an equal sex incidence and no familial grouping of cases.[95] Chondrosarcomas develop in approximately 15% of cases, and other cancers have also been reported.[95] The condition appears to be a generalized disorder of mesenchymal tissues.[96]

VERRUCOUS HAEMANGIOMA

This is a vascular malformation which appears to arise at birth or in childhood and enlarges and spreads in later life.[97,98] Lesions occur predominantly on the legs and consist of bluish-red soft papules and nodules which become wart-like as the patient ages or following trauma. Satellite nodules may develop. Recurrence is frequent after removal of the lesions because of involvement of the deeper tissues. An eruptive form with multiple disseminated cutaneous lesions has also been described.[99]

Histopathology

Fully evolved lesions consist of dermal and subcutaneous foci of capillary and cavernous haemangioma with overlying verrucous hyperplasia of the epidermis. There is irregular papillomatosis with acanthosis and hyperkeratosis. Angiokeratomatous areas may be present; however, unlike angiokeratomas, which are ectasias of superficial vessels (see p. 945), verrucous haemangiomas contain true areas of haemangioma and involve deeper levels.[97,98]

LOBULAR CAPILLARY HAEMANGIOMAS

This term refers to a group of vascular tumours characterized by the presence of capillary-sized vessels arranged in lobules.[100,101] Included in this category are pyogenic granuloma and its variants and angioblastoma and acquired tufted angioma (progressive capillary haemangioma).[100] The infection-related angiomatoses (bacillary epithelioid angiomatosis and verruga peruana) may also have a lobular pattern.

Pyogenic granuloma and variants

Pyogenic granuloma is a common benign vascular tumour of mucous membranes and skin. Recent studies imply that it represents a haem-

angioma and not simply a florid proliferation of granulation tissue.[102] Common sites include the gingiva, lips, fingers and face.[103] These tumours are commonly polypoid and pedunculated but they may be sessile. Most are red or red-brown in colour. Some darker lesions may clinically mimic nodular malignant melanoma. The lesions typically evolve rapidly over a period of weeks to maximum size. In one series this varied from 0.5 to 4 cm, with a mean diameter of 1.1 cm.[104] The surface is often ulcerated and bleeds easily.

Spontaneous involution of lesions is uncommon but has been reported in cases of *disseminated pyogenic granuloma*[105] and post partum in women who developed lesions during pregnancy (*epulis gravidarum*).[106] The lesions may develop at any age and both sexes are affected. There is a female predominance in some reports.[107] In one series of oral and nasal mucosal lesions there was a marked male predominance in the first two decades and a female predominance during the child-bearing years.[102] Occasionally, these tumours may be multiple or disseminated.[105,108,108a] *Multiple satellite recurrences* sometimes occur after treatment of the primary lesion, particularly when the latter was on the trunk, an uncommon site for pyogenic granuloma.[109,110] Pyogenic granulomas have been reported in a pre-existing naevus flammeus[111] and in a 'spider' angioma.[112]

In the majority of cases there is no apparent cause for these lesions; a minority follow trauma.[102,104] The higher incidence in women during child-bearing years, the occurrence in pregnancy, an association with use of the oral contraceptive pill and the spontaneous regression of lesions following parturition suggest that a hormonal factor is involved in their genesis.[106] It has been suggested that pyogenic granulomas represent small acquired arteriovenous fistulae.[113] Immunohistochemical and ultrastructural studies have confirmed that pyogenic granulomas are tumours of vessels and endothelial cells.[114]

Histopathology

Pyogenic granulomas are lobular capillary haemangiomas (Fig. 38.7).[102] The lobular arrange-

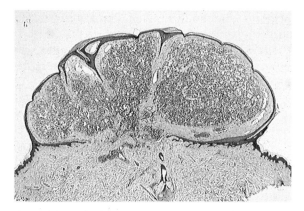

Fig. 38.7 Pyogenic granuloma. There is a well-developed collarette at the margins of this lobular vascular proliferation. Haematoxylin — eosin

ment of the lesions is distinct from the pattern of capillaries in granulation tissue and, unlike granulation tissue, the capillaries do not usually involute with time. The underlying morphology is often obscured by secondary ulceration, oedema, haemorrhage and inflammatory changes. In uncomplicated lesions there is a lobulated proliferation of capillary-sized vessels. The deep lobules are compact and cellular with small indistinct lumina. Occasional mitotic figures may be seen within the cellular lobules. Towards the surface the lobules are larger and less tightly packed and have distinct capillaries with larger branching lumina. The lobules are separated by myxoid or fibrous connective tissue septa.[115]

The surface epithelium is attenuated, and at the margins of the lesion there is often an epidermal collarette formed by elongated rete ridges or sweat ducts. Surface ulceration and inflammation are secondary events and sometimes lead to the formation of true granulation tissue near the surface of the lesions.

Lesions with the same lobular haemangiomatous pattern have also been described within veins[116] and in subcutaneous tissues.[117] *Intravenous pyogenic granuloma* occurs predominantly in the neck, arms and hands.[116] *Subcutaneous pyogenic granuloma* occurs predominantly on the upper extremities.[117]

Acquired tufted angioma

Wilson Jones first gave this name to an unusual acquired vascular proliferation which consisted of slowly spreading erythematous macules and plaques, predominantly on the neck and upper trunk of children and young adults.[118,119] A similar lesion had previously been called progressive capillary haemangioma.[120] The condition known in Japan as 'angioblastoma (Nakagawa)' appears to be identical to acquired tufted angioma.[121] Raised papules resembling pyogenic granulomas are sometimes seen within the area of the lesion.[100] There is one report of this condition in an elderly adult in whom the lesion appeared to have arisen from a naevus flammeus of the neck.[122] Unlike 'strawberry naevi' of infancy and childhood these lesions show no tendency to regress.

Histopathology

There are multiple separated cellular lobules within the dermis and subcutis. Some lobules bulge the walls of dilated thin-walled vascular channels which are within the lobules or at their periphery. This sometimes gives the vessels a semilunar profile.[100] These larger vessels have a distinct endothelial lining.

Each lobule is composed of cells with spindle-shaped and oval nuclei (Fig. 38.8). Mitotic figures may be seen but there is no cellular

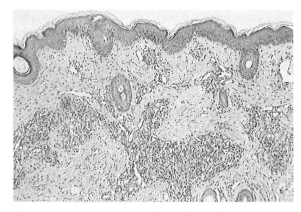

Fig. 38.8 Acquired tufted angioma. The multiple vascular lobules are composed of spindle-shaped and polygonal cells. Haematoxylin — eosin

atypia. Small capillary-sized vascular lumina are present in these areas. The morphology of the lobules resembles those seen in pyogenic granulomas. Haemosiderin may be present in the lesions; inflammation and oedema are not usually seen.

The pattern of cellular nodules with a peripheral dilated channel superficially resembles Kaposi's sarcoma but the lobules lack the characteristic interlacing bundles of spindle cells and slit-like vessels, and usually lack an inflammatory infiltrate with plasma cells. In endovascular papillary angioendothelioma of childhood (see p. 969), papillary processes lined by atypical endothelial cells protrude into vascular lumina. In Masson's 'vegetant intravascular haemangioendothelioma' (see p. 957), papillary processes, composed of hyperplastic endothelium supported by fibrous stalks, are confined within vascular lumina.

Electron microscopy. Ultrastructural studies have confirmed cell-marker studies which have shown that these lesions consist of endothelial cells and pericytes with small lumina.[119] In one study of 'angioblastoma (Nakagawa)' crystalloid inclusions were seen in endothelial cells.[121]

BACILLARY ANGIOMATOSIS

Vascular lesions, distinct from Kaposi's sarcoma, have been reported in association with human immunodeficiency virus infection.[123–125] These lesions, which may clinically mimic Kaposi's sarcoma, present as single or multiple red, purple or skin-coloured papules or nodules on any part of the body. They have been referred to as bacillary angiomatosis,[125a] epithelioid angiomatosis,[123] AIDS-related angiomatosis[125b] and epithelioid haemangioma-like vascular proliferation.[124] Mucosal surfaces and viscera may also be involved.

Clusters of bacilli are present in the lesions and there is some evidence that these organisms are the same as the bacillus of cat-scratch disease[125c] or are organisms related to *Bartonella bacilliformis*.[125d]

Death may result from visceral involvement,

although lesions will clear with erythromycin therapy.[124,125]

Recently, bacillary angiomatosis was reported in an immunocompetent individual.[125e]

Histopathology

The vessels are arranged in a lobular pattern, similar to that seen in pyogenic granuloma. A collarette is often present. The vascular channels are lined by cuboidal ('epithelioid') endothelial cells. There are no fascicles of spindle cells as seen in Kaposi's sarcoma. Neutrophils, nuclear dust and clumps of granular purplish material representing bacteria are also present (Fig. 38.9).[124a,125] The bacilli are Gram-negative, and they stain with the Warthin–Starry method.[124] They stain positively with antisera to the bacillus of cat-scratch disease using immunoperoxidase techniques.[124]

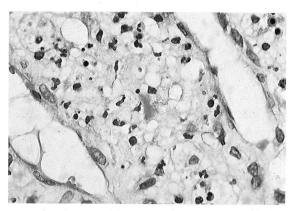

Fig. 38.9 Bacillary angiomatosis in a patient with AIDS. Neutrophils, nuclear dust and a clump of granular material (representing bacteria) are present in the stroma between the small vascular channels.
Haematoxylin — eosin
Microscopic slide provided by Dr Philip LeBoit, Department of Pathology and Dermatology, University of California, San Francisco, USA.

VERRUGA PERUANA

The skin lesion of the eruptive phase of Carrión's disease (bartonellosis), caused by *Bartonella bacilliformis*, is known as verruga peruana (Peruvian wart).[126,127] Carrión's disease is endemic at altitudes between 800 and 2500 metres in parts of Peru, Ecuador and Colombia. Multiple, miliary, superficial, haemangioma-like lesions or larger, deeper, sometimes ulcerated lesions occur in this condition. They resolve spontaneously over weeks to months.[126,127]

Histopathology

Superficial lesions consist of a proliferation of capillary-like vessels in the papillary dermis, with the formation of a collarette. There is an associated inflammatory infiltrate composed of lymphocytes and plasma cells. In nodular lesions there is a multilobular proliferation or more solid aggregation of cells in the dermis and sometimes also in the subcutis. Vascular lumina are fewer and smaller. The 'tumour cells' are large and epithelioid; groups of them are surrounded by a reticulum network. Mitotic figures are frequent. A spindle cell element is occasionally seen which may make distinction from Kaposi's sarcoma extremely difficult. Immunohistochemical studies have identified these cells as endothelial in nature as they are positive for both factor-VIII-associated antigen and *Ulex europaeus* 1 lectin.[126] In regressing lesions there is involution and necrosis of the vascular elements, associated with a heavy infiltrate of lymphocytes, histiocytes and neutrophils. There is subsequent fibrosis.

The causative organism is not seen by light microscopy but may be found on ultrastructural examination, predominantly in an extracellular location but occasionally in phagosomes.[126] Rocha Lima inclusions, consisting of conglomerates of apparently intracellular cytoplasmic granules that are coloured red by Romanowsky–Giemsa stains, may be seen within the endothelial cells. Ultrastructurally these appear to consist of phagosomes containing organisms and interstitial matrix-like material as well as a labyrinth of cisternal channels with similar contents.[126]

ARTERIOVENOUS HAEMANGIOMA

Arteriovenous haemangioma (acral arteriovenous tumour) presents as a solitary, red or purple papule with a predilection for the lips, the perioral skin, the nose and the eyelids of middle-aged to elderly men.[128–130] It is usually asymptomatic.

Histopathology[128,129]

There is a well-circumscribed, non-encapsulated collection of large, thick-walled vessels in the upper and mid dermis (Fig. 38.10). These vessels are lined by endothelium and have a fibromuscular wall which contains elastic fibres but no definite elastic laminae. In approximately one-third of cases there are thin-walled, dilated, angiomatous capillaries superficial to the large tumour vessels.

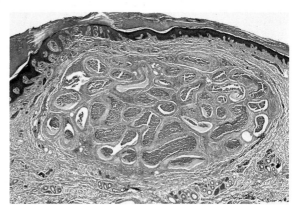

Fig. 38.10   Arteriovenous haemangioma. It is composed of thick-walled vascular channels.
Haematoxylin — eosin

ANGIOLYMPHOID HYPERPLASIA WITH EOSINOPHILIA

This is an incompletely characterized tumour of skin and subcutaneous tissues composed of vessels, a proliferation of a distinctive type of endothelial cell and a variable component of inflammatory cells.[131] Whether it is a true neoplasm or a reactive process is at present undecided. It appears to be identical to the lesions known as pseudo-pyogenic granuloma, atypical pyogenic granuloma, epithelioid haemangioma, histiocytoid haemangioma, intravenous atypical vascular proliferation and nodular angioblastic hyperplasia with eosinophilia and lympho-folliculosis.[132-136] Kimura's disease,[137,138] although previously included by some in this group of conditions, appears to be a separate entity.[138a,138b] Kimura's disease is clinically different and lacks the characteristic vascular proliferation.[134,139,140]

The lesions involve the subcutaneous tissue or the dermis or both. Single or multiple pink to red-brown papules or nodules occur, predominantly on the face, scalp and ears; they are uncommon on the limbs and trunk. One case has been reported involving the vulva.[140a] Symptomatic lesions may be painful, pruritic or pulsatile.[141] In some series there is a female predominance.[142] Young to middle-aged people are most commonly affected. Some cases are associated with a blood eosinophilia. Lesions may remain for years without evidence of involution and they may recur after excision.[136]

Histopathology

These lesions consist of circumscribed collections of vessels and inflammatory cells. The vascular component comprises thick-walled and thin-walled vessels lined by plump endothelial cells (Fig. 38.11). These cells also occur in clumps that appear solid or sometimes contain small lumina. They have been described as epithelioid or histiocytic and are characteristic of this condition. They have a large nucleus and abundant eosinophilic cytoplasm. Prominent cytoplasmic vacuoles are seen in some. Mitotic figures are sometimes present; they are of normal configuration. Intravascular proliferations of these cells may be seen in the lumina of larger vessels.[135] Associated with the vascular and endothelial proliferations there is a stromal cellular infiltrate which varies in intensity and consists of lymphocytes (sometimes with lymphoid follicle formation), eosinophils and mast cells. The stroma may be fibrous or myxoid in character.

The true nature of these lesions is uncertain. A few examples appear to be associated with trauma or pregnancy.[141] Rosai has called this condition 'a primary proliferation with neoplastic qualities'.[134] He has included these lesions in his unifying concept of histiocytoid haemangiomas in which the characteristic proliferating cell is an endothelial cell with histiocytic features.[143] Although these cells share some enzymes with histiocytes[144] they do not contain lysozyme; they have ultrastructural features of endothelial cells, including Weibel–Palade bodies.[141] The cells also contain factor-VIII-related antigen, a marker for endothelial cells.[145] The vacuoles in their cytoplasm possibly represent primitive vascular lumina.

INTRAVASCULAR PAPILLARY ENDOTHELIAL HYPERPLASIA

Pierre Masson first described this vascular proliferation in haemorrhoidal veins; he regarded it as a neoplastic process. He named it *'hémangioendothéliome végétant intravasculaire'*.[146] Its importance lies in its histological resemblance to angiosarcoma: the name 'Masson's pseudoangiosarcoma' has also been proposed.[147-151] The condition is now generally regarded as an unusual pattern of organization of a thrombus within a vein,[148,150,151a] or within one or more of the component vessels of various vascular abnormalities. These include cavernous

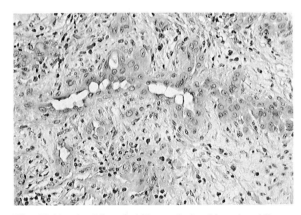

Fig. 38.11 Angiolymphoid hyperplasia with eosinophils. The vascular channels are lined by plump, partly vacuolated endothelial cells. There are scattered eosinophils in the stroma.
Haematoxylin — eosin

haemangiomas,[147,149] pyogenic granulomas[147] and lymphangiomas.[152] In most cases there is a single lesion, but multiple lesions have also been described.[153] They usually present clinically as firm, sometimes painful nodules which appear blue or purple through the overlying skin.[150] On section, typical lesions appear encapsulated and cystic; they contain variable amounts of thrombus. Although lesions can occur at any site, including the tongue,[151] they are most commonly found on the fingers, head and neck, and trunk.[147,150] There is a female predominance in most series.[147,150] Local excision is curative.

Histopathology

In most examples the proliferation is limited to the lumen of an identifiable vein or vessel in a vascular abnormality. Occasionally there is only a fibrous capsule lacking definite features of a vessel wall. Rarely, the proliferation extends outside the lumen, possibly due to rupture of the wall of the vessel. Masses of papillary processes are present within the lumen and they are almost always associated with some thrombus. Each papillary frond is covered by a single layer of plump endothelial cells. Mitotic figures may be present but they are never frequent. There is no multi-layering of the cells, and solid cellular areas, cellular tufts, atypia and necrosis are not evident. The core of the papillae consists of fibrin or collagenous connective tissue, depending on the stage of organization.

Electron microscopy. This confirms the endothelial nature of the cells and demonstrates that they lie on a basement membrane, outside which are pericytes.[154]

ACRO-ANGIODERMATITIS

This vasoproliferative disorder resembles Kaposi's sarcoma clinically and histologically, and has been termed 'pseudo-Kaposi sarcoma'.[155] The lesions arise in a background of increased venous pressure due to chronic venous insufficiency,[156] paralysis of a limb,[157] congenital arteriovenous malformation[158] or acquired arteriovenous fistula.[158a,159] It has also been reported in an above-knee amputation stump.[159a] The majority occur on the lower part of the legs and on the feet; in cases associated with arteriovenous malformations they are found over the site of the malformation. In most cases affecting the legs there is also stasis dermatitis. The lesions consist of purple papules and nodules with variable surface scale. Those cases associated with venous insufficiency or paralysis of the legs have a characteristic distribution, occupying a triangular region on the extensor surface of the foot and toes, with the most prominent lesions on the first and second toes.[156] Lesions may be unilateral or bilateral, depending on the cause. There is a male preponderance.[160]

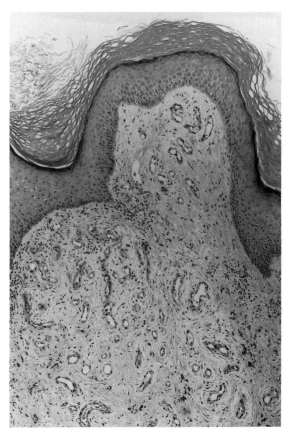

Fig. 38.12 Acro-angiodermatitis. There is a proliferation of small vessels in an oedematous dermis. Fibroblasts are also increased.
Haematoxylin — eosin

Histopathology[161,162]

The papules and nodules consist of a proliferation of small dilated vessels in an oedematous dermis (Fig. 38.12). The vessels have fairly regular profiles and lack the jagged outline and 'promontory' sign seen in early lesions of Kaposi's sarcoma (see p. 964).[161] Plump endothelial cells, without atypia, line the vessels. A slight perivascular fibroblastic proliferation is also seen but is not marked. Some lesions show nodular collections of vessels with narrow lumina (Fig. 38.13).[162] Extravasated red blood cells, haemosiderin and a variable round cell infiltrate are seen around the vascular proliferation. Plasma cells are usually not present. The overlying epidermis may show hyperkeratosis.

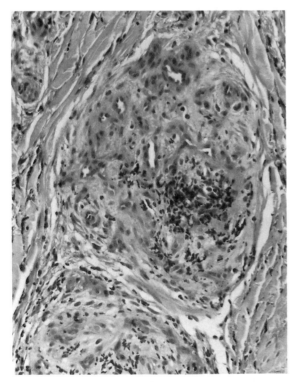

Fig. 38.13   Acro-angiodermatitis. In this variant of the condition there is a nodular collection of small blood vessels with narrow lumina. A mild lymphocytic infiltrate is also present within the nodule. The endothelial cells are not atypical.
Haematoxylin — eosin

PAPULAR ANGIOPLASIA

The two recorded cases of this condition were in elderly patients who presented with vascular papules of the face and scalp in which the dermal vascular proliferation contained atypical bizarre endothelial cells.[163] The lesions, which were termed papular angioplasia, were thought of as a 'pseudo-malignancy'. Their relationship to pyogenic granuloma and angiolymphoid hyperplasia is uncertain.

MULTINUCLEATE CELL ANGIOHISTIOCYTOMA

This entity is characterized by grouped, red-brown papules with a predilection for the distal extremities of middle-aged women.[163a,163b]

Histopathology

There is a proliferation of small blood vessels in the upper and mid dermis. The endothelial cells have enlarged nuclei, some of which are hyperchromatic and protrude into the lumen. There are large, bizarre basophilic cells within the collagen between the vessels. These cells, many of which are multinucleate, have an irregular shape. Immunohistochemical and ultrastructural studies suggest that these cells are fibroblastic in differentiation.[163b]

GLOMUS TUMOUR

Glomus tumours are variably regarded as hamartomas or neoplasms which resemble elements of the glomus apparatus in the skin. Although they almost always occur in the skin, rare lesions have been described at other sites. The glomus apparatus contains a central coiled canal, the Sucquet–Hoyer canal, which is lined by endothelium and several layers of glomus cells. Glomus tumours consist of cells resembling glomus cells combined with vascular structures.

There are two main types of glomus tumour: they have different distributions and clinical features.[164]

those of blood vessels. There are two specific clinicopathological entities, lymphangioma (with a superficial and deep form) and acquired progressive lymphangioma.

LYMPHANGIOMA

Lymphangiomas are uncommon benign tumours of lymphatic vessels; the majority appear to be developmental abnormalities. Most are present at birth or arise in infancy or early in childhood.[169,170] It has been suggested that lymphangiomas represent sequestrated lymphatic vessels which have failed to link up with the rest of the lymphatic system or with the venous system during embryological development.[171,172] Histologically identical lesions which arise because of acquired obstruction of lymphatics, often in association with lymphoedema, are classified as lymphangiectases. There have been several attempts to classify lymphangiomas; the classification used here is that of Flanagan and Helwig,[169] which divides them into superficial and deep types.

Superficial lymphangioma. The superficial lymphangioma is also known as lymphangioma circumscriptum. Although these lesions may occur on almost any part of the body, they are most common on the proximal parts of the limbs and in the limb girdle regions.[170] Typically, there are multiple, scattered or grouped, translucent vesicles and papulovesicles in an area of skin; single small lesions composed of a group of vessels also occur.[170] The lesions have been likened to frog spawn. Secondary haemorrhage and thrombus formation in vesicles may produce red or purple colouration in the lesions. Some lesions have a warty appearance due to epidermal hyperplasia and hyperkeratosis. There may be an underlying deep lymphangioma or other abnormality of lymphatic drainage, resulting in lymphoedema and enlargement of the limb.[173,174] Most of the lesions are present at birth or develop in early infancy or in childhood. Occasionally the lesions appear first in adult life: this is most common in the small

localized form.[170] In the typical extensive lesion, the superficial vessels communicate through deep vessels with large closed lymphatic cisterns in the subcutaneous tissues; the superficial ectatic lymphatic vessels appear to result from raised pressure in these cisterns.[171] This underlying abnormality may explain the tendency of the lesions to recur after superficial excision. Lesions may enlarge and spread with time and they may persist indefinitely. The development of lymphangiosarcoma has been reported in an area of superficial lymphangioma treated with radiotherapy.[175]

Deep lymphangioma. This group includes the lesions known as lymphangioma cavernosum and cystic hygroma.[169] The term *cystic hygroma* is generally used for large deep lymphangiomas in the neck or axilla which consist of single or multiloculate fluid-filled cavities. Cystic hygromas of the posterior triangle of the neck are associated with hydrops fetalis and fetal death.[176] There is an association with the 45 XO karyotype (Turner's syndrome), other congenital malformation syndromes and several varieties of chromosomal aneuploidy.[176] It is thought that these lesions represent failed connection between the jugular lymph sac and the internal jugular vein.[172,176] There is no clear-cut distinction between other deep lymphangiomas and classic cystic hygromas[169] and it has been suggested that the appearance of the tumour is determined by the site and nature of the tissues in which it arises.[177] Deep lymphangiomas present as soft swellings in the skin and subcutaneous tissues. Progressive extension into deeper structures, such as muscle, is said to be an unfavourable sign.[169] The overlying epidermis is normal except in those cases in which there is an associated superficial lymphangioma. When cut across, these tumours vary from a spongy mass of small vascular spaces to large 'multicystic' tumours. Most are present at birth or arise in the first few years of life.[169,177]

Histopathology

Superficial lymphangiomas. The epidermis is

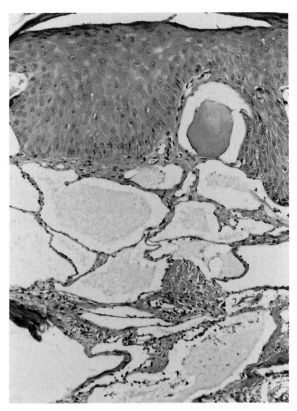

Fig. 38.18 Superficial lymphangioma. It is composed of ectatic lymphatic channels, situated in the upper dermis. Haematoxylin — eosin

elevated above the general level of the skin by solitary or grouped ectatic lymphatics located in the papillary dermis (Fig. 38.18). This accounts for the raised vesicles seen clinically. These channels abut closely on the overlying epidermis and are thin walled, consisting predominantly of an endothelial lining. The vessels may contain eosinophilic proteinaceous lymph or blood or thrombus and occasionally foamy histiocytes or multinucleate giant cells.[171] Scattered lymphoid cells are sometimes seen in the dermis. There is atrophy of the epidermis directly over the vessels with elongation of the rete ridges such that the vessels may appear to be intraepidermal, the picture resembling that of angiokeratoma. Deep irregular lymphatics are sometimes seen beneath the surface vessels in the dermis and subcutis, particularly in the extensive lesions.[171]

Deep lymphangiomas. The histological picture of these tumours is inconstant. There are irregular dilated lymphatic channels of variable size in the dermis, subcutis and deeper tissues. These vary from an endothelium-lined channel with no obvious supporting stroma to vessels with thick fibromuscular walls. The intervening dermis or subcutis may be unaltered or there may be loose or compact fibrous stroma.[169] Blood may be present in some channels. In larger lesions collections of lymphocytes are sometimes present in the stroma and cause the endothelium to bulge into the vascular lumen.

ACQUIRED PROGRESSIVE LYMPHANGIOMA

Acquired progressive lymphangioma is a rare vascular proliferative lesion of presumptive lymphatic origin.[178] It has also been called benign lymphangioendothelioma.[178a] Although there are histological similarities to cutaneous angiosarcoma, the course of the few reported cases has been benign. The lesions present as erythematous patches or plaques which gradually enlarge. They have occurred on the limbs, trunk and head. Both children and adults may be affected.[178–180]

Histopathology

The reported cases have shown anastomosing channels which dissect the dermal collagen bundles.[178a,180] These vessels are lined by a single layer of endothelial cells which may be plump and mildly atypical. Histologically, the lesions resemble the early vascular changes of Kaposi's sarcoma or of a low-grade angiosarcoma. Cellular atypia is not usually seen in Kaposi's sarcoma, in which there is often haemorrhage, haemosiderin deposition and an inflammatory infiltrate which includes plasma cells. Clinical features should distinguish these lesions from cutaneous angiosarcoma, which is usually a disease of the elderly. (see p. 970). The nature and origin of this tumour is as yet undecided. One ultrastructural study has failed to show specific lymphatic features in the vessels.[179]

TUMOURS WITH VARIABLE BEHAVIOUR

The following tumours have a variable behaviour and outcome:

Kaposi's sarcoma
Haemangiopericytoma
Spindle cell haemangioendothelioma
Endovascular papillary angioendothelioma of
  childhood
Epithelioid haemangioendothelioma.

KAPOSI'S SARCOMA

This tumour, composed of vessels and spindle-shaped cells, was first described by Kaposi in 1872 as 'idiopathic multiple pigment-sarcoma of the skin'.[181] The epidemic type of Kaposi's sarcoma, associated with the acquired immunodeficiency syndrome (AIDS), first reported in the United States of America in 1981, has provoked considerable interest in this previously uncommon condition.[182] There are four clinicopathological types: the classic type, the African type (endemic type), a variant associated with immunosuppressive therapy, and the AIDS-associated type (epidemic type).

Classic type. The classic type affects predominantly men in the fifth to seventh decades. There is an increased incidence in Jews and in people of Mediterranean origin.[183] In most cases the lesions are limited to the skin of the extremities, particularly the lower part of the legs and feet; occasionally lymph nodes and other organs are involved. Oedema sometimes precedes or follows the appearance of the lesions.[184] This type of Kaposi's sarcoma has a chronic course, with the development of more lesions; death is usually due to other causes. There is an increased risk of developing other tumours, particularly malignant lymphomas.[185,186] Spontaneous regression of the lesions may occur.

African type. The African type of Kaposi's sarcoma is endemic in parts of tropical Africa,

with the highest prevalence in eastern Zaire and western Uganda.[187] There are three main subtypes.[188] The most common is *nodular disease*, similar to classic Kaposi's sarcoma with a benign clinical course. A more *aggressive subtype* is characterized by extensive florid and infiltrative skin lesions, which may involve soft tissues and underlying bone. A *lymphadenopathic subtype* occurs predominantly in children: in this variety there is involvement of lymph nodes, often without cutaneous lesions; prognosis is poor.[189] There is a marked male predominance in endemic African Kaposi's sarcoma.[190]

Kaposi's sarcoma associated with immunosuppressive therapy. This is a rare complication of organ transplantation, chemotherapy for tumours, and long-term corticosteroid treatment for a variety of dermatological and other conditions.[186,191,192] Renal transplant recipients are particularly at risk. The male preponderance of cases is less marked than in the other types of the disease; younger age groups are also affected. Tumours may appear within a short time of commencement of immunosuppressive therapy and may regress spontaneously following cessation of therapy.[192] There may be a more aggressive clinical course than in classic Kaposi's sarcoma. Death may follow widespread disease, particularly from gastrointestinal haemorrhage.

Epidemic type. The epidemic type of Kaposi's sarcoma is associated with the acquired immunodeficiency syndrome (AIDS), now known to be caused by retroviruses.[193,194] Most cases of AIDS are caused by human immunodeficiency virus (HIV).[195] A second virus, HIV type 2, is associated with AIDS in West Africa. Kaposi's sarcoma also occurs in this group.[196] AIDS-associated HIV infection is now occurring in many parts of Africa.[197] Areas with a high prevalence of endemic Kaposi's sarcoma have a marked increase in atypical forms associated with AIDS.[198] The endemic African type itself is not associated with HIV infection (see above).[198]

In AIDS patients in the USA, the prevalence of the tumour is not equal among the various risk groups, and is most common in homosexual men. It is uncommon in haemophiliacs with AIDS and in recipients of blood transfusion who develop the disease.[198a] There is an intermediate risk in intravenous drug users.[199] Children with AIDS may also develop Kaposi's sarcoma.[200] In the USA and in Australia, Kaposi's sarcoma is the presenting diagnosis in 18% of AIDS patients.[201]

There is a different distribution of lesions in this form compared with classic Kaposi's sarcoma. The trunk, arms, head and neck are frequently involved. Lesions are usually multiple. There is frequent involvement of mucosal surfaces and internal organs. In one autopsy study, the lungs were involved in 37% of cases, the gastrointestinal tract in 50% and lymph nodes in 50%. Twenty-nine per cent had evidence of visceral lesions without skin lesions.[202] The extent of cutaneous involvement does not correlate well with the extent of visceral disease.[203] The clinical course ranges from chronic to rapidly progressive. Most patients die from opportunistic infections or other complications of AIDS rather than from Kaposi's sarcoma. In one large series of AIDS patients, survival was best in those whose only manifestation was Kaposi's sarcoma.[204] The lesions may regress spontaneously.[205]

Skin lesions are similar in all groups but in the epidemic form they tend to occur earlier and to be smaller and more subtle. Early lesions are brown to red macules or patches which may resemble a bruise. Papules, nodules and plaques may be bluish or purple in colour and may ulcerate. Current evidence based on ultrastructural and immunohistochemical studies suggests that Kaposi's sarcoma is a proliferation of vessels and that the spindle cell component shows endothelial differentiation.[206,207] Whether this represents blood vessel or lymphatic endothelium is controversial.[208–210] It appears at present that disseminated Kaposi's sarcoma represents a multifocal process rather than metastasis.[211] Biopsies of clinically uninvolved skin from AIDS patients have shown early vascular changes.[212,213] It is not clear if Kaposi's sarcoma represents a reactive vascular proliferation or a true neoplastic proliferation.[211]

Cox and Helwig have described malignant transformation with changing histological appearance of the tumour and the presence of tumour within vessels, suggesting a capacity for metastasis.[184]

The pathogenesis of Kaposi's sarcoma is at present unknown. An element of immune dysfunction is present in some cases of classic disease[214] and in immunosuppressed patients and patients with AIDS. In renal transplant recipients with Kaposi's sarcoma who are on maintenance immunosuppressive therapy, cessation of this therapy may result in regression of the Kaposi lesions.[192] Studies of HLA subtypes in patients with AIDS-associated and classic Kaposi's sarcoma have suggested that there is a significant association with HLA-DR5 antigen;[215,216] other antigen types have also been implicated in AIDS patients with Kaposi's sarcoma.[216] The significance of these findings is inconclusive and in AIDS patients may reflect a susceptibility to AIDS rather than to Kaposi's sarcoma.[216,217]

The part played by potentially oncogenic viruses in the pathogenesis of this tumour is at present unknown. Although HIV infection is present in AIDS patients, its absence from patients with other forms of Kaposi's sarcoma suggests that it is not the primary causative agent. There is much serological and molecular epidemiological evidence pointing to a specific association between cytomegalovirus (CMV) and Kaposi's sarcoma in classic, African and AIDS-associated forms and in some renal transplant recipients.[218] Cytomegalovirus DNA and RNA have been identified in tumour cells from Kaposi's sarcoma.[219] The difference in prevalence of this tumour in different groups with AIDS suggests that another as yet unknown factor may be involved. The use of the so-called recreational drugs (particularly amyl nitrite and butyl nitrite) by homosexual men has been proposed as a possible explanation for the difference in prevalence of Kaposi's sarcoma in patients with AIDS.[220] These nitrites may have immunosuppressant activity.

Histopathology

The microscopic appearance of the lesions is identical in the different types of Kaposi's sarcoma.[221,222] The earliest lesions, corresponding to the flat macule or patch stage, are predominantly vascular in nature. Within the dermis there is a proliferation of irregular vascular channels which partly surround pre-existing blood vessels in some areas. This characteristic appearance has been termed the 'promontory sign' (Fig. 38.19).[161] The vascular proliferation is also present about appendages and between collagen bundles. The vessels are thin walled and the endothelial lining consists of plump cells which are atypical. Scattered groups of perivascular lymphocytes and plasma cells may also be present (Fig. 38.20). Extravasated

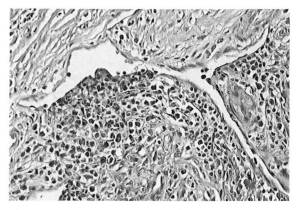

Fig. 38.20   Kaposi's sarcoma. Lymphocytes and plasma cells are present in the stroma adjacent to an irregularly-shaped vascular channel.
Haematoxylin — eosin

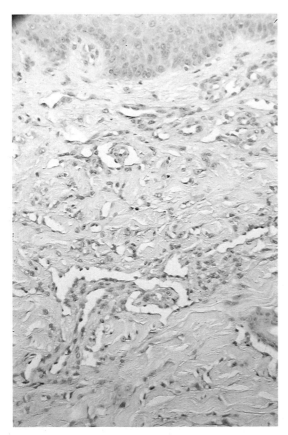

Fig. 38.19   Kaposi's sarcoma. Dilated, irregular vascular channels surround a preexisting vessel ('promontory sign').
Haematoxylin — eosin

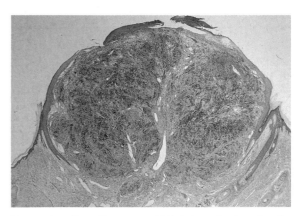

Fig. 38.21   Kaposi's sarcoma. This haemorrhagic variant is composed of vascular spaces and spindle-shaped cells.
Haematoxylin — eosin

erythrocytes and deposits of haemosiderin are also found in the dermis.

The papules, nodules and plaques consist of a dermal proliferation of interlacing bundles of spindle cells and intimately related, poorly defined slit-like vessels (Fig. 38.21). The proportion of vessels and spindle cells varies. There is an associated inflammatory cell infiltrate consisting predominantly of lymphocytes and plasma cells. Dilated thin-walled vessels are found at the periphery of the tumour. The spindle cell component shows variable nuclear pleomorphism (Fig. 38.22).

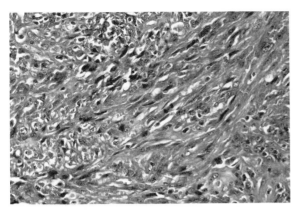

Fig. 38.22 Kaposi's sarcoma. Several of the spindle-shaped cells are in mitosis. Haematoxylin — eosin

Mitotic figures are present but not usually frequent. Erythrocytes can be seen within vascular lumina and extravasated in and around the lesion.

Clusters of eosinophilic hyaline globules, varying in size from those just visible with the light microscope to larger than an erythrocyte, may be seen within spindle cells and macrophages or in an extracellular location. These were first described in African cases but are also seen in classic Kaposi's sarcoma and in the epidemic form.[211,223] They resemble Russell bodies and are PAS positive, stain bright red with Mallory's trichrome stain (Fig. 38.23) and

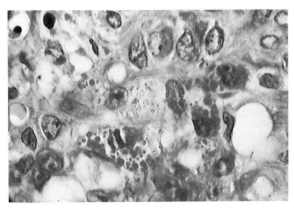

Fig. 38.23 Kaposi's sarcoma. Small hyaline globules are present in the cytoplasm of some macrophages and spindle-shaped cells. Masson trichrome × 600

are autofluorescent.[224] They are seen in early patch lesions in some cases.[211] They appear to represent effete red blood cell fragments which have been phagocytosed.[224a] Erythrophagocytosis by tumour cells has been described in all stages of Kaposi's sarcoma.[225]

An anaplastic form has been reported in African and sporadic cases.[188,226] The anaplastic lesions exhibit greater cellularity, nuclear pleomorphism and more frequent mitotic figures, and may have areas resembling angiosarcoma or fibrosarcoma.[184,226] Epidermal changes vary with the lesion and include atrophy and ulceration over raised lesions. A peripheral epidermal collarette is sometimes present about papules and nodules.

Differential diagnosis. The early vascular lesions are subtle and must be differentiated from telangiectases, pigmented purpuric dermatosis (see p. 238), acro-angiodermatitis (see p. 958) and low grade angiosarcoma (see p. 970). The vessels in Kaposi's sarcoma are usually more irregular than in most developmental or acquired telangiectases, pigmented purpuric dermatosis or acro-angiodermatitis.[162] An inflammatory infiltrate which includes plasma cells is found in some early lesions of Kaposi's sarcoma. In low grade angiosarcoma there is usually some evidence of cellular atypia. Small intravascular endothelial buds are sometimes seen. Irregular jagged vessels, dissection of collagen bundles by vascular structures and an inflammatory cell infiltrate may all be seen in low grade angiosarcoma.

Lesions with a spindle cell component must be differentiated from cutaneous smooth muscle tumours, some forms of dermatofibroma (fibrous histiocytoma)[227] and the recently described spindle cell haemangioendothelioma (see p. 968).[228] Smooth muscle tumours lack the intimate mingling of spindle cells, slit-like vessels and eosinophilic globules, and are usually positive for desmin intermediate filaments on immunoperoxidase staining. Vascular dermatofibromas can usually be differentiated from Kaposi's sarcoma because of the presence of foamy macrophages, multinucleate giant cells and the overlying epidermal changes which range from epidermal hyperplasia to basal budding resembling hair differentiation.

The lesions of spindle-cell haemangioendothelioma closely mimic Kaposi's sarcoma but the component vessels are usually more cavernous and, focally, the endothelial cells are epithelioid and vacuolated. Eosinophilic globules have not been reported in these tumours.

HAEMANGIOPERICYTOMA

Enzinger and Smith have divided cases of this uncommon tumour into two groups.[229] The usual form of haemangiopericytoma (*adult type*) occurs in adults and rarely in children.[229,230] These are tumours of deep soft tissues, particularly the lower extremities, pelvis and retroperitoneum, and occasionally other organs. They rarely arise in the subcutis.[229–231] A second group (*congenital or infantile haemangiopericytoma*) is present at birth or arises in the first year of life.[232,233] The tumours of this group are multilobulate and arise almost exclusively in the subcutis. They may also arise in the dermis.[229] More than one tumour may be present.[232,234] Conventional haemangiopericytomas have an unpredictable course and may recur after treatment; they may metastasize, predominantly to the lungs and skeleton.[229] Congenital and infantile tumours have a benign clinical course.[229]

Histopathology[229]

The *adult type* exhibits the characteristic pattern of tightly packed cellular areas surrounding endothelium-lined ramifying vessels. The cell boundaries are poorly defined; the nuclei are round or oval. Tumour cells are separated from the endothelial cells by a basement membrane and are themselves surrounded by a meshwork of reticulin fibres. Histological variations include myxoid areas, fibrotic areas and, rarely, osseous and cartilaginous metaplasia.[229] Several studies have stressed the difficulty in predicting the behaviour of these tumours from their histological appearance, but frequent mitotic figures, necrosis, haemorrhage and increased cellularity are features that indicate a poor prognosis.[230] Many soft tissue tumours may have haemangiopericytoma-like areas.

Congenital and infantile haemangiopericytomas have the typical pattern of cells and vessels described above, but they are multilobulate, with perivascular and intravascular tumour outside the main tumour mass.[229,234] Endothelial proliferation within vascular lumina has been described.[229] Mitotic figures and necrosis may be seen but do not indicate a bad prognosis as these tumours have a benign course.[232] Haemangiopericytoma-like areas are sometimes seen in infantile myofibromatosis (see p. 881), which affects infants and children and may involve the skin and subcutis.[235]

Electron microscopy. Ultrastructurally, the tumour cells are partially or completely surrounded by well-formed basement membranes. Pinocytotic vesicles and cytoplasmic filaments, sometimes with dense-body formation, are seen within the cells.[236]

SPINDLE CELL HAEMANGIOENDOTHELIOMA

This lesion, first described by Weiss and Enzinger in 1986,[228] has histological features resembling Kaposi's sarcoma and cavernous haemangioma. It appears to be a vascular tumour of low grade malignancy. Although it may occur in any age group, approximately 50% of cases arise before the age of 25. The lesions are sometimes single but are usually multiple and, if multiple, tend to occur in the same area. Most tumours are sited in the dermis or subcutis. The hands and feet are the commonest sites.[228,237] The tumours are circumscribed, haemorrhagic nodules which may contain phlebolith-like calcified bodies. Tumour size and the number of lesions increase with time, often over a long period. Local recurrence of lesions is common after removal; metastasis has been reported.[228] Two cases have occurred in patients with Maffucci's syndrome (see p. 952).[228,237]

Histopathology

There are two components to this tumour, a vascular component consisting of large thin-walled cavernous channels, and a spindle cell element. The cavernous vascular spaces sometimes contain thrombi or phlebolith-like bodies. Spindle cells may line slit-like vessels. Nuclear atypia is minimal and mitotic figures are seen only occasionally. A feature which is not seen in Kaposi's sarcoma is the presence of plump, sometimes vacuolated, endothelial cells, either in groups or lining vascular channels. Lymphocytes and siderophages may be associated with the lesions but eosinophilic globules, as described in Kaposi's sarcoma, have not been reported.

Immunohistochemical studies have confirmed the endothelial nature of the cells lining vascular spaces. The exact nature of the spindle cells is unclear: they are negative for *Ulex europaeus* 1 lectin and ultrastructural studies have not shown differentiating features.[237]

ENDOVASCULAR PAPILLARY ANGIOENDOTHELIOMA OF CHILDHOOD

Dabska, in the first report of this very rare vascular tumour, described it as malignant endovascular papillary angioendothelioma because it was locally invasive and appeared to have the potential to metastasize.[238] More recently, others have suggested that this lesion should be classified as of borderline malignancy because of its good long-term prognosis, minimal cellular atypia and controversial metastatic potential.[239,240]

All but one of the patients whose cases have been published were children.[241] In the majority the lesions were present at birth and occurred in a variety of sites, either as a diffuse swelling of the skin or as an intradermal tumour. The tumours enlarged and eventually, in some cases in Dabska's series, invaded deeper soft tissues and bone and metastasized to regional lymph nodes.[238] Despite these features no deaths have been reported from this condition.

Histopathology

There is some variability in histological features.[238,242] Irregular vascular channels are present in the dermis and subcutis. They are lined by endothelial cells ranging from flattened to columnar in shape. Some cells have a 'hobnail' appearance. Within the lumina of these vessels are papillary structures covered by similar cells. The cores of the papillae are avascular and consist of fibrous tissue or peculiar eosinophilic hyaline globules, some with central clearing.

Some of the vascular structures have a glomeruloid appearance. Lymphocytes are seen both within the lumina of the vascular channels, in intimate association with the endothelial cells, and also in the extravascular stroma. There is nuclear hyperchromatism and mitotic figures are present.[238]

Immunohistochemical and ultrastructural studies have confirmed the endothelial nature of the tumour cells and identified the hyaline globules as basal-lamina-like material.[239,240] It has been suggested that the cells of this lesion may differentiate towards the appearances typical of the high endothelial cells seen in post-capillary venules of lymph nodes and of mucosal lymphoid tissue, a view that finds support in their apparently close relationship to the lymphocytes within the lumina.[240]

EPITHELIOID HAEMANGIOENDOTHELIOMA

This rare tumour has a clinical course which is intermediate between haemangioma and angiosarcoma. Although most cases occur in soft tissues and other organs, including bone and liver, they have also been reported in the skin.[243–245] Skin lesions have been reported with underlying bone lesions.[246] These tumours have low grade or borderline malignant potential and may metastasize. They are less aggressive tumours than conventional angiosarcomas.

Histopathology

There is a proliferation of nests and cords of

plump, epithelioid to spindle-shaped endothelial cells in a fibromyxoid stroma. Many of the cells contain cytoplasmic vacuoles. Well-formed vascular channels are not a feature of this tumour.[243] Slight cellular pleomorphism and occasional mitotic figures are sometimes present. These tumours may be difficult to distinguish from secondary adenocarcinoma but the cells stain for *Ulex europaeus* agglutinin-1 and factor-VIII-related antigen with immunoperoxidase techniques. There is one report of tumour cells also expressing cytokeratin.[247] An epithelioid variant of angiosarcoma has also been described but in this tumour there are largely confluent sheets of tumour cells with greater cellular atypia and areas of necrosis.[248,249]

MALIGNANT TUMOURS

ANGIOSARCOMA AND LYMPHANGIOSARCOMA

The nomenclature of malignant neoplasms reportedly showing blood vessel endothelial differentiation includes the terms haemangiosarcoma, malignant angioendothelioma and malignant haemangioendothelioma. The distinction between malignant tumours showing blood vessel differentiation (angiosarcoma) and those showing lymphatic differentiation (lymphangiosarcoma) is often unclear or controversial and it is convenient to discuss both types together.

There are three main clinicopathological subtypes: idiopathic cutaneous angiosarcoma of the head and neck, angiosarcoma complicating lymphoedema, and post-irradiation angiosarcoma.

Idiopathic cutaneous angiosarcoma of the head and neck.[250–252] These tumours most commonly involve the upper part of the face or the scalp of elderly people. Men are affected more frequently than women.[253] The lesions are single or multifocal, bluish or violaceous nodules, plaques or flat infiltrating areas; they occasionally may bleed or ulcerate. Extensive local growth is common and margins are difficult to define surgically. Metastasis to regional lymph nodes and to the lungs occurs, often after repeated surgical excision of the primary growth. The prognosis is poor. In one series only 15% survived for 5 years or more after diagnosis.[253] This may reflect the fact that clinical diagnosis is often delayed until the lesions are advanced.

Lymphangiosarcoma arising in chronic lymphoedematous limbs. Since 1948, when Stewart and Treves recognized the syndrome of post-mastectomy lymphangiosarcoma, the association of such tumours with chronic lymphoedema has become well known.[254] In their original series they described the appearance of purplish-red, raised, macular or polypoid tumours in the chronically oedematous arm of women who had undergone radical mastectomy on that side. The tumours appeared on average 12.5 years after surgery. Similar tumours have been reported in men after mastectomy. They have also occurred in cases without lymph node dissection and without preceding oedema. Much less commonly, similar tumours arise in the limbs of patients with chronic lymphoedema due to other causes. These include congenital lymphoedema (Milroy's disease), lymphoedema following other types of surgery, and chronic venous stasis.[255–257] Lymphangiosarcoma has also been reported in association with chronic filarial lymphoedema but appears to be a rare complication of this condition.[258]

Post-irradiation angiosarcoma. These tumours are very rare and occur many years (average 23.3 years) after X-irradiation for various conditions.[259,260]

Angiosarcomas have been reported to arise in pre-existing benign vascular tumours, including lymphangioma[261] and 'port wine' stains.[262] They have also occurred as a complication of varicose ulceration.[263]

Histopathology

The appearances are similar in the three groups.[250–252,254] The lesions are poorly circumscribed dermal tumours which infiltrate subcutaneous fat and other tissues and often have a multifocal distribution. Angiomatous and solid patterns may be seen. In the angiomatous areas a meshwork of anastomosing dilated vessels extends between pre-existing dermal collagen bundles and around skin appendages. The vessels are irregular and lined by crowded endothelial cells which range in appearance from virtually normal-looking endothelial cells to plump atypical protuberant cells with enlarged hyperchromatic nuclei (Fig. 38.24). Papillary processes may extend into the lumen of the vessel. In the solid areas of the poorly differentiated tumours the cells vary from spindle-shaped to polygonal epithelioid cells. Some areas may resemble Kaposi's sarcoma. Cytoplasmic vacuoles resembling primitive vascular lumina may be seen in some cells. Reticulin stains show that the cellular proliferation is on the luminal side of the reticulin fibres in the angiomatous areas. Generally, as architectural differentiation decreases cytological atypia and cell size tend to increase.[251] Lymphocytic infiltrates are commonly seen in the tumours and may obscure the underlying lesion, particularly in well-differentiated tumours with minimal cellular atypia.[251] Distinguishing the well differentiated angiomatous areas from benign vascular proliferations depends on the recognition of cellular atypia, the presence of crowding of lining cells and of solid papillary

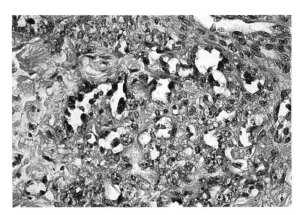

Fig. 38.24 Angiosarcoma. The vascular channels are lined by atypical endothelial cells.
Haematoxylin — eosin

clusters of cells, and an irregular interconnecting pattern of vessels. The differentiation of early lesions from early lesions of Kaposi's sarcoma may be dependent on clinicopathological correlation.

Poorly differentiated tumours with polygonal and epithelioid cells can resemble carcinomas and even amelanotic melanoma. Immuno-histochemical markers for keratins and S100 protein will help to distinguish between these tumours.

Many immunohistochemical markers for endothelial cells have been reported, including the well-known factor-VIII-related antigen and *Ulex europaeus* 1 lectin.[264,265] Poorly differentiated tumours are unfortunately less likely to stain with immunohistochemical markers than well-differentiated tumours, in which the vascular differentiation is already more obvious. In some cases, the use of frozen sections instead of paraffin sections[266] and special fixation techniques[267] may facilitate positive reactions.

Whether immunohistochemical markers such as factor-VIII-related antigen and anti-basement-membrane antibodies can distinguish tumours showing blood vessel differentiation from lymphatic differentiation is controversial.[268,269] The presence of factor-VIII-related antigen in endothelium of blood vessels and its absence in that of lymphatics has been reported by some[268] but not by others.[270] More specific markers such as PAL-E monoclonal antibody, which stains blood vessel endothelium but not lymphatic endothelium, are now being used to investigate tumour differentiation.[271]

Ultrastructural features of blood vessel endothelium include well-formed junctional complexes of the zonula adherens type, a well-developed basal lamina and Weibel–Palade bodies.[272] Lymphatic endothelial cells are said to lack Weibel–Palade bodies, to have cell junctions that are inconspicuous, and to have incomplete, if any, basal laminae.

Ultrastructural and immunohistochemical studies have confirmed that post-mastectomy lymphangiosarcomas are of endothelial origin[268,273,274] and not secondary breast carcinoma as has been suggested.[275] As alluded to in the introduction, the distinction between angiosarcoma and lymphangiosarcoma has become, in some cases, blurred with the use of modern investigative techniques. Immuno-histochemical studies have suggested that tumours arising in oedematous extremities are angiosarcomas rather than lymphangio-sarcomas.[268,276] A recent study of angiosarcoma of the face and scalp suggested that these tumours are more akin to lymphangiosarcomas than angiosarcomas.[267] As noted above, poorly differentiated tumours tend to lose the characteristic cell markers that would indicate their nature.

MALIGNANT ANGIOENDOTHELIOMATOSIS

This is a rare disorder characterized by an intravascular proliferation of cytologically malignant cells involving vessels of the skin and other organs. Early studies concluded that this was a neoplastic proliferation of endothelial cells. However, there is now convincing evidence, both histochemical and ultrastructural, that this is a peculiar form of malignant lymphoma. This entity is discussed in further detail on page 1046.

MALIGNANT GLOMUS TUMOUR

Rare cases have been described in which a spindle cell sarcomatous element has been identified in tumours otherwise showing the features of a glomus tumour.[277] Most of these tumours have not metastasized. Others have metastasized, the metastasis showing the histological features of a glomus tumour.

REFERENCES

Introduction

1. Metzker A. Cutaneous vascular lesions. Semin Dermatol 1988; 7: 9–16.

Telangiectases

1a. Jacobs AH, Walton RG. The incidence of birthmarks in the neonate. Pediatrics 1976; 58: 218–222.
2. Barsky SH, Rosen S, Geer DE, Noe JM. The nature and evolution of port wine stains: a computer-assisted study. J Invest Dermatol 1980; 74: 154–157.
3. Finley JL, Noe JM, Arndt KA, Rosen S. Port-wine stains. Morphologic variations and developmental lesions. Arch Dermatol 1984; 120: 1453–1455.
4. Braverman IM, Keh-Yen A. Ultrastructure and three-dimensional reconstruction of several macular and papular telangiectases. J Invest Dermatol 1983; 81: 489–497.
5. Finley JL, Clark RAF, Colvin RB et al. Immunofluorescent staining with antibodies to Factor VIII, fibronectin, and collagenous basement membrane protein in normal human skin and port wine stains. Arch Dermatol 1982; 118: 971–975.
6. Smoller BR, Rosen S. Port-wine stains. A disease of altered neural modulation of blood vessels? Arch Dermatol 1986; 122: 177–179.
7. Enjolras O, Riche MC, Merland JJ. Facial port-wine stains and Sturge-Weber syndrome. Pediatrics 1985; 76: 48–51.
8. Baskerville PA, Ackroyd JS, Browse NL. The etiology of the Klippel-Trenaunay syndrome. Ann Surg 1985; 202: 624–627.
9. Viljoen D, Saxe N, Pearn J, Beighton P. The cutaneous manifestations of the Klippel-Trenaunay-Weber syndrome. Clin Exp Dermatol 1987; 12: 12–17.
10. Servelle M. Klippel and Trenaunay's syndrome. 768 operated cases. Ann Surg 1985; 201: 365–373.
11. Jessen RT, Thompson S, Smith EB. Cobb syndrome. Arch Dermatol 1977; 113: 1587–1590.
12. Smith MA, Manfield PA. The natural history of salmon patches in the first year of life. Br J Dermatol 1962; 74: 31–33.
13. Tan KL. Nevus flammeus of the nape, glabella and eyelids. Clin Pediatrics 1972; 11: 112–118.
14. Bean WB. Vascular spiders and related lesions of the skin. Oxford: Blackwell Scientific Publications, 1958; 3.
15. Wenzl JE, Burgert EO Jr. The spider nevus in infancy and childhood. Pediatrics 1964; 33: 227–232.
16. Bean WB, Walsh JR. Venous lakes. Arch Dermatol 1956; 74: 459–463.
17. Epstein E, Novy FG Jr, Allington HV. Capillary aneurysms of the skin. Arch Dermatol 1965; 91: 335–341.
18. Imperial R, Helwig EB. Angiokeratoma. A clinicopathological study. Arch Dermatol 1967; 95: 166–175.
19. Haye KR, Rebello DJA. Angiokeratoma of Mibelli. Acta Derm Venereol 1961; 41: 56–60.
20. Imperial R, Helwig EB. Angiokeratoma of the scrotum (Fordyce type). J Urol 1967; 98: 379–387.
21. Bean WB. Vascular spiders and related lesions of the skin. Oxford: Blackwell Scientific Publications, 1958; 262–264.
22. Agger P, Osmundsen PE. Angiokeratoma of the scrotum

(Fordyce). A case report on response to surgical treatment of varicocele. Acta Derm Venereol 1970; 50: 221–224.

23. Imperial R, Helwig E. Angiokeratoma of the vulva. Obstet Gynecol 1967; 29: 307–312.

24. Novick NL. Angiokeratoma vulvae. J Am Acad Dermatol 1985; 12: 561–563.

25. Lynch PJ, Kosanovich M. Angiokeratoma circumscriptum. Arch Dermatol 1967; 96: 665–668.

26. Holmes RC, Fensom AH, McKee P et al. Angiokeratoma corporis diffusum in a patient with normal enzyme activities. J Am Acad Dermatol 1984; 10: 384–387.

27. Clarke JTR, Knaack J, Crawhall JC, Wolfe JS. Ceramide trihexosidosis (Fabry's disease) without skin lesions. N Engl J Med 1971; 284: 233–235.

28. Wallace HJ. Anderson-Fabry disease. Br J Dermatol 1973; 88: 1–23.

29. Epinette WW, Norins AL Drew AL et al. Angiokeratoma corporis diffusum with α-L-fucosidase deficiency. Arch Dermatol 1973; 107: 754–757.

30. Ishibashi A, Tsuboi R, Shinmei M. β-galactosidase and neuraminidase deficiency associated with angiokeratoma corporis diffusum. Arch Dermatol 1984; 120: 1344–1346.

31. Nakamura T, Kaneko H, Nishino I. Angiokeratoma corporis diffusum (Fabry disease): ultrastructural studies of the skin. Acta Derm Venereol 1981; 61: 37–41.

32. Bean WB. Vascular spiders and related lesions of the skin. Oxford: Blackwell Scientific Publications, 1958; 228.

32a. Tuder RM, Young R, Karasek M, Bensch K. Adult cutaneous hemangiomas are composed of nonreplicating endothelial cells. J Invest Dermatol 1987; 89: 594–597.

33. Barker LP, Sachs PM. Angioma serpiginosum. Arch Dermatol 1965; 92: 613–620.

34. Marriott PJ, Munro DD, Ryan T. Angioma serpiginosum — familial incidence. Br J Dermatol 1975; 93: 701–706.

35. Kumakiri M, Katoh N, Miura Y. Angioma serpiginosum. J Cutan Pathol 1980; 7: 410–421.

36. Michalowski R, Urban J. Atypical angioma serpiginosum: a case report. Dermatologica 1982; 164: 331–337.

37. Bean WB. Vascular spiders and related lesions of the skin. Oxford: Blackwell Scientific Publications, 1958; 132.

38. Daly JJ, Schiller AL. The liver in hereditary hemorrhagic telangiectasia (Osler-Weber-Rendu disease). Am J Med 1976; 60: 723–726.

39. Chandler D. Pulmonary and cerebral arteriovenous fistula with Osler's disease. Arch Intern Med 1965; 116: 277–282.

40. Dines DE, Arms RA, Bernatz PE, Gomes MR. Pulmonary arteriovenous fistulas. Mayo Clin Proc 1974; 49: 460–465.

41. Hashimoto K, Pritzker MS. Hereditary hemorrhagic telangiectasia. An electron microscopic study. Oral Surg 1972; 34: 751–758.

42. Menefee MG, Flessa HC, Glueck HI, Hogg SP. Hereditary hemorrhagic telangiectasia (Osler-Weber-Rendu disease). An electron microscopic study of the vascular lesions before and after therapy with hormones. Arch Otolaryngol 1975; 101: 246–251.

43. McGrae JD Jr, Winkelmann RK. Generalized essential telangiectasia. Report of a clinical and histochemical study of 13 patients with acquired cutaneous lesions. JAMA 1963; 185: 909–913.

43a. Ryan TJ, Wells RS. Hereditary benign telangiectasia. Trans St John's Hosp Dermatol Soc 1971; 57: 148–156.

43b. Gold MH, Eramo L, Prendiville JS. Hereditary benign telangiectasia. Pediatr Dermatol 1989; 6: 194–197.

44. Wagner RF Jr, Grande DJ, Bhawan J et al. Unilateral dermatomal superficial telangiectasia overlapping Becker's melanosis. Int J Dermatol 1989; 28: 595–596.

45. Wilkin JK, Smith JG Jr, Cullison DA et al. Unilateral dermatomal superficial telangiectasia. J Am Acad Dermatol 1983; 8: 468–477.

46. Uhlin SR, McCarty KS Jr. Unilateral nevoid telangiectatic syndrome. The role of estrogen and progesterone receptors. Arch Dermatol 1983; 119: 226–228.

47. Smith LL, Conerly SL. Ataxia-telangiectasia or Louis-Bar syndrome. J Am Acad Dermatol 1985; 12: 681–696.

48. Way BH, Hermann J, Gilbert EF et al. Cutis marmorata telangiectatica congenita. J Cutan Pathol 1974; 1: 10–25.

49. Rogers M, Poyzer KG. Cutis marmorata telangiectatica congenita. Arch Dermatol 1982; 118: 895–899.

50. South DA, Jacobs AH. Cutis marmorata telangiectatica congenita (congenital generalized phlebectasia). J Pediatrics 1978; 93: 944–947.

51. Picascia DD, Esterly NB. Cutis marmorata telangiectatica congenita: Report of 22 cases. J Am Acad Dermatol 1989; 20: 1098–1104.

52. Nicholls DSH, Harper JI. Cutis marmorata telangiectatica congenita with soft-tissue herniations on the lower legs. Clin Exp Dermatol 1989; 14: 369–370.

53. Lewis-Jones MS, Evans S, Graham-Brown RAC. Cutis marmorata telangiectatica congenita — a report of two cases occurring in male children. Clin Exp Dermatol 1988; 13: 97–99.

54. Lynch PJ, Zelickson AS. Congenital phlebectasia. A histopathologic study. Arch Dermatol 1967; 95: 98–101.

55. Miko T, Adler P, Endes P. Simulated cancer of the lower lip attributed to a 'caliber persistent' artery. J Oral Pathol 1980; 9: 137–144.

56. Miko TL, Molnar P, Vereckei L. Interrelationships of calibre persistent artery, chronic ulcer and squamous cancer of the lower lip. Histopathology 1983; 7: 595–599.

57. Marshall RJ, Leppard BJ. Ulceration of the lip associated with a 'calibre- persistent artery'. Br J Dermatol 1985; 113: 757–760.

Lymphangiectases

58. Prioleau PG, Santa Cruz DJ. Lymphangioma circumscriptum following radical mastectomy and radiation therapy. Cancer 1978; 42: 1989–1991.

59. Leshin B, Whitaker DC, Foucar E. Lymphangioma circumscriptum following mastectomy and radiation therapy. J Am Acad Dermatol 1986; 15: 1117–1119.

59a. Ziv R, Schewach-Millet M, Trau H. Lymphangiectasia. A complication of thoracotomy for bronchial carcinoid. Int J Dermatol 1988; 27: 123.

60. Weakley DR, Juhlin EA. Lymphangiectases and lymphangiomata. Arch Dermatol 1961; 84: 574–578.

61. Fisher I, Orkin M. Acquired lymphangioma (lymphangiectasis). Report of a case. Arch Dermatol 1970; 101: 230–234.

61a. Ambrojo P, Cogolludo EF, Aguilar A et al. Cutaneous lymphangiectases after therapy for carcinoma of the cervix — a case with unusual clinical and histological features. Clin Exp Dermatol 1990; 15: 57–59.

62. LaPolla J, Foucar E, Leshin B et al. Vulvar lymphangioma circumscriptum: a rare complication of therapy for squamous cell carcinoma of the cervix. Gynecol Oncol 1985; 22: 363–366.

Benign blood vessel proliferations

63. Storino WD, Engel GH. Multiple capillary hemangiomatosis. Acquired case with adult onset. Arch Dermatol 1973; 107: 739–740.

64. Norwood OT, Everett MA. Cardiac failure due to endocrine dependent hemangiomas. Arch Dermatol 1964; 89: 759–760.

65. Kaplan EN. In: Williams HB, ed. Symposium on vascular malformations and melanotic lesions. St Louis: CV Mosby, 1983; 144.

66. Höpfel-Kreiner I. Histogenesis of hemangiomas — an ultrastructural study on capillary and cavernous hemangiomas of the skin. Path Res Pract 1980; 170: 70–90.

67. Pesce C, Colacino R. Morphometric analysis of capillary and cavernous hemangiomas. J Cutan Pathol 1986; 13: 216–221.

68. Mulliken JB, Glowacki J. Hemangiomas and vascular malformations in infants and children: a classification based on endothelial characteristics. Plast Reconstr Surg 1982; 69: 412–420.

69. Hidano A, Nakajima S. Earliest features of the strawberry mark in the newborn. Br J Dermatol 1972; 87: 138–144.

70. Bowers RE, Graham EA, Tomlinson KM. The natural history of the strawberry nevus. Arch Dermatol 1960; 82: 667–680.

71. Walsh TS Jr, Tompkins VN. Some observations on the strawberry nevus of infancy. Cancer 1956; 9: 869–904.

72. Williams HB. Hemangiomas of the parotid gland in children. Plast Reconstr Surg 1975; 56: 29–34.

73. Jacobs AH. Vascular nevi. Pediatr Clin North Am 1983; 30: 465–482.

74. Wallace HJ. Conservative treatment of haemangiomatous naevi. Br J Plast Surg 1953; 6: 78–82.

75. Williams HB. Hemangiomas and lymphangiomas. Adv Surg 1981; 15: 317–349.

76. Wilkin JK. Unilateral dermatomal cavernous hemangiomatosis. Dermatologica 1980; 161: 347–354.

77. Steinway DM, Fretzin DF. Acquired zosteriform cavernous hemangiomas: brief clinical observation. Arch Dermatol 1977; 113: 848–849.

78. Baker ER, Manders E, Whitney CW. Growth of cavernous hemangioma with puberty. Clin Pediatr 1985; 24: 596–598.

79. Glowacki J, Mulliken JB. Mast cells in hemangiomas and vascular malformations. Pediatrics 1982; 70: 48–51.

80. Waldo ED, Vuletin JC, Kaye GI. The ultrastructure of vascular tumors: additional observations and a review of the literature. Pathol Annu 1977; 12 (part 2): 279–308.

81. Furusato M, Fukunaga M, Kikuchi Y et al. Two- and three-dimensional ultrastructural observations of angiogenesis in juvenile hemangioma. Virchows Arch [B] 1984; 46: 229–237.

82. Pasyk KA, Grabb WC, Cherry GW. Crystalloid inclusions in endothelial cells of cellular and capillary hemangiomas. A possible sign of cellular immaturity. Arch Dermatol 1983; 119: 134–137.

83. Holden KR, Alexander F. Diffuse neonatal hemangiomatosis. Pediatrics 1970; 46: 411–421.

84. Burke EC, Winkelmann RK, Strickland MK. Disseminated hemangiomatosis. The newborn with central nervous system involvement. Am J Dis Child 1964; 108: 418–424.

85. Cooper AG, Bolande RP. Multiple hemangiomas in an infant with cardiac hypertrophy. Postmortem angiographic demonstration of the arteriovenous fistulae. Pediatrics 1965; 35: 27–35.

86. Stern JK, Wolf JE Jr, Jarratt M. Benign neonatal hemangiomatosis. J Am Acad Dermatol 1981; 4: 442–445.

87. Keller L, Bluhm JF III. Diffuse neonatal hemangiomatosis. A case with heart failure and thrombocytopenia. Cutis 1979; 23: 295–297.

88. Bean WB. Vascular spiders and related lesions of the skin. Oxford: Blackwell Scientific Publications, 1958; 178.

89. Rice JS, Fischer DS. Blue rubber-bleb nevus syndrome. Arch Dermatol 1962; 86: 503–511.

90. Fine RM, Derbes VJ, Clark WH Jr. Blue rubber bleb nevus. Arch Dermatol 1961; 84: 802–805.

91. Berlyne GM, Berlyne N. Anaemia due to "blue rubber-bleb" naevus disease. Lancet 1960; 2: 1275–1277.

92. Talbot S, Wyatt EH. Blue rubber bleb naevi. (Report of a family in which only males were affected). Br J Dermatol 1970; 82: 37–39.

93. Suringa DWR, Ackerman AB. Cutaneous lymphangiomas with dyschondroplasia (Maffucci's syndrome). A unique variant of an unusual syndrome. Arch Dermatol 1970; 101: 472–474.

94. Bean WB. Dyschondroplasia and hemangiomata (Maffucci's syndrome). Arch Intern Med 1955; 95: 767–778.

95. Lewis RJ, Ketcham AS. Maffucci's syndrome: functional and neoplastic significance. J Bone Joint Surg [A] 1973; 55: 1465–1479.

96. Loewinger RJ, Lichtenstein JR, Dodson WE, Eisen AZ. Maffucci's syndrome: a mesenchymal dysplasia and multiple tumour syndrome. Br J Dermatol 1977; 96: 317–322.

97. Imperial R, Helwig EB. Verrucous hemangioma. A clinicopathologic study of 21 cases. Arch Dermatol 1967; 96: 247–253.

98. Rossi A, Bozzi M, Barra E. Verrucous hemangioma and angiokeratoma circumscriptum: clinical and histologic differential characteristics. J Dermatol Surg Oncol 1989; 15: 88–91.

99. Cruces MJ, De la Torre C. Multiple eruptive verrucous hemangiomas: a variant of multiple hemangiomatosis. Dermatologica 1985; 171: 106–111.

100. Padilla RS, Orkin M, Rosai J. Acquired "tufted"

angioma (progressive capillary hemangioma). A distinctive clinicopathologic entity related to lobular capillary hemangioma. Am J Dermatopathol 1987; 9: 292–300.

101. LeBoit PE. Lobular capillary proliferation: the underlying process in diverse benign cutaneous vascular neoplasms and reactive conditions. Semin Dermatol 1989; 8: 298–310.

102. Mills SE, Cooper PH, Fechner RE. Lobular capillary hemangioma: The underlying lesion of pyogenic granuloma. A study of 73 cases from the oral and nasal mucous membranes. Am J Surg Pathol 1980; 4: 471–479.

103. Kerr DA. Granuloma pyogenicum. Oral Surgery 1951; 4: 158–176.

104. Leyden JL, Master GH. Oral cavity pyogenic granuloma. Arch Dermatol 1973; 108: 226–228.

105. Nappi O, Wick MR. Disseminated lobular capillary hemangioma (pyogenic granuloma). A clinicopathologic study of two cases. Am J Dermatopathol 1986; 8: 379–385.

106. Mussalli NG, Hopps RM, Johnson NW. Oral pyogenic granuloma as a complication of pregnancy and the use of hormonal contraceptives. Int J Gynaecol Obstet 1976; 14: 187–191.

107. Ronchese F. Granuloma pyogenicum. Am J Surg 1965; 109: 430–431.

108. Juhlin L, Hjertquist S-O, Ponten J, Wallin J. Disseminated granuloma pyogenicum. Acta Derm Venereol 1970; 50: 134–136.

108a. Wilson BB, Greer KE, Cooper PH. Eruptive disseminated lobular capillary hemangioma (pyogenic granuloma). J Am Acad Dermatol 1989; 21: 391–394.

109. Warner J, Wilson Jones E. Pyogenic granuloma recurring with multiple satellites. A report of 11 cases. Br J Dermatol 1968; 80: 218–227.

110. Blickenstaff RD, Roenigk RK, Peters MS, Goellner JR. Recurrent pyogenic granuloma with satellitosis. J Am Acad Dermatol 1989; 21: 1241–1244.

111. Swerlick RA, Cooper PH. Pyogenic granuloma (lobular capillary hemangioma) within port-wine stains. J Am Acad Dermatol 1983; 8: 627–630.

112. Okada N. Solitary giant spider angioma with an overlying pyogenic granuloma. J Am Acad Dermatol 1987; 16: 1053–1054.

113. Rusin LJ, Harrell ER. Arteriovenous fistula. Cutaneous manifestations. Arch Dermatol 1976; 112: 1135–1138.

114. Marsch W Ch. The ultrastructure of eruptive hemangioma ('pyogenic granuloma'). J Cutan Pathol 1981; 8: 144–145.

115. Davies MG, Barton SP, Atai F, Marks R. The abnormal dermis in pyogenic granuloma. Histochemical and ultrastructural observations. J Am Acad Dermatol 1980; 2: 132–142.

116. Cooper PH, McAllister HA, Helwig EB. Intravenous pyogenic granuloma. A study of 18 cases. Am J Surg Pathol 1979; 3: 221–228.

117. Cooper PH, Mills SE. Subcutaneous granuloma pyogenicum. Lobular capillary hemangioma. Arch Dermatol 1982; 118: 30–33.

118. Wilson Jones E. Malignant vascular tumours. Clin Exp Dermatol 1976; 1: 287–312.

119. Wilson Jones E, Orkin M. Tufted angioma (angioblastoma). A benign progressive angioma, not to be confused with Kaposi's sarcoma or low-grade angiosarcoma. J Am Acad Dermatol 1989; 20: 214–225.

120. Macmillan A, Champion RH. Progressive capillary haemangioma. Br J Dermatol 1971; 85: 492–493.

121. Kumakiri M, Muramoto F, Tsukinaga I et al. Crystalline lamellae in the endothelial cells of a type of hemangioma characterized by the proliferation of immature endothelial cells and pericytes — angioblastoma (Nakagawa). J Am Acad Dermatol 1983; 8: 68–75.

122. Alessi E, Bertani E, Sala F. Acquired tufted angioma. Am J Dermatopathol 1986; 8: 426–429.

123. Cockerell CJ, Whitlow MA, Webster GF, Friedman-Kien AE. Epithelioid angiomatosis: a distinct vascular disorder in patients with the acquired immunodeficiency syndrome or AIDS-related complex. Lancet 1987; 2: 654–656.

123a. Szaniawski WK, Don PC, Bitterman SR, Schachner JR. Epithelioid angiomatosis in patients with AIDS. Report of seven cases and review of the literature. J Am Acad Dermatol 1990; 23: 41–48.

124. LeBoit PE, Berger TG, Egbert BM et al. Epithelioid haemangioma-like vascular proliferation in AIDS: manifestation of cat scratch disease bacillus infection? Lancet 1988; 1: 960–963.

124a. Walford N, Van der Wouw PA, Das PK et al. Epithelioid angiomatosis in the acquired immunodeficiency syndrome: morphology and differential diagnosis. Histopathology 1990; 16: 83–88.

125. Berger TG, Tappero JW, Kaymen A, LeBoit PE. Bacillary (epithelioid) angiomatosis and concurrent Kaposi's sarcoma in acquired immunodeficiency syndrome. Arch Dermatol 1989; 125: 1543–1547.

125a. Cockerell CJ, LeBoit PE. Bacillary angiomatosis: A newly characterized, pseudoneoplastic, infectious, cutaneous vascular disorder. J Am Acad Dermatol 1990; 22: 501–512.

125b. Axiotis CA, Schwartz R, Jennings TA, Glaser N. AIDS-related angiomatosis. Am J Dermatopathol 1989; 11: 177–181.

125c. Koehler JE, LeBoit PE, Egbert BM, Berger TG. Cutaneous vascular lesions and disseminated cat-scratch disease in patients with the acquired immunodeficiency syndrome (AIDS) and AIDS-related complex. Ann Intern Med 1988; 109: 449–455.

125d. LeBoit PE, Berger TG, Egbert BM et al. Bacillary angiomatosis. The histopathology and differential diagnosis of a pseudoneoplastic infection in patients with human immunodeficiency virus disease. Am J Surg Pathol 1989; 13: 909–920.

125e. Cockerell CJ, Bergstresser PR, Myrie-Williams C, Tierno PM. Bacillary epithelioid angiomatosis occurring in an immunocompetent individual. Arch Dermatol 1990; 126: 787–790.

126. Arias-Stella J, Lieberman PH, Erlandson RA, Arias-Stella J Jr. Histology, immunohistochemistry, and ultrastructure of the verruga in Carrion's disease. Am J Surg Pathol 1986; 10: 595–610.

127. Arias-Stella J, Lieberman PH, Garcia-Caceres U et al. Verruga peruana mimicking neoplasms. Am J Dermatopathol 1987; 9: 279–291.

128. Girard C, Graham JH, Johnson WC. Arteriovenous

hemangioma (arteriovenous shunt). A clinicopathological and histochemical study. J Cutan Pathol 1974; 1: 73–87.

129. Connelly MG, Winkelmann RK. Acral arteriovenous tumor. A clinicopathologic review. Am J Surg Pathol 1985; 9: 15–21.

130. Neumann RA, Knobler RM, Schuller-Petrovic S et al. Giant arteriovenous hemangioma (cirsoid aneurysm) of the nose. J Dermatol Surg Oncol 1989; 15: 739–742.

131. Wells GC, Whimster IW. Subcutaneous angiolymphoid hyperplasia with eosinophilia. Br J Dermatol 1969; 81: 1–15.

132. Wilson Jones E, Bleehen SS. Inflammatory angiomatous nodules with abnormal blood vessels occurring about the ears and scalp (pseudo or atypical pyogenic granuloma). Br J Dermatol 1969; 81: 804–816.

133. Enzinger FM, Weiss SW. Soft tissue tumors. St Louis: CV Mosby, 1983; 391–397.

134. Rosai J. Angiolymphoid hyperplasia with eosinophilia of the skin. Am J Dermatopathol 1982; 4: 175–184.

135. Rosai J, Akerman LR. Intravenous atypical vascular proliferation. A cutaneous lesion simulating a malignant blood vessel tumor. Arch Dermatol 1974; 109: 714–717.

136. Bendl BJ, Asano K, Lewis RJ. Nodular angioblastic hyperplasia with eosinophilia and lymphofolliculosis. Cutis 1977; 19: 327–329.

137. Kimura T, Yoshimura S, Ishikawa E. Unusual granulation combined with hyperplastic change of lymphatic tissue. Trans Soc Path Jap 1948; 37: 179–180.

138. Kawada A, Takahashi H, Anzai T. Eosinophilic lymphofolliculosis of the skin (Kimura's disease). Jpn J Dermatol 1966; 76: 61–72.

138a. Kuo T-T, Shih L-Y, Chan H-L. Kimura's disease. Involvement of regional lymph nodes and distinction from angiolymphoid hyperplasia with eosinophilia. Am J Surg Pathol 1988; 12: 843–854.

138b. Chan JKC, Hui PK, Ng CS et al. Epithelioid haemangioma (angiolymphoid hyperplasia with eosinophilia) and Kimura's disease in Chinese. Histopathology 1989; 15: 557–574.

139. Kung ITM, Gibson JB, Bannatyne PM. Kimura's disease: a clinico-pathological study of 21 cases and its distinction from angiolymphoid hyperplasia with eosinophilia. Pathology 1984; 16: 39–44.

140. Googe PB, Harris NL, Mihm MC Jr. Kimura's disease and angiolymphoid hyperplasia with eosinophilia: two distinct histopathological entities. J Cutan Pathol 1987; 14: 263–271.

140a. Aguilar A, Ambrojo P, Requena L et al. Angiolymphoid hyperplasia with eosinophilia limited to the vulva. Clin Exp Dermatol 1990; 15: 65–67.

141. Olsen TG, Helwig EB. Angiolymphoid hyperplasia with eosinophilia. A clinicopathologic study of 116 patients. J Am Acad Dermatol 1985; 12: 781–796.

142. Henry PG, Burnett JW. Angiolymphoid hyperplasia with eosinophilia. Arch Dermatol 1978; 114: 1168–1172.

143. Rosai J, Gold J, Landy R. The histiocytoid hemangiomas. Hum Pathol 1979; 10: 707–730.

144. Eady RAJ, Wilson Jones E. Pseudopyogenic granuloma: enzyme histochemical and ultrastructural study. Hum Pathol 1977; 8: 653–668.

145. Burgdorf WHC, Mukai K, Rosai J. Immunohistochemical identification of factor VIII-related antigen in endothelial cells of cutaneous lesions of alleged vascular nature. Am J Clin Pathol 1981; 75: 167–171.

146. Masson P. Hémangioendothéliome végétant intravasculaire. Bull Soc Anat (Paris) 1923; 93: 517–532.

147. Kuo T-T, Sayers CP, Rosai J. Masson's "vegetant intravascular hemangioendothelioma:" a lesion often mistaken for angiosarcoma. Cancer 1976; 38: 1227–1236.

148. Salyer WR, Salyer DC. Intravascular angiomatosis: development and distinction from angiosarcoma. Cancer 1975; 36: 995–1001.

149. Kumakiri M, Fukaya T, Miura Y. Blue rubber-bleb nevus syndrome with Masson's vegetant intravascular hemangioendothelioma. J Cutan Pathol 1981; 8: 365–373.

150. Clearkin KP, Enzinger FM. Intravascular papillary endothelial hyperplasia. Arch Pathol Lab Med 1976; 100: 441–444.

151. Escasany RT, Millet PU. Masson's pseudoangiosarcoma of the tongue: report of two cases. J Cutan Pathol 1985; 12: 66–71.

151a. Albrecht S, Kahn HJ. Immunohistochemistry of intravascular papillary endothelial hyperplasia. J Cutan Pathol 1990; 17: 16–21.

152. Kuo T-T, Gomez LG. Papillary endothelial proliferation in cystic lymphangiomas. Arch Pathol Lab Med 1979; 103: 306–308.

153. Reed CN, Cooper PH, Swerlick RA. Intravascular papillary endothelial hyperplasia. Multiple lesions simulating Kaposi's sarcoma. J Am Acad Dermatol 1984; 10: 110–113.

154. Kreutner A Jr, Smith RM, Trefny FA. Intravascular papillary endothelial hyperplasia. Light and electron microscopic observations of a case. Cancer 1978; 42: 2304–2310.

155. Earhart RN, Aeling JA, Nuss DD, Mellette JR. Pseudo-Kaposi sarcoma. A patient with arteriovenous malformation and skin lesions simulating Kaposi sarcoma. Arch Dermatol 1974; 110: 907–910.

156. Mali JWH, Kuiper JP, Hamers AA. Acro-angiodermatitis of the foot. Arch Dermatol 1965; 92: 515–518.

157. Meynadier J, Malbos S, Guilhou J-J, Barneon G. Pseudo-angiosarcomatose de Kaposi sur membre paralytique. Dermatologica 1980; 160: 190–197.

158. Bluefarb SM, Adams LA. Arteriovenous malformation with angiodermatitis. Stasis dermatitis simulating Kaposi's sarcoma. Arch Dermatol 1967; 96: 176–181.

158a. Landthaler M, Stolz W, Eckert F et al. Pseudo-Kaposi's sarcoma occurring after placement of arteriovenous shunt. A case report with DNA content analysis. J Am Acad Dermatol 1989; 21: 499–505.

159. Goldblum OM, Kraus E, Bronner AK. Pseudo-Kaposi's sarcoma of the hand associated with an acquired, iatrogenic arteriovenous fistula. Arch Dermatol 1985; 121: 1038–1040.

159a. Kolde G, Worheide J, Baumgartner R, Brocker E-B. Kaposi-like acroangiodermatitis in an above-knee amputation stump. Br J Dermatol 1989; 120: 575–580.

160. Rüdlinger R. Kaposiforme Akroangiodermatitiden (Pseudokaposi). Hautarzt 1985; 36: 65–68.
161. Gottlieb GJ, Ackerman AB. Kaposi's sarcoma: an extensively disseminated form in young homosexual men. Hum Pathol 1982; 13: 882–892.
162. Strutton G, Weedon D. Acro-angiodermatitis. A simulant of Kaposi's sarcoma. Am J Dermatopathol 1987; 9: 85–89.
163. Wilson-Jones E, Marks R. Papular angioplasia. Vascular papules of the face and scalp simulating malignant vascular tumors. Arch Dermatol 1970; 102: 422–427.
163a. Smith NP, Wilson Jones E. Multinucleate cell angiohistiocytoma: a new entity. J Cutan Pathol 1986; 13: 77.
163b. Smolle J, Auboeck L, Gogg-Retzer et al. Multinucleate cell angiohistiocytoma: a clinicopathological, immunohistochemical and ultrastructural study. Br J Dermatol 1989; 121: 113–121.
164. Pepper MC, Laubenheimer R, Cripps DJ. Multiple glomus tumors. J Cutan Pathol 1977; 4: 244–257.
165. Slater DN, Cotton DWK, Azzopardi JG. Oncocytic glomus tumour: a new variant. Histopathology 1987; 11: 523–531.
165a. Dervan PA, Tobbia IN, Casey M et al. Glomus tumours: an immunohistochemical profile of 11 cases. Histopathology 1989; 14: 483–491.
166. Miettinen M, Lehto V-P, Virtanen I. Glomus tumor cells: Evaluation of smooth muscle and endothelial cell properties. Virchows Arch [B] 1983; 43: 139–149.
167. Kishimoto S, Nagatani H, Miyashita A, Kobayashi K. Immunohistochemical demonstration of substance P-containing nerve fibres in glomus tumours. Br J Dermatol 1985; 113: 213–218.
168. Tsuneyoshi M, Enjoji M. Glomus tumor. A clinicopathologic and electron microscopic study. Cancer 1982; 50: 1601–1607.
168a. Bolton-Maggs PHB, Rustin MHA. Diffuse angioma-like changes associated with chronic DIC. Clin Exp Dermatol 1988; 13: 180–182.
168b. Hunt SJ, Santa Cruz DJ, Barr RJ. Microvenular hemangioma. J Cutan Pathol 1991; 18: 235–240.
168c. Santa Cruz DJ, Aronberg J. Targetoid hemosiderotic hemangioma. J Am Acad Dermatol 1988; 19: 550–558.

Benign lymphatic proliferations

169. Flanagan BP, Helwig EB. Cutaneous lymphangioma. Arch Dermatol 1977; 113: 24–30.
170. Peachey RDG, Lim C-C, Whimster IW. Lymphangioma of skin. A review of 65 cases. Br J Dermatol 1970; 83: 519–527.
171. Whimster IW. The pathology of lymphangioma circumscriptum. Br J Dermatol 1976; 94: 473–486.
172. Singh RP, Carr DH. The anatomy and histology of XO human embryos and fetuses. Anat Rec 1966; 155: 369–383.
173. Burstein JH. Lymphangioma circumscriptum with congenital unilateral lymphedema. Arch Dermatol 1956; 74: 689.
174. Palmer LC, Strauch WG, Welton WA.
Lymphangioma circumscriptum. A case with deep lymphatic involvement. Arch Dermatol 1978; 114: 394–396.
175. King DT, Duffy DM, Hirose FM, Gurevitch AW. Lymphangiosarcoma arising from lymphangioma circumscriptum. Arch Dermatol 1979; 115: 969–972.
176. Chervenak FA, Isaacson G, Blakemore KJ et al. Fetal cystic hygroma. Cause and natural history. N Engl J Med 1983; 309: 822–825.
177. Bill AH Jr, Sumner DS. A unified concept of lymphangioma and cystic hygroma. Surg Gynecol Obstet 1965; 120: 79–86.
178. Gold SC. Angioendothelioma (lymphatic type). Br J Dermatol 1970; 82: 92–93.
178a. Wilson Jones E, Winkelmann RK, Zachary CB, Reda AM. Benign lymphangioendothelioma. J Am Acad Dermatol 1990; 23: 229–235.
179. Tadaki T, Aiba S, Masu S, Tagami H. Acquired progressive lymphangioma as a flat erythematous patch on the abdominal wall of a child. Arch Dermatol 1988; 124: 699–701.
180. Watanabe M, Kishiyama K, Ohkawara A. Acquired progressive lymphangioma. J Am Acad Dermatol 1983; 8: 663–667.

Tumours with variable behaviour

181. Kaposi M. Idiopathisches multiple Pigmentsarkom der Haut. Arch Dermatol Syphilol 1872; 4: 265–273.
182. Centers for Disease Control. Kaposi's sarcoma and Pneumocystis pneumonia among homosexual men — New York City and California. MMWR 1981; 30: 305–308.
183. Rothman S. Remarks on sex, age and racial distribution of Kaposi's sarcoma and on possible pathogenetic factors. Acta Un Int Cancer 1962; 18: 326–329.
184. Cox FH, Helwig EB. Kaposi's sarcoma. Cancer 1959; 12: 289–298.
185. Safai B, Mike V, Giraldo G et al. Association of Kaposi's sarcoma with second primary malignancies. Possible etiopathogenic implications. Cancer 1980; 45: 1472–1479.
186. Piette WW. The incidence of second malignancies in subsets of Kaposi's sarcoma. J Am Acad Dermatol 1987; 16: 855–861.
187. Templeton AC. Kaposi's sarcoma. Pathol Annu 1981; 16 (part 2): 315–336.
188. Taylor JF, Templeton AC, Vogel CL et al. Kaposi's sarcoma in Uganda: a clinico-pathological study. Int J Cancer 1971; 8: 122–135.
189. Slavin G, Cameron HMcD, Forbes C, Smith RM. Kaposi's sarcoma in East African children: a report of 51 cases. J Pathol 1970; 100: 187–199.
190. Taylor JF, Smith PG, Bull D. Kaposi's sarcoma in Uganda. Geographic and ethnic distribution. Br J Cancer 1972; 26: 483–497.
191. Gange RW, Wilson Jones E. Kaposi's sarcoma and immunosuppressive therapy: an appraisal. Clin Exp Dermatol 1978; 3: 135–146.
192. Harwood AR, Osoba D, Hofstader SL et al. Kaposi's sarcoma in recipients of renal transplants. Am J Med 1979; 67: 759–765.
193. Barre-Sinoussi F, Chermann JC, Rey F et al. Isolation of a T-lymphotropic retrovirus from a patient at risk

for acquired immune deficiency syndrome (AIDS). Science 1983; 220: 868–871.

194. Gallo RC, Wong-Staal F. A human T-lymphotropic retrovirus (HTLV-III) as the cause of the acquired immunodeficiency syndrome. Ann Intern Med 1985; 103: 679–689.

195. Coffin J, Haase A, Levy JA et al. Human immunodeficiency viruses. Science 1986; 232: 697.

196. Chavel F, Masinho K, Chamaret S et al. Human immunodeficiency virus type 2 infection associated with AIDS in West Africa. N Engl J Med 1987; 316: 1180–1185.

197. Biggar RJ. The AIDS problem in Africa. Lancet 1986; 1: 79–82.

198. Bayley AC, Dowing RG, Cheingsong-Popov R et al. HTLV-III serology distinguishes atypical and endemic Kaposi's sarcoma in Africa. Lancet 1985; 1: 359–361.

198a. Padilla S, Rivera-Perlman Z, Solomon L. Kaposi's sarcoma in transfusion-associated acquired immunodeficiency syndrome. A case report and review of the literature. Arch Pathol Lab Med 1990; 114: 40–42.

199. Haverkos HW, Drotman DP, Morgan M. Prevalence of Kaposi's sarcoma among patients with AIDS. N Engl J Med 1985; 312: 1518.

200. Buck BE, Scott GB, Valdes-Dapena M, Parks WP. Kaposi sarcoma in two infants with acquired immune deficiency syndrome. J Pediatr 1983; 103: 911–913.

201. Whyte BM, Gold J, Dobson AJ, Cooper DA. Epidemiology of acquired immunodeficiency syndrome in Australia. Med J Aust 1987; 146: 65–69.

202. Lemich G, Schwan L, Lebwohl M. Kaposi's sarcoma and acquired immunodeficiency syndrome. Postmortem findings in twenty-four cases. J Am Acad Dermatol 1987; 16: 319–325.

203. Gottlieb MS, Groopman JE, Weinstein WM et al. The acquired immunodeficiency syndrome. Ann Intern Med 1983; 99: 208–220.

204. Rothenberg R, Woelfel M, Stoneburner R et al. Survival with the acquired immunodeficiency syndrome. Experience with 5833 cases in New York City. N Engl J Med 1987; 317: 1297–1302.

205. Real FX, Krown SE. Spontaneous regression of Kaposi's sarcoma in patients with AIDS. N Engl J Med 1985; 313: 1659.

206. Russell Jones R, Wilson Jones E. The histogenesis of Kaposi's sarcoma. Am J Dermatopathol 1986; 8: 369–370.

207. Nadji M, Morales AR, Ziegles-Weissman J, Penneys NS. Kaposi's sarcoma. Immunohistologic evidence for an endothelial origin. Arch Pathol Lab Med 1981; 105: 274–275.

208. Rutgers JL, Wieczorek R, Bonetti F et al. The expression of endothelial cell surface antigens by AIDS-associated Kaposi's sarcoma. Evidence for a vascular endothelial cell origin. Am J Pathol 1986; 122: 493–499.

208a. Holden CA, Histogenesis of Kaposi's sarcoma and angiosarcoma of the face and the scalp. J Invest Dermatol 1989; 93: 119s–124s.

209. Russell Jones R, Spaull J, Spry C, Wilson Jones E. Histogenesis of Kaposi's sarcoma in patients with and without acquired immune deficiency syndrome (AIDS). J Clin Pathol 1986; 39: 742–749.

209a. Witte MH, Stuntz M, Witte CL. Kaposi's sarcoma. A lymphologic perspective. Int J Dermatol 1989; 28: 561–570.

210. Beckstead JH, Wood GS, Fletcher V. Evidence for the origin of Kaposi's sarcoma from lymphatic endothelium. Am J Pathol 1985; 119: 294–300.

211. Dorfman RF. Kaposi's sarcoma with special reference to its manifestations in infants and children and to the concepts of Arthur Purdy Stout. Am J Surg Pathol (Suppl) 1986; 1: 68–77.

212. Schwartz JL, Muhlbauer JE, Steigbigel RT. Pre-Kaposi's sarcoma. J Am Acad Dermatol 1984; 11: 377–380.

213. De Dobbeleer G, Godfrine S, André J, et al. Clinically uninvolved skin in AIDS: evidence of atypical dermal vessels similar to early lesions observed in Kaposi's sarcoma. Ultrastructural study in four patients. J Cutan Pathol 1987; 14: 154–157.

214. Mittelman A, Wong G, Safai B et al. Analysis of T cell subsets in different clinical subgroups of patients with the acquired immune deficiency syndrome. Comparison with the "classic" form of Kaposi's sarcoma. Am J Med 1985; 78: 951–956.

215. Pollack MS, Safai B, Myskowski PL et al. Frequencies of HLA and Gm immunogenetic markers in Kaposi's sarcoma. Tissue Antigens 1983; 21: 1–8.

216. Prince HE, Schroff RW, Ayoub G et al. HLA studies in acquired immune deficiency syndrome patients with Kaposi's sarcoma. J Clin Immunol 1984; 4: 242–245.

217. Safai B, Johnson KG, Myskowski PL et al. The natural history of Kaposi's sarcoma in the acquired immunodeficiency syndrome. Ann Intern Med 1985; 103: 744–750.

218. Giraldo G, Beth E, Kyalwazi SK. Role of cytomegalovirus in Kaposi's sarcoma. IARC Sci Publ 1984; 63: 583–606.

219. Boldogh I, Beth E, Huang E-S et al. Kaposi's sarcoma. IV. Detection of CMV DNA, CMV RNA and CMNA in tumor biopsies. Int J Cancer 1981; 28: 469–474.

220. Jorgensen KA, Lawesson S-O. Amyl nitrite and Kaposi's sarcoma in homosexual men. N Engl J Med 1982; 307: 893–894.

221. Leu HJ, Odermatt B. Multicentric angiosarcoma (Kaposi's sarcoma). Virchows Arch [A] 1985; 408: 29–41.

222. Chow JWM, Lucas SB. Endemic and atypical Kaposi's sarcoma in Africa — histopathological aspects. Clin Exp Dermatol 1990; 15: 253–259.

223. Murray JF, Lothe F. The histopathology of Kaposi's sarcoma. Acta Un Int Cancer 1962; 18: 413–428.

224. Senba M. Autofluorescence of eosinophilic globules in Kaposi's sarcoma. Arch Pathol Lab Med 1985; 109: 703.

224a. Kao GF, Johnson FB, Sulica VI. The nature of hyaline (eosinophilic) globules and vascular slits of Kaposi's sarcoma. Am J Dermatopathol 1990; 12: 256–267.

225. Waldo E. Subtle clues to diagnosis by electron microscopy. Kaposi's sarcoma. Am J Dermatopathol 1979; 1: 177–180.

226. O'Connell KM. Kaposi's sarcoma: histopathological study of 159 cases from Malawi. J Clin Pathol 1977; 30: 687–695.

227. Blumenfeld W, Egbert BM, Sagebiel RW. Differential

diagnosis of Kaposi's sarcoma. Arch Pathol Lab Med 1985; 109: 123–127.

228. Weiss SW, Enzinger FM. Spindle cell hemangioendothelioma. A low-grade angiosarcoma resembling a cavernous hemangioma and Kaposi's sarcoma. Am J Surg Pathol 1986; 10: 521–530.

229. Enzinger FM, Smith BH. Hemangiopericytoma. An analysis of 106 cases. Hum Pathol 1976; 7: 61–82.

230. McMaster MJ, Soule EH, Ivins JC. Hemangiopericytoma. A clinicopathologic study and long-term followup of 60 patients. Cancer 1975; 36: 2232–2244.

231. Angervall L, Kindblom L-G, Nielsen JM et al. Hemangiopericytoma. A clinicopathologic, angiographic and microangiographic study. Cancer 1978; 42: 2412–2427.

232. Kauffman SL, Purdy Stout A. Hemangipericytoma in children. Cancer 1960; 13: 695–710.

233. Tulenko JF. Congenital hemangiopericytoma: case report. Plast Reconstr Surg 1968; 41: 276–277.

234. Hayes MMM, Dietrich BE, Uys CJ. Congenital hemangiopericytomas of skin. Am J Dermatopathol 1986; 8: 148–153.

235. Chung EB, Enzinger FM. Infantile myofibromatosis. Cancer 1981; 48: 1807–1818.

236. Nunnery EW, Kahn LB, Reddick RL, Lipper S. Hemangiopericytoma: a light microscopic and ultrastructural study. Cancer 1981; 47: 906–914.

237. Scott GA, Rosai J. Spindle cell hemangioendothelioma. Report of seven additional cases of a recently described vascular neoplasm. Am J Dermatopathol 1988; 10: 281–288.

238. Dabska M. Malignant endovascular papillary angioendothelioma of the skin in childhood. Clinicopathologic study of 6 cases. Cancer 1969; 24: 503–510.

239. Patterson K, Chandra RS. Malignant endovascular papillary angioendothelioma. Cutaneous borderline tumor. Arch Pathol Lab Med 1985; 109: 671–673.

240. Manivel JC, Wick MR, Swanson PE et al. Endovascular papillary angioendothelioma of childhood: a vascular lesion possibly characterized by "high" endothelial cell differentiation. Hum Pathol 1986; 17: 1240–1244.

241. de Dulanto F, Armijo-Moreno M. Malignant endovascular papillary hemangioendothelioma. Acta Derm Venereol 1973; 53: 403–407.

242. Morgan J, Robinson MJ, Rosen LB et al. Malignant endovascular papillary angioendothelioma (Dabska tumor). A case report and review of the literature. Am J Dermatopathol 1989; 11: 64–68.

243. Weiss SW, Enzinger FM. Epithelioid hemangioendothelioma. Cancer 1982; 50: 970–981.

244. Tsunugoshi M, Dorfman HD, Bauer TW. Epithelioid hemangioendothelioma of bone: a clinicopathologic, ultrastructural and immunohistochemical study. Am J Surg Pathol 1986; 10: 754–764.

245. Ishak KG, Sesterhenn IA, Goodman ZD et al. Epithelioid hemangioendothelioma of the liver. Hum Pathol 1984; 15: 839–852.

246. Tyring S, Guest P, Lee P et al. Epithelioid hemangioendothelioma of the skin and femur. J Am Acad Dermatol 1989; 20: 362–366.

247. Gray MH, Rosenberg AE, Dickersin GR, Bhan AK. Cytokeratin expression in epithelioid vascular neoplasms. Hum Pathol 1990; 21: 212–217.

248. Weiss SW, Ishak KG, Dail DH et al. Epithelioid hemangioendothelioma and related lesions. Semin Diagn Pathol 1986; 3: 259–287.

249. Marrogi AJ, Hunt SJ, Santa Cruz DJ. Cutaneous epithelioid angiosarcoma. Am J Dermatopathol 1990; 12: 350–356.

Malignant tumours

250. Wilson Jones E. Malignant angioendothelioma of the skin. Br J Dermatol 1964; 76: 21–39.

251. Cooper PH. Angiosarcomas of the skin. Semin Diagn Pathol 1987; 4: 2–17.

252. Rosai J, Sumner HW, Major MC et al. Angiosarcoma of the skin. A clinicopathologic and fine structural study. Hum Pathol 1976; 7: 83–109.

253. Holden CA, Spittle MF, Wilson Jones E. Angiosarcoma of the face and scalp, prognosis and treatment. Cancer 1987; 59: 1046–1057.

254. Stewart FW, Treves N. Lymphangiosarcoma in postmastectomy lymphedema. A report of six cases in elephantiasis chirurgica. Cancer 1948; 1: 64–81.

255. Alessi E, Sala F, Berti E. Angiosarcomas in lymphedematous limbs. Am J Dermatopathol 1986; 8: 371–378.

256. Woodward AH, Ivins JC, Soule EH. Lymphangiosarcoma arising in chronic lymphedematous extremities. Cancer 1972; 30: 562–572.

257. Maddox JC, Evans HL. Angiosarcoma of skin and soft tissue: A study of forty-four cases. Cancer 1981; 48: 1907–1921.

258. Muller R, Hajdu SI, Brennan MF. Lymphangiosarcoma associated with chronic filarial lymphedema. Cancer 1987; 59: 179–183.

259. Goette DK, Detlefs RL. Postirradiation angiosarcoma. J Am Acad Dermatol 1985; 12: 922–926.

260. Handfield-Jones SE, Kennedy CTC, Bradfield JB. Angiosarcoma arising in an angiomatous naevus following irradiation in childhood. Br J Dermatol 1988; 118: 109–112.

261. King DT, Duffy DM, Hirose FM, Gurevitch AW. Lymphangiosarcoma arising from lymphangioma circumscriptum. Arch Dermatol 1979; 115: 969–972.

262. Girard C, Johnson WC, Graham JH. Cutaneous angiosarcoma. Cancer 1970; 26: 868–883.

263. Al-Najjar AA-W, Harrington CI, Slater DN. Angiosarcoma: a complication of varicose leg ulceration. Acta Derm Venereol 1986; 66: 167–170.

264. Miettinen M, Holthofer H, Lehto V-P. Ulex europaeus 1 lectin as a marker for tumors derived from endothelial cells. Am J Clin Pathol 1983; 79: 32–36.

265. Burgdorf WHC, Mukai K, Rosai J. Immunohistochemical identification of factor VIII-related antigen in endothelial cells of cutaneous lesions of alleged vascular nature. Am J Clin Pathol 1981; 75: 167–171.

266. Perez-Atayde AR, Achenbach H, Lack EE. High-grade epithelioid angiosarcoma of the scalp. An immunohistochemical and ultrastructural study. Am J Dermatopathol 1986; 8: 411–418.

267. Holden CA, Spaull J, Das AK et al. The histogenesis of angiosarcoma of the face and scalp: an

immunohistochemical and ultrastructural study. Histopathology 1987; 11: 37–51.

268. Capo V, Ozzello L, Fenoglio CM et al. Angiosarcomas arising in edematous extremities: Immunostaining for factor VIII-related antigen and ultrastructural features. Hum Pathol 1985; 16: 144–150.

269. Barsky SH, Togo S, Baker A et al. Use of anti-basement membrane antibodies to distinguish blood vessel capillaries from lymphatic capillaries. Am J Surg Pathol 1983; 7: 667–677.

270. Svanholm H, Nielsen K, Hauge P. Factor VIII-related antigen and lymphatic collecting vessels. Virchows Arch [A] 1984; 404: 223–228.

271. Schlingemann RO, Dingjan GM, Emeis JJ. Monoclonal antibody PAL-E specific for endothelium. Lab Invest 1985; 52: 71–76.

272. Carstens PHB. The Weibel–Palade Body in the diagnosis of endothelial tumors. Ultrastruct Pathol 1981; 2: 315–325.

273. Kanitakis J, Bendelac A, Marchand C et al. Stewart-Treves syndrome: an histogenetic (ultrastructural and immunohistological) study. J Cutan Pathol 1986; 13: 30–39.

274. McWilliam LJ, Harris M. Histogenesis of post-mastectomy angiosarcoma — an ultrastructural study. Histopathology 1985; 9: 331–343.

275. Schafler K, McKenzie CG, Salm R. Postmastectomy lymphangiosarcoma: a reappraisal of the concept — a critical review and report of an illustrative case. Histopathology 1979; 3: 131–152.

276. Hultberg BM. Angiosarcomas in chronically lymphedematous extremities. Two cases of Stewart-Treves syndrome. Am J Dermatopathol 1987; 9: 406–412.

277. Aiba M, Hirayama A, Kuramochi S. Glomangiosarcoma in a glomus tumor. An immunohistochemical and ultrastructural study. Cancer 1988; 61: 1467–1471.

Cutaneous metastases

INTRODUCTION

Metastasis represents the end stage of a complex series of interreactions between the tumour cells and the tissues of the host.[1] There are many factors which influence the localization of metastases other than the natural lymphatic and vascular connections of the primary tumour. In the past, the concept of 'favourable soil' and 'unfavourable soil' was invoked in an attempt to explain why certain organs were only rarely involved by metastases. There are now some scientific explanations available to account for the 'unfavourable soil' of some organs, although none has been advanced that explains satisfactorily why the skin generally is an uncommon site for visceral metastases. The vascularity of the scalp may explain why this is sometimes a favoured site. The tumour cells may reach the skin by direct invasion from an underlying tumour, by accidental implantation during a surgical or diagnostic procedure and by lymphatic and haematogenous spread.

Based on several large autopsy series of patients with visceral cancer, the incidence of cutaneous metastases is about 2% of all cases.[1] The usually quoted range from several different studies is 1.2–4.4%.[2,3] In one series, the skin was the 18th most frequent metastatic site for all tumour types.[4]

There are many generalizations that can be made about cutaneous metastases. These relate to the time interval between their manifestation and the diagnosis of the primary tumour, their clinical appearance, their location, the site of origin of the primary tumour and their prognostic significance. These aspects will be considered below, followed by an account of the cutaneous metastases derived from various viscera.

CLINICAL AND MORPHOLOGICAL FEATURES

Time of development

Cutaneous metastases may be the first indication of a visceral cancer,[5] the incidence in one series being 0.8%.[5a] These *precocious metastases* are particularly likely to present at the umbilicus, or less frequently on the scalp. The kidney,[6] lung,[7] thyroid,[8] and ovary[5] are organs whose tumours may present in this way.[9]

With most tumours, the metastases develop some months or years after the primary malignancy has been diagnosed,[5] so-called *metachronous metastases*. In about 7% of cases, this interval exceeds five years. Tumours of the breast and kidney and malignant melanomas may give rise to delayed metastases.[10]

The term *synchronous metastasis* is used when the cutaneous metastasis and the primary tumour are diagnosed simultaneously.[11] This sometimes occurs with tumours of the breast and oral cavity.

Clinical aspects

Cutaneous metastases are more likely to be found in older individuals.[12] In neonates, they are usually derived from a neuroblastoma. Metastases from germ cell and trophoblastic tumours, although rare in the skin, develop there particularly in young adults.

Cutaneous metastases usually present as multiple, discrete, painless, freely movable nodules of sudden onset.[9,13] Sometimes there are several small nodules localized to one area.[14] Solitary metastases occur in about 10% of cases. The nodules are usually 1–3 cm in diameter. They vary in colour from red to bluish-purple to light brown or flesh coloured. Occasionally plaques are formed. One variant of this form develops in the scalp as patches of alopecia (alopecia neoplastica), sometimes resembling

alopecia areata.[15,16] Cicatricial plaques also form: metastases from the breast,[15,16] lung and kidney may give this pattern on rare occasions.

There are isolated reports of other patterns of cutaneous metastases.[3] For example, they may resemble erythema annulare,[3] a chancre,[17] an epidermal cyst,[18] a condyloma,[3] or an ulcer.[3] They may present in a zosteriform pattern[10,19–20a] or produce elephantiasis of the lower limbs due to lymphatic obstruction.[21] Metastases have also been reported in an area of radiation dermatitis.[22]

There are three clinical patterns of metastasis which are almost exclusively related to carcinomas of the breast — carcinoma erysipelatoides ('inflammatory carcinoma'), carcinoma telangiectaticum and carcinoma en cuirasse.[12,23] The inflammatory pattern presents as a large, tender, warm plaque which may resemble erysipelas.[10,23,24] It is found in less than 2% of all breast carcinomas. Some would regard this as due to direct extension from the underlying carcinoma and not a true metastasis.[9] Rarely, this pattern is seen with metastases from carcinomas of the stomach, pancreas,[25] rectum[26] and lung.[20,27] It follows the obstruction of lymphatics at all levels of the dermis with resulting oedema.[24] There are often some perivascular and perilymphatic inflammatory cells. Carcinoma telangiectaticum presents as a telangiectatic sclerotic plaque often studded with pink papules and pseudovesicles.[23,28] There is massive subepidermal oedema resulting from obstruction by tumour of small blood vessels and lymphatics in the upper dermis. Other vessels are congested. Rarely, metastases from the lung will give this picture. Carcinoma en cuirasse is a diffuse induration of the breast resulting from some dermal fibrosis and a diffuse infiltrate of tumour cells between collagen bundles, sometimes in an Indian file pattern.[23]

Location of metastases

Metastases tend to occur on the cutaneous surfaces near the site of the primary tumour, although there are many exceptions. Metastases from tumours of the lung often involve the chest wall and proximal parts of the upper extremities,

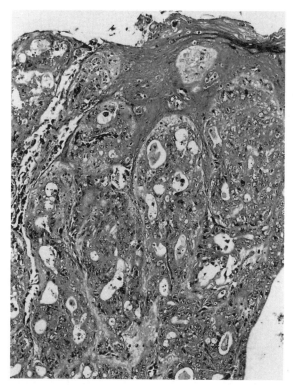

Fig. 39.1 Umbilicus: Sister Mary Joseph nodule. The dermis is replaced by metastatic adenocarcinoma of colonic origin. Haematoxylin — eosin

while those from the oral cavity and oesophagus may metastasize to the head and neck, and those from the gastrointestinal and genitourinary systems to the abdominal wall.[14,29] Approximately 5% of metastases involve the scalp.[5]

Metastasis to the umbilicus is also quite common.[30,31] The lesion that results has been called the Sister Mary Joseph nodule, in recognition of a nursing superintendent at the Mayo Clinic, Rochester, Minn., who is credited with recognizing the clinical significance of these nodules.[31] The underlying primary tumour is usually an adenocarcinoma of the stomach, large bowel, ovary, pancreas, endometrium or breast (Fig. 39.1).[30,31] Rare primary tumours have included a carcinoid and a leiomyosarcoma of the intestine. Sister Mary Joseph nodules are usually solitary and firm, sometimes with surface fissuring. In 12 of a series of 85 cases reported in 1984, the umbilical nodule was the initial presentation of the tumour.[31] There are various routes by which tumour cells can reach the umbilicus. These include contiguous extension and spread by lymphatic and venous channels, often associated with embryological vestiges in this region.[31]

The penis may be the site of metastases from the bladder and prostate.[32,33] The deposits are usually multiple. Sometimes they are associated with priapism.[32]

The lower extremities, excluding the thighs, are uncommonly involved with metastases.[5] Other rare sites of metastases include the nail bed, thumb, scrotum, eyebrow and ear.[1,3,34]

Cutaneous metastases may develop at the site of a surgical or diagnostic procedure.[1] Metastases are sometimes seen in abdominal, perineal, mastectomy and nephrectomy scars, around colostomy sites, and along the track produced by a thoracentesis needle. However, seeding along the needle track is unexpectedly rare following percutaneous biopsy of prostatic carcinomas.[35]

Sites of the primary tumour

The detailed studies of Brownstein and Helwig (1972) provided valuable information regarding the most frequent sites of origin of the tumours that give rise to cutaneous metastases.[29] They studied 724 patients in whom there was histopathological confirmation of both the primary tumour and the secondary deposit in the skin. Their studies complement the earlier report by Gates in 1937.[34]

The most frequent primary tumours in men were carcinoma of the lung (24%), carcinoma of the large intestine (19%), melanoma (13%), and squamous cell carcinoma of the oral cavity (12%).[29] In women they were carcinoma of the breast (69%), carcinoma of the large intestine (9%), melanoma (5%), and carcinoma of the ovary (4%).[29] A more recent study from India (1988) show the lung and oesophagus to be the most common sites of the primary tumour in men and the breast and ovary in women.[35a]

Prognostic aspects

The development of cutaneous metastases is

usually a grave prognostic feature, as dissemination to other organs has usually occurred. The average survival time after the appearance of cutaneous metastases is three to six months.[14] However, there are many reports of patients with carcinoma of the breast, neuroblastoma, and other tumours[8] who survived many years after the appearance of the cutaneous metastases.

Histopathological features

More than 60% of metastases are adenocarcinomas, usually arising in the large intestine, lung or breast.[10,14] If the glandular structures are well differentiated, the colon or rectum should be suspected as the primary site. Tumours from the breast usually have a very undifferentiated pattern with sheets of cells or sometimes columns between the collagen bundles. Signet-ring cells can be found in some metastases of mammary origin, but they are more usual in secondary deposits of gastric origin.

About 15% of metastases are of squamous cell type. They usually arise from the oral cavity, lung or oesophagus. The remainder of cutaneous metastases are melanomas, anaplastic tumours, or other rare specific patterns.

Metastases usually resemble the primary tumour, although the features are sometimes more anaplastic.[14] The metastases from a renal clear cell carcinoma can appear disarmingly benign:[36] a mistaken diagnosis of a benign appendage tumour may be made in these circumstances (Fig. 39.2).

Metastases are centred on the dermis, although there is sometimes extension into the subcutis. The epidermis is usually intact and there is an underlying narrow zone of compressed collagen separating the tumour from the epidermis (grenz zone). Occasionally a metastatic squamous cell carcinoma will touch the undersurface of the epidermis, making distinction from a primary carcinoma difficult.[37] Dermal sclerosis is uncommon, but this can be seen with some breast carcinomas.

Lymphatic permeation is a prominent feature of the so-called inflammatory carcinomas (see p. 982). It is sometimes present at the edge of a

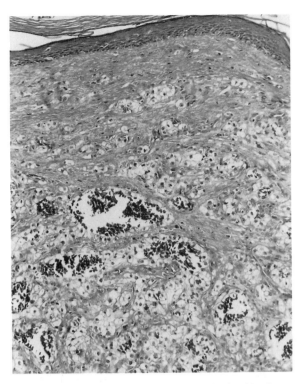

Fig. 39.2   Metastatic renal cell carcinoma in the skin. A mistaken diagnosis of eccrine hidradenoma is sometimes made in such a case.
Haematoxylin — eosin

cutaneous metastasis. Uncommonly, lymphatic channels throughout the dermis are involved (Fig. 39.3).

Immunohistochemistry is of increasing value in the interpretation of cutaneous metastases.[38] Monoclonal antibodies against thyroglobulin, calcitonin, prostatic antigens, leucocyte common antigen (CD45), epithelial membrane antigen, S 100 protein, neuron-specific enolase, various cytokeratins, vimentin and desmin can be used to elucidate or confirm the nature of the primary tumour that gave rise to the cutaneous metastasis. This investigative field is expanding rapidly with many new markers appearing.

SPECIFIC METASTASES

Breast

The anterior chest wall is commonly involved by recurrences of carcinoma of the breast, although

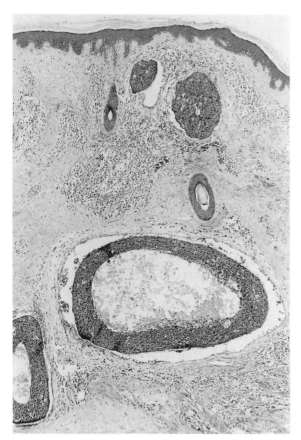

Fig. 39.3 Metastatic adenocarcinoma with widespread lymphatic permeation. Haematoxylin — eosin

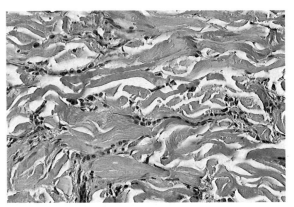

Fig. 39.4 Metastatic carcinoma of breast origin. The tumour cells are arranged in an 'Indian file' pattern. Haematoxylin — eosin

distant cutaneous metastases are uncommon.[39] In his review of cutaneous metastases, Rosen mentions two autopsy series of carcinoma of the breast where cutaneous metastases were found in 18.6 and 37.7% of cases respectively.[1] Brownstein and Helwig in their study of 724 patients with cutaneous metastases recorded 168 cases in women with carcinoma of the breast (69% of the total number of women in the series) and 9 in men.[29] In 20 of these there were single, distant metastases; in 3 there were multiple metastases.[29] In the remainder, only the chest wall was involved.

The scalp is a favoured site of distant metastases.[39] Patches of alopecia resembling alopecia areata (alopecia neoplastica) may result.[15,16,40–42] Other clinical patterns found on the chest wall include the so-called inflammatory carcinoma, carcinoma telangiectaticum and carcinoma en cuirasse.[23] Prolonged survival has been recorded after the appearance of the cutaneous lesions.[41]

Carcinoma of the inframammary crease is an uncommon but distinctive pattern of presentation which results from early invasion of the skin by a peripherally situated tumour.[43,44] It is exophytic and fissured and may simulate a primary epidermal tumour both clinically and microscopically.[45]

Histopathology

The histopathology is usually that of a poorly differentiated adenocarcinoma (Fig. 39.4). There may be sheets or large clusters of tumour cells in the dermis. Sometimes the cells are in linear array between the collagen bundles, resulting in an 'Indian file' pattern.[29] Rarely, the cells resemble those seen in a granular cell tumour.[45a] Lymphatic permeation may be prominent, particularly in those with an inflammatory or telangiectatic clinical pattern. Sclerosis of dermal collagen is sometimes present, particularly in the scalp lesions associated with alopecia neoplastica.[16]

Occasionally only scattered small tumour cells are present in the dermis, and these may be difficult to distinguish from inflammatory cells.[29] Epithelial membrane antigen is detectable on these cells by immunoperoxidase methods. It should be remembered that an occasional carcinoma of the breast will have S100-positive cells, which could lead to a mistaken diagnosis of malignant melanoma.

Lung

Cutaneous metastases are found in 4% or less[46] of patients with carcinoma of the lung. In a small number of cases these are precocious metastases.[7] The chest wall and abdomen are the usual sites, although 'oat cell' carcinomas appear to have a predilection for metastasizing to the back.[11] Rarely, an inflammatory or zosteriform pattern is produced. Death usually occurs within three months of the development of the skin lesions. The histopathological pattern is squamous cell carcinoma in 40%, adenocarcinoma in 20%, and undifferentiated carcinoma in 40%.[11] One bronchiolar and one mucoepidermoid bronchial carcinoma were among the tumours of lung reported by Brownstein and Helwig in their review on cutaneous metastases.[29]

Oral cavity and gastrointestinal system

Tumours of the *oral cavity* usually spread to the face or neck.[29] In some instances this results from direct extension of the tumour rather than true metastasis.[9] The tumours are usually squamous cell carcinomas.

Less than 2% of *oesophageal carcinomas* metastasize to the skin.[11] The primary lesion is usually a squamous cell carcinoma in the lower oesophagus.[11] The metastases are multiple nodules with a predilection for the upper part of the trunk and the neck.

Brownstein and Helwig reported 29 cases of *gastric carcinoma* with metastasis to skin.[29] The trunk, particularly the umbilical area, is a favoured site.[31,47,48] The tumours are usually poorly differentiated adenocarcinomas. Signet-ring cells and extracellular mucin pools may be present.

The *colon* is a common source of cutaneous metastases. Brownstein and Helwig recorded 90 males and 22 females in this category.[29] This makes it the second most common primary site

in both males and females. Brady reported a 3.5% incidence of cutaneous metastases in patients coming to autopsy with adenocarcinoma of the colon and rectum.[11] The metastases are usually multiple and metachronous and most often are in the skin of the abdominal wall or perineal region.[11,29] The umbilicus may be involved.[31,49,50] The appearance of multiple metastases is a bad prognostic sign. The deposits are usually composed of well-differentiated adenocarcinoma, although mucinous, less well differentiated variants are found.

Liver, pancreas and gallbladder

Cutaneous metastases occur in nearly 3% of patients with malignant *hepatomas*.[51,52] Rarely, it is the presenting manifestation,[53] although death still follows in several weeks.[52] A 12-year-old child with cutaneous metastases on the thorax and epigastrium has been reported.[54] The histopathological pattern may be either a chol-angiocarcinoma or a hepatocellular carcinoma.[52]

Brownstein and Helwig recorded 15 cases of metastatic *pancreatic carcinoma* involving the skin.[29] The umbilicus is a favoured site for these metastases.[30,55,56] Rarely, an inflammatory pattern is present.[25]

There are several reports in which the primary tumour was in the *gallbladder*.[57,58] Rarely, the metastasis in such cases is to the umbilicus.[31]

Kidney

Metastases have been reported in the skin in from 2.8–6.3% of renal carcinomas.[11] They accounted for 6% of the cutaneous metastases in males, and 0.5% in females in the series of Brownstein and Helwig.[29] As such, they rank after breast, lung, gastrointestinal tract and melanoma in order of frequency.[29] The metastases are solitary in from 15–20% of cases.[36,59] The head, particularly the scalp, is a common site of involvement.[36,59] They may also be found in nephrectomy scars and the external genitalia.[59] The metastases are sometimes precocious. Metachronous metastases usually appear within three years of the nephrectomy,[29] although an interval of 23 years has been recorded.[36] The deposits can be quite vascular and even resemble a pyogenic granuloma[60] or Kaposi's sarcoma.[61]

Most cases are clear cell carcinomas in which the cells contain considerable glycogen and some fat.[36] Mitoses are sparse. There is usually extravasation of blood with subsequent deposition of haemosiderin in the stroma. Metastasis of a Wilms' tumour to the skin is rarely reported.[36]

Bladder and urethra

Cutaneous metastases from *carcinomas of the urinary bladder* are rare,[62,63] ranging from 0.18%[64] to 1.8%.[11] Brownstein and Helwig reported only 10 cases in their review of 724 patients with cutaneous metastases.[29] The *urethra* is more rarely the primary site.[62,65]

Metastases from the bladder are usually multiple, and at a single site.[11] The upper extremities, trunk, abdomen and penis are the usual sites.[62,66] The tumours are transitional cell carcinomas or anaplastic carcinomas which may show areas of squamous differentiation.[65]

Male genital system

In one study of 321 metastatic lesions in 176 autopsy cases of carcinoma of the *prostate*, 4 lesions metastatic to the skin were found.[67] Brownstein and Helwig recorded only 5 cases in their large series.[29] The metastases are usually firm violaceous nodules, although unusual clinical patterns[32] such as Sister Mary Joseph nodules (see p. 983),[31] penile deposits,[32,33,68,69] a zosteriform pattern[19] and a nodule simulating a sebaceous cyst[18] have been recorded. The primary tumour is usually an adenocarcinoma,[70] but one transitional cell carcinoma has been documented.[71] Immunoperoxidase staining for prostate-specific antigen is a useful technique for confirming the prostatic origin of the metastatic adenocarcinomas.[71a]

There are only few reports of cutaneous metastases from *testicular tumours*.[72] The histopathological pattern has included seminoma,[72] teratocarcinoma[73] and choriocarcinoma.[14]

Squamous cell carcinomas of the *penis* rarely give rise to cutaneous metastases.[10]

Female genital system

Cutaneous metastases are found in approximately 2% of patients with fatal *ovarian carcinoma*.[11] Brownstein and Helwig recorded 10 cases, which represent 4% of the cutaneous metastatic lesions in females.[29] There are usually multiple nodules at a solitary site on the chest or abdomen. The umbilicus may be involved.[74] The pattern is usually that of a well-differentiated adenocarcinoma, sometimes having a papillary configuration with psammoma bodies.[29] A carcinoma of mucinous pattern and a Brenner tumour[75] have also been reported.

Cutaneous metastases are unusual in carcinoma of the *cervix*[76] *and uterine body*,[77,78] even in the terminal phases.[79,80] They usually involve the lower abdomen, groin, upper thighs[81] or umbilicus.[31,74,78,82,83] Endometrial tumours are adenocarcinomas,[77] while those from the cervix may be squamous cell carcinomas[76,81] or adenosquamous in type.[13,14] In a review of the literature of genital carcinomas with metastases to the umbilicus, Galle recorded 18 of ovarian origin, 12 from the uterine body, 1 squamous cell carcinoma from the cervix, and 2 adenocarcinomas from the *fallopian tube*.[74]

Skin metastases are an unfavourable prognostic sign in *gestational trophoblastic disease*. They occur only in association with widespread disease.[84] Gluteal metastases[85] and a solitary nodule in the scalp[86] have been reported. There have been several cases of placental choriocarcinoma metastasizing to the skin of a neonate.[87] The histopathology is usually similar to the primary lesion with large syncytial trophoblastic cells and much haemorrhage.[86] Chorionic gonadotrophin can be demonstrated using immunoperoxidase techniques.

Thyroid

Brownstein and Helwig recorded only 4 cases of metastatic thyroid tumours.[29] In one autopsy study, cutaneous metastases were noted in 2 of 12 medullary carcinomas and 4 of 12 giant cell

REFERENCES

Introduction

1. Rosen T. Cutaneous metastases. Med Clin North Am 1980; 64: 885–900.
2. Krumerman MS, Garret R. Carcinomas metastatic to skin. NY State J Med 1977; 77: 1900–1903.
3. Su WPD, Powell FC, Goellner JR. In: Wick MR. Pathology of unusual malignant cutaneous tumors. New York: Marcel Dekker, 1985; 357–397.
4. Abrams HL, Spiro R, Goldstein N. Metastases in carcinoma: Analysis of 1,000 autopsied cases. Cancer 1950; 3: 74–85.

Clinical and morphological features

5. Brownstein MH, Helwig EB. Patterns of cutaneous metastasis. Arch Dermatol 1972; 105: 862–868.
5a. Lookingbill DP, Spangler N, Sexton FM. Skin involvement as the presenting sign of internal carcinoma. A retrospective study of 7316 cancer patients. J Am Acad Dermatol 1990; 22: 19–26.
6. Jevtic AP. Skin metastasis from renal carcinoma presenting as an inflammatory lesion. Australas J Dermatol 1987; 28: 18–20.
7. Camiel MR, Aron BS, Alexander LL et al. Metastases to palm, sole, nailbed, nose, face and scalp from unsuspected carcinoma of the lung. Cancer 1969; 23: 214–220.
8. Pitlik S, Kitzes R, Ben-Bassat M, Rosenfeld JB. Thyroid carcinoma presenting as a solitary skin metastasis. Cutis 1983; 31: 532–536.
9. White JW Jr. Evaluating cancer metastatic to the skin. Geriatrics 1985; 40: 67–73.
10. Brownstein MH, Helwig EB. Spread of tumors to the skin. Arch Dermatol 1973; 107: 80–86.
11. Brady LW, O'Neill EA, Farber SH. Unusual sites of metastases. Semin Oncol 1977; 4: 59–64.
12. McKee PH. Cutaneous metastases. J Cutan Pathol 1985; 12: 239–250.
13. Taboada CF, Fred HL. Cutaneous metastases. Arch Intern Med 1966; 117: 516–519.
14. Reingold IM. Cutaneous metastases from internal carcinoma. Cancer 1966; 19: 162–168.
15. Cohen I, Levy E, Schreiber H. Alopecia neoplastica due to breast carcinoma. Arch Dermatol 1961; 84: 490–492.
16. Baum EM, Omura EF, Payne RR, Little WP. Alopecia neoplastica — a rare form of cutaneous metastasis. J Am Acad Dermatol 1981; 4: 688–694.
17. Markson LS, Stoops CW, Kanter J. Metastatic transitional cell carcinoma of the penis simulating a chancre. Arch Dermatol 1949; 59: 50–54.
18. Peison B. Metastasis of carcinoma of the prostate to the scalp. Simulation of a large sebaceous cyst. Arch Dermatol 1971; 104: 301–303.
19. Bluefarb SM, Wallk S, Gecht M. Carcinoma of the prostate with zosteriform cutaneous lesions. Arch Dermatol 1957; 76: 402–407.
20. Hodge SJ, Mackel S, Owen LG. Zosteriform inflammatory metastatic carcinoma. Int J Dermatol 1979; 18: 142–145.
20a. Matarasso SL, Rosen T. Zosteriform metastasis: case presentation and review of the literature. J Dermatol Surg Oncol 1988; 14: 774–778.
21. Lillis PJ, Zuehlke RL. Cutaneous metastatic carcinoma and elephantiasis symptomatica. Arch Dermatol 1979; 115: 83–84.
22. Marley NF. Skin metastases in an area of radiation dermatitis. Arch Dermatol 1982; 118: 129–131.
23. Leavell UW Jr, Tillotson FW. Metastatic cutaneous carcinoma from the breast. Arch Dermatol 1951; 64: 774–782.
24. Siegel JM. Inflammatory carcinoma of the breast. Arch Dermatol 1952; 66: 710–716.
25. Edelstein JM. Pancreatic carcinoma with unusual metastasis to the skin and subcutaneous tissue simulating cellulitis. N Engl J Med 1950; 242: 779–781.
26. Graham BS, Wong SW. Cancer cellulitis. South Med J 1984; 77: 277–278.
27. Hazelrigg DE, Rudolph AH. Inflammatory metastatic carcinoma. Arch Dermatol 1977; 113: 69–70.
28. Ingram JT. Carcinoma erysipelatoides and carcinoma telangiectaticum. Arch Dermatol 1958; 77: 227–231.
29. Brownstein MH, Helwig EB. Metastatic tumors of the skin. Cancer 1972; 29: 1298–1307.
30. Steck WD, Helwig EB. Tumors of the umbilicus. Cancer 1965; 18: 907–915.
31. Powell FC, Cooper AJ, Massa MC et al. Sister Mary Joseph's nodule: A clinical and histologic study. J Am Acad Dermatol 1984; 10: 610–615.
32. Powell FC, Venencie PY, Winkelmann RK. Metastatic prostate carcinoma manifesting as penile nodules. Arch Dermatol 1984; 120: 1604–1606.
33. Abeshouse BS, Abeshouse GA. Metastatic tumors of the penis: a review of the literature and a report of two cases. J Urol 1961; 86: 99–109.
34. Gates O. Cutaneous metastases of malignant disease. Am J Cancer 1937; 30: 718–730.
35. Burkholder GV, Kaufman JJ. Local implantation of carcinoma of the prostate with percutaneous needle biopsy. J Urol 1966; 95: 801–804.
35a. Tharakaram S. Metastases to the skin. Int J Dermatol 1988; 27: 240–242.
36. Connor DH, Taylor HB, Helwig EB. Cutaneous metastasis of renal cell carcinoma. Arch Pathol 1963; 76: 339–346.
37. Weidner N, Foucar E. Epidermotropic metastatic squamous cell carcinoma. Arch Dermatol 1985; 121: 1041–1043.
38. Kahn H, Baumal R, From L. Role of immunohistochemistry in the diagnosis of undifferentiated tumors involving the skin. J Am Acad Dermatol 1986; 14: 1063–1072.

Specific metastases

39. Peled IJ, Okon E, Weschler Z, Wexler MR. Distant, late metastases to skin of carcinoma of the breast. J Dermatol Surg Oncol 1982; 8: 192–195.
40. Schorr WF, Swanson PM, Gomez F, Reyes CN. Alopecia neoplastica. Hair loss resembling alopecia areata caused by metastatic breast cancer. JAMA 1970; 213: 1335–1337.
41. Nelson CT. Alopecia neoplastica (possibly of 28 years' duration). Arch Dermatol 1972; 105: 120.

42. Ronchese F. Alopecia due to metastases from adenocarcinoma of the breast. Arch Dermatol 1949; 59: 329–332.

43. Waisman M. Carcinoma of the inframammary crease. Arch Dermatol 1978; 114: 1520–1521.

44. Watson JR, Watson CG. Carcinoma of the mammary crease. A neglected clinical entity. JAMA 1969; 209: 1718–1719.

45. Dowlati Y, Nedwich A. Carcinoma of mammary crease "simulating basal cell epithelioma". Arch Dermatol 1973; 107: 628–629.

45a. Franzblau MJ, Manwaring J, Plumhof C et al. Metastatic breast carcinoma mimicking granular cell tumor. J Cutan Pathol 1989; 16: 218–222.

46. Ariel IM, Avery EE, Kanter L et al. Primary carcinoma of the lung. A clinical study of 1205 cases. Cancer 1950; 3: 229–239.

47. Flynn VT, Spurrett BR. Sister Joseph's nodule. Med J Aust 1969; 1: 728–730.

48. Samitz MH. Umbilical metastasis from carcinoma of the stomach. Sister Joseph's nodule. Arch Dermatol 1975; 111: 1478–1479.

49. Zeligman I, Schwilm A. Umbilical metastasis from carcinoma of the colon. Arch Dermatol 1974; 110: 911–912.

50. Jager RM, Max MH. Umbilical metastasis as the presenting symptom of cecal carcinoma. J Surg Oncol 1979; 12: 41–45.

51. Eppstein S. Primary carcinoma of the liver. Am J Med Sci 1964; 247: 137–144.

52. Reingold IM, Smith BR. Cutaneous metastases from hepatomas. Arch Dermatol 1978; 114: 1045–1046.

53. Kahn JA, Sinhamohapatra SB, Schneider AF. Hepatoma presenting as a skin metastasis. Arch Dermatol 1971; 104: 299–300.

54. Helson L, Garcia EJ. Skin metastases and hepatic cancer in childhood. NY State J Med 1975; 75: 1728–1730.

55. Chakraborty AK, Reddy AN, Grosberg SJ, Wapnick S. Pancreatic carcinoma with dissemination to umbilicus and skin. Arch Dermatol 1977; 113: 838–839.

56. Chatterjee SN, Bauer HM. Umbilical metastasis from carcinoma of the pancreas. Arch Dermatol 1980; 116: 954–955.

57. Padilla RS, Jarmillo M, Dao A, Chapman W. Cutaneous metastatic adenocarcinoma of gallbladder origin. Arch Dermatol 1982; 118: 515–517.

58. Tongco RC. Unusual skin metastases from carcinoma of the gallbladder. Am J Surg 1961; 102: 90–93.

59. Rosenthal AL, Lever WF. Involvement of the skin in renal carcinoma. Arch Dermatol 1957; 76: 96–102.

60. Batres E, Knox JM, Wolf JE Jr. Metastatic renal cell carcinoma resembling a pyogenic granuloma. Arch Dermatol 1978; 114: 1082–1083.

61. Rogow L, Rotman M, Roussis K. Renal metastases simulating Kaposi sarcoma. Arch Dermatol 1975; 111: 717–719.

62. Scott LS, Head MA, Mack WS. Cutaneous metastases from tumours of the bladder, urethra, and penis. Br J Urol 1954; 26: 387–400.

63. Beautyman EJ, Garcia CJ, Sibulkin D, Snyder PB. Transitional cell bladder carcinoma metastatic to the skin. Arch Dermatol 1983; 119: 705–707.

64. McDonald JH, Heckel NJ, Kretschmer HL. Cutaneous metastases secondary to carcinoma of urinary bladder. Report of two cases and review of the literature. Arch Dermatol 1950; 61: 276–284.

65. Schwartz RA, Fleishman JS. Transitional cell carcinoma of the urinary tract presenting with a cutaneous metastasis. Arch Dermatol 1981; 117: 513–515.

66. Hollander A, Grots IA. Oculocutaneous metastases from carcinoma of the urinary bladder. Case report and review of the literature. Arch Dermatol 1968; 97: 678–684.

67. Arnheim FK. Carcinoma of the prostate: a study of the postmortem findings in one hundred and seventy-six cases. J Urol 1948; 60: 599–603.

68. Tan HT, Vishniavsky S. Carcinoma of the prostate with metastases to the prepuce. J Urol 1971; 106: 588–589.

69. Oka M, Nakashima K. Carcinoma of the prostate with metastases to the skin and glans penis. Br J Urol 1982; 54: 61.

70. Schellhammer PF, Milsten R, Bunts RC. Prostatic carcinoma with cutaneous metastases. Br J Urol 1973; 45: 169–172.

71. Razvi M, Firfer R, Berkson B. Occult transitional cell carcinoma of the prostate presenting as skin metastasis. J Urol 1975; 113: 734–735.

71a. Scupham R, Beckman E, Fretzin D. Carcinoma of the prostate metastatic to the skin. Am J Dermatopathol 1988; 10: 178–180.

72. Schiff BL. Tumors of testis with cutaneous metastases to scalp. Arch Dermatol 1955; 71: 465–467.

73. Price NM, Kopf AW. Metastases to skin from occult malignant neoplasms. Cutaneous metastases from a teratocarcinoma. Arch Dermatol 1974; 109: 547–550.

74. Galle PC, Jobson VW, Homesley HD. Umbilical metastasis from gynecologic malignancies: a primary carcinoma of the fallopian tube. Obstet Gynecol 1981; 57: 531–533.

75. Beck H, Raahave D, Boiesen P. A malignant Brenner tumour of the ovary with subcutaneous metastases. Acta Pathol Microbiol Scand (A) 1977; 85: 859–863.

76. Freeman CR, Rozenfeld M, Schopflocher P. Cutaneous metastases from carcinoma of the cervix. Arch Dermatol 1982; 118: 40–41.

77. Debois JM. Endometrial adenocarcinoma metastatic to the scalp. Report of two cases. Arch Dermatol 1982; 118: 42–43.

78. Bukovsky I, Lifshitz Y, Langer R et al. Umbilical mass as a presenting symptom of endometrial adenocarcinoma. Int J Gynaecol Obstet 1979; 17: 229–230.

79. Rasbach D, Hendricks A, Stoltzner G. Endometrial adenocarcinoma metastatic to the scalp. Arch Dermatol 1978; 114: 1708–1709.

80. Damewood MD, Rosenshein NB, Grumbine FC, Parmley TH. Cutaneous metastasis of endometrial carcinoma. Cancer 1980; 46: 1471–1475.

81. Tharakaram S, Rajendran SS, Premalatha S et al. Cutaneous metastasis from carcinoma cervix. Int J Dermatol 1985; 24: 598–599.

82. Daw E, Riley S. Umbilical metastasis from squamous carcinoma of the cervix. Case report. Br J Obstet Gynecol 1982; 89: 1066.

83. Hsu C-T, Sai Y-S. Skin metastases from genital cancer. Report of 2 cases. Obstet Gynecol 1962; 19: 69–75.

84. Park WW, Lees J. Choriocarcinoma. Arch Pathol 1950; 49: 205–241.

85. Ertungealp E, Axelrod J, Stanek A et al. Skin

metastases from malignant gestational trophoblastic disease: Report of two cases. Am J Obstet Gynecol 1982; 143: 843–846.

86. Cosnow I, Fretzin DF. Choriocarcinoma metastatic to skin. Arch Dermatol 1974; 109: 551–553.

87. Avril MF, Mathieu A, Kalifa C, Caillou C. Infantile choriocarcinoma with cutaneous tumors. An additional case and review of the literature. J Am Acad Dermatol 1986; 14: 918–927.

88. Ibanez ML, Russell WO, Albores-Saavedra J et al. Thyroid carcinoma — biologic behavior and mortality. Cancer 1966; 19: 1039–1052.

89. Barr R, Dann F. Anaplastic thyroid carcinoma metastatic to the skin. J Cutan Pathol 1974; 1: 201–206.

90. Rico MJ, Penneys NS. Metastatic follicular carcinoma of the thyroid to the skin: a case confirmed by immunohistochemistry. J Cutan Pathol 1985; 12: 103–105.

91. Horiguchi Y, Takahashi C, Imamura S. Cutaneous metastasis from papillary carcinoma of the thyroid. Report of two cases. J Am Acad Dermatol 1984; 10: 988–992.

92. Hamilton D. Cutaneous metastases from a follicular thyroid carcinoma. J Dermatol Surg Oncol 1980; 6: 116–117.

93. Hoie J, Stenioig AE, Kullmann G, Lindegaard M. Distant metastases in papillary thyroid cancer. A review of 91 patients. Cancer 1988; 61: 1–6.

94. Auty RM. Dermal metastases from a follicular carcinoma of the thyroid. Arch Dermatol 1977; 113: 675–676.

95. Ordonez NG, Samaan NA. Medullary carcinoma of the thyroid metastatic to the skin: report of two cases. J Cutan Pathol 1987; 14: 251–254.

96. Rudner EJ, Lentz C, Brown J. Bronchial carcinoid tumor with skin metastases. Arch Dermatol 1965; 92: 73–75.

97. Keane J, Fretzin DF, Jao W, Shapiro CM. Bronchial carcinoid metastatic to skin. Light and electron microscopic findings. J Cutan Pathol 1980; 7: 43–49.

98. van Dijk C, Ten Seldam REJ. A possible primary cutaneous carcinoid. Cancer 1975; 36: 1016–1020.

98a. Bart RS, Kamino H, Waisman J et al. Carcinoid tumor of skin: Report of a possible primary case. J Am Acad Dermatol 1990; 22: 366–370.

99. Norman JL, Cunningham PJ, Cleveland BR. Skin and subcutaneous metastases from gastrointestinal carcinoid tumors. Arch Surg 1971; 103: 767–769.

100. Brody HJ, Stallings WP, Fine RM, Someren A. Carcinoid in an umbilical nodule. Arch Dermatol 1978; 114: 570–572.

101. Archer CB, Wells RS, MacDonald DM. Metastatic cutaneous carcinoid. J Am Acad Dermatol 1985; 13: 363–366.

102. Reingold IM, Escovitz WE. Metastatic cutaneous carcinoid. Arch Dermatol 1960; 82: 971–975.

103. Bean SF, Fusaro RM. An unusual manifestation of the carcinoid syndrome. Arch Dermatol 1968; 98: 268–269.

104. Castiello RJ, Lynch PJ. Pellagra and the carcinoid syndrome. Arch Dermatol 1972; 105: 574–577.

105. Lucky AW, McGuire J, Komp DM. Infantile neuroblastoma presenting with cutaneous blanching nodules. J Am Acad Dermatol 1982; 6: 389–391.

106. Nguyen TQ, Fisher GB Jr, Tabbarah SO et al. Stage IV-S metastatic neuroblastoma presenting as skin nodules at birth. Int J Dermatol 1988; 27: 712–713.

107. Hawthorne HC Jr, Nelson JS, Witzleben CL, Giangiacomo J. Blanching subcutaneous nodules in neonatal neuroblastoma. J Pediatr 1970; 77: 297–300.

108. Shown TE, Durfee MF. Blueberry muffin baby: neonatal neuroblastoma with subcutaneous metastases. J Urol 1970; 104: 193–195.

109. Shapiro L. Neuroblastoma with multiple cutaneous metastases. Arch Dermatol 1969; 99: 502–504.

110. Schneider KM, Becker JM, Krasna IH. Neonatal neuroblastoma. Pediatrics 1965; 36: 359–366.

111. Balch CM, Milton GW. In: Balch CM, Milton GW, Shaw HM, Soong S-J. Cutaneous melanoma. Clinical management and treatment results worldwide. Philadelphia: JB Lippincott, 1985; 221–250.

112. Stehlin JS Jr, Hills WJ, Rufino C. Disseminated melanoma. Biologic behavior and treatment. Arch Surg 1967; 94: 495–501.

113. Karakousis CP, Temple DF, Moore R, Ambrus JL. Prognostic parameters in recurrent malignant melanoma. Cancer 1983; 52: 575–579.

114. Patel JK, Didolkar MS, Pickren JW, Moore RH. Metastatic pattern of malignant melanoma. A study of 216 autopsy cases. Am J Surg 1978; 135: 807–810.

115. Beardmore GL, Davis NC, McLeod R et al. Malignant melanoma in Queensland: a study of 219 deaths. Aust J Dermatol 1969; 10: 158–168.

116. Das Gupta T, Brasfield R. Metastatic melanoma. A clinicopathological study. Cancer 1964; 17: 1323–1339.

117. Baab GH, McBride CM. Malignant melanoma. The patient with an unknown site of primary origin. Arch Surg 1975; 110: 896–900.

118. Balch CM, Urist MM, Maddox WA et al. In: Balch CM, Milton GW, Shaw HM, Soong S-J. Cutaneous melanoma. Clinical management and treatment results worldwide. Philadelphia: JB Lippincott 1985; 93–130.

119. Unger SW, Wanebo HJ, Cooper PH. Multiple cutaneous malignant melanomas with features of primary melanoma. Ann Surg 1981; 193: 245–250.

120. Kornberg R, Harris M, Ackerman AB. Epidermotropically metastatic malignant melanoma. Arch Dermatol 1978; 114: 67–69.

121. Warner TFCS, Gilbert EF, Ramirez G. Epidermotropism in melanoma. J Cutan Pathol 1980; 7: 50–54.

122. Vinod SU, Gay RM. Adenoid cystic carcinoma of the minor salivary glands metastatic to the hand. South Med J 1979; 72: 1483–1485.

123. White RM, Patterson JW. Distant skin metastases in a long-term survivor of malignant ameloblastoma. J Cutan Pathol 1986; 13: 383–389.

124. Bedford GU. A case of carcinoma of the thymus with extensive metastases in a new-born child. Can Med Assoc J 1930; 23: 197–202.

125. Nakada JR. Primary carcinoma of the adrenals with metastases in the skin and myocardium. J Miss State Med Assoc 1930; 27: 367–371.

126. Schultz BM, Schwartz RA. Hypopharyngeal squamous cell carcinoma metastatic to skin. J Am Acad Dermatol 1985; 12: 169–172.

127. Cawley EP, Hsu YT, Weary PE. The evaluation of

neoplastic metastases to the skin. Arch Dermatol 1964; 90: 262–265.

128. Kleinman GM, Hochberg FH, Richardson EP Jr. Systemic metastases from medulloblastoma. Report of two cases and review of the literature. Cancer 1981; 48: 2296–2309.

129. Campbell AN, Chan HSL, Becker LE et al. Extracranial metastases in childhood primary intracranial tumors. A report of 21 cases and review of the literature. Cancer 1984; 53: 974–981.

130. Youngberg GA, Berro J, Young M, Leicht SS. Metastatic epidermotropic squamous carcinoma histologically simulating primary carcinoma. Am J Dermatopathol 1989; 11: 457–465.

131. Broderick PA, Connors RC. Unusual manifestation of metastatic uterine leiomyosarcoma. Arch Dermatol 1981; 117: 445–446.

132. Powell FC, Cooper AJ, Massa MC et al. Leiomyosarcoma of the small intestine metastatic to the umbilicus. Arch Dermatol 1984; 120: 402–406.

133. Cerroni L, Soyer HP, Smolle J, Kerl H. Cutaneous

134. King DT, Gurevitch AW, Hirose FM. Multiple cutaneous metastases of a scapular chondrosarcoma. Arch Dermatol 1978; 114: 584–586.

135. Leal-Khouri SM, Barnhill RL, Baden HP. An unusual cutaneous metastasis from a chondrosarcoma. J Cutan Pathol 1989; 16: 315 (abstract).

136. Cartwright LE, Steinman HK. Malignant papillary mesothelioma of the tunica vaginalis testes: Cutaneous metastases showing pagetoid epidermal invasion. J Am Acad Dermatol 1987; 17: 887–890.

137. Berkowitz RK, Longley J, Buchness MR et al. Malignant mesothelioma: Diagnosis by skin biopsy. J Am Acad Dermatol 1989; 21: 1068–1073.

138. Feldman AR, Keeling JH III. Cutaneous manifestation of atrial myxoma. J Am Acad Dermatol 1989; 21: 1080–1084.

139. Reed RJ, Utz MP, Terezakis N. Embolic and metastatic cardiac myxoma. Am J Dermatopathol 1989; 11: 157–165.

metastases of a giant cell tumor of bone: case report. J Cutan Pathol 1990; 17: 59–63.

cytoplasm ('hypodense eosinophils') which corresponds with activation of the cell.[8,9] This activation of eosinophils appears to be under the influence of several factors — eosinophil-activating factor (EAF), eosinophil-stimulation promoter (ESP) and eosinophil-cytotoxicity-enhancing factor (ECEF).[4] The best studied of these is EAF, which stimulates degranulation of the eosinophil.[4] It is now thought to be derived from mononuclear cells, although until recently it was regarded as a lymphokine produced by T lymphocytes.[4]

Diseases with conspicuous eosinophils

Eosinophils are a conspicuous component of the inflammatory cell infiltrate in Wells' syndrome (p. 959), eosinophilic pustular folliculitis (p. 440), parasitic infestations (Chs 29 & 30), the hypereosinophilic syndrome (p. 1000), some cases of eosinophilic fasciitis (p. 332), and angio-lymphoid hyperplasia with eosinophilia and Kimura's disease (p. 956). Eosinophils are also prominent in allergic contact dermatitis (p. 102), urticaria (p. 217), drug reactions (Ch. 20), some cases of hypersensitivity vasculitis (p. 219), allergic granulomatosis (p. 246), allergic necrotizing eosinophilic granulomatosis,[10] some dermatophyte infections (p. 643), eosinophilic panniculitis (p. 510), juvenile xanthogranuloma (p. 1009), Langerhans cell histiocytosis (p. 1022), the rare eosinophilic variant of lymphomatoid papulosis (p. 1032) and the first stage of incontinentia pigmenti (p. 317). Various vesiculobullous diseases may have numerous eosinophils in the infiltrate: these include dermatitis herpetiformis (p. 154), bullous pemphigoid (p. 150), cicatricial pemphigoid (p. 158), herpes gestationis (p. 153), linear IgA bullous dermatosis (p. 157), eosinophilic spongiosis (p. 97), toxic erythema of the newborn (p. 133) and pemphigus vegetans (p. 138). Nodular infiltrates of eosinophils have been reported in the skin in a patient with an islet cell tumour of the pancreas.[11] Eosinophils may be present in the stroma of some cutaneous tumours, particularly squamous cell carcinomas (p. 752), keratoacanthomas (p. 759) and, rarely, malignant melanomas (p. 798).

Eosinophils are a minor component of the inflammatory infiltrate in many other cutaneous diseases. These conditions will not be considered further in this section; mention is made of the presence of eosinophils in the discussion of the histopathological findings of the various entities.

The distribution of the eosinophils within the skin may be characteristic. This is referred to in the discussion of the various entities listed above. One pattern of distribution of eosinophils within the dermis — interstitial eosinophils — is characteristic of certain diseases. 'Interstitial eosinophils' refers to the presence of eosinophils between collagen bundles in the intervascular dermis. Eosinophils are invariably present in a perivascular location as well. Interstitial eosinophils are characteristic of various parasitic infestations, particularly arthropod bites (p. 721), but they are also found in certain drug reactions (Ch. 20), urticaria (p. 217), Wells' syndrome (see below), the urticarial stage of bullous pemphigoid (p. 151) and 'dermal hypersensitivity'. This latter term, which does not correlate with any defined clinical entity, is used by some dermatopathologists for the morphological finding of a mixed infiltrate of lymphocytes and eosinophils in the upper and mid dermis with perivascular and interstitial eosinophils. There is a resemblance to the picture seen in arthropod bites, although the infiltrate is not usually as heavy nor does it extend as deeply in the dermis. This morphological pattern is sometimes seen in patients with an internal cancer who have a non-specific cutaneous eruption. In other cases this pattern appears to be related to food or drug allergies.

A detailed discussion of Wells' syndrome and the hypereosinophilic syndrome follows.

WELLS' SYNDROME (EOSINOPHILIC CELLULITIS)

Wells' syndrome (eosinophilic cellulitis)[12–16] is a disorder of unknown pathogenesis characterized by the tissue reaction pattern known as 'eosinophilic cellulitis with flame figures' (see p. 25).

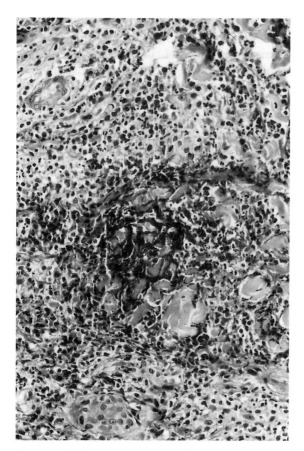

Fig. 40.1 Wells' syndrome. A flame figure is shown. There are many eosinophils in the surrounding dermis. Haematoxylin — eosin

Clinically, there are oedematous, infiltrated plaques resembling cellulitis, often with blister formation. This is followed by the development of slate-grey morphoea-like induration which resolves, usually without trace, over 4–8 weeks.[14,17,18] Recurrent lesions may develop over a period of months to years. Milder cases have annular or circinate erythematous plaques.[19] There is a predilection for the extremities and trunk; rarely, the face is involved as a major clinical feature.[20]

Wells' syndrome may occur at any age, although onset in childhood is uncommon.[18,21,22] Several cases of Wells' syndrome occurring in the same family have been documented.[23]

Although most cases of Wells' syndrome are idiopathic, some cases are associated with arthropod bites, parasitic infestation, drug allergy or an atopic history.[14,16]

Histopathology[13,24,25]

In early lesions of Wells' syndrome there is dermal oedema and massive infiltration of eosinophils, both interstitial and angiocentric. Subepidermal blisters containing eosinophils may form. After one week, scattered histiocytes and characteristic 'flame figures' are found. The 'flame figures' are surrounded, in part, by a palisade of histiocytes and a few multinucleate giant cells. Uncommonly, there are numerous multinucleate giant cells present.[26]

The inflammatory process involves the entire thickness of the dermis and often the subcutis as well. Localization to the subcutis has been reported as eosinophilic panniculitis (see p. 510). Extensive necrotizing granulomas have been reported in the subcutis in this condition.[21] Rarely, the inflammatory infiltrate extends into the fascia and muscle.[27]

The 'flame figures' consist of eosinophil granule major basic protein encrusted on otherwise normal collagen.[17] There is no mucopolysaccharide or lipid, but sometimes basophilic fibrillar material may be seen at the periphery of the eosinophilic material (Fig. 40.1). There is a superficial resemblance to the Splendore–Hoeppli phenomenon which may develop around metazoal parasites in the tissues (see p. 662).

The tissue reaction pattern of eosinophilic cellulitis with flame figures may be seen in a number of disparate conditions,[13,24,28] including arthropod reactions,[24,29,30] other parasitic infestations,[31] internal cancers,[32] dermatophyte infections,[13] bullous pemphigoid,[13] herpes gestationis,[13] allergic eczemas[13] and eosinophilic ulcer of the tongue.[33] It is an uncommon reaction pattern in all of these conditions, except eosinophilic ulcer of the tongue. This reaction pattern has also been reported in association with eosinophilic folliculitis, as a manifestation of a drug reaction.[34] The clinical setting and other histopathological features allow the conditions listed above to be distinguished from Wells' syndrome.

early infancy with thickening of the skin, which may be erythematous or yellow-brown in colour.[140] Pruritus and blistering are common, and the bullae which form are more persistent than in urticaria pigmentosa of childhood.[141] Nodules may develop within the thickened skin but this does not necessarily indicate a bad prognosis.[142] Systemic involvement is common.

TMEP. This is the universally accepted short designation for *telangiectasia macularis eruptiva perstans*, a rare adult form of mastocytosis with a high incidence of systemic involvement.[143] Erythema and telangiectasia are found in faintly pigmented macules on the trunk and proximal parts of the extremities.[109] Facial involvement has been reported.[144]

Systemic mastocytosis. In systemic mastocytosis there is a proliferation of mast cells in various tissues apart from or in addition to the skin.[145] Systemic mastocytosis may develop in childhood cases of urticaria pigmentosa which persist beyond puberty, and in approximately 40% of adults with urticaria pigmentosa, usually of long standing.[122,131,146] It may also be associated with TMEP.[147]

The bone marrow is the tissue most frequently involved in systemic mastocytosis, followed by the liver, spleen, gastrointestinal tract, lymph nodes and, rarely, other organs.[145] Sometimes bone is the only tissue involved besides the skin. Systemic mast cell disease without skin involvement is quite uncommon, and often difficult to diagnose.[143,145] However, the urinary excretion of the histamine metabolite methylimidazoleacetic acid is increased in cases of systemic mastocytosis.[118,148]

Systemic mastocytosis may progress to malignant mastocytosis and/or mast cell leukaemia. Various lymphoproliferative and myeloproliferative conditions may sometimes eventuate,[149] particularly myelogenous leukaemia.[143,150] It has been claimed that up to one-third of individuals with systemic mastocytosis may progress to malignancy, but this seems unduly pessimistic in the light of other studies, one of which showed that the clinical course of systemic

mastocytosis was stable over a period of 10 years in all those followed.[131]

Malignant mast cell disease.[151] There may be a progressive proliferation of atypical mast cells leading to the enlargement of various organs. This usually follows systemic mastocytosis and has been called malignant mastocytosis and mast cell reticulosis.[151] The extremely rare mast cell sarcoma is a localized mass of malignant mast cells in the soft tissues.[151] Mast cell leukaemia may develop in any of these settings or as a progression of systemic mastocytosis.[151] There is extensive bone marrow infiltration and atypical mast cells circulating in the peripheral blood.[152] It has a poor prognosis.[109]

Histopathology[109]

The histological pattern of mastocytosis is similar regardless of the clinical type, although there are major variations in the number of mast cells present.[152] The infiltrate is predominantly in the upper third of the dermis, at times in proximity to the dermo–epidermal junction (Fig. 40.3).[152] In the usual macular lesions of urticaria pigmentosa the infiltrate may vary from sparse and perivascular to larger aggregates of mast cells. Perivascular mast cells may be cuboidal or fusiform in shape while those in larger aggregates tend to be cuboidal (Fig. 40.4). A scattering of eosinophils is usually present and there may be superficial oedema in lesions that are rubbed prior to removal. Basal hyperpigmentation is a useful clue to the diagnosis of urticaria pigmentosa and some other types of mastocytosis.

In *solitary mastocytoma* there are dense aggregates of mast cells in the dermis, sometimes extending into its deeper levels and even into the subcutis.[109] In *TMEP*, there may be only subtle alterations in mast cell numbers; the cells tend to be fusiform and loosely arranged around the dilated vessels of the superficial plexus (Fig. 40.5). Eosinophils are usually absent. In *disseminated cutaneous mastocytosis* there are loosely arranged mast cells throughout the dermis.[142] The mast cells are deeper in the dermis in the xanthomatous form.

Superficial oedema leading to subepidermal

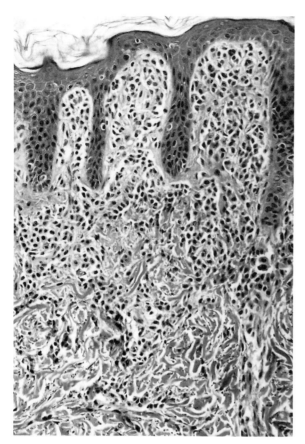

Fig. 40.3   Urticaria pigmentosa. Mast cells fill the papillary dermis.
Haematoxylin — eosin

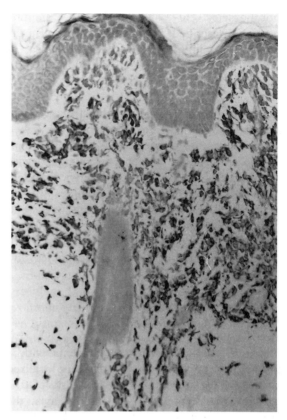

Fig. 40.4   Urticaria pigmentosa. Numerous mast cells are present in the upper dermis. There is also mild hyperpigmentation of the basal layer.
Toluidine blue

vesiculobullous changes is common with mast cell lesions of infancy and childhood.[129] There may be eosinophils, mast cells and occasional neutrophils within the bullae and a diffuse aggregate of mast cells in the upper dermis below the band of oedema or the blister cavity.

Quantitative studies have shown that the number of mast cells in the cutaneous lesions of mastocytosis is from 2–160 times that in the adjacent normal skin.[112,153] Normal skin may contain up to 10 mast cells per high power ($\times$ 40) field. In TMEP, in which the increase may be subtle, it is often useful to have some normal skin at one end of the biopsy for comparison with lesional skin.[109] Qualitatively, the mast cells in mastocytosis resemble normal mast cells, with little atypia and only minor changes detected by

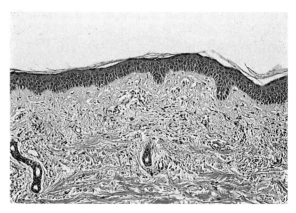

Fig. 40.5   Telangiectasia macularis eruptiva perstans (TMEP). The mast cells are predominantly perivascular in location. The blood vessels are not as telangiectatic as usual.
Haematoxylin — eosin

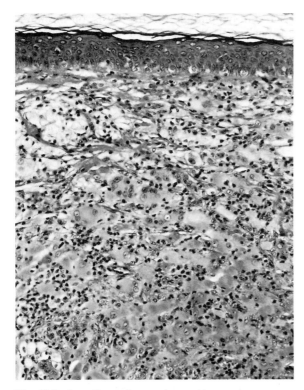

Fig. 40.7　Juvenile xanthogranuloma with many large histiocytic cells.
Haematoxylin — eosin

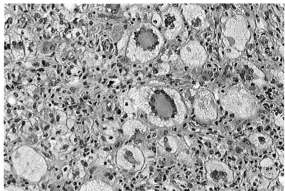

Fig. 40.8　Juvenile xanthogranuloma. The Touton giant cells, which are unusually large, are admixed with lymphocytes and histiocytes.
Haematoxylin — eosin

also scattered lymphocytes and neutrophils, rare plasma cells and sometimes eosinophils. Lesions of longer duration will show interstitial fibrosis and proliferating fibroblasts. Fat stains confirm the presence of some lipid. Haemosiderin has been demonstrated in a few cases.[194] The histiocytes are often positive for lysozyme and α_1-antichymotrypsin,[178] but they are negative for S100 protein.[181] Approximately 1–10% of the other cells are S100 positive. Such cells are elongated or dendritic in appearance.[185]

Electron microscopy.[177] Ultrastructural examination of mature lesions has shown lipid vacuoles (often without a limiting membrane),[195] lysosomes, cholesterol clefts[196] and myeloid bodies, but no Birbeck granules. Early lesions have only a few lipid-laden cells and there are complex interdigitations of the cell membrane.[197] Fibroblastic cells have also been noted in some lesions.[198,199]

PROGRESSIVE NODULAR HISTIOCYTOMA

This term has been used for a normolipaemic, histioxanthomatous syndrome in which multiple yellowish-brown papules and nodules develop on the skin and mucous membranes.[200,201] Similar lesions have been noted in a patient with acute myelomonocytic leukaemia.[202] It has been suggested that these cases are variants of juvenile xanthogranuloma.[203] Another confusing feature is the use of the term 'progressive nodular histiocytosis' for cases with morphological features of multicentric reticulohistiocytosis but an absence of the usual systemic symptoms of this disorder (see below).[177] Leonine facies has been present in the latter condition.[177,204]

Histopathology[165,201,202]

The nodules have a similar appearance to the cellular and fibrous patterns seen in a dermatofibroma. There are histiocytes, foam cells and fibrous areas, sometimes having a storiform appearance. Touton cells may be present. There are usually no other inflammatory cells. Fat and haemosiderin can be demonstrated in the histiocytes with special stains.

No monoclonal antibody studies have been reported.

NECROBIOTIC XANTHOGRANULOMA

This is a rare, chronic disorder, first delineated by Kossard and Winkelmann in 1980.[205,206] Examples had been included in earlier reports of atypical necrobiosis lipoidica, atypical multicentric reticulohistiocytosis, and even xanthoma disseminatum.[207] Necrobiotic xanthogranuloma is characterized by the presence of multiple, sharply demarcated nodules and large indurated plaques.[208] These are violaceous to red with a partly xanthomatous hue. Central atrophy, ulceration and telangiectasia may develop. There is a predilection for the periorbital area, but other areas of the face, as well as the trunk and limbs, are often involved.

Paraproteinaemia has been present in nearly all the reported cases.[207,209] Other less frequent findings include leucopenia, bone marrow plasmacytosis and, occasionally, hyperlipidaemia. Normolipaemic plane xanthomas were reported in one patient.[210] Ophthalmic complications are common and include scleritis, episcleritis and keratitis.

Histopathology[211]

The distinctive changes are found both in the dermis and subcutis, and consist of broad zones of hyaline necrobiosis and granulomatous foci composed of histiocytes, foam cells and multinucleate giant cells (Fig. 40.9). These are of both Touton and foreign body type, the latter often having bizarre features with irregular size, shape and distribution of the nuclei. The multinucleate cells may be present in the granulomas and dispersed near the zones of necrobiosis. Sometimes the Touton cells are prominent in the subcutis ('Touton cell panniculitis'). Blood vessels may be secondarily involved in the granulomatous process.

The amount of xanthomatization is variable, and sometimes the foam cell population is small. Aggregates of histiocytes may extend into the papillary dermis and there may be ulceration. Other less constant changes include the presence of cholesterol clefts,[212] rarely with surrounding palisaded granuloma formation, the presence of lymphoid nodules, sometimes with germinal

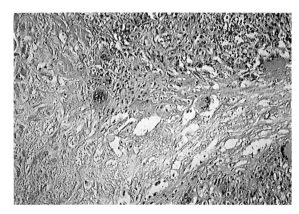

Fig. 40.9 Necrobiotic xanthogranuloma. A zone of necrobiosis is surrounded by multinucleate giant cells and some histiocytes.
Haematoxylin — eosin

centres, and plasma cell collections. Eosinophils are rare. Transepithelial elimination of cholesterol crystals and cellular debris has also been documented.[209] The process is more cellular, and has more atypical and prominent giant cells than necrobiosis lipoidica (see p. 192).

Histochemical findings include scant mucin in areas of necrobiosis, sparse or absent elastic fibres, focal lipid droplets in giant cells and histiocytes and in some areas of necrobiosis, and PAS-positive, diastase-resistant granules in giant cells. The histiocytes do not stain for S100 protein.

Electron microscopy has not contributed any useful further information.

MULTICENTRIC RETICULOHISTIOCYTOSIS

This uncommon normolipaemic histiocytosis is characterized by the presence of an extensive papulonodular cutaneous eruption and a severe, sometimes destructive arthropathy, the onset of which may precede, follow, or accompany the eruption of skin lesions.[213–215a] The interphalangeal joints of the hands are usually affected. Oral, nasal and pharyngeal mucosae are often involved. There are isolated reports of infiltrates in lymph nodes, lungs,[216] bone marrow, endocardium, stomach,[217] salivary gland[218] and perirenal fat.[217] Xanthelasmas of the eyelids are also common.[214]

The cutaneous lesions, which preferentially involve the face and distal parts of the upper extremities, are multiple brown-yellow papules and nodules which measure 0.3–2 cm in diameter.[219] Onset of the disease is usually in middle life, and there is a predilection for females.[220] The clinical course is variable, with eventual spontaneous regression of the skin lesions after 5–10 years or more.[220] There may be residual joint impairment. Malignancies of various types may develop in up to 25% of cases.[215,220–222] Systemic vasculitis is rarely associated with multicentric reticulohistiocytosis.

A related entity is *diffuse cutaneous reticulohistiocytosis* in which multiple cutaneous lesions, identical histologically to those seen in multicentric reticulohistiocytosis, develop in the absence of arthritis or systemic lesions.[223,224] The terms reticulohistiocytoma and reticulohistiocytic granuloma have been used for solitary cutaneous lesions of similar histology (see below).

Histopathology[213,218,225]

There is a circumscribed, non-encapsulated dermal and synovial infiltrate of mononuclear and multinucleate histiocytes with an eosinophilic, finely granular, 'ground-glass' cytoplasm. The hallmark of the disease is the presence of the multinucleate cells which measure 50 μm or more in diameter (Fig. 40.10). They have 3–10 or more nuclei which may be placed haphazardly, or along the periphery, or clustered in the centre of the giant cell. Mitoses are infrequent. Some giant cells may have foamy cytoplasm at the periphery of the cell. Phagocytosis of nuclear debris is uncommon. Transition from mononucleate to multinucleate forms can be seen.[226] Giant cells may be sparse in early lesions.[227] The cytoplasm of the histiocytes contains PAS-positive, diastase-resistant material, which usually stains with Sudan black as well.[213,228] The cells in one case were S100 and OKT6 (CD1) negative, and OKM1 (CD11b) and Leu-M3 (CD14) positive,[223] while in another case there were numerous T lymphocytes admixed with macrophages which

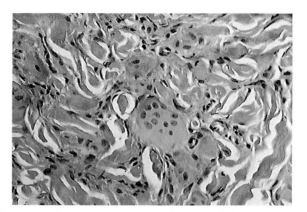

Fig. 40.10 Multicentric reticulohistiocytosis. The characteristic multinucleate giant cells are scattered through the collagen of the dermis. Haematoxylin — eosin

were Leu-M5 positive (CD11c).[229] Reticulin fibres can be demonstrated around individual cells.

In addition to the histiocytes there are small numbers of lymphocytes scattered through the infiltrate. There may be some perivascular cuffing by lymphocytes in early lesions.[177] The walls of small blood vessels sometimes show 'onion-skin' thickening.[214]

Epidermal changes are variable. There is sometimes thinning of the epidermis overlying the lesion, with loss of rete ridges; ulceration is uncommon. Usually there is a narrow grenz zone of uninvolved collagen which separates the undersurface of the epidermis from the tumour nodule below.

Electron microscopy. The cytoplasm of the histiocytes is rich in organelles. A characteristic feature is the presence of innumerable, rounded, dense bodies with the morphological structure of lysosomes.[226] Lipid vacuoles are sometimes present, but there are no Birbeck granules.[218] Elastin and collagen in various stages of degeneration may be seen in the cytoplasm of some of the giant cells.[230,231]

RETICULOHISTIOCYTOMA

Reticulohistiocytomas (reticulohistiocytic granulomas) are nodular lesions 0.5–2 cm in diameter, with similar histology to the lesions of multicentric reticulohistiocytosis but without associated arthritis or systemic lesions.[215a,232–234] They are usually solitary, but several may be present.[234,235] There is a predilection for the head and neck, but they may occur anywhere on the skin. Paraproteinaemia accompanied several cutaneous nodules in one reported case.[235]

Histopathology[234]

There is a circumscribed dermal nodule, often with overlying epidermal thinning. Like multicentric reticulohistiocytosis, there is an irregular admixture of histiocytes, multinucleate giant cells and inflammatory cells (Fig. 40.11). Phagocytosis of leucocytes is sometimes seen. A few Touton giant cells may be present and these may contain lipid. Reticulin fibres are increased and surround individual cells.

There is usually more of a neutrophilic infiltrate than in multicentric reticulohistiocytosis,

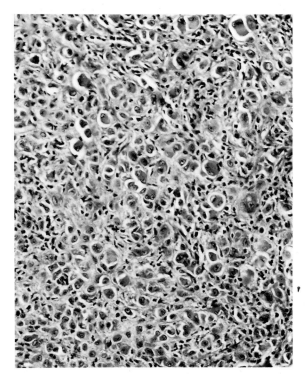

Fig. 40.11 Solitary reticulohistiocytoma. It is composed of multinucleate giant cells, histiocytes and lymphocytes. There is some fibrosis of the stroma.
Haematoxylin — eosin

and a further point of distinction is the greater propensity for the stroma in reticulohistiocytoma to have many spindle-shaped cells.

FAMILIAL HISTIOCYTIC DERMATOARTHRITIS

This exceedingly rare disorder presents in childhood or adolescence as a papulonodular eruption on the face and limbs associated with a symmetrical destructive arthritis and ocular lesions.[236] A closely related entity is the autosomal recessive dermo-chondro-corneal dystrophy reported in the French literature.[237]

Histopathology

There is a dermal infiltrate of mononuclear histiocytes admixed with some lymphocytes and plasma cells.[236] There is no stored lipid or PAS-positive cytoplasmic material. Fibrosis is conspicuous in older lesions. Recently, two cases were reported in which multinucleate histiocytes were present. PAS-positive material was present in the cytoplasm. The authors suggested that these two cases had features overlapping with both familial histiocytic dermatoarthritis and multicentric reticulohistiocytosis, which probably form part of a spectrum of dermatoarthritides.[237]

XANTHOMA DISSEMINATUM

This rare histiocytic proliferation of unknown cause presents with papules, nodules and plaques with a predilection for flexural areas, the proximal parts of the extremities and the trunk.[238] The lesions are initially reddish-brown in colour but become yellow with time.[177] Mucosal lesions and transitory diabetes insipidus are present in approximately 40% of affected individuals.[239] The condition runs a chronic but benign course.

Xanthoma disseminatum appears to be a distinctive disorder in which there is a primary proliferation of histiocytes with subsequent accumulation of lipid.[240,241] The lipid profile of the serum is normal.

Histopathology[239]

Histiocytes predominate in the early stages, but in established lesions there are histiocytes, foam cells, fibroblasts, Touton cells and a moderate number of chronic inflammatory cells.[177] There may be phagocytosis of elastic fibres and sometimes of collagen by macrophages.[240] Siderosis is often observed and this is quite prominent in the rare variant known as xanthosiderohistiocytosis.[242]

Immunohistochemical characterization of the cells has shown HLA-DR positivity but no staining for S100 protein, OKT4 (CD4) or OKT6 (CD1).[243]

Electron microscopy. The cells are similar to those seen in papular xanthoma and juvenile xanthogranuloma but the plasma membranes of the foamy cells show many microvilli.[177] There are no Birbeck granules.

BENIGN CEPHALIC HISTIOCYTOSIS

Benign cephalic histiocytosis is a clinically distinct, non-lipid, 'non-X' histiocytic proliferation in children.[244–245a] It is characterized by the development of asymptomatic red-brown maculopapules, 2–5 mm or more in diameter, on the face, whence the condition may evolve to affect the neck, upper part of the trunk, arms, and other parts of the body.[246] The palmoplantar regions, mucous membranes and viscera are spared.[244] Spontaneous regression, complete or partial, occurs during childhood, without scarring.[244,247]

Histopathology[244]

There is a diffuse infiltrate of histiocytes, mainly in the upper dermis and in close apposition to the undersurface of the epidermis. The cells have an oval or reniform vesicular nucleus and ill-defined pale cytoplasm.[245] There are no cytoplasmic lipids at any stage of evolution of the lesions. Occasional multinucleate histiocytes are present. There are scattered or grouped lymphocytes within the infiltrate, and occasional

eosinophils in some lesions. The histiocytes are negative for S100 and CD1 (OKT6), but positive for CD11b (OKM1) and CD14b (Leu-M3).[244,247]

The absence of Touton cells and foam cells and the presence of only a small number of admixed inflammatory cells help distinguish the lesions of benign cephalic histiocytosis from those of juvenile xanthogranuloma.[248]

Electron microscopy.[244] The most characteristic feature of the histiocytes is the presence of many coated vesicles, 500–1500 nm in diameter, in the cytoplasm. Comma-shaped inclusion bodies are present in 5–30% of the histiocytes.[249] No Birbeck granules or lipid droplets are present. Desmosome-like junctions are present between the histiocytes in densely cellular areas.[244]

GENERALIZED ERUPTIVE HISTIOCYTOMA

This rare, non-lipid, 'non-X' histiocytosis is characterized clinically by the development of recurrent crops of hundreds of small reddish papules which are distributed symmetrically on the trunk and on the extensor surfaces of the extremities.[250–259] Lesions usually subside spontaneously, leaving macular hyperpigmentation or no residual features. It has been reported in children as well as in adults.[253,254]

Histopathology[258,259]

There is an infiltrate of histiocyte-like cells in the upper and mid dermis. Sometimes the cells are arranged in nests around blood vessels. They have pale cytoplasm and an oval nucleus. No lipid, iron or PAS-positive material is demonstrable in the cytoplasm.[260] A few lymphocytes, and sometimes fibroblasts, are intermingled but there are usually no giant cells. The histiocytes are negative for S100 protein and CD1 (OKT6), but are positive for CD11b (OKM1) and CD14b (Leu-M3).[254]

Benign cephalic histiocytosis and a case reported recently as 'benign non-X histiocytosis'[168] have features on light microscopy that are similar to those of generalized eruptive histiocytoma but they differ clinically and ultrastructurally.[254–256] Benign cephalic histiocytosis and eruptive histiocytoma may be different expressions of the same histiocytosis.[257]

Electron microscopy. There are many dense bodies, some with myelin laminations, in the cytoplasm.[256,258] There are also occasional comma-shaped bodies and lipid droplets, but no Birbeck granules.[254,259]

CUTANEOUS ATYPICAL HISTIOCYTOSIS

Only a few cases of this entity have been reported.[261,262] It is characterized clinically by the presence of one or more nodular lesions resembling cutaneous lymphoma. There has been a good response to various modes of treatment in the cases reported so far.

Histopathology

There is a monomorphous infiltrate of medium-sized histiocytoid cells with occasional cytoplasmic vacuoles and scattered mitoses.

Electron microscopy. The distinctive feature is the presence in the cells of giant multivesicular bodies and pleomorphic granules.

ROSAI–DORFMAN DISEASE

The eponymous designation Rosai–Dorfman disease[263] is more appropriate than 'sinus histiocytosis with massive lymphadenopathy', because it is now recognized that in some instances extranodal lesions, including lesions in the skin, may be the sole manifestation of this condition.[264–268a] The typical presentation is with painless cervical lymphadenopathy, accompanied by fever, anaemia, an elevated erythrocyte sedimentation rate and hypergammaglobulinaemia which has been polyclonal in all but one case.[269,270] Any age may be affected but 80% of cases develop in the first two decades of life.[271]

Extranodal lesions occur in almost one-third of cases, while the skin has been involved in approximately 10% of the 400 or so cases reported.[264,270]

Cutaneous lesions, which are usually multiple, have been varied in their clinical appearance.[264] There may be nodules up to 4 cm or more in diameter,[272] papules which are erythematous or xanthomatous,[264] plaques, pigmented macules,[265] and even a transient panniculitis.[273] The eyelids and the malar regions are the sites of predilection.[265]

The disease usually runs a benign, albeit protracted, clinical course, sometimes with significant morbidity.[270] Death may sometimes result from infiltration of organs or from immunological disturbances.[265,274–276] The aetiology is unknown.

Histopathology[264]

The pathological changes in the lymph nodes are characteristic, and include expansion of the sinuses by large foamy histiocytes admixed with plasma cells. Cutaneous lesions are not diagnostically specific. There is usually a dense dermal infiltrate of large histiocytes with abundant, lightly eosinophilic cytoplasm and vesicular nuclei.[264] Scattered multinucleate cells and Touton cells and collections of neutrophils may be present.[269] Plasma cells are invariably present, and sometimes contain prominent Russell bodies. Nodular lymphoid aggregates may be conspicuous.

Other features which may be present include phagocytosis of lymphocytes, fibrosis, increased vascularity and focal necrosis.[264] A mixed septal and lobular panniculitis with some features of cytophagic histiocytic panniculitis (see p. 505) was present in one case.[273]

Recent reports suggest that the histiocyte of Rosai–Dorfman disease is S100 positive and negative for CD1 (OKT6).[266,277,278] There are isolated reports suggesting that the cells are negative for CD45 (leucocyte common antigen)[273] and positive for CD11b (OKM1) and CD14b (Leu-M3).[266] Another study showed that the cells were positive for S100 protein, CD11c (Leu-M5) and α_1-chymotrypsin, suggesting that they coexpress phenotypic characteristics of histiocytes of the mononuclear phagocytic system and of histiocytes of the interdigitating reticulum cell and Langerhans cell lineages.[279] There are no Birbeck (Langerhans) inclusions in the histiocytes.[266]

MALIGNANT HISTIOCYTOSIS

Malignant histiocytosis, formerly known as histiocytic medullary reticulosis, is a rare and usually fatal systemic proliferation of atypical histiocytes and their precursors.[280] Clinical features include fever, generalized lymphadenopathy, hepatosplenomegaly, pancytopenia, and sometimes disseminated intravascular coagulation, night sweats and abdominal pain.[281]

The skin is involved in 10–15% of cases, and in some this is the presenting feature.[282–284] Lesions take the form of papules, nodules or plaques anywhere on the body, but with a predilection for the extremities and buttocks.[285,286] Sometimes only a solitary nodule is present initially. Spontaneous healing of individual lesions may occur.

Malignant histiocytosis occurs at all ages, but significant numbers have been reported in childhood.[287–289] The prognosis at all ages is poor, although patients presenting with skin lesions form a subgroup with a more favourable outlook.[281,282] At autopsy there is usually involvement of many organs.

Malignant histiocytosis was thought to originate from the macrophage-monocyte system but T-zone histiocytes, positive for S100 protein, may be another cell of origin.[280,290] It has been claimed that some cases may be of Langerhans cell[166] or T-cell origin.[291]

Histopathology

Two patterns of cutaneous involvement may be seen.[284] In one there is a dense, predominantly periadnexal and perivascular infiltrate of atypical histiocytes; in the other there is a diffuse infiltrate of similar cells in the deep dermis and subcutis, with focal necrosis.[292] The papillary dermis is usually spared, but if there are cells in this region, there is no associated epidermotropism such as is seen in Langerhans cell histiocytosis (histiocytosis X; see p. 1022).[293]

The cells in the infiltrate show variable pleomorphism which increases with the passage of time.[294] The cells measure 15–25 μm in diameter and have an oval or reniform nucleus and abundant eosinophilic cytoplasm. Occasional binucleate cells are present. Phagocytosis of erythrocytes and nuclear debris may be seen, but it is not a universal feature.[286] There are also some small lymphocytes and plasma cells in the infiltrate.[293]

The nuclear atypia in malignant histiocytosis allows it to be distinguished from the virus-associated haemophagocytic syndrome, histiocytosis X and cytophagic panniculitis.[282] It seems likely that cytophagic panniculitis is merely a low grade form of malignant histiocytosis that preferentially involves the subcutis.[281,295]

Receptors for Concanavalin A, a new histochemical marker for macrophages/histiocytes, were present in all cases in one series.[280] Approximately half the cases have S100-positive histiocytes,[289] a finding that is more likely in children than in adults.[280] The subset of cases which are S100 negative may be positive for NCS (non-specific cross-reacting antigen).[280] Approximately 50% of the cells stain for lysozyme and for α_1-antitrypsin.[296]

Electron microscopy. The histiocytes are non-cohesive and sometimes have irregular surface projections.[281,297] There are many cytoplasmic organelles including lysosomes and lipid droplets.[297] There are no Birbeck granules.[298,299] Phagocytosis is sometimes seen in the more differentiated histiocytes.[300]

REACTIVE HISTIOCYTOSIS

The term 'reactive histiocytosis', also known as secondary histiocytosis, refers to the increased number of histiocytes that may be seen in a variety of cutaneous infections. These include histoplasmosis, toxoplasmosis, brucellosis, tuberculosis, leprosy, rubella and certain infections with the Epstein–Barr virus.[165] Histiocytes are also prominent in actinic reticuloid, and they are a major component in the haemophagocytic syndromes, although their cutaneous manifestations are usually non-specific. In susceptible hosts, particularly those with various immunodeficiency syndromes, infections may trigger idiopathic histiocytic proliferations indistinguishable from Langerhans cell histiocytosis.[165]

XANTHOMATOUS INFILTRATES

Xanthomas represent the accumulation of lipid-rich macrophages known as foam cells.[301] They present clinically as yellow or yellow-brown papules, nodules or plaques, the colour depending on the amount of lipid present and its depth below the surface. They are usually associated with disorders of lipoprotein metabolism, although only a minority of individuals with such disorders develop xanthomas.[301–303]

Xanthomas can be further subdivided on the basis of their clinical morphology, anatomical distribution and mode of development into the following types: eruptive, tuberous, tendinous, planar, verruciform and papular.[301,303] In addition, there are isolated reports in the literature of xanthomas which cannot be fitted into an orderly classification.[304–310a] Specifically excluded, perhaps arbitrarily so, are the xanthogranulomas (which are not related to disorders of lipoprotein metabolism and which usually possess an admixture of cell types) and the histiocytic, dendrocytic and Langerhans cell proliferations in which lipid accumulation (xanthomatization) may be a secondary phenomenon.[303,306,310b] Tangier disease (see p. 528) and disseminated lipogranulomatosis (Farber's disease; see p. 522), which also possess some xanthoma cells, are not usually included with the xanthomas. The various diseases featuring the presence of xanthoma cells in the skin are summarized in Table 40.2.

Aetiology and pathogenesis of xanthomas

Several of the xanthoma types mentioned above are associated with specific abnormalities of lipoprotein metabolism; more than one type of

Table 40.2 Diseases with xanthoma cells in the skin

Eruptive xanthoma
Tuberous xanthoma
Tendinous xanthoma
Planar xanthoma
Verruciform xanthoma
Papular xanthoma
Facial xanthomatosis
Subcutaneous xanthomatosis
Juvenile xanthogranuloma
Progressive nodular histiocytoma
Necrobiotic xanthogranuloma
Xanthoma disseminatum
Tangier disease
Disseminated lipogranulomatosis
Langerhans cell histiocytosis (histiocytosis X)
Congenital self-healing histiocytosis
Lepromatous leprosy
Rhinoscleroma
Malakoplakia
Scars
Arthropod bites
Lymphoedema
Dermatofibroma (histiocytoma)
Hamartoma of dermal dendrocytes
Mycosis fungoides
Erythroderma

xanthoma may be present in a particular lipoprotein disorder.[303] The lipids in xanthomas are primarily free and esterified cholesterol, but occasionally other sterols and even triglycerides accumulate. This is usually the result of a high plasma concentration with subsequent permeation of lipoproteins through the walls of dermal capillaries.[301,311] The lipid is then taken up by dermal macrophages which evolve into foam cells.[301,311]

There are several possible explanations for the formation of xanthomas in normolipaemic states.[311] There may be altered lipoprotein content or structure, or an underlying lymphoproliferative disease with xanthomatization of cells infiltrating the dermis.[311] Finally, local tissue factors may play a role in those cases of xanthoma developing in chronic eczema, photosensitive eruptions,[312] erythroderma[313] and lymphoedema,[314] and at sites of injury such as bites, scars and striae and in some regressing tumours.[315] The term *dystrophic xanthoma* has been used for the accumulation of lipid-rich foam cells within an area of abnormal or damaged skin in both normolipaemic and hyperlipoproteinaemic states.[316]

The various types of xanthoma will now be considered.

ERUPTIVE XANTHOMA

In this variant of xanthoma, multiple small red-yellow papules with an erythematous halo develop in crops.[301] There is a predilection for the buttocks and thighs and the extensor surfaces of the arms and legs.[303] The lesions become progressively more yellow and they eventually resolve spontaneously over several weeks.

Eruptive xanthomas occur in a setting of elevated plasma chylomicrons such as may occur in uncontrolled diabetes mellitus or following the ingestion of alcohol or the use of exogenous oestrogens.[303,317] Rare associations include lipoprotein lipase deficiency,[303] types IV and V hyperlipoproteinaemia,[318,319] normolipaemia,[320] the nephrotic syndrome,[321] hypothyroidism, the use of intravenous miconazole[322] and the oral ingestion of 13-cis-retinoic acid.[323]

Histopathology[324]

The architecture of the reticular dermis is disturbed by an infiltrate of cells and extravascular lipid deposits in the form of lace-like eosinophilic material between the collagen bundles. The cellular infiltrate cuffs capillaries and extends throughout the dermis.[324] Initially it is composed of neutrophils and lymphocytes, and histiocytes with a finely stippled cytoplasm.[324] Neutrophils may be quite prominent in early lesions and the absence of foam cells makes the diagnosis difficult on histopathological grounds alone. In established lesions, the lipidization of cells is more obvious, although foam cells are never as obvious as in the other variants of xanthoma (Fig. 40.12).[325]

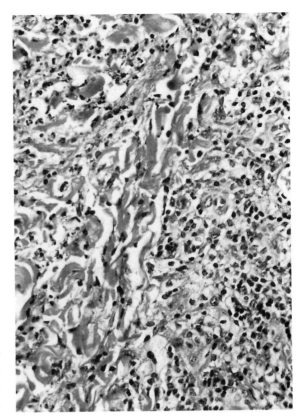

Fig. 40.12 Eruptive xanthoma. Small foam cells are admixed with lymphocytes, macrophages and neutrophils. Haematoxylin — eosin

In some stages of their evolution, eruptive xanthomas may mimic the changes seen in granuloma annulare, but close inspection for the features mentioned above allows the distinction to be made.[324] Furthermore, doubly-refractile lipid can be seen between foam cells in formalin-fixed material in some cases of eruptive xanthoma, but not in granuloma annulare.[326]

TUBEROUS XANTHOMA

Tuberous xanthomas present a spectrum which ranges from small inflammatory lesions at one end (tuberoeruptive xanthomas) to large nodular lesions at the other. Tuberous xanthomas often form by coalescence of smaller lesions.[301] They are yellowish in colour, and are found particularly on the elbows, knees and buttocks.

With treatment of the underlying hyper-lipidaemia there is usually slow resolution over many months.

Tuberous xanthomas are most characteristic of familial dysbetalipoproteinaemia (type III), but they can be seen rarely in homozygous and heterozygous familial hypercholesterolaemia, hepatic cholestasis,[327] cerebrotendinous xan-thoma and β-sitosterolaemia.[303] Tendinous xanthomas are also present in these latter two conditions. Tuberous xanthomas have also been reported in a normolipidaemic subject.[328]

Histopathology

There are large aggregates of foam cells throughout the dermis but usually no Touton giant cells or other inflammatory cells. Fibroblasts are increased in number in older lesions, leading to the progressive deposition of collagen.[328] In one case, concentric layers of xanthoma cells surrounded a cutaneous nerve.[329]

The lipid within the foam cells can be stained with oil red O in frozen sections, or examined polariscopically to confirm its doubly-refractile property.

TENDINOUS XANTHOMA

In this variant of xanthoma, lesions of varying size develop in ligaments, fasciae and tendons, especially the extensor tendons of the hands and feet and the Achilles tendon.[303] They are firm to hard, flesh-coloured nodules which develop slowly over decades.

Tendinous xanthomas are most commonly associated with heterozygous familial hypercholes-terolaemia, but they have also been reported in cerebrotendinous xanthoma, β-sitosterolaemia, familial dysbetalipoproteinaemia (type III) and hepatic cholestasis, and rarely in normolipidaemic individuals.[303,328,330]

Histopathology

The appearances are similar to those seen in tuberous xanthomas, except for the different tissue substrate.

PLANAR XANTHOMA

Planar xanthomas are yellow, soft macules or slightly elevated plaques which are further subdivided on the basis of their location into xanthelasmas, intertriginous xanthomas,[303,331] xanthoma striatum palmaris[318,332,333] and dif-fuse (generalized) plane xanthomas.[301,303] A further variant, planar xanthoma of cholestasis, is sometimes recognized.[303]

Xanthelasma. This is the best known and most common form of xanthoma and is characterized by one or more yellowish plaques on the eyelids or in periorbital skin. Lipid levels are normal in approximately 50% of affected individuals, although in young affected persons there is a higher incidence of hypercholesterolaemia.[301] Abnormalities in the apoprotein moiety of lipoproteins have been detected in some of those with normal levels of lipid in the blood.[334]

Intertriginous xanthoma. This variant, with localization in intertriginous areas, is patho-gnomonic of homozygous familial hypercholes-terolaemia.[303,331]

Xanthoma striatum palmaris. The lesions in this variant, which is characteristic of familial dysbetalipoproteinaemia (type III), are present on the palms and volar surfaces of the fingers.[318,332,335] They are sometimes subtle, requiring proper lighting for their recognition.

Diffuse (generalized) plane xanthomas. This rare condition is associated with macular, yellowish discoloration of the skin, involving particularly the trunk and neck, and sometimes the face. It usually runs a protracted course. The majority of patients are normolipidaemic,[336–338] although several hyperlipoproteinaemic states have been associated with this variant.[339] There is a significant association with lymphoreticular neoplasms, particularly myeloma, although these

Ultrastructurally, Langerhans cells possess many organelles, the most characteristic of which is the Birbeck (Langerhans) granule. This is a rod or tennis-racquet-shaped organelle of variable length and a constant width of 33 nm.[362] Similar dendritic cells without Birbeck granules are known as indeterminate cells.[362]

Langerhans cells show esterase, acid phosphatase and ATPase activity.[370] They express certain antigens such as CD1 (OKT6), S100 protein and HLA-DR, and they bind peanut lectin.[370,374] Another marker is Lag, an antigen present in the membranes of the Birbeck granules.[375]

Langerhans cells play an important role in the pathogenesis of allergic contact dermatitis, and a lesser role in various other inflammatory dermatoses such as lichen planus.[362] However, significant infiltrates of Langerhans cells are found only in Langerhans cell histiocytosis (formerly known as histiocytosis X) and congenital self-healing histiocytosis, which is now regarded as a self-limited variant of Langerhans cell histiocytosis.[376]

LANGERHANS CELL HISTIOCYTOSIS

Langerhans cell histiocytosis, formerly known as histiocytosis X,[377] is the collective designation for a clinical spectrum of diseases which includes Letterer–Siwe disease, Hand–Schüller–Christian disease, and eosinophilic granuloma of bone, as well as intermediate and poorly elucidated forms.[378–380] It is a rare disease with a prevalence of approximately 0.5/100 000 children/year.[381] In general, Letterer–Siwe disease occurs in the first two years of life, Hand–Schüller–Christian disease in older children, and eosinophilic granuloma in older children and adults.[382] However, there are isolated reports of older adults being affected by all three major clinical types of the disease.[383–389a]

Letterer–Siwe disease. Cutaneous lesions are common and extensive in this acute disseminated form of Langerhans cell histiocytosis.[390] They consist of yellow-brown, scaly papules on the scalp, face, trunk and buttocks which can coalesce to form a weeping erythematous eruption resembling seborrhoeic dermatitis.[177] Sometimes there is a haemorrhagic component. Cutaneous lesions are accompanied by fever, anaemia, lymphadenopathy, osteolytic lesions[391] and often hepatosplenomegaly.

Hand–Schüller–Christian disease. This chronic multisystem form of the disease is characterized by the triad of bone lesions, diabetes insipidus and exophthalmos, although it is uncommon for all three to be seen together in the same patient.[177] The skin is involved in one-third or more of cases: the cutaneous manifestations may resemble the lesions of Letterer–Siwe disease or take the form of papulonodular lesions or granulomatous ulceration in intertriginous areas.[392–394]

Eosinophilic granuloma. Cutaneous lesions are quite uncommon in this form,[390] but when they occur they take the form of nodulo-ulcerative lesions in the mouth[395] or in the perineal, perivulvar or retroauricular region.[177,382]

In some instances of Langerhans cell histiocytosis the presentations are atypical and do not conform to the three patterns listed above. Rare cutaneous presentations have included recurrent cutaneous ulcerations resembling pyoderma gangrenosum,[396] scattered papular lesions resembling bites,[397] lesions resembling cherry angiomas,[398] verruca plana[399] or Darier's disease,[400] and a solitary lesion on the buttock[401] or eyelid.[402] Cutaneous lesions are rarely the only manifestation of the disease.[403] Many of the cases that were reported as 'familial histiocytosis X'[404] appear to have been immunodeficiency syndromes associated with an idiopathic proliferation of histiocytes.[165,170]

The prognosis in Langerhans cell histiocytosis depends on the age of the patient, the extent of the disease and the presence of organ dysfunction. Children under the age of two years with multisystem disease and organ dysfunction have a mortality of 50% or more.[405] Spontaneous healing has been reported in several instances,[406] even with multisystem disease,[407–409] leading to the suggestion that Langerhans cell histiocytosis is a reactive rather than a malignant neoplastic process.[410,411] Flow cytometric studies support this view.[412]

Histopathology

Langerhans cell histiocytosis is characterized by clusters and sheets of large ovoid cells, 15–25 μm in diameter, with abundant eosinophilic cytoplasm and a nucleus which is indented or reniform and sometimes eccentric (Fig. 40.15).[413] The cells are found immediately beneath the epidermis and usually show little tendency to extend into the reticular dermis.[414] Focally, the cells invade the epidermis, sometimes forming small aggregates in the upper epidermis (Fig. 40.16). A few lipidized cells may be present in the papillary dermis, but more marked xanthomatous changes are exceedingly rare,[415] usually being confined to the Hand–Schüller–Christian variant. Occasional binuclear cells are present and there are scattered mitoses.

There is a variable admixture of other inflammatory cells; this will depend on the type of lesion biopsied and, to some extent, the clinical variant of the disease. The cells include neutrophils, eosinophils, lymphocytes and mast cells.[416] In Letterer–Siwe disease the infiltrate is largely of Langerhans cells with the admixture of relatively few neutrophils, eosinophils and lymphocytes, while in eosinophilic granuloma

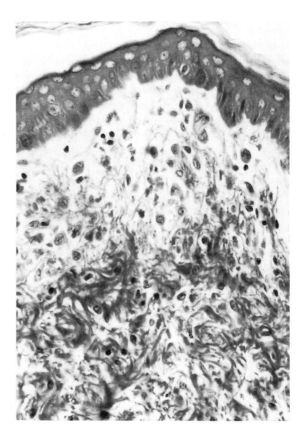

Fig. 40.16 Langerhans cell histiocytosis. Scattered Langerhans cells are present in the oedematous papillary dermis.
Haematoxylin — eosin

clusters of eosinophils may form a prominent component of the infiltrate. Multinucleate giant cells may be prominent in both eosinophilic granuloma and Hand–Schüller–Christian disease. Other microscopic changes that are sometimes present include focal necrosis and fibrosis in older lesions.[411] It should be noted that the outcome cannot be predicted from the histopathological appearances.[411]

Immunohistochemical markers are those discussed above for the Langerhans cell and include CD1 (OKT6), HLA-DR and S100 protein.[383,417–418a] There appears to be some immunophenotypic heterogeneity, not all cells staining with a particular marker in an individual case.[419] In one report, one group of Langerhans cells stained positively for ferritin and for α_2–macroglobulin while others were negative for these markers.[420]

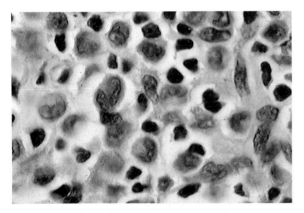

Fig. 40.15 Langerhans cell histiocytosis. The cells have a characteristic reniform nucleus.
Haematoxylin — eosin

Electron microscopy. The cells are the same in all three clinical variants and more or less resemble normal Langerhans cells. Birbeck granules may be absent in a proportion of cells. Interestingly, these granules are relatively resistant to destruction by formalin fixation and paraffin embedding, and accordingly may be seen in material removed from paraffin blocks and reprocessed for electron microscopy.[380]

CONGENITAL SELF-HEALING HISTIOCYTOSIS

This rare infiltrative disorder of the skin was described in 1973 by Hashimoto and Pritzker.[421] It is now regarded as a self-limited form of Langerhans cell histiocytosis (histiocytosis X).[376,422-424a]

The usual clinical presentation is with numerous, firm, red-violaceous or brown papulonodules, 1–10 mm in diameter, scattered over the scalp, face and, to a lesser extent, the trunk and extremities.[422,425] Only a solitary lesion was present in several reported cases.[426,427] The tumours are usually present at birth, although early postnatal onset has also been recorded.[428] The lesions all regress by three months of age, usually leaving residual hyperpigmentation. There are usually no systemic manifestations although hepatomegaly, haematological abnormalities[425] and a case with pulmonary nodules and lytic lesions of the tibia[429] have been reported.

Histopathology

The histological picture may be indistinguishable from Langerhans cell histiocytosis.[422,425] There is usually a dense infiltrate of large histiocytes in the mid and lower dermis. Extension into the subcutis and papillary dermis may occur; there is usually no significant epidermotropism.[430] The histiocytes have abundant eosinophilic cytoplasm with a variable number of PAS-positive granules. Some cells have foamy cytoplasm. The nuclei are oval or reniform. Multinucleate giant cells are invariably present. There are also lymphocytes and some eosinophils in the infiltrate. Focal necrosis[430] and extravasation of erythrocytes

have also been reported.[426] Abundant reticulin fibres are often present around groups of cells and sometimes between individual cells.[431]

The tumour cells usually express CD1 (OKT6) and S100 protein[422,424a] although in one reported case only 30% of the cells were S100 positive.[424] In this latter case none of the cells contained Birbeck granules.[424] In congenital self-healing histiocytosis the histiocytes and giant cells are sometimes larger than in Langerhans cell histiocytosis, and some of these cells may have foamy cytoplasm.[425]

Electron microscopy. Contrasting with their immunophenotype, only 5–25% of tumour cells contain Birbeck (Langerhans) granules.[426,431,432] The finding of concentrically laminated dense core bodies in the same cells that contain Birbeck granules has been proposed as a specific marker for this disease.[433] Other cytoplasmic inclusions of unusual shape may also be present, as well as lipid droplets.[433]

LYMPHOCYTIC INFILTRATES

Lymphocytes are an important component of the inflammatory cell infiltrate in many dermatoses and of the infiltrate in cutaneous lymphomas. In most inflammatory dermatoses lymphocytes are admixed with varying numbers of other cells including histiocytes, macrophages, Langerhans cells, mast cells and, sometimes, plasma cells, eosinophils and even neutrophils. The term 'lymphocytic infiltrate' is usually restricted to those conditions in which there is an almost pure population of lymphocytes in the skin.

Aspects of the development and function of normal lymphocytes will be discussed before consideration of the classification of lymphocytic infiltrates.

Lymphocytes

The human immune system comprises about 2 x 10^{12} lymphocytes.[434] They are concentrated in lymph nodes, the spleen, and lymphoid tissue associated with various mucosal surfaces.[434] Some lymphocytes circulate in the blood and in lymphatics. In comparison, normal skin contains only a few lymphocytes, most of which are scattered around the post-capillary venules of the papillary dermis or adjacent to cutaneous appendages.[435]

There are two major types of lymphocytes, T cells and B cells, both of which originate from a progenitor cell in the bone marrow.[434] They are indistinguishable by light microscopy although on scanning electron microscopy B cells have long microvilli on the surface whereas T cells have a relatively smooth surface.[436] T cells are so named because their maturation takes place in the thymus. They play an important role in cell-mediated immune reactions, particularly in the defence against viruses and certain bacteria. B lymphocytes are the functional equivalent of the lymphocytes produced in the avian bursa of Fabricius;[434] they produce antibodies against specific antigens. T lymphocytes comprise approximately 70–80% of blood lymphocytes while most of the remainder express B-cell markers. The small number of lymphocytes found in normal skin is almost exclusively of T-cell phenotype.[435]

In recent years, lymphocytes have been further categorized by the identification of various antigens (mostly glycoproteins) on the cell surface.[437] Some of these antigens are specific for subpopulations of lymphocytes within the B-cell and T-cell categories. Other antigens are expressed only at certain stages in the maturation of lymphocytes or on activation. The various antigens, known as cluster designations (CD), have been allocated numbers by international agreement.[437] The CD system replaces earlier designations applied by the manufacturers of particular monoclonal antibodies. In tissue sections the various lymphocytic antigens are best detected using frozen sections. A limited number of antigens can be demonstrated in paraffin sections using monoclonal antibodies which are commercially available.[438] CD45 (leucocyte common antigen, L200) is expressed by all lymphocytes,[439] whereas CD2 and CD3 are antigens unique to T lymphocytes.[440] B-cell antigens include CD19, CD20 and CD72.[437] In practice, B cells are usually identified by the demonstration of

surface or cytoplasmic immunoglobulin (see below). Monoclonality of a B-cell infiltrate is considered to be present if the great majority of B cells in the infiltrate express the same light chain. More sophisticated techniques involving gene-receptor studies have been developed for this purpose. In the case of T cells this involves the identification of an identical T-cell receptor in all T cells in an infiltrate. CD typing does not establish monoclonality. However, in some monoclonal (malignant) T-cell infiltrates there may be loss of one or more of the CD antigens that are expressed by normal T lymphocytes. It should also be noted that malignant infiltrates of lymphoid cells may be accompanied by a reactive (polyclonal) component of lymphocytes; in some circumstances the reactive component may comprise up to 40% of the infiltrate.

Various aspects of T-cell and B-cell function, and their subtypes, will now be considered.

T lymphocytes. T lymphocytes leave the bone marrow and migrate to the thymus where they proliferate, mature and undergo selection.[441] The process of selection involves the elimination of self-reactive T cells and the positive selection for proliferation of lymphocytes with receptors that can recognize antigens associated with major histocompatibility complex (MHC) molecules.[442,443] T cells emerge from the thymus as immunocompetent cells expressing the antigens CD2 (the E-rosette receptor), CD3 (associated with the T-cell receptor),[440,444] CD7 (also a marker of acute lymphocytic leukaemia) and, usually, CD5.[445] Approximately 60% of circulating lymphocytes also express CD4 while approximately 35% are CD8 positive.[444] A small number of lymphocytes express both antigens or neither. There is an approximately equal number of CD4-positive and CD8-positive lymphocytes in normal skin.[435] The CD4 and CD8 glycoproteins play an important role in T-cell activation by binding to MHC class II or class I molecules respectively.[443] Endogenously-synthesized antigens (e.g. viral proteins produced by infected cells) are presented in the context of MHC class I, whereas protein antigens which enter antigen-presenting cells through endocytosis are presented to CD4-positive cells in the context of MHC class II molecules.[442,446,447] In addition to their recognition of antigens attached to MHC molecules, CD4-positive cells also help other cells to divide and/or differentiate. Accordingly, they are also known as T-helper/inducer cells.[448] However, there is recent evidence to suggest that some cells with this phenotype may have cytolytic and suppressor functions, a role previously regarded as the exclusive domain of the CD8-positive lymphocytes;[441,449] the latter cells are known as T-suppressor/cytotoxic lymphocytes. A few CD8-positive cells appear to have a helper function. It is now known that CD4 is the cellular ligand to which the human immunodeficiency virus (HIV) attaches.[439,447]

Engagement of the T-cell receptor (TCR) by a foreign antigen is the primary signal for T-cell activation.[450] The TCR in most T cells is composed of α and β chains which are the products of the recombination of a large number of independent gene segments.[451,452] This recombination occurs in the thymus and conveys the unique specificity to each T cell.[441]

T lymphocytes release various biological molecules into the extracellular milieu.[453,454] These substances, known as lymphokines, are rapidly consumed at the reaction site. They include the interleukins, colony-stimulating factors, tumour necrosis factors and interferons.[453] Lymphokines are not antigen specific, nor dependent on antigen for many of their actions. Various lymphokines selectively stimulate different stages of T- and B- cell development.[453]

B lymphocytes. B lymphocytes arise first in the fetal yolk sac, then in the fetal liver and finally in the bone marrow.[451] The earliest identified cell of B-cell lineage is the pre-B cell which is characterized by small amounts of intracytoplasmic IgM. It lacks surface immunoglobulin whereas mature B lymphocytes synthesize and express immunoglobulins on their cell surfaces.[455] The immunoglobulin functions as an antigen receptor.

Maturation of B lymphocytes takes place in the lymph nodes, spleen and mucosa-associated lymphoid tissue. In lymphoid tissue B lymphocytes respond to antigen by proliferating and developing into plasmablasts and antibody-secreting plasma cells (see page 1000). Some B lymphocytes differentiate into long-lived B-memory cells.[456] Either of these processes may be accompanied by further DNA rearrangement, contributing to the generation of the B-cell repertoire.

Subsets of B lymphocytes have been defined on the basis of the class of immunoglobulin produced (both heavy chain and light chain), the presence of various glycoproteins (CD-subset) on the surface, their tissue location, and their ability to respond to particular antigens. A distinctive subpopulation of B lymphocytes expresses CD5 antigen.[451] This class of B cells has a propensity to produce certain autoantibodies, for example, rheumatoid factor.[456] CD5-positive B lymphocytes are generated from precursors in fetal tissue but not in adult bone marrow.[451]

Although the above account has focussed on the specific features of B lymphocytes, it should be noted that an interaction between T and B lymphocytes is necessary for a complete antibody response to most antigens.

Classification of the lymphocytic infiltrates

Currently there is no universally acceptable classification of the lymphocytic infiltrates of the skin. The pragmatic approach is a subdivision into *pseudolymphomas* and *lymphomas*. This categorization, which has obvious prognostic implications, can usually be achieved by the examination of biopsy material stained with haematoxylin and eosin. Both categories of lymphocytic infiltrates can be further subdivided into T-cell and B-cell subtypes on the basis of the predominant cell, ascertained by the use of various monoclonal antibodies specific for either T cells or B cells. Still further categorization of pseudolymphomas and lymphomas can be made using aetiological, clinical or histological features.

Cutaneous pseudolymphomas

Pseudolymphomas are benign proliferations of lymphocytes which simulate malignant lymphomas clinically and histologically.[457] The histological pattern may be that of a superficial, band-like infiltrate of lymphocytes in the upper dermis (the so-called T-cell pattern) or a nodular or diffuse infiltrate throughout the dermis (the so-called B-cell pattern). However, there are well-documented cases of T-cell pseudolymphoma having a nodular pattern of dermal infiltration.[458,459]

Pseudolymphomas are best categorized as follows:

B-cell pseudolymphoma

T-cell pseudolymphoma
Jessner's lymphocytic infiltrate
Lymphomatoid papulosis
Lymphomatoid contact dermatitis
Lymphomatoid drug reactions.

B-cell pseudolymphoma is regarded as a distinct clinicopathological entity whereas T-cell pseudolymphoma is a heterogeneous group of diseases, rather than a disease sui generis. The term T-cell pseudolymphoma has been used for the rare cases of pseudolymphoma resembling B-cell pseudolymphoma (see above) but with an infiltrate of T cells.[458,459] Arthropod bites may produce a nodular infiltrate composed of either T cells or B cells, as may drugs.[457]

B-cell pseudolymphoma, Jessner's lymphocytic infiltrate and lymphomatoid papulosis are considered in detail in this section. Lymphomatoid contact dermatitis (see p. 104) is a little-studied variant of contact dermatitis in which there is a heavy dermal infiltrate with a so-called T-cell pattern of distribution of the inflammatory cells. Lymphomatoid drug reactions may present as plaques or nodules. They have followed the ingestion of phenytoin sodium, penicillin, griseofulvin and atenolol.[460–462] Many of the pseudolymphomatous drug reactions were reported prior to the introduction of lymphocyte subtyping. This applies also to the nodular infiltrates reported in association with the wearing of gold earrings.[463–465]

Cutaneous lymphomas

Cutaneous lymphomas are relatively rare. Controversy surrounds their classification as none of the currently used classifications of nodal lymphomas has been generally adopted for cutaneous lymphomas.[466–469]

The simplest classification of cutaneous non-Hodgkin's lymphomas is into T-cell and B-cell variants, as for pseudolymphomas. The cells in some lymphomas express neither B-cell nor T-cell markers; they have been called null-cell lymphomas: gene-rearrangement studies suggest that most of these lymphomas are in fact poorly-differentiated B-cell lymphomas.[470]

The following classification of non-Hodgkin's lymphomas will be used here:

T-cell lymphomas
Mycosis fungoides
Sézary syndrome
Pagetoid reticulosis
Adult T-cell leukaemia/lymphoma
Pleomorphic lymphoma
Large cell anaplastic lymphoma
Regressing atypical histiocytosis
Granulomatous slack skin
Lennert's lymphoma
Angiocentric T-cell lymphoma
Miscellaneous T-cell lymphomas

B-cell lymphomas
Cutaneous B-cell lymphoma
Crosti's lymphoma
Malignant angioendotheliomatosis
Gamma heavy chain disease

Miscellaneous lymphomas
Lymphoblastic lymphoma.

If mycosis fungoides is excluded, T-cell lymphomas and B-cell lymphomas are approximately equal in incidence.[471,472] Malignant lymphomas, other than mycosis fungoides and its variants, may be either primary in the skin or secondary to nodal or non-cutaneous extranodal lymphomas.[472,473] Some T-cell lymphomas arise in a pre-existing dermatosis such as large plaque parapsoriasis (see p. 1032), lymphomatoid papulosis (see p. 1031), actinic reticuloid (see p. 584)[474] and, rarely, atopic dermatitis.[475] Recent work suggests that cases with a high proportion of Leu-8-negative and Leu-9-negative T cells may represent a subset of benign lymphoid infiltrates at high risk for transformation into mycosis fungoides.[476] Progression of a B-cell pseudolymphoma to a lymphoma has also been recorded (see below).

T-cell lymphomas are a clinically and prognostically heterogeneous group. Most are of T-helper phenotype. B-cell lymphomas mimic stages in normal B-cell differentiation. They may have surface or cytoplasmic immunoglobulin, depending on their stage of maturation.

Cellular monomorphism coupled with cytological atypia is the histological hallmark of cutaneous lymphomas.[477,478] The great majority of cutaneous lymphomas are of diffuse type.[468,479] Large cells predominate in both types of lymphoma (excluding mycosis fungoides).[477]

The various pseudolymphomas and lymphomas of the skin are discussed below.

B-CELL PSEUDOLYMPHOMA

A plethora of terms has been used in the past for the entity described below as cutaneous B-cell pseudolymphoma.[480] The terms include lymphocytoma cutis, lymphadenosis benigna cutis,[481] cutaneous lymphoplasia,[482,483] cutaneous lymphoid hyperplasia[484,485] and Speigler–Fendt sarcoid.[486] Just as cutaneous lymphomas are now being characterized on the basis of the lineage of the constituent lymphocytes, so too should pseudolymphomas, even though this approach makes comparisons with histologically similar cases in the earlier literature difficult. Furthermore, it must be recognized that B-cell pseudolymphomas are not composed entirely of B cells; T lymphocytes are also present between the nodular collections of B lymphocytes.[487]

Evidence is accumulating that pseudolymphomas with a high proportion of B cells have a diffuse or nodular pattern of lymphocytic infiltration throughout the dermis, in contrast to pseudolymphomas with a predominance of T lymphocytes, in which the infiltrate is usually confined to the upper dermis.[485] An exception is Jessner's lymphocytic infiltrate (see p. 1030), in which the lymphocytes occupy the entire thickness of the dermis, although it does have a predominantly perivascular localization.[485] This entity was included in some of the earlier reports of 'cutaneous lymphoplasia'.[482] Uncommonly, nodular lymphocytic infiltrates in the skin have a predominance of T lymphocytes.

Notwithstanding these exceptions, it seems safe to assume that the entity described below correlates with a significant proportion of the cases described in the earlier literature under the terms listed above.

B-cell pseudolymphomas usually present as asymptomatic, red-brown or violaceous papules or nodules which vary in diameter from 3 mm–5 cm or more.[488] The lesions may be solitary, grouped, or numerous and widespread.[485,488] Solitary lesions occur predominantly on the head, while the grouped and multiple lesions tend to involve the trunk and lower extremities, although any site can be involved.[488,489] Females are affected more often than males. Lesions may resolve spontaneously after months to many years, but there is a tendency for some to recur.[488] Progression to a malignant lymphoma has been reported, but some of these cases may represent an initial misdiagnosis of an early cutaneous lymphoma rather than malignant transformation of a pseudolymphoma.[490–492]

Pseudolymphomas have been reported in the past (without marker studies) in association with tick and other arthropod bites,[484] antigen injections, gold earrings,[493] tattoos (particularly the red areas)[494–496] and following the ingestion of drugs such as phenytoin sodium.[497] In Europe, cutaneous lymphoid hyperplasia has been associated with *Borrelia* infection.[498] In this latter circumstance, the lymphocytic infiltrate involves the ears, the areolae of the nipples or the axillary folds.[498] In most cases, the aetiology of cutaneous pseudolymphomas is unknown, although the condition is thought to represent an exaggerated immune response to antigens of various types.

Histopathology[484,485]

By definition, cutaneous B-cell pseudolymphomas are composed of nodular collections of B lymphocytes (Fig. 40.17). The lymphocytes are polyclonal, in contrast to malignant lymphomas of B-cell type in which there is monotypic light chain expression.[499] The infiltrate in B-cell pseudolym-

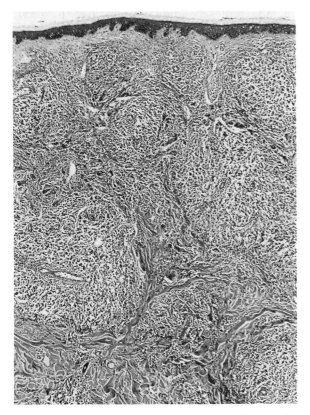

Fig. 40.17 B-cell pseudolymphoma. Nodular infiltrates of mature lymphocytes involve the dermis.
Haematoxylin — eosin

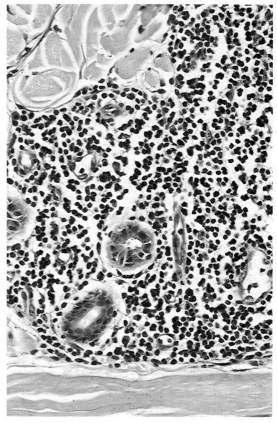

Fig. 40.18 B-cell pseudolymphoma. The infiltrate of lymphocytes surrounds but does not destroy the eccrine glands.
Haematoxylin — eosin

phomas is polymorphous with variable numbers of T lymphocytes, predominantly of helper type, between the B-cell collections.[487,499] There are also macrophages, Langerhans cells, follicular dendritic cells and, usually, a few plasma cells and eosinophils.[499,500]

B-cell pseudolymphomas are composed of a relatively dense infiltrate of lymphocytes throughout the entire dermis. The infiltrate often shows perivascular and periadnexal accentuation but the surrounded structures are not destroyed (Fig. 40.18). A narrow grenz zone is often present. The infiltrate may extend into the subcutaneous fat, but even in these circumstances there is not the 'bottom-heavy' pattern of infiltration that characterizes many cases of cutaneous lymphoma.

Follicular structures are present in approximately 10% of cases.[489] 'Tingible body' macrophages are usually present within the germinal centres of follicles, a feature which is usually lacking in follicular lymphomas.[501] Furthermore, the follicles in pseudolymphomas may be surrounded by a mantle of small lymphocytes. Immunohistochemical studies have demonstrated a follicular pattern of B cells in many cases in which this is not discernible in sections stained with haematoxylin and eosin.[480,489] Rarely, the follicular structures are composed of large pleomorphic lymphocytes with frequent mitoses. These cases have been reported as *large cell lymphocytomas*.[502,503] The relationship of this entity to Crosti's lymphoma (see p. 1045) and follicular centre cell lymphoma (see p. 1044) awaits elucidation. The three conditions appear to form part of a spectrum.

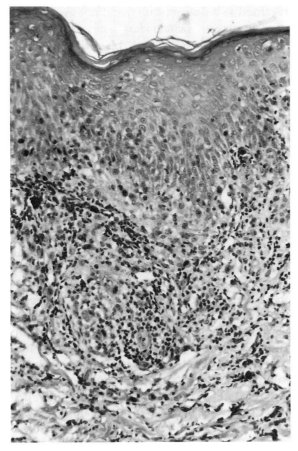

Fig. 40.20 Lymphomatoid papulosis. The dermal infiltrate includes atypical lymphocytes with hyperchromatic nuclei ('chunks of coal').
Haematoxylin — eosin

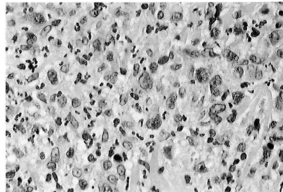

Fig. 40.21 Lymphomatoid papulosis. Large 'histiocytic' cells are admixed with small lymphocytes and some neutrophils.
Haematoxylin — eosin

large 'histiocytic' cells with a pale-staining nucleus and a prominent nucleolus (Fig. 40.21).[560] These cells may express the Ki-1 antigen (CD30), an antigen possessed by some activated T and B lymphocytes and by Reed–Sternberg cells.[546,547] Eosinophils are prominent in the variant of type A lymphomatoid papulosis known as *eosinophilic histiocytosis*.[561,562] In *type B lymphomatoid papulosis* (lymphocytic type) the atypical cells have a cerebriform nucleus which is often hyperchromatic. The cells are of varying size and express antigens for T-helper cells. The dermal infiltrate is usually more dense in type B than in type A lesions. Mitoses are quite common in both histological types, and

sometimes these are atypical. A small amount of nuclear dust is sometimes present.

In resolving lesions there is some dermal fibrosis, particularly in lesions that have ulcerated. There are only a few atypical cells in late lesions. It has been suggested that cell-mediated immune reactions involving the small lymphocytes in the infiltrate may play a role in the spontaneous regression of lesions of lymphomatoid papulosis.[563]

Electron microscopy.[539,564] There is a mixture of cells present, the proportions depending on the histological type. Some cells have a cerebriform nucleus with deep indentations. Small and large lymphocytes, some with a folded nucleus, are present. Langerhans cells can be found in both the epidermis and the dermis, and in the latter situation they are often in close contact with lymphocytes.[565]

LARGE PLAQUE PARAPSORIASIS

Large plaque parapsoriasis (atrophic parapsoriasis, retiform parapsoriasis, poikiloderma atrophicans vasculare) is a controversial entity (see page 83 for a discussion on the concept of 'parapsoriasis'). It is regarded by many authorities as synonymous with the patch stage of mycosis fungoides.[566-568] Alternative views are that it is a low grade T-cell lymphoproliferative process or a preneoplastic disorder — a T-cell 'dysplasia'.[569] As only 10–30% of cases progress to an overt T-cell lymphoma[568] there is some justification for the retention of this diagnosis. Nuclear DNA studies on the cutaneous infiltrate may help to predict the cases likely to progress to lymphoma.

Large plaque parapsoriasis is characterized by the development of irregular erythematous patches and plaques, with minimal scale, on the trunk and in the major flexures.[570,571] The lesions are some 10 cm or more in diameter. With time, atrophic (poikilodermatous) changes may supervene in a proportion of cases.[572] Progression to mycosis fungoides is usually restricted to cases that have evolved through this atrophic stage.[570] Atrophic large plaque parapsoriasis, as this stage is called, is now regarded by a majority of dermatologists and pathologists as early mycosis fungoides, even in centres that retain the concept of parapsoriasis for the preceding non-atrophic stages.[566]

Histopathology[572]

The appearances in early plaques may resemble those of chronic superficial dermatitis (small plaque parapsoriasis — see p. 115). That is, there is mild psoriasiform hyperplasia (psoriasiform acanthosis), sometimes with overlying mild orthokeratosis or spotty parakeratosis. The dermal infiltrate may be sparse and perivascular or band-like and ·a little heavier. It extends upwards into the dermal papillae. There is usually mild exocytosis of lymphocytes, but unlike early mycosis fungoides these do not form a 'horizontal band' in the lower epidermis. Pautrier abscesses are not seen. Occasional large lymphocytes, with mild nuclear atypia, are present.

In atrophic lesions, there is epidermal atrophy and a band-like infiltrate of lymphocytes in the papillary dermis.[573] These may obscure the interface by extending into the lower epidermis.[574] Telangiectasia of superficial vessels and melanin incontinence are further features. Some of the lymphocytes in the infiltrate have convoluted nuclei. These changes are identical to those described for the atrophic patch stage of mycosis fungoides (see p. 1035).

MYCOSIS FUNGOIDES

Mycosis fungoides is a clinically and pathologically distinct form of cutaneous T-cell lymphoma characterized by infiltration of the skin by neoplastic lymphocytes.[575] The infiltrating cells usually have the immunophenotype of mature T-helper lymphocytes; monoclonality is not detectable until the late stages of the disease.[576]

Mycosis fungoides is uncommon, with an annual incidence in the USA of one new case per one million population. It usually begins in mid to late adulthood but earlier onset has been recorded.[577,578] There is a definite male predominance. Lesions tend to develop on the lower part of the trunk and the thighs, and on the breasts in females.[579] In advanced stages, the entire body may be affected, including the face and scalp. The palms and soles have been involved in some cases in which the infiltrating cells had the immunophenotype of T-suppressor cells.[580]

Although it is accepted that mycosis fungoides usually evolves through three clinical stages[581] — patch, plaque and tumour stages — there is still considerable controversy as to the existence of a preceding stage (premycotic eruption) and its nature.[582,583] Large plaque parapsoriasis (see opposite) is regarded by some as a premycotic condition, while others regard it as being synonymous with the patch stage of mycosis fungoides (see below). As only 10–30% of such cases progress to overt mycosis fungoides there is some justification for the retention of large plaque parapsoriasis as an entity. Even more controversy surrounds the use of the term poikiloderma atrophicans vasculare, which has variously been regarded as a premycotic eruption, as synonymous with the atrophic form of large plaque parapsoriasis, as a distinct variant of mycosis fungoides, and as an atrophic form of the patch stage of mycosis fungoides.[584,585] It is best regarded as a reaction pattern, associated with a variety of disorders including parapsoriasis, collagen diseases, radiation dermatitis, graft-versus-host disease and certain genodermatoses (see p. 54).

The *patch stage* (eczematous stage) consists of ill-defined patches of varying hue, often with a fine scale. They are irregular in size and shape and have a random distribution, usually on the trunk. This stage may persist for many years before progression occurs.[586]

The *plaque stage* (infiltrative stage) is characterized by well-demarcated lesions which are often annular or arciform in appearance. They are red to violaceous and occasionally scaly.[585] The plaques may develop de novo or from patches. In the early stages, lesions are often limited to less than 10% of the skin surface but they may be more widespread, particularly in the late plaque stage.[585] Intractable pruritus is sometimes present.

Tumours usually develop in pre-existing lesions.[581] Rarely, they develop without a preceding patch or plaque stage (the d'emblee form).[581] The tumours are violaceous to deep red in colour with a tense shiny surface. Ulceration may occur. They measure from 1 cm in diameter to much larger lesions.

Erythroderma can develop at any stage in the evolution of mycosis fungoides.[581] In contrast to the Sézary syndrome (see p. 1038), in which erythroderma is a universal feature, there are no circulating 'Sézary cells' in the peripheral blood in the erythrodermic form of mycosis fungoides. Rarely, patients with mycosis fungoides develop a clinical picture indistinguishable from the Sézary syndrome, leading to the view that the latter is a leukaemic phase of mycosis fungoides.[586]

Rare clinical presentations of mycosis fungoides include hypopigmented patches and plaques,[587–592] bullae,[593,594] pustules, acneiform lesions, hyperkeratotic and verrucous lesions[595] and plaques resembling acanthosis nigricans.[596] Unilesional forms, resembling those seen in pagetoid reticulosis (see p. 1038) have also been reported.[597] Acquired epidermal cysts,[598] nail dystrophy[599] and second malignancies,[600–603] including skin cancers thought to have resulted from previous topical therapy, have been reported.[604,605] Follicular mucinosis (see p. 394) occurs in approximately 10–15% of cases.[606]

Although mycosis fungoides primarily involves the skin, it is not uncommon to find involvement of lymph nodes and other organs as the disease progresses.[607] Lymphadenopathy in the early stages of mycosis fungoides is due in most cases to dermatopathic lymphadenopathy, a reactive condition which may be seen in lymph nodes draining skin affected by a variety of inflammatory dermatoses as well as mycosis fungoides.[608] Visceral involvement is frequently found at autopsy.[609,610] The lungs,[611] spleen, liver[612] and kidneys are most frequently involved but every organ of the body can be infiltrated by tumour cells.[613–617]

The clinical course of mycosis fungoides is quite variable. It may progress slowly through the various clinical stages (see above) or it may evolve rapidly with extension to the viscera. Spontaneous resolution of an individual lesion may occur at any time during the disease. The median survival in one series was 7.8 years.[618] Extensive involvement of the skin with the development of tumours, lymph node involvement and organomegaly are bad prognostic signs.[619–625]

The aetiopathogenesis of mycosis fungoides is unknown. It has been regarded as a selective proliferation of a subpopulation of lymphocytes undergoing blast transformation, the result of the persistence of a specific antigen.[626] The disease has also been regarded as an abnormal immunological response to an environmental allergen[627] but a case control study in 1987 failed to give evidence of any environmental association.[628] Recently, attention has focussed on the possible role of a retrovirus. The human T-lymphotropic virus (HTLV-I), the causative agent of adult T-cell leukaemia/lymphoma, has been detected in a small number of patients with mycosis fungoides, particularly in endemic regions.[629,630] In T-cell leukaemia/lymphoma (see p. 1039) there is a clonal proliferation of virus-infected cells, a finding which has not been made, to date, in cases of mycosis fungoides associated with HTLV-I.[631] Another retrovirus, HTLV-V, has been associated with some cases,[632] but further studies are needed to elucidate its pathogenic role. A few cases of cutaneous T-cell lymphoma have been reported in association with the acquired immuno-deficiency syndrome.[633] Finally, it should be mentioned that a mycosis fungoides-like picture has been associated with the therapeutic ingestion of carbamazepine,[634] captopril[473] and phenytoin;[635,636] the eruption cleared in each instance following cessation of the drug.[636]

Histopathology[637,638]

Mycosis fungoides is characterized by the presence of a variably dense infiltrate of mononuclear cells in the papillary dermis, with extension of these cells into the epidermis, a characteristic known as epidermotropism. In establishing the diagnosis in the early stages of the disease these architectural abnormalities are more important than cytological atypia of the infiltrating lymphocytes, which is usually quite mild.[638-640] The histological appearances vary in the different clinical stages of the disease. They may also be altered by treatment with corticosteroids and ultraviolet A radiation which diminishes the amount of epidermotropism and the density of the infiltrate.[641]

Patch stage. In the patch stage of mycosis fungoides there is a relatively sparse infiltrate of lymphocytes spread along the slightly expanded papillary dermis. The infiltrate shows little tendency to aggregate around the vessels of the superficial plexus. Rather, the cells extend upwards in the papillary dermis and 'colonize' the lower layers of the epidermis, either singly or in small collections. This epidermotropism differs in subtle ways from the random exocytosis of lymphocytes and other inflammatory cells seen in some inflammatory dermatoses. Epidermotropic lymphocytes tend to be confined to the lower layers of the epidermis. They are often surround-ed by a clear halo but there is usually little or no spongiosis.[638] In epidermotropism there is a tendency for the cells to aggregate, a feature not seen in inflammatory exocytosis in which the cells are found singly and at all levels of the epidermis. Pautrier microabscesses (sharply marginated, discrete clusters of lymphocytes in

close apposition with one another, within the epidermis) are not usually seen in the patch stage.[637] As already mentioned, atypia of the cells is usually slight in the early stages, although cytological abnormalities may be seen in thin plastic sections that are not apparent in conventional haematoxylin and eosin stained sections.[473] Rare mitoses may be seen in lymphocytes in the papillary dermis. Other changes seen in patch stage lesions include an increase in collagen in the papillary dermis and epidermal changes.[473] The epidermis may show mild acanthosis; in poikilodermatous and atrophic lesions the epidermis is thin.[638] Basal vacuolar change and pigment incontinence are also present in these lesions.[642]

Plaque stage. In plaques of mycosis fungoides the infiltrate is more dense and atypical lymphocytes are more common. The lympho-cytes measure 10–30 μm in diameter and their nuclei are often indented.[479] A small number have prominent convolutions imparting a cerebriform appearance, best appreciated in thin sections. Small collections of cells may aggregate around vessels of the superficial plexus and, less often, the deep plexus. They also extend around the adnexae, particularly pilosebaceous follicles.[643] In addition to lymphocytes, the infiltrate usually contains a small number of eosinophils and sometimes plasma cells.[637] Epidermotropism is still a conspicuous feature (Fig. 40.22). Pautrier microabscesses are seen in more than 50% of biopsies; this proportion increases if step sections are examined (Fig. 40.23). Epidermal changes include parakeratosis, usually of confluent type, mild to moderate psoriasiform hyperplasia and epidermal muci-nosis.[637,644] Mild spongiosis does not exclude the diagnosis of mycosis fungoides, as sometimes claimed,[638] but spongiotic microvesiculation does not occur. Spongiotic foci resembling Pautrier microabscesses sometimes develop in certain spongiotic diseases such as allergic contact dermatitis.[645] Follicular mucinosis (see p. 394) is present in a small percentage of cases.

Tumour stage. In the tumour stage, the infiltrate has a more monomorphous appearance.

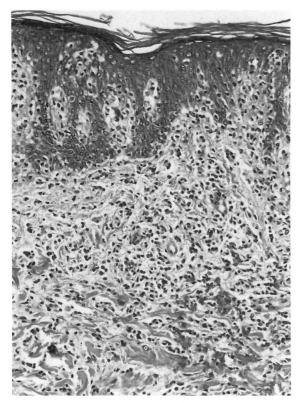

Fig. 40.22   Mycosis fungoides. Epidermotropism is a conspicuous feature in this plaque-stage lesion. Haematoxylin — eosin

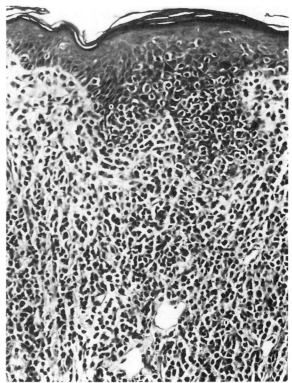

Fig. 40.24   Mycosis fungoides (tumour stage). The infiltrate is heavy and extends below the papillary dermis. Haematoxylin — eosin

It is dominated by large, atypical cells.[646] Mitoses are easily seen. The entire dermis is often involved and extension into the subcutis

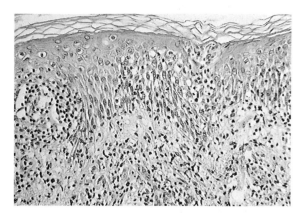

Fig. 40.23   Mycosis fungoides with epidermotropism and the formation of Pautrier microabscesses. Haematoxylin — eosin

may occur (Fig. 40.24). Deep dermal and subcutaneous nodules are particularly likely to occur if electron beam therapy has been used on a preceding plaque lesion in the same region.[647] Epidermotropism and Pautrier microabscesses are uncommon in the tumour stage.

Granulomas are a rare finding in mycosis fungoides.[648-650] They are usually small and tuberculoid in type but they may be palisaded and mimic granuloma annulare. At other times the granulomas are poorly formed and consist of small collections of multinucleate 'histiocytes'. The granulomas are more localized than in granulomatous slack skin, a rare variant of cutaneous lymphoma in which granulomas and multinucleate giant cells extend throughout the dermis, resulting in elastolysis (see p. 1042).[650] Granulomas in mycosis fungoides should also be distinguished from small collections of lipidized macrophages (dystrophic xanthomatosis) which are a rare finding in the dermis in mycosis fungoides.[650]

Other rare histological changes include the presence of a vasculitis[651] and the formation of bullae. In bullous lesions the split may occur at any level of the epidermis. The majority of cases have been subepidermal in location with negative immunofluorescence.[594] In hypopigmented lesions of mycosis fungoides there is a reduction in melanin in the basal layer and, sometimes, melanin incontinence.[652]

Immunohistochemistry. This technique must be performed on frozen sections of biopsy material as only a few lymphocyte monoclonal antibodies give satisfactory results on paraffin-embedded tissue.[653] Most patch and plaque lesions of mycosis fungoides are composed of T lymphocytes expressing the immunophenotype of mature T-helper cells (CD4+).[654] They usually express CD2 and CD3.[655,656] Being of memory subtype they are also CDw29 positive and CD45RA negative.[657] A deficiency of the T-cell antigens Leu 8 and Leu 9 (CD7) has been established in most lesions studied.[569,656,658–660] While isolated Leu-8 deficiency is seen in the lymphocytes in some inflammatory dermatoses, a combined deficiency of these two antigens is quite uncommon in benign conditions, although it does occur in atrophic forms of large plaque parapsoriasis.[569] It has been postulated that a cell lacking the antigens Leu 8 and Leu 9 (CD7) may be the precursor cell of mycosis fungoides.[476] With advancing disease, loss of mature T-cell antigens may occur.[661–663] A predominance of CD8-positive cells (suppressor/cytotoxic lymphocytes) has been observed in some plaques and tumours in patients with mycosis fungoides.[587,664–666] The patients in these circumstances have heterogeneous clinical manifestations.[580,667] Rapid progression was observed, in one series, in patients in whom the dermal lymphocytes were CD8 positive, CD7 positive and CD2 negative.[580] In addition to lymphocytes, the dermal infiltrate in mycosis fungoides includes numerous dendritic cells that are CD1 (OKT-6) positive. B lymphocytes are sometimes present in small numbers.[668]

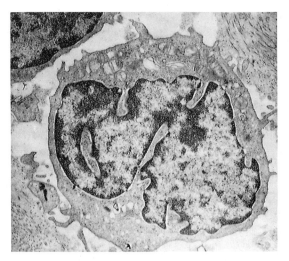

Fig. 40.25 Mycosis fungoides. A mycosis cell with its characteristic indented nucleus. Electron micrograph × 5000

Electron microscopy. There is a great diversity in the morphology of the atypical lymphocytes in mycosis fungoides.[669] The characteristic cell has a highly convoluted (cerebriform) nucleus with heterochromatin located predominantly beneath the nuclear membrane (Fig. 40.25). The cytoplasm contains multivesicular bodies and mitochondria which are sometimes clumped. Some authors use the term *Sézary cell* for a small to medium-sized lymphocyte with a highly convoluted nucleus, and the term *mycosis cell* for a cell which is slightly larger with fewer nuclear indentations.[639,670] Most authors use the terms Sézary cell, mycosis cell and Lutzner cell interchangeably for the various atypical cells, recognizing that intermediate forms also exist.[586,671,672] A much larger cell, sometimes called the *pleomorphic cell*, is seen in the tumour stage. It has a vesicular nucleus and a conspicuous nucleolus.[670,673] The nucleus of the pleomorphic cell may be variably convoluted.

Quantitative electron microscopy has been used to characterize the atypical lymphocytes in mycosis fungoides.[674–676] There are more lymphocytes with sharply-indented nuclear invaginations in mycosis fungoides than in benign disorders.

Langerhans cells are also present in the skin and lymph nodes in mycosis fungoides.[607,677]

Interdigitating cells are present in the dermis and may be in close association with lymphocytes.[575]

SÉZARY SYNDROME

The Sézary syndrome is an uncommon form of cutaneous T-cell lymphoma that is generally considered to represent a leukaemic stage of mycosis fungoides.[678] It is characterized by generalized erythroderma, intractable pruritus and a circulating Sézary cell count that usually exceeds $1.0 \times 10^9/l$ (see below). Less constant clinical features include cutaneous oedema, alopecia, nail dystrophy, palmar and plantar keratoderma and lymphadenopathy.[679,680] Visceral involvement may eventuate, resulting in a shorter survival than the median of 2.5 years for all cases.[678] Rarely, bullous lesions,[681] plane xanthomas,[682] vitiligo[683] or a monoclonal gammopathy[684] may develop.

The Sézary syndrome usually develops in late adult life. It may be preceded by an inflammatory dermatosis of some duration. The term pre-Sézary syndrome has been used for patients with erythroderma and a Sézary cell count of less than $1.0 \times 10^9/l$,[685] although others believe that the presence of any number of circulating Sézary cells is significant.[678] However, Sézary cells can sometimes be found in the peripheral blood of patients with various inflammatory dermatoses.[686]

Sézary cells can be recognized in blood films stained with the Giemsa or Wright methods.[687] The cells have a high nucleocytoplasmic ratio, deep nuclear indentations giving a cerebriform appearance, and condensed chromatin at the nuclear membrane.[688] Some Sézary cells are the size of normal lymphocytes; others are much larger.

The aetiology of the syndrome is unknown, although environmental factors and retrovirus infection have been suggested.[678,689]

Histopathology[682,690,691]

There is great variability in the histological findings. The most frequently observed pattern in the Sézary syndrome is a band-like infiltrate involving the papillary dermis and, sometimes, the upper reticular dermis as well.[691] Epidermotropism is present in some of these cases and Pautrier abscesses may be found, particularly if several sections are examined.[691] The infiltrate is of varying density; it is composed of small lymphocytes admixed with some larger cells with an indented nucleus. The use of ultrathin sections enhances the detection of cells with a hyperconvoluted nucleus.

In approximately one-third of all cases the biopsy appearances are non-specific with an infiltrate of lymphocytes in the upper dermis, mostly in a perivascular location. A few larger lymphocytes and macrophages are usually present. Eosinophils and plasma cells may be found in small numbers. Epidermotropism is usually mild. When present, the lymphocytes are not localized to the lower epidermis as in mycosis fungoides.

In both patterns mentioned above there is usually irregular acanthosis of the epidermis with focal parakeratosis. Spongiosis is sometimes present, although it is usually mild.[690] The papillary dermis contains scattered melanophages and some thickened collagen bundles. Occasional giant cells have been recorded.

The lymphocytes in the dermis usually express the T-helper phenotype (CD4-positive).[692,693]

Electron microscopy.[694,695] The Sézary cells have a convoluted nucleus with deep and narrow indentations. The cytoplasm contains a number of fibrils.[695] Ultrastructural morphometry has been used to distinguish Sézary cells in the blood from normal and reactive lymphocytes.[696] Dendritic cells, devoid of Birbeck granules, have been reported in the upper dermis, dispersed between the lymphocytes.[697]

PAGETOID RETICULOSIS

Pagetoid reticulosis (Woringer–Kolopp disease) is a rare, chronic dermatosis of slow evolution and disputed histogenesis[698] which presents clinically as a large, usually solitary, erythematous, scaly or verrucous plaque.[699] It preferentially involves the distal parts of the limbs of males. Most authors deny the existence of disseminated lesions (Ketron–Goodman disease) or visceral involvement,[699] and believe that recorded cases purporting to show these features[700–702] are examples of mycosis fungoides with prominent epidermotropism.[703] Nevertheless, a case of pagetoid reticulosis progressing to a large cell anaplastic lymphoma has been reported.[704]

Although marker studies have produced variable results,[705] probably due, in part, to the inclusion of some cases of mycosis fungoides, a trend is beginning to emerge. It seems that the epidermal infiltrate is of T-cell origin, probably of cytotoxic/suppressor cell type (CD8-positive) in contrast to the T-helper-cell (CD4-positive) origin of the infiltrate in mycosis fungoides.[706,707] In some cases the lymphocytes in the epidermis have been negative for both CD8 and CD4.[708] The cells show a variable loss of pan-T-cell antigens, such as CD45R/UCHL1.[708] The cells are activated and accordingly express CD25 and CD30.[708] Of interest is the finding of cytotoxic/suppressor cells in one case of epidermotropic mycosis fungoides.[707] There are several reports suggesting a monocyte/macrophage origin for the cells of pagetoid reticulosis,[709,710] but it now seems likely that this component represents part of the immune reaction to the abnormal T cells.[711]

Histopathology[699]

The epidermis is markedly acanthotic with overlying hyperkeratosis and patchy parakeratosis. The epidermis is infiltrated by large, atypical mononuclear cells with lightly eosinophilic cytoplasm, a large nucleus and a prominent nucleolus.[702,712] The cells have a pagetoid appearance. They are present at all levels of the epidermis but are most prominent in the lower third.[699] Cells in the upper layers of the epidermis may show subtle degenerative changes.[702] There are scattered mitoses.

Unlike mycosis fungoides there are no atypical cells in the dermis, which contains a dense, banal infiltrate of non-activated lymphocytes, histiocytes and some plasma cells.[702,713] There are usually no eosinophils.

Electron microscopy. Although not made clear in most studies, there appear to be two cell populations in the epidermis — histiocytes and stimulated T lymphocytes.[706,714] The latter cell is the major component.[699]

ADULT T-CELL LEUKAEMIA/LYMPHOMA

Adult T-cell leukaemia/lymphoma (ATLL) is a variant of peripheral T-cell lymphoma resulting from infection with human T-cell lymphotropic virus type I (HTLV-I), a type C retrovirus.[631,715] The virus is endemic in southwestern Japan and the Caribbean but there are now reports of its emergence in parts of Europe, Africa and the south-eastern USA.[716,717] HTLV-I differs from the human immunodeficiency virus (HIV) — formerly known as HTLV-III — which causes the acquired immunodeficiency syndrome (AIDS), by causing leukaemic transformation of the infected T lymphocytes and their 'immortalization', whereas HIV causes dysfunction of infected lymphocytes and their eventual destruction.[716] HTLV-I appears to be transmitted by sexual contact, by breast-feeding of infants and by infected blood products.[716]

ATLL has variable clinical manifestations which include a cutaneous eruption, bone marrow and peripheral blood involvement, lymphadenopathy, hepatosplenomegaly, pulmonary infiltrates and hypercalcaemia. Onset of the disease occurs in early adult life. It usually runs a rapid course, the median survival time being approximately 1 year.[718] Cases with a 'smouldering' course have been reported.[719,720]

Skin lesions, which may be the initial manifestation of the disease, occur in 50–70% of cases and are often widespread.[721,722] They take the form of erythematous or purpuric papules, nodules and plaques. Erythroderma and a pompholyx-like vesicular eruption are less common cutaneous manifestations.

Atypical lymphocytes are found in the peripheral blood in 50–80% of patients at presentation; virtually all develop a leukaemic phase eventually.[718] The leukaemic cells have a distinctive convoluted or clover-shaped appearance. They express a T-helper-cell phenotype (CD4-positive).[723] They also express certain antigens — CD25 (the interleukin 2 receptor), CD30 (Ki-1), CD38 and Leu 8 — which are not commonly found in the cells of mycosis fungoides.[724] There are some deficiencies of the major T-cell antigens, most commonly CD5 and CD7.[715] Although of T-helper type, the cells comprising the clonal proliferation of lymphocytes in ATLL exhibit suppressor activity.[722]

Histopathology[722]

The cutaneous lesions of ATLL share some features with mycosis fungoides in having an infiltrate of atypical lymphocytes in the upper dermis with variable epidermotropism and occasional Pautrier microabscesses (Fig. 40.26). The infiltrate in some cases is more massive than in mycosis fungoides while in others it conforms to a papular outline, an uncommon pattern in mycosis fungoides.[473]

The infiltrating cells may be medium-sized, large or pleomorphic, or a mixture of these types.[716,721] Other elements, such as small lymphocytes, macrophages, dendritic cells, eosinophils and plasma cells, are less common than in mycosis fungoides.

Atypical lymphocytes are sometimes found in the lumen of blood vessels in the dermis. They occasionally involve the walls of the vessels, leading to their damage and the extravasation of erythrocytes.[724] Angiocentric and angiodestructive lesions resembling those of lymphomatoid granulomatosis (see p. 245) are a rare manifestation of ATLL.[722]

Electron microscopy.[721] The tumour cells show slight to marked nuclear irregularity with a convoluted shape and a speckled chromatin pattern. The degree of nuclear indentation is much less than in the cells of mycosis fungoides and the Sézary syndrome. The cells in ATLL have lysosomal granules and glycogen in their cytoplasm.

PLEOMORPHIC T-CELL LYMPHOMA

This variant of cutaneous T-cell lymphoma shares many features with adult T-cell leukaemia/lymphoma (see above), although antibodies to HTLV-I are not present.[725,726] Similar cases have been included in reports of Lennert's lymphoma (see p. 1042), T-cell immunoblastic lymphoma, large cell lymphoma and multilobate T-cell lymphoma.[725,727–729]

Histopathology[725]

Pleomorphic T-cell lymphoma is characterized by a dense infiltrate of small and medium-sized lymphocytes in the upper and mid dermis and around adnexal structures. Epidermotropism is unusual. There is pronounced nuclear pleomorphism. In some cases, the nuclei have been multilobate but they are not cerebriform.

Most of the tumour cells express the activation markers CD25 and CD30.[725] The cells are usually of T-helper type but they may lack the CD5 antigen.

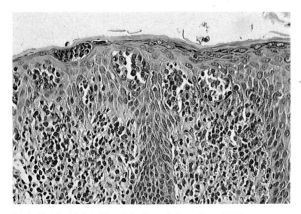

Fig. 40.26　Adult T-cell leukaemia/lymphoma. There are atypical lymphocytes in the upper dermis with epidermotropism of these cells and the formation of Pautrier microabscesses.
Haematoxylin — eosin
Photograph supplied by Drs Tetsunori and Kimura, Section of Dermatology, Sapporo General Hospital, Sapporo, Japan.

LARGE CELL ANAPLASTIC LYMPHOMA

Large cell anaplastic lymphoma is a recently delineated, morphologically distinct variant of lymphoma that is usually of T-cell lineage.[730–732] Most of the neoplastic cells express the Ki-1 (CD30) antigen, although this antigen is also present on a considerable proportion of cells in angioimmunoblastic lymphadenopathy, pleomorphic T-cell lymphoma, pagetoid reticulosis and lymphomatoid papulosis.[704,730,732–734]

Three different clinical types of large cell anaplastic lymphoma occur.[730] The first is found in children and adolescents.[735] Cutaneous lesions are often painful and they sometimes ulcerate. Spontaneous regression of individual lesions may occur and the outcome is often favourable.[735] Similar cases have been reported in the earlier literature as regressing atypical histiocytosis (see below). The second clinical type is the rare occurrence of primary cutaneous lesions in older patients, and the third is the development of the large cell anaplastic lymphoma of the skin as a complication of mycosis fungoides or of some other cutaneous T-cell lymphoma, or of an antecedent lymph node infiltration.[736]

Histopathology[725]

There is a diffuse infiltrate of large lymphocytes which extends through the entire dermis and sometimes into the subcutaneous fat. Usually there is no epidermotropism. Small foci of necrosis are often present. The cells, which may have a cohesive growth pattern, have an oval or kidney-shaped nucleus with dense chromatin around the nuclear membrane. The cytoplasm is abundant and pale staining. Numerous mitotic figures, some atypical, are usually present. A few neutrophils and eosinophils may also be present, as well as small and medium-sized lymphocytes in varying numbers.[730] Giant cells with a variable resemblance to Sternberg–Reed cells are always present. A subgroup with a high content of reactive histiocytes has been defined.[737]

Marker studies show that the cells are positive for Ki-1 (CD30), but there is variable expression of leucocyte common antigen (CD45).[738] The monoclonal antibody Ber-H2 has the advantage of recognizing the CD30 antigen in paraffin sections.[739] The tumour cells often express markers of activation such as CD25 and Ki-67.

In the majority of reported cases the cells have shown the phenotype of T-helper cells,[730,740] but in a few cases they have been of B-cell or null type.[736] In childhood cases, T-cell markers may be lost; the T-cell lineage has been confirmed in some of these cases by gene-receptor analysis.[730]

Electron microscopy. Multivesicular bodies have been present in the cytoplasm of the cells in the few cases in which electron microscopy has been performed.[725] Some tumour cells may show sharp indentations of the nucleus.

REGRESSING ATYPICAL HISTIOCYTOSIS

Regressing atypical histiocytosis is an extremely rare, primary cutaneous neoplasm composed of atypical 'histiocytes'.[741–745] It presents with solitary or multiple, nodulo-ulcerative lesions, 2–10 cm in diameter, which develop over several weeks.[744] There is a predilection for the extremities.

Despite the appearances of a high grade malignancy, the disease has a chronic clinical course of many years, typified by regression of individual lesions.[743] However, long-term follow-up suggests a probable substantial risk of the development of systemic lymphoma.[744,745]

The suggestion that this tumour has a histiocytic origin was based on non-specific cytochemistry, as well as on the presence of Fc and complement receptors.[741] Based on immunological phenotyping and the finding of a rearrangement of T-cell receptor genes, a T cell lineage has recently been proposed.[743,744] Similar cases have been included as a variant of large cell anaplastic lymphoma (see above).

Histopathology[744]

There is a polymorphous cellular infiltrate throughout the dermis composed of large, highly atypical mononuclear cells admixed with small lymphocytes and occasional neutrophils and plasma cells, and sometimes eosinophils. The large cells have a round, oval or slightly reniform nucleus with one or more prominent nucleoli and a perinuclear clear zone.[742] The cytoplasm is well defined, and lightly eosinophilic. Occasional multinucleate cells are present. Mitoses are frequent, with occasional atypical forms. Erythrophagocytosis is present but rare. Other features that may be present include perilesional fibrosis, tumour necrosis, and ulceration with bordering epidermal hyperplasia.

In one case, the majority of the cells were positive for leucocyte common antigen, OKT II (CD2) (a pan-T-cell marker) and Ki-1 (CD30).[743] (CD30).[743]

Electron microscopy. The large cells have a highly folded nucleus with large, often multiple nucleoli.[742] There are no Birbeck granules or other distinctive features to permit unequivocal identification.[742]

GRANULOMATOUS SLACK SKIN

Granulomatous slack skin is a very rare condition in which pendulous folds of skin develop in large, pre-existing, erythematous plaques.[746–748] There is a predilection for flexural areas, particularly the axillae and groins.[749] The condition is regarded as a chronic form of cutaneous T-cell lymphoma of helper-cell phenotype, with associated granulomatous inflammation that mediates dermal elastolysis.[750] Long survival is the usual outcome although progression to disseminated lymphoma has been reported in a few cases.[650]

Histopathology[650]

There is permeation of the entire dermis and the subcutis by lymphocytes, some of which are large and atypical with a hyperconvoluted nucleus. Epidermotropism is present. The cutaneous infiltrate also includes multinucleate giant cells and there is granuloma formation. The giant cells may have up to 30 nuclei; their cytoplasm may contain lymphocytes and elastic fibres. Foam cells and dendritic cells have also been reported in the infiltrate.[650,751] Stains for elastic tissue show a complete absence of elastic fibres from the dermis.

LENNERT'S LYMPHOMA

Lennert's lymphoma (lymphoepithelioid lymphoma) is an uncommon variant of peripheral T-cell lymphoma. It is a low-grade lymphoma although sometimes it runs a rapid course.[752] There have been comparatively few reports of this entity in recent years, as its status has been disputed.[753,754] Cutaneous involvement is rare.[754–756] Various skin infections have been reported in patients with this lymphoma.[757]

Histopathology

There is usually a predominantly dermal infiltrate of malignant lymphoid cells without the high content of epithelioid histiocytes which characterize the lymph node changes.[754,755] The abnormal lymphocytes are of T-helper phenotype.[754]

ANGIOCENTRIC T-CELL LYMPHOMA

Angiocentric T-cell lymphoma is a subset of peripheral T-cell lymphoma with an angiocentric infiltrate of atypical lymphocytes involving the dermis and subcutis.[758,759] It has an aggressive course with eventual visceral involvement. Angiocentric T-cell lymphoma is closely related to lymphomatoid granulomatosis (see p. 245); both conditions are angiocentric immunoproliferative diseases.[760] On the basis of recent reports it seems likely that lymphomatoid granulomatosis will eventually be reclassified as angiocentric T-cell lymphoma.[758] Cases reported as angiocentric T-cell lymphoma have presented with nodular cutaneous lesions, most often on the lower extremities.[759] Pulmonary involvement is present in some advanced cases, in contrast to lymphomatoid granulomatosis in which it is a common feature at the time of presentation.

Antibodies to the virus HTLV-I were detected in two cases reported recently as angiocentric T-cell lymphoma.[758] The clinical and histological features of both cases were more those of lymphomatoid granulomatosis, as currently defined.

Histopathology[759]

There is a lymphomatous infiltrate in the lower dermis and subcutis. Epidermotropism is not usually present.[761] The infiltrate shows perivascular and periadnexal accentuation and it extends into the walls of small and large blood vessels. Local necrosis is sometimes present. The infiltrate also invades small nerves in the lower dermis.

The cells in the infiltrate are medium-sized and large with stippled chromatin in the nucleus and a prominent nucleolus. Some nuclear folding is often present but there are no cerebriform cells. The cytoplasm is pale to clear. In contrast, the infiltrate in lymphomatoid granulomatosis tends to be more polymorphous, with an admixture of other cell types, including many small lymphocytes and some plasma cells and histiocytes.[759] In malignant angio-endotheliomatosis (see p. 1046), the infiltrate is predominantly intravascular in location, in contrast to the extravascular and intramural location in angiocentric T-cell lymphoma.[759]

Although the T-cell nature of the infiltrate has been confirmed, it should be noted that there is often loss of one or more of the pan-T-cell markers (CD2, CD3, CD5 and CD7).[759]

MISCELLANEOUS T-CELL LYMPHOMAS

This category refers to those peripheral T-cell lymphomas which do not fit into any of the categories already discussed. They usually present as one or more indurated, red or purple nodules. Uncommonly, non-scaling plaques are formed. Lesions may occur primarily in the skin or during the course of a nodal lymphoma.[762]

Histopathology[763]

In contrast to mycosis fungoides, the infiltrate in this category of T-cell lymphoma is non-epidermotropic.[467,764] The infiltrate may be massive, with diffuse involvement of the dermis and subcutis, or less dense, with perivascular and periadnexal accentuation (Fig. 40.27).[765] Lymphomas of most categories within the Kiel

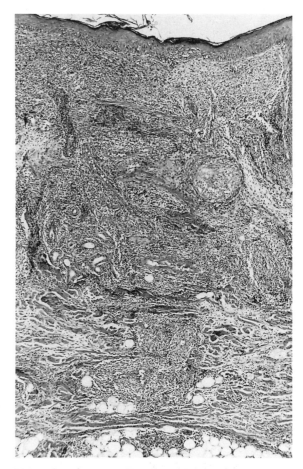

Fig. 40.27 Cutaneous T-cell lymphoma with a heavy infiltrate of small and large lymphocytes in the dermis and in the upper subcutis.
Haematoxylin — eosin

classification and the Working Formulation may be represented. The cells do not usually have a cerebriform nucleus.

In the majority of cases the cells express the T-helper phenotype.

CUTANEOUS B-CELL LYMPHOMA

The term 'cutaneous B-cell lymphoma' can be used as a group generic term to describe all cutaneous lymphomas of B-cell lineage, and as a designation for B-cell tumours which do not fit neatly into any of the distinct clinicopathological subtypes such as Crosti's lymphoma (see p. 1045) and malignant angioendotheliomatosis (see p. 1046).

Although the skin is not a preferential site of localization for B lymphocytes, cutaneous B-cell lymphomas are almost as common as cutaneous T-cell lymphomas if mycosis fungoides is excluded.[471,766] Cutaneous B-cell lymphomas may be primary in the skin or develop during the course of a nodal lymphoma.[763] The skin is eventually involved in approximately 10% of all B-cell lymphomas.[767,768]

The condition presents clinically as a solitary nodule or as a few nodules or plaques localized to one area of the body.[769] The forehead, trunk and the proximal parts of the limbs are favoured sites.[763,770] The nodules, which are pink or violaceous, measure from 0.5–5 cm or more in diameter.

Rare clinical associations have included the presence of paraproteinaemia[771] and of antibodies to the retrovirus HTLV-I.[772] The prognosis depends on the clinical stage of the disease and the histological subtype. Patients with the variant of B-cell lymphoma known as Crosti's lymphoma have a good prognosis (see opposite).

Histopathology[773,774]

The infiltrate usually involves the mid and deep dermis in the form of coalescent nodules or of a perivascular and periadnexal infiltrate (so-called 'bottom heavy' infiltrate).[532] Extension into the subcutis is common. There is usually an uninvolved subepidermal zone (grenz zone). Appendages, vessel walls and nerves are often infiltrated but not destroyed.[775,776] In a small proportion of cases follicular structures are present (Fig. 40.28).[775,777] Sometimes this pattern can be seen in immunohistochemical preparations but not in sections stained with haematoxylin and eosin.[775] It should be remembered that most cutaneous lymphoid infiltrates with a follicular pattern are benign pseudolymphomas.[775]

B-cell lymphomas comprise a wide spectrum of cell types, reflecting the various steps in the differentiation of B lymphocytes from the pre-B lymphocyte to the mature plasma cell.[470,773]

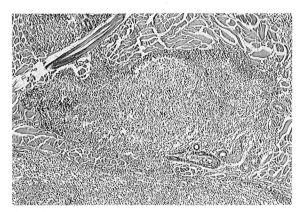

Fig. 40.28 Malignant lymphoma of B-cell type. A follicular structure is just discernible.
Haematoxylin — eosin

Tumours composed of plasma cells (plasmacytomas) have been considered earlier in this chapter (see p. 1001). Most B-cell lymphomas are diffuse large cell lymphomas composed of cleaved or non-cleaved cells;[532] immunoblastic lymphoma of B-cell type is included in this category.[773,778] Others are composed of small round or cleaved lymphocytes or a mixture of small and large cells. Included within these categories are tumours derived from follicular centre cells, known as centroblasts and centrocytes in the Kiel classification.[779–781] Crosti's lymphoma (see below) is now thought to be derived from follicular centre cells.[782]

Uncommon variants of B-cell lymphoma include the lymphoplasmacytoid lymphoma,[75,783–786] the 'signet-ring' cell lymphoma[775,787] and the variant with multilobate nuclei.[729,788] T-cell variants of these latter two types have also been described.[789]

Lymphomatous infiltrates must be distinguished from benign lymphocytic infiltrates.[790] These aspects are discussed on page 1030.

The tumour cells have surface or cytoplasmic immunoglobulin in the majority of cases, although the proportion is lower for cutaneous B-cell lymphomas than for nodal lymphomas. Those that are immunoglobulin positive are monotypic, expressing the same light chain.[775] IgM kappa is the most frequently expressed immunoglobulin.[776] Cytoplasmic immunoglobulin is detectable using monoclonal antibodies and paraffin-processed tissue, whereas surface immunoglobulin can be demonstrated only in frozen sections.[776]

B-cell lineage is best confirmed by demonstrating one or other of the B-cell surface antigens — CD19, CD20, CD21, CD22, and CD37.[776] Monoclonal antibodies that can be used on paraffin sections include MB-1 (detects CD20), MB-2 (detects CD21) and LN-1 (detects CD75).[776] From 10–40% or more of the cells in B-cell lymphomas of the skin are T lymphocytes, particularly in the lymphomas of mixed centroblastic/centrocytic type.[472,776,791–793] T cells are a minor component of the immunoblastic variant.[793] Occasionally, T lymphocytes may obscure a minority population of neoplastic B cells. Gene-rearrangement studies are rarely necessary to establish monoclonality in B-cell lymphomas.[794] Langerhans cells and dendritic reticulum cells may also be present, particularly in the lymphomas with a follicular structure.[778,795]

CROSTI'S LYMPHOMA

There is now some evidence to suggest that Crosti's lymphoma (reticulohistiocytoma of the dorsum), hitherto regarded as a histiocytic disorder[796,797] or T-cell lymphoma,[798] is in fact a primary cutaneous B-cell lymphoma of follicular centre cell origin.[799] It is considered here as a distinct clinicopathological entity for prognostic and historical reasons. Over 50 cases have now been recorded in the literature.

This variant of cutaneous lymphoma, which has an indolent course, presents with one or more large, figurate, erythematous plaques or nodules localized to the back or the lateral aspects of the thorax.[799] Lesions are markedly sensitive to radiation therapy. Systemic involvement is uncommon, even after many years of follow-up.[799]

Histopathology[799]

An uninvolved zone (grenz zone) separates a normal epidermis from a dense, dermal infiltrate

of lymphocytes and large histiocyte-like cells. The infiltrate is predominantly perivascular and periadnexal in location, although there is a tendency for the infiltrate in these situations to coalesce in the lower dermis.[799] The small lymphocytes form a rim around nodular masses of the larger cells (Fig. 40.29). Mitoses, sometimes atypical, are readily found.[798] Using the Kiel classification the appearances are those of a mixed centroblastic/centrocytic lymphoma which is follicular and/or diffuse. Within the Working Formulation, cases may be follicular or diffuse and of mixed small and large cell type; less commonly, they may be of diffuse large cell type.

The large cells react with B-cell-associated

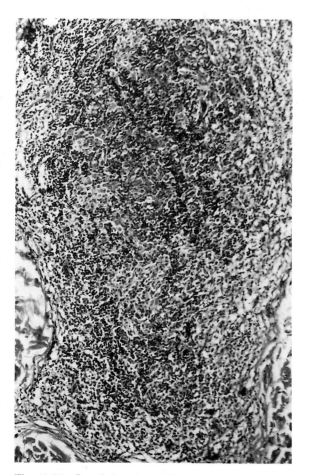

Fig. 40.29 Crosti's lymphoma. The large cells are found towards the centre of the nodular masses. Haematoxylin — eosin

monoclonal antisera while the mantle of small lymphocytes includes some T cells.[799]

Morphologically identical lymphomas occur in the skin which do not have the favourable prognosis of Crosti's lymphoma. Several such tumours (interestingly, all situated on the leg), were included, along with cases identical to Crosti's lymphoma, in a series reported as 'primary cutaneous large cell lymphomas of follicular center cell origin'.[781] It is worth mentioning here that the skin may be secondarily involved in 5% or more of cases of generalized follicular lymphoma.[775,781] Such cases do not usually have a good prognosis.

There are morphological similarities between Crosti's lymphoma and the cases reported as large cell lymphocytoma (see p. 1029).[686,800] Clinically, the latter condition is characterized by single or multiple nodules involving mainly the head or extremities and by a benign course.[686] The two entities are very similar: further studies are required to ascertain their exact relationship.[800]

Electron microscopy.[799] A range of cell types has been described. These include centrocytic cells with nuclear indentation, binucleate centroblastic cells, plasmacytic cells, cells with cerebriform nuclei and cells with cytoplasmic cellular debris.[797,799] Cell membranes are frequently villous and intertwined.[799]

MALIGNANT ANGIOENDOTHELIOMATOSIS

Malignant angioendotheliomatosis (intravascular lymphomatosis, angiotropic large cell lymphoma) is a rare disorder characterized by an intravascular proliferation of cytologically malignant lymphoid cells involving vessels of the skin and other organs.[801-804] Early studies concluded that it was a neoplastic proliferation of endothelial cells.[805-807] However, there is now convincing evidence, both histochemical and ultrastructural, that this condition is a peculiar form of malignant lymphoma.[801,808-810] All cases reported recently have been of B-cell type.[802,804,811] Wick and his colleagues have

suggested that malignant angioendotheliomatosis should be reclassified as 'intravascular lymphomatosis'.[801,802]

Most patients present with multiple neurological defects, including dementia.[812] Skin lesions, seen initially in about one-third of the cases, take the form of erythematous to blue plaques and nodules on the extremities, trunk or face.[812] There may be an associated extravascular large cell lymphoma, either nodal or extranodal. The condition is almost uniformly fatal despite treatment.

Histopathology

There is an increase in the number of vessels within the dermis and subcutis. These vessels are dilated and tortuous and they are partially or completely occluded by large atypical cells. The cells are several times larger than endothelial cells and have a high nucleocytoplasmic ratio. Their nuclei are round to oval, and nucleoli are often prominent. Mitoses are frequent and sometimes atypical. Fibrin thrombi are often present in the vessels, either with or without the atypical cells. Extravascular neoplastic cells may also be found.

The tumour cells express the leucocyte common antigen (CD45) and various B-cell markers.[802,804,811,813] Focal staining for factor-VIII-related antigen can be demonstrated in cells entrapped in fibrin-platelet thrombi in affected vessels.[802,814]

GAMMA HEAVY-CHAIN DISEASE

Gamma heavy-chain disease is a biochemical expression of a mutant clone of B cells which produce abnormal, incomplete, gamma heavy chains, devoid of light chains.[815] It is usually associated with a lymphoplasmacytic proliferative disorder, although the associated clinical and histological findings are varied.[816] Cutaneous involvement is rare, being present in less than 5% of the reported cases.[815] The usual skin lesions are erythematous, infiltrated plaques on the trunk and extremities.

Histopathology

In the few reported cases of gamma heavy-chain disease with cutaneous involvement, there has been a dermal infiltrate of lymphoplasmacytic cells, immunoblasts and mature plasma cells.[815] In one case vascular proliferation and the presence of eosinophils led to an initial diagnosis of angiolymphoid hyperplasia with eosinophilia.[816,817] Sometimes the cells have a conspicuous periadnexal distribution.

LYMPHOBLASTIC LYMPHOMA

Lymphoblastic lymphoma, a tumour of lymphoid precursors, may, rarely, present in the skin.[467,818] It occurs primarily in adolescents and young adults.[819] The mediastinum is commonly involved at an early stage. The cells may be of B-cell, T-cell or non-B, non-T type.[532,820]

Histopathology

There is a diffuse growth pattern in the dermis with extension into the subcutis.[763] The lymphoid cells are medium-sized to large. The nucleus is often convoluted, with a fine chromatin pattern and inconspicuous cytoplasm.[818] A number of cells show PAS-positive material in the perinuclear region. In some areas there are many tingible body macrophages leading to a 'starry-sky' pattern.[763]

MISCELLANEOUS AND MIXED INFILTRATES

This category of cutaneous infiltrates includes:

    Extramedullary haematopoiesis
    Leukaemic infiltrates
    Hodgkin's disease.

EXTRAMEDULLARY HAEMATOPOIESIS

Haematopoiesis takes place in the skin in early embryonic life. This process has also been reported in neonates as a consequence of intrauterine viral infection (rubella, cytomegalovirus and coxsackievirus[821]) and of congenital haematological dyscrasias (haemolytic disease of the newborn and the 'twin transfusion' syndrome).[822] In adults it is an extremely rare complication of myelofibrosis, particularly following splenectomy.[823–826]

The clinical features of extramedullary haematopoiesis are quite variable and include solitary lesions, plaque-like lesions, leg ulcers,[827] and bullae and erythema in the margins of a surgical wound.[823] In neonates there are often multiple, violaceous papulonodular lesions (the so-called 'blueberry muffin' eruption).[822,828]

Histopathology

Extramedullary haematopoiesis presents as a polymorphic dermal infiltrate consisting predominantly of myeloid and erythroid elments;[829] sometimes megakaryocytes are a conspicuous component of the infiltrate.[826,828,830] Cells in all stages of maturation can usually be found. The infiltrate is present in the superficial and deep dermis, particularly in a perivascular position (Fig. 40.30).[824]

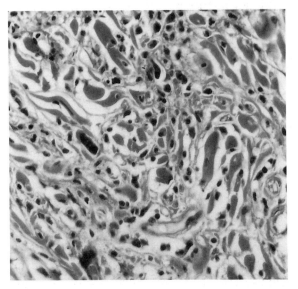

Fig. 40.30 Extramedullary haematopoiesis. The polymorphous infiltrate includes haematopoietic cells in various stages of maturation.
Haematoxylin — eosin

The Leder stain can be used to confirm the presence of the myeloid elements in the infiltrate.

LEUKAEMIC INFILTRATES

Leukaemia cutis refers to infiltration of the skin by leukaemic cells, resulting in lesions which are clinically identifiable.[831] It represents dissemination to the skin and is associated with a poor prognosis.[831,832] The deposits are thought to result from local proliferation of the leukaemic cells within the skin rather than from constant egress of cells from blood vessels in the region.[831]

Cutaneous manifestations of leukaemia have been divided into specific lesions (leukaemia cutis) and non-specific lesions.[833] The *specific lesions* take the form of violaceous, or reddish-brown and haemorrhagic, papules, nodules or plaques of varying size.[832] In acute leukaemias and chronic lymphocytic leukaemia the lesions have a predilection for the face and extremities, in chronic myeloid leukaemia for the trunk, and in monocytic leukaemia the entire body may be involved.[832,834] Marked thickening of the gums and oral petechiae are further manifestations of monocytic leukaemia.[832] Specific skin lesions usually occur late in the course of the disease, although sometimes they antedate by months the detection of leukaemic cells in the blood or bone marrow. The term *aleukaemic leukaemia cutis* is used for this uncommon event, which is seen more often with myeloid leukaemia than with the other types.[835-840]

The incidence of leukaemia cutis varies with the type of leukaemia.[833,841] It occurs in 10–50% of cases of monocytic leukaemia, in 4–20% of cases of chronic lymphocytic leukaemia and in less than 10% of cases of acute lymphocytic leukaemia, myeloid leukaemia and hairy-cell leukaemia.[841-843] These figures are based on series published some time ago. They may need to be revised in the light of current treatment regimens.

Unusual clinical presentations of leukaemia cutis have included eczematous lesions, penile[844] or scrotal ulcers,[845] erythema nodosum-like lesions,[846] acral lividosis,[847] induration of the lower part of the leg resembling stasis dermatitis,[848] localization to the scar at the site of insertion of a catheter,[849] figurate erythema,[850] annular purpuric plaques,[851] haemorrhagic bullae[852,853] and paronychia.[854] Exceptionally, the condition has been present at birth.[855] In one case of congenital monoblastic leukaemia the neonate presented with a 'blueberry muffin' appearance[856] (see p. 988). Another rare clinical presentation seen in acute myeloid leukaemia and, rarely, in other myelodysplastic states, is the *granulocytic sarcoma*, a soft tissue mass composed of tumour cells.[857-862] It occurs most often in the orbit but it can arise in any part of the body. The term 'chloroma' was previously applied to this tumour mass because of the greenish colour that some examples develop on exposure to light.[860]

Non-specific cutaneous manifestations of leukaemia are more common than specific leukaemic infiltration of the skin and occur in up to 40% or more of leukaemic patients.[833] The most frequent of these are the haemorrhagic manifestations, which include petechiae, purpura and ecchymoses.[833] *Candida albicans*, *Trichophyton rubrum* and *Cryptococcus neoformans* are the commonest causes of cutaneous fungal infections complicating leukaemia. Ecthyma gangrenosum (see p. 598) has resulted from severe *Pseudomonas* infection.[863] Herpes zoster is particularly common in patients with chronic lymphocytic leukaemia.[833] Other non-specific cutaneous findings include pyoderma gangrenosum (see p. 242), Sweet's syndrome (see p. 229), erythroderma (see p. 554), erythema multiforme (see p. 43), urticaria (see p. 216), cutaneous hyperpigmentation, xanthomas[864] and pruritus.[865]

Histopathology[866]

There is a wide spectrum of changes in leukaemia cutis that depends on the type of leukaemia and the degree of differentiation of the constituent cells. The usual picture is a diffuse infiltrate of cells in the dermis with accentuation around blood vessels and adnexae (Fig. 40.31). Involvement of the subcutis is common, but the

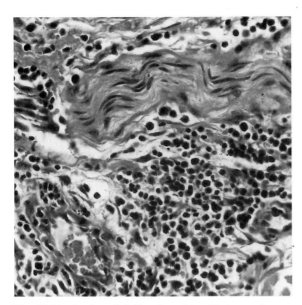

Fig. 40.31 Leukaemic infiltration of the skin in a patient with chronic lymphocytic leukaemia. Haematoxylin — eosin

epidermis is usually spared and there is a subepidermal grenz zone. Sometimes the infiltrate is nodular and perivascular. Myeloid cells typically infiltrate collagen bundles and the subcutaneous fibrous septa. Any variety of leukaemic cells may infiltrate the walls of blood vessels; they are often seen in the lumen of vessels.[866]

The cells composing the infiltrate vary greatly in the different types of leukaemia.[866] In acute myeloid leukaemia the cells are large, with a round or oval vesicular nucleus and basophilic cytoplasm. Mitoses are quite common. In chronic myeloid leukaemia the cell population is more pleomorphic, with granulocytes in varying stages of differentiation. Eosinophils may be present. The infiltrate in acute lymphocytic leukaemia is composed of medium to large blast-like cells with scanty cytoplasm, while in chronic lymphocytic leukaemia the infiltrate is composed of small mature lymphocytes.[866] The cells in monocytic leukaemia are monocytoid, with a fine chromatin pattern and prominent nucleoli.[866] They can be mistaken for the cells of a large cell lymphoma should the cutaneous lesions be the presenting feature of the

leukaemia.[867,868] In granulocytic sarcomas (chloromas) there is a dense infiltrate of myeloblasts and myelocytes with some more mature cells.[860] Focal necrosis may also be present.

Other features may include haemorrhage and the presence of macrophages which have ingested nuclear debris.[838] Nodules of extramedullary haematopoiesis (see p. 1047) may be found in chronic myeloid leukaemia.[866] Erythrophagocytosis was present in the skin in one case of the myelodysplastic syndrome.[869]

Histochemical techniques may be used to confirm the nature of the leukaemic infiltrate. Cells in myeloid leukaemias and acute monocytic leukaemia contain lysozyme while the cells in myeloid leukaemias and granulocytic sarcomas stain with naphthol AS-D chloroacetate esterase (NASD).[860,866,870] The degree of cellular maturation will determine the number of cells staining by this method. In hairy-cell leukaemia, which is of B-cell lineage, the cells stain with tartrate-resistant acid phosphatase.[871,872] Finally, an array of mono-clonal antibodies can be used to characterize the cells.[868] Using these techniques one study found a few cases of presumptive leukaemia cutis in which the cutaneous infiltrate showed T-cell markers, yet the circulating lymphocytes were of B-cell lineage.[873] The reasons for this disparity are still unresolved.

HODGKIN'S DISEASE

Infiltration of the skin is usually a late manifestation of Hodgkin's disease and develops in from 0.5–7.5% of patients.[874,875] Lesions often occur in a localized area of the trunk or of the proximal part of the extremities in the vicinity of involved lymph nodes, suggesting retrograde lymphatic spread.[874,876] Haematogenous and in-continuity direct spread are less common routes of dissemination to the skin.

Cutaneous lesions may be papules, nodules or plaques, although rare clinical presentations have included multiple ulcers on the scalp,[877] a bullous eruption,[878] and widespread lesions.

Paradoxically, two of the cases with widespread skin deposits had a more prolonged survival than is usually seen with cutaneous disease.[879,880] Spontaneous regression of skin lesions has also been reported.[881]

Skin lesions may rarely be the initial manifestation of Hodgkin's disease, with lymph node involvement appearing some months later.[882–884] Those cases reported as primary cutaneous Hodgkin's disease without the subsequent development of nodal lesions probably in fact represent another diagnosis — for example, lymphomatoid papulosis.[885,886]

A variety of non-specific manifestations are commonly found in the skin in Hodgkin's disease. They include pruritus, herpes zoster and acquired ichthyosis.[887] Less common associations[878,887,888] have included urticaria, erythema multiforme, drug eruptions, bullous pemphigoid, dermatitis herpetiformis, pemphigus,[889,890] acquired epidermolysis bullosa, lymphomatoid papulosis,[891–892a] follicular mucinosis, alopecia, lymphoedema, dermatomyositis and granuloma annulare.[893]

There is a wealth of contradictory data concerning the histogenesis of the Reed–Sternberg cells and the mononuclear cells in the infiltrate in Hodgkin's disease. Many studies have shown a predominance of T-helper lymphocytes in tissues affected with Hodgkin's disease, although an origin of the Reed–Sternberg cells from an interdigitating reticulum cell or a monocyte/macrophage lineage has not been excluded.[894]

Histopathology[874,883]

There is a diffuse infiltrate of cells involving the dermis and upper subcutis. A thin grenz zone is usually present. Skin appendages and blood vessels are frequently invaded.[883] There is a mixed infiltrate which includes mononuclear cells with large eosinophilic nucleoli, lymphocytes, eosinophils and, sometimes, neutrophils and plasma cells. Reed–Sternberg cells are usually present.[895] Fibrosis is another common feature. The histology may resemble that of a nodular sclerosing or mixed pattern; lymphocyte depletion may be present in advanced cases.[874] The Reed–Sternberg cells and their mononuclear counterparts react with the antibody Ki-1 (CD30).[896] In one study, the majority of the cells infiltrating the skin were of CD8-positive phenotype.[894] Variable numbers of cells reacted with markers for mononuclear-phagocytic cells.[894]

Non-specific changes that have been reported in the skin include the presence of small epithelioid cell granulomas[897,898] and, in one case, palisading necrobiotic granulomas.[899]

REFERENCES

Neutrophil infiltrates

1. Wade BH, Mandell GL. Polymorphonuclear leukocytes: dedicated professional phagocytes. Am J Med 1983; 74: 686–693.
2. Cannistra SA, Griffin JD. Regulation of the production and function of granulocytes and monocytes. Semin Hematol 1988; 25: 173–188.
3. Metcalf D. Peptide regulatory factors. Haemopoietic growth factors 1. Lancet 1989; 1: 825–827

Eosinophil infiltrates

4. Gleich GJ, Adolphson CR. The eosinophilic leukocyte: structure and function. Adv Immunol 1986; 39: 177–253.
4a. Leiferman KM, Peters MS, Gleich GJ. The eosinophil and cutaneous edema. J Am Acad Dermatol 1986; 15: 513–517.
4b. Wolf C, Pehamberger H, Breyer S et al. Episodic angioedema with eosinophilia. J Am Acad Dermatol 1989; 20: 21–27.
4c. Gleich GJ, Schroeter AL, Marcoux JP et al. Episodic angioedema associated with eosinophilia. N Engl J Med 1984; 310: 1621–1626.
5. Berretty PJM, Cormane RH. The eosinophilic granulocyte. Int J Dermatol 1978; 17: 776–784.
6. Peters MS, Winkelmann RK, Greaves MW et al. Extracellular deposition of eosinophil granule major basic protein in pressure urticaria. J Am Acad Dermatol 1987; 16: 513–517.
7. Leiferman KM, Ackerman SJ, Sampson HA et al. Dermal deposition of eosinophil-granule major basic

protein in atopic dermatitis. Comparison with onchocerciasis. N Engl J Med 1985; 313: 282–285.

8. Spry CJF. New properties and roles for eosinophils in disease: discussion paper. J R Soc Med 1985; 78: 844–848.

9. Fukuda T, Gleich GJ. Heterogeneity of human eosinophils. J Allergy Clin Immunol 1989; 83: 369–373.

10. Gaffney MG, Hanke CW. Allergic necrotizing eosinophilic granulomatosis. J Dermatol Surg Oncol 1988; 14: 1282–1285.

11. Kniffin WD Jr, Spencer SK, Memoli VA, LeMarbre PJ. Metastatic islet cell amphicrine carcinoma of the pancreas. Association with an eosinophilic infiltration of the skin. Cancer 1988; 62: 1999–2004.

12. Wells GC. Recurrent granulomatous dermatitis with eosinophilia. Trans St John's Hosp Dermatol Soc 1971; 57: 46–56.

13. Wells GC, Smith NP. Eosinophilic cellulitis. Br J Dermatol 1979; 100: 101–109.

14. Dijkstra JWE, Bergfeld WF, Steck WD, Tuthill RJ. Eosinophilic cellulitis associated with urticaria. A report of two cases. J Am Acad Dermatol 1986; 14: 32–38.

15. Fisher GB, Greer KE, Cooper PH. Eosinophilic cellulitis (Wells' syndrome). Int J Dermatol 1985; 24: 101–107.

16. Aberer W, Konrad K, Wolff K. Wells' syndrome is a distinctive disease entity and not a histologic diagnosis. J Am Acad Dermatol 1988; 18: 105–114.

17. Peters MS, Schroeter AL, Gleich GJ. Immunofluorescence identification of eosinophil granule major basic protein in the flame figures of Wells' syndrome. Br J Dermatol 1983; 109: 141–148.

18. Nielsen T, Schmidt H, Sogaard H. Eosinophilic cellulitis (Wells' syndrome) in a child. Arch Dermatol 1981; 117: 427–429.

19. Marks R. Eosinophilic cellulitis — a response to treatment with dapsone: case report. Australas J Dermatol 1980; 21: 10–12.

20. Mitchell AJ, Anderson TF, Headington JT, Rasmussen JE. Recurrent granulomatous dermatitis with eosinophilia. Wells' syndrome. Int J Dermatol 1984; 23: 198–202.

21. Lindskov R, Illum N, Weismann K, Thomsen OF. Eosinophilic cellulitis: five cases. Acta Derm Venereol 1988; 68: 325–330.

22. Saulsbury FT, Cooper PH, Bracikowski A, Kennaugh JM. Eosinophilic cellulitis in a child. J Pediatr 1983; 102: 266–269.

23. Kamani N, Lipsitz PJ. Eosinophilic cellulitis in a family. Pediatr Dermatol 1987; 4: 220–224.

24. Wood C, Miller AC, Jacobs A et al. Eosinophilic infiltration with flame figures. A distinctive tissue reaction seen in Wells' syndrome and other diseases. Am J Dermatopathol 1986; 8: 186–193.

25. Stern JB, Sobel HJ, Rotchford JP. Wells' syndrome: is there collagen damage in the flame figures? J Cutan Pathol 1984; 11: 501–505.

26. Newton JA, Greaves MW. Eosinophilic cellulitis (Wells' syndrome) with florid histological changes. Clin Exp Dermatol 1988; 13: 318–320.

27. Spigel GT, Winkelmann RK. Wells' syndrome. Recurrent granulomatous dermatitis with eosinophilia. Arch Dermatol 1979; 115: 611–613.

28. Steffen C. Eosinophilic cellulitis. Am J Dermatopathol 1986; 8: 185.

29. Schorr WF, Tauscheck AL, Dickson KB, Melski JW. Eosinophilic cellulitis (Wells' syndrome): Histologic and clinical features in arthropod bite reactions. J Am Acad Dermatol 1984; 11: 1043–1049.

30. Burket JM. Wells' syndrome: recurrent granulomatous dermatitis with eosinophilia. Arch Dermatol 1981; 117: 759.

31. Van Den Hoogenband HM. Eosinophilic cellulitis as a result of onchocerciasis. Clin Exp Dermatol 1983; 8: 405–408.

32. Murray D, Eady RAJ. Migratory erythema and eosinophilic cellulitis associated with nasopharyngeal carcinoma. J R Soc Med 1981; 74: 845–847.

33. Burgess GH, Mehregan AH, Drinnan AJ. Eosinophilic ulcer of the tongue. Report of two cases. Arch Dermatol 1977; 113: 644–645.

34. Andreano JM, Kantor GR, Bergfeld WF et al. Eosinophilic cellulitis and eosinophilic pustular folliculitis. J Am Acad Dermatol 1989; 20: 934–936.

35. Hardy WR, Anderson RE. The hypereosinophilic syndromes. Ann Intern Med 1968; 68: 1220–1229.

36. Chusid MJ, Dale DC, West BC, Wolff SM. The hypereosinophilic syndrome: Analysis of fourteen cases with review of the literature. Medicine 1975; 54: 1–27.

37. Kazmierowski JA, Chusid MJ, Parrillo JE et al. Dermatologic manifestations of the hypereosinophilic syndrome. Arch Dermatol 1978; 114: 531–535.

38. Leiferman KM, O'Duffy JD, Perry HO et al. Recurrent incapacitating mucosal ulcerations. A prodrome of the hypereosinophilic syndrome. JAMA 1982; 247: 1018–1020.

39. Shelley WB, Shelley ED. Erythema annulare centrifugum as the presenting sign of the hypereosinophilic syndrome: observations on therapy. Cutis 1985; 35: 53–55.

40. Fitzpatrick JE, Johnson C, Simon P, Owenby J. Cutaneous microthrombi: a histologic clue to the diagnosis of hypereosinophilic syndrome. Am J Dermatopathol 1987; 9: 419–422.

41. Van Den Hoogenband HM. Skin lesions as the first manifestation of the hypereosinophilic syndrome. Clin Exp Dermatol 1982; 7: 267–272.

42. Katzen DR, Leiferman KM, Weller PF, Leung DYM. Hypereosinophilia and recurrent angioneurotic edema in a 2½-year-old girl. Am J Dis Child 1986; 140: 62–64.

43. Stanley J, Perez D, Gigli I et al. Hyperimmunoglobulin E syndrome. Arch Dermatol 1978; 114: 765–767.

44. Zachary CB, Atherton DJ. Hyper IgE syndrome — case history. Clin Exp Dermatol 1986; 11: 403–408.

45. Nir MA, Westfield M. Hypereosinophilic dermatitis. A distinct manifestation of the hypereosinophilic syndrome with response to dapsone. Dermatologica 1981; 162: 444–450.

46. Sanchez JL, Padilla MA. Hypereosinophilic syndrome. Cutis 1982; 29: 490–494.

47. Songsiridej V, Peters MS, Dor PJ et al. Facial edema and eosinophilia. Evidence for eosinophil degranulation. Ann Intern Med 1985; 103: 503–506.

Plasma cell infiltrates

48. Torres SM, Sanchez JL. Cutaneous plasmacytic infiltrates. Am J Dermatopathol 1988; 10: 319–329.

49. Erlach E, Gebhart W, Niebauer G. Ultrastructural

investigations on the morphogenesis of Russell bodies. J Cutan Pathol 1976; 3: 145 (abstract).

50. Patterson JW. An extracellular body of plasma cell origin in inflammatory infiltrates within the dermis. Am J Dermatopathol 1986; 8: 117–123.

51. Weedon D. Unpublished observations.

52. Boehncke W-H, Schulte-Rebbelmund H, Sterry W. Plasma cells in the dermal infiltrate of mycosis fungoides are of polyclonal origin. Acta Derm Venereol 1989; 69: 166–169.

52a. Hurt MA, Santa Cruz DJ. Cutaneous inflammatory pseudotumor. Am J Surg Pathol 1990; 14: 764–773.

53. Shelley WB, Rawnsley HM. Plasma cell granulomas in non-lipemic xanthomatosis: apparent induction by indomethacin. Acta Derm Venereol 1975; 55: 489–492.

54. Lupton GP, Goette DK. Lichen planus with plasma cell infiltrate. Arch Dermatol 1981; 117: 124–125.

55. Jorizzo JL, Gammon WR, Briggaman RA. Cutaneous plasmacytomas. A review and presentation of an unusual case. J Am Acad Dermatol 1979; 1: 59–66.

56. Wiltshaw E. The natural history of extramedullary plasmacytoma and its relation to solitary myeloma of bone and myelomatosis. Medicine (Baltimore) 1976; 55: 217–238.

57. Newman W, Diefenbach WCL, Quinn M, Meyer LM. A case of acute plasma-cell leukemia supports the concept of unity of plasmacellular neoplasia. Cancer 1952; 5: 514–520.

58. Stankler L, Davidson JF. Multiple extra-medullary plasmacytomas of the skin. Case report with a note on prognosis. Br J Dermatol 1974; 90: 217–221.

59. Patterson JW, Parsons JM, White RM et al. Cutaneous involvement of multiple myeloma and extramedullary plasmacytoma. J Am Acad Dermatol 1988; 19: 879–890.

60. Edwards GA, Zawadzki ZA. Extraosseous lesions in plasma cell myeloma. A report of six cases. Am J Med 1967; 43: 194–205.

61. River GL, Schorr WF. Malignant skin tumors in multiple myeloma. Arch Dermatol 1966; 93: 432–438.

62. Alberts DS, Lynch P. Cutaneous plasmacytomas in myeloma. Relationship to tumor cell burden. Arch Dermatol 1978; 114: 1784–1787.

63. Wuepper KD, MacKenzie MR. Cutaneous extramedullary plasmacytomas. Arch Dermatol 1969; 100: 155–164.

64. La Perriere RJ, Wolf JE, Gellin GA. Primary cutaneous plasmacytoma. Arch Dermatol 1973; 107: 99–100.

65. Gomez EC, Margulies M, Rywlin A et al. Cutaneous involvement by IgD myeloma. Arch Dermatol 1978; 114: 1700–1703.

66. Swanson NA, Keren DF, Headington JT. Extramedullary IgM plasmacytoma presenting in skin. Am J Dermatopathol 1981; 3: 79–83.

67. Johnson WH Jr, Taylor BG. Solitary extramedullary plasmacytoma of the skin. Cancer 1970; 26: 65–68.

68. Burke WA, Merritt CC, Briggaman RA. Disseminated extramedullary plasmacytomas. J Am Acad Dermatol 1986; 14: 335–339.

69. Klein M, Grishman E. Single cutaneous plasmacytoma with crystalloid inclusions. Arch Dermatol 1977; 113: 64–68.

70. Mikhail GR, Spindler AC, Kelly AP. Malignant plasmacytoma cutis. Arch Dermatol 1970; 101: 59–62.

71. Canlas MS, Dillon ML, Loughrin JJ. Primary cutaneous plasmacytoma. Report of a case and review of the literature. Arch Dermatol 1979; 115: 722–724.

72. Prost C, Reyes F, Wechsler J et al. High-grade malignant cutaneous plasmacytoma metastatic to the central nervous system. Am J Dermatopathol 1987; 9: 30–36.

73. Kyle RA. Multiple myeloma. Review of 869 cases. Mayo Clin Proc 1975; 50: 29–40.

74. Hoss DM, Clendenning WE. Cutaneous plasmacytoma causing macroglobulinemia. J Cutan Pathol 1988; 15: 314 (abstract).

75. van der Putte SCJ, Go DMDS, de Kreek EJ, van Unnik JAM. Primary cutaneous lymphoplasmacytoid lymphoma (immunocytoma). Am J Dermatopathol 1984; 6: 15–24.

76. Vincendeau P, Claudy A, Thivolet J et al. Bullous dermatosis and myeloma. Monoclonal anticytoplasmic antibody activity. Arch Dermatol 1980; 116: 681–682.

77. Piette WW. Myeloma, paraproteinemias, and the skin. Med Clin North Am 1986; 70: 155–176.

78. Ishikawa O, Nihei Y, Ishikawa H. The skin changes of POEMS syndrome. Br J Dermatol 1987; 117: 523–526.

79. Fishel B, Brenner S, Weiss S, Yaron M. POEMS syndrome associated with cryoglobulinemia, lymphoma, multiple seborrheic keratosis, and ichthyosis. J Am Acad Dermatol 1988; 19: 979–982.

80. Feddersen RM, Burgdorf W, Foucar K et al. Plasma cell dyscrasia: A case of POEMS syndrome with a unique dermatologic presentation. J Am Acad Dermatol 1989; 21: 1061–1068.

81. Janier M, Bonvalet D, Blanc M-F et al. Chronic urticaria and macroglobulinemia (Schnitzler's syndrome): Report of two cases. J Am Acad Dermatol 1989; 20: 206–211.

82. Orengo IF, Kettler AH, Bruce S et al. Cutaneous Waldenström's macroglobulinemia. A report of a case successfully treated with radiotherapy. Cancer 1987; 60: 1341–1345.

83. Feiner HD. Pathology of dysproteinemia: light chain amyloidosis, non-amyloid immunoglobulin deposition disease, cryoglobulinemia syndromes, and macroglobulinemia of Waldenström. Hum Pathol 1988; 19: 1255–1272.

84. Nishijima S, Hosokawa H, Yanase K et al. Primary macroglobulinemia presenting as multiple ulcers of the legs. Acta Derm Venereol 1983; 63: 173–175.

85. Jones RR. The cutaneous manifestations of paraproteinaemia. I. Br J Dermatol 1980; 103: 335–345.

86. Mascaro JM, Montserrat E, Estrach T et al. Specific cutaneous manifestations of Waldenström's macroglobulinaemia. A report of two cases. Br J Dermatol 1982; 106: 217–222.

87. Tichenor RE, Rau JM, Mantz FA. Macroglobulinemia cutis. Arch Dermatol 1978; 114: 280–281.

88. Hanke CW, Steck WD, Bergfeld WF et al. Cutaneous macroglobulinosis. Arch Dermatol 1980; 116: 575–577.

89. Bureau Y, Barrière H, Bureau B et al. Les localisations cutanées de la macroglobulinémie de Waldenström. Ann Dermatol Syphiligr 1968; 95: 125–137.

90. Swanson NA, Keren DF, Headington JT. Extramedullary IgM plasmacytoma presenting in skin. Am J Dermatopathol 1981; 3: 79–83.

91. Bergroth V, Reitamo S, Konttinen YT, Wegelius O.

Skin lesions in Waldenström's macroglobulinaemia. Acta Med Scand 1981; 209: 129–131.

92. Mozzanica N, Finzi AF, Facchetti G, Villa ML. Macular skin lesions and monoclonal lymphoplasmacytoid infiltrates. Arch Dermatol 1984; 120: 778–781.

93. Perks WH, Green F, Gleeson MH. A case of purpura hyperglobulinaemica of Waldenström studied by skin immunofluorescence. Br J Dermatol 1974; 91: 563–568.

94. Watanabe S, Ohara K, Kukita A, Mori S. Systemic plasmacytosis. Arch Dermatol 1986; 122: 1314–1320.

95. Garnier G. Benign plasma-cell erythroplasia. Br J Dermatol 1957; 69: 77–81.

96. Baughman RD, Berger P, Pringle WM. Plasma cell cheilitis. Arch Dermatol 1974; 110: 725–726.

97. White JW JR, Olsen KD, Banks PM. Plasma cell orificial mucositis. Report of a case and review of the literature. Arch Dermatol 1986; 122: 1321–1324.

98. Aiba S, Tagami H. Immunoglobulin-producing cells in plasma cell orificial mucositis. J Cutan Pathol 1989; 16: 207–210.

99. Perry HO, Deffner NF, Sheridan PJ. Atypical gingivostomatitis. Nineteen cases. Arch Dermatol 1973; 107: 872–878.

100. Leonforte JF. Balanitis circumscripta plasmacellularis: case report with ultrastructural study. Acta Derm Venereol 1982; 62: 352–356.

101. Souteyrand P, Wong E, MacDonald DM. Zoon's balanitis (balanitis circumscripta plasmacellularis). Br J Dermatol 1981; 105: 195–199.

102. Brodin MB. Balanitis circumscripta plasmacellularis. J Am Acad Dermatol 1980; 2: 33–35.

102a. Nishimura M, Matsuda T, Muto M, Hori Y. Balanitis of Zoon. Int J Dermatol 1990; 29: 421–423.

103. Stern JK, Rosen T. Balanitis plasmacellularis circumscripta (Zoon's balanitis plasmacellularis). Cutis 1980; 25: 57–60.

104. Sonnex TS, Dawber RPR, Ryan TJ, Ralfs IG. Zoon's (plasma-cell) balanitis: treatment by circumcision. Br J Dermatol 1982; 106: 585–588.

105. Toonstra J, van Wichen DF. Immunohistochemical characterization of plasma cells in Zoon's balanoposthitis and (pre)malignant skin lesions. Dermatologica 1986; 172: 77–81.

106. Morioka S, Nakajima S, Yaguchi H et al. Vulvitis circumscripta plasmacellularis treated successfully with interferon alpha. J Am Acad Dermatol 1988; 19: 947–950.

107. Davis J, Shapiro L, Baral J. Vulvitis circumscripta plasmacellularis. J Am Acad Dermatol 1983; 8: 413–416.

108. Nedwich JA, Chong KC. Zoon's vulvitis. Australas J Dermatol 1987; 28: 11–13.

Mast cell infiltrates

109. Mihm MC, Clark WH, Reed RJ, Caruso MG. Mast cell infiltrates of the skin and the mastocytosis syndrome. Hum Pathol 1973; 4: 231–239.

110. Markey AC, Churchill LJ, MacDonald DM. Human cutaneous mast cells — a study of fixative and staining reactions in normal skin. Br J Dermatol 1989; 120: 625–631.

111. Leder L-D. Subtle clues to diagnosis by histochemistry. Mast cell disease. Am J Dermatopathol 1979; 1: 261–266.

112. Kasper CS, Freeman RG, Tharp MD. Diagnosis of mastocytosis subsets using a morphometric point counting technique. Arch Dermatol 1987; 123: 1017–1021.

113. Olafsson JH, Roupe G, Enerback L. Dermal mast cells in mastocytosis: fixation, distribution and quantitation. Acta Derm Venereol 1986; 66: 16–22.

113a. Omerod D, Herriot R, Davidson RJL, Sewell HF. Adult mastocytosis: an immunophenotypic and flow-cytometric investigation. Br J Dermatol 1990; 122: 737–744.

114. Green RM, Cordero A, Winkelmann RK. Epidermal mast cells. Arch Dermatol 1977; 113: 166–169.

115. Leder LD. Intraepidermal mast cells and their origin. Am J Dermatopathol 1981; 3: 247–250.

116. Fine JD. Mastocytosis. Int J Dermatol 1980; 19: 117–123.

117. Atkins FM, Clark RAF. Mast cells and fibrosis. Arch Dermatol 1987; 123: 191–193.

118. Roupe G. Urticaria pigmentosa and systemic mastocytosis. Semin Dermatol 1987; 6: 334–341.

119. Eady RAJ. The mast cells: distribution and morphology. Clin Exp Dermatol 1976; 1: 313–321.

120. Okun MR. Mast cells and melanocytes. Int J Dermatol 1976; 15: 711–722.

121. Stein DH. Mastocytosis: A review. Pediatr Dermatol 1986; 3: 365–375.

122. Tharp MD. Southwestern Internal Medical Conference: The spectrum of mastocytosis. Am J Med Sci 1985; 289: 117–132.

123. Melman SA. Mast cells and their mediators. Int J Dermatol 1987; 26: 335–344.

124. Basler RSW, Harrell ER. Urticaria pigmentosa associated with scleroderma. Arch Dermatol 1974; 109: 393–394.

125. Jackson N, Burt D, Crocker J, Boughton B. Skin mast cells in polycythaemia vera: relationship to the pathogenesis and treatment of pruritus. Br J Dermatol 1987; 116: 21–29.

126. Klein LR, Klein JB, Hanno R, Callen JP. Cutaneous mast cell quantity in pruritic and nonpruritic hemodialysis patients. Int J Dermatol 1988; 27: 557–559.

127. Caplan RM. The natural course of urticaria pigmentosa. Arch Dermatol 1963; 87: 146–157.

128. Kettelhut BV, Parker RI, Travis WD, Metcalfe DD. Hematopathology of the bone marrow in pediatric cutaneous mastocytosis. A study of 17 patients. Am J Clin Pathol 1989; 91: 558–562.

129. Orkin M, Good RA, Clawson CC et al. Bullous mastocytosis. Arch Dermatol 1970; 101: 547–562.

130. Poterack CD, Sheth KJ, Henry DP, Eisenberg C. Shock in an infant with bullous mastocytosis. Pediatr Dermatol 1989; 6: 122–125.

131. Czarnetzki BM, Kolde G, Schoemann A et al. Bone marrow findings in adult patients with urticaria pigmentosa. J Am Acad Dermatol 1988; 18: 45–51.

132. Fenske NA, Lober CW, Pautler SE. Congenital bullous urticaria pigmentosa. Arch Dermatol 1985; 121: 115–118.

133. Griffiths WAD, Daneshbod K. Pseudoxanthomatous mastocytosis. Br J Dermatol 1975; 93: 91–95.

134. Rasmussen JE. Xanthelasmoidea. An unusual case of

urticaria pigmentosa. Arch Dermatol 1976; 112: 1270–1271.

135. Stanoeva L, Konstantinov D. A case of systemic multinodular mastocytosis. Br J Dermatol 1973; 88: 509–515.

136. Niemi K-M, Karvonen J. A case of pseudoxanthomatous mastocytosis. Br J Dermatol 1976; 94: 343–344.

137. Ruiz-Maldonado R, Tamayo L, Ridaura C. Diffuse dermographic mastocytosis without visible skin lesions. Int J Dermatol 1975; 14: 126–128.

138. Kendall ME, Fields JP, King LE Jr. Cutaneous mastocytosis without clinically obvious skin lesions. J Am Acad Dermatol 1984; 10: 903–905.

139. Fowler JF Jr, Parsley WM, Cotter PG. Familial urticaria pigmentosa. Arch Dermatol 1986; 122: 80–81.

140. Harrison PV, Cook LJ, Lake HJ, Shuster S. Diffuse cutaneous mastocytosis: a report of neonatal onset. Acta Derm Venereol 1979; 59: 541–543.

141. Meneghini CL, Angelini G. Systemic mastocytosis with diffuse crocodile-like pachydermic skin, pedunculated pseudofibromas and comedones. Br J Dermatol 1980; 102: 329–334.

142. Willemze R, Ruiter DJ, Scheffer E, van Vloten WA. Diffuse cutaneous mastocytosis with multiple cutaneous mastocytomas. Br J Dermatol 1980; 102: 601–607.

143. Bruning RD, McKenna RW, Rosai J et al. Systemic mastocytosis. Extracutaneous manifestations. Am J Surg Pathol 1983; 7: 425–438.

144. Fried SZ, Lynfield YL. Unilateral facial telangiectasia macularis eruptiva perstans. J Am Acad Dermatol 1987; 16: 250–252.

145. Webb TA, Li C-Y, Yam LT. Systemic mast cell disease: A clinical and hematopathologic study of 26 cases. Cancer 1982; 49: 927–938.

146. Travis WD, Li C-Y, Su WPD. Adult-onset urticaria pigmentosa and systemic mast cell disease. Am J Clin Pathol 1985; 84: 710–714.

147. Monheit GD, Murad T, Conrad M. Systemic mastocytosis and the mastocytosis syndrome. J Cutan Pathol 1979; 6: 42–52.

148. Granerus G, Olafsson JH, Roupe G. Studies on histamine metabolism in mastocytosis. J Invest Dermatol 1983; 80: 410–416.

149. Fromer JL, Jaffe N. Urticaria pigmentosa and acute lymphoblastic leukemia. Arch Dermatol 1973; 107: 283–284.

150. Travis WD, Li C-Y, Bergstralh EJ. Solid and hematologic malignancies in 60 patients with systemic mast cell disease. Arch Pathol Lab Med 1989; 113: 365–368.

151. Lennert K, Parwaresch MR. Mast cells and mast cell neoplasia: a review. Histopathology 1979; 3: 349–365.

152. DiBacco RS, Deleo VA. Mastocytosis and the mast cell. J Am Acad Dermatol 1982; 7: 709–722.

153. Olafsson JH. Cutaneous and systemic mastocytosis in adults. Acta Derm Venereol (Suppl) 1985; 115: 1–43.

154. Tharp MD, Glass MJ, Seelig LL Jr. Ultrastructural morphometric analysis of lesional skin: Mast cells from patients with systemic and nonsystemic mastocytosis. J Am Acad Dermatol 1988; 18: 298–306.

155. Tharp MD, Glass MJ, Seelig LL Jr. Ultrastructural morphometric analysis of human mast cells in normal

156. James MP, Eady RAJ. Familial urticaria pigmentosa with giant mast cell granules. Arch Dermatol 1981; 117: 713–718.

157. Kruger PG, Nyfors A. Phagocytosis by mast cells in urticaria pigmentosa. Acta Derm Venereol 1984; 64: 373–377.

158. Okun MR, Bhawan J. Combined melanocytoma-mastocytoma in a case of nodular mastocytosis. J Am Acad Dermatol 1979; 1: 338–347.

159. Waisman M. Solar pruritus of the elbows (brachioradial summer pruritus). Arch Dermatol 1968; 98: 481–485.

160. Walcyk PJ, Elpern DJ. Brachioradial pruritus: a tropical dermopathy. Br J Dermatol 1986; 115: 177–180.

161. Heyl T. Brachioradial pruritus. Arch Dermatol 1983; 119: 115–116.

162. Weedon D. Unpublished observations.

163. Kestenbaum T, Kalivas J. Solar pruritus. Arch Dermatol 1979; 115: 1368.

Histiocytic infiltrates

164. Winkelmann RK. Cutaneous syndromes of non-X histiocytosis. A review of the macrophage-histiocyte diseases of the skin. Arch Dermatol 1981; 117: 667–672.

165. Roper SS, Spraker MK. Cutaneous histiocytosis syndromes. Pediatr Dermatol 1985; 3: 19–30.

166. Turner RR, Wood GS, Beckstead JH et al. Histiocytic malignancies. Morphologic, immunologic, and enzymatic heterogeneity. Am J Surg Pathol 1984; 8: 485–500.

167. Headington JT. The histiocyte. In memoriam. Arch Dermatol 1986; 122: 532–533.

168. Coldiron BM, Cruz PD Jr, Freeman RG, Sontheimer RD. Benign non-X histiocytosis: A unique case bridging several of the non-X histiocytic syndromes. J Am Acad Dermatol 1988; 18: 1282–1289.

168a. Foucar K, Foucar E. The mononuclear phagocyte and immunoregulatory effector (M-PIRE) system: evolving concepts. Semin Diagn Pathol 1990; 7: 4–18.

168b. Weber-Matthiesen K, Sterry W. Organization of the monocyte/macrophage system of normal human skin. J Invest Dermatol 1990; 95: 83–89.

169. Cerio R, Spaull J, Wilson Jones E. Histiocytoma cutis: a tumour of dermal dendrocytes (dermal dendrocytoma). Br J Dermatol 1989; 120: 197–206.

170. van der Valk P, Meijer CJLM. Cutaneous histiocytic proliferations. Dermatol Clin 1985; 3: 705–717.

171. Groopman JE, Golde DW. The histiocytic disorders: A pathophysiologic analysis. Ann Intern Med 1981; 94: 95–107.

172. Horiguchi Y, Tanaka T, Toda K et al. Regressing ulcerative histiocytosis. Am J Dermatopathol 1989; 11: 166–171.

173. Shimizu H, Komatsu T, Harada T et al. An immunohistochemical and ultrastructural study of an unusual case of multiple non-X histiocytoma. Arch Dermatol 1988; 124: 1254–1257.

174. Bork K, Hoede N. Hereditary progressive mucinous histiocytosis in women. Report of three members in a

family. Arch Dermatol 1988; 124: 1225–1229.

175. Berti E, Gianotti R, Alessi E. Unusual cutaneous histiocytosis expressing an intermediate immunophenotype between Langerhans' cells and dermal macrophages. Arch Dermatol 1988; 124: 1250–1253.

176. Helwig EB, Hackney VC. Juvenile xanthogranuloma (nevoxanthoendothelioma). Am J Pathol 1954; 30: 625–626.

177. Gianotti F, Caputo R. Histiocytic syndromes: A review. J Am Acad Dermatol 1985; 13: 383–404.

178. Sonoda T, Hashimoto H, Enjoji M. Juvenile xanthogranuloma. Clinicopathologic analysis and immunohistochemical study of 57 patients. Cancer 1985; 56: 2280–2286.

179. Esterly NB, Sahihi T, Medenica M. Juvenile xanthogranuloma. An atypical case with study of ultrastructure. Arch Dermatol 1972; 105: 99–102.

180. Grice K. Juvenile xanthogranuloma (nevoxanthoendothelioma). Clin Exp Dermatol 1978; 3: 327–329.

181. Flach DB, Winkelmann RK. Juvenile xanthogranuloma with central nervous system lesions. J Am Acad Dermatol 1986; 14: 405–411.

182. Torok E, Daroczy J. Juvenile xanthogranuloma: An analysis of 45 cases by clinical follow-up, light- and electron microscopy. Acta Derm Venereol 1985; 65: 167–169.

183. Davies MG, Marks R. Multiple xanthogranulomata in an adult. Br J Dermatol (Suppl) 1977; 97: 70–72.

184. Rodriguez J, Ackerman AB. Xanthogranuloma in adults. Arch Dermatol 1976; 112: 43–44.

185. Tahan SR, Pastel-Levy C, Bhan AK, Mihm MC Jr. Juvenile xanthogranuloma. Clinical and pathologic characterization. Arch Pathol Lab Med 1989; 113: 1057–1061.

185a. Cohen BA, Hood A. Xanthogranuloma: report on clinical and histologic findings in 64 patients. Pediatr Dermatol 1989; 6: 262–266.

186. Chu AC, Wells RS, MacDonald DM. Juvenile xanthogranuloma with recurrent subdural effusions. Br J Dermatol 1981; 105: 97–101.

187. Webster SB, Reister HC, Harman LE. Juvenile xanthogranuloma with extracutaneous lesions. Arch Dermatol 1966; 93: 71–76.

188. Jensen NE, Sabharwal S, Walker AE. Naevoxanthoendothelioma and neurofibromatosis. Br J Dermatol 1971; 85: 326–330.

189. Sibulkin D, Olichney JJ. Juvenile xanthogranuloma in a patient with Niemann-Pick disease. Arch Dermatol 1973; 108: 829–831.

190. Wood WS, Dimmick JE, Dolman CL. Niemann-Pick disease and juvenile xanthogranuloma. Are they related? Am J Dermatopathol 1987; 9: 433–437.

191. De Villez RL, Limmer BL. Juvenile xanthogranuloma and urticaria pigmentosa. Arch Dermatol 1975; 111: 365–366.

192. Garvey WT, Grundy SM, Eckel R. Xanthogranulomatosis in an adult: Lipid analysis of xanthomas and plasma. J Am Acad Dermatol 1987; 16: 183–187.

193. Hurt MA, Janney C, Santa Cruz DJ. Deep juvenile xanthogranuloma. Subcutaneous and intramuscular forms. J Cutan Pathol 1988; 15: 315 (abstract).

194. Gallant CJ, From L. Juvenile xanthogranuloma and xanthoma disseminatum — variations on a single theme. J Am Acad Dermatol 1986; 15: 108–109.

195. Gonzalez-Crussi F, Campbell RJ. Juvenile xanthogranuloma: Ultrastructural study. Arch Pathol 1970; 89: 65–72.

196. Mortensen T, Weismann K, Kobayasi T. Xanthogranuloma juvenile: A case report. Acta Derm Venereol 1983; 63: 79–81.

197. Seifert HW. Membrane activity in juvenile xanthogranuloma. J Cutan Pathol 1981; 8: 25–33.

198. Niizuma K. Solitary adult xanthogranuloma: a case report with new observation on lipid droplet formation. Acta Derm Venereol 1980; 60: 477–483.

199. Seo IS, Min KW, Mirkin LD. Juvenile xanthogranuloma. Ultrastructural and immunocytochemical studies. Arch Pathol Lab Med 1986; 110: 911–915.

200. Taunton OD, Yeshurun D, Jarratt M. Progressive nodular histiocytoma. Arch Dermatol 1978; 114: 1505–1508.

201. Burgdorf WHC, Kusch SL, Nix TE Jr, Pitha J. Progressive nodular histiocytoma. Arch Dermatol 1981; 117: 644–649.

202. Statham BN, Fairris GM, Cotterill JA. Atypical eruptive histiocytosis — a marker of underlying malignancy? Br J Dermatol 1984; 110: 103–105.

203. Winkelmann RK, Hu C-H, Kossard S. Response of nodular non-X histiocytosis to vinblastine. Arch Dermatol 1982; 118: 913–917.

204. Rodriguez HA, Saul A, Galloso de Bello L et al. Nodular cutaneous reactive histiocytosis caused by an unidentified microorganism: report of a case. Int J Dermatol 1974; 13: 248–260.

205. Kossard S, Winkelmann RK. Necrobiotic xanthogranuloma with paraproteinemia. J Am Acad Dermatol 1980; 3: 257–270.

206. Kossard S, Winkelmann RK. Necrobiotic xanthogranuloma. Australas J Dermatol 1980; 21: 85–88.

207. Finan MC, Winkelmann RK. Necrobiotic xanthogranuloma with paraproteinemia. A review of 22 cases. Medicine (Baltimore) 1986; 65: 376–388.

208. Holden CA, Winkelmann RK, Wilson Jones E. Necrobiotic xanthogranuloma: a report of four cases. Br J Dermatol 1986; 114: 241–250.

209. Dupre A, Viraben R. Necrobiotic xanthogranuloma: a case without paraproteinemia but with transepithelial elimination. J Cutan Pathol 1988; 15: 116–119.

210. Macfarlane AW, Verbov JL. Necrobiotic xanthogranuloma with paraproteinaemia. Br J Dermatol 1985; 113: 339–343.

211. Finan MC, Winkelmann RK. Histopathology of necrobiotic xanthogranuloma with paraproteinemia. J Cutan Pathol 1987; 14: 92–99.

212. Gibson LE, Reizner GT, Winkelmann RK. Necrobiosis lipoidica diabeticorum with cholesterol clefts in the differential diagnosis of necrobiotic xanthogranuloma. J Cutan Pathol 1988; 15: 18–21.

213. Barrow MV, Holubar K. Multicentric reticulohistiocytosis. A review of 33 patients. Medicine (Baltimore) 1969; 48: 287–305.

214. Lesher JL Jr, Allen BS. Multicentric reticulohistiocytosis. J Am Acad Dermatol 1984; 11: 713–723.

215. Lotti T, Santucci M, Casigliani R et al. Multicentric

reticulohistiocytosis. Report of three cases with the evaluation of tissue proteinase activity. Am J Dermatopathol 1988; 10: 497–504.

215a. Oliver GF, Umbert I, Winkelmann RK. Reticulohistiocytoma cutis — review of 15 cases and an association with systemic vasculitis in two cases. Clin Exp Dermatol 1990; 15: 1–6.

216. Fast A. Cardiopulmonary complications in multicentric reticulohistiocytosis. Arch Dermatol 1976; 112: 1139–1141.

217. Ehrlich GE, Young I, Nosheny SZ, Katz WA. Multicentric reticulohistiocytosis (lipoid dermatoarthritis). Am J Med 1972; 52: 830–840.

218. Furey N, Di Mauro J, Eng A, Shaw J. Multicentric reticulohistiocytosis with salivary gland involvement and pericardial effusion. J Am Acad Dermatol 1983; 8: 679–685.

219. Orkin M, Goltz RW, Good RA et al. A study of multicentric reticulohistiocytosis. Arch Dermatol 1964; 89: 640–654.

220. Catterall MD. Multicentric reticulohistiocytosis a review of eight cases. Clin Exp Dermatol 1980; 5: 267–279.

221. Coupe MO, Whittaker SJ, Thatcher N. Multicentric reticulohistiocytosis. Br J Dermatol 1987; 116: 245–247.

222. Catterall MD, White JE. Multicentric reticulohistiocytosis and malignant disease. Br J Dermatol 1978; 98: 221–224.

223. Caputo R, Ermacora E, Gelmetti C. Diffuse cutaneous reticulohistiocytosis in a child with tuberous sclerosis. Arch Dermatol 1988; 124: 567–570.

224. Goette DK, Odom RB, Fitzwater JE Jr. Diffuse cutaneous reticulohistiocytosis. Arch Dermatol 1982; 118: 173–176.

225. Heathcote JG, Guenther LC, Wallace AC. Multicentric reticulohistiocytosis: a report of a case and a review of the pathology. Pathology 1985; 17: 601–608.

226. Coode PE, Ridgway H, Jones DB. Multicentric reticulohistiocytosis: report of two cases with ultrastructure, tissue culture and immunology studies. Clin Exp Dermatol 1980; 5: 281–293.

227. Flam M, Ryan SC, Mah-Poy GL et al. Multicentric reticulohistiocytosis. Report of a case, with atypical features and electron microscopic study of skin lesions. Am J Med 1972; 52: 841–848.

228. Tani M, Hori K, Nakanishi T et al. Multicentric reticulohistiocytosis. Electron microscopic and ultracytochemical studies. Arch Dermatol 1981; 117: 495–499.

229. Kuramoto Y, Iizawa O, Aiba S et al. Multicentric reticulohistiocytosis in a child with sclerosing lesion of the leg. Immunohistopathologic studies and therapeutic trial with systemic cyclosporine. J Am Acad Dermatol 1989; 20: 329–335.

230. Heenan PJ, Quirk CJ, Spagnolo DV. Multicentric reticulohistiocytosis: A light and electron microscopic study. Australas J Dermatol 1983; 24: 122–126.

231. Caputo R, Alessi E, Berti E. Collagen phagocytosis in multicentric reticulohistiocytosis. J Invest Dermatol 1981; 76: 342–346.

232. Zak FG. Reticulohistiocytoma of the skin. Br J Dermatol 1950; 62: 351–355.

233. Davies BT, Wood SR. The so-called reticulohistiocytoma of the skin. A comparison of two distinct types. Br J Dermatol 1955; 67: 205–211.

234. Purvis WE III, Helwig EB. Reticulohistiocytic granuloma ("reticulohistiocytoma") of the skin. Am J Clin Pathol 1954; 24: 1005–1015.

235. Rendall JRS, Vanhegan RI, Robb-Smith AHT et al. Atypical multicentric reticulohistiocytosis with paraproteinemia. Arch Dermatol 1977; 113: 1576–1582.

236. Zayid I, Farraj S. Familial histiocytic dermatoarthritis. A new syndrome. Am J Med 1973; 54: 793–800.

237. Valente M, Parenti A, Cipriani R, Peserico A. Familial histiocytic dermatoarthritis. Am J Dermatopathol 1987; 9: 491–496.

238. Altman J, Winkelmann RK. Xanthoma disseminatum. Arch Dermatol 1962; 86: 582–596.

239. Maize JC, Ahmed AR, Provost TT. Xanthoma disseminatum and multiple myeloma. Arch Dermatol 1974; 110: 758–761.

240. Kumakiri M, Sudoh M, Miura Y. Xanthoma disseminatum. Report of a case, with histological and ultrastructural studies of skin lesions. J Am Acad Dermatol 1981; 4: 291–299.

241. Mishkel MA, Cockshott WP, Nazir DJ et al. Xanthoma disseminatum. Clinical, metabolic, pathologic, and radiologic aspects. Arch Dermatol 1977; 113: 1094–1100.

242. Battaglini J, Olsen TG. Disseminated xanthosiderohistiocytosis, a variant of xanthoma disseminatum, in a patient with a plasma cell dyscrasia. J Am Acad Dermatol 1984; 11: 750–755.

243. Szekeres E, Tiba A, Korom I. Xanthoma disseminatum: A rare condition with non-x, non-lipid cutaneous histiocytopathy. J Dermatol Surg Oncol 1988; 14: 1021–1024.

244. Gianotti F, Caputo R, Ermacora E, Gianni E. Benign cephalic histiocytosis. Arch Dermatol 1986; 122: 1038–1043.

245. Commens C, Jaworski R. Benign cephalic histiocytosis. Australas J Dermatol 1987; 28: 56–61.

245a. Godfrey KM, James MP. Benign cephalic histiocytosis: a case report. Br J Dermatol 1990; 123: 245–248.

246. Eisenberg EL, Bronson DM, Barsky S. Benign cephalic histiocytosis. A case report and ultrastructural study. J Am Acad Dermatol 1985; 12: 328–331.

247. Larralde de Luna M, Glikin I, Goldberg J et al. Benign cephalic histiocytosis: report of four cases. Pediatr Dermatol 1989; 6: 198–201.

248. Barsky BL, Lao I, Barsky S, Rhee HL. Benign cephalic histiocytosis. Arch Dermatol 1984; 120: 650–655.

249. Ayala F, Balato N, Iandoli R et al. Benign cephalic histiocytosis. Acta Derm Venereol 1988; 68: 264–266.

250. Winkelmann RK, Muller SA. Generalized eruptive histiocytoma: A benign papular histiocytic reticulosis. Arch Dermatol 1963; 88: 586–595.

251. Pegum JS. Generalized eruptive histiocytoma. Proc R Soc Med 1973; 56: 1175–1178.

252. Sohi AS, Tiwari VD, Subramanian CSV, Chakraborty M. Generalized eruptive histiocytoma. Dermatologica 1979; 159: 471–475.

253. Winkelmann RK, Kossard S, Fraga S. Eruptive histiocytoma of childhood. Arch Dermatol 1980; 116: 565–570.

254. Caputo R, Ermacora E, Gelmetti C et al. Generalized eruptive histiocytoma in children. J Am Acad Dermatol 1987; 17: 449–454.

255. Aliaga A, Alegre VA, Hernandez M et al. Benign cephalic histiocytosis VS. generalized eruptive histiocytoma. J Cutan Pathol 1989; 16: 293 (abstract).

256. Alliaga A, Martinez-Aparicio A, Alegre V et al. Generalized eruptive histiocytoma. J Cutan Pathol 1988; 15: 292 (abstract).

257. Umbert IJ, Winkelmann RK. Eruptive histiocytoma. J Am Acad Dermatol 1989; 20: 958–964.

258. Caputo R, Alessi E, Allegra F. Generalized eruptive histiocytoma. A clinical, histologic, and ultrastructural study. Arch Dermatol 1981; 117: 216–221.

259. Shimizu N, Ito M, Sato Y. Generalized eruptive histiocytoma: an ultrastructural study. J Cutan Pathol 1987; 14: 100–105.

260. Muller SA, Wolff K, Winkelmann RK. Generalized eruptive histiocytoma. Enzyme histochemistry and electron microscopy. Arch Dermatol 1967; 96: 11–17.

261. Furukawa F, Taniguchi S, Oguchi M et al. True histiocytic lymphoma. Arch Dermatol 1980; 116: 915–918.

262. Maier H, Burg G, Schmoeckel C, Braun-Falco O. Primary cutaneous atypical histiocytosis with possible dissemination. Am J Dermatopathol 1985; 7: 373–382.

263. Rosai J, Dorfman RF. Sinus histiocytosis with massive lymphadenopathy. Arch Pathol 1969; 87: 63–70.

264. Thawerani H, Sanchez RL, Rosai J, Dorfman RF. The cutaneous manifestations of sinus histiocytosis with massive lymphadenopathy. Arch Dermatol 1978; 114: 191–197.

265. Wright DH, Richards DB. Sinus histiocytosis with massive lymphadenopathy (Rosai-Dorfman disease): report of a case with widespread nodal and extra nodal dissemination. Histopathology 1981; 5: 697–709.

266. Lazar AP, Esterly NB, Gonzalez-Crussi F. Sinus histiocytosis clinically limited to the skin. Pediatr Dermatol 1987; 4: 247–253.

267. Viraben R, Dupre A, Gorguet B. Pure cutaneous histiocytosis resembling sinus histiocytosis. Clin Exp Dermatol 1988; 13: 197–199.

268. Nawroz IM, Wilson-Storey D. Sinus histiocytosis with massive lymphadenopathy (Rosai-Dorfman disease). Histopathology 1989; 14: 91–99.

268a. Foucar E, Rosai J, Dorfman R. Sinus histiocytosis with massive lymphadenopathy (Rosai-Dorfman disease): review of the entity. Semin Diagn Pathol 1990; 7: 19–73.

269. Olsen EA, Crawford JR, Vollmer RT. Sinus histiocytosis with massive lymphadenopathy. Case report and review of a multisystemic disease with cutaneous infiltrates. J Am Acad Dermatol 1988; 18: 1322–1332.

270. Foucar E, Rosai J, Dorfman RF. Sinus histiocytosis with massive lymphadenopathy. Current status and future directions. Arch Dermatol 1988; 124: 1211–1214.

271. Lampert F, Lennert K. Sinus histiocytosis with massive lymphadenopathy. Fifteen new cases. Cancer 1976; 37: 783–789.

272. Penneys NS, Ahn YS, McKinney EC et al. Sinus histiocytosis with massive lymphadenopathy. Cancer 1982; 49: 1994–1998.

273. Suster S, Cartagena N, Cabello-Inchausti B, Robinson MJ. Histiocytic lymphophagocytic panniculitis. An unusual extranodal presentation of sinus histiocytosis with massive lymphadenopathy (Rosai-Dorfman disease). Arch Dermatol 1988; 124: 1246–1249.

274. Buchino JJ, Byrd RP, Kmetz DR. Disseminated sinus histiocytosis with massive lymphadenopathy. Arch Pathol Lab Med 1982; 106: 13–16.

275. Foucar E, Rosai J, Dorfman RF, Eyman JM. Immunologic abnormalities and their significance in sinus histiocytosis with massive lymphadenopathy. Am J Clin Pathol 1984; 82: 515–525.

276. Foucar E, Rosai J, Dorfman RF. Sinus histiocytosis with massive lymphadenopathy. An analysis of 14 deaths occurring in a patient registry. Cancer 1984; 54: 1834–1840.

277. Bonetti F, Chilosi M, Menestrina F et al. Immunohistological analysis of Rosai-Dorfman histiocytosis. A disease of S-100 + CD1-histiocytes. Virchows Arch (A) 1987; 411: 129–135.

278. Miettinen M, Paljakka P, Haveri P, Saxen E. Sinus histiocytosis with massive lymphadenopathy. A nodal and extranodal proliferation of S-100 protein positive histiocytes? Am J Clin Pathol 1987; 88: 270–277.

279. Lopez P, Estes ML. Immunohistochemical characterization of the histiocytes in sinus histiocytosis with massive lymphadenopathy: analysis of an extranodal case. Hum Pathol 1989; 20: 711–715.

280. Hibi S, Esumi N, Todo S, Imashuku S. Malignant histiocytosis in childhood: Clinical, cytochemical, and immunohistochemical studies of seven cases. Hum Pathol 1988; 19: 713–719.

281. Ducatman BS, Wick MR, Morgan TW et al. Malignant histiocytosis: A clinical, histologic, and immunohistochemical study of 20 cases. Hum Pathol 1984; 15: 368–377.

282. Dodd HJ, Stansfeld AG, Chambers TJ. Cutaneous malignant histiocytosis — a clinicopathological review of five cases. Br J Dermatol 1985; 113: 455–461.

283. Kojiro M, Isomura T, Ohtsu N et al. Atypical malignant histiocytosis. Its appearance as a single meningeal tumor or as multiple skin tumors. Arch Pathol Lab Med 1981; 105: 317–321.

284. Wick MR, Sanchez NP, Crotty CP, Winkelmann RK. Cutaneous malignant histiocytosis: A clinical and histopathologic study of eight cases, with immunohistochemical analysis. J Am Acad Dermatol 1983; 8: 50–62.

285. Abele DC, Griffin TB. Histiocytic medullary reticulosis. Report of two cases and review of the literature. Arch Dermatol 1972; 106: 319–329.

286. Marshall ME, Farmer ER, Trump DL. Cutaneous involvement in malignant histiocytosis. Case report and review of the literature. Arch Dermatol 1981; 117: 278–281.

287. Zucker JM, Caillaux JM, Vanel D, Gerard-Marchant R. Malignant histiocytosis in childhood. Clinical study

and therapeutic results in 22 cases. Cancer 1980; 45: 2821–2829.

288. Jurco S III, Starling K, Hawkins EP. Malignant histiocytosis in childhood: Morphologic considerations. Hum Pathol 1983; 14: 1059–1065.

289. Esumi N, Hashida T, Matsumura T et al. Malignant histiocytosis in childhood. Clinical features and therapeutic results by combination chemotherapy. Am J Pediatr Hematol Oncol 1986; 8: 300–307.

290. Watanabe S, Nakajima T, Shimosato Y et al. Malignant histiocytosis and Letterer-Siwe disease. Neoplasms of T-zone histiocyte with S 100 protein. Cancer 1983; 51: 1412–1424.

291. Ishii E, Hara T, Okamura J et al. Malignant histiocytosis in infants: surface marker analysis of malignant cells in two cases. Med Pediatr Oncol 1987; 15: 102–108.

292. Pinol-Aguade J, Ferrando J, Tomas JM et al. Necropsy and ultrastructural findings in histiocytic medullary reticulosis. Br J Dermatol 1976; 95: 35–44.

293. Morgan NE, Fretzin D, Variakojis D, Caro WA. Clinical and pathologic cutaneous manifestations of malignant histiocytosis. Arch Dermatol 1983; 119: 367–372.

294. Warnke RA, Kim H, Dorfman RF. Malignant histiocytosis (histiocytic medullary reticulosis). I. Clinicopathologic study of 29 cases. Cancer 1975; 35: 215–230.

295. Barron DR, Davis BR, Pomeranz JR et al. Cytophagic histiocytic panniculitis. A variant of malignant histiocytosis. Cancer 1985; 55: 2538–2542.

296. Nemes Z, Thomazy V. Diagnostic significance of histiocyte-related markers in malignant histiocytosis and true histiocytic lymphoma. Cancer 1988; 62: 1970–1980.

297. Tubbs RR, Sheibani K, Sebek BA, Savage RA. Malignant histiocytosis. Ultrastructural and immunocytochemical characterization. Arch Pathol Lab Med 1980; 104: 26–29.

298. Huhn D, Meister P. Malignant histiocytosis. Morphologic and cytochemical findings. Cancer 1978; 42: 1341–1349.

299. Rausch PG, Herion JC, Carney CN, Weinstein P. Malignant histiocytosis. A cytochemical and electron microscopic study of an unusual case. Cancer 1979; 44: 2158–2164.

300. Risdall RJ, Brunning RD, Sibley RK et al. Malignant histiocytosis. A light- and electron-microscopic and histochemical study. Am J Surg Pathol 1980; 4: 439–450.

Xanthomatous infiltrates

301. Parker F. Xanthomas and hyperlipidemias. J Am Acad Dermatol 1985; 13: 1–30.

302. Polano MK. Xanthomatosis and hyperlipoproteinemia. A review. Dermatologica 1974; 149: 1–9.

303. Cruz PD Jr, East C, Bergstresser PR. Dermal, subcutaneous, and tendon xanthomas: Diagnostic markers for specific lipoprotein disorders. J Am Acad Dermatol 1988; 19: 95–111.

304. Hall-Smith P. Unusual facial xanthoma. Clin Exp Dermatol 1978; 3: 451–453.

305. Smoller BR, McNutt NS, Kline M et al. Xanthomatous infiltrate of the face. J Cutan Pathol 1989; 16: 277–280.

306. Vail JT Jr, Adler KR, Rothenberg J. Cutaneous xanthomas associated with chronic myelomonocytic leukemia. Arch Dermatol 1985; 121: 1318–1320.

307. Caputo R, Ermacora E, Gelmetti C, Gianni E. Fatal nodular xanthomatosis in an infant. Pediatr Dermatol 1987; 4: 242–246.

308. Archer CB, Sharvill DE, Smith NP. Normolipemic subcutaneous xanthomatosis. J Cutan Pathol 1988; 15: 293 (abstract).

309. Winkelmann RK, Oliver GF. Subcutaneous xanthogranulomatosis: An inflammatory non-X histiocytic syndrome (subcutaneous xanthomatosis). J Am Acad Dermatol 1989; 21: 924–929.

310. Fleischmajer R, Schaefer EJ, Gal AE et al. Normolipemic subcutaneous xanthomatosis. Am J Med 1983; 75: 1065–1070.

310a. Archer CB, Sharvill DE, Smith NP. Subcutaneous xanthomatosis. Br J Dermatol 1990; 123: 107–112.

310b. Bork K, Gabbert H, Knop J. Fat-storing hamartoma of dermal dendrocytes. Clinical, histologic, and ultrastructural study. Arch Dermatol 1990; 126: 794–796.

311. Parker F. Normocholesterolemic xanthomatosis. Arch Dermatol 1986; 122: 1253–1257.

312. James MP, Warin AP. Plane xanthoma developing in photosensitive eczema. Clin Exp Dermatol 1978; 3: 307–314.

313. Walker AE, Sneddon IB. Skin xanthoma following erythroderma. Br J Dermatol 1968; 80: 580–587.

314. Berger BW, Kantor I, Maier HS. Xanthomatosis and lymphedema. Arch Dermatol 1972; 105: 730–733.

315. Rosen T. Dystrophic xanthomatosis in mycosis fungoides. Arch Dermatol 1978; 114: 102–103.

316. McCradden ME, Glick AD, King LE Jr. Mycosis fungoides associated with dystrophic xanthomatosis. Arch Dermatol 1987; 123: 91–94.

317. Brunzell JD, Bierman EL. Chylomicronemia syndrome. Med Clin North Am 1982; 66: 455–468.

318. Vermeer BJ, Van Gent CM, Goslings B, Polano MK. Xanthomatosis and other clinical findings in patients with elevated levels of very low density lipoproteins. Br J Dermatol 1979; 100: 657–666.

319. Borrie P, Slack J. A clinical syndrome characteristic of primary Type IV-V hyperlipoproteinaemia. Br J Dermatol 1974; 90: 245–253.

320. Caputo R, Monti M, Berti E, Gasparini G. Normolipemic eruptive cutaneous xanthomatosis. Arch Dermatol 1986; 122: 1294–1297.

321. Teltscher J, Silverman RA, Stock J. Eruptive xanthomas in a child with the nephrotic syndrome. J Am Acad Dermatol 1989; 21: 1147–1149.

322. Barr RJ, Fujita WH, Graham JH. Eruptive xanthomas associated with intravenous miconazole therapy. Arch Dermatol 1978; 114: 1544–1545.

323. Dicken CH, Connolly SM. Eruptive xanthomas associated with isotretinoin (13-cis-retinoic acid). Arch Dermatol 1980; 116: 951–952.

324. Cooper PH. Eruptive xanthoma: a microscopic simulant of granuloma annulare. J Cutan Pathol 1986; 13: 207–215.

325. Archer CB, MacDonald DM. Eruptive xanthomata in type V hyperlipoproteinaemia associated with diabetes mellitus. Clin Exp Dermatol 1984; 9: 312–316.

326. Poomeechaiwong S, Golitz LE, Brownstein MH. Eruptive xanthomas: evaluation of nineteen cases by polarized light microscopy. J Cutan Pathol 1988; 15: 338 (abstract).
327. Weston CFM, Burton JL. Xanthomas in the Watson-Alagille syndrome. J Am Acad Dermatol 1987; 16: 1117–1121.
328. Fleischmajer R, Tint GS, Bennett HD. Normolipemic tendon and tuberous xanthomas. J Am Acad Dermatol 1981; 5: 290–296.
329. Nakayama H, Mihara M, Shimao S. Perineural xanthoma. Br J Dermatol 1986; 115: 715–720.
330. Vega GL, Illingworth R, Grundy SM et al. Normocholesterolemic tendon xanthomatosis with overproduction of apolipoprotein B. Metabolism 1983; 32: 118–125.
331. Elias P, Goldsmith LA. Intertriginous xanthomata in type 2 hyperbetalipoproteinemia. Arch Dermatol 1973; 107: 761–762.
332. Friedman SJ, Martin TW. Xanthoma striatum palmare associated with multiple myeloma. J Am Acad Dermatol 1987; 16: 1272–1274.
333. Polano MK, Baes H, Hulsmans HAM et al. Xanthomata in primary hyperlipoproteinemia. Arch Dermatol 1969; 100: 387–399.
334. Gomez JA, Gonzalez MJ, de Moragas JM et al. Apolipoprotein E phenotypes, lipoprotein composition, and xanthelasmas. Arch Dermatol 1988; 124: 1230–1234.
335. Abrams JJ, Grundy SM, Kane JP, Chang C-M. Normocholesterolemic dysbetalipoproteinemia with xanthomatosis. Metabolism 1979; 28: 113–124.
336. Weber G, Pilgrim M. Contribution to the knowledge of normolipaemic plane xanthomatosis. Br J Dermatol 1974; 90: 465–469.
337. Fleischmajer R, Hyman AB, Weidman AI. Normolipemic plane xanthomas. Arch Dermatol 1964; 89: 319–323.
338. Bovenmyer DA, Caplan RM. Generalized normolipemic plane xanthoma. Report of a case associated with Ehlers-Danlos syndrome. Arch Dermatol 1963; 87: 158–163.
339. Russell Jones R, Baughan ASJ, Cream JJ et al. Complement abnormalities in diffuse plane xanthomatosis with paraproteinaemia. Br J Dermatol 1979; 101: 711–716.
340. Lynch PJ, Winkelmann RK. Generalized plane xanthoma and systemic disease. Arch Dermatol 1966; 93: 639–646.
341. Marien KJC, Smeenk G. Plane xanthomata associated with multiple myeloma and hyperlipoproteinaemia. Br J Dermatol 1975; 93: 407–415.
342. Taylor JS, Lewis LA, Battle JD Jr et al. Plane xanthoma and multiple myeloma with lipoprotein-paraprotein complexing. Arch Dermatol 1978; 114: 425–431.
343. Moschella SL. Plane xanthomatosis associated with myelomatosis. Arch Dermatol 1970; 101: 683–687.
344. Neville B. The verruciform xanthoma. A review and report of eight new cases. Am J Dermatopathol 1986; 8: 247–253.
345. Buchner A, Hansen S, Merrell PW. Verruciform xanthoma of the oral mucosa. Arch Dermatol 1981; 117: 563–565.
346. Santa Cruz DJ, Martin SA. Verruciform xanthoma of the vulva. Report of two cases. Am J Clin Pathol 1979; 71: 224–228.
347. Griffel B, Cordoba M. Verruciform xanthoma in the anal region. Am J Proctol 1980; 32 (4): 24–25.
348. Kimura S. Verruciform xanthoma of the scrotum. Arch Dermatol 1984; 120: 1378–1379.
349. Al-Nafussi AI, Azzopardi JG, Salm R. Verruciform xanthoma of the skin. Histopathology 1985; 9: 245–252.
350. Kraemer BB, Schmidt WA, Foucar E, Rosen T. Verruciform xanthoma of the penis. Arch Dermatol 1981; 117: 516–518.
351. Ronan SG, Bolano J, Manaligod JR. Verruciform xanthoma of penis. Light and electron-microscopic study. Urology 1984; 23: 600–603.
352. Duray PH, Johnston YE. Verruciform xanthoma of the nose in an elderly male. Am J Dermatopathol 1986; 8: 237–240.
353. Cooper TW, Santa Cruz DJ, Bauer EA. Verruciform xanthoma. Occurrence in eroded skin in a patient with recessive dystrophic epidermolysis bullosa. J Am Acad Dermatol 1983; 8: 463–467.
354. Mountcastle EA, Lupton GP. Verruciform xanthomas of the digits. J Am Acad Dermatol 1989; 20: 313–317.
355. Grosshans E, Laplanche G. Verruciform xanthoma or xanthomatous transformation of inflammatory epidermal nevus. J Cutan Pathol 1981; 8: 382–384.
356. Palestine RF, Winkelmann RK. Verruciform xanthoma in an epithelial nevus. Arch Dermatol 1982; 118: 686–691.
357. Barr RJ, Plank CJ. Verruciform xanthoma of the skin. J Cutan Pathol 1980; 7: 422–428.
358. Chyu J, Medenica M, Whitney DH. Verruciform xanthoma of the lower extremity — report of a case and review of literature. J Am Acad Dermatol 1987; 17: 695–698.
359. Travis WD, Davis GE, Tsokos M et al. Multifocal verruciform xanthoma of the upper aerodigestive tract in a child with a systemic lipid storage disease. Am J Surg Pathol 1989; 13: 309–316.
360. Meyrick Thomas RH, Miller NE, Rowland Payne CME et al. Papular xanthoma associated with primary dysbetalipoproteinaemia. J R Soc Med 1982; 75: 906–908.
360a. Caputo R, Gianni E, Imondi D et al. Papular xanthoma in children. J Am Acad Dermatol 1990; 22: 1052–1056.
361. Sanchez RL, Raimer SS, Peltier F. Papular xanthoma. A clinical, histologic, and ultrastructural study. Arch Dermatol 1985; 121: 626–631.

Langerhans cell infiltrates

362. Breathnach SM. The Langerhans cell. Br J Dermatol 1988; 119: 463–469.
363. Dezutter-Dambuant C. Role of Langerhans cells in cutaneous immunologic processes. Semin Dermatol 1988; 7: 163–170.
364. Hui PK, Feller AC, Kaiserling E et al. Skin tumors of T accessory cells (interdigitating reticulum cells) with high content of T lymphocytes. Am J Dermatopathol 1987; 9: 129–137.
365. Kolde G, Brocker E-B. Multiple skin tumors of indeterminate cells in an adult. J Am Acad Dermatol 1986; 15: 591–597.

366. Wood GS, Hu C-H, Beckstead JH et al. The indeterminate cell proliferative disorder: report of a case manifesting as an unusual cutaneous histiocytosis. J Dermatol Surg Oncol 1985; 11: 1111–1119.

367. Fowler JF, Callen JP, Hodge SJ, Verdi G. Cutaneous non-X histiocytosis: Clinical and histologic features and response to dermabrasion. J Am Acad Dermatol 1985; 13: 645–649.

368. Miracco C, Raffaelli M, Margherita de Santi M et al. Solitary cutaneous reticulum cell tumor. Enzyme-immunohistochemical and electron-microscopic analogies with IDRC sarcoma. Am J Dermatopathol 1988; 10: 47–53.

368a. Contreras F, Fonseca E, Gamallo C, Burgos E. Multiple self-healing indeterminate cell lesions of the skin in an adult. Am J Dermatopathol 1990; 12: 396–401.

369. Stingl G. New aspects of Langerhans' cell function. Int J Dermatol 1980; 19: 189–213.

370. Ishii E, Watanabe S. Biochemistry and biology of the Langerhans cell. Hematol Oncol Clin North Am 1987; 1: 99–118.

371. Thiers BH. The Langerhans cell. J Am Acad Dermatol 1982; 6: 519–522.

372. Horton JJ, Allen MH, MacDonald DM. An assessment of Langerhans cell quantification in tissue sections. J Am Acad Dermatol 1984; 11: 591–593.

373. Ashworth J, Turbitt ML, Mackie R. The distribution and quantification of the Langerhans cell in normal human epidermis. Clin Exp Dermatol 1986; 11: 153–158.

374. Writing group of the Histiocyte Society. Histiocytosis syndromes in children. Lancet 1987; 1: 208–209.

375. Kashihara-Sawami M, Horiguchi Y, Ikai K et al. Letterer-Siwe disease: Immunopathologic study with a new monoclonal antibody. J Am Acad Dermatol 1988; 18: 646–654.

376. Lee CW, Park MH, Lee H. Recurrent cutaneous Langerhans cell histiocytosis in infancy. Br J Dermatol 1988; 119: 259–265.

377. Lichtenstein L. Histiocytosis X. Arch Pathol 1953; 56: 84–102.

378. Osband ME, Pochedly C. Histiocytosis-X: an overview. Hematol Oncol Clin North Am 1987; 1: 1–7.

379. Osband ME. Histiocytosis X. Langerhans' cell histiocytosis. Hematol Oncol Clin North Am 1987; 1: 737–751.

380. Favara BE, Jaffe R. Pathology of Langerhans cell histiocytosis. Hematol Oncol Clin North Am 1987; 1: 75–97.

381. Bingham EA, Bridges JM, Kelly AMT et al. LettererSiwe disease: a study of thirteen cases over a 21-year period. Br J Dermatol 1982; 106: 205–209.

382. Cavender PA, Bennett RG. Perianal eosinophilic granuloma resembling condyloma latum. Pediatr Dermatol 1988; 5: 50–55.

383. Neumann C, Kolde G, Bonsmann G. Histiocytosis X in an elderly patient. Ultrastructure and immunocytochemistry after PUVA photochemotherapy. Br J Dermatol 1988; 119: 385–391.

384. Caputo R, Berti E, Monti M et al. Letterer-Siwe disease in an octogenarian. J Am Acad Dermatol 1984; 10: 226–233.

385. Feuerman EJ, Sandbank M. Histiocytosis X with skin lesions as the sole clinical expression. Acta Derm Venereol 1976; 56: 269–277.

386. Benisch B, Peison B, Carter H. Histiocytosis X of the skin in an elderly man. Am J Clin Pathol 1977; 67: 36–40.

387. Eady RAJ. Letterer-Siwe disease in an elderly patient: histological and ultrastructural findings. Clin Exp Dermatol 1979; 4: 413–420.

388. Novice FM, Collison DW, Kleinsmith DM et al. Letterer-Siwe disease in adults. Cancer 1989; 63: 166–174.

389. Claudy AL, Larbre B, Colomb M et al. Letterer-Siwe disease and subacute monocytic leukemia. J Am Acad Dermatol 1989; 21: 1105–1106.

389a. McLelland J, Chu AC. Multi-system Langerhans-cell histiocytosis in adults. Clin Exp Dermatol 1990; 15: 79–82.

390. Winkelmann RK. The skin in histiocytosis X. Mayo Clin Proc 1969; 44: 535–549.

391. Esterly NB, Maurer HS, Gonzalez-Crussi F. Histiocytosis X: A seven-year experience at a children's hospital. J Am Acad Dermatol 1985; 13: 481–496.

392. Zachary CB, MacDonald DM. Hand-Schüller-Christian disease with secondary cutaneous involvement. Clin Exp Dermatol 1983; 8: 177–183.

393. Fitzpatrick R, Rapaport MJ, Silva DG. Histiocytosis X. Arch Dermatol 1981; 117: 253–257.

394. Dolezal JF, Thomson ST. Hand-Schüller-Christian disease in a septuagenarian. Arch Dermatol 1978; 114: 85–87.

395. Hashimoto K, Takahashi S, Fligiel A, Savoy LB. Eosinophilic granuloma. Presence of OKT6-positive cells and good response to intralesional steroid. Arch Dermatol 1985; 121: 770–774.

396. Norris JFB, Marshall TL, Byrne JPH. Histiocytosis X in an adult mimicking pyoderma gangrenosum. Clin Exp Dermatol 1984; 9: 388–392.

397. Eng AM. Papular histiocytosis X. Am J Dermatopathol 1981; 3: 203–206.

398. Messenger GG, Kamei R, Honig PJ. Histiocytosis X resembling cherry angiomas. Pediatr Dermatol 1985; 3: 75–78.

399. Nagy-Vezekenyi K, Makai A, Ambro I, Nagy E. Histiocytosis X with unusual skin symptoms. Acta Derm Venereol 1981; 61: 447–451.

400. Vollum DI. Letterer-Siwe disease in the adult. Clin Exp Dermatol 1979; 4: 395–406.

401. Taieb A, de Mascarel A, Surleve-Bazeille JE et al. Solitary Langerhans cell histiocytoma. Arch Dermatol 1986; 122: 1033–1037.

402. Warner TFCS, Hafez GR. Langerhans' cell tumor of the eyelid. J Cutan Pathol 1982; 9: 417–422.

403. Wolfson SL, Botero F, Hurwitz S, Pearson HA. "Pure" cutaneous histiocytosis-X. Cancer 1981; 48: 2236–2238.

404. Schoeck VW, Peterson RDA, Good RA. Familial occurrence of Letterer-Siwe disease. Pediatrics 1963; 32: 1055–1063.

405. Greenberger JS, Crocker AC, Vawter G et al. Results of treatment of 127 patients with systemic histiocytosis (Letterer-Siwe syndrome, Schüller-Christian syndrome

and multifocal eosinophilic granuloma). Medicine (Baltimore) 1981; 60: 311–338.

406. Corbeel L, Eggermont E, Desmyter J et al. Spontaneous healing of Langerhans cell histiocytosis (histiocytosis X). Eur J Pediatr 1988; 148: 32–33.

407. Meenan FO, Cahalane SF. Spontaneous resolution of histiocytosis X. Report of a case. Arch Dermatol 1967; 96: 532–535.

408. Broadbent V, Davies EG, Heaf D et al. Spontaneous remission of multi-system histiocytosis X. Lancet 1984; 1: 253–254.

409. Freeman S. A benign form of Letterer-Siwe disease. Aust J Dermatol 1971; 12: 165–171.

410. Kragballe K, Zachariae H, Herlin T, Jensen J. Histiocytosis X — an immune deficiency disease? Studies on antibody-dependent monocyte-mediated cytotoxicity. Br J Dermatol 1981; 105: 13–18.

411. Risdall RJ, Dehner LP, Duray P et al. Histiocytosis X (Langerhans' cell histiocytosis). Arch Pathol Lab Med 1983; 107: 59–63.

412. McLelland J, Newton JA, Malone M et al. A flow cytometric study of Langerhans cell histiocytosis. Br J Dermatol 1989; 120: 485–491.

413. Harrist TJ, Bhan AK, Murphy GF et al. Histiocytosis-X. In situ characterization of cutaneous infiltrates with monoclonal antibodies. Am J Clin Pathol 1983; 79: 294–300.

414. Wells GC. The pathology of adult type Letterer-Siwe disease. Clin Exp Dermatol 1979; 4: 407–412.

415. Altman J, Winkelmann RK. Xanthomatous cutaneous lesions of histiocytosis X. Arch Dermatol 1963; 87: 164–170.

416. Foucar E, Piette WW, Tse DT et al. Urticating histiocytosis: A mast cell-rich variant of histiocytosis X. J Am Acad Dermatol 1986; 14: 867–873.

417. Rowden G, Connelly EM, Winkelmann RK. Cutaneous histiocytosis X. The presence of S-100 protein and its use in diagnosis. Arch Dermatol 1983; 119: 553–559.

418. Iwatsuki K, Tsugiki M, Yoshizawa N et al. The effect of phototherapies on cutaneous lesions of histiocytosis X in the elderly. Cancer 1986; 57: 1931–1936.

418a. Rabkin MS, Kjeldsberg CR, Wittwer CT, Marty J. A comparison study of two methods of peanut agglutinin staining with S100 immunostaining in 29 cases of histiocytosis X (Langerhans' cell histiocytosis). Arch Pathol Lab Med 1990; 114: 511–515.

419. Groh V, Gadner H, Radaszkiewicz T et al. The phenotypic spectrum of histiocytosis X cells. J Invest Dermatol 1988; 90: 441–447.

420. Wakuya J. Immunohistochemical and ultrastructural studies on histiocytosis in children. Acta Pathol Jpn 1987; 37: 901–913.

421. Hashimoto K, Pritzker MS. Electron microscopic study of reticulohistiocytoma. An unusual case of congenital, self-healing reticulohistiocytosis. Arch Dermatol 1973; 107: 263–270.

422. Kanitakis J, Zambruno G, Schmitt D et al. Congenital self-healing histiocytosis (Hashimoto-Pritzker). An ultrastructural and immunohistochemical study. Cancer 1988; 61: 508–516.

423. Herman LE, Rothman KF, Harawi S, Gonzalez-Serva A. Congenital self-healing reticulohistiocytosis. A new entity in the differential diagnosis of neonatal papulovesicular eruptions. Arch Dermatol 1990; 126: 210–212.

424. Oranje AP, Vuzevski VD, de Groot R, Prins MEF. Congenital self-healing non-Langerhans cell histiocytosis. Eur J Pediatr 1988; 148: 29–31.

424a. Whitehead B, Michaels M, Sahni R et al. Congenital self-healing Langerhans cell histiocytosis with persistent cellular immunological abnormalities. Br J Dermatol 1990; 122: 563–568.

425. Hashimoto K, Bale GF, Hawkins HK et al. Congenital self-healing reticulohistiocytosis (Hashimoto-Pritzker type). Int J Dermatol 1986; 25: 516–523.

426. Berger TG, Lane AT, Headington JT et al. A solitary variant of congenital self-healing reticulohistiocytosis: solitary Hashimoto-Pritzker disease. Pediatr Dermatol 1986; 3: 230–236.

427. Jordaan HF, Drusinsky SF. Congenital self-healing reticulohistiocytosis: report of a case. Pediatr Dermatol 1986; 3: 473–475.

428. Hashimoto K, Griffin D, Kohsbaki M. Self-healing reticulohistiocytosis: A clinical, histologic, and ultrastructural study of the fourth case in the literature. Cancer 1982; 49: 331–337.

429. Hawkins HK, Langston C. Self-healing reticulohistiocytosis with apparent visceral involvement. Lab Invest 1985; 52: 5P (abstract).

430. Kapila PK, Grant-Kels JM, Alfred C et al. Congenital, spontaneously regressing histiocytosis: case report and review of the literature. Pediatr Dermatol 1985; 2: 312–317.

431. Bonifazi E, Caputo R, Ceci A, Meneghini C. Congenital self-healing histiocytosis. Clinical, histologic, and ultrastructural study. Arch Dermatol 1982; 118: 267–272.

432. Timpatanapong P, Rochanawutanon M, Siripoonya P, Nitidandhaprabhas P. Congenital self-healing reticulohistiocytosis: report of a patient with a strikingly large tumor mass. Pediatr Dermatol 1989; 6: 28–32.

433. Hashimoto K, Takahashi S, Lee RG, Krull EA. Congenital self-healing reticulohistiocytosis. Report of the seventh case with histochemical and ultrastructural studies. J Am Acad Dermatol 1984; 11: 447–454.

Lymphocytic infiltrates

434. Holborow EJ, Papamichail M. The lymphoid system and lymphocyte subpopulations. In: Holborow EJ, Reeves WG, eds. Immunology in medicine. 2nd ed. London: Grune & Stratton, 1983: 17–34.

435. Bos JD, Zonneveld I, Das PK et al. The skin immune system (SIS): distribution and immunophenotype of lymphocyte subpopulations in normal human skin. J Invest Dermatol 1987; 88: 569–573.

436. Burg G, Braun-Falco O. Cutaneous lymphomas, pseudolymphomas, and related disorders. Berlin: Springer-Verlag, 1983; 3–5.

437. Knapp W, Rieber P, Dörken B, et al. Towards a better definition of human leucocyte surface molecules. Immunol Today 1989; 10: 253–258.

438. West KP, Warford A, Fray L, Allen M. The demonstration of B-cell, T-cell and myeloid antigens in paraffin sections. J Pathol 1986; 150: 89–101.

439. Clark EA, Ledbetter JA. Leukocyte cell surface enzymology: CD45 (LCA, T200) is a protein tyrosine phosphatase. Immunol Today 1989; 10: 225–228.

440. Samelson LE. Lymphocyte activation. Current Opinion in Immunology 1989; 2: 210–214.

441. MacDonald HR. T cell repertoire selection during development. Current Opinion in Immunology 1989; 2: 199–203.

442. Kyewski B. Editorial. A closer look at T cell differentiation. Lab Invest 1988; 59: 561–563.

443. Hackett CJ. Cell-mediated processing and presentation of T cell antigenic determinants. Current Opinion in Immunology 1989; 2: 117–122.

444. Acuto O, Reinherz EL. The human T-cell receptor. Structure and function. N Engl J Med 1985; 312: 1100–1111.

445. Haynes BF, Denning SM, Singer KH, Kurtzberg J. Ontogeny of T-cell precursors: a model for the initial stages of T-cell development. Immunol Today 1989; 10: 87–92.

446. Otten G. Antigen processing and presentation. Current Opinion in Immunology 1989; 2: 204–209.

447. Janeway CA Jr. The role of CD4 in T-cell activation: accessory molecule or co-receptor? Immunol Today 1989; 10: 234–238.

448. Mustelin T, Altman A. Do CD4 and CD8 control T-cell activation via a specific tyrosine protein kinase? Immunol Today 1989; 10: 189–192.

449. Lanzavecchia A. Is suppression a function of class II-restricted cytotoxic T cells? Immunol Today 1989; 10: 157–159.

450. Wagner H, Eichmann K. T-cell receptors and cellular interactions. Immunol Today 1989; 10: S25–S27.

451. Miller JFAP. Immune response. Editorial overview. Current Opinion in Immunology 1989; 2: 187–188.

452. Danska JS. The T cell receptor: structure, molecular diversity and somatic localization. Current Opinion in Immunology 1989; 2: 81–86.

453. Kelso A. Cytokines: structure, function and synthesis. Current Opinion in Immunology 1989; 2: 215–225.

454. Balkwill FR, Burke F. The cytokine network. Immunol Today 1989; 10: 299–304.

455. Dorshkind K. Hemopoietic stem cells and B-lymphocyte differentiation. Immunol Today 1989; 10: 399–401.

456. Hardy RR. B cell ontogeny and B cell subsets. Current Opinion in Immunology 1989; 2: 189–198.

457. Smolle J, Torne R, Soyer HP, Kerl H. Immunohistochemical classification of cutaneous pseudolymphomas: delineation of distinct patterns. J Cutan Pathol 1990; 17: 149–159.

458. van der Putte SCJ, Toonstra J, Felten PC, van Vloten WA. Solitary nonepidermotropic T cell pseudolymphoma of the skin. J Am Acad Dermatol 1986; 14: 444–453.

459. van Hale HM, Winkelmann RK. Nodular lymphoid disease of the head and neck: Lymphocytoma cutis, benign lymphocytic infiltrate of Jessner, and their distinction from malignant lymphoma. J Am Acad Dermatol 1985; 12: 455–461.

460. Kardaun SH, Scheffer E, Vermeer BJ. Drug-induced pseudolymphomatous skin reactions. Br J Dermatol 1988; 118: 545–552.

461. Schreiber MM, McGregor JG. Pseudolymphoma syndrome. A sensitivity to anticonvulsant drugs. Arch Dermatol 1968; 97: 297–300.

462. Henderson CA, Shamy HK. Atenolol-induced pseudolymphoma. Clin Exp Dermatol 1990; 15: 119–120.

463. Iwatsuki K, Tagami H, Moriguchi T, Yamada M. Lymphadenoid structure induced by gold hypersensitivity. Arch Dermatol 1982; 118: 608–611.

464. Iwatsuki K, Yamada M, Takigawa M et al. Benign lymphoplasia of the earlobes induced by gold earrings: Immunohistologic study on the cellular infiltrates. J Am Acad Dermatol 1987; 16: 83–88.

465. Comaish S. A case of contact hypersensitivity to metallic gold. Arch Dermatol 1969; 99: 720–723.

466. Rywlin AM. Non-Hodgkin's malignant lymphomas. Brief historical review and simple unifying classification. Am J Dermatopathol 1980; 2: 17–25.

467. Garvin AJ. The histopathologic classification of cutaneous lymphomas. Dermatol Clin 1985; 3: 587–591.

468. Mukai K, Sato Y, Watanabe S et al. Non-Hodgkin's lymphoma of the skin excluding mycosis fungoides and cutaneous involvement of adult T-cell leukemia/lymphoma. J Cutan Pathol 1988; 15: 193–200.

469. Ralfkiaer E, Saati TA, Bosq J et al. Immunocytochemical characterisation of cutaneous lymphomas other than mycosis fungoides. J Clin Pathol 1986; 39: 553–563.

470. McNutt NS, Balin AK, Placek E. B-cell lymphoma. J Dermatol Surg Oncol 1989; 15: 716–720.

471. Braun-Falco O, Burg G, Schmoeckel C. Recent advances in the understanding of cutaneous lymphoma. Clin Exp Dermatol 1981; 6: 89–109.

472. Wood GS, Burke JS, Horning S et al. The immunologic and clinicopathologic heterogeneity of cutaneous lymphomas other than mycosis fungoides. Blood 1983; 62: 464–472.

473. LeBoit PE. Cutaneous lymphomas and their histopathologic imitators. Semin Dermatol 1986; 5: 322–333.

474. Ashinoff R, Buchness MR, Lim HW. Lymphoma in a black patient with actinic reticuloid treated with PUVA: Possible etiologic considerations. J Am Acad Dermatol 1989; 21: 1134–1137.

475. Lange-Vejlsgaard G, Ralfkiaer E, Larsen JK et al. Fatal cutaneous T cell lymphoma in a child with atopic dermatitis. J Am Acad Dermatol 1989; 20: 954–958.

476. Payne CM, Spier CM, Grogan TM et al. Nuclear contour irregularity correlates with Leu-9-, Leu-8- cells in benign lymphoid infiltrates of skin. Am J Dermatopathol 1988; 10: 377–389.

477. Burke JS, Hoppe RT, Cibull ML, Dorfman RF. Cutaneous malignant lymphoma. A pathologic study of 50 cases with clinical analysis of 37. Cancer 1981; 47: 300–310.

478. Burke JS. Malignant lymphomas of the skin: their differentiation from lymphoid and nonlymphoid cutaneous infiltrates that simulate lymphoma. Semin Diagn Pathol 1985; 2: 169–182.

479. Saxe N, Kahn LB, King H. Lymphoma of the skin. A comparative clinico-pathologic study of 50 cases including mycosis fungoides and primary and secondary cutaneous lymphoma. J Cutan Pathol 1977; 4: 111–122.

480. Wirt DP, Grogan TM, Jolley CS et al. The immunoarchitecture of cutaneous pseudolymphoma. Hum Pathol 1985; 6: 492–510.

481. Bafverstedt B. Lymphadenosis benigna cutis. Acta Derm Venereol 1968; 48: 1–6.

482. Mach KW, Wilgram GF. Characteristic histopathology of cutaneous lymphoplasia (lymphocytoma). Arch Dermatol 1966; 94: 26–32.

483. Clark WH, Mihm MC Jr, Reed RJ, Ainsworth AM. The lymphocytic infiltrates of the skin. Hum Pathol 1974; 5: 25–43.

484. Caro WA, Helwig EB. Cutaneous lymphoid hyperplasia. Cancer 1969; 24: 487–502.

485. Brodell RT, Santa Cruz DJ. Cutaneous pseudolymphomas. Dermatol Clin 1985; 3: 719–734.

486. Cerio R, MacDonald DM. Benign cutaneous lymphoid infiltrates. J Cutan Pathol 1985; 12: 442–452.

487. Ralfkaier E, Lange Wantzin G, Mason DY et al. Characterization of benign cutaneous lymphocytic infiltrates by monoclonal antibodies. Br J Dermatol 1984; 111: 635–645.

488. Lange Wantzin G, Hou-Jensen K, Nielsen M et al. Cutaneous lymphocytomas: clinical and histological aspects. Acta Derm Venereol 1982; 62: 119–124.

489. Torne R, Roura M, Umbert P. Generalized cutaneous B-cell pseudolymphoma. Report of a case studied by immunohistochemistry. Am J Dermatopathol 1989; 11: 544–548.

490. Shelley WB, Wood MG, Wilson JF, Goodman R. Premalignant lymphoid hyperplasia preceding and coexisting with malignant lymphoma in the skin. Arch Dermatol 1981; 117: 500–503.

491. Halevy S, Sandbank M. Transformation of lymphocytoma cutis into a malignant lymphoma in association with the sign of Leser-Trélat. Acta Derm Venereol 1987; 67: 172–175.

492. Lange Wantzin G, Thomsen K, Ralfkiaer E. Evolution of cutaneous lymphoid hyperplasia to cutaneous T-cell lymphoma. Clin Exp Dermatol 1988; 13: 309–313.

493. Petros H, Macmillan AL. Allergic contact sensitivity to gold with unusual features. Br J Dermatol 1973; 88: 505–508.

494. Blumental G, Okun MR, Ponitch JA. Pseudolymphomatous reaction to tattoos. Report of three cases. J Am Acad Dermatol 1982; 6: 485–488.

495. Zinberg M, Heilman E, Glickman F. Cutaneous pseudolymphoma resulting from a tattoo. J Dermatol Surg Oncol 1982; 8: 955–958.

496. Rijlaarsdam JU, Bruynzeel DP, Vos W et al. Immunohistochemical studies of lymphadenosis benigna cutis occurring in a tattoo. Am J Dermatopathol 1988; 10: 518–523.

497. Adams JD. Localized cutaneous pseudolymphoma associated with phenytoin therapy: a case report. Australas J Dermatol 1981; 22: 28–29.

498. Duray PH, Luger S. Cutaneous manifestations of Lyme disease — 1988 update. J Cutan Pathol 1988; 15: 304 (abstract).

499. Medeiros LJ, Picker LJ, Abel EA et al. Cutaneous lymphoid hyperplasia. Immunologic characteristics and assessment of criteria recently proposed as diagnostic of malignant lymphoma. J Am Acad Dermatol 1989; 21: 929–942.

500. Cerroni L, Smolle J, Soyer HP et al. Immunophenotyping of cutaneous lymphoid infiltrates in frozen and paraffin-embedded tissue sections: A comparative study. J Am Acad Dermatol 1990; 22: 405–413.

501. Mach KW, Wilgram GF. Cutaneous lymphoplasia with giant follicles. Arch Dermatol 1966; 94: 749–756.

502. Duncan SC, Evans HL, Winkelmann RK. Large cell lymphocytoma. Arch Dermatol 1980; 116: 1142–1146.

503. Winkelmann RK, Banks PM. Paraffin section light-chain immunostaining of large-cell lymphocytoma. Acta Derm Venereol 1988; 68: 356–365.

504. Eckert F, Schmid U. Identification of plasmacytoid T cells in lymphoid hyperplasia of the skin. Arch Dermatol 1989; 125: 1518–1524.

505. Eckert F, Schmid U, Kaudewitz P et al. Follicular lymphoid hyperplasia of the skin with high content of Ki-1 positive lymphocytes. Am J Dermatopathol 1989; 11: 345–352.

506. Evans HL, Winkelmann RK, Banks PM. Differential diagnosis of malignant and benign cutaneous lymphoid infiltrates. A study of 57 cases in which malignant lymphoma had been diagnosed or suspected in the skin. Cancer 1979; 44: 699–717.

507. MacDonald DM. Histopathological differentiation of benign and malignant cutaneous lymphoid infiltrates. Br J Dermatol 1982; 107: 715–718.

508. Connors RC, Ackerman AB. Histologic pseudomalignancies of the skin. Arch Dermatol 1976; 112: 1767–1780.

509. Pierard GE, Pierard-Franchimont C. Pattern of distribution and intensity of lymphoblastogenesis as an aid to distinguishing pseudolymphomas from lymphomas. Br J Dermatol 1983; 109: 253–259.

510. Stolz W, Vogt T, Braun-Falco O et al. Differentiation between lymphomas and pseudolymphomas of the skin by computerized DNA-image cytometry. J Invest Dermatol 1990; 94: 254–260.

511. Bass J, Elgart G, Pomeranz J, Kish S. Progression of cutaneous lymphoid hyperplasia to cutaneous lymphoma: histopathology, immunohistochemistry, and gene rearrangement studies. J Cutan Pathol 1988; 15: 297 (abstract).

512. Jessner M, Kanof NB. Lymphocytic infiltration of the skin. Arch Dermatol 1953; 68: 447–449.

513. Calnan CD. Lymphocytic infiltration of the skin (Jessner). Br J Dermatol 1957; 69: 169–173.

514. Toonstra J, Wildschut A, Boer J et al. Jessner's lymphocytic infiltration of the skin. A clinical study of 100 patients. Arch Dermatol 1989; 125: 1525–1530.

515. Mullen RH, Jacobs AH. Jessner's lymphocytic infiltrate in two girls. Arch Dermatol 1988; 124: 1091–1093.

516. Konttinen YT, Reitamo S, Ranki A, Segerberg-Konttinen M. T lymphocytes and mononuclear phagocytes in the skin infiltrate of systemic and discoid lupus erythematosus and Jessner's lymphocytic infiltrate. Br J Dermatol 1981; 104: 141–145.

517. Willemze R, Dijkstra A, Meijer CJLM. Lymphocytic infiltration of the skin (Jessner): a T-cell lymphoproliferative disease. Br J Dermatol 1984; 110: 523–529.

518. Willemze R, Vermeer BJ, Meijer CJLM. Immunohistochemical studies in lymphocytic infiltration of the skin (Jessner) and discoid lupus erythematosus. A comparative study. J Am Acad Dermatol 1984; 11: 832–840.

519. Konttinen YT, Bergroth V, Johansson E et al. A long-

term clinicopathologic survey of patients with Jessner's lymphocytic infiltration of the skin. J Invest Dermatol 1987; 89: 205–208.

520. Cerio R, Oliver GF, Wilson Jones E, Winkelmann RK. The heterogeneity of Jessner's lymphocytic infiltration of the skin. J Am Acad Dermatol 1990; 23: 63–67.

521. Abele DC, Anders KH, Chandler FW. Benign lymphocytic infiltration (Jessner-Kanof): Another manifestation of borreliosis? J Am Acad Dermatol 1989; 21: 795–797.

522. Facchetti F, Boden G, de Wolf-Peeters C et al. Plasmacytoid monocytes in Jessner's lymphocytic infiltration of the skin. Am J Dermatopathol 1990; 12: 363–369.

523. Gottlieb B, Winkelmann RK. Lymphocytic infiltration of skin. Arch Dermatol 1962; 86: 626–633.

524. Ashworth J, Turbitt M, Mackie R. A comparison of the dermal lymphoid infiltrates in discoid lupus erythematosus and Jessner's lymphocytic infiltrate of the skin using the monoclonal antibody Leu 8. J Cutan Pathol 1987; 14: 198–201.

525. Rijlaarsdam JU, Nieboer C, de Vries E, Willemze R. Characterization of the dermal infiltrates in Jessner's lymphocytic infiltrate of the skin, polymorphous light eruption and cutaneous lupus erythematosus: differential diagnostic and pathogenetic aspects. J Cutan Pathol 1990; 17: 2–8.

526. Merot Y, French L, Saurat J-H. Leu 8-positive cells in discoid lupus erythematosus and Jessner-Kanof's lymphocytic infiltrate of the skin. J Cutan Pathol 1988; 15: 412–413.

527. Viljaranta S, Ranki A, Kariniemi A-L et al. Distribution of natural killer cells and lymphocyte subclasses in Jessner's lymphocytic infiltration of the skin and in cutaneous lesions of discoid and systemic lupus erythematosus. Br J Dermatol 1987; 116: 831–838.

528. Macaulay WL. Lymphomatoid papulosis. A continuing self-healing eruption, clinically benign — histologically malignant. Arch Dermatol 1968; 97: 23–30.

529. Macaulay WL. Lymphomatoid papulosis. Int J Dermatol 1978; 17: 204–212.

530. Macaulay WL. Lymphomatoid papulosis update. A historical perspective. Arch Dermatol 1989; 125: 1387–1389.

531. Willemze R. Lymphomatoid papulosis. Dermatol Clin 1985; 3: 735–757.

532. Wood GS, Strickler JG, Deneau DG et al. Lymphomatoid papulosis expresses immunophenotypes associated with T cell lymphoma but not inflammation. J Am Acad Dermatol 1986; 15: 444–458.

533. Sanchez NP, Pittelkow MR, Muller SA et al. The clinicopathologic spectrum of lymphomatoid papulosis: Study of 31 cases. J Am Acad Dermatol 1983; 8: 81–94.

534. Whittaker SJ, Russel Jones R, Spry CJF. Lymphomatoid papulosis and its relationship to 'idiopathic' hypereosinophilic syndrome. J Am Acad Dermatol 1988; 18: 339–344.

535. Madison JF, O'Keefe TE, Meier FA, Clendenning WE. Lymphomatoid papulosis terminating as cutaneous T cell lymphoma (mycosis fungoides). J Am Acad Dermatol 1983; 9: 743–747.

536. Scheen SR III, Doyle JA, Winkelmann RK. Lymphoma-associated papulosis: Lymphomatoid papulosis associated with lymphoma. J Am Acad Dermatol 1981; 4: 451–457.

537. Tucker WFG, Leonard JN, Smith N et al. Lymphomatoid paulosis progressing to immunoblastic lymphoma. Clin Exp Dermatol 1984; 9: 190–195.

538. Lange Wantzin G, Thomsen K, Brandrup F, Larsen JK. Lymphomatoid papulosis. Development into cutaneous T-cell lymphoma. Arch Dermatol 1985; 121: 792–794.

539. Espinoza CG, Erkman-Balis B, Fenske NA. Lymphomatoid papulosis: A premalignant T cell disorder. J Am Acad Dermatol 1985; 13: 736–743.

540. Harrington DS, Braddock SW, Blocher KS et al. Lymphomatoid papulosis and progression to T cell lymphoma: An immunophenotypic and genotypic analysis. J Am Acad Dermatol 1989; 21: 951–957.

541. Marques Pinto G, Goncalves L, Goncalves H et al. A case of lymphomatoid papulosis and Hodgkin's disease. J Am Acad Dermatol 1989; 21: 1051–1056.

542. Kardashian JL, Zackheim HS, Egbert BM. Lymphomatoid papulosis associated with plaque-stage and granulomatous mycosis fungoides. Arch Dermatol 1985; 121: 1175–1180.

543. Thomsen K, Wantzin GL. Lymphomatoid papulosis. A follow-up study of 30 patients. J Am Acad Dermatol 1987; 17: 632–636.

544. Weiss LM, Wood GS, Trela M et al. Clonal T-cell populations in lymphomatoid papulosis. N Engl J Med 1986; 315: 475–479.

545. Kadin M, Nasu K, Sako D et al. Lymphomatoid papulosis. A cutaneous proliferation of activated helper T cells expressing Hodgkin's disease-associated antigens. Am J Pathol 1985; 119: 315–325.

546. Kadin ME. Characteristic immunologic profile of large atypical cells in lymphomatoid papulosis. Arch Dermatol 1986; 122: 1388–1390.

547. Tokura Y, Takigawa M, Oku T, Yamada M. Lymphomatoid papulosis. Histologic and immunohistochemical studies in a patient with a scaly pigmented eruption. Arch Dermatol 1986; 122: 1400–1405.

548. el Azhary RA, Gibson LE, Gonchoroff NJ, Muller SA. Lymphomatoid papulosis: histologic review of 24 cases with immunophenotyping, DNA flow cytometry and gene rearrangement. J Cutan Pathol 1989; 16: 301 (abstract).

549. Matsuyoshi N, Horiguchi Y, Tanaka T et al. Lymphomatoid papulosis: ultrastructural, immunohistochemical and gene analytical studies. Br J Dermatol 1989; 121: 381–389.

550. Tanaka T, Takahashi K, Ideyama S et al. Demonstration of clonal proliferation of T lymphocytes in early neoplastic disease. J Am Acad Dermatol 1989; 21: 218–223.

551. Muller SA, Schulze TW Jr. Mucha-Habermann disease mistaken for reticulum cell sarcoma. Arch Dermatol 1971; 103: 423–427.

552. Valentino LA, Helwig EB. Lymphomatoid papulosis. Arch Pathol 1973; 96: 409–416.

553. Black MM. Lymphomatoid papulosis and pityriasis lichenoides: are they related? Br J Dermatol 1982; 106: 717–721.

554. Weinman VF, Ackerman AB. Lymphomatoid papulosis. A critical review and new findings. Am J Dermatopathol 1981; 3: 129–163.

555. Pierard GE, Ackerman AB, Lapiere CM. Follicular lymphomatoid papulosis. Am J Dermatopathol 1980; 2: 173–180.

556. Sexton FM, Maize JC. Follicular lymphomatoid papulosis. Am J Dermatopathol 1986; 8: 496–500.

557. Requena L, Sanchez M, Coca S, Sanchez Yus E. Follicular lymphomatoid papulosis. Am J Dermatopathol 1990; 12: 67–75.

558. Willemze R, Meyer CJLM, Van Vloten WA, Scheffer E. The clinical and histological spectrum of lymphomatoid papulosis. Br J Dermatol 1982; 107: 131–144.

559. Willemze R, Scheffer E, Ruiter DJ et al. Immunological, cytochemical and ultrastructural studies in lymphomatoid papulosis. Br J Dermatol 1983; 108: 381–394.

560. Willemze R, Scheffer E. Clinical and histologic differentiation between lymphomatoid papulosis and pityriasis lichenoides. J Am Acad Dermatol 1985; 13: 418–428.

561. McLeod WA, Winkelmann RK. Eosinophilic histiocytosis: A variant form of lymphomatoid papulosis or a disease sui generis? J Am Acad Dermatol 1985; 13: 952–958.

562. Tuneu A, Moreno A, Pujol RM, de Moragas JM. Eosinophilic histiocytosis. A subset of lymphomatoid papulosis. Dermatologica 1988; 176: 95–100.

563. Agnarsson BA, Kadin ME. Host response in lymphomatoid papulosis. Hum Pathol 1989; 20: 747–752.

564. Sina B, Burnett JW. Lymphomatoid papulosis. Case reports and literature review. Arch Dermatol 1983; 119: 189–197.

565. Horiguchi Y, Horiguchi M, Toda K-I et al. The ultrastructural observation of a case of lymphomatoid papulosis. Acta Derm Venereol 1984; 64: 308–315.

566. Jones RE Jr. Questions to the Editorial Board and other authorities. Am J Dermatopathol 1986; 8: 534–545.

567. Bluefarb SM. The clinical implications of parapsoriasis. Int J Dermatol 1980; 19: 556–557.

568. Lazar AP, Caro WA, Roenigk HH Jr, Pinski KS. Parapsoriasis and mycosis fungoides: The Northwestern University experience, 1970 to 1985. J Am Acad Dermatol 1989; 21: 919–923.

569. Lindae ML, Abel EA, Hoppe RT, Wood GS. Poikilodermatous mycosis fungoides and atrophic large-plaque parapsoriasis exhibit similar abnormalities of T-cell antigen expression. Arch Dermatol 1988; 124: 366–372.

570. Lambert WC, Everett MA. The nosology of parapsoriasis. J Am Acad Dermatol 1981; 5: 373–395.

571. Samman PD. The natural history of parapsoriasis en plaques (chronic superficial dermatitis) and prereticulotic poikiloderma. Br J Dermatol 1972; 87: 405–411.

572. Altman J. Parapsoriasis: a histopathologic review and classification. Semin Dermatol 1984; 3: 14–21.

573. Everett MA, Headington JT. Parapsoriasis. JCE Dermatology 1978; 17(12): 12–24.

574. McMillan EM, Wasik R, Martin D et al. Immuno-electron microscopy of "T" cells in large plaque parapsoriasis. J Cutan Pathol 1981; 8: 385–392.

575. Bani D, Pimpinelli N, Moretti S, Giannotti B. Langerhans cells and mycosis fungoides — a critical overview of their pathogenic role in the disease. Clin Exp Dermatol 1990; 15: 7–12.

576. Dosaka N, Tanaka T, Fujita M et al. Southern blot analysis of clonal rearrangements of T-cell receptor gene in plaque lesion of mycosis fungoides. J Invest Dermatol 1989; 93: 626–629.

577. Koch SE, Zackheim HS, Williams ML et al. Mycosis fungoides beginning in childhood and adolescence. J Am Acad Dermatol 1987; 17: 563–570.

578. Peters MS, Thibodeau SN, White JW Jr, Winkelmann RK. Mycosis fungoides of childhood and adolescents. J Am Acad Dermatol 1990; 22: 1011–1018.

579. Schwartz JG, Clark EGI. Fine-needle aspiration biopsy of mycosis fungoides presenting as an ulcerating breast mass. Arch Dermatol 1988; 124: 409–413.

580. Agnarsson BA, Vonderheid EC, Kadin ME. Cutaneous T cell lymphoma with suppressor/cytotoxic (CD8) phenotype: Identification of rapidly progressive and chronic subtypes. J Am Acad Dermatol 1990; 22: 569–577.

581. Grekin DA, Zackheim HS. Mycosis fungoides. Med Clin North Am 1980; 64: 1005–1016.

582. Lambert WC. Premycotic eruptions. Dermatol Clin 1985; 3: 629–645.

583. Brehmer-Andersson E. Mycosis fungoides and its relation to Sézary's syndrome, lymphomatoid papulosis, and primary cutaneous Hodgkin's disease. Acta Derm Venereol (Suppl) 1976; 75: 1–142.

584. Samman PD. Mycosis fungoides and other cutaneous reticuloses. Clin Exp Dermatol 1976; 1: 197–214.

585. Abel EA. Clinical features of cutaneous T-cell lymphoma. Dermatol Clin 1985; 3: 647–664.

586. Thiers BH. Controversies in mycosis fungoides. J Am Acad Dermatol 1982; 7: 1–16.

587. Rustin MHA, Griffiths M, Ridley CM. The immunopathology of hypopigmented mycosis fungoides. Clin Exp Dermatol 1986; 11: 332–339.

588. Smith NP, Samman PD. Mycosis fungoides presenting with areas of cutaneous hypopigmentation. Clin Exp Dermatol 1978; 3: 213–216.

589. Misch KJ, Maclennan KA, Marsden RA. Hypopigmented mycosis fungoides. Clin Exp Dermatol 1987; 12: 53–55.

590. Sigal M, Grossin M, Laroche L et al. Hypopigmented mycosis fungoides. Clin Exp Dermatol 1987; 12: 453–454.

591. Goldberg DJ, Schinella RS, Kechijian P. Hypopigmented mycosis fungoides. Speculations about the mechanism of hypopigmentation. Am J Dermatopathol 1986; 8: 326–330.

592. Zackheim HS. Cutaneous T-cell lymphomas. A review of the recent literature. Arch Dermatol 1981; 117: 295–304.

593. Roenigk HH Jr, Castrovinci AJ. Mycosis fungoides bullosa. Arch Dermatol 1971; 104: 402–406.

594. Kartsonis J, Brettschneider F, Weissmann A, Rosen L. Mycosis fungoides bullosa. Am J Dermatopathol 1990; 12: 76–80.

595. Price NM, Fuks ZY, Hoffman TE. Hyperkeratotic and

verrucous features of mycosis fungoides. Arch Dermatol 1977; 113: 57–60.

596. Willemze R, Scheffer E, van Vloten WA. Mycosis fungoides simulating acanthosis nigricans. Am J Dermatopathol 1985; 7: 365–371.

597. Oliver GF, Winkelmann RK. Unilesional mycosis fungoides: A distinct entity. J Am Acad Dermatol 1989; 20: 63–70.

598. Radeff B, Merot Y, Saurat J-H. Acquired epidermal cysts and mycosis fungoides. A possible pitfall in clinical staging. Am J Dermatopathol 1988; 10: 424–429.

599. Dalziel KL, Telfer NR, Dawber RPR. Nail dystrophy in cutaneous T-cell lymphoma. Br J Dermatol 1989; 120: 571–574.

600. Donald D, Green JA, White M. Mycosis fungoides associated with nodular sclerosing Hodgkin's disease: a case report. Cancer 1980; 46: 2505–2508.

601. Lofgren RK, Wiltsie JC, Winkelmann RK. Mycosis fungoides evolving to myelomonocytic leukemia. Arch Dermatol 1978; 114: 916–920.

602. Caya JG, Choi H, Tieu TM et al. Hodgkin's disease followed by mycosis fungoides in the same patient. Case report and literature review. Cancer 1984; 53: 463–467.

603. Olsen EA, Delzell E, Jegasothy BV. Second malignancies in cutaneous T cell lymphoma. J Am Acad Dermatol 1984; 10: 197–204.

604. Al-Rawi HA, Duff GW. Mycosis fungoides with squamous cell carcinoma. Clin Exp Dermatol 1979; 4: 353–355.

605. Abel EA, Sendagorta E, Hoppe RT. Cutaneous malignancies and metastatic squamous cell carcinoma following topical therapies for mycosis fungoides. J Am Acad Dermatol 1986; 14: 1029–1038.

606. Knobler RM, Edelson RL. Cutaneous T cell lymphoma. Med Clin North Am 1986; 70: 109–138.

607. Slater DN, Rooney N, Bleehen S, Hamed A. The lymph node in mycosis fungoides: a light and electron microscopy and immunohistological study supporting the Langerhans' cell-retrovirus hypothesis. Histopathology 1985; 9: 587–621.

608. Scheffer E, Meijer CJLM, van Vloten WA. Dermatopathic lymphadenopathy and lymph node involvement in mycosis fungoides. Cancer 1980; 45: 137–148.

609. Rappaport H, Thomas LB. Mycosis fungoides: the pathology of extracutaneous involvement. Cancer 1974; 34: 1198–1229.

610. Long JC, Mihm MC. Mycosis fungoides with extracutaneous dissemination: a distinct clinicopathologic entity. Cancer 1974; 34: 1745–1755.

611. Stein RS. Mycosis fungoides with pulmonary involvement. A complete remission. Arch Dermatol 1978; 114: 247–249.

612. Huberman MS, Bunn PA Jr, Matthews MJ et al. Hepatic involvement in the cutaneous T-cell lymphomas. Results of percutaneous biopsy and peritoneoscopy. Cancer 1980; 45: 1683–1688.

613. Camisa C, Goldstein A. Mycosis fungoides. Small-bowel involvement complicated by perforation and peritonitis. Arch Dermatol 1981; 117: 234–237.

614. Greer KE, Legum LL, Hess CE. Multiple osteolytic lesions in a patient with mycosis fungoides. Arch Dermatol 1977; 113: 1242–1244.

615. Lundberg WB, Cadman EC, Skeel RT. Leptomeningeal mycosis fungoides. Cancer 1976; 38: 2149–2153.

616. Zackheim HS, Lebo CF, Wasserstein P et al. Mycosis fungoides of the mastoid, middle ear, and CNS. Literature review of mycosis fungoides of the CNS. Arch Dermatol 1983; 119: 311–318.

617. Epstein EH Jr, Levin DL, Croft JD Jr, Lutzner MA. Mycosis fungoides. Survival, prognostic features, response to therapy, and autopsy findings. Medicine (Baltimore) 1972; 15: 61–72.

618. Weinstock MA, Horm JW. Population-based estimate of survival and determinants of prognosis in patients with mycosis fungoides. Cancer 1988; 62: 1658–1661.

619. Hamminga L, Hermans J, Noordijk EM et al. Cutaneous T-cell lymphoma: clinicopathological relationships, therapy and survival in ninety-two patients. Br J Dermatol 1982; 107: 145–156.

620. Green SB, Byar DP, Lamberg SI. Prognostic variables in mycosis fungoides. Cancer 1981; 47: 2671–2677.

621. Redmond WJ, Rahbari H. Mycosis fungoides: A retrospective study. J Am Acad Dermatol 1979; 1: 431–436.

622. Cohen SR, Stenn KS, Braverman IM, Beck GJ. Mycosis fungoides. Clinicopathologic relationships, survival, and therapy in 59 patients with observations on occupation as a new prognostic factor. Cancer 1980; 46: 2654–2666.

623. Sausville EA, Worsham GF, Matthews MJ et al. Histologic assessment of lymph nodes in mycosis fungoides/Sézary syndrome (cutaneous T-cell lymphoma): clinical correlations and prognostic import of a new classification system. Hum Pathol 1985; 16: 1098–1109.

624. Sausville EA, Eddy JL, Makuch RW et al. Histopathologic staging at initial diagnosis of mycosis fungoides and the Sézary syndrome. Definition of three distinct prognostic groups. Ann Intern Med 1988; 109: 372–382

625. Yamamura T, Aozasa K, Sano S. The cutaneous lymphomas with convoluted nucleus. Analysis of thirty-nine cases. J Am Acad Dermatol 1984; 10: 796–803.

626. Tan RS-H, Butterworth CM, McLaughlin H et al. Mycosis fungoides — a disease of antigen persistence. Br J Dermatol 1974; 91: 607–616.

627. Norris DA. The pathogenesis of mycosis fungoides. Clin Exp Dermatol 1981; 6: 77–87.

628. Tuyp E, Burgoyne A, Aitchison T, Mackie R. A case-control study of possible causative factors in mycosis fungoides. Arch Dermatol 1987; 123: 196–200.

629. Lange Wantzin G, Thomsen K, Nissen NI et al. Occurrence of human T cell lymphotropic virus (type 1) antibodies in cutaneous T cell lymphoma. J Am Acad Dermatol 1986; 15: 598–602.

630. Peterman A, Jerdan M, Staal S et al. Evidence for HTLV-1 associated with mycosis fungoides and B-cell chronic lymphocytic leukemia. Arch Dermatol 1986; 122: 568–571.

631. Yamada M, Takigawa M, Iwatsuki K, Inoue F. Adult T-cell leukemia/lymphoma and cutaneous T-cell lymphoma. Are they related? Int J Dermatol 1989; 28: 107–113.

632. Fine RM. HTLV-V: A new human retrovirus

associated with cutaneous T-cell lymphoma (mycosis fungoides). Int J Dermatol 1988; 27: 473–474.

633. Longacre TA, Foucar K, Koster F, Burgdorf W. Atypical cutaneous lymphoproliferative disorder resembling mycosis fungoides in AIDS. Am J Dermatopathol 1989; 11: 451–456.

634. Welykyj S, Gradini R, Nakao J, Massa M. Carbamazepine induced drug eruption mimicking mycosis fungoides. J Cutan Pathol 1988; 15: 350 (abstract).

635. Wolf R, Kahane E, Sandbank M. Mycosis fungoides-like lesions associated with phenytoin therapy. Arch Dermatol 1985; 121: 1181–1182.

636. Rosenthal CJ, Noguera CA, Coppola A, Kapelner SN. Pseudolymphoma with mycosis fungoides manifestations, hyperresponsiveness to diphenylhydantoin, and lymphocyte disregulation. Cancer 1982; 49: 2305–2314.

637. Nickoloff BJ. Light-microscopic assessment of 100 patients with patch/plaque-stage mycosis fungoides. Am J Dermatopathol 1988; 10: 469–477.

638. Sanchez JL, Ackerman AB. The patch stage of mycosis fungoides. Criteria for histologic diagnosis. Am J Dermatopathol 1979; 1: 5–26.

639. Eng AM, Blekys I, Worobec SM. Clinicopathologic correlations in Alibert-type mycosis fungoides. Arch Dermatol 1981; 117: 332–337.

640. Lefeber WP, Robinson JK, Clendenning WE et al. Attempts to enhance light microscopic diagnosis of cutaneous T-cell lymphoma (mycosis fungoides). Arch Dermatol 1981; 117: 408–411.

641. Mackie RM, Foulds IS, McMillan EM, Nelson HM. Histological changes observed in the skin of patients with mycosis fungoides receiving photochemotherapy. Clin Exp Dermatol 1980; 5: 405–413.

642. Everett MA. Early diagnosis of mycosis fungoides: vacuolar interface dermatitis. J Cutan Pathol 1985; 12: 271–278.

643. Kim SY. Follicular mycosis fungoides. Am J Dermatopathol 1985; 7: 300.

644. Nickoloff BJ. Epidermal mucinosis in mycosis fungoides. J Am Acad Dermatol 1986; 15: 83–86.

645. Ackerman AB, Breza TS, Capland L. Spongiotic simulants of mycosis fungoides. Arch Dermatol 1974; 109: 218–220.

646. Horiuchi Y, Tone T, Umezawa A, Takezaki S. Large cell mycosis fungoides at the tumor stage. Unusual T8, T4, T6 phenotypic expression. Am J Dermatopathol 1988; 10: 54–58.

647. Proctor MS, Price NM, Cox AJ, Hoppe RT. Subcutaneous mycosis fungoides. Arch Dermatol 1978; 114: 1326–1328.

648. Ackerman AB, Flaxman BA. Granulomatous mycosis fungoides. Br J Dermatol 1970; 82: 397–401.

649. Flaxman BA, Koumans JAD, Ackerman AB. Granulomatous mycosis fungoides. A 14-year follow-up of a case. Am J Dermatopathol 1983; 5: 145–151.

650. LeBoit PE, Zackheim HS, White CR Jr. Granulomatous variants of cutaneous T-cell lymphoma. The histopathology of granulomatous mycosis fungoides and granulomatous slack skin. Am J Surg Pathol 1988; 12: 83–95.

651. Granstein RD, Soter NA, Haynes HA. Necrotizing vasculitis within cutaneous lesions of mycosis fungoides. J Am Acad Dermatol 1983; 9: 128–133.

652. Goldberg DJ, Schinella RS, Kechijian P. Hypopigmented mycosis fungoides. Speculations about the mechanism of hypopigmentation. Am J Dermatopathol 1986; 8: 326–330.

653. Sterry W, Hauschild A. Use of monoclonal antibodies (UCHL1, Ki-B3) against T and B cell antigens in routine paraffin-embedded skin biopsy specimens. J Am Acad Dermatol 1989; 21: 98–107.

654. Vonderheid EC, Tan E, Sobel EL et al. Clinical implications of immunologic phenotyping in cutaneous T cell lymphoma. J Am Acad Dermatol 1987; 17: 40–52.

655. Michie SA, Abel EA, Hoppe RT et al. Expression of T-cell receptor antigens in mycosis fungoides and inflammatory skin lesions. J Invest Dermatol 1989; 93: 116–120.

656. Wood NL, Kitces EN, Blaylock WK. Depressed lymphokine activated killer cell activity in mycosis fungoides. A possible marker for aggressive disease. Arch Dermatol 1990; 126: 907–913.

657. Sterry W, Mielke V. CD4+ cutaneous T-cell lymphomas show the phenotype of helper/inducer T cells (CD45RA−, CDw29+). J Invest Dermatol 1989; 93: 413–416.

658. Wood GS, Abel EA, Hoppe RT, Warnke RA. Leu-8 and Leu-9 antigen phenotypes: Immunologic criteria for the distinction of mycosis fungoides from cutaneous inflammation. J Am Acad Dermatol 1986; 14: 1006–1013.

659. Wood GS, Hong SR, Sasaki DT et al. Leu-8/CD7 antigen expression by CD3+ T cells: Comparative analysis of skin and blood in mycosis fungoides/Sézary syndrome relative to normal blood values. J Am Acad Dermatol 1990; 22: 602–607.

660. Turbitt ML, Mackie RM. An assessment of the diagnostic value of the monoclonal antibodies Leu 8, OKT9, OKT10 and Ki67 in cutaneous lymphocytic infiltrates. Br J Dermatol 1986; 115: 151–158.

661. Willemze R, de Graaff-Reitsma CB, Cnossen J et al. Characterization of T-cell subpopulations in skin and peripheral blood of patients with cutaneous T-cell lymphomas and benign inflammatory dermatoses. J Invest Dermatol 1983; 80: 60–66.

662. van der Putte SCJ, Toonstra J, van Wichen DF et al. Aberrant immunophenotypes in mycosis fungoides. Arch Dermatol 1988; 124: 373–380.

663. McMillan EM, Wasik R, Beeman K, Everett MA. In situ immunologic phenotyping of mycosis fungoides. J Am Acad Dermatol 1982; 6: 888–897.

664. Piepkorn M, Marty J, Kjeldsberg CR. T cell subset heterogeneity in a series of patients with mycosis fungoides and Sézary syndrome. J Am Acad Dermatol 1984; 11: 427–432.

665. Beuchner SA, Winkelmann RK, Banks PM. T cells and T-cell subsets in mycosis fungoides and parapsoriasis. Arch Dermatol 1984; 120: 897–905.

666. Reinhold U, Pawelec G, Fratila A et al. Phenotypic and functional characterization of tumor infiltrating lymphocytes in mycosis fungoides: continuous growth of CD4+ CD45R+ T-cell clones with suppressor-inducer activity. J Invest Dermatol 1990; 94: 304–309.

667. Caputo R, Monti M, Berti E, Cavicchini S. A verrucoid epidermotropic OKT8-positive lymphoma. Am J Dermatopathol 1983; 5: 159–164.

668. van der Putte SCJ, Toonstra J, van Wichen DF. B cells

and plasma cells in mycosis fungoides. A study including cases with B cell follicle formation or a monotypical plasma cell component. Am J Dermatopathol 1989; 11: 509–516.

669. Sandbank M. Mycosis fungoides. Ultrastructural study with demonstration of atypical cells and nuclear bodies. Arch Dermatol 1971; 103: 206–214.

670. Tykocinski M, Schinella R, Greco A. The pleomorphic cells of advanced mycosis fungoides. An ultrastructural study. Arch Pathol Lab Med 1984; 108: 387–391.

671. Rosas-Uribe A, Variakojis D, Molnar Z, Rappaport H. Mycosis fungoides: an ultrastructural study. Cancer 1974; 34: 634–645.

672. van der Putte SCJ, van der Meer JB. Mycosis fungoides: a morphological study. Clin Exp Dermatol 1981; 6: 57–76.

673. Vonderheid EC, Tam DW, Johnson WC et al. Prognostic significance of cytomorphology in the cutaneous T-cell lymphomas. Cancer 1981; 47: 119–125.

674. Payne CM, Nagle RB, Lynch PJ. Quantitative electron microscopy in the diagnosis of mycosis fungoides. A simple analysis of lymphocytic nuclear convolutions. Arch Dermatol 1984; 120: 63–75.

675. Payne CM, Grogan TM, Lynch PJ. An ultrastructural morphometric and immunohistochemical analysis of cutaneous lymphomas and benign lymphocytic infiltrates of skin. Useful criteria for diagnosis. Arch Dermatol 1986; 122: 1139–1154.

676. Rieger E, Smolle J, Hoedl S et al. Morphometrical analysis of mycosis fungoides on paraffin-embedded sections. J Cutan Pathol 1989; 16: 7–13.

677. McMillan EM, Beeman K, Wasik R, Everett MA. Demonstration of OKT6-reactive cells in mycosis fungoides. J Am Acad Dermatol 1982; 6: 880–887.

678. Wieselthier JS, Koh HK. Sézary syndrome: Diagnosis, prognosis, and critical review of treatment options. J Am Acad Dermatol 1990; 22: 381–401.

679. Winkelmann RK. Clinical studies of T-cell erythroderma in the Sézary syndrome. Mayo Clin Proc 1974; 49: 519–525.

680. Buzzanga J, Banks PM, Winkelmann RK. Lymph node histopathology in Sézary syndrome. J Am Acad Dermatol 1984; 11: 880–888.

681. Zina G, Bernengo MG, Zina AM. Bullous Sézary syndrome. Dermatologica 1981; 163: 25–33.

682. Holdaway DR, Winkelmann RK. Histopathology of Sézary syndrome. Mayo Clin Proc 1974; 49: 541–547.

683. Alcalay J, David M, Shohat B, Sandbank M. Generalized vitiligo following Sézary syndrome. Br J Dermatol 1987; 116: 851–855.

684. Venencie PY, Winkelmann RK, Puissant A, Kyle RA. Monoclonal gammopathy in Sézary syndrome. Report of three cases and review of the literature. Arch Dermatol 1984; 120: 605–608.

685. Winkelmann RK, Buechner SA, Diaz-Perez JL. Pre-Sézary syndrome. J Am Acad Dermatol 1984; 10: 992–999.

686. Duncan SC, Winkelmann RK. Circulating Sézary cells in hospitalized dermatology patients. Br J Dermatol 1978; 99: 171–178.

687. Flandrin G, Brouet J-C. The Sézary cell: cytologic, cytochemical, and immunologic studies. Mayo Clin Proc 1974; 49: 575–583.

688. Hamminga L, Hartgrink-Groeneveld CA, van Vloten WA. Sézary's syndrome: a clinical evaluation of eight patients. Br J Dermatol 1979; 100: 291–296.

689. Ikai K, Uchiyama T, Maeda M, Takigawa M. Sézary-like syndrome in a 10-year-old girl with serologic evidence of human T-cell lymphotropic virus type I infection. Arch Dermatol 1987; 123: 1351–1355.

690. Buechner SA, Winkelmann RK. Sézary syndrome. A clinicopathologic study of 39 cases. Arch Dermatol 1983; 119: 979–986.

691. Sentis HJ, Willemze R, Scheffer E. Histopathologic studies in Sézary syndrome and erythrodermic mycosis fungoides: A comparison with benign forms of erythroderma. J Am Acad Dermatol 1986; 15: 1217–1226.

692. Piepkorn M, Marty J, Kjeldsberg CR. T cell subset heterogeneity in a series of patients with mycosis fungoides and Sézary syndrome. J Am Acad Dermatol 1984; 11: 427–432.

693. Hofman FM, Rea TH, Meyer PR et al. Demonstration of a subpopulation of $1a^+$ and T-helper cells in mycosis fungoides and the Sézary syndrome. Am J Dermatopathol 1983; 5: 135–143.

694. Edelson RL, Lutzner MA, Kirkpatrick CH et al. Morphologic and functional properties of the atypical T lymphocytes of the Sézary syndrome. Mayo Clin Proc 1974; 49: 558–566.

695. Zucker-Franklin D. Properties of the Sézary lymphoid cell. An ultrastructural analysis. Mayo Clin Proc 1974; 49: 567–574.

696. Payne CM, Glasser L. Ultrastructural morphometry in the diagnosis of Sézary syndrome. Arch Pathol Lab Med 1990; 114: 661–671.

697. Romagnoli P, Moretti S, Fattorossi A, Giannotti B. Dendritic cells in the dermal infiltrate of Sézary syndrome. Histopathology 1986; 10: 25–36.

698. Zackheim HS. Is "localized epidermotropic reticulosis" (Woringer–Kolopp disease) benign? J Am Acad Dermatol 1984; 11: 276–279.

699. Mandojana RM, Helwig EB. Localized epidermotropic reticulosis (Woringer–Kolopp disease). A clinicopathologic study of 15 new cases. J Am Acad Dermatol 1983; 8: 813–829.

700. Braun-Falco O, Schmoeckel C, Burg G, Ryckmanns F. Pagetoid reticulosis. A further case report with a review of the literature. Acta Derm Venereol (Suppl) 1979; 85: 11–21.

701. Ioannides G, Engel MF, Rywlin AM. Woringer-Kolopp disease (pagetoid reticulosis). Am J Dermatopathol 1983; 5: 153–158.

702. Wood WS, Killby VAA, Stewart WD. Pagetoid reticulosis (Woringer–Kolopp disease). J Cutan Pathol 1979; 6: 113–123.

703. Ringel E, Medenica M, Lorincz A. Localized mycosis fungoides not manifesting as Woringer–Kolopp disease. Arch Dermatol 1983; 119: 756–760.

704. Ralfkiaer E, Thomsen K, Agdal N et al. The development of a Ki-1-positive large cell non-Hodgkin's lymphoma in pagetoid reticulosis. Acta Derm Venereol 1989; 69: 206–211.

705. Deneau DG, Wood GS, Beckstead J et al. Woringer-Kolopp disease (pagetoid reticulosis). Arch Dermatol 1984; 120: 1045–1051.

706. Mackie RM, Turbitt ML. A case of Pagetoid reticulosis bearing the T cytotoxic suppressor surface marker on the lymphoid infiltrate: further evidence that

Pagetoid reticulosis is not a variant of mycosis fungoides. Br J Dermatol 1984; 110: 89–94.

707. Tan RS-H, Macleod TIF, Dean SG. Pagetoid reticulosis, epidermotropic mycosis fungoides and mycosis fungoides: a disease spectrum. Br J Dermatol 1987; 116: 67–77.

708. Mielke V, Wolff HH, Winzer M, Sterry W. Localized and disseminated pagetoid reticulosis. Diagnostic immunophenotypical findings. Arch Dermatol 1989; 125: 402–406.

709. Kerdel FA, MacDonald DM. Pagetoid reticulosis. Histiocyte marker studies. Arch Dermatol 1984; 120: 76–79.

710. Chu AC, MacDonald DM. Pagetoid reticulosis: a disease of histiocytic origin. Br J Dermatol 1980; 103: 147–157.

711. MacDonald DM. Pagetoid reticulosis — is it a disease entity? Br J Dermatol 1982; 107: 603–604.

712. Lever WF. Localized mycosis fungoides with prominent epidermotropism. Woringer–Kolopp disease. Arch Dermatol 1977; 113: 1254–1256.

713. Medenica M, Lorincz AL. Pagetoid reticulosis (Woringer-Kolopp disease). Arch Dermatol 1978; 114: 262–268.

714. Russell Jones R, Chu A. Pagetoid reticulosis and solitary mycosis fungoides. Distinct clinicopathological entities. J Cutan Pathol 1981; 8: 40–51.

715. Wood GS, Weiss LM, Warnke RA, Sklar J. The immunopathology of cutaneous lymphomas: immunophenotypic and immunogenotypic characteristics. Semin Dermatol 1986; 5: 334–345.

716. Gross DJ, Kavanaugh A. HTLV-I. Int J Dermatol 1990; 29: 161–165.

717. Knobler RM, Rehle T, Grossman M et al. Clinical evolution of cutaneous T cell lymphoma in a patient with antibodies to human T-lymphotropic virus type I. J Am Acad Dermatol 1987; 17: 903–909.

718. Jaffe ES. The morphologic spectrum of T-cell lymphoma. Am J Surg Pathol 1988; 12: 158–159.

719. Chan H-L, Su I-J, Kuo T-t et al. Cutaneous manifestations of adult T cell leukaemia/lymphoma. Report of three different forms. J Am Acad Dermatol 1985; 13: 213–219.

720. Takahashi K, Tanaka T, Fujita M et al. Cutaneous-type adult T-cell leukaemia/lymphoma. A unique clinical feature with monoclonal T-cell proliferation detected by Southern blot analysis. Arch Dermatol 1988; 124: 399–404.

721. Zimbow K, Takami T. Cutaneous T-cell lymphoma and related disorders. Int J Dermatol 1986; 25: 485–497.

722. Manabe T, Hirokawa M, Sugihara K et al. Angiocentric and angiodestructive infiltration of adult T-cell leukaemia/lymphoma (ATLL) in the skin. Report of two cases. Am J Dermatopathol 1988; 10: 487–496.

723. Tanaka T, Takahashi K, Ideyama S et al. Demonstration of clonal proliferation of T lymphocytes in early neoplastic disease. J Am Acad Dermatol 1989; 21: 218–223.

724. Maeda K, Takahashi M. Characterization of skin infiltrating cells in adult T-cell leukaemia/lymphoma (ATLL): clinical, histological and immunohistochemical studies on eight cases. Br J Dermatol 1989; 121: 603–612.

725. Sterry W, Korte B, Schubert C. Pleomorphic T-cell lymphoma and large-cell anaplastic lymphoma of the skin. Am J Dermatopathol 1989; 11: 112–123.

726. Bendelac A, Lesavre P, Boitard C et al. Cutaneous pleomorphic T cell lymphoma. Immunologic, virologic, and T-cell receptor gene rearrangement studies in one European case with initial pseudolymphoma presentation. J Am Acad Dermatol 1986; 15: 657–664.

727. Brisbane JU, Berman LD, Nieman RS. Peripheral T-cell lymphoma. A clinicopathologic study of nine cases. Am J Clin Pathol 1983; 79: 285–293.

728. Grogan TM, Fielder K, Rangel C et al. Peripheral T-cell lymphoma: aggressive disease with heterogeneous immunotypes. Am J Clin Pathol 1985; 83: 279–288.

729. Weinberg DS, Pinkus GS. Non-Hodgkin's lymphoma of large multilobated cell type. Am J Clin Pathol 1981; 76: 190–196.

730. Feller AC, Sterry W. Large cell anaplastic lymphoma of the skin. Br J Dermatol 1989; 121: 593–602.

731. Bitter MA, Franklin WA, Larson RA et al. Morphology in Ki-1 (CD30)-positive non-Hodgkin's lymphoma is correlated with clinical features and the presence of a unique chromosomal abnormality, t(2;5)(p 23; q35). Am J Surg Pathol 1990; 14: 305–316.

732. Leake J, Kellie SJ, Pritchard J et al. Peripheral T-cell lymphoma in childhood. A clinicopathological study of six cases. Histopathology 1989; 14: 255–268.

733. Sugimoto H, Nakayama F, Yamauchi T et al. Ki-1$^+$ cutaneous lymphoma. Gene rearrangement analysis of tumor cells in tissue and short-term culture of a patient. Arch Dermatol 1988; 124: 405–408.

734. Lindholm JS, Barron DR, Williams ME, Swerdlow SH. Ki-1-positive cutaneous large cell lymphoma of T cell type: Report of an indolent subtype. J Am Acad Dermatol 1989; 20: 342–348.

735. Kadin ME, Sako D, Berliner N et al. Childhood Ki-1 lymphoma presenting with skin lesions and peripheral lymphadenopathy. Blood 1986; 68: 1042–1049.

736. Chan JKC, Ng CS, Hui PK et al. Anaplastic large cell Ki-1 lymphoma. Delineation of two morphological types. Histopathology 1989; 13: 11–34.

737. Pileri S, Falini B, Delsol G et al. Lymphohistiocytic T-cell lymphoma (anaplastic large cell lymphoma CD30+/Ki-1+ with a high content of reactive histiocytes). Histopathology 1990; 16: 383–391.

738. Falini B, Pileri S, Stein H et al. Variable expression of leucocyte-common (CD45) antigen in CD30 (Ki1)-positive anaplastic large-cell lymphoma: implications for the differential diagnosis between lymphoid and nonlymphoid malignancies. Hum Pathol 1990; 21: 624–629.

739. Pallesen G. The diagnostic significance of the CD30 (Ki-1) antigen. Histopathology 1990; 16: 409–413.

740. Chott A, Kaserer K, Augustin I et al. Ki-1-positive large cell lymphoma. A clinicopathologic study of 41 cases. Am J Surg Pathol 1990; 14: 439–448.

741. Flynn KJ, Dehner LP, Gajl-Peczalska KJ et al. Regressing atypical histiocytosis: A cutaneous proliferation of atypical neoplastic histiocytes with unexpectedly indolent biologic behavior. Cancer 1982; 49: 959–970.

742. McCormick S, Stenn KS, Nelligan D. Regressing atypical histiocytosis. Report of a case. Am J Dermatopathol 1984; 6: 259–263.

743. Headington JT, Roth MS, Ginsburg D et al. T-cell

receptor gene rearrangement in regressing atypical histiocytosis. Arch Dermatol 1987; 123: 1183–1187.

744. Headington JT, Roth MS, Schnitzer B. Regressing atypical histiocytosis: A review and critical appraisal. Semin Diagnostic Pathol 1987; 4: 28–37.

745. Ringel E, Moschella S. Primary histiocytic dermatoses. Arch Dermatol 1985; 121: 1531–1541.

746. Convit J, Kerdel F, Goihman M et al. Progressive, atrophying, chronic granulomatous dermohypodermitis. Autoimmune disease? Arch Dermatol 1973; 107: 271–274.

747. Ackerman AB. Histologic diagnosis of inflammatory skin diseases. Philadelphia: Lea & Febiger, 1978; 483–485.

748. Kauffman CL, Nigra TP, Friedman KJ. A case of granulomatous slack skin. J Cutan Pathol 1988; 15: 319 (abstract).

749. Alessi E, Crosti C, Sala F. Unusual case of granulomatous dermohypodermitis with giant cells and elastophagocytosis. Dermatologica 1986; 172: 218–221.

750. LeBoit PE, Beckstead JH, Bond B et al. Granulomatous slack skin: clonal rearrangement of the T-cell receptor β gene is evidence for the lymphoproliferative nature of a cutaneous elastolytic disorder. J Invest Dermatol 1987; 89: 183–186.

751. Balus L, Bassetti F, Gentili G. Granulomatous slack skin. Arch Dermatol 1985; 121: 250–252.

752. Weis JW, Winter MW, Phyliky RL, Banks PM. Peripheral T-cell lymphomas: histologic, immunohistologic and clinical characterization. Mayo Clin Proc 1986; 61: 411–426.

753. Kim H, Nathwani BN, Rappaport H. So-called 'Lennert's lymphoma'. Is it a clinicopathologic entity? Cancer 1980; 45: 1379–1399.

754. Kiesewetter F, Haneke E, Lennert K et al. Cutaneous lymphoepithelioid lymphoma (Lennert's lymphoma). Combined immunohistological, ultrastructural, and DNA-flow-cytometric analysis. Am J Dermatopathol 1989; 11: 549–554.

755. Roundtree JM, Burgdorf W, Harkey MR. Cutaneous involvement in Lennert's lymphoma. Arch Dermatol 1980; 116: 1291–1294.

756. Kim H, Jacobs C, Warnke RA, Dorfman RF. Malignant lymphoma with a high content of epithelioid histiocytes. Cancer 1978; 41: 620–635.

757. Zamora I, Nunez C, Hu C-H. Lennert's lymphoma presenting with clusters of cutaneous infection. J Am Acad Dermatol 1981; 5: 450–454.

758. McNutt NS, Smoller BR, Kline M et al. Angiocentric T-cell lymphoma associated with human T-cell lymphotropic virus type I infection. Arch Pathol Lab Med 1990; 114: 170–175.

759. Chan JKC, Ng CS, Ngan KC et al. Angiocentric T-cell lymphoma of the skin. An aggressive lymphoma distinct from mycosis fungoides. Am J Surg Pathol 1988; 12: 861–876.

760. Lipford EH Jr, Margolick JB, Longo DL et al. Angiocentric immunoproliferative lesions: a clinicopathologic spectrum of post-thymic T-cell proliferations. Blood 1988; 72: 1674–1681.

761. Fujiwara Y, Abe Y, Kuyama M et al. CD8+ cutaneous T-cell lymphoma with pagetoid epidermotropism and angiocentric and angiodestructive infiltration. Arch Dermatol 1990; 126: 801–804.

762. Armitage JO, Greer JP, Levine AM et al. Peripheral T-cell lymphoma. Cancer 1989; 63: 158–163.

763. Holbert JM Jr, Chesney T McC. Malignant lymphoma of the skin: a review of recent advances in diagnosis and classification. J Cutan Pathol 1982; 9: 133–168.

764. Edelson RL. Cutaneous T-cell lymphoma. J Dermatol Surg Oncol 1980; 6: 358–368.

765. Fisher ER, Park EJ, Wechsler HL. Histologic identification of malignant lymphoma cutis. Am J Clin Pathol 1976; 65: 149–158.

766. Burg G, Kerl H, Przybilla B, Braun-Falco O. Some statistical data, diagnosis, and staging of cutaneous B-cell lymphoma. J Dermatol Surg Oncol 1984; 10: 256–262.

767. Sterry W, Kruger GRF, Steigleder G-K. Skin involvement of malignant B-cell lymphomas. J Dermatol Surg Oncol 1984; 10: 276–277.

768. Oliver GF, Dabski K, Cerio R, Winkelmann RK. Systemic follicular lymphoma with cutaneous manifestations: an immunohistochemical study. J Cutan Pathol 1988; 15: 333 (abstract).

769. Wilkel CS, Grant-Kels JM. Cutaneous B-cell lymphoma. An unusual presentation. Arch Dermatol 1987; 123: 1362–1367.

770. Krishnan J, Li C-Y, Su WPD. Cutaneous lymphomas: correlation of histochemical and immunohistochemical characteristics and clinicopathologic features. Am J Clin Pathol 1983; 79: 157–165.

771. Horton JJ, Cairns RJ, MacDonald DM. Cutaneous B cell lymphocytic lymphoma associated with paraproteinaemia. Clin Exp Dermatol 1984; 9: 384–387.

772. Burg G, von der Helm D, Kaudewitz P et al. Antihuman T-cell leukemia/lymphoma virus antibodies in three patients with primary cutaneous B-cell lymphoma. J Dermatol Surg Oncol 1988; 14: 653–656.

773. Burg G, Kaudewitz P, Klepzig K et al. Cutaneous B-cell lymphoma. Dermatol Clin 1985; 3: 689–704.

774. Kerl H, Burg G. Histomorphology and cytomorphology of cutaneous B-cell lymphomas. J Dermatol Surg Oncol 1984; 10: 266–270.

775. Garcia CF, Weiss LM, Warnke RA, Wood GS. Cutaneous follicular lymphoma. Am J Surg Pathol 1986; 10: 454–463.

776. Faure P, Chittal S, Gorguet B et al. Immunohistochemical profile of cutaneous B-cell lymphoma on cryostat and paraffin sections. Am J Dermatopathol 1990; 12: 122–133.

777. Kwittken J, Goldberg AF. Follicular lymphoma of the skin. Arch Dermatol 1966; 93: 177–183.

778. Willemze R, de Graaff-Reitsma CB, van Vloten WA, Meijer CJLM. The cell population of cutaneous B-cell lymphomas. Br J Dermatol 1983; 108: 395–409.

779. Kerl H, Kresbach H. Germinal centre cell-derived lymphomas of the skin. J Dermatol Surg Oncol 1984; 10: 291–295.

780. Willemze R, Meijer CJLM, Scheffer E et al. Diffuse large cell lymphomas of follicular center cell origin presenting in the skin. A clinicopathologic and immunologic study of 16 patients. Am J Pathol 1987; 126: 325–333.

781. Willemze R, Meijer CJLM, Sentis HJ et al. Primary cutaneous large cell lymphomas of follicular center cell origin. A clinical follow-up study of nineteen patients. J Am Acad Dermatol 1987; 16: 518–526.

782. Pimpinelli N, Santucci M, Bosi A et al. Primary cutaneous follicular centre-cell lymphoma — a lymphoproliferative disease with favourable prognosis. Clin Exp Dermatol 1989; 14: 12–19.

783. Burg G, Kerl H, Kaudewitz P et al. Immunoenzymatic typing of lymphoplasmacytoid skin infiltrates. J Dermatol Surg Oncol 1984; 10: 284–290.

784. Patsouris E, Noel H, Lennert K. Lymphoplasmacytic/lymphoplasmacytoid immunocytoma with a high content of epithelioid cells. Histologic and immunohistochemical findings. Am J Surg Pathol 1990; 14: 660–670.

785. Aloi FG, Appino A, Puiatti P. Lymphoplasmacytoid lymphoma arising in herpes zoster scars. J Am Acad Dermatol 1990; 22: 130–131.

786. Marti RM, Estrach T, Palou J et al. Primary cutaneous lymphoplasmacytic lymphoma. J Am Acad Dermatol 1987; 16: 1106–1110.

787. Hanna W, Kahn HJ, From L. Signet ring lymphoma of the skin: ultrastructural and immunohistochemical features. J Am Acad Dermatol 1986; 14: 344–350.

788. Eckert F, Hefner H, Kaudewitz F, Burg G. Multilobated B-cell lymphoma of the skin — a variant of follicular center cell lymphoma. J Cutan Pathol 1989; 16: 301 (abstract).

789. van der Putte SCJ, Toonstra J, Bruns HM et al. T-cell signet-ring cell proliferation in the skin simulating true histiocytic lymphoma. Am J Dermatopathol 1987; 9: 120–128.

790. Burg G, Kerl H, Schmoeckel C. Differentiation between malignant B-cell lymphomas and pseudolymphomas of the skin. J Dermatol Surg Oncol 1984; 10: 271–275.

791. Willemze R, Meijer CJLM. Analysis of non-neoplastic cells in cutaneous B-cell lymphomas. J Dermatol Surg Oncol 1984; 10: 315–318.

792. Kaudewitz P, Burg G, Klepzig K et al. Cells reactive with anti-T-cell monoclonal antibodies in malignant cutaneous B-cell lymphomas and pseudolymphomas. J Dermatol Surg Oncol 1984; 10: 313–314.

793. Smolle J, Kerl H. Immunohistologic analysis of cutaneous B-cell lymphomas. Arch Dermatol 1984; 120: 1615 (abstract).

794. Liang G, Pardo RJ, Voigt W et al. Studies of immunoglobulin and T cell receptor gene rearrangement in cutaneous B and T cell lymphomas. J Am Acad Dermatol 1989; 21: 457–460.

795. Pimpinelli N, Romagnoli P, Moretti S, Giannotti B. Non-lymphoid accessory cells in the cutaneous infiltrate of B cell lymphomas. An immunohistochemical and ultrastructural study. Br J Dermatol 1988; 118: 353–362.

796. Forestier J-Y, Schmitt D, Thivolet J. Histiocytosarcome cutané: aspects cliniques, immunohistochimiques et ultrastructuraux; difficultés d'étude et problèmes nosologiques. Ann Dermatol Venereol 1980; 107: 7–19.

797. Zala L, Zimmermann A, Armagni C, Krebs A. Morbus Crosti (Retikulohistiozytom Typ Crosti). Hautarzt 1981; 32: 499–504.

798. Rowland Payne CME, Meyrick Thomas RH, Black MM. Crosti's indolent lymphoma and persistent superficial dermatitis. Clin Exp Dermatol 1984; 9: 303–308.

799. Berti E, Alessi E, Caputo R et al. Reticulohistiocytoma

800. Winkelmann RK, Dabski K. Large cell lymphocytoma: follow up, immunopathology studies, and comparison to cutaneous follicular and Crosti lymphoma. Arch Dermatol Res 1987; 279: s81–s87.

801. Wick MR, Mills SE, Scheithauer BW et al. Reassessment of malignant "angioendotheliomatosis". Evidence in favor of its reclassification as "intravascular lymphomatosis". Am J Surg Pathol 1986; 10: 112–123.

802. Wick MR, Rocamora A. Reactive and malignant 'angioendotheliomatosis': a discriminant clinicopathological study. J Cutan Pathol 1988; 15: 260–271.

803. Cooper PH. Angioendotheliomatosis: two separate diseases. Hum Pathol 1988; 15: 259.

804. Willemze R, Kruyswijk MRJ, de Bruin CD et al. Angiotropic (intravascular) large cell lymphoma of the skin previously classified as malignant angioendotheliomatosis. Br J Dermatol 1987; 116: 393–399.

805. Braverman IM, Lerner AB. Diffuse malignant proliferation of vascular endothelium. A possible new clinical and pathological entity. Arch Dermatol 1961; 84: 22–30.

806. Petito CK, Gottlieb GJ, Dougherty JH, Petito FA. Neoplastic angioendotheliosis: ultrastructural study and review of the literature. Ann Neurol 1978; 3: 393–399.

807. Scott PWB, Silvers DN, Helwig EB. Proliferating angioendotheliomatosis. Arch Pathol 1975; 99: 323–326.

808. Sheibani K, Battifora H, Winberg CD et al. Further evidence that "malignant angioendotheliomatosis" is an angiotropic large-cell lymphoma. N Engl J Med 1986; 314: 943–948.

809. Bhawan J, Wolff SM, Ucci AA, Bhan AK. Malignant lymphoma and malignant angioendotheliomatosis: one disease. Cancer 1985; 55: 570–576.

810. Bhawan J. Angioendotheliomatosis proliferans systemisata: an angiotropic neoplasm of lymphoid origin. Semin Diagn Pathol 1987; 4: 18–27.

811. Petroff N, Koger O'NW, Fleming MG et al. Malignant angioendotheliomatosis: An angiotropic lymphoma. J Am Acad Dermatol 1989; 21: 727–733.

812. Berger TG, Dawson N A. Angioendotheliomatosis. J Am Acad Dermatol 1988; 18: 407–412.

813. Mori S, Itoyama S, Mohri N et al. Cellular characteristics of neoplastic angioendotheliosis. An immunohistochemical marker study of 6 cases. Virchows Arch (A) 1985; 407: 167–175.

814. Dominguez FE, Rosen LB, Kramer HC. Malignant angioendotheliomatosis proliferans. Report of an autopsied case studied with immunoperoxidase. Am J Dermatopathol 1986; 8: 419–425.

815. Kanoh T, Takigawa M, Niwa Y. Cutaneous lesions in γ heavy-chain disease. Arch Dermatol 1988; 124: 1538–1540.

816. Wester SM, Banks PM, Li C-Y. The histopathology of γ heavy-chain disease. Am J Clin Pathol 1982; 78: 427–436.

817. Kyle RA, Greipp PR, Banks PM. The diverse picture of gamma heavy-chain disease. Report of seven cases

and review of the literature. Mayo Clin Proc 1981; 56: 439–451.

818. Willemze R, van Vloten WA, van der Loo EM, Meyer CJLM. Primary lymphoblastic non-Hodgkin's lymphoma of the skin. Br J Dermatol 1981; 104: 333–338.

819. Zaatari GS, Chan WC, Kim TH et al. Malignant lymphoma of the skin in children. Cancer 1987; 59: 1040–1045.

820. Vaillant L, Lorette G, Colombat P, Monegier du Sorbier C. Primary cutaneous lymphoblastic lymphoma of non-B, non-T phenotype. J Am Acad Dermatol 1990; 126: 400–402.

Miscellaneous and mixed infiltrates

821. Brough AJ, Jones D, Page RH, Mizukami I. Dermal erythropoiesis in neonatal infants. A manifestation of intra-uterine viral disease. Pediatrics 1967; 40: 627–635.

822. Bowden JB, Hebert AA, Rapini RP. Dermal hematopoiesis in neonates: Report of five cases. J Am Acad Dermatol 1989; 20: 1104–1110.

823. Hocking WG, Lazar GS, Lipsett JA, Busuttil RW. Cutaneous extramedullary hematopoiesis following splenectomy for idiopathic myelofibrosis. Am J Med 1984; 76: 956–958.

824. Sarma DP. Extramedullary hemopoiesis of the skin. Arch Dermatol 1981; 117: 58–59.

825. Mizoguchi M, Kawa Y, Minami T et al. Cutaneous extramedullary hematopoiesis in myelofibrosis. J Am Acad Dermatol 1990; 22: 351–355.

826. Schofield JK, Shun JLK, Cerio R, Grice K. Cutaneous extramedullary hematopoiesis with a preponderance of atypical megakaryocytes in myelofibrosis. J Am Acad Dermatol 1990; 22: 334–337.

827. Kuo T. Cutaneous extramedullary hematopoiesis presenting as leg ulcers. J Am Acad Dermatol 1981; 4: 592–596.

828. Tagami H, Tashima M, Uehara N. Myelofibrosis with skin lesions. Br J Dermatol 1980; 102: 109–112.

829. Ortonne JP, Jeune R, Perrot H. Myeloid metaplasia of the skin in two patients suffering from primary myelofibrosis. Arch Dermatol 1977; 113: 1459.

830. Pedro-Botet J, Feliu E, Rozman C et al. Cutaneous myeloid metaplasia with dysplastic features in idiopathic myelofibrosis. Int J Dermatol 1988; 27: 179–180.

831. Shaikh BS, Frantz E, Lookingbill DP. Histologically proven leukemia cutis carries a poor prognosis in acute nonlymphocytic leukemia. Cutis 1987; 39: 57–60.

832. Su WPD, Buechner SA, Li C-Y. Clinicopathologic correlations in leukemia cutis. J Am Acad Dermatol 1984; 11: 121–128.

833. Stawiski MA. Skin manifestations of leukemias and lymphomas. Cutis 1978; 21: 814–818.

834. Bonvalet D, Foldes C, Civatte J. Cutaneous manifestations in chronic lymphocytic leukemia. J Dermatol Surg Oncol 1984; 10: 278–282.

835. Ohno S, Yokoo T, Ohta M et al. Aleukemic leukemia cutis. J Am Acad Dermatol 1990; 22: 374–377.

836. Hansen RM, Barnett J, Hanson G et al. Aleukemic leukemia cutis. Arch Dermatol 1986; 122: 812–814.

837. Yoder FW, Schuen RL. Aleukemic leukemia cutis. Arch Dermatol 1976; 112: 367–369.

838. Heskel NS, White CR, Fryberger S et al. Aleukemic leukemia cutis: Juvenile chronic granulocytic leukemia presenting with figurate cutaneous lesions. J Am Acad Dermatol 1983; 9: 423–427.

839. Cochrane T, Milne JA. Aleukaemic acute lymphoblastic leukaemia presenting with cutaneous lesions. Br J Dermatol 1974; 91: 587–589.

840. Horlick HP, Silvers DN, Knobler EH, Cole JT. Acute myelomonocytic leukemia presenting as a benign-appearing cutaneous eruption. Arch Dermatol 1990; 126: 653–656.

841. Boggs DR, Wintrobe MM, Cartwright GE. The acute leukemias. Analysis of 322 cases and review of the literature. Medicine (Baltimore) 1962; 41: 163–225.

842. Lawrence DM, Sun NCJ, Mena R, Moss R. Cutaneous lesions in hairy-cell leukemia. Case report and review of the literature. Arch Dermatol 1983; 119: 322–325.

843. Finan MC, Su WPD, Li C-Y. Cutaneous findings in hairy cell leukemia. J Am Acad Dermatol 1984; 11: 788–797.

844. Czarnecki DB, O'Brien TJ, Rotstein H, Brenan J. Leukaemia cutis mimicking primary syphilis. Acta Derm Venereol 1981; 61: 368–369.

845. Zax RH, Kulp-Shorten CL, Callen JP. Leukemia cutis presenting as a scrotal ulcer. J Am Acad Dermatol 1989; 21: 410–413.

846. Sumaya CV, Babu S, Reed RJ. Erythema nodosum-like lesions of leukemia. Arch Dermatol 1974; 110: 415–418.

847. Frankel DH, Larson RA, Lorincz AL. Acral lividosis — a sign of myeloproliferative diseases. Hyperleukocytosis syndrome in chronic myelogenous leukemia. Arch Dermatol 1987; 123: 921–924.

848. Butler DF, Berger TG, Rodman OG. Leukemia cutis mimicking stasis dermatitis. Cutis 1985; 35: 47–48.

849. Baden TJ, Gammon WR. Leukemia cutis in acute myelomonocytic leukemia. Preferential localization in a recent Hickman catheter scar. Arch Dermatol 1987; 123: 88–90.

850. Warin AP, Roberts MM. Chronic lymphocytic leukaemia with cutaneous involvement. Clin Exp Dermatol 1979; 4: 241–246.

851. Logan RA, Smith NP. Cutaneous presentation of prolymphocytic leukaemia. Br J Dermatol 1988; 118: 553–558.

852. Côté J, Trudel M, Gratton D. T cell chronic lymphocytic leukemia with bullous manifestations. J Am Acad Dermatol 1983; 8: 874–878.

853. Eubanks SW, Patterson JW. Subacute myelomonocytic leukemia — an unusual skin manifestation. J Am Acad Dermatol 1983; 9: 581–584.

854. High DA, Luscombe HA, Kauh YC. Leukemia cutis masquerading as chronic paronychia. Int J Dermatol 1985; 24: 595–597.

855. Francis JS, Sybert VP, Benjamin DR. Congenital monocytic leukemia: report of a case with cutaneous involvement, and review of the literature. Pediatr Dermatol 1989; 6: 306–311.

856. Gottesfeld E, Silverman RA, Coccia PF et al. Transient blueberry muffin appearance of a newborn

with congenital monoblastic leukemia. J Am Acad Dermatol 1989; 21: 347–351.

857. Sadick N, Edlin D, Myskowski PL et al. Granulocytic sarcoma. A new finding in the setting of preleukemia. Arch Dermatol 1984; 120: 1341–1343.

858. Meis JM, Butler JJ, Osborne BM, Manning JT. Granulocytic sarcoma in nonleukemic patients. Cancer 1986; 58: 2697–2709.

859. Nieman RS, Barcos M, Berard C et al. Granulocytic sarcoma: A clinicopathologic study of 61 biopsied cases. Cancer 1981; 48: 1426–1437.

860. Choi H-SH, Orentreich D, Kornblee L, Muhlfelder TW. Granulocytic sarcoma presenting as a solitary nodule of skin in a patient with Waldenström's macroglobulinemia. An immunohistochemical and electron-microscopic study. Am J Dermatopathol 1989; 11: 51–57.

861. Sun NCJ, Ellis R. Granulocytic sarcoma of the skin. Arch Dermatol 1980; 116: 800–802.

862. Raman BKS, Janakiraman N, Raju UR et al. Osteomyelosclerosis with granulocytic sarcoma of chest wall. Morphological, ultrastructural, immunologic, and cytogenetic study. Arch Pathol Lab Med 1990; 114: 426–429.

863. Koriech OM, Al-Dash FZ. Skin and bone necrosis following ecthyma gangrenosum in acute leukaemia — report of three cases. Clin Exp Dermatol 1988; 13: 78–81.

864. Mays JA, Neerhout RC, Bagby GC, Koler RD. Juvenile chronic granulocytic leukemia. Emphasis on cutaneous manifestations and underlying neurofibromatosis. Am J Dis Child 1980; 134: 654–658.

865. Peterson AO Jr, Jarratt M. Pruritus and nonspecific nodules preceding myelomonocytic leukemia. J Am Acad Dermatol 1980; 2: 496–498.

866. Buechner SA, Li C-Y, Su WPD. Leukemia cutis. A histopathologic study of 42 cases. Am J Dermatopathol 1985; 7: 109–119.

867. Burg G, Schmoeckel C, Braun-Falco O, Wolff HH. Monocytic leukemia. Clinically appearing as 'malignant reticulosis of the skin'. Arch Dermatol 1978; 114: 418–420.

868. Blaustein JC, Narang S, Palutke M, Karanes C. Extramedullary (skin) presentation of acute monocytic leukemia resembling cutaneous lymphoma: morphological and immunological features. J Cutan Pathol 1987; 14: 232–237.

869. Horn TD, Hines HC, Farmer ER. Erythrophagocytosis in the skin: case report. J Cutan Pathol 1988; 15: 399–403.

870. Leder L-D. The chloroacetate esterase reaction. A useful means of histological diagnosis of hematological disorders from paraffin sections of skin. Am J Dermatopathol 1979; 1: 39–42.

871. Anderson KC, Boyd AW, Fisher DC et al. Hairy cell leukemia: A tumor of pre-plasma cells. Blood 1985; 65: 620–629.

872. Arai E, Ikeda S, Itoh S, Katayama I. Specific skin lesions as the presenting symptom of hairy cell leukemia. Am J Clin Pathol 1988; 90: 459–464.

873. Greenwood R, Barker DJ, Tring FC et al. Clinical and immunohistological characterization of cutaneous lesions in chronic lymphocytic leukaemia. Br J Dermatol 1985; 113: 447–453.

874. Smith JL Jr, Butler JJ. Skin involvement in Hodgkin's disease. Cancer 1980; 45: 354–361.

875. Benninghoff DL, Medina A, Alexander LL, Camiel MR. The mode of spread of Hodgkin's disease to the skin. Cancer 1970; 26: 1135–1140.

876. Heyd J, Weissberg N, Gottschalk S. Hodgkin's disease of the skin. A case report. Cancer 1989; 63: 924–929.

877. Misra RS, Mukherjee A, Ramesh V et al. Specific skin ulcers in Hodgkin's disease. Cutis 1987; 39: 247–248.

878. Hanno R, Bean SF. Hodgkin's disease with specific bullous lesions. Am J Dermatopathol 1980; 2: 363–366.

879. Rubins J. Cutaneous Hodgkin's disease. Indolent course and control with chemotherapy. Cancer 1978; 42: 1219–1221.

880. Gordon RA, Lookingbill DP, Abt AB. Skin infiltration in Hodgkin's disease. Arch Dermatol 1980; 116: 1038–1040.

881. Williams MV. Spontaneous regression of cutaneous Hodgkin's disease. Br Med J 1980; 280: 903.

882. O'Bryan-Tear CG, Burke M, Coulson IH, Marsden RA. Hodgkin's disease presenting in the skin. Clin Exp Dermatol 1987; 12: 69–71.

883. Silverman CL, Strayer DS, Wasserman TH. Cutaneous Hodgkin's disease. Arch Dermatol 1982; 118: 918–921.

884. Hayes TG, Rabin VR, Rosen T, Zubler MA. Hodgkin's disease presenting in the skin: Case report and review of the literature. J Am Acad Dermatol 1990; 22: 944–947.

885. Szur L, Harrison CV, Levene GM, Samman PD. Primary cutaneous Hodgkin's disease. Lancet 1970; 1: 1016–1020.

886. Brehmer-Andersson E. The validity of the concept of primary cutaneous Hodgkin's disease. Acta Derm Venereol (Suppl) 1976; 75: 124–125.

887. Ultmann JE, Moran EM. Clinical course and complications in Hodgkin's disease. Arch Intern Med 1973; 131: 332–353.

888. Samman PD. Cutaneous manifestations. Proc R Soc Med 1967; 60: 736–737.

889. Sood VD, Pasricha JS. Pemphigus and Hodgkin's disease. Arch Dermatol 1974; 90: 575–578.

890. Naysmith A, Hancock DW. Hodgkin's disease and pemphigus. Br J Dermatol 1976; 94: 695–696.

891. Chen KTK, Flam MS. Hodgkin's disease complicating lymphomatoid papulosis. Am J Dermatopathol 1985; 7: 555–561.

892. Lederman JS, Sober AJ, Harrist TJ, Lederman GS. Lymphomatoid papulosis following Hodgkin's disease. J Am Acad Dermatol 1987; 16: 331–335.

892a. Kaudewitz P, Stein H, Plewig G et al. Hodgkin's disease followed by lymphomatoid papulosis. J Am Acad Dermatol 1990; 22: 999–1006.

893. Harman RRM. Hodgkin's disease, seminoma of testicle and widespread granuloma annulare. Br J Dermatol (Suppl) 1977; 15: 50–51.

894. Moretti S, Pimpinelli N, Di Lollo S et al. In situ immunologic characterization of cutaneous involvement in Hodgkin's disease. Cancer 1989; 63: 661–666.

895. Torne R, Umbert P. Hodgkin's disease presenting with superficial lymph nodes and tumors of the scalp. Dermatologica 1986; 172: 225–228.

896. Jones DB. The histogenesis of the Reed-Sternberg cell and its mononuclear counterparts. J Pathol 1987; 151: 191–195.

897. Brincker H. Epithelioid-cell granulomas in Hodgkin's disease. Acta Pathol Microbiol Scand 1970; 78A: 19–32.

898. Randle HW, Banks PM, Winkelmann RK. Cutaneous granulomas in malignant lymphoma. Arch Dermatol 1980; 116: 441–443.

899. Peltier FA, Pursley TV, Apisarnthanarax P, Raimer SS. Necrobiotic granulomas of the skin associated with Hodgkin's disease. Arch Dermatol 1981; 117: 123–124.

Glossary

Acantholysis: loss of cohesion between keratinocytes leading to the formation of clefts or vesicles.

Acanthosis: increased thickness of the spinous layer of the epidermis. This is usually associated with enlargement and downgrowth of the rete pegs.

Acrosyringium: the intraepidermal portion of the eccrine sweat duct. It is lined by keratinocytes which are smaller than those of the adjacent epidermis. The keratinocytes lining this part of the duct are attached to the adjoining larger keratinocytes by desmosomes in the usual way.

Acrotrichium: the intraepidermal portion of the follicular infundibulum. It is composed of keratinocytes that are morphologically similar to the keratinocytes of the adjacent epidermis. However, unlike the latter, the cells of the acrotrichium may be unaffected in solar keratoses and Bowen's disease.

Anagen: the growth phase of the hair cycle (p. 455).

Apoptosis: a mode of cell death which is morphologically distinct from necrosis (p. 31). It usually involves single cells (rather than sheets of cells, as in necrosis). The dying cells shrink and bud into smaller fragments, some of which are beyond the resolution of the light microscope. In contrast to necrosis, the cytoplasmic organelles are still intact at this stage, but some redistribution occurs during the budding phase. The small fragments are phagocytosed by adjacent parenchymal cells (keratinocytes, tumour cells etc., as the case may be) or macrophages. In the case of keratinocytes undergoing apoptosis, the tonofilaments are redistributed into an area of the cell which is incapable of budding into fragments small enough to be phagocytosed by adjacent keratinocytes. Such larger fragments are usually extruded into the dermis where they are known as colloid bodies (see below). Some filamentous fragments are phagocytosed by macrophages.

Ballooning degeneration: pronounced swelling and vacuolation of keratinocytes leading to the detachment of affected cells from neighbouring ones (acantholysis). It is characteristic of certain viral infections of the epidermis, particularly herpes simplex, herpes zoster and varicella.

Birefringence: the property of some materials which enables them to be visualized on microscopic examination using polarized light. The birefringent material, which is said to be 'doubly refractile', appears white against a dark background. This property is shown by some normal tissues (collagen, keratin and bone) and also by uric acid crystals and by various materials foreign to the skin.

Bulla: a fluid-filled lesion (blister) which forms within the epidermis or just beneath it. A bulla may also contain inflammatory cells, fibrin and detached keratinocytes. Blisters less than 1 cm

1075

(some authors say 0.5 cm) in diameter are known as vesicles.

Catagen: the involutionary stage of the hair cycle which results from the spontaneous death, by apoptosis, of the cells forming the lower part of the hair follicle (p. 455).

Civatte body: see colloid body (below).

Colloid body: an eosinophilic cytoid body found in the basal layer of the epidermis or in the upper papillary dermis. It represents the tonofilament-rich remnant of a keratinocyte which has undergone death, usually by apoptosis (see above). The filamentous structure of colloid bodies is responsible for their trapping of immunoglobulins, particularly the large IgM molecule; this can be detected by direct immunofluorescence. The term 'Civatte body' has been used both for a shrunken apoptotic keratinocyte containing a nuclear remnant and for an intraepidermal colloid body. Sometimes the term colloid body is restricted to cytoid bodies in the papillary dermis.

Corps ronds: literally, 'round bodies' — a form of dyskeratotic cell in which the cytoplasm is densely basophilic rather than deeply eosinophilic as in most dyskeratotic cells. An unstained zone is usually present surrounding the nucleus (perinuclear halo). The cells eventually become detached from adjacent keratinocytes: that is, they become acantholytic.

Dyskeratosis: a term which lacks precision. It is generally used to describe keratinocytes with hypereosinophilic cytoplasm and a shrunken, hyperchromatic nucleus. It refers to abnormal keratinization of keratinocytes, usually associated with an abnormal accumulation of filaments in the cytoplasm. Such dyskeratotic cells usually die by the process of apoptosis but the filamentous nature of their cytoplasm prevents the cell from breaking down into multiple small fragments as occurs in other cells of the body undergoing death by apoptosis.

Epidermotropism: the presence of mononuclear cells, usually large lymphocytes, within the epidermis but not accompanied by significant spongiosis. The cells are usually confined to the lower half of the epidermis where they may aggregate to form a Pautrier microabscess. They are often surrounded by a clear halo. Epidermotropism is characteristic of large plaque parapsoriasis, mycosis fungoides and some drug reactions. The term is sometimes applied to invasion of the epidermis by tumour cells in the dermis.

Exocytosis: the presence of inflammatory cells within the epidermis. In contrast to epidermotropism the cells are randomly distributed at all levels of the epidermis, often in association with spongiosis.

Fibrinoid necrosis: the extravasation of fibrin into the wall of a blood vessel or its immediate surrounding. The term fibrinoid degeneration is used for a wider permeation of collagen with fibrin.

Grenz zone: derived from the German word for boundary. The term refers to an uninvolved zone separating the epidermis from an underlying inflammatory cell infiltrate or tumour. Sometimes the term is used for any uninvolved zone separating one tissue component from another.

Horn cyst: a keratin-filled space within the centre of a squamous epithelial island.

Hyperkeratosis: increased thickness of the stratum corneum. The term is usually applied when the keratin is anucleate (orthokeratosis, orthokeratotic hyperkeratosis) in contra-distinction to parakeratosis which refers to an altered, usually thickened stratum corneum containing nuclear remnants. In hyperkeratosis the normal basket-weave pattern of the stratum corneum is seldom retained; more often the keratin is compact or laminated.

Koebner phenomenon: the induction or development of lesions characteristic of a particular disease at the site of physical trauma or some other noxious stimulus (isomorphic reaction).

Leucocytoclasis: the disintegration of white cells, usually neutrophils, resulting in small pyknotic nuclear fragments (nuclear dust). The process is a feature of some forms of hypersensitivity vasculitis (p. 219) and of the neutrophilic dermatoses (p. 228).

Lichenoid infiltrate: a term sometimes used to refer to a band-like infiltrate of inflammatory cells confined to the papillary dermis, comparable to that seen in lichen planus. In most instances it is associated with the lichenoid reaction pattern in which there is basal cell damage (p. 31).

Metachromasia: the phenomenon in which certain dyes in solution react with a tissue component to produce a colour that is different from that of the original dye. This property is limited to a relatively few basic dyes. The mechanism is assumed to be related to polymerization of the dye when it reacts with the tissue component. Toluidine blue is the best known metachromatic dye. It colours most tissues blue but will stain certain components (e.g. mast cell granules) purple.

Microabscess: a collection of neutrophils admixed with some cell debris and fibrin. The term is usually restricted to three circumstances, in all of which the lesions are smaller than pustules (see below): the Munro microabscess develops in the parakeratotic layer in psoriasis; the Pautrier 'microabscess', which occurs in mycosis fungoides, consists of three or more large lymphocytes (not neutrophils as the definition of a microabscess requires) aggregated within the malpighian layer; and papillary microabscesses in which numerous neutrophils, admixed with variable numbers of eosinophils, fill the dermal papillae (in dermatitis herpetiformis, cicatricial pemphigoid, etc.).

Naevus: this term is used for benign tumours of melanocyte-derived naevus cells (naevocellular naevi) and also for a variety of hamartomatous lesions of the epidermis, cutaneous appendages or connective tissue elements. The word needs qualification to indicate the context in which it is being used (e.g. naevocellular naevus, connective tissue naevus, epidermal naevus, etc.).

Necrobiosis: a controversial word, used in dermatopathology to refer to the accumulation of acid mucopolysaccharides in the interstitium of the dermis associated with some 'smudging' of the collagen fibres and, sometimes, loss of fibroblasts. Zones of necrobiosis are usually surrounded by an increased number of fibroblasts, dendrocytes, macrophages and epithelioid cells. The concept of 'necrobiosis of collagen' is disparaged because collagen is not a vital substance and the word necrobiosis, as originally defined, referred to cell death, particularly the physiological death of individual cells.

Papillomatosis: projections of the dermal papillae and the epidermis overlying them above the surface of the surrounding skin. This process produces undulations of the surface. Diseases associated with papillomatosis are listed on page 25.

Parakeratosis: an alteration of the stratum corneum, with retention of nuclei; the nuclei are usually flattened. It results from the rapid transit of keratinocytes to the surface (as seen, for example, in psoriasis and solar keratoses) and from altered maturation of the epidermis resulting from a variety of processes, particularly spongiosis. Hypogranulosis almost invariably underlies areas of parakeratosis.

Pigment incontinence: the deposition of melanin in the upper dermis, both within macrophages (melanocytes) and lying free. It is a common complication of the lichenoid reaction pattern which is characterized by damage to the basal layer of the epidermis.

Pseudoepitheliomatous hyperplasia: pronounced hyperplasia of the epidermis with irregular expansion and downgrowth of the rete pegs in contrast to the regular nature of this process in psoriasiform hyperplasia. Enlargement of the follicular infundibula is usually present. At times, pseudoepitheliomatous hyperplasia may mimic a well-differentiated squamous cell carcinoma.

Psoriasiform hyperplasia: epidermal hyperplasia in which there is elongation of the rete pegs in a regular fashion. Its presence is indicative of the psoriasiform reaction pattern (see Ch. 4).

Pustule: a localized collection of neutrophils and their breakdown products, usually within the epidermis or within a pilosebaceous follicle. The term eosinophilic pustule refers to the accumulation of eosinophils in similar locations. A spongiform pustule is another variant of pustule, characteristic of pustular psoriasis. It is a multilocular pustule in the upper epidermis: neutrophils are present between the keratinocytes and are surrounded by clear spaces. The appearances give the misleading impression of vacuolation of keratinocytes and the presence of neutrophils within their cytoplasm.

Scale crust: localized areas of altered stratum corneum composed of serum, variable numbers of inflammatory cells and parakeratotic cells.

Spongiosis: intraepidermal intercellular oedema leading to widening of the space between keratinocytes. If the accumulation of oedema fluid becomes pronounced the desmosomal attachments rupture, leading to vesicle formation (spongiotic vesiculation). The presence of spongiosis is indicative of the spongiotic reaction pattern (p. 95).

Sporotrichoid: the distribution of lesions in the line of the superficial lymphatics (usually involving the arms), in a pattern resembling that seen in the lymphangitic form of sporotrichosis (p. 655).

Squamous eddies: concentric layers of keratinocytes (squamous cells) surrounding an area of keratinization.

Telogen: the resting phase of the hair cycle which follows catagen (involution of the follicle). This period may last up to several months. It is usually followed by a new cycle of growth of the hair follicle (anagen).

Vesicle: a small fluid-filled cavity within the epidermis or immediately below it and less than 1 cm (some authors say 0.5 cm) in diameter. Larger blisters are known as bullae.

Zosteriform: the localization of a disease process to a circumscribed area, usually on one side of the body only. The distribution may conform to that of one or more specific dermatomes, as in herpes zoster.

Index